Geriatric Practice

Audrey Chun
Editor

Geriatric Practice

A Competency Based Approach to Caring for Older Adults

Springer

Editor
Audrey Chun
Department of Geriatrics and Palliative Medicine
Icahn School of Medicine at Mount Sinai
New York, NY
USA

ISBN 978-3-030-19624-0 ISBN 978-3-030-19625-7 (eBook)
https://doi.org/10.1007/978-3-030-19625-7

This Springer imprint is published by the registered company Springer Nature Switzerland AG
The registered company address is: Gewerbestrasse 11, 6330 Cham, Switzerland

Preface

It is an honor and privilege to write the preface to this first edition of *Practicing Geriatrics: A Competency Based Approach to Caring for Older Adults.* Conceived as a practical resource for care providers and trainees, the goal of this book is to advance the care of older adults by providing a comprehensive reference for the basic principles of caring for an older population. Chapters are grounded in the student competencies as well as in cases to provide context to the clinical reasoning underlying the competency.

By 2030, more than 20% of Americans will be over the age of 65 years and will account for a large proportion of health system utilization. Due to age, increased rates of multimorbidity, polypharmacy, functional changes, and cognitive impairment, older adults require specific considerations that should be incorporated into practice for all medical specialties. There is immense heterogeneity in the aging process between individuals, and lack of recognition of this phenomenon can lead to overtreatment for some and undertreatment for others. Function becomes the best predictor of morbidity and mortality with advancing age, with the frailest being at highest risk for bad outcomes and adverse events from tests and treatments. Geriatrics is the ultimate "personalized" medicine by matching treatment plans to patients' goals/wishes anchored in communications around both the likely benefit and burdens of different management options.

Training in these principles of geriatric medicine is critical to improving the care for all older adults. The following chapters will facilitate the knowledge required for the safe and appropriate care of older adults required by all providers serving an aging population – from primary to surgical and other specialty care. It is organized to introduce the reader to the framework for geriatrics care, followed by common conditions encountered with older adults, and includes models and sites of care important to managing health across the spectrum of aging needs. There is also a focus on common geriatric syndromes, identifying unique considerations for older adults with common diseases, as well as functional assessment and safety.

I want to take this opportunity to thank those who made this book possible. My mentors, colleagues, and family provided tremendous support in the creation and completion of this work. The authors committed countless hours and ideas to the formation of this project. Their enthusiasm and experiences are the heart of this book. Finally, I am immensely grateful for the patients and their families who have allowed me to be part of their lives. Their stories inspire and challenge me each day.

Audrey Chun
New York, NY, USA

Contents

IV Medication Management (MEDICATIONS)

V Cognitive and Behavioral Disorders (MENTATION)

VI Functional Assessment/Self-Care Ability (MOBILITY)

Contributors

Nabila Ahmed-Sarwar, PharmD, BCPS, CDE, BC-ADM
St. John Fisher College, Wegmans School of Pharmacy
University of Rochester, Highland Family Medicine
Rochester, NY, USA

Amy S. Aloysi, MD, MPH
Departments of Psychiatry and Neurology,
Mount Sinai Hospital
New York, NY, USA

Allen D. Andrade, MD DM(Lon) MRCP(UK)
Brookdale Department of Geriatrics and Palliative
Medicine at the Icahn School of Medicine at Mount Sinai
The Mount Sinai Hospital
New York, NY, USA

Claire K. Ankuda, MD, MPH
Hertzberg Palliative Care Institute, Brookdale
Department of Geriatrics and Palliative Medicine
Icahn School of Medicine at Mount Sinai
New York, NY, USA

Olusegun Apoeso, MD
Hertzberg Palliative Care Institute, Brookdale
Department of Geriatrics and Palliative Medicine
Icahn School of Medicine at Mount Sinai
New York, NY, USA

Shahla Baharlou, MD
Brookdale Department of Geriatrics
and Palliative Medicine
Icahn School of Medicine at Mount Sinai
New York, NY, USA

Melissa Bakar, MD
Brookdale Department of Geriatrics
and Palliative Medicine
Icahn School of Medicine at Mount Sinai
New York, NY, USA

Sheila Barton, MA, LCSW
Mount Sinai Hospital, Brookdale Department
of Geriatrics and Palliative Medicine
New York, NY, USA

Mollie A. Biewald, MD
Brookdale Department of Geriatrics
and Palliative Medicine
Mount Sinai Hospital
New York, NY, USA

Michael Bogaisky, MD, MPH
Division of Geriatrics
Montefiore Medical Center and Albert Einstein College
Of Medicine
Bronx, NY, USA

Sara M. Bradley, MD, FACP
Division of General Internal Medicine and Geriatrics
Northwestern Feinberg School of Medicine
Chicago, IL, USA

Gary H. Brandeis, MD, CMD
Department of Geriatric and Palliative Medicine
Icahn School of Medicine at Mount Sinai
New York, NY, USA

Medical Department, Mount Sinai Services,
Elmhurst Hospital Center
New York, NY, USA

Nicole J. Brandt, PharmD, MBA, BCGP, BCPP, FASCP
Peter Lamy Center on Drug Therapy and Aging,
University of Maryland School of Pharmacy
Department of Pharmacy Practice and Science
Baltimore, MD, USA

MedStar Good Samaritan Hospital,
Center for Successful Aging
Baltimore, MD, USA

Eileen H. Callahan, MD
Brookdale Department of Geriatrics
and Palliative Medicine
Icahn School of Medicine at Mount Sinai
New York, NY, USA

Kathryn E. Callahan, MD, MS
Section on Gerontology and Geriatric Medicine,
Department of Internal Medicine
Wake Forest School of Medicine
Wake Forest, NC, USA

Denise Cauble, PhD, BSN
University of Texas at Arlington, College of Nursing
and Health Innovation
Arlington, TX, USA

Emily J. Chai, MD
Brookdale Department of Geriatrics
and Palliative Medicine
Mount Sinai Hospital, Icahn School of Medicine
at Mount Sinai
New York, NY, USA

Christine Chang, MD, AGSF
Department of Geriatrics and Palliative Medicine
Icahn School of Medicine at Mount Sinai Hospital
New York, NY, USA

Steven Y. Chao, MD
Department of Surgery,
Weill Cornell Medicine, New York Presbyterian – Queens
Flushing, NY, USA

Serena Hsiou-Ling Chao, MD, MSc, AGSF
Geriatrics Division, CHA House Calls Program
Cambridge Health Alliance
Cambridge, MA, USA

Department of Medicine, Harvard School of Medicine
Boston, MA, USA

Erica Y. Chu, MD
Division of Geriatrics and Palliative Medicine,
Department of Internal Medicine
New York-Presbyterian Hospital/
Weill Cornell Medical Center
New York, NY, USA

Stephanie W. Chow, MD, MPH
Brookdale Department of Geriatrics
and Palliative Medicine
New York, NY, USA

Kelly Cummings, MD
Brookdale Department of Geriatrics and Palliative Medicine
Icahn School of Medicine at Mount Sinai
New York, NY, USA

Kathryn M. Daniel, PhD, MSN
University of Texas at Arlington
College of Nursing and Health Innovation
Arlington, TX, USA

Claire Davenport, MD, MS
Department of Geriatrics and Palliative Medicine
Icahn School of Medicine at Mount Sinai
New York, NY, USA

Kristen DeCarlo, MD
Division of General Internal Medicine and Geriatrics
Northwestern University Feinberg School of Medicine
Chicago, IL, USA

Linda V. DeCherrie, MD
Brookdale Department of Geriatrics
and Palliative Medicine
Mount Sinai Hospital
New York, NY, USA

Ogechi N. Dike, MD
Division of Hospital Medicine
UT Southwestern Medical Center,
Department of Medicine
Dallas, TX, USA

Clements University Hospital
Dallas, TX, USA

Komal D'Souza, MD
Departments of Geriatrics and Palliative Medicine
Mount Sinai Hospital
New York, NY, USA

Grace Farris, MD
Mount Sinai West Division of Hospital Medicine,
Icahn School of Medicine at Mount Sinai,
Department of Medicine
New York, NY, USA

Helen Fernandez, MD, MPH
Brookdale Department of Geriatrics and Palliative Medicine
Icahn School of Medicine at Mount Sinai
New York, NY, USA

Jean Y. Guan, MD
Division of Geriatrics
University of California, San Diego
San Diego, CA, USA

Roopali Gupta, MD
Division of Geriatrics
University of California, San Diego
La Jolla, CA, USA

Nami Safai Haeri, MD
Brookdale Department of Geriatrics and Palliative
Medicine at the Icahn School of Medicine at Mount
Sinai, The Mount Sinai Hospital
New York, NY, USA

Gregory A. Hinrichsen, PhD, ABPP
Brookdale Department of Geriatrics
and Palliative Medicine
Icahn School of Medicine at Mount Sinai
New York, NY, USA

Annette M. Hintenach, MSSW
James J. Peters VA Medical Center, VISN 2 Geriatric
Research, Education & Clinical Center
Bronx, NY, USA

Judith L. Howe, PhD, MPA
Brookdale Department of Geriatrics and Palliative Medicine, VISN 2 GRECC at James J. Peters, Icahn School of Medicine at Mount Sinai
Bronx, NY, USA

Noelle Marie Javier, MD
Brookdale Department of Geriatrics and Palliative Medicine, Mount Sinai Hospital
New York, NY, USA

Joanna Jimenez-Mejia, DNP, MSN, AGPCNP-BC
Brookdale Department of Geriatrics and Palliative Medicine
Mount Sinai Health System
New York, NY, USA

Parham Khalili, MD, MAPP, MA
Division of Geriatrics and Palliative Medicine
New York Presbyterian Hospital
New York, NY, USA

Stephanie Le, MD
Brookdale Department of Geriatrics and Palliative Medicine at the Icahn School of Medicine at Mount Sinai
The Mount Sinai Hospital
New York, NY, USA

Michele Lee, MD
Brookdale Department of Geriatrics and Palliative Medicine
Icahn School of Medicine at Mount Sinai
New York, NY, USA

Rosanne M. Leipzig, MD, PhD
Brookdale Department of Geriatrics and Palliative Medicine, Icahn School of Medicine at Mount Sinai
Riverdale, NY, USA

Kenneth L. Lichstein, PhD
Department of Psychology, University of Alabama
Tuscaloosa, AL, USA

Cynthia Lien, MD
Department of Medicine/Geriatrics
Weill Cornell Medical Center
New York, NY, USA

Matthew Majeske, MD
Department of Psychiatry, Icahn School of Medicine at Mount Sinai
New York, NY, USA

Elizabeth Mann, MD, MPH
Geriatrics and Palliative Care, Gallup Indian Medical Center
Gallup, NM, USA

Daniel Z. Mansour, PharmD, BCGP, FASCP
Peter Lamy Center on Drug Therapy and Aging, University of Maryland School of Pharmacy
Department of Pharmacy Practice and Science
Baltimore, MD, USA

Michelle Martinchek, MD, MPH
Department of Medicine, Section of Geriatrics and Palliative Medicine, University of Chicago
Chicago, IL, USA

Hylton E. Molzof, MPH
Department of Psychology, University of Alabama
Tuscaloosa, AL, USA

Barbara Morano, MPH, LCSW
Brookdale Department of Geriatrics and Palliative Medicine, Icahn School of Medicine at Mount Sinai
New York, NY, USA

Carmen Morano, PhD, MSW
School of Social Welfare, The University at Albany
Albany, NY, USA

Lizette Muñoz, MSW
Brookdale Department of Geriatrics and Palliative Medicine
Mount Sinai Health System
New York, NY, USA

Neha Naik, MD
Department of Medicine/Geriatrics
Weill Cornell Medical Center
New York, NY, USA

Erika Diaz Narvaez, MD
Departments of Geriatrics and Palliative Medicine; Family and Community Medicine; and Medical Education
Mount Sinai Hospital
New York, NY, USA

Bernard F. Ortega, MPA
Department of Ambulatory Care
Mount Sinai Health System
New York, NY, USA

Karin Ouchida, MD
Division of Geriatrics and Palliative Medicine
New York Presbyterian Hospital
New York, NY, USA

Jennifer A. Ouellet, MD
Section of Geriatrics, Internal Medicine
Yale School of Medicine
New Haven, CT, USA

Amanda N. Overstreet, DO
Medical University of South Carolina,
General Internal Medicine
Charleston, SC, USA

Khusbu Patel, PharmD
Assistant Clinical Professor, St. John's University
College of Pharmacy and Health Sciences
Queens, NY, USA

Ayla Pelleg, MD
Brookdale Department of Geriatrics
and Palliative Medicine
Icahn School of Medicine at Mount Sinai
New York, NY, USA

Lisa A. Perez, A/GNP-BC, MSN, RN, CWOCN-AP
Wound Ostomy and Continence of North Texas
Crowley, TX, USA

Megan E. Petrov, PhD
College of Nursing & Health Innovation
Arizona State University
Phoenix, AZ, USA

Ravishankar Ramaswamy, MD
Brookdale Department of Geriatrics
and Palliative Medicine
Icahn School of Medicine at Mount Sinai
New York, NY, USA

Savitri Ramdial, MBBS, MD
Department of Family Medicine/Geriatric Medicine
Archbold Memorial Hospital
Thomasville, GA, USA

Megan E. Rau, MD, MPH
Division of Geriatric Medicine and Palliative Care,
Department of Medicine
New York University School of Medicine
New York, NY, USA

Alan Remde, MD, FAAFP, DAIHM
SLUHN Department of Family Medicine
Family Medicine Residency - Warren Coventry Family
Practice
Phillipsburg, NJ, USA

Veronica Rivera, MD
Departments of Geriatrics and Palliative Medicine; Family
and Community Medicine; and Medical Education
Mount Sinai Hospital
New York, NY, USA

Vanessa Rodriguez, MD
Brookdale Department of Geriatrics
and Palliative Medicine
Icahn School of Medicine at Mount Sinai Hospital
New York, NY, USA

Katherine Roza, MD
Brookdale Department of Geriatrics
and Palliative Medicine
Mount Sinai Medical Center
New York, NY, USA

Nisha Rughwani, BSc, MBBS (MD)
Brookdale Department of Geriatrics
and Palliative Medicine
Mount Sinai Medical Center
New York, NY, USA

Martine Sanon, MD
Brookdale Department of Geriatrics
and Palliative Medicine
Department of Medicine – Division of Hospital Medicine
Mount Sinai Hospital
New York, NY, USA

Adora Tricia V. Santos, DO
Department of Surgery, NewYork-Presbyterian/Queens
Flushing, NY, USA

Sharon See, PharmD, BCPS, FCCP
St. John's University College of Pharmacy
and Health Sciences
Queens, NY, USA

Brookdale Department of Geriatrics
and Palliative Medicine,
Mobile Acute Care for the Elderly Team (MACE),
Icahn School of Medicine at Mount Sinai
New York, NY, USA

Belinda Setters, MD, MS, AGSF, FACP
Inpatient Geriatrics, Robley Rex VAMC
Louisville, KY, USA

Departments of Internal Medicine and Family
& Geriatric Medicine, University of Louisville
Louisville, KY, USA

Amit Shah, MD
Division of Community Internal Medicine
Mayo Clinic School of Medicine
Scottsdale, AZ, USA

Kriti Sharma, MBBS, MD, MPH
Peter Lamy Center on Drug Therapy and Aging,
University of Maryland School of Pharmacy
Department of Pharmaceutical Health Services Research
Baltimore, MD, USA

Ruth M. Spinner, MD
Brookdale Department of Geriatrics and
Palliative Medicine, Mount Sinai Hospital
New York, NY, USA

The New Jewish Home, Manhattan
New York, NY, USA

Rebecca J. Stetzer, MD
Department of Geriatrics and Palliative Care,
Albany Stratton VA, Department of Family and
Community Medicine, Albany Medical College
Albany, NY, USA

Dustin E. Suanino, MD
Division of Palliative Medicine & Bioethics
NYU Winthrop Hospital
New York, NY, USA

Sara Suleman, MD
Brookdale Department of Geriatrics
and Palliative Medicine
Icahn School of Medicine at Mount Sinai
New York, NY, USA

David Sundel, MIA
Columbia University School of International
and Public Affairs
New York, NY, USA

Siobhan Sundel, DNP, GNP-BC, ANP
Retired Business Analyst, Brookdale Department of
Geriatrics and Palliative Medicine
Mount Sinai Hospital
New York, NY, USA

Raymond Teets, MD
Family Medicine and Community Health,
Icahn School of Medicine at Mount Sinai,
Mount Sinai & Institute for Family Health
New York, NY, USA

Katherine Thompson, MD
Department of Medicine, Section of Geriatrics
and Palliative Medicine, University of Chicago
Chicago, IL, USA

Kristen Thornton, MD
Family Medicine, Internal Medicine (Division of Geriatrics
& Aging), University of Rochester Medical Center
Rochester, NY, USA

Ania Wajnberg, MD
Department of Medicine,
Icahn School of Medicine at Mount Sinai
New York, NY, USA

Lisa M. Walke, MD, MSHA, AGSF
Division of Geriatrics, Internal Medicine
University of Pennysylvania, Perelman
School of Medicine
Philadelphia, PA, USA

Katherine Wang, MD
Brookdale Department of Geriatrics
and Palliative Medicine
Icahn School of Medicine at Mount Sinai
New York, NY, USA

Lindsey C. Yourman, MD
Division of Geriatrics, Department of Medicine
University of California, San Diego
La Jolla, CA, USA

Abbreviations

ADE	Adverse Drug Event
AGS	American Geriatric Society
AUR	acute urinary retention
B.C.G.P	Borad Certified in Geriatric Pharmacy
B.C.P.P.	Board Certified in Psychiatry Pharmacy
BID	2 times per day
BOO	bladder outlet obstruction
BP	Blood Pressure
BPH	benign prostatic hyperplasia
C.R.N.P.	Certified Registered Nurse Practitioner
CA-UTI	catheter-associated urinary tract infection
CBC	complete blood count
CBI	continuous bladder irrigation
CHF	Congestive heart failure
CIC	clean intermittent catheterization
CMP	comprehensive metabolic panel
CNS	Central nervous system
COPD	Chronic Obstructive Pulmonary Disease
CrCl	Creatinine Clearance
CV	Cardiovascular
D.O.	Doctor of Osteopathy
DHIC	detrusor hyperactivity with impaired contractility
DRE	digital rectal exam
DTCA	Direct To Consumer Advertising
EF	Ejection Fraction
F.A.S.C.P.	Fellow of the American Society of Consultant Pharmacists
FBG	Fasting Blood Glucose
FDA	Food and Drug Administration
GERD	Gastrointestinal reflux disease
GI	Gastrointestinal
GU	Genitourinary
HbA1c	Hemoglobin A 1c
HR	Heart Rate
IPEC 2016	Interprofessional Education Collaborative 2016
LUTS	lower urinary tract symptoms
LVHF	Left Ventricular Heart Failure
M.B.A.	Masters in Business Administration
M.D.	Doctor of Medicine
M.P.H.	Masters in Public Health
MBSR	Mindfulness-based stress reduction
NREM	Non-rapid eye movement sleep
NSAID	Non-Steroidal Anti-Inflammatory Drug
OA	Osteoarthritis
OAWI	Older adults with insomnia
OTC	Over The Counter
P.A.	Physician Assistant
Pharm.D.	Doctor of Pharmacy
PLMD	Periodic limb movement disorder
PO	by mouth
PRN	as needed
PSA	prostate specific antigen
REM	Rapid eye movement sleep
SOL	Sleep onset latency
TST	Total sleep time
TURP	transurethral resection of the prostate
TWOC	trial without catheter
UTI	urinary tract infection
WASO	Wake after sleep onset

Introduction and Approach to Caring for Older Adults

Contents

History and Trends

Jennifer A. Ouellet and Lisa M. Walke

A. Chun (ed.), *Geriatric Practice*, https://doi.org/10.1007/978-3-030-19625-7_1

1

Key Points
- Older adults make up an increasingly large share of the US and global populations due to increased life expectancy and reduced fecundity.
- Due to improvements in the treatment of many acute illnesses, a greater percentage of patients are living with chronic illnesses including hypertension, diabetes, ischemic heart disease, Alzheimer's disease and other dementias, and cancer.
- Older adults rely heavily on public health insurance programs including Medicare and Medicaid and spend more on healthcare costs than younger Americans.
- The unique needs of older adults have necessitated changes over time within healthcare policy, clinical practice, research, and education.

1.1 Background/Introduction

Over the last century, significant medical advances have greatly prolonged the average life expectancy. Life expectancy in the United States at birth in 1900 was 46.3 years; in contrast, life expectancy at birth in 2000 was 73.8. This increase has resulted in a rapid growth in the number of older adults in the United States and globally. The number of adults 65 and older in the United States rose from 150 million in 1950 to 300 million in 2010, and is projected to continue to increase. Growth in this segment of the population has caused a demographic shift such that it is predicted that 1 in 5 Americans will be 65 and older by 2030 [1]. Similarly, the global population of older adults has increased dramatically, with projections for continued growth (an estimated 1.4 billion persons by 2030 and 2.1 billion persons in 2050) [2]. The magnitude of this population growth, coupled with the unique health and social needs of older adults, has resulted in the realization of the need for a number of societal changes.

1.2 Historical Perspectives and Clinical Context

Geriatrics is a healthcare specialty aimed at promoting the health of adults over the age of 65, by optimizing quality of life and patient-centered care. The geriatric approach to clinical care is a departure from the disease-focused diagnosis and treatment paradigm that has long dominated medical care, allowing for nuance and not forcing a "one size fits all" solution. Tailoring care to the individual is essential, as the potential benefits and harms of guideline-based care are uncertain for older adults with a variety of potential vulnerabilities including frailty, multiple chronic conditions, and functional disabilities [3]. Furthermore, these patients may differ in the outcomes that they most hope to achieve from their healthcare.

The term "geriatrics" was coined in 1909, when a mere 4% of the population was over the age of 65, by Ignatz Leo Nascher, who wrote a number of books and articles regarding "diseases of old age and their treatment" [4]. He suggested the term as "an addition to our vocabulary, to cover the same field in old age that is covered by the term pediatrics in childhood, to emphasize the necessity of considering senility and its diseases apart from maturity and to assign it a separate place in medicine."

After the Great Depression led to an increase in the number of older adults living in poverty (30% in 1930 and 66% by 1940), the social issues unique to the aging population and the implications on healthcare costs and overall outcomes became apparent. As a result, President Franklin D. Roosevelt passed the Social Security Act of 1935 in order to provide aid to older adults, children, and unemployed persons. Healthcare professionals also sought to identify ways to improve the health, independence, and quality of life of older adults, and in 1942, the American Geriatrics Society was established. In 1950, President Harry S. Truman convened the first National Conference on Aging, with a purpose of addressing policy changes to meet the needs of an aging population. The value of geriatric principles has become increasingly recognized over time, prompting changes within healthcare policy, clinical practice, research, and education.

1.2.1 Policy Changes: Social Security Act of 1965 and the Affordable Care Act

1.2.1.1 Social Security Act of 1965

In 1965, the US government passed the Social Security Act of 1965, legislation designed to improve access to acute healthcare for old, disabled, or poor people. This led to the creation of Medicare and Medicaid, federal health insurance programs. During the decades that followed, the resulting Medicare and Medicaid programs have expanded and evolved to meet the needs of eligible beneficiaries.

Medicare (Title XVIII) is a federal insurance program run by the Center for Medicare & Medicaid Services (CMS), which pays health professionals and organizations to provide healthcare for Americans who are 65 years old or older, disabled, or suffering from end-stage renal disease and amyotrophic lateral sclerosis after 2 years. As originally enacted, Medicare comprises two separate fee-for-service (FFS) plans (Part A and Part B), each of which pays predetermined amounts for specified health-related goods and services: Part A covering hospital and hospice care and Part B covering ambulatory health services. More than 55 million Americans are covered by both plans, which is 15% of the total US population.

Medicaid (Title XIX) is a joint federal and state program that provides health insurance to people of all ages who have low income and limited savings. The exact criteria for Medicaid eligibility and the benefit packages provided by Medicaid programs vary from state to state because of state contributions to the program. Medicaid also pays for long-term custodial care in nursing homes for those who qualify.

1.2.1.2 Patient Protection and Affordable Care Act (ACA) 2010

The areas of the ACA affecting older adults and those providing their care are primarily focused on increasing access and changing the current fee-for-service (FFS) reimbursement system. The ACA increases access to Medicare beneficiaries by eliminating out-of-pocket expenditures for many preventive screening studies, reducing the Medicare Part D (prescription drug coverage) coverage gap, and expanding Medicaid coverage. The ACA also has initiated changes in reimbursement from the current FFS system to systems that improve outcomes including bundling reimbursement, and pay-for-performance which reimburses for quality measures as opposed to fee-for-service.

1.2.2 Clinical Practice: Development of Models of Care and Reimbursement Incentives

The field of geriatrics, focusing on the principles of care in treating older adults, has witnessed groundbreaking work in healthcare delivery models, many of which are widely disseminated including Acute Care of the Elderly (ACE) Unit [7], Geriatric Resources for Assessment and Care of Elders [8], Program of All-inclusive Care for the Elderly [9], Hospital Elder Life Program [10], and Nurses Improving Care for Health System Elders [11]. Other specialties have also recognized the value in the geriatric approach and as such, there has been a proliferation of comanagement interventions, in particular with surgical subspecialties (e.g., combined orthogeriatric hospital services) [12].

As recent growth in healthcare costs is unsustainable, policymakers seeking to inject value into the system have begun to appreciate the wisdom of geriatric principles. For example, readmission of persons with multiple chronic conditions has become a quality measure, as have assessment and management of several geriatric syndromes [13–15]. The Centers for Medicare and Medicaid Services (CMS) now provide modest payment for home visits, transitional care, and care coordination, and payment for advanced care planning discussion has been introduced [16–18].

1.2.3 Research

The National Institute of Health (NIH), first established in 1887, is the primary agency of the US Government responsible for biomedical and public health research, allocating federal funding to researchers in a variety of medical fields. In 1974, Congress granted the authority to create the National Institute on Aging to provide leadership in aging research, training, health information dissemination, and other programs relevant to aging and older people.

Over the last 30 years, the field of geriatrics has built an impressive research base and has begun to contribute its unique knowledge to the mainstream medical community. Understanding the multifactorial nature of many geriatric syndromes has led to strong, targeted interventions which have shown improved outcomes. Furthermore, principles that were once championed by few other than geriatricians have entered the clinical mainstream. For example, function has always played a large role in the geriatric assessment and is now finally being appreciated as a "worthy" outcome in clinical research and quality measure.

1.2.4 Education

Growth in the population of older adults with identification of their unique healthcare needs led to the realization of a need for specialized training within Geriatrics. In 1962, the American Nurses Association held focus groups on gerontologic nursing practice, and the first geriatric nursing standards were established in 1968. The first fellowship in Medical Geriatrics was started in 1966 by Leslie Libow at City Hospital Center (an Icahn School of Medicine at Mount Sinai, formerly Mount Sinai School of Medicine, affiliate) [19], and the first department of Geriatrics was established at Icahn School of Medicine at Mount Sinai in 1982. In 1988, the first certifying examination in Geriatrics was offered, and 62 internal medicine and 16 family practice programs were accredited by the Accreditation Council for Graduate Medical Education to offer Geriatrics fellowship programs.

A growing population of older adults has led to a need for robust education for all medical trainees. Most medical trainees will end up in careers where they treat older adults and, as such, should have a basic training in the unique needs and general principles of care for this population. The objectives for the education of medical trainees should ideally be uniform across disciplines and institutions, providing a challenge to medical educators across the country.

The Association of American Medical Colleges (AAMC) and the John A. Hartford Foundation (JAHF) hosted a National Consensus Conference on the Competencies in Geriatric Education in 2007. The goal of this conference was to develop a set of minimum set of graduating medical student competencies to assure competent care to patients. The metrics that individual medical schools utilize to measure student achievement of each competency varies, but the minimum competencies provide a basic benchmark and have been endorsed by the American Geriatrics Society (AGS) and the Association of Directors of Geriatric Academic Programs (ADGAP) [20].

1.2.5 Call for Value-Based Care

For complex older adults, care in our current system is often fragmented and geared toward achieving outcomes which may not be relevant to patients. With growing consensus about the need to improve the value of clinical care, the Institute for Healthcare Improvement introduced the ambitious Triple Aim in 2008 [5], i.e., improving population health, improving patient experience, and reducing costs. The National Academy of Medicine, formerly known as the Institute of Medicine (IoM), a non-profit, non-governmental agency, provides national advice on the healthcare of the United States. In 1978, they recommended that geriatrics be developed in various disciplines and in 2008 put out a report entitled, "Retooling for an aging America: Building the Healthcare Workforce." This report described the healthcare workforce as critically unprepared for the unique needs of the aging population [6] and called for broadening the responsibilities of trained workers, preparing for the needs of caregivers, and development of new models of healthcare delivery.

At this juncture there remains controversy among policymakers about relevant outcomes for reimbursement. Geriatric principles have informed some progress in this area including changes to Medicare coverage of advanced care planning and transitional care models (see below in clinical care). However, many quality metrics are still tied to mortality or to disease-specific outcomes or laboratory measures which may not be relevant to medically complex older adults. As such, there is significant opportunity for geriatrics to contribute to a much wider sphere of influence through national health policy.

1.3 Trends in Demographic Statistics

As discussed, there has been rapid growth in the population of older adults within the last several decades. There have been shifts in demographics and statistics resulting in the need for many of the policy, clinical care, research, and education changes discussed above.

1.3.1 Demographics

1.3.1.1 Age

According to the US Census Bureau, the total number of older adults (persons aged 65 and older) was 47.8 million, up 1.6 million from the year prior in 2014 [21, 22]. This number is projected to double by 2060 to total 98.2 million older adults (◘ Fig. 1.1). The number of people aged 85 and older is growing at an even more rapid rate, and is expected to more than triple from 5.8 million in 2010 to over 19 million by 2060 [23]. The total number of centenarians, or people aged 100 years or older, has also increased over time; from 32,000 in 1980 to more than 53,000 in 2010, with projections of more than 600,000 in 2060 [24].

Worldwide, there were 901 million older adults in 2015, an increase of 48 percent from 607 million older persons in 2000. Echoing the projected trends within the United States, this number is expected to continue to grow exponentially, with a projected population of older adults of 1.4 billion in 2030 and 2.1 billion in 2050. The number of people aged 80 years and older worldwide is growing even faster than the number of older persons overall, with a projected increase from 71 million in 2000 to 202 million in 2030 and 434 million in 2050 [2]. The growth in the number of older adults was greatest in the upper-middle-income countries between 2010 and 2015, and this group of countries is expected to see the greatest growth over the next several decades as well.

1.3.1.2 Sex

Female life expectancy has historically exceeded male life expectancy, resulting in higher proportions of women aged 65 and older in the general population. In 2012, 56.4% of those over the age of 65 were female, projected to decline slightly to 55.1 percent in 2050. In 2012, 66.6% of those aged 85 and older were female, projected to decline to 61.9% in 2050. The decline in proportion of female older adults with

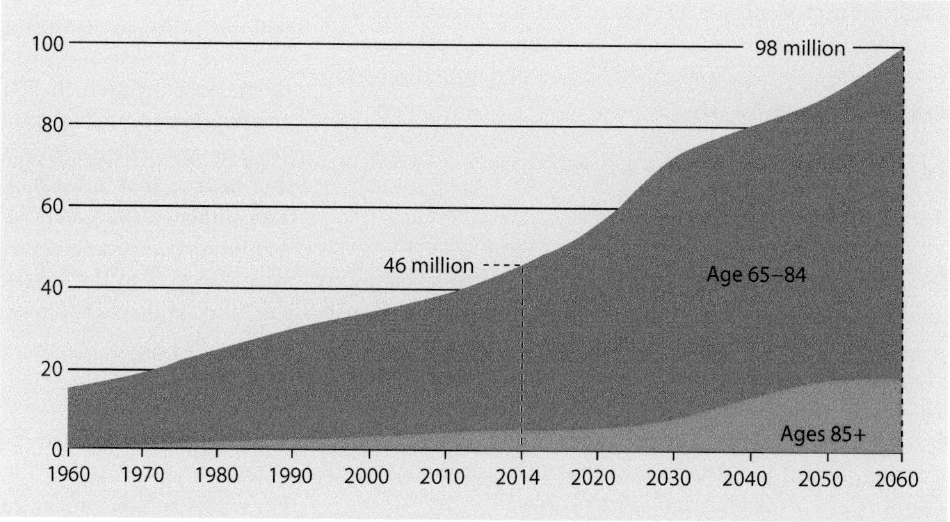

◘ **Fig. 1.1** The population of older adults in the United States will more than double by 2060 [22]. (Modified from: Mather et al. [42])

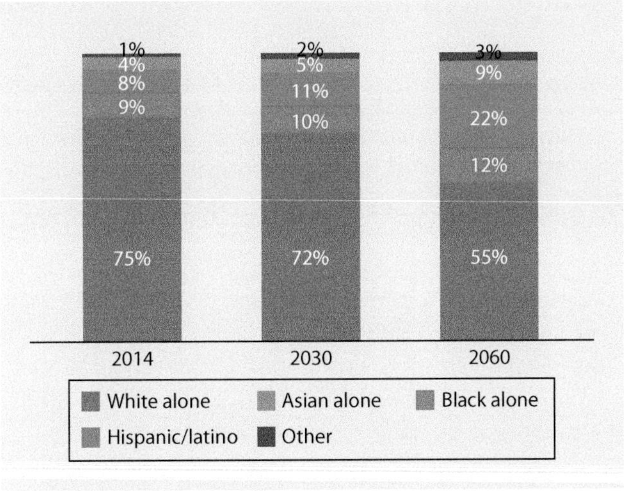

Fig. 1.2 Expected decline in diversity gap in older adults by 2060 [22]. (Modified from: Mather et al. [42])

time is expected due to a rapid increase in male life expectancy over the next several decades [25].

Globally, there are also a higher proportion of female older adults as compared to male, which is also attributed to longer life expectancies in females. During the 2010–2015 time period, women outlived men by an average of 4.5 years [2].

1.3.1.3 Race and Ethnicity

The US population is becoming more racially and ethnically diverse; however, currently, most of this diversity is accounted for in the younger age groups. In 2014, more than 75% of older adults were non-Hispanic white, while only 50% of children under 18 were non-Hispanic white. This gap in the diversity of the older adult population is expected to shrink; in 2060, the proportion of older adults who are non-Hispanic white is expected to drop to 55% (Fig. 1.2) [22]. This shift has and will continue to prompt the training of healthcare professionals to include cultural competency education in addition to the development of public health programs designed for wide ranges of audiences.

1.3.1.4 Marital Status and Living Arrangements

Studies have shown that approximately half of caregivers for older adults are spouses [26], resulting in changes in their ability to continue outside employment and seek care for themselves. Given an increase in the life expectancy of men over the last several decades, the proportion of women over the age of 65 who are married has increased, while the number of women over the age of 65 who are widowed has decreased. Despite this trend, over half of women over the age of 65 are not married, compared to 25% of men over the age of 65. Older men are less likely to be widowed, both due to longer life expectancy of women and due to men over the age of 65 being more like to remarry compared to women [22]. Marital trends are expected to shift over the next several decades due to delays in marriage and childbearing, increasing divorce rates, and increased rates of cohabitation and unmarried childbearing. These trends will have important implications to the care of older adults.

More older adults live in the community (96.6%) than in institutional or group (nursing home and group home) settings (3.4%). There are more women than men living in nursing homes, likely reflective of increased life expectancy. The proportion of older adults in nursing homes increases with increasing age, [21, 22] with most nursing home residents (40.7%) being aged 85 or older.

This is likely a factor of increasing functional impairments, as studies have demonstrated that 67% of nursing home residents need assistance with three or more activities of daily living (ADLs) [27]. ADLs include bathing, dressing, grooming, toileting, and eating. Of the total population of nursing home residents, 16% are 65–74 years old, 26.8% are 75–84 years old, and 40.7% are ≥85 years old. Women 65 years and older make up 69.4% older adult population living in nursing homes.

1.3.1.5 Educational Attainment

Over the last several decades, the proportion of older adults receiving higher education has increased. The majority of older adults in 1950 had less than high school education (82.3%) and very few obtained college education (3.7%). These statistics have changed considerably over the last six decades. By 2016, 85.4% of older adults had completed high school and 28.1% had obtained college education. The percentage of older adult high school graduates varied by race or ethnicity as follows: 90% white (non-Hispanic), 79.5% Asian (non-Hispanic), 76.7% black or African-American (non-Hispanic), 71.6% American Indian and Alaska native (non-Hispanic), 73.8% Native Hawaiian and Other Pacific Islander (non-Hispanic), 85.3% two or more races (non-Hispanic), and 54.4% Hispanic.

1.3.2 Life Expectancy and Mortality

In 2014, life expectancy in the United States was 78.8 years. Life expectancy in the United States has been increasing for decades, with additional life expectancy at age 65 rising from 15.2 years in 1972 to 19.1 years in 2010—a net gain of 3.9 years. At age 85 in 1972, additional life expectancy was 5.5 years, rising to 6.5 years by 2010 and 6.6 years in 2014. Over the past several decades, there has been a narrowing in the gap in life expectancy differences between males and females. In 2014, the Centers for Disease Control and Prevention (CDC) reported that life expectancy at age 65 was 18 years for men and 20.5 years for women [28].

Globally, all regions have experienced substantial increases in life expectancy since 1950. In 2015, global life expectancy was 70.5 years, having risen from 46.8 years in 1955. Life expectancy at birth in 2015 was highest in North America (79.2 years) and shortest in Africa (59.5 years).

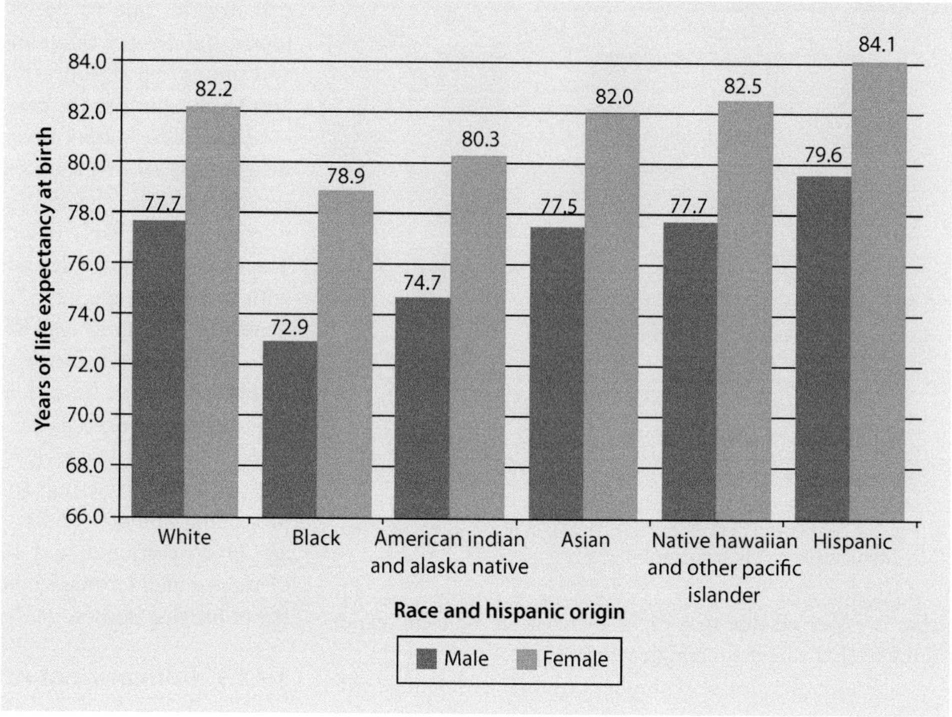

Fig. 1.3 Life expectancy at birth, by sex and race. (Modified from [31])

Life expectancy, though increasing in the United States over time, has lagged behind that of many other high-income countries. In 2012, the United States ranked 27th out of 34 Organization for Economic Cooperation and Development (OECD) countries in overall life expectancy [29]. This is thought to be due to early deaths in the United States related to obesity and higher rates of tobacco use [6, 30]. In addition, there are wide gaps in life expectancy across different racial/ethnic groups. Hispanic women and men have the highest life expectancy at birth when compared to other races, followed by white and Native Hawaiian and other Pacific Islander (Fig. 1.3).

The age-adjusted death rate in the United States declined to a record low in 2014: with statistics of deaths per 100,000 for persons aged 65 to 74 of 1786.3, 75–84 of 4564.2, and 85 and over of 13,407.9. The three leading causes of death in older adults are the same as those for younger adults: heart disease, cancer, and chronic lower respiratory disease. Though these conditions accounted for approximately half of all deaths in 2014, the overall mortality rate for each condition is slowly declining over the last several years. The age-adjusted death rates for unintentional injuries, stroke, Alzheimer's disease, suicide, and chronic liver disease, however, have increased over the last several years [32]. In 2012, the three leading causes of death in men and women globally were ischemic heart disease, stroke, and COPD [2].

1.3.3 Comorbidities and Healthcare Expenditures

Older adults are more likely than younger adults to have chronic medical conditions and disabilities. In 1999, 82% of Medicare Beneficiaries had one or more chronic condition, and 65% had two or more chronic conditions [33]. These statistics have remained relatively stable over time, with 65% of Medicare Beneficiaries having 2 or more chronic conditions in 2007 and 2015 as well. Among fee-for-service beneficiaries, the prevalence of chronic conditions in patients aged 65 years and older is not surprisingly higher compared to patients aged 65 and younger (Fig. 1.4).

According to the CDC, in 2015, 34.5% of older adults had one or more disabilities; 15.3% had hearing difficulty, 9.4% had vision difficulty, 9% had cognitive difficulty, 16.3% had difficulty with physical function, and 12% had self-care difficulty [35]. Studies have shown, however, that the rates of disability in the United States have been declining and the number of years a person can expect to live disability free has been increasing [36]. These changes are thought to be due to improvements in preventive care and in treatment of conditions including cardiovascular disease and diabetes.

As chronic conditions increase, health costs have also drastically increased. Most older adults (98.9%) have some type of health insurance with Medicare covering the majority (93.3%). Despite insurance coverage, out of pocket medical expenses are estimated at over 12% for older adults. The majority of these expenses are for insurance premiums, but also include medications, equipment and appointment copayments. The appropriate living environment is essential for older adults for safety, including the potential need for assistance with daily activities. The average annual cost of residing in a nursing home in the United States is $89,000-$100,000. By contrast the annual cost of residing in an assisted living is $48,000, which is equivalent to the average cost of out of pocket home health and home maker services [37].

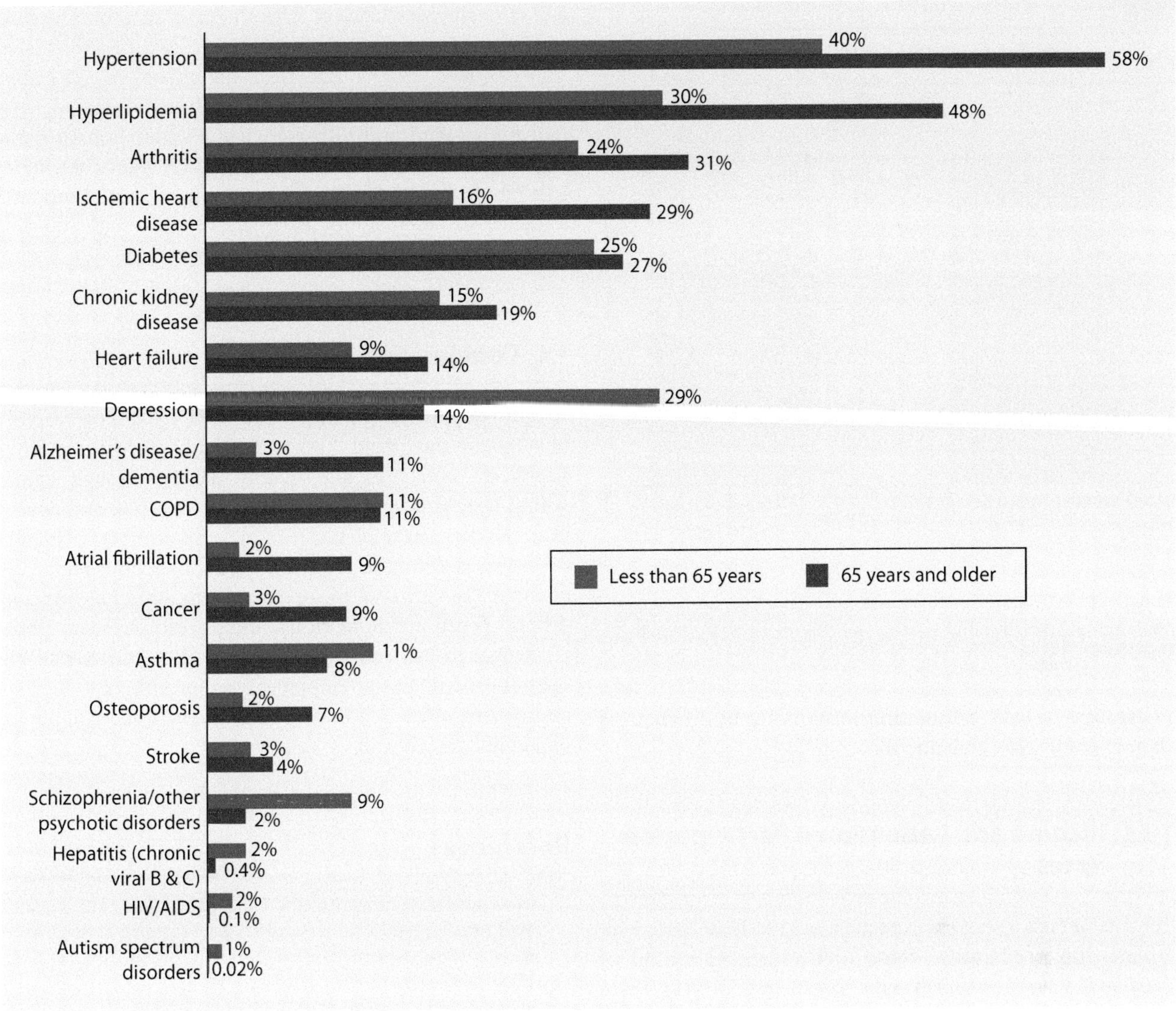

Fig. 1.4 Proportion of fee-for-service beneficiaries with chronic conditions by age. (Modified from [34])

Spending on healthcare has increased exponentially over time within the United States, reaching $3.3 trillion or $10,348 annually per person and accounting for 17.9% of the nation's Gross Domestic Product (GDP) in 2016. Not surprisingly, healthcare costs increase in older adults with multiple chronic conditions. The proportion of increase, however, is substantial. Of the per capita Medicare expenditures in 2012, 51% were attributed to the 15% of beneficiaries with 6 or more chronic conditions (Fig. 1.5) [34]. The unsustainable growth in healthcare costs, along with the unequal distribution of costs among those with the most chronic conditions, will continue to necessitate the development of healthcare policy and models of healthcare delivery aimed at cost reductions.

1.3.4 Distribution of Older Adults

Though older adults live throughout the United States, more than half of all older adults live in only 10 states: California, Florida, Texas, New York, Pennsylvania, Ohio, Illinois, Michigan, North Carolina and New Jersey [38]. As available resources and funding for support services for older adults vary considerably from state to state, attention to state policies, in addition to federal policies, is necessary to ensure optimal care of older adults. Florida has the highest proportion of older adults, with 19.4% of its total state population aged 65 and older, while less than 10% of Alaska population is over the age of 65. The state with the highest total number of older adults is California, with approximately 5 million (10.9%) of the total population of older adults living there. Alaska has the fewest total number of older adults, with less than 1% of the total population of older adults residing there. In 2015, older adults made up 18% of the population in rural areas and 14.1% of the population of urban areas. Older adults residing in rural areas may have limited access to healthcare resources due to longer lengths of travel necessary and rural hospital closures [22].

According to World Population Ageing, in 2015, 75% of the world's population of older adults lived in just 20 countries and 50% lived in just 5 countries: China, India, the United States, Japan, and the Russian Federation. The

1

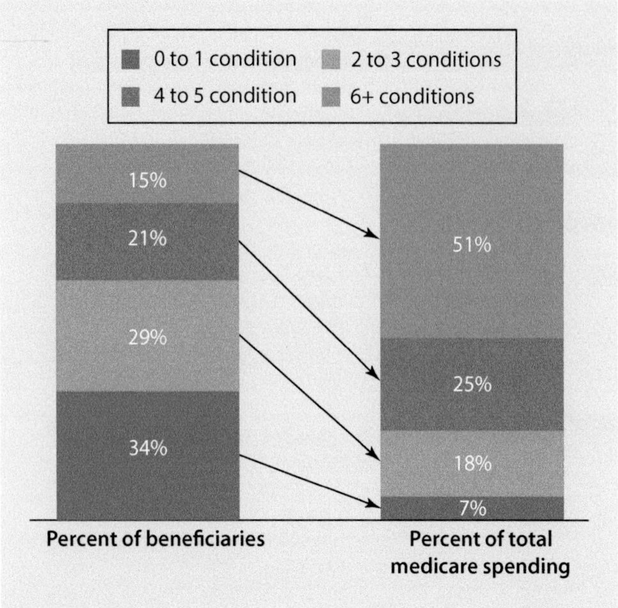

Fig. 1.5 Distribution of Medicare fee-for-service beneficiaries and Medicare spending by number of chronic conditions: 2015. (Modified from [34])

population of older adults is growing faster in urban areas than in rural areas globally [2].

1.3.5 Income and Labor Force Participation Rates

The median income of older adults was $38,515 in 2015, with a wide disparity between those with an annual income of $20,000 (24.3%) or $70,000 and over (27.3%). [40, 41]. There is even wider disparity between annual income by race. Most older adults (84%) receive some income from Social Security, and this income makes up more than half of the total income for many beneficiaries [39].

In 2016, 18.6% of people over the age of 65 were employed [39]. A larger percentage of men aged 65 years and older were working (23.1%) compared to women (14.9%) aged 65 years and older. Globally, in 2015, more than 30% of men and 14% of women were employed, with older adults in developed regions being more likely to be employed than their peers in less-developed regions [2].

1.3.6 Poverty

In 2016, the US poverty threshold for an older adult living alone was set at $11,511. Based on this figure, it was estimated that about 8.8% of older adults (10.3% of women and 7% of men) were living in poverty, down from nearly 30% in 1966. Increasing costs of medical care contribute greatly to the financial strain of many older adults, as out-of-pocket medical expenses alone place 5.65% of the older population in the poverty threshold. The proportion according to race and ethnicity were black or African-American non-Hispanic (18.2%), Asian non-Hispanic (11.8%), two or more races non-Hispanic (10.9%), American Indian and Alaska Native non-Hispanic (19.6%), white non-Hispanic (6.6%), and native Hawaiian and Other Pacific Islander non-Hispanic (7.7%) [22]. This disparity among poverty rates contributes to a number of health disparities and to the social supports available to older adults, particularly those with multiple chronic conditions.

1.4 Conclusions

As the population of older adults is expanding rapidly throughout the world, efforts must be made to improve healthcare outcomes and quality of life through efforts within healthcare policy, clinical care, research, and education. Geriatric principles have informed a number of changes over time resulting in many positive trends both nationally and globally. However, the presence of multiple chronic conditions, functional limitations, and poverty presents global challenges to the well-being of older adults. Geriatrics will continue to lead the development of innovative, cost-effective approaches which will improve health and quality of life for older adults worldwide.

References

1. Projected future growth of the older population 2017 [updated April 26 2017; cited 2018 January 31]. Available from: https://www.acl.gov/news-and-events/announcements/subject-profile-older-americans-2016.
2. United Nations DoEaSA. World population ageing 2015. New York: 2015 ST/ESA/SER.A/390.
3. Fried TR, Tinetti ME, Iannone L, O'Leary JR, Towle V, Van Ness PH. Health outcome prioritization as a tool for decision making among older persons with multiple chronic conditions. Arch Intern Med. 2011;171(20):1854–6.
4. JE M. A Brief History of Geriatrics. Gerontology. 2004;59(11):1132–52.
5. Berwick DM, Nolan TW, Whittington J. The triple aim: care, health, and cost. Health affairs (Project Hope). 2008;27(3):759–69.
6. National Research C, Institute of M. The National Academies Collection: reports funded by National Institutes of Health. In: Woolf SH, Aron L, editors. US health in international perspective: shorter lives, poorer health. Washington, DC: National Academies Press (US) National Academy of Sciences; 2013.
7. Landefeld CS, Palmer RM, Kresevic DM, Fortinsky RH, Kowal J. A randomized trial of care in a hospital medical unit especially designed to improve the functional outcomes of acutely ill older patients. N Engl J Med. 1995;332(20):1338–44.
8. Counsell SR, Callahan CM, Clark DO, Tu W, Buttar AB, Stump TE, et al. Geriatric care management for low-income seniors: a randomized controlled trial. JAMA. 2007;298(22):2623–33.
9. Eng C, Pedulla J, Eleazer GP, McCann R, Fox N. Program of All-inclusive Care for the Elderly (PACE): an innovative model of integrated geriatric care and financing. J Am Geriatr Soc. 1997;45(2):223–32.
10. Inouye SK, Bogardus ST Jr, Charpentier PA, Leo-Summers L, Acampora D, Holford TR, et al. A multicomponent intervention to prevent delirium in hospitalized older patients. N Engl J Med. 1999;340(9):669–76.

11. Capezuti E, Boltz M, Cline D, Dickson VV, Rosenberg MC, Wagner L, et al. Nurses improving care for healthsystem elders – a model for optimising the geriatric nursing practice environment. J Clin Nurs. 2012;21(21–22):3117–25.
12. Combined orthopaedic-geriatric care. Lancet. 1985;1(8424):349–50.
13. Accountable Care Organization 2015 Program analyis quality performance standards narrative measures specifications: RTI International; 2015 [cited 2018 January 31]. Available from: https://www.cms.gov/Medicare/Medicare-Fee-for-Service-Payment/sharedsavingsprogram/Downloads/RY2015-Narrative-Specifications.pdf.
14. 2015 Physician Quality Reporting System M (PQRS): implementation guide: CMS; 2015 [cited 2018 January 31]. Available from: https://www.cms.gov/Medicare/Quality-Initiatives-Patient-Assessment-Instruments/PQRS/Downloads/2015_PQRS_ImplementationGuide.pdf.
15. Skilled Nursing Facility Quality Reporting Program – Specifications for the quality measures adopted through the fiscal year 2016 final rule: RTI International; 2015 [cited 2018 January 31]. Available from: https://www.cms.gov/Medicare/Quality-Initiatives-Patient-Assessment-Instruments/NursingHomeQualityInits/Downloads/SNF-specs.pdf.
16. Quality measures used in the Home Health Quality Reporting Program: CMS; 2018 [cited 2018 January 31]. Available from: https://www.cms.gov/Medicare/Quality-Initiatives-Patient-Assessment-Instruments/HomeHealthQualityInits/Home-Health-Quality-Reporting-Requirements.html.
17. Chronic Care Management Services: CMS; 2015 [cited 2018 January 31]. Available from: https://www.cms.gov/Outreach-and-Education/Medicare-Learning-Network-MLN/MLNProducts/Downloads/ChronicCareManagement.pdf.
18. Proposed Policy, payment, and quality provisions changes to the medication physician fee schedule for calendar year 2016: CMS; 2016 [cited 2018 January 31]. Available from: https://www.cms.gov/Newsroom/MediaReleaseDatabase/Fact-sheets/2016-Fact-sheets-items/2016-07-07-2.html.
19. Libow LS. The birth of geriatrics in America. J Am Geriatr Soc. 2014;62(7):1369–76.
20. AAMC Geriatric competencies for medical students: the portal of geriatrics online education; [updated 2018; cited 2018 January 31]. Available from: https://www.pogoe.org/Minimum_Geriatric_Competencies.
21. The United States Census Bureau [updated 2017; cited 2018 January 31]. Available from: https://www.census.gov/.
22. Mather MJL, Pallard KM. Aging in the United States. 2015.
23. Vincent GKVV. The next four decades, the older population in the United States: 2010 to 2050. 2010 2010. Report No.: Contract No.: P25–1138.
24. J M. Centenarians 2010: 2010 Census Special Reports. 2010 May 2010. Report No.: Contract No.: CS2010SR-03.
25. Ortman JMVV, Hogan H. An aging nation: the older population in the United States; 2014. p. P25–1140.
26. Wolff JL, Mulcahy J, Huang J, Roth DL, Covinsky K, Kasper JD. Family caregivers of older adults, 1999–2015: trends in characteristics, circumstances, and role-related appraisal. The Gerontologist. 2017.
27. Older Americans 2016: key indicators of well-being. Available from: https://agingstats.gov/.
28. Older person' health: Centers for Disease Control and Prevention; 2017 [cited 2018 January 31]. Available from: https://www.cdc.gov/nchs/fastats/older-american-health.htm.
29. (OECD) OfECaD. How does the United States compare? OECD health statistics 2014: Oganization for Economic Cooperation and Development (OECD); 2014 [cited 2018 January 31]. Available from: www.oecd.org/unitedstates/Briefing-Note-UNITED-STATES-2014.pdf.
30. National Research Council Panel on Understanding Divergent Trends in Longevity in High-Income C. The national academies collection: reports funded by National Institutes of Health. In: Crimmins EM, Preston SH, Cohen B, editors. International differences in mortality at older ages: dimensions and sources. Washington, DC: National Academies Press (US). National Academy of Sciences; 2010.
31. Bureau USC. Population Division 2014 [cited 2018 January 31]. National Population Projections as Reported in Table 17]. Available from: https://census.gov/data/tables/2014/demo/popproj/2014-summary-tables.html.
32. Kochanek KD, Xu J, Tejada-Vera B. Deaths: final data for 2014. 2016.
33. Wolff JL, Starfield B, Anderson G. Prevalence, expenditures, and complications of multiple chronic conditions in the elderly. Arch Intern Med. 2002;162(20):2269–76.
34. CMS Chronic Conditions Chartbook. Available from: https://www.cms.gov/Research-Statistics-Data-and-Systems/Statistics-Trends-and-Reports/Chronic-Conditions/Chartbook_Charts.html.
35. National Center for Health Statistics, Disability and Functioning Centers for Disease Control and Prevention. Available from: https://www.cdc.gov/nchs/fastats/disability.htm.
36. Crimmins EM, Hayward MD, Hagedorn A, Saito Y, Brouard N. Change in disability-free life expectancy for Americans 70 years old and older*. Demography. 2009;46(3):627–46.
37. The United States Social Security Administration 2017 [cited 2018 January 31]. Available from: https://www.ssa.gov/news/press/fact-sheets/basicfact-alt.pdf.
38. Calculate the cost of Care in Your Area. Available from: Genworth.com.
39. Medina-Walpole A, Pacala JT, Potter JF, eds. Geriatrics Review Syllabus: A core Curriculum in geriatric Medicine. 9th Edition. New York: American Geriatrics Society; 2016.
40. US Bureau of Labor Statistics. Available from: https://www.bls.gov/bls/newsrels.htm-OEUS.
41. L F. The Supplemental Poverty Measure: 2010. 2017 P60–261 (RV).
42. Mather M, Jacobsen LA, Pollard KM. "Aging in the United States," Population Bulletin 70, no. 2. Washington, DC: Population Reference Bureau; 2015

Identifying the Unique Needs of the Aging Population

Amit Shah

A. Chun (ed.), *Geriatric Practice*, https://doi.org/10.1007/978-3-030-19625-7_2

2.1 Are Older Adults Really Different? Why Geriatric Medicine?

Should there be a field of geriatrics? Are older adults really that different from younger adults? There was a time when children were regarded, medically, as "little adults," and the field of pediatrics did not exist. Gradually, there was recognition that children suffered from different diseases, had different problems, and needed a different approach than adults, and finally by the 1930s, the specialty of pediatrics was established. The same had been said about the care of the older patient. For many years, the care of the older adult was not felt to be so different from that of younger adults, and many questioned the need for a separate specialty of geriatric medicine. Over several decades, the contributions of researchers in ***gerontology*** (the multidisciplinary study of aging) and ***geriatrics*** (the study of health and disease in later life) left no doubt that the care of the older adult was a distinctive specialty. By the late 1970s, the field of geriatrics was established as a specialty of medicine. However, unlike pediatrics, geriatrics is not yet a mandatory part of medical training in the United States at most institutions.

Unfortunately, in part due to the lack of required teaching in geriatric medicine in many health professional training programs, many students find their first experiences caring for complex older patients to be overwhelming [1]. In fact, such experiences can result in negative attitudes toward the older patient and a desire to avoid having to care for such patients [1, 2]. However, studies have shown that if a trainee learns how to manage these patients, the care of the older patient can be seen not as overwhelming but rewarding [3]. The remainder this book will teach you how the care of the older patient is different and some approaches to help you when you encounter an older patient in your future practice of medicine.

Let's preview some of what you'll learn in this book by going over some of the following 15 aphorisms which many geriatricians use in their teaching and highlight some of what you will learn in more detail in this book.

Care of the Older Patient: 15 Pearls of Wisdom

1. **If You've Seen One 80-Year-Old, You've Seen One 80-Year-Old**
2. **Aging Is Not a Disease**
3. **It Takes a Lot of Energy to Tread Water!**
4. **The Atypical Presentation of Illness Is Typical**
5. **A Patient May Have as Many Diseases as He Pleases**
6. **A Single Presenting Symptom May Have Many Contributing Etiologies**
7. **Multifactorial Syndromes Need Multifactorial Solutions**
8. **Watch Them Walk!**
9. **Start Low, Go Slow... But Get There!**
10. **You Can Cure More Diseases by Stopping Medicines than by Starting Them**
11. **It Takes a Village**
12. **Hazards of Hospitalization: You Can Win the Battle but Lose the War**
13. **Transitions Are the Danger Zone**
14. **Screen the Strong and Will the Weak**
15. **Death and Dying Are Not 4-Letter Words**

2.2 "If You've Seen One 80-Year-Old, You've Seen One 80-Year-Old"

There are varying definitions of what age delineates "younger" and "older" adults. In the United States, due to the age, a person qualifies for Medicare insurance coverage; the age 65 has often been used as an arbitrary dividing line defining "geriatric." However, there are substantial differences between the average 65-year-old and average 85-year-old. Many geriatricians split the age over 65 group into two and define these as "young-old" and "old-old," often with age 80 or 85 as the dividing line between these two groups. The "old-old" group is particularly vulnerable to frailty. One of the most striking features of taking care of a group of older patients is how much heterogeneity there is compared to a population of younger patients. For example, an 80-year-old patient you see could be in perfect health, on no medications, and still working. The next 80-year-old patient you see could be in a nursing home, completely dependent on care due to a stroke, and on multiple medications. This heterogeneity is the norm in geriatric medicine, and decisions must be made taking into account patient preferences, goals of care, life expectancy, functional status, and degree of frailty. Frailty can be defined as a condition of increased vulnerability to adverse outcomes from stressors due to the decline in physiologic reserves [4]. Frailty is often associated with weight loss, weakness (measured by grip strength), exhaustion, poor endurance, slowness (measured by gait speed), and low physical activity [4].

2.3 "Aging Is Not a Disease"

Aging by itself is not a disease. In ▶ Chap. 4, we will review some of the changes which occur with aging in all of the organ systems. In addition to these changes affecting how you interpret findings on history, physical exam, imaging, and labs, these changes significantly affect the older patient's ability to respond to illness and stressors and maintain homeostasis. Unfortunately, many older patients will underreport symptoms thinking they are just a part of getting older rather than a disease that could be intervened upon. Urinary incontinence and cognitive problems such as dementia are two examples of common diseases in older patients that are not a normal part of aging as you will learn about in ▶ Sects. 2.3 and 2.5.

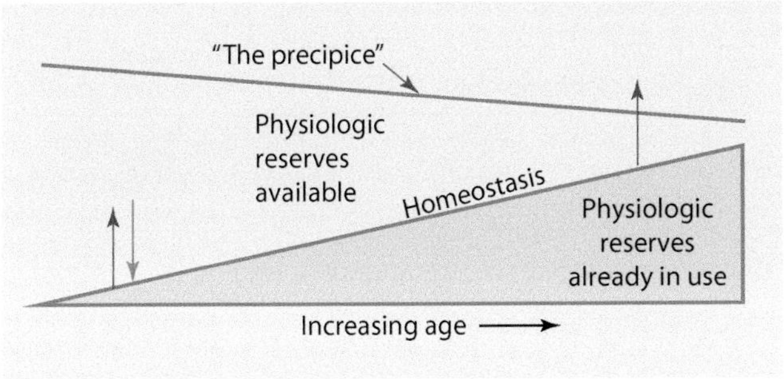

Fig. 2.1 Homeostenosis module. (Modified from Taffet [20])

2.4 "It Takes a Lot of Energy to Tread Water!"

When treading water in a pool, it takes considerable effort and energy expenditure just to stay afloat and remain in one place. Similarly, the maintenance of homeostasis requires more and more use of our physiological reserves as we age due to the cumulative effects of aging. This means that there is a decrease in the physiological reserves that are available to respond to a given stressor. This process is called ***homeostenosis***, as illustrated in Fig. 2.1. The "precipice" in the figure is the point beyond which an individual is in physiologic "trouble," has major symptoms, or dies. For example, a woman may have a urinary tract infection at age 25 which affects her homeostasis (depicted by the first red arrow), but since she has ample physiologic reserves she is able to fight the infection and return to homeostasis (depicted by the green arrow down) without any major symptoms other than dyuria affecting her. At age 85, the same woman can have the same urinary tract infection with the same organism, but due to homeostenosis, end up severely ill, delirious, and be admitted to the hospital, having crossed the "precipice" (second red arrow in the figure below) due to lack of available physiologic reserves.

2.5 "The Atypical Presentation of Illness Is Typical"

Indeed, due to these changes of aging, the classic or "textbook" illness presentation you may have learned is often not how the older person will present with a disease. For example, it is quite common for the 90-year-old nursing home resident to have only altered mental status as the presenting symptom of pneumonia rather than the classic pneumonia symptoms of fever and cough. This non-classic presentation of pneumonia has clinical implications, as failure to recognize that the cause of the patient's altered mental status is pneumonia results in delayed time to antibiotics in the emergency room or inpatient setting, which is associated with worse outcomes, including increased mortality [5]. Indeed, the "atypical" presentation of diseases is so typical that many geriatricians teach that the "atypical presentation of illness is typical." Due to this fact, providers must take careful and comprehensive histories and physical exams when an older person presents with a symptom, especially when delayed diagnosis may substantially affect morbidity or mortality, such as infection, myocardial infarction, or stroke.

2.6 "A Patient May Have as Many Diseases as He or She Pleases"

The clinical reasoning espoused by Dr. William Osler and in traditional teaching of clinical reasoning is to take all of a patient's signs and symptoms and try to come up with a single unifying diagnosis. This is called *Occam's razor* or "the simplest explanation is the likely correct explanation." Although there is utility to this type of clinical reasoning in making diagnoses, this "diagnostic parsimony" can often cause problems in older patients due to the fact that older patients often have multiple chronic diseases, a condition called "multimorbidity" which we will discuss in ▶ Sect. 2.3. For some older patients, *Hickam's Dictum* that "a patient may have as many diseases as he damn well pleases" is more appropriate [6] as it is quite common for the ill older person to have multiple diseases simultaneously or that one acute illness can cause worsening of the patient's chronic diseases. For example, an 85-year-old patient may come to the hospital with a severe pneumonia, but due to his preexisting coronary artery disease, he may have a myocardial infraction during the hospitalization caused by hypotension from the pneumonia. The heart attack may be missed as the patient may have only worsening shortness of breath as a symptom (not have chest pain), and this symptom could be mistakenly attributed to the pneumonia. Indeed, this has been shown in the literature, with ~20% of older patients admitted for pneumonia at one hospital suffering either a myocardial infarction, congestive heart failure exacerbation, or new-onset arrhythmia during a pneumonia hospitalization [7].

2.7 A Presenting Symptom May Have Many Contributing Etiologies: The Geriatric Syndrome

In addition to the possibility that the patient may have a few simultaneous illnesses, the older patient often presents with only one problem, but this problem may actually have multiple causes. These types of conditions are called ***geriatric syndromes.*** In a typical disease, such as influenza (see Fig. 2.2), there are a constellation of signs and symptoms which all have one underlying etiology with a known pathogenesis. In contrast, with geriatrics syndromes, just one presenting symptom, such as delirium (see Fig. 2.3), may be due to many possible etiologies, including the possibility that a patient could have two or more causes which may be interacting with one another to result in the final symptom of delirium. The approach to a patient with a geriatric syndrome presentation such as delirium or falls should be one which evaluates for multiple precipitating and predisposing factors as we will discuss in ▶ Sects. 2.5 and 2.6.

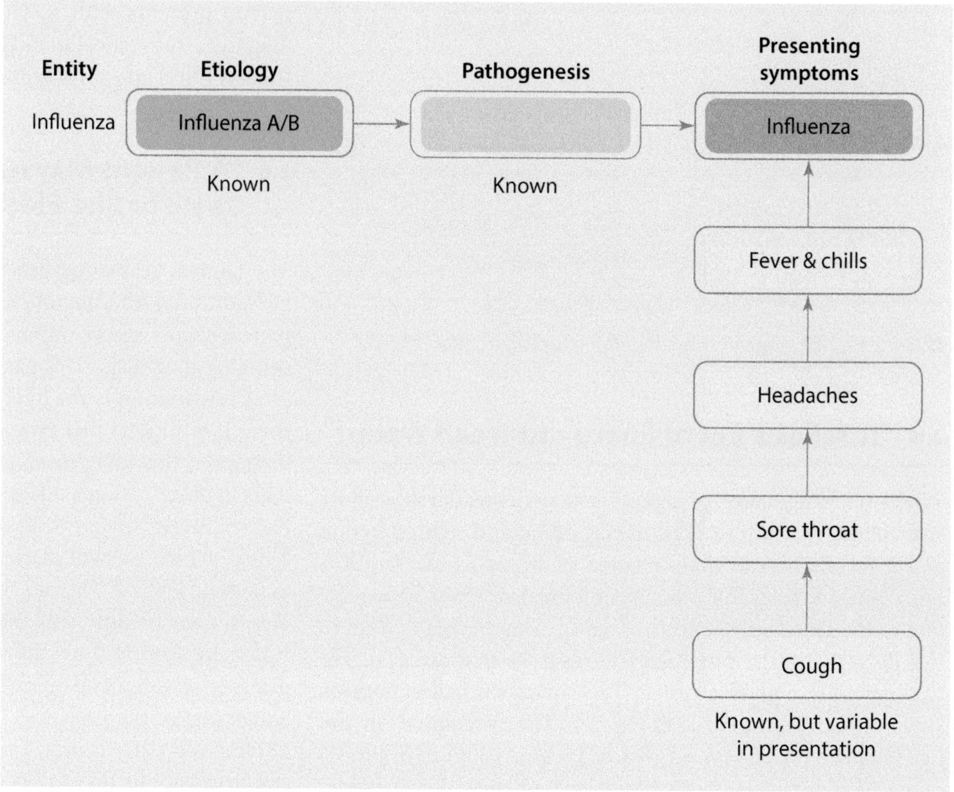

Fig. 2.2 Classic disease orientation presentation of an illness

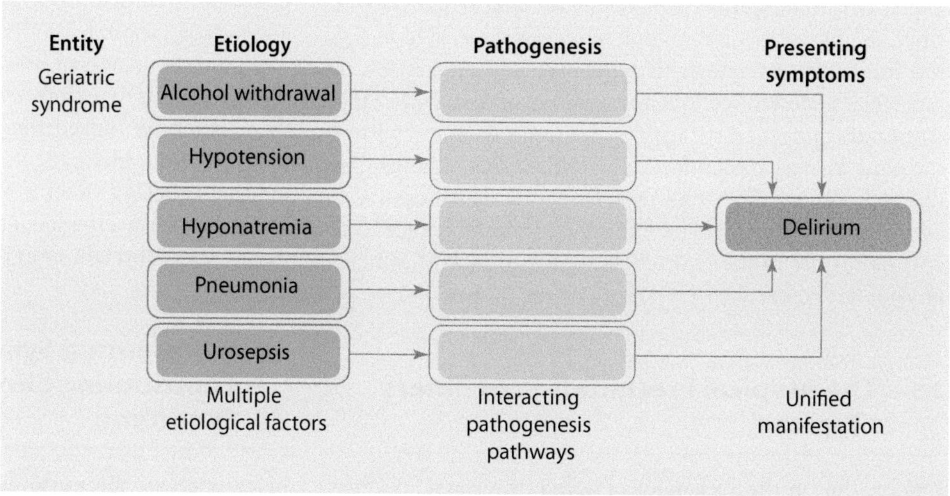

Fig. 2.3 Geriatric syndrome

2.8 "Multifactorial Syndromes Need Multifactorial Solutions"

If a patient has a multifactorial geriatric syndrome, such as falls, it is unlikely that addressing just one contributing factor will be successful. Multifactorial etiologies need to be addressed by a multifaceted approach or the solution may not be effective. For example, for interventions to help nursing home patients with recurrent falls, a meta-analysis showed that multifactorial interventions significantly reduced falls by 33% and number of recurrent fallers by 21%, whereas single-intervention-type trials which addressed just one cause or risk factor for falling did not reduce falls [8]. Another example is delirium in hospitalized inpatients. As will be discussed in ► Sect. 2.5, delirium can be prevented in hospitalized older patients with multifactorial interventions which include addressing sleep, hydration, immobility, and visual/hearing impairment all at the same time [9].

2.9 "Watch Them Walk!"

Maintenance of independence and function is a key goal of the aging patient. For this reason, assessment of functional status and mobility is very important. Two simple tests can be very helpful. The Timed Get-Up-and-Go test involves watching a patient get up from a chair to a standing position and then walking 3 meters and sitting back down. The second test is measurement of the person's gait speed. Decreased gait speed is a marker of frailty and has been correlated with increased perioperative mortality after cardiac surgery [10]. Simple gait speed measurements can help surgeons make decisions about who might be too frail for an operation and help patients make informed decisions about the risk for elective, non-emergent surgeries. Poor performance on the Get-Up-And-Go test can identify those who are frail and those who are at risk for falls and also has been correlated with risk for functional decline after an emergency room visit [11–13]. The importance of functional assessment, self-care ability, and assessment of home safety will be discussed in ▶ Sect. 2.6.

2.10 "Start Low, Go Slow.... But Get There!"

When starting a new medication, this adage is a good one to follow. When starting a patient on medications such as thyroid hormone or warfarin, it is better to start at a lower dose and monitor frequently until therapeutic range has been achieved. The traditional starting dose may be too high for the older patient with decreased renal function and altered body composition and volume of distribution of drug, as will be discussed in ▶ Sect. 2.6.

2.11 "You Can Cure More Diseases by Stopping Medicines than by Starting Them"

This adage is a bit of an overstatement, but it is true that polypharmacy and medication side effects are common problems for the older patient, as will be reviewed in ▶ Sect. 2.4. It is important to carefully review all of the medications a patient takes, including over-the-counter medications and supplements. It is estimated that one-third of all older patients have polypharmacy (are on 5 or more prescription medications) and about two-thirds are on 5 or more medications of all types (prescription/over-the-counter/supplements). In a nationally representative sample, about 15% of the adults were on medication combinations with the potential for a major drug-drug interaction [14]. Older adults have over three times as many emergency room visits as the general population for adverse drug events, with common medications such as diabetes medications and anticoagulants as the main offenders [15, 16]. Of course, many of these medications are indicated and beneficial. However, others can cause side effects or may have been started to treat the side effects of another medication (called the "prescribing cascade"). ◻ Figure 2.4 shows an example of this in which a patient is started on a non-steroidal anti-inflammatory drug (NSAID) for arthritis, which causes salt retention and worsening blood pressure. A calcium-channel blocker (CCB) is then added which then causes the patient to have ankle swelling and edema, for which a diuretic is started. This results in increased uric acid level and episodes of gout, and eventually, the patient ends up on allopurinol.

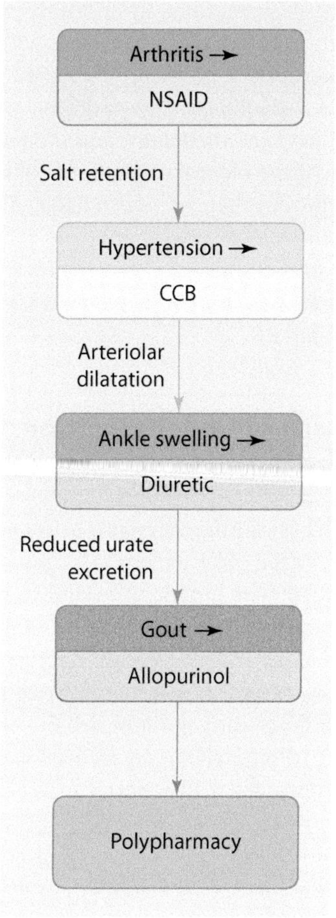

◻ **Fig. 2.4** The prescribing cascade (NSAID non-steroidal anti-inflammatory drug, CCB calcium-channel blocker)

In other cases, a medication may be a poor choice for the altered physiology of the older patient. For example, use of a long-acting sulfonylurea such as glyburide should not be used due to the significantly increased risk for hypoglycemia compared to a shorter half-life medication such as glipizide. Sometimes, appropriate medications or medication doses can become inappropriate as the patient ages. For example, a patient may have needed digoxin 0.25 mg (a high dose), but after as the patient's renal function declines over time, the patient can become toxic on this medicine without dose adjustment. Careful medication "deprescribing" or "medication debridement" can often help the older patient. Use of non-pharmacologic measures to treat common geriatric problems, such as insomnia and urinary incontinence, can also help to reduce polypharmacy and medication side effects by avoiding medication initiation in the first place.

2.12 "It Takes a Village"

Care of a complex, frail, geriatric patient almost never can be done successfully without an interdisciplinary approach. This interdisciplinary approach has been at the heart of geriatrics since its inception. In addition to physicians in other specialties, geriatricians often work with nurses, social workers, pharmacists, physical therapists, occupational therapists, speech therapists, care coordinators, home health aides, hospice workers, dieticians, and others to provide for the care needs of the older patient. Some older patients will end up moving from their homes to assisted living facilities or nursing homes for ongoing care. It is very important to work with the interdisciplinary teams at these institutions to provide the optimal care for your patient as will be discussed in ▶ Sects. 2.8 and 2.9.

2.13 "Hazards of Hospitalization: You Can Win the Battle but Lose the War"

Hospitalization has long been recognized as a particularly dangerous period for the older patient [17]. Take, for example, a 95-year-old patient with hip fracture. Unfortunately, although the medical team may be successful in "winning the battle" by successfully fixing the patient's hip fracture, the functional decline caused by bedrest and immobility may result in "losing the war" and a downward spiral of debility and dependency from which the patient may never recover, in spite of the primary problem being fixed. In ▶ Sect. 2.8, we will discuss some of the hazards of hospitalization such as pressure ulcers and use of physical and pharmacological restraints. Methods to reduce or prevent some of the risks of hospitalization will be discussed along with care models to avoid hospitalization in the first place, such as hospital-in-home.

2.14 "Transitions Are the Danger Zone"

A time of particular vulnerability for the older patient is when the patient changes sites of care, such as upon discharge from the hospital. The older patient often faces many changes in location of care. For example, after a hospitalization, a patient may experience significant loss of function and go to a subacute rehabilitation facility before being able to go back home. In ▶ Sects. 2.8 and 2.9, you will learn how to help patients navigate these transitions, including the importance of discharge planning and medication reconciliation during care transitions.

2.15 "Screen the Strong and Will the Weak"

The approach to the preventative care and decision making about invasive interventions may not differ that much from younger patients when the older patient is in good health, has good functional status, and is not frail. For example, a top-quartile 80-year-old male has an average life expectancy of greater than 10 years, and so a procedure such as a screening colonoscopy or elective knee replacement surgery would be reasonable and likely well-tolerated. In contrast, a bottom-quartile 80-year-old male has a life expectancy of about 3 years, and so cancer screening or an elective procedure could result in significant harm [18]. When caring for a frail older patient with limited life expectancy, it is more important to discuss goals of care, advance care planning, and patient preferences about the intensity of medical intervention he or she would like.

2.16 "Death and Dying Are Not 4-letter Words"

Geriatric medicine also includes caring for patients who are nearing the end of life. Doing so in a skilled way can result in the patient experiencing end-of-life without unwanted aggressive interventions or needless suffering. This requires those caring for the older patient to be comfortable addressing goals of care, prognostication, and skill at transitioning the patient from preventative or curative intent care to care focused on the patient's symptoms and quality of life. As will be discussed in ▶ Sect. 2.10, in addition to addressing medical problems and physical pain, the holistic care of the patient's psychological, social, and spiritual needs is required to help patients achieve a "good death." Finally, the older person is often cared for by others in his/her last years, and addressing the needs and expectations of family and caregivers is a key skill in the care of the geriatric patient as caregiver burnout can adversely affect the patient.

2.17 Geriatric Practice: Mastering Subtlety and Complexity

Geriatricians have been described as masters of subtlety and complexity who work in interdisciplinary teams to care for older patients by respecting and addressing the physical, social, and psychological factors to make them unique individuals [19]. You too can provide such competent and masterful care of the older patient you encounter in your practice by using the approaches discussed in this book and remembering some of the key "pearls of geriatric wisdom" described in this chapter.

References

1. Bagri AS, Tiberius R. Medical student perspectives on geriatrics and geriatric education. J Am Geriatr Soc. 2010;58(10):1994–9.
2. Meiboom AA, de Vries H, Hertogh CM, Scheele F. Why medical students do not choose a career in geriatrics: a systematic review. BMC Med Educ. 2015;15:101.
3. Drickamer MA, Levy B, Irwin KS, Rohrbaugh RM. Perceived needs for geriatric education by medical students, internal medicine residents and faculty. J Gen Intern Med. 2006;21(12):1230–4.
4. Fried LP, Tangen CM, Walston J, Newman AB, Hirsch C, Gottdiener J, et al. Frailty in older adults: evidence for a phenotype. J Gerontol A Biol Sci Med Sci. 2001;56(3):M146–56.
5. Waterer GW, Kessler LA, Wunderink RG. Delayed administration of antibiotics and atypical presentation in community-acquired pneumonia. Chest. 2006;130(1):11–5.

6. Mani N, Slevin N, Hudson A. What Three Wise Men have to say about diagnosis. B Med J. 2011;343:d7769.
7. Musher DM, Rueda AM, Kaka AS, Mapara SM. The association between pneumococcal pneumonia and acute cardiac events. Clin Infect Dis. 2007;45(2):158–65.
8. Vlaeyen E, Coussement J, Leysens G, Van der Elst E, Delbaere K, Cambier D, et al. Characteristics and effectiveness of fall prevention programs in nursing homes: a systematic review and meta-analysis of randomized controlled trials. J Am Geriatr Soc. 2015;63(2):211–21.
9. Inouye SK, Bogardus ST Jr, Charpentier PA, Leo-Summers L, Acampora D, Holford TR, et al. A multicomponent intervention to prevent delirium in hospitalized older patients. N Engl J Med. 1999;340(9):669–76.
10. Afilalo J, Kim S, O'Brien S, Brennan JM, Edwards FH, Mack MJ, et al. Gait speed and operative mortality in older adults following cardiac surgery. JAMA Cardiol. 2016;1(3):314–21.
11. Ansai JH, Farche ACS, Rossi PG, de Andrade LP, Nakagawa TH, Takahashi ACM. Performance of different timed up and go subtasks in frailty syndrome. J Geriatr Phys Ther. 2017.
12. Eagles D, Perry JJ, Sirois MJ, Lang E, Daoust R, Lee J, et al. Timed Up and Go predicts functional decline in older patients presenting to the emergency department following minor trauma. Age Ageing. 2017;46(2):214–8.
13. Savva GM, Donoghue OA, Horgan F, O'Regan C, Cronin H, Kenny RA. Using timed up-and-go to identify frail members of the older population. J Gerontol A Biol Sci Med Sci. 2013;68(4):441–6.
14. Qato DM, Wilder J, Schumm LP, Gillet V, Alexander GC. Changes in prescription and over-the-counter medication and dietary supplement use among older adults in the United States, 2005 vs 2011. JAMA Intern Med. 2016;176(4):473–82.
15. Shehab N, Lovegrove MC, Geller AI, Rose KO, Weidle NJ, Budnitz DS. US Emergency Department visits for outpatient adverse drug events, 2013-2014. JAMA. 2016;316(20):2115–25.
16. Budnitz DS, Shehab N, Kegler SR, Richards CL. Medication use leading to emergency department visits for adverse drug events in older adults. Ann Intern Med. 2007;147(11):755–65.
17. Creditor MC. Hazards of hospitalization of the elderly. Ann Intern Med. 1993;118(3):219–23.
18. Walter LC, Covinsky KE. Cancer screening in elderly patients: a framework for individualized decision making. JAMA. 2001;285(21):2750–6.
19. Hazzard WR. I am a geriatrician. J Am Geriatr Soc. 2004;52(1):161.
20. Taffet GE. Physiology of aging. In: Cassel CK, Leipzig RM, Cohen HJ, et al., editors. Geriatric medicine: an evidence-based approach. 4th ed. New York: Springer; 2003.

Education of Current and Future Providers

Kathryn E. Callahan and Rosanne M. Leipzig

A. Chun (ed.), *Geriatric Practice*, https://doi.org/10.1007/978-3-030-19625-7_3

> *It is far more important to know what patient the disease has than to know what disease the patient has. –Attributed to Hippocrates*

What's so different about older people that they warrant having their own medical specialty? Some healthcare providers argue that older people suffer the same diseases as middle-aged people; they simply have more of them. This approach can lead to over- and underdiagnosis and over- and under-treatment for older adults, since the presentation, diagnosis, and treatment of diseases may be different, causing excess burden, morbidity, and mortality.

In this chapter, we will:

- Define the core features of geriatric medicine and a "Function First" approach to care [1], using the Geriatrics 5 M's [2].
- Discuss assessment of physical and cognitive function, and illustrate its implications for prognostication and personalized medicine for older adults.
- Review areas of competence needed by healthcare providers caring for older adults.
- Discuss what older adults need from their healthcare [3].

3.1 Core Features of Geriatric Medicine: "Function First" and "The Geriatrics 5 M's"

So what is unique about geriatric medicine? Firstly, older adults differ greatly one from the other, a phenomenon called the ***heterogeneity of aging***. Median life expectancy for an 80-year-old woman is 88.6; however, one in four will live to be over 93 years old, while another one in four will die before they are 85 [4]. Not taking this into account means you may be overtreating, putting someone through diagnostic tests and treatment for a condition they're unlikely to ever get sick from. Secondly, function is the primary driver of life expectancy and certainly the highest priority of older adults themselves [1]. There is also significant heterogeneity in function, and function is the best predictor of morbidity and mortality. Older adults can be stratified into those who are fit, vulnerable (also called pre-frail), and frail, and the more frail they are, the more likely that they will have bad outcomes and suffer adverse events from tests and treatments. Not taking this into account means you might recommend treatment for someone when their risk of a bad treatment outcome exceeds their likelihood of benefit from treatment.

Many other factors also argue against a solely disease-focused approach for older adults, including the age-related loss of physiological and functional reserve, the prevalence of multiple conditions (also called multimorbidity), and high rates of functional impairment. Further, the heterogeneity of aging demands individualized care: that is, an understanding of what the individual really needs and wants their medical care to focus on.

Table 3.1 The Geriatric 5 M's

Mind	Mentation Dementia Depression Delirium
Mobility	Gait and balance Falls prevention
Medications	Polypharmacy De-prescribing and optimal prescribing Adverse medication effects
Multicomplexity	Multimorbidity Frailty Complex psychosocial situations
What matters most	Individual's health goals and preferences

The **Geriatrics 5 M's** (Table 3.1) is a mnemonic focusing on five domains that are important in caring for older persons [2]. Specialty geriatricians are masters in these areas, not only by identifying these concerns but by providing comprehensive evaluation and integration of these into each patient's care. Making a review of the 5 M's a regular part of your practice will aid in your ability to tailor care for your older patients recognizing the heterogeneity of aging.

3.2 Geriatric Medicine Is Personalized Medicine

In medicine, we often teach that before you order a diagnostic test, you should know how the results would change your patient management; if they would not, why do the test? In a disease-based care model, it may be difficult to see how applying the principles of geriatric medicine would change management. To illustrate this, the next section provides case scenarios of older adults who are *fit*, *vulnerable*, or *frail*. There are several validated tools for stratifying older adults into these categories. What they have in common are measures of disease damage and dysregulation, physical function (muscle mass and strength, unintentional weight loss, exhaustion, slowness, loss of Activities of Daily Living (ADLs)), and cognitive function [5]. Frailty and vulnerability, or pre-frailty, identify people with decreased resiliency and more poor health outcomes than those who are fit, with the frail having the worst outcomes. Each case scenario is augmented by patient-specific answers to the 5 M's, demonstrating how this knowledge affects the patient's care plan.

Case Scenario One

Ms. DeAngelo is an 82-year-old woman with hypertension, type 2 diabetes mellitus (DM) without complications, and a history of colon polyps, who drove herself to her Annual Wellness Visit. She wants to discuss what her target goals should be for her blood pressure (BP) and her hemoglobin a1c, whether she should undergo any cancer screening, and if she needs all the medications she is currently taking (Table 3.2).

In Case Scenario One, Ms. DeAngelo would be considered a "**fit**" older person, so we would recommend:

- **Hypertension target goal**: Recent guidelines suggest a target BP of 130/80 for this community-dwelling older woman with increased risk of cardiovascular outcomes due to her DM [6]. Even though she is fit, she should still be checked for orthostatic hypotension since treatment may exacerbate this and her target BP should be based on her standing BP.
- **Diabetes target goal**: A hemoglobin a1c level between 7 and 8 will keep her from developing hypo- or hyperglycemia. Considering her excellent function, prognostication models would estimate she likely has at least another 5–10 years of life remaining, and would be unlikely to develop complications of diabetes during this time with this level of glucose control. If her hemoglobin a1c is ≤6.5, we would recommend de-escalating medications by tapering her metformin dose and monitoring [7].
- **Cancer screening**: Recommendations for cancer screening often have an upper age limit, since it takes years for a screen-detected cancer to clinically affect patients. The American Geriatrics Society recommends *offering breast cancer screening* every 2 years for those patients like Ms. DeAngelo with a life expectancy of 10 years or more, which would be reasonable given her good physical and cognitive function [8]. Colon cancer screening would depend on her prior screening and the polyp types previously found. It would be reasonable to *offer colon cancer screening* if her prior polyps were pre-cancerous and if she were due for a colonoscopy before she is age 85 [9]. After 85, the risk of colonic perforation increases while the risk of dying from a new colon cancer decreases, so screening colonoscopy may not be appropriate.
- **Medications**: Although she is taking eight medications, each has an appropriate indication, so she does not have polypharmacy. However, two of these medications should be used with caution in older adults. Tylenol PM contains diphenhydramine which is very anticholinergic and can cause delirium in elders, while ibuprofen can increase BP and cause congestive heart failure (CHF), acute kidney injury, and gastric ulcers. Alternative treatments, including nonpharmacological ones, should be discussed with her.
- She is interested in medications for urinary incontinence (UI). Nonpharmacological interventions are more effective and longer lasting than medications for UI. You should determine the type of UI (see ▶ Chap. 36) and then discuss her options for treatment. Many of the medications for treating UI are anticholinergic, which increase concerns for dry mouth and confusion.
- **Function**: Ms. DeAngelo is able to complete all her ADLs and gets exercise working in her garden. She does not have cognitive impairment; you could recommend a walking program with some strength training to further enhance her physical and cognitive function [13, 14]. It is important to determine if she is socially isolated, and if so, encouraging social connections within and outside the family may enhance her quality of life.
- **Advance care planning**: As she approaches 85 years old, an overall discussion of her goals of care is appropriate [10]. While she does not have a single dominant disease, she is at increased risk of death by age alone, and a better understanding of her healthcare priorities and end of life wishes can help guide much of her overall care.

Table 3.2 The Geriatric 5 M's of Case Scenario One

Mind	No cognitive concerns per patient/family. *Independent in her Instrumental Activities of Daily Living (IADLs), including finances.* Dementia screening (75+): negative (Mini-Cog) Depression screening: negative (PHQ-2) No delirium *Extended grief following husband's death; now no evidence mood disorder, memory loss*
Mobility	Timed up and go: 10 seconds (low risk for falls ≤11 seconds) 3-chair rise: 9 seconds (normal <10 seconds) One fall—tripped over garden hose; no injury *Lives in split-level home. Does all her own gardening and lawn maintenance (4+ hour stretches) 3 seasons out of the year*
Medications	For HTN: hydrochlorothiazide; losartan; amlodipineFor DM: metformin For arthritis: acetaminophen For osteoporosis: alendronate Occasional Tylenol PM, ibuprofen *She asks about treatment for urinary incontinence*
Multicomplexity	Multimorbidity: HTN, DM, OA, OP *Lives alone; son travels and stays weekends; granddaughter comes by twice a week*
What matters most	Independence is most important—cognition and physical function Advance care planning: full code *Will not consider a "rest home" and would prefer to stay home. Believes she can afford nursing home or home care if needed. Sons hold her healthcare powers of attorney*

Case Scenario Two

Ms. DeAngelo is an 82-year-old woman with hypertension, type 2 diabetes mellitus without complications, urinary incontinence, and a history of colon polyps, whose granddaughter drove her to her Annual Wellness Visit. They want to discuss her blood pressure and diabetes treatment, whether she should undergo any cancer screening, and if she needs all the medications she is currently taking (◘ Table 3.3).

In Case Scenario Two, Ms. DeAngelo would be considered "**vulnerable or pre-frail**," so we would recommend:

- **Hypertension target goal**: Recent guidelines suggest a target BP of 130–150/80 for this community-dwelling older woman with moderate dementia, functional impairment, and increased risk of cardiovascular outcomes due to her DM [6]. It is important to be sure that none of her symptoms are due to these medications. The target BP goal would be an ideal subject for shared decision making with her and her family based on her concern for stroke (which could be devastating to her physical and cognitive function) versus the side effects and burdens of the four antihypertensive medications she is currently taking.
- **Diabetes target goal**: A hemoglobin a1c level of 8–9 should keep her from developing hypo- or hyperglycemia. Tight control of her diabetes will not improve her survival and is unlikely to improve her quality of life. Taking glipizide puts her at greater risk of hypoglycemia with subsequent falls or delirium. As discussed above, she is less cognitively and functionally intact as compared with Scenario One. While she is likely to live another 5 or more years, it is most likely that her trajectory will be a continued functional decline.
- **Cancer screening**: It is unlikely that breast cancer or colon cancer screening would help Ms. DeAngelo live longer or better. The preparation for colon cancer screening could cause dehydration, falls, or delirium—similar to her recent hospitalization. She may respond poorly to sedation for the colonoscopy. Screening cessation should be discussed with her and her granddaughter.
- **Medications:** Ms. DeAngelo has polypharmacy: she is on multiple medications which have unclear indications, and some that are high risk for older people. She may need fewer antihypertensives, and glipizide and naproxen should be stopped (older adults are at increased risk of bleeding and acute kidney injury from NSAIDs). Her risks of bleeding from aspirin are likely greater than any prevention benefits on cardiac disease or colon cancer at this stage of her life. The esomeprazole was likely prescribed as gastric protection from the aspirin and naproxen, and so can be discontinued if these are stopped. There should be a discussion with the family and patient as to whether the citalopram has helped her depression and if the oxybutynin has helped her incontinence. Was the sleeping problem new during hospitalization, and does she need help with sleeping now that she is home? Her initial questions suggest she would rather be on fewer medications, and we want her to only be on medications that will benefit her. She is at high risk

◘ **Table 3.3** The Geriatric 5 M's of Case Scenario Two

Mind	Cognitive concerns per patient/family. *Son has taken over her finances, and granddaughter does pill box weekly* *Dementia* case-finding: positive screens (Mini-Cog; follow-up MOCA 23/30) *Depression* screening: PHQ-2 positive for anhedonia. *Frustrated and tearful over loss of function and "independence." Fears further losses and ambivalent about family help* *Delirium*: recent hospitalization for pneumonia with mild delirium; this "revealed her memory problems," per granddaughter
Mobility	Timed up and go: 15 seconds (at risk for falls >11 seconds) 3-chair rise: 15 seconds (at risk for falls >10 seconds) *Fell when diagnosed with pneumonia—orthostatic and dehydrated—worked with physical therapy, but gave up many activities like lawn maintenance, and with fear or falling, she fears restarting gardening, too*
Medications	For HTN: hydrochlorothiazide; losartan; amlodipine; hydralazine For DM: metformin; glipizide For arthritis: acetaminophen, naproxen For osteoporosis: alendronate For incontinence: oxybutynin **New post-hospitalization**: esomeprazole; trazodone as needed for insomnia; citalopram; aspirin
Multicomplexity	Multimorbidity: HTN, DM, OA, OP, UI, likely depression *Lives alone; one son travels for work and stays weekends; granddaughter comes by twice a week but worries patient needs more. Patient fearful of going out by herself, doesn't want to move from her home (split level) to an assisted living facility but worries she is burdening family by staying home*
What matters most	Independence is most important, being able to do what she wants Advance care planning: DNR; would still want aggressive care in the event of a potentially reversible illness, but not to be "on a machine" long-term *She feels she is no different than she ever has been, except that she's slower and her memory is not as sharp. Would prefer to live at home. She has good insight into her physical challenges and early cognitive changes and feels she can hire in help as needed. Sons hold her healthcare powers of attorney*

for a hip fracture, so it makes sense to continue the alendronate (depending on how long she has been taking it and her bone mineral density).

- **Function:** Ms. DeAngelo's function has declined since prior to her hospitalization; despite completing PT, she has "fear of falling" and has concerns about trips outside her home. She is also depressed and becoming more physically isolated. Physical therapy should be reinstated with a goal of increasing her confidence walking outside. Her depression needs to be proactively treated with additional medications, talk therapy, or both. Consultation with a social worker could provide connections with Meals on Wheels and friendly visitors to aid with socialization. Once her depression lifts, she may be open to referral to community-based resources that could help her overcome her fear of falling, start a walking program, increase her strength, limit further functional decline, and enhance socialization. Depending on her cognitive testing, and a careful history with her family surrogates, she may need to give up driving. These conversations will be challenging, especially since insight and judgment are among the earliest losses in dementia. However, since she is early in her cognitive decline, discussing parameters for cessation of driving and other responsibilities are important. Plans for social and familial support will be critical to next steps as her dementia progresses.
- **Advance care planning**: She is approaching 85 years old with moderate dementia, multimorbidity, and functional decline. Her insight is fair, and she may be able to tell you her healthcare priorities and end of life wishes, and in particular, her wishes if she is no longer able to care for herself. Since dementia is progressive, she will never be better able to have this discussion.

Case Scenario Three

Ms. DeAngelo, an 82-year-old woman with hypertension, type 2 diabetes mellitus, and a history of colon polyps, declines to come for an Annual Wellness Visit—her son and granddaughter note, "She's not well – and it's hard to get her in even to go over all her problems." She sees you for a follow-up after falling, accompanied by her granddaughter (◘ Table 3.4).

From these findings, Ms. DeAngelo would be considered a "frail" older person, so we would recommend:

- **Hypertension target goal**: 150/80. She is frail with dementia and recent falls, so you need to be sure that none of her symptoms are actually side effects of the three antihypertensive medications

◘ Table 3.4 The Geriatric 5 M's of Case Scenario Three

Mind	Strong cognitive concerns per family. *One son handles her finances and healthcare needs, and the other is using the Family Medical Leave Act (FMLA) to help care for her; granddaughter helps when she can. Needs help with IADLs* *Dementia* case-finding: positive (Mini-Cog; MOCA 14/30.) Has had some hallucinations that scare her (children in the living room, knocking at the door during the night) *Depression* screening: PHQ-2 positive for anhedonia. *Feels as though she just "sits around." Recognizes need for help but tearful about moving from her home. Poor insight into cognition, frailtyDelirium*: Recent hospitalization for aspiration pneumonia with delirium; "she was a totally different person," per granddaughter, and has not recovered her pre-hospitalization baseline cognition and function
Mobility	Timed up and go: 25 seconds (at risk of losing an ADL in the next year) 3-chair rise: cannot stand without using her arms to get up from the chair *Fell yesterday when got up from couch—"legs just went out from under me." Needs prompting to use walker*
Medications	For HTN: hydrochlorothiazide; losartan; amlodipine For DM: metformin; lantus insulin For arthritis: acetaminophen For osteoporosis: alendronate For dementia: donepezil, memantine; risperidone prn hallucinations post-hospital For depression: citalopram
Multicomplexity	Multimorbidity: HTN, DM, OA, OP, UI (uses diapers), depression, moderate–severe dementia, lost 5% body weight over the last year *Lives with youngest son who has taken FMLA to stay with her. Granddaughter comes by three times a week to assist. All are concerned she may need more care than they can provide at home, but are distressed that she never wanted to live in a nursing home*
What matters most	She reports her family is most important—she cannot be more specific. Son and granddaughter recall that she has always been avid reader and a "wit"; now she cannot track a conversation or a novel. They worry her current life is not a quality of life she would value Advance care planning: DNR; no intubation/escalation to critical care *Family is struggling with home* versus *SNF. Patient is tearful through conversation and cannot understand why she should leave home but defers decision to her family. Sons hold her healthcare powers of attorney and durable power of attorney*

she is taking. Eliminating some of these medications may help her avoid future falls. Although she is community-dwelling, she would meet requirements for SNF/nursing home living and therefore guidelines intended for this population. Despite some evidence that tight BP control may reduce strokes and cardiovascular mortality even in frail individuals, those with dementia were not included in these trials, and her decreased life expectancy (see below) and history of falls and dementia suggest that the risk of tight control is greater than benefit.

- **Diabetes target goal**: Considering her function, life expectancy, and weight loss, diabetes control should focus on avoiding the symptoms of hyperglycemia and hypoglycemia. Therefore, we would recommend de-escalating medications, in particular tapering the insulin [7]. A target hemoglobin a1c of, for instance, 8–9, may achieve this.
- **Cancer screening and other prevention**: Cancer screening will not help her to live longer or better, so should not be recommended. Continued treatment of osteoporosis is reasonable depending on how long she has been taking alendronate, as avoiding a fracture is important. Since she is having difficulty swallowing, and alendronate has very specific instructions for use to avoid esophageal ulcerations, may need to change to a different osteoporosis medication.
- **Medications**: As discussed above, her hypertension and diabetes can be managed with fewer medications, and she may need a medication to maintain bone density. There is no clear answer as to whether she should continue with donepezil and memantine—a discussion about pill burden, costs, and possible side effects is reasonable. There should be a discussion with the family as to whether the citalopram has helped her depression. Her episode of aspiration pneumonia suggests she is having some dysphagia, in which case taking medications with liquids could exacerbate this and it would be reasonable to decrease the numbers of medications and give them in food as opposed to sipping water.
- **Function:** She is sedentary, with dementia and increasing physical functional dependence. If she is able to participate, a chair yoga or walking program may help regulate her sleep-wake cycles and assist with behavioral and psychiatric symptoms of dementia. Her life-space is narrow [11]. She would benefit from a residential or community day program with a focus on care for memory impaired individuals or a memory care unit with potential for SNF level care, unless her family is able to provide 24-hour care soon.
- **Advance care planning**: First episodes of pneumonia and eating difficulties, especially dysphagia and aspiration, are "red flags" in people with dementia signaling an increased likelihood of dying over the next 2 years [12]. It's time to readdress her end-of-life care with her family, beginning discussions on whether, for example, she develops serious infections or stops eating, she would have wanted to be re-hospitalized, given a feeding tube, or receive antibiotics. It is always better to have these conversations in the office rather than in the midst of a crisis.

These three case scenarios illustrate how geriatrics medicine has to be personalized medicine and how using the 5 M's can help you work with your patient and their families to develop care plans that match their concerns and values.

3.3 Training Requirements and National Need

So how much geriatrics do you need to learn? And does every older person need a geriatrician's care? No, but every doctor who cares for older people needs to be competent in the care of older adults. What does this mean? First, comfort and facility with diagnosing and managing the diseases common to older adults that affect care across all specialties and subspecialties of medicine, as well as those unique to your discipline. Specific skills have been identified by the Institute of Medicine (now the National Academies of Sciences, Engineering, and Medicine (NASEM), the public policy arm of American medicine) [13]. Publications include expertise in cognition and dementia, physical function, frailty, chronic illness and multimorbidity, promoting community and social connectedness, and meeting older adults' preferences in the dying process. Each of these topics and skills represents a key component in the effective care of older adults. Each report has also demonstrated significant need for skills development.

This book is based on the AAMC/John A. Hartford Foundation medical student geriatrics competencies, and covers these domains: Medication Management; Cognitive and Behavioral Disorders; Self-Care Capacity; Falls, Balance, and Gait Disorders; Health Care Planning, Promotion, and Prevention; Atypical Presentation of Disease; Palliative Care; and Hospital Care. Competencies for Internal Medicine and Family Medicine also include Complex and Chronic Illnesses, and Transitions of Care. The public policy and educational arms of medicine are remarkably similar in their description of what healthcare providers must do to provide effective, person-centered care of older adults.

As reviewed in the first chapter of this book, the population of older adults is growing rapidly. In recognition of the changing demographics, the Institute of Medicine (now NASEM) released a guide for workforce development [14], entitled "Retooling for an Aging America." This call for "gerontologizing" the existing and upcoming healthcare workforce informed the financial support of foundations and government entities to support the career development of geriatrics educators, to incorporate geriatrics education into undergraduate and graduate medical education [15], and to define competencies in geriatrics care for students [16], generalists (Internal Medicine (IM) and Family Medicine (FM) residents) [17], specialists [18–20], and multidisciplinary care teams [21].

3.4 What Do Older Adults Need From Healthcare?

There are, fundamentally, three care needs of older adults: first, they need providers competent to care for most of them (so-called "little g" geriatricians) in primary care, specialty care, and surgical care; second, specialty geriatricians are needed to provide care for the most complex and frailest older adults and those with dementia (so-called "big G" board-certified geriatricians); and finally, the healthcare system must embrace person-centered care, optimizing personal goals and minimizing iatrogenic harm for older adults.

By integrating the geriatric principles taught and demonstrated in this book into the care of your older adult patients, you can help assure that your grandparents, parents, and eventually even you will get healthcare that enhances rather than burdens old age.

References

1. Kritchevsky SB, Williamson J. Putting function first. J Nutr Health Aging. 2014;18:467–8.
2. Tinetti M, Huang A, Molnar F. The Geriatrics 5M's: a new way of communicating what we do. J Am Geriatr Soc. 2017;65:2115.
3. Callahan KE, Tumosa N, Leipzig RM. Big 'G' and Little 'g' Geriatrics education for physicians. J Am Geriatr Soc. 2017;65:2313–7.
4. Walter LC, Covinsky KE. Cancer screening in elderly patients: a framework for individualized decision making. JAMA. 2001;285(21):1750–6.
5. Junius-Walker U, Onder G, Soleymani D, et al. The essence of frailty: a systematic review and qualitative synthesis on frailty concepts and definitions. Eur J Intern Med. 2018; epub ahead of press.
6. Whelton PK, Carey RM, Aronow WS, et al. ACC/AHA/AAPA/ABC/ACPM/AGS/APhA/ASH/ASPC/NMA/PCNA guideline for the prevention, detection, evaluation, and management of high blood pressure in adults: a report of the American College of Cardiology/American Heart Association Task Force on Clinical Practice Guidelines. J Am Coll Cardiol. 2018;71:e127–248.
7. Qaseem A, Wilt TJ, Kansagara D, et al. Hemoglobin A1c targets for glycemic control with pharmacologic therapy for nonpregnant adults with Type 2 Diabetes Mellitus: a guidance statement update from the American College of Physicians. Ann Intern Med. 2018;168(8):569–76.
8. American Geriatrics Society Clinical Practice Committee. Breast cancer screening in older women. J Am Geriatr Soc. 2000;48:842–4.
9. Calonge N, Petitti DB, DeWitt TG, et al. Screening for colorectal cancer: U.S. Preventive Services Task Force recommendation statement. Ann Intern Med. 2008;149(9):627–37.
10. Smith AK, Williams BA, Lo B. Discussing overall prognosis with the very elderly. N Engl J Med. 2011;365:2149–51.
11. Peel C, Baker PS, Roth DL, et al. Assessing mobility in older adults: the UAB study of aging life-space assessment. Phys Ther. 2005;85(10):1008–19.
12. Mitchell SL, Teno JM, Kiely DK, et al. The clinical course of advanced dementia. N Engl J Med. 2009;361(16):1529–38.
13. The National Academics of Sciences, Engineering, and Medicine. http://www.nationalacademies.org/hmd/ Accessed 14 Sept 2018.
14. Institute of Medicine. Retooling for an aging America: building the health care workforce. Washington, DC: The National Academies Press; 2008.
15. Boult C, Counsell SR, Leipzig RM, Berenson RA. The urgency of preparing primary care physicians to care for older people with chronic illnesses. Health Aff (Project Hope). 2010;29:811–8.
16. Leipzig RM, Granville L, Simpson D, Anderson MB, Sauvigne K, Soriano RP. Keeping granny safe on July 1: a consensus on minimum geriatrics competencies for graduating medical students. Acad Med. 2009;84:604–10.
17. Williams BC, Warshaw G, Fabiny AR, et al. Medicine in the 21st century: recommended essential geriatrics competencies for internal medicine and family medicine residents. J Grad Med Educ. 2010;2:373–83.
18. Lee AG, Burton JA, Lundebjerg NE. Geriatrics-for-specialists initiative: an eleven-specialty collaboration to improve care of older adults. J Am Geriatr Soc. 2017;65:2140.
19. Bell RH Jr, Drach GW, Rosenthal RA. Proposed competencies in geriatric patient care for use in assessment for initial and continued board certification of surgical specialists. J Am Coll Surg. 2011;213:683–90.
20. Hogan TM, Losman ED, Carpenter CR, et al. Development of geriatric competencies for emergency medicine residents using an expert consensus process. Acad Emerg Med. 2010;17:316–24.
21. Semla TP, Barr JO, Beizer JL et al. Multidisciplinary competencies in the care of older adults at the completion of the entry-level health professional degree. Partnership for health in aging, 2008.

Disease Presentations in Older Adults

Contents

Physiology of Aging

Katherine Roza and Nisha Rughwani

A. Chun (ed.), *Geriatric Practice*, https://doi.org/10.1007/978-3-030-19625-7_4

4.1 Introduction

Our population is aging at an astonishing rate. According to the US census, the US population totaled about 321 million in 2015, and 14.9% were over the age of 65. By the year 2050, this percentage is expected to grow to 22.1% [1]. The explosive growth of the older population is attributable to the aging of the baby boomers, increasing longevity, and declining fertility rates. In 2008, older adults accounted for 26% of physician office visits and 35% of hospital stays. That same year, the geriatrician physician workforce only numbered about 7100 [2]. We are staggeringly underprepared to care for our aging population.

You will likely care for older adults in whatever specialty you choose to practice and will need to be able to distinguish between the changes expected with normal aging and changes that indicate underlying pathology. The difference between normal and pathological aging is often a subtle one. In his piece titled "The Way We Age Now," Atul Gawande reflected on the changes of normal aging:

> Even as our bones and teeth soften, the rest of our body hardens. Blood vessels, joints, the muscle and valves of the heart, and even the lungs pick up substantial deposits of calcium and turn stiff… As we age, it's as if the calcium flows out of our skeletons and into our tissues [3].

The aging body experiences a number of changes that may increase vulnerability to disease. Individuals, and even different organ systems within the same person, age at varying rates depending on various lifestyle and environmental factors [4].

A key concept in understanding aging is homeostenosis, which refers to the reduced physiologic reserve available to respond to stress in older adults. Due to the changes of aging, the older adult uses more physiologic resources simply to maintain homeostasis. With depleted reserves, the older adult may experience a greater frequency and severity of illness [4]. This chapter reviews the expected physiology of aging by organ system.

4.2 Aging of the Cardiovascular System

This section will discuss the effects of aging on the structure and physiology of the vasculature, including the arteries and veins, and the heart.

4.2.1 Arteries

Reviewing the anatomy of the arteries is helpful in understanding the changes of the aging arterial system. Arteries consist of three layers, aptly called tunics, from the outermost to the innermost layer:

1. Tunica adventitia (outermost layer)—Composed of proteins, collagen, and elastin. Adventitia simply means an "additional" layer.
2. Tunica media (middle layer)—Consists largely of smooth muscle cells that propel blood through the arteries.
3. Tunica intima (innermost layer)—Contains the endothelium, a protective and dynamic inner layer that helps regulate arterial dilation and constriction, angiogenesis (creation of new arteries), thrombosis (clotting), and thrombolysis (clot-busting) [5].

The makeup of arterial walls changes over time. They continually stretch and recoil to circulate blood, causing elastin to fray and wear out much like a used rubber band. Collagen takes the place of elastin in the tunica intima (inner layer), and the number of smooth muscle cells in the tunica media (middle layer) becomes fewer. The loss of elastin and smooth muscle cells causes the arterial wall to become less elastic and pliant [5]. With the loss of elasticity, large arteries become stretched out over time, much like your favorite winter sweater, and increase in diameter and length [6] (Fig. 4.1). Additionally, even in the absence of atherosclerosis, the thickness of the intimal and medial arterial layers triples between 20 and 90 years of age [7]. Age-related thickening of the arterial wall is a risk factor for atherosclerosis. Lastly, healthy endothelial cells release nitric oxide to help arteries relax. Over time, endothelial cells malfunction and produce less nitric oxide, further stiffening the arteries.

All of these age-related structural changes harden and stiffen the large arteries, leading to increased systolic and decreased diastolic blood pressures and predisposing older people to atherosclerosis, particularly in developed countries. Hypertension and atherosclerosis increase the risk of heart disease, myocardial infarction, stroke, and renal disease. Common risk factors of diabetes, high cholesterol, smoking, obesity, and physical inactivity compound the effects of aging on the vascular system.

4.2.2 Veins

Like arteries, veins stretch over time and become less elastic. One-way valves in healthy veins prevent backward blood flow. However, as these valves weaken with age, blood pools and engorges the veins, causing varicose veins. Venous insufficiency, combined with the downward pull of gravity, causes edema in the legs.

4.2.3 Cardiac Changes

4.2.3.1 Left Ventricular Hypertrophy

As noted earlier, the stiffening of large arteries contributes to hypertension. Hypertension increases cardiac afterload. The heart has to work harder during systole (period in the cardiac

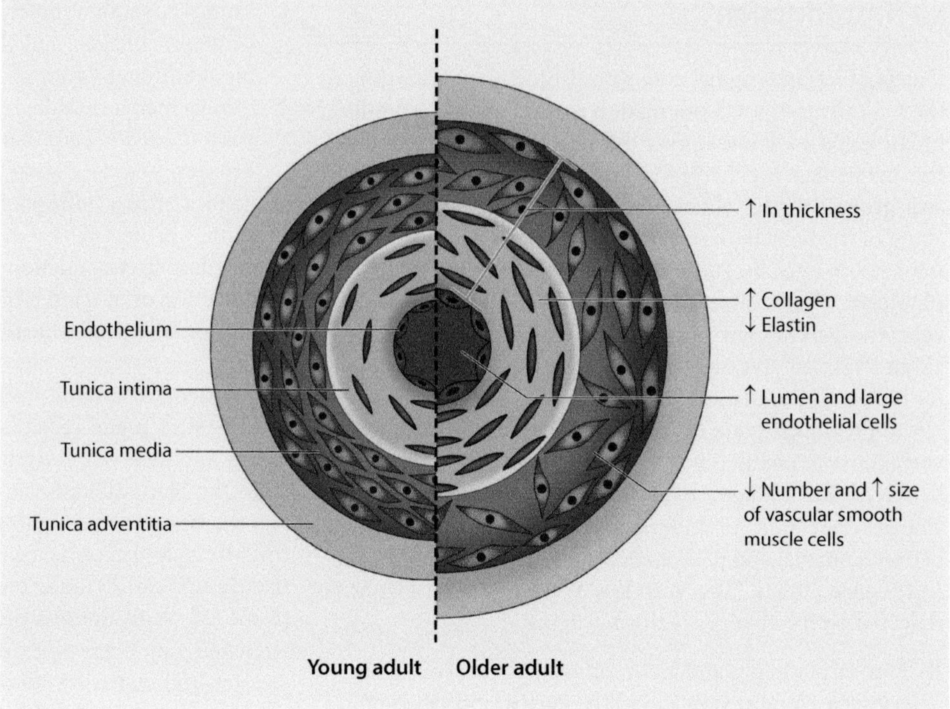

Fig. 4.1 Shows remodeling of central arteries with age. There are significant changes in each of the layers of the arterial wall. The intimal and medial layers thicken. In the intimal layer, collagen replaces elastin. The number of smooth muscle cells in the medial layer decreases. (Modified from: Fillit et al. [29])

cycle when the ventricles contract) to push blood through stiff arteries. Working harder causes the heart muscle to enlarge and stiffen, resulting in left ventricular hypertrophy (Fig. 4.2a, b). As the left ventricular walls hypertrophy, they do not gain healthy muscle, but instead fibrose, calcify, and acquire fatty deposits. S4, also known as an atrial gallop, is actually a normal finding on the physical exam of an older patient. It represents blood forced from the left atrium slapping against the stiffened walls of the left ventricle.

Now, let's talk about what happens in diastole with aging and the development of left ventricular hypertrophy. During diastole, the left ventricle relaxes and fills with blood. Due to hypertrophy, the left ventricular cavity stiffens and shrinks in size. It is no longer able to relax or stretch to accommodate blood from the left atrium. Blood then backs up in the left atrium and overspills into the lungs, causing pulmonary edema and shortness of breath. In short, heart failure results. Depending on the severity of heart failure, the right side of the heart may also fail. Because of left ventricular diastolic dysfunction, older adults are prone to more frequent and severe heart failure exacerbations.

4.2.3.2 Decreased Heart Rate and Cardiac Output in Response to Stress

The maximal heart rate achieved in response to exercise or stress also decreases with age, partly because the heart becomes less sensitive to the beta-adrenergic stimulation of the sympathetic nervous system (which regulates the body's "fight-or-flight" response). In fact, the target maximal heart rate is calculated as "220-age" [8]. We learn in physiology that cardiac output, the blood volume pumped out by the left ventricle each minute, is the product of stroke volume and heart rate (CO = SV × HR). Due to decreased heart rate, the older heart is less able to increase cardiac output in response to physiologic stress [9].

4.2.3.3 Orthostatic Hypotension

When someone stands, gravity causes blood to pool in the legs, resulting in decreased blood supply to the heart and brain. Usually, baroreceptors (sensors that detect changes in blood pressure) respond to drops in blood pressure by constricting arteries and increasing heart rate in order to maintain blood pressure. Many older adults, however, have a blunted baroreceptor response such that the body is not able to adapt to decreases in blood pressure.

Orthostatic hypotension (an abnormal decrease in blood pressure that occurs with standing) becomes more common among older adults due to decreases in baroreceptor sensitivity, arterial and cardiac compliance, plasma volume, and vasopressin (also known as antidiuretic hormone) response. This decreases cerebral perfusion, resulting in syncope (transient loss of consciousness) and falling [6].

4.2.3.4 Valvular Disease

The aortic and mitral valves thicken and calcify over time, increasing prevalence of valvular diseases, such as aortic and mitral regurgitation and stenosis.

4.2.3.5 Atrial Fibrillation

The left atrium stretches to accommodate the backup of blood from a failing and hypertrophied left ventricle or malfunctioning mitral valve (Fig. 4.2a, b). The stretching of the left atrial walls may disrupt the heart's electrical circuits, increasing the risk of atrial fibrillation.

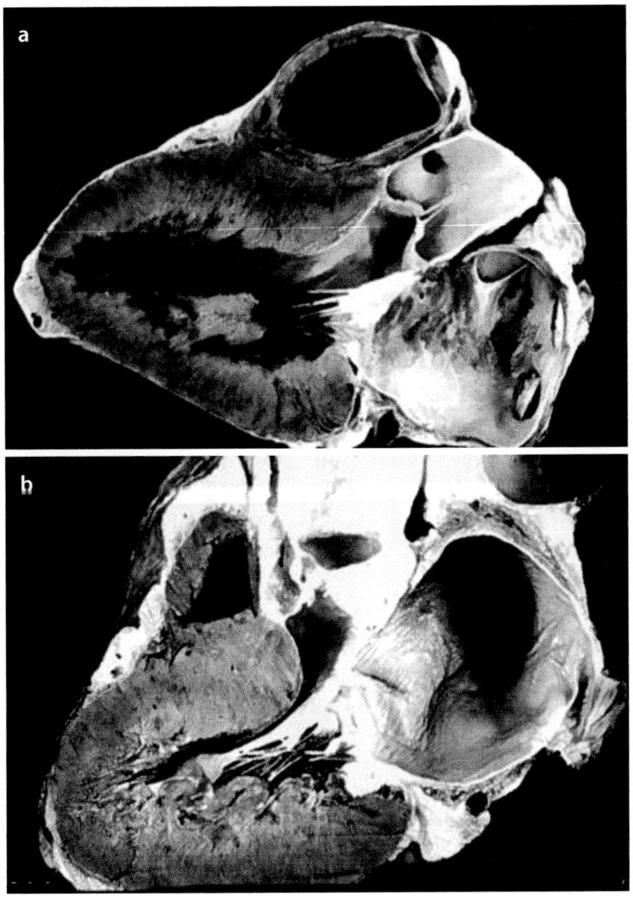

Fig. 4.2 **a** Normal heart from an 18-year-old for comparison (left ventricular long axis view). **b** Normal heart from an 84-year-old man shows decreased size of left ventricular cavity, dilated aortic root, and left atrial dilatation. (Reprinted with permission from: Halter et al. [30])

4.2.3.6 Sick Sinus Syndrome

By age 75, only 10% of pacemaker cells in the sinus node (the heart's primary pacemaker) remain [9]. Due to the loss of pacemaker cells, older adults are more prone to sick sinus syndrome. This syndrome causes abnormal heart rates and is also known as tachycardia-bradycardia syndrome (Table 4.1).

4.3 Aging of the Pulmonary System

Ever wonder why older adults become so ill when they get pneumonia and may even need to be admitted to the hospital?

The respiratory changes caused by aging may not be clinically significant in the healthy older adult. However, as the lungs age, they are less able to compensate for respiratory stresses, such as pneumonia. This section will describe the impact of aging on three components of respiration [10]:

1. Lung parenchyma
2. Chest wall compliance
3. Respiratory muscles

Table 4.1 Aging of the cardiovascular system

Changes in structure	
Age-associated changes	*Possible consequences*
↑ Vascular intimal thickening	Atherosclerosis
↑ Vascular stiffness	Systolic hypertension Atherosclerosis
↑ Left ventricular wall thickness → ↓ Cardiac diastolic filling	Pulmonary edema Heart failure
↑ Left atrial size → disrupts electrical circuits	Atrial fibrillation
Changes in function	
Age-associated changes	*Possible consequences*
Altered regulation of vascular tone Vascular stiffening	Hypertension
↓ Cardiovascular reserve	↑ Frequent heart failure exacerbation ↑ Severity of heart failure

4.3.1 Changes in Structure and Function of the Pulmonary System

1. Lung Parenchyma

Over time, lung mass decreases because the number of alveoli (small sacs responsible for gas exchange between the lungs and bloodstream) dwindles. The lungs lose elasticity and are less able to expand and recoil. When the lungs are not able to fully open, intrathoracic negative pressure drops, causing airway collapse and decrease in alveolar surface area by as much as 20% [7, 11]. This collapse is known as atelectasis, which then leads to a ventilation-perfusion (V/Q) mismatch. In this case, a V/Q mismatch means that inadequate air is available in the alveoli for gas exchange with the blood, causing lower blood oxygen levels.

Due to the loss of elastic recoil, the lungs also hyperinflate over time, mimicking the disease process of chronic obstructive pulmonary disease (COPD) [10, 12]. In fact, this process of aging is also known as "senile emphysema."

Pulmonary function test parameters change with aging. Forced expiratory volume (FEV), the total volume of air exhaled after maximum inspiration, and forced expiratory volume in 1 second (FEV1), the volume of air exhaled after maximum inspiration in 1 second, both decrease. Consequently, the residual volume (amount of remaining air in the lungs after maximal expiration) increases about 10% per decade [4]. Due to hyperinflation of the lungs, older people have smaller tidal volumes and consequently may have a higher respiratory rate [11]. As a result of these changes in pulmonary function parameters, functional reserve decreases, and older people are less able to compensate for physiologic stress.

Diffusion capacity of carbon monoxide (DLCO), a measure of the efficiency of gas exchange, becomes less effective due to both structural changes and V/Q mismatch, as previously described [11].

2. Chest Wall Compliance

Chest wall compliance decreases with age due to both stiffening of the chest wall and altered shape of the thoracic cavity. The chest wall becomes less compliant as rib cartilage ossifies. The spine shortens due to the loss of intervertebral space and the compression of vertebral bodies, shrinking and stiffening the thoracic cage. Osteoporosis may cause vertebral collapse [11]. These skeletal changes result in kyphosis, or a rounded upper back, and a barrel-shaped chest, limiting the capacity of the lungs to expand and recoil.

3. Respiratory Muscles

Respiratory muscles, including intercostal muscles and the diaphragm, weaken over time. Due to the shrinking of the thoracic cage, the diaphragm flattens and generates less force. Because of the increased effort needed to breathe, the older person may expend 120% more energy than a young adult needs to breathe [11].

4.3.1.1 Increased Susceptibility to Pneumonia

Older adults may be less able to perceive respiratory symptoms due to reduced sensation, impaired cognition, or even deconditioning, leading to more subtle and delayed presentations of respiratory problems.

They may lose the strength needed to generate an effective cough, or may develop impaired swallowing ability (dysphagia) in the setting of stroke or neurological disease. A weaker cough or dysphagia increases the risk of aspiration pneumonia.

Glandular epithelial cells decrease in number and produce less mucous, which traps bacteria. Cilia (hair-like structures in the respiratory tract) are less able to clear the respiratory tract effectively. The combination of a weaker cough, less mucous, and less effective ciliary action means that older people are less able to defend against respiratory infections [11] (◘ Table 4.2).

◘ **Table 4.2** Aging of the pulmonary system

Changes in structure	
Age-associated changes	*Possible consequences*
Chest wall stiffening and ↓ elasticity of parenchymal fibers ↓ elastic recoil of the lungs → lung hyperinflation ↓ Alveoli → ↓ lung mass	↓ Pulmonary reserve
↓ Effectiveness of ciliary action → ↓ Ability to clear secretions	↑ Respiratory infections
Respiratory muscles (including diaphragm) weaken	↓ Effectiveness of cough ↑ Shortness of breath ↑ Atelectasis

4.4 Aging of the Gastrointestinal System

This section will describe the age-associated changes of the gastrointestinal system by considering the gastrointestinal tract from the mouth to the colon and then concluding with a brief description of age-related changes in the liver, pancreas, and gallbladder.

4.4.1 Mouth

As we age, saliva glands in the mouth atrophy and produce less saliva. Due to the decreased production of saliva and the prevalent use of medications that cause xerostomia (dry mouth) as a side effect, up to 40% of healthy older adults experience xerostomia [13]. Dryness renders the mouth more vulnerable to cavities, oral infections, and gum disease [14].

The gums recede, causing teeth to loosen and fall out and increasing the risk of malnutrition. Jaw muscles weaken such that older adults are less able to chew foods of a hard or tough consistency. Further, the combination of dry mouth, poorly fitted dentures, and weakened chewing power may contribute to dysphagia (swallowing difficulties) in older adults [15].

4.4.2 Esophagus

With age, food moves more slowly from the mouth to the esophagus. The slowed movement of food occurs both because the oropharyngeal muscles slow and the upper esophageal sphincter takes longer to relax. The prolonged transit time of food increases the risk for silent aspiration. However, these changes usually only become clinically significant in the presence of pathology, such as dementia, neurodegenerative disease, or neck radiation or surgery [15].

In the aging esophagus, peristaltic contractions may become weaker. In addition, the esophagus dilates in size. The lower esophageal sphincter weakens and is also less able to fully relax [15]. When the lower esophageal sphincter does not fully open, the esophagus is less able to clear gastric acid, leading to gastroesophageal reflux disease (GERD) and damage to the esophageal mucosa. Because of decreased acid clearance, GERD symptoms may last longer in older adults [13]. GERD-related damage to the esophageal mucosa may cause a benign esophageal stricture.

The weakness of the lower esophageal sphincter may allow a part of the stomach to protrude through the hiatus (opening) in the diaphragm, exacerbating GERD. Up to 60% of people over age 60 have hiatal hernias [13].

Odynophagia (painful swallowing) in older adults may arise due to GERD, chemotherapy, radiation, and medications, such as NSAIDs, aspirin, and alendronate.

4.4.3 Stomach

- *Delayed gastric emptying*: The stomach empties more slowly, meaning that older people may experience satiety more quickly and have longer periods of abdominal distention. Delayed gastric emptying may both decrease appetite and increase exposure to toxic medications, such as NSAIDs.
- *Decreased production of prostaglandin*: The production of prostaglandin (a substance responsible for lowering acid levels in the stomach) decreases with age, meaning that older people may be more susceptible to gastritis or to gastric irritants, such as NSAIDs. NSAIDs further lower prostaglandin levels by blocking the cyclooxygenase assembly pathway that produces prostaglandin [4].
- *Helicobacter pylori*: *Helicobacter pylori* infection in the stomach and duodenum becomes more common with age [4]. In fact, more than 50% of older people have *H. pylori* infection. The reason for increased *H. pylori* prevalence among older people is unknown. *H. pylori* is associated with gastric ulcers, pernicious anemia (anemia that results from the inability of gastric parietal cells to produce intrinsic factor, preventing the absorption of vitamin B12 and leading to the underproduction of red blood cells), and gastric lymphoma [15]. Gastric ulcers in older adults are more likely to bleed and may take longer to heal.
- *Stress ulcers*: The stress of hospitalization in older adults results in a higher production of cortisol (stress hormone), which, in turn, heightens the risk for stomach ulcers. Proton pump inhibitors (PPIs) are routinely given to older hospitalized patients to decrease gastric acid production and protect against stomach ulcers. PPIs are most effective for short-term treatment of uncomplicated GERD (up to 8 weeks) and should be discontinued after hospitalization [16].

4.4.4 Small Intestine

- *Decreased calcium absorption*: The small intestine absorbs less calcium with age due to lower levels of vitamin D in the blood and fewer vitamin D receptors in the small intestine [4]. Reduced calcium absorption contributes to bone loss in the older adult.
- *Bacterial overgrowth*: Bacterial overgrowth in the small intestine is more common in older adults. It is unclear if small bowel bacterial overgrowth is attributable to medications that slow bowel transit time, immobility, comorbidities such as diabetes, or advancing age [13]. Bacterial overgrowth further exacerbates the malabsorption of nutrients [4].

4.4.5 Colon

- *Slowed colonic transit*: The effect of aging on motility of the colon is unknown. It appears that colonic peristaltic contractions may weaken with age. The time required for fecal matter to pass through the colon may increase over time. However, it is thought that prolonged colonic transit time may be due to medications, comorbidities, and immobility, rather than aging [13].
- *Diverticulosis*: Parts of the colonic wall weaken over time due to increased intraluminal pressure caused by constipation and consequent straining during bowel movements as well as decreased muscle strength. The weak spots in the colonic wall form pouches known collectively as diverticulosis. More than 65% of those over age 65 have diverticulosis [4]. Diverticulitis occurs when one or more of these pouches become inflamed (◘ Fig. 4.3).

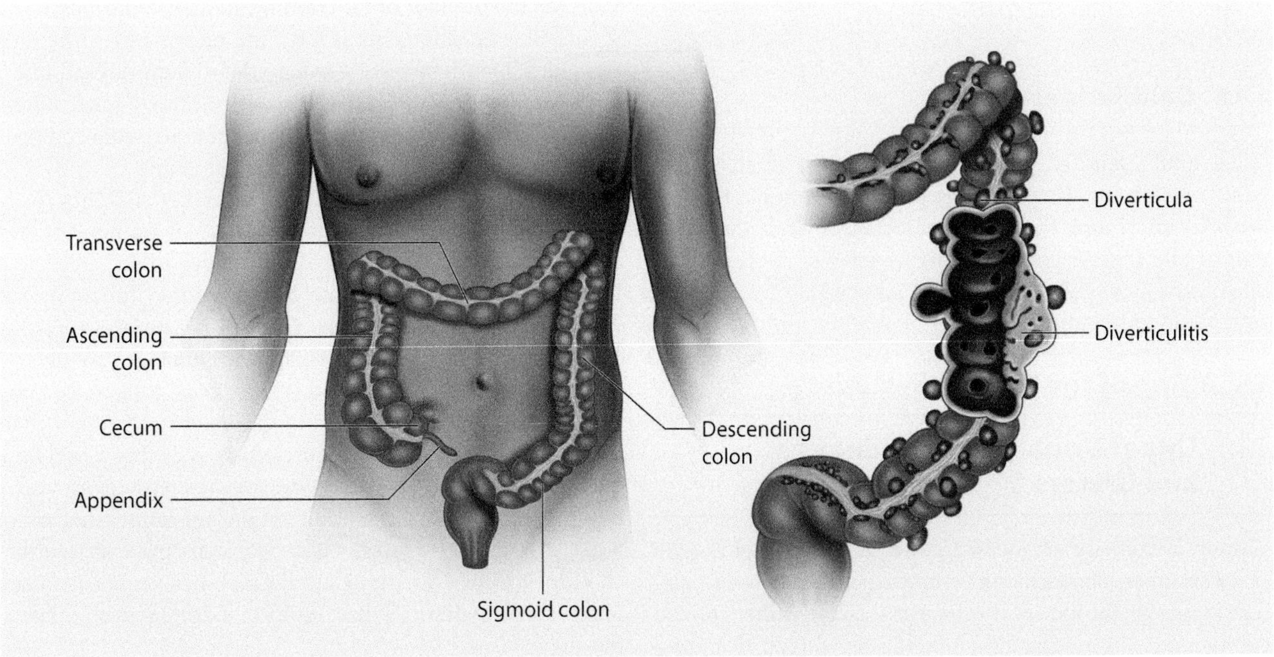

◘ **Fig. 4.3** Diverticulosis and diverticulitis. (Modified from: Mayo Clinic [31])

- *Constipation*: Constipation becomes more common among older adults. Over time, colonic contractions weaken and rectal sensation diminishes. Older adults are more likely to have risk factors for constipation, such as immobility, low-fiber diet, and use of constipating medications.
- *Hernias and hemorrhoids*: Older adults experience greater prevalence of hernias due to the weakening of the abdominal wall over time. Hemorrhoids (engorged veins in the anus or rectum) also become more common due to increased pressure in the rectum caused by constipation.
- *Intestinal ischemia*: Blood flow to the splanchnic vessels decreases over time partly due to atherosclerosis and may lead to chronic intestinal ischemia.
- *Decreased anorectal sphincter tone*: The resting anorectal sphincter tone decreases in both older men and women. It has been observed that older women are more prone to fecal incontinence due to pelvic floor dysfunction and decreased maximal anorectal sphincter tone, rectal compliance, and sensation [13].

4.4.6 Liver

With age, liver size and hepatic blood supply decrease. Older adults are more sensitive to the side effects of medications and toxins in part because the liver is less able to quickly metabolize them [13].

4.4.7 Pancreas

The pancreas shrinks over time and produces less insulin, thereby leading to insulin resistance and increasing the risk of diabetes.

4.4.8 Gallbladder

Older adults tend to have larger bile duct diameters than younger adults do. They are more prone to gallstones because the biliary secretion of cholesterol increases while the secretion of bile acids decreases. A higher level of cholesterol in bile means more gallstones [15] (◻ Table 4.3).

◻ **Table 4.3** Aging of the gastrointestinal system

Changes in structure	
Age-associated changes	*Possible consequences*
↓ Saliva production	↑ Oral infections ↑ Gum disease
↓ Liver size and blood flow	Impaired drug clearance (i.e., acetaminophen)
↓ Pancreatic mass	Insulin resistance
Changes in function	
Age-associated changes	*Possible consequences*
↓ Prostaglandin	Gastritis
↑ *Helicobacter pylori*	Gastric ulcers Pernicious anemia Gastric lymphoma
Impaired acid clearance	Gastroesophageal reflux disease (GERD)
Slowed gastric emptying	Prolonged gastric distention ↑ Postprandial satiety
↓ Calcium absorption	↑ Bone loss
↓ Rectal wall sensitivity Weaker colonic contractions	Constipation
↓ Strength in smooth muscles of colon wall	↑ Diverticulosis
↓ Insulin secretion	↑ Insulin resistance

4.5 Aging of the Urinary System

4.5.1 Upper Urinary Tract: Kidneys and Ureters

Kidneys become smaller with age. Because 30% of glomeruli (network of capillaries in the nephron that filters blood) sclerose by age 75, the kidneys become less selective filters [4]. To compensate, the remaining glomeruli are forced to filter a greater volume of blood. This compensatory mechanism is known as hyperfiltration. The increased blood flow creates shear stress that damages the glomeruli, causing further sclerosis. As the number of functioning glomeruli decreases, the glomerular filtration rate (GFR), the rate at which the kidneys filter blood, falls [17]. Due to their compromised filtering capacity, the kidneys are less able to excrete medications and toxins. Therefore, it is crucial to consider renal compromise when dosing medications for older adults.

Creatinine becomes a less reliable marker of kidney function in older adults. Muscle produces small amounts of creatinine. As muscle mass decreases in older adults, creatinine levels fall and do not accurately reflect kidney function. The Modification of Renal Diet (MDRD) study equation is commonly used to accurately calculate GFR in older patients.

Like the rest of the arterial system, renal arteries become less elastic and stiffen over time. They constrict rather than dilate and often develop atherosclerosis, reducing blood flow to the kidneys. Renal blood flow may decrease from about 600 mL/min in a young adult to 300 mL/min in an older adult [18]. For this reason, older people are more susceptible to kidney injury during acute illness, such as sepsis, heart failure, or dehydration, that results in a decreased circulating plasma volume.

Renal tubules decrease in number and length and lose the ability to concentrate urine over time, such that fluid and electrolyte abnormalities are more common, particularly with physiologic stress.

Dehydration and hypernatremia are common among older adults because they may have decreased sensation of thirst and less urge to drink water. For example, people who have dementia are less likely to feel thirsty and those who are immobile do not have access to water [19].

Further contributing to the risk of dehydration, older kidneys are less responsive to water or salt depletion [19]. The renin-angiotensin-aldosterone (RAA) system regulates the body's sodium and fluid balance and blood pressure. Renin, angiotensin, and aldosterone levels decrease over time, meaning that the older adult is more at risk for volume depletion and hyperkalemia.

At the same time, antidiuretic hormone (ADH) baroreceptors (pressure sensors) become less sensitive to decreased circulating plasma volumes and fail to release enough ADH. In turn, the kidneys become less sensitive to ADH and are thus less able to retain sodium and water in response to volume depletion.

Hyponatremia is more common among older adults. As the GFR declines, the proximal tubule has more time to reabsorb free water. Less free water reaches the distal tubules, meaning that the kidneys are less able to dilute urine or excrete free water. Hyponatremia results. Although usually mild and asymptomatic in older people, hyponatremia is associated with higher mortality, falls, fractures, cognitive impairment, hospitalization, and nursing home placement [19].

Older kidneys also activate less vitamin D, contributing to vitamin D deficiency (◘ Table 4.4).

◘ **Table 4.4** Aging of the upper urinary tract

Changes in structure	
Age-associated changes	*Possible consequences*
↓ Kidney size, mass, and number of functional glomeruli	↓ Renal function
↓ Number/length of functional renal tubules	↑ Fluid and electrolyte abnormalities
↓ Renal blood vessel elasticity	↓ Renal blood flow
Changes in function	
Age-associated changes	*Possible consequences*
↓ Creatinine clearance and glomerular filtration rate (GFR)	↓ Excretion of drugs and toxins
↓ Concentrating/diluting capacity	↑ Fluid and electrolyte abnormalities
↓ Serum renin and aldosterone	Volume depletion ↑ Risk of hyperkalemia
↓ Vitamin D activation	Vitamin D deficiency

4.5.2 Lower Urinary Tract: Bladder and Outlet

The lower urinary tract consists of the bladder and urethra. It stores and voids urine and also protects the kidneys from external infectious agents [18]. A healthy adult usually has voluntary control over urination. However, the aging of the nervous system and the lower urinary tract results in decreased voluntary control of voiding (◘ Fig. 4.4).

It is important to understand lower urinary tract symptoms as manifestations of a syndrome [18]. The process of urination is complex and requires the coordination of multiple systems. Let's review the components of successful urination in a healthy adult. The detrusor muscle (muscular wall of the bladder) generates the force needed to empty the bladder. The parasympathetic nervous system stimulates urination. Pelvic nerves release acetylcholine, which stimulates the muscarinic receptors in the bladder and signals the detrusor muscle to contract and void [18]. At the same time, the urethral sphincter relaxes in order to allow urine to pass. The older adult also needs to have intact cognition and mobility to be able to respond to the urge to urinate.

Any number of these components may fail in the older adult, resulting in lower urinary tract symptoms. The number of muscarinic receptors decreases with age, such that the detrusor muscle does not receive the signal to contract [18]. In the presence of cognitive impairment and degenerative disease, older brains have decreased sensitivity to bladder volume and ability to coordinate urination. Due to limited mobility, some older people may not reach the toilet in time and may experience urinary incontinence.

Urinary symptoms fall into the following three categories:

1. *Irritability*: The hallmarks of an overactive, or irritable, bladder include nocturia and increased urge and frequency. An older adult with an overactive bladder makes more trips to the bathroom during the night, increasing the risk of falls.
2. *Retention*: Symptoms of hesitancy, incomplete emptying, and pelvic discomfort indicate an underactive bladder.
3. *Incontinence*: Older people are more likely to experience urinary incontinence due to decreased detrusor muscle strength, bladder elasticity and capacity, sensitivity to bladder volume, and ability to control the timing of voiding. For instance, if an older person experiences a delay in sensing bladder fullness due to impaired cognition or sensory nerves, he or she may have less time between the initial urge to urinate and the leakage of urine, resulting in an episode of incontinence. Urinary incontinence alone may lead to caregiver strain and increase the risk of nursing home placement [18].

Women and men have different risk factors for developing lower urinary tract symptoms. In women, lower estrogen lev-

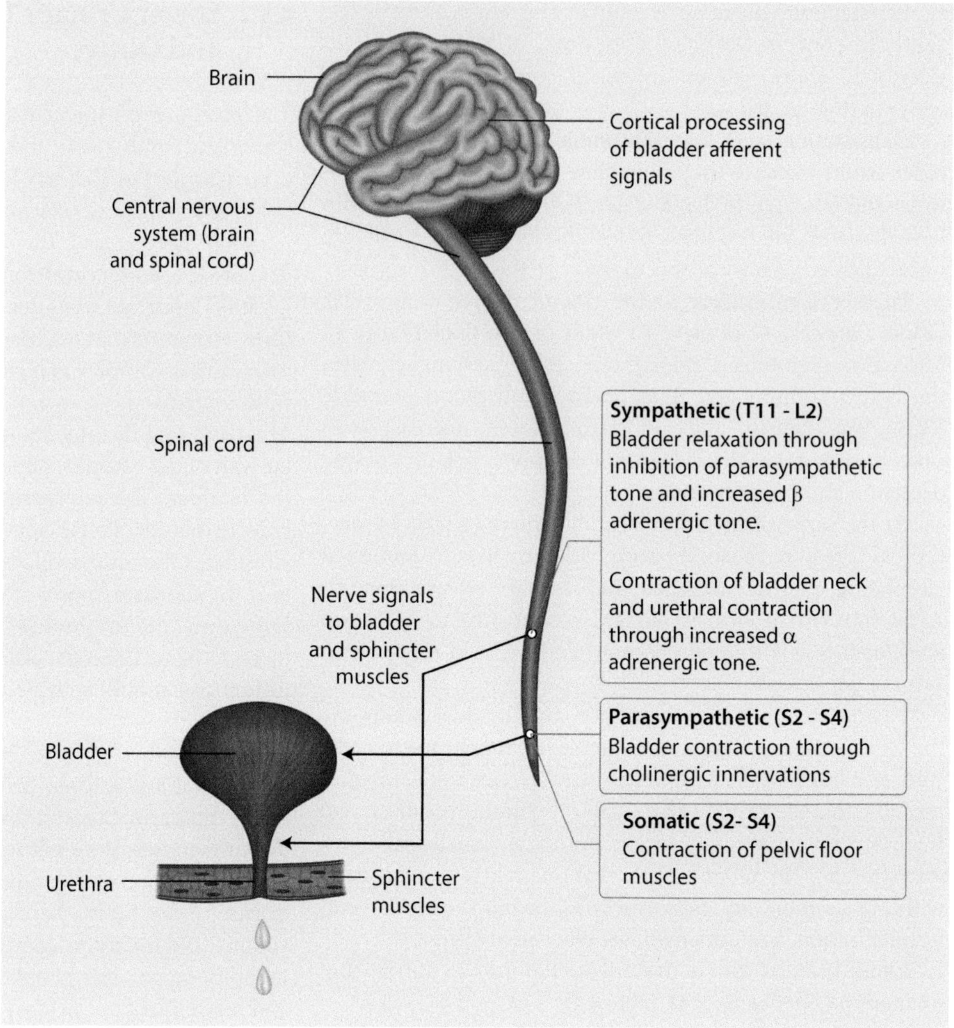

Fig. 4.4 Shows involvement of central and peripheral nervous system in urination. (Reprinted with permission from: Halter et al. [30])

els lead to urethral shortening, increasing exposure to bacteria. Pelvic organ prolapse is also common due to the weakening of pelvic floor muscles, particularly if a woman has a history of multiple vaginal births. Vaginal prolapse in women may cause irritative or obstructive symptoms. In men, benign prostatic hypertrophy (BPH) may cause urinary hesitancy and retention and nocturia.

Other disease processes may exacerbate urinary incontinence. Fecal impaction can increase pressure on the bladder, causing incontinence. Obesity, dementia, and diabetic neuropathy also increase risk of urinary incontinence (Table 4.5).

Table 4.5 Aging of the lower urinary tract

Changes in structure	
Age-associated changes	*Possible consequences*
↓ Detrusor muscle strength ↓ Bladder capacity ↓ Bladder elasticity	↑ Urinary incontinence
Changes in function	
Age-associated changes	*Possible consequences*
↑ Cognitive impairment ↑ Neurodegenerative disease ↓ Mobility	↓ Voluntary control of urination ↑ Urinary incontinence

4.6 Aging of the Endocrine System

The levels of most hormones decrease with age, starting at around 30 years of age, and continue to decline at about 1% per year [20] (Fig. 4.5). The body secretes most hormones in a circadian rhythm, which becomes more irregular with age [20]. Older people are also more likely to have autoimmune diseases that result in decreased hormone levels.

4.6.1 Pineal Gland

The pineal gland is a small endocrine organ beneath the thalamus that makes melatonin. The name of the gland arises from the Latin word for "pine cone" and refers to the gland's shape. The diurnal rhythm of melatonin secretion changes with time and may cause disruptions in sleep-wake

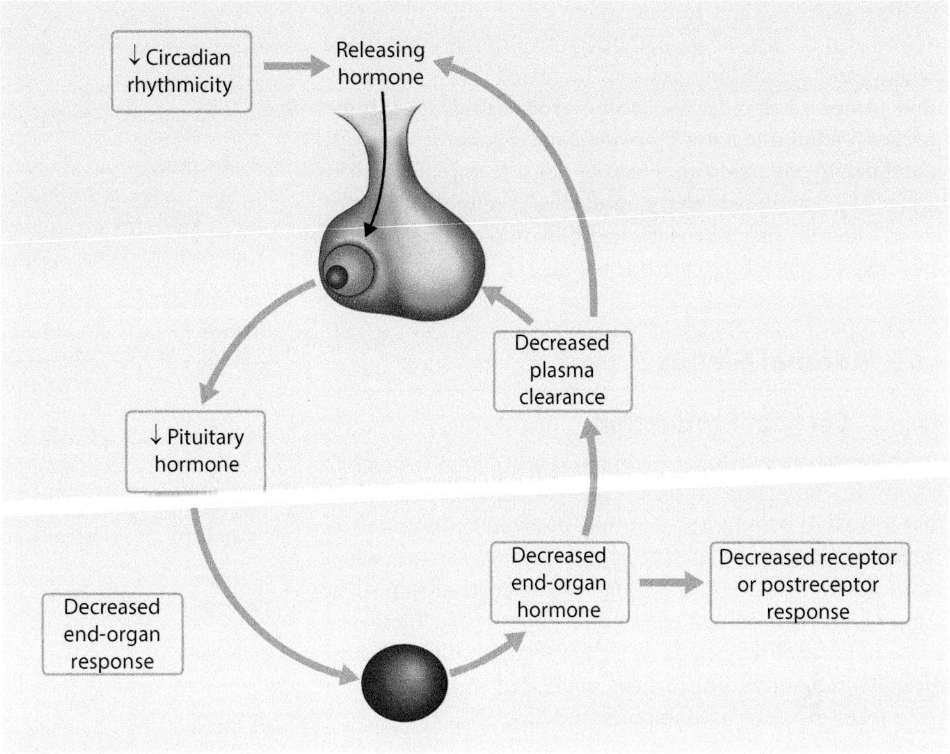

Fig. 4.5 Shows hormonal changes of aging. Hormone levels generally decline with aging. Circadian rhythm also declines. The response of receptors and post-receptors is less robust. (Reprinted with permission from: Fillit et al. [29])

cycles, such as insomnia. Reduced exposure to bright daylight in the older population may decrease secretion of melatonin [21].

4.6.2 Thyroid

The older thyroid may develop nodules and fibrosis, requiring thyroid hormone replacement therapy such as levothyroxine. Older people are also more prone to acquire both clinical and subclinical hypothyroidism and hyperthyroidism. The presentations of these syndromes are both atypical and have similar characteristics in the older population. Symptoms of fatigue, constipation, cognitive impairment, depression, and weight loss are not only more common among older people but are also symptoms of both hypothyroidism and hyperthyroidism, rendering diagnosis challenging [20, 21]. What is known as "apathetic hyperthyroidism," for instance, may present with depression in the older adult [21].

4.6.3 Female Gonads

A woman is born with a limited number of oocytes, which deplete over time until menopause. Menopause begins after 1 year of amenorrhea. On average, women undergo menopause at about 52 years of age [22].

Follicle-stimulating hormone (FSH), produced in the pituitary, stimulates a dwindling number of oocytes to produce estrogen, resulting in declining estrogen levels. In response to lower estrogen levels, FSH level increases prior to and during menopause and is a hallmark laboratory finding of menopause. Decreased production of estrogen causes common menopausal symptoms, including hot flashes, vaginal dryness and dyspareunia, and increasing fracture risk.

4.6.4 Male Gonads

Dehydroepiandrosterone (DHEA) and its sulfated form (DHEA-S), the precursors of female and male sex hormones such as estradiol, progesterone, and testosterone, decrease with age. Production of androgens over time decreases in part due to declining adrenal output.

Testosterone levels decrease with age due a decline in the functioning of the hypothalamic-pituitary axis. The hypothalamus secretes less gonadotropin-releasing hormone (GnRH), consequently decreasing the amount of luteinizing hormone (LH) produced by the pituitary gland. LH stimulates Leydig cells in the testes to produce testosterone. Less LH stimulation of declining Leydig cells means less testosterone production. Once testosterone is released into the bloodstream, it binds to sex hormone-binding globulin (SHBG). With age, SHBG increases such that less free testosterone is available.

The number of seminiferous tubules (where sperm are produced) and Sertoli cells (which nourish developing sperm in the seminiferous tubules) decreases. Overall sperm production decreases, and the number of abnormal sperm increases [21]. These changes in testicular function tend to occur slowly.

Testosterone levels in older men are usually mildly low, resulting in decreased strength, cognitive functioning, bone density, and sexual function, and increased frailty and fractures. Among frail older men, testosterone deficiency is more marked, and as much as 45% of male nursing home residents may have hypogonadism, which is not a feature of healthy aging [21]. It is thought that central obesity may also contribute to lower testosterone levels and that, in some, weight loss may help to correct testosterone levels [21].

4.6.5 Adrenal Glands

4.6.5.1 Cortisol Production

The hypothalamic-pituitary-adrenal axis becomes overactive over time, increasing cortisol levels [20]. It is hypothesized that increased adipose tissue results in greater conversion of corticosterone to cortisol. The aging body also clears cortisol more slowly. In older adults, stress causes cortisol to peak at higher levels and remain elevated for longer [21]. Increased levels of cortisol may cause muscle wasting, frailty, physical disability, cognitive impairment, increased obesity, insulin resistance, and decreased immune function [20].

4.6.5.2 Renin-Angiotensin-Aldosterone System

Due to the decline of the renin-aldosterone-angiotensin (RAA) system, the body produces less angiotensin, decreasing renin by 50% and aldosterone by 30% in older adults compared to younger adults [21]. The body is less able to mount an appropriate response to low sodium levels or orthostatic hypotension as the RAA system declines.

Sympathetic receptors lose sensitivity over time, rendering older persons at higher risk of orthostatic hypotension [20]. For instance, the aging heart may not be able to strengthen contractions in response to hypoxia. Stimulation of alpha-adrenergic receptors may result in less vasoconstriction.

4.6.6 Osteoporosis

Vitamin D promotes the absorption of calcium from the small intestine. However, aging kidneys produce less vitamin D. The intestines also become less sensitive to Vitamin D and thus absorb less calcium. As a result of decreased calcium levels, parathyroid hormone (PTH) increases. PTH indirectly stimulates osteoclasts to release calcium from the bone to compensate for decreased calcium levels and, in so doing, lowers bone density.

In women, estrogen acts on receptors in osteoblasts and osteoclasts to repress bone turnover. Lower estrogen levels in older women cause decreased inhibition of bone turnover, increased bone loss, and greater risk of osteoporosis. Decreasing levels of estrogen in older men also predict age-related bone loss [22] (◘ Table 4.6).

◘ **Table 4.6** Aging of the endocrine system

Glands	Age-associated changes	Possible consequences
Pineal gland	↓ Circadian rhythm of melatonin	Insomnia
Thyroid	Atrophy ↑ Fibrosis and nodule formation	↑ Rate of hypo- and hyperthyroidism
Parathyroid glands	↑ Parathyroid hormone (PTH) ↓ 1,25 (OH) Vitamin D levels Changes in bone mineral homeostasis	Vitamin D deficiency Osteoporosis
Adrenal glands	↓ Aldosterone secretion	Orthostatic hypotension
Female gonads	↓ Estrogen	Menopause Bone loss
Male gonads	↓ DHEA, DHEA-S, and testosterone levels Changes in diurnal rhythm	Changes in skin, hair, muscle, and bone

4.7 Aging of the Nervous System

Healthy older adults may experience mild cognitive and sensorimotor deficits. Mobility, coordination, and strength may decrease. However, the presence of more significant deficits may signify neurologic disease, such as stroke, Parkinson's disease, or Alzheimer disease, all of which are more common among older adults. Thorough neurological exam and assessment of baseline mental status are crucial in order to differentiate between changes associated with healthy aging and pathology.

4.7.1 Central Nervous System

The aging brain undergoes a number of changes. Brain mass decreases (◘ Fig. 4.6). Brain neuron membranes also stiffen. Neurofibrils (filaments) and lipofuscin (lipid pigment that represents wear and tear) deposit in the neurons. Baroreceptors that help maintain blood flow to the brain deteriorate. Due to these changes, nutrient supply to the nerves wanes, and nerve impulses slow.

Cognitive changes of normal aging include decreases in cognitive flexibility, visual-spatial perception, working memory, and attention span [23]. The ability to learn does stay intact; however, processing speed decreases over time [4]. The response time of an older adult is about 1.5 times slower than that of a younger adult [24]. Executive functioning and working memory also deteriorate, particularly after age 70 [4].

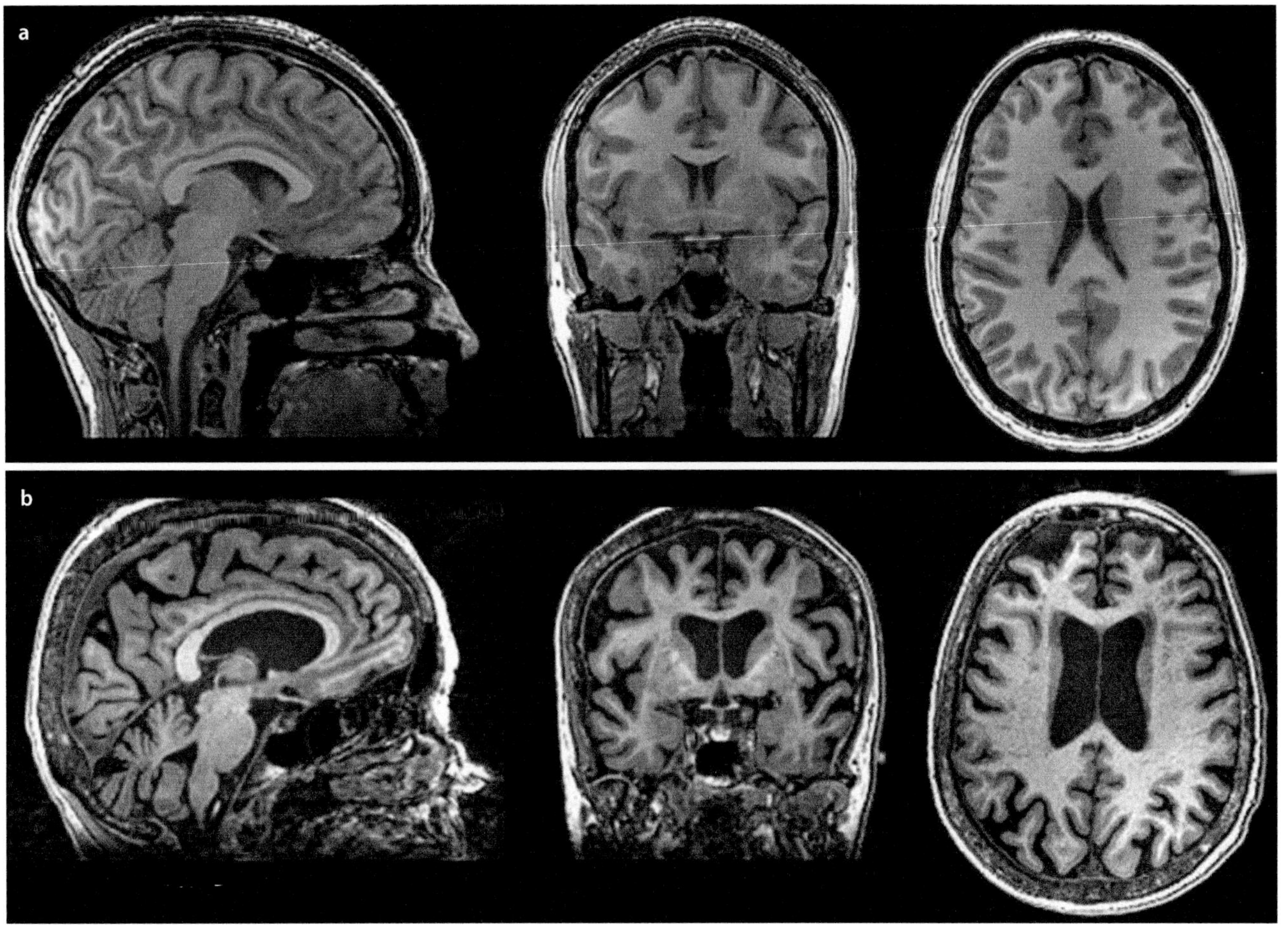

Fig. 4.6 Shows decreasing volume of human brain over time. **a** Magnetic resonance imaging (MRI) sections from a healthy 24-year-old woman. **b** MRI images of brain from a healthy 80-year-old woman without dementia (mini-mental status examination 30). Note the brain atrophy, larger sulci, and ventricles and different shapes of the ventricles due to brain tissue loss. (Reprinted with permission from: Halter et al. [30])

Other factors, such as fatigue, stress, medications, delirium, and depression, also compromise cognitive function. Decreased cognitive function often entails loss of independence for the older adult.

4.7.2 Peripheral Nervous System

Autonomic dysfunction may occur due to failure of the peripheral nervous system or the presence of comorbidities such as diabetes. Autonomic dysfunction may result in urinary retention or incontinence, constipation, impotence, gastroparesis, or anhidrosis (absence of sweating) [25]. Autonomic failure also thwarts the body's blood pressure regulation system, leading to orthostasis and increased risks of falls.

The number of spinal neurons decreases, and spinal nerve conduction slows, resulting in delayed transmission of sensory information, slowed motor movements, and prolonged response times (Table 4.7).

Table 4.7 Aging of the nervous system

Central nervous system (CNS)	
Age-associated changes	*Possible consequences*
↓ Brain weight ↓ Cerebral blood flow ↓ Number and functioning of CNS neurons ↑ Neurofibrillary tangles and lipofuscin Altered neurotransmitters	Slower processing speed → tasks take longer to perform ↓ Cognitive flexibility ↓ Visual-spatial perception ↓ Working memory ↓ Attention span
Peripheral nervous system	
Age-associated changes	*Possible consequences*
↓ Spinal motor neurons Nerve conduction slows	Delayed transmission of sensory information Slowed motor movements Delayed response times

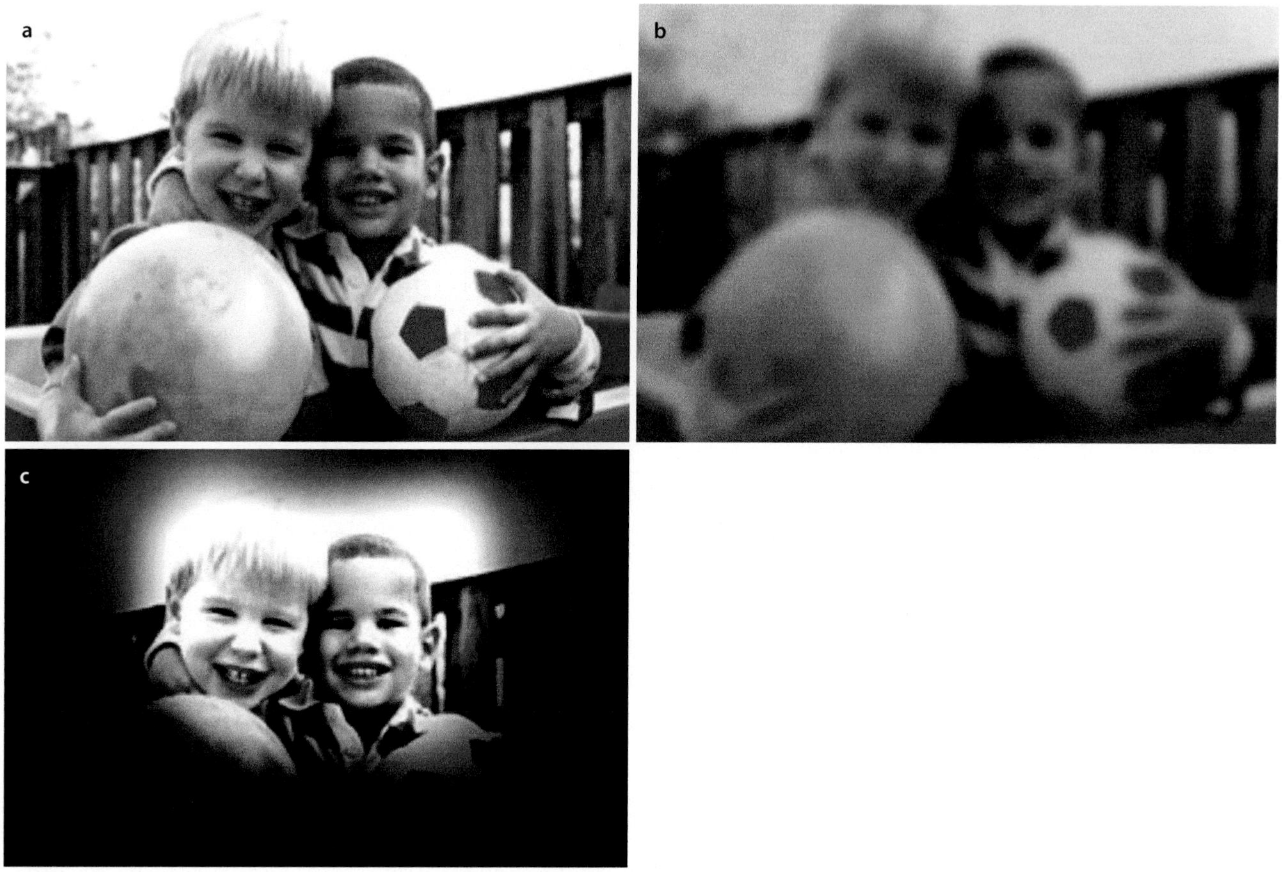

Fig. 4.7 a Normal vision. b Blurry vision due to cataracts. c Loss of peripheral vision, leading to "tunnel-like" vision, due to glaucoma. (Reprinted with permission from: National Eye Institute, National Institutes of Health [32, 33])

4.8 Sensory Changes of Aging

4.8.1 Sight

Changes in vision occur due to structural changes of the aging eye. Pupil size shrinks (senile miosis), and pupillary reflexes lag, requiring more time to constrict and dilate and slowing responses to changes in lighting and glare. The number of photoreceptors decreases, leading to compromised visual acuity, particularly when lighting is dim or scarce. This is why older people often have difficulty driving at night. With age, people lose the ability to gaze upward and may have difficulty seeing traffic lights and street signs [23].

The lenses of the eyes stiffen due to the constant formation of epithelial cells at the lens, causing both blurry vision and presbyopia (loss of nearsightedness). This is why more older adults need reading glasses.

Cataracts (opacification of the lens), glaucoma (increased intraocular pressure), and macular degeneration (deterioration of the macula of the retina) are more frequent in the older population and also contribute to compromised visual acuity (Fig. 4.7). Diabetes and hypertension, both common among older people, affect the blood vessels of the retina, further distorting vision.

Hearing loss in the elderly is known as presbycusis. Older people may acquire sensorineural hearing loss and decreased auditory acuity for high-frequency sounds due to loss of cochlear hair cells and stiffening of the ossicles. Loss of high-frequency sounds compromises their ability to comprehend speech. Older adults may also develop conductive hearing loss and decreased auditory acuity for low-frequency sounds due to thickening of the eardrum.

4.8.2 Smell and Taste

The senses of smell and taste wane with age. Older adults have greater difficulty distinguishing between different odors. Decreased sense of smell may be due to anatomical changes of the upper airway or the olfactory nerve. Alzheimer and Parkinson's diseases are both associated with decreased smell [23]. Taste lessens as the sense of smell and the number and sensitivity of taste buds decline [14]. This may partially account for diminished appetite among older adults, causing weight loss and malnutrition.

4.8.3 Vibration and Proprioception

Older adults have a decreased sense of vibration and proprioception, both of which depend on the dorsal column of the spinal cord. The decline in these senses may be due to degen-

Table 4.8 Aging of the senses

Changes in vision	
Age-associated changes	*Possible consequences*
↓ Pupil diameter Slowed pupillary reflexes ↓ Number of photoreceptors	↓ Visual acuity
↑ Lens rigidity due to formation of central epithelial cells at the front of lens	Inability to focus on near objects (Presbyopia) ↓ Visual acuity
Changes in hearing	
Age-associated changes	*Possible consequences*
↓ Number of cochlear hair cells ↓ Stiffening of ossicles	↑ Sensorineural hearing loss (high-frequency sounds)
Thickened eardrum	↑ Conductive deafness (low-frequency range)
Changes in smell	
Age-associated changes	*Possible consequences*
↓ Sense of smell	↓ Ability to enjoy food ↓ Appetite, leading to potential weight loss
Changes in taste	
Age-associated changes	*Possible consequences*
↓ Number and sensitivity of taste buds	↓ Taste Weight loss Malnutrition

erative changes in the dorsal column nerve fibers and atherosclerosis of arteries supplying the dorsal column. Due to decreased proprioception, older adults may have a mild sway on the Romberg test, increasing their risk for falls [23] (Table 4.8).

4.9 Aging of the Musculoskeletal System

4.9.1 Muscle

Muscle mass decreases over time. This loss in muscle mass among older adults is called sarcopenia. It is especially common in the hands, feet, and shoulders and occurs due to the loss of muscle fibers and infiltration of fat cells. The weakening of abdominal muscles may exacerbate lumbar lordosis (abnormal inward curve of the lower back) and low back pain and increase the risk of umbilical and inguinal hernias.

Older people move more slowly. One study found that older people tap their hands and feet 20% more slowly [23]. Another study found that Parkinsonian signs, such as rigidity, bradykinesia, tremor, and gait disturbance, were present in 14.9% of those 65–74 years of age and in 52.4% of those 85 years of age or older. These symptoms hinder the ability to perform activities of daily living, such as dressing and eating.

Older people have greater difficulty with balance and maintaining an upright posture, both of which are needed for a steady gait. Gait instability increases the risk of mortality twofold [23].

Older adults fall more often and have a higher risk of hip fracture due to increased bone fragility. Hip fractures are associated with increased morbidity and mortality, and many older people do not return to their prior level of functioning after a hip fracture.

Table 4.9 Aging of the musculoskeletal system

Components of musculoskeletal system	Age-associated changes	Possible disease outcomes
Muscle	↓ Muscle fibers → ↓ Muscle mass (sarcopenia) Infiltration of fat into muscle	Weakness Lumbar lordosis (abnormal inward curve of the low back) ↓ Mobility ↓ Functional independence
Bone	↓ Number of osteoblasts ↓ Vitamin D → ↓ Calcium levels → ↓ Bone formation ↑ Bone loss	Osteoporosis Kyphosis Loss of height
Joints	↓ Thickness of cartilage ↓ Chondrocytes	Osteoarthritis

4.9.2 Bone

Bone loss starts at about 35–40 years of age for both women and men as the number of osteoblasts (cells that produce bone) decreases [22]. Decreased weight-bearing exercise and vitamin D deficiency also contribute to bone loss. In postmenopausal women, lower levels of estrogen exacerbate this bone loss. Bone loss increases the risk for osteoporosis.

Height decreases because intervertebral discs lose fluid and vertebrae lose mineral content, shortening the spinal column and causing posture to become stooped [7].

4.9.3 Cartilage

Friction causes cartilage in the joints to erode, leading to osteoarthritis [7]. Chondrocytes (cells that regenerate cartilage) also decrease over time. Joint cartilage never regenerates (Table 4.9).

4

4.10 Aging of the Skin

Skin atrophies with age. Wrinkles form and skin sags due to loss of skin elasticity from increased collagen and decreased elastin. Skin may become paler and hair becomes gray because melanocytes dwindle. Hair thins due to decreased hair follicles [7].

Understanding the layers of the skin is important in order to understand how the skin ages. The skin consists of two layers as well as a basement membrane:
1. Epidermis, the outer layer
2. Dermis, the inner layer
3. Dermo-epidermal junction, basement membrane that connects the epidermis and dermis

The epidermis and the dermo-epidermal junction thin, making the skin more fragile and susceptible to shear stress. Taking off an adhesive bandage may result in skin tears in older adults as the adhesiveness of the bandage is stronger than the bond between the epidermis and the dermo-epidermal junction. Bleeding between the epidermis and dermis also becomes more common [4].

Because the dermo-epidermal junction loses its unevenness, there is less surface area for nutrient exchange, leading to xerosis (dry skin). Blood vessels in the dermis decrease, delaying and altering wound healing, which may lead to chronic ulcers. Dendritic cells (antigen-presenting cells that stimulate the immune system to help repair cells) malfunction, increasing risk for skin cancer [26].

Thermoregulation of the skin also decreases, making older people more susceptible to cold.

Photoaging, which occurs due to exposure to UV rays, results in skin yellowing, wrinkles, and hyperpigmentation (called lentigines, or sun spots) or hypopigmentation. Due to the loss of melanocytes and melanin in the skin, aging skin has less protection against UV rays and becomes more susceptible to skin cancers [27].

Immobility in the older adult increases susceptibility to pressure ulcers and wound infections (▫ Table 4.10).

▫ **Table 4.10** Aging of the skin

Changes in structure	
Age-associated changes	*Possible consequences*
↓ Melanocytes ↑ Lentigines (sun spots) Epidermis thins	Pale skin ↑ Susceptibility to skin tears Skin cancer
Dermal changes ↑ Collagen ↓ Elastin	Wrinkles Lax skin
↓ Melanocytes at base of hair follicles	Gray hair
Changes in function	
Age-associated changes	*Possible consequences*
↓ Effectiveness of thermoregulation	Vulnerability to heat and cold
Impaired wound healing	Chronic ulcers Persistent wounds

4.11 Aging of the Immune System

Due to immune senescence (the process of immune system aging), an older person is less able to protect against infection and malignancy. Poor nutrition, poor dentition, muscle atrophy, dementia, and polypharmacy compromise the ability of an older person to compensate for infection. The number of autoimmune cells increases, weakening the immune system and increasing the prevalence of autoimmune diseases.

4.11.1 T Cells

The thymus is an organ in the mediastinum that produces T cells, a type of lymphocyte or white blood cell. With age, the thymus atrophies. The production of naïve T cells decreases, increasing susceptibility to new infections. The thymus also produces fewer natural killer cells and fewer of the cytokines essential for the growth and maturation of B cells (lymphocytes that produce antibodies). There is also an expansion of differentiated T cells, resulting in a more homogenous and less versatile T-cell population. Decreased ability to repair DNA damage and combat oxidants increases cancer risk.

4.11.2 B Cells

Like T cells, there is a decreased production of naïve B cells and expansion of antigen-differentiated B cells, resulting in a smaller and less diverse B-cell population. This results in a declining antibody response to vaccinations and foreign antigens, such as microbes. The formation of germinal centers, which are B-cell-producing factories, also decreases over time. Due to immune system dysregulation, production of autoimmune antibodies increases and may underlie the higher prevalence of autoimmune disease in older adults [4].

After receiving the influenza vaccine, 70–90% of people younger than 65 years of age are protected; however, only 10–30% of older frail adults are protected due to the aging of the immune system [28].

All of these changes mean that an aging immune system is less able to defend against infections. Influenza, pneumococcal pneumonia, and urinary tract infections become more common. Older adults manifest atypical presentations of infections. A subtle change in mental status or behavior, loss of appetite, falls, incontinence, or fatigue may be the only signs of an infection. Signs, such as leukocytosis or fevers, may not be present in the older adult with an infection because the immune system is less able to mount a response to foreign antigens (▫ Table 4.11).

Table 4.11 Aging of the immune system

Age-associated changes	Possible consequences
↑ Autoimmune antibodies	↓ Immune functioning ↑ Autoimmune disease
↓ T-cell function ↓ Naïve cells ↑ Differentiated T cells	↓ Response to new pathogens ↑ Susceptibility to infection ↑ Susceptibility to malignancy
Atrophy of thymus → ↓ T cells, natural killer cells	↑ Susceptibility to infection ↑ Susceptibility to malignancy

Table 4.12 Aging of the hematological system

Age-associated changes	Possible consequences
↓ Hematopoietic tissue in bone marrow	Anemia
↑ Fat infiltration of bone marrow	Myelodysplastic syndrome
↓ Stem cells in bone marrow	Leukemia
↓ Incorporation of iron into RBC → slowed erythropoiesis	
↓ (slightly) Average hemoglobin/hematocrit	

4.12 Aging of the Hematological System

Stem cells and hematopoietic tissue in the bone marrow diminish as fat takes their place. Infiltrated by fat, the bone marrow is less able to regenerate blood cells. Greater amounts of iron are incorporated into red blood cells, slowing erythropoiesis. Consequently, the average hemoglobin and hematocrit of the older patient decreases slightly. The prevalence of anemia in the elderly may also be due to inflammation, hence the term anemia of chronic disease.

Damaged DNA increases with age perhaps both due to increased reactive oxygen species (ROS) and malfunction of DNA repair mechanisms, contributing to the risk of hematologic malignancy. Shortening of telomeres, the end section of chromosomal DNA, may also contribute to bone marrow failure [28]. Bone marrow failure leads to myelodysplastic syndromes (MDS). The hallmarks of myelodysplastic syndromes (MDS) include a diminished capacity to produce blood cells, progressive bone marrow failure, and risk of transformation to acute myeloid leukemia (AML) (Table 4.12).

4.13 Conclusion

It is important to recognize typical physiologic changes in aging as reviewed in this chapter and to be able to distinguish them from pathology in older adults. Toward that goal, the following chapters will describe disease in the older population.

Learning to care for a vulnerable population of older adults offers unique challenges and rewards. We hope this textbook will serve as a reference for you as you learn more about this population.

References

1. He W, Goodkind D, Kowal P. An aging world:2015 [Internet]. Washington, D.C.: U.S. Government Publishing Office; 2016 [cited 2018 January 12]. Available from: https://www.census.gov/content/dam/Census/library/publications/2016/demo/p95-16-1.pdf.
2. Committee on the Future Healthcare Workforce for Older Americans, Board on Healthcare Services. Retooling for an aging America: building the healthcare workforce [Internet]. Washington D.C: The National Academies Press; 2008 [cited 2018 January 12]. Available from: https://www.nap.edu/read/12089/chapter/1.
3. Gawande A. The way we age now. The New Yorker. 2007:50–9.
4. Taffett GE. 2017. [cited 2018 January 12]. Normal aging [Internet]. UpToDate. Topic 14605 Version 23.0. Available from: https://www.uptodate.com/contents/normal-aging?search=normal%20aging&source=search_result&selectedTitle=1~150&usage_type=default&display_rank=1.
5. Howlett SE. Effects of aging on the cardiovascular system. In: Fillit H, Rockwood K, Young J, editors. Brocklehurst's textbook of geriatric medicine and gerontology [Internet]. Philadelphia: Elsevier; 2017. [cited 2018 January 12]. Available from: EBook library.
6. Taffett GE. Physiology of aging. In: Cassel CK, editor. Geriatric medicine: an evidence-based approach [Internet]. New York: Springer; 2003. [cited 2018 January 12]. Available from: EBook library.
7. Fedarko NS, McNabney MK. Biology. In: Medina-Walpole A, Pacala JT, Potter JF, editors. Geriatrics review syllabus. 9th ed. New York: American Geriatrics Society; 2016. p. 13.
8. Braun LT, Rosenson RS. 2017 [cited 2018 January 12]. Exercise assessment and measurement of exercise capacity in patients with coronary heart disease. UpToDate. Topic 1475 Version 10.0. Available from: https://www.uptodate.com/contents/exercise-assessment-and-measurement-of-exercise-capacity-in-patients-with-coronary-heart-disease?search=maximum%20heart%20rate&sectionRank=1&usage_type=default&anchor=H5&source=machineLearning&selectedTitle=1~84&display_rank=1#H5.
9. Aronow WS. Cardiac arrhythmias. In: Fillit H, Rockwood K, Young J, editors. Brocklehurst's textbook of geriatric medicine and gerontology [Internet]. Philadelphia: Elsevier; 2017. [cited 2018 January 12]. Available from: EBook library.
10. Shanker S, Rojas M, Caufield C. Aging of the respiratory system. In: Halter J, Ouslander J, Studenski S, High KP, Asthana S, Supiano MA, Ritchie C, editors. Hazzard's geriatric medicine and gerontology. 7th ed [Internet]. New York: McGraw-Hill; 2017. [cited 2018 January 12]. Available from: EBook library.
11. Davies GA, Bolton CE. Age-related changes in the respiratory system. In: Fillit H, Rockwood K, Young J, editors. Brocklehurst's textbook of geriatric medicine and gerontology [Internet]. Philadelphia: Elsevier; 2017. [cited 2018 January 12]. Available from: EBook library.
12. Kevorkian RT, Morley JE. The physiology of aging. In: Sinclair A, Morley JE, Vellas BJ, Pathy MSJ, editors. Pathy's principles and practice of geriatric medicine. 5th ed [Internet]: Wiley-Blackwell; 2012 [cited 2018 January 12]. Available from: EBook library.
13. Feldstein R, Beyda DJ, Katz S. Aging and the gastrointestinal system. In: Fillit H, Rockwood K, Young J, editors. Brocklehurst's textbook of geriatric medicine and gerontology [Internet]. Philadelphia: Elsevier; 2017 [cited 2018 January 12]. Available from: EBook library.
14. Kane RL, Ouslander JG, Abrass IB, Resnick B. Essential of clinical geriatrics. 7th ed. [Internet]. New York: McGraw Hill; 2013 [cited 2018 January 12]. Available from: EBook library.

15. Hall KE. Aging of the gastrointestinal system. In: Halter J, Ouslander J, Studenski S, High KP, Asthana S, Supiano MA, Ritchie C, editors. Hazzard's geriatric medicine and gerontology. 7th ed [Internet]. New York: McGraw-Hill; 2017. [cited 2018 January 12]. Available from: EBook library.
16. Fick DM, Semla TP, Beizer J, Brandt N, Dombrowski R, DuBeau CE, Eisenberg W, Epplin JJ, Flanagan N, Giovannetti E, Hanlon J, Hollmann P, Laird R, Linnebur S, Sandhu S, Steinman M. American Geriatrics Society 2015 updated Beers Criteria for potentially inappropriate medication use in older adults. J Am Geriatr Soc. 2015;63(11):2227–46.
17. Fedarko NS, McNabney MK. Biology. In: Medina-Walpole A, Pacala JT, Potter JF, editors. Geriatrics review syllabus. 9th ed. New York: American Geriatrics Society; 2016. p. 15.
18. Smith PP, Kuchel GA. Aging of the urinary tract. In: Fillit H, Rockwood K, Young J, editors. Brocklehurst's textbook of geriatric medicine and gerontology [Internet]. Philadelphia: Elsevier; 2017. [cited 2018 January 12]. Available from: EBook library.
19. Wiggins J, Patel SR. Aging of the kidney. In: Halter J, Ouslander J, Studenski S, High KP, Asthana S, Supiano MA, Ritchie C, editors. Hazzard's geriatric medicine and gerontology. 7th ed [Internet]. New York: McGraw-Hill; 2017. [cited 2018 January 12]. Available from: EBook library.
20. Morley JE, McKee A. Endocrinology of aging. In: Fillit H, Rockwood K, Young J, editors. Brocklehurst's textbook of geriatric medicine and gerontology [Internet]. Philadelphia: Elsevier; 2017. [cited 2018 January 12]. Available from: EBook library.
21. Gruenewald DA, Matsumoto AM. Aging of the endocrine system and selected endocrine disorders. In: Halter J, Ouslander J, Studenski S, High KP, Asthana S, Supiano MA, Ritchie C, editors. Hazzard's geriatric medicine and gerontology. 7th ed [Internet]. New York: McGraw-Hill; 2017. [cited 2018 January 12]. Available from: EBook library.
22. Brinton RD. Neuroendocrinology of aging. In: Fillit H, Rockwood K, Young J, editors. Brocklehurst's textbook of geriatric medicine and gerontology [Internet]. Philadelphia: Elsevier; 2017. [cited 2018 January 12]. Available from: EBook library.
23. Galvin JE. Neurologic signs in older adults. In: Fillit H, Rockwood K, Young J, editors. Brocklehurst's textbook of geriatric medicine and gerontology [Internet]. Philadelphia: Elsevier; 2017. [cited 2018 January 12]. Available from: EBook library.
24. Martin J, Li C. Normal cognitive aging. In: Fillit H, Rockwood K, Young J, editors. Brocklehurst's textbook of geriatric medicine and gerontology [Internet]. Philadelphia: Elsevier; 2017. [cited 2018 January 12]. Available from: EBook library.
25. Kenny RA, Bhangu J. Syncope. In: Fillit H, Rockwood K, Young J, editors. Brocklehurst's textbook of geriatric medicine and gerontology [Internet]. Philadelphia: Elsevier; 2017 [cited 2018 January 12]. Available from: EBook library.
26. Sinclair A, Morley JE, Vellas BJ, Pathy MSJ, editors. Pathy's principles and practice of geriatric medicine. 5th ed [Internet]: Wiley-Blackwell; 2012 [cited 2018 January 12]. Available from: EBook library.
27. Tobin DJ, Veysey EC, Finlay AJ. In: Fillit H, Rockwood K, Young J, editors. Brocklehurst's textbook of geriatric medicine and gerontology [Internet]. Philadelphia: Elsevier; 2017 [cited 2018 January 12]. Available from: EBook library.
28. McDevitt MA. Aging and the blood. In: Fillit H, Rockwood K, Young J, editors. Brocklehurst's textbook of geriatric medicine and gerontology [Internet]. Philadelphia: Elsevier; 2017 [cited 2018 January 12]. Available from: EBook library.
29. Fillit H, Rockwood K, Young J. Brocklehurst's textbook of geriatric medicine and gerontology [Internet]. Philadelphia: Elsevier; 2017 [cited 2018 January 12]. Available from: EBook library.
30. Halter J, Ouslander J, Studenski S, High KP, Asthana S, Supiano MA, Ritchie C, editors. Hazzard's geriatric medicine and gerontology. 7th ed [Internet]. New York: McGraw-Hill, 2017 [cited 2018 January 12]. Available from: EBook library.
31. Mayo Clinic. Diverticulitis [Internet]. 2015 [cited 2018 January 12]. Available from: https://www.mayoclinic.org/diseases-conditions/diverticulitis/symptoms-causes/syc-20371758.
32. National Eye Institute, National Institutes of Health. Facts about cataracts [Internet]. 2015 [cited 2018 January 12]. Available from: https://nei.nih.gov/health/cataract/cataract_facts.
33. National Eye Institute, National Institutes of Health. Facts about glaucoma [Internet]. 2015 [cited 2018 January 12]. Available from: https://nei.nih.gov/health/glaucoma/glaucoma_facts. Hearing.

4

Normal Versus Abnormal Physical Exam

Vanessa Rodriguez and Melissa Bakar

A. Chun (ed.), *Geriatric Practice*, https://doi.org/10.1007/978-3-030-19625-7_5

5.1 Introduction

During your training, you will find that there are aspects of taking a history and performing a physical exam that are unique to older adult patients. As discussed in ▶ Chap. 4, older adult patients experience physiologic changes that may require adaptation of your standard history and physical exam. Some of these changes are a normal part of the aging process, but others can be clues to underlying issues that may negatively impact the health and function of your older adult patients.

5

One of the challenges in taking care of older adult patients is that older adults frequently do not present with one symptom or "chief complaint" which points directly to one diagnosis. Older adults are also frequently prone to the development of geriatric syndromes such as delirium and incontinence, which require a high index of suspicion to properly assess and diagnose them. Their symptoms are often atypical, multiple, vague, and nonspecific. Older adults can present very differently from younger people with similar medical problems, and findings can be subtle or undifferentiated [1]. The classic teaching of Occam's Razor that there is a single diagnosis that unites all of the patient's symptoms and complaints has been found to be less likely for older adult patients who often have multiple comorbid conditions [2]. Furthermore, older adults may suffer from more severe illness or unanticipated complications due to the process of homeostenosis. Homeostenosis is the inability to compensate in the presence of stressors because of a decline in the physiologic reserve of several systems [3].

5.2 General Approach

While the content of the examination of older patients generally includes the same medical domains you have learned for younger patients, there are additional nonmedical domains that play a crucial role in developing an understanding of your older adult patient. This multidimensional assessment provides a more complete and relevant problem list that also includes functional impairments and psychosocial issues [4]. This approach allows us to prevent disability and increase safety. When disability is detected, the knowledge of how to conduct a thoughtful history and physical examination will enable you to develop a patient-centered plan that focuses on reducing disability and improving quality of life.

Your approach to the older adult patient may also differ from the approach you use with younger patients due to sensory impairments, physical limitations, or cognitive deficits. It also should be modified when appropriate to avoid causing undue discomfort, embarrassment, or stress. ◘ Table 5.1 identifies considerations such as impaired hearing, slower response times, and diminished mobility that you must take into account when providing care to older adults [5].

◘ **Table 5.1** Changes that occur with aging and their impact on conducting a history and physical exam

Changes that may occur with aging	Effect on history and physical exam	Adaptations that may be required
Hearing impairment	Difficulty hearing examiner may result in misunderstanding	Hearing aids or amplification devices Limit background noise Be sure you have patient's attention Position yourself closer to the good ear if there is one Speak slowly and clearly Use a lower than normal pitch Allow the patient to see your mouth Ask patient to confirm understanding
Visual impairment	Interferes with aspects such as cognitive testing that require visual input	Magnification devices Large print forms Ensure adequate lighting
Slowed responses	Prolongs encounter	Allow additional time for patient response
Mobility limitations	Makes disrobing and positioning during physical examination challenging	Provide assistance as needed in disrobing, transferring, and positioning Minimize position changes during exam
Cognitive impairment	May affect patient's comprehension of questions Can make answering open ended questions challenging Can impair recall of medical history and symptoms	Use short, simple questions; do not combine multiple questions Minimize distractions and interruptions Use more direct questions Provide a list of options (was your chest pain, sharp, dull, stabbing, or crushing?) Obtain collateral information from caregivers, family
Family/caregivers accompanying patient	Decreases patient privacy and sense of autonomy	Speak to patient directly Ask patient's permission to speak with family members Ensure you have time alone with the patient and with caregivers if desired Address the concerns of both the patient and the caregivers

5.3 Taking the History

- Taking an accurate and comprehensive history from your older adult patients is often the key to identifying the issues underlying your patients' health concerns. Many older adults have complex medical histories that can be seem overwhelming. So it is important to obtain a complete history in an organized manner, while allowing time for the patient and accompanying family or caregivers to express their concerns.
- For all but the most cognitively impaired, it is always important to speak directly to the older adult and to ask the patient's permission to speak with the accompanying family member or caregiver. If there is an especially complex history or there are numerous concerns, multiple sessions may be required to adequately address all of the issues.
- The routine parts of the history including the chief complain, history of present illness, past medical and surgical history including hospitalizations, medications, allergies, family history, social history, and review of systems must all be included. In addition to the common questions that are typically included in the social history, we can further supplement our understanding of the older adult patient by inquiring about:
  - Education level
  - Employment history
  - Religious or spiritual beliefs
  - Living situation
  - Hobbies
  - Need for assistive device
  - Need for unpaid or paid caregiver
  - Marital status
  - Healthcare proxy

Table 5.2 provides an expanded review of systems for an older adult patient that highlights questions related to common geriatric syndromes.

Table 5.2 Review of systems for the older adult

General	Memory loss Weight loss/gain Fatigue Weakness Fever Chills Loss of appetite Snores Night sweats Swollen lymph nodes Pain	Eyes	Visual loss Blurry vision Double vision Eye pain Itchy/burning eyes
Ears	Hearing loss Ear discharge Ear pain Room spinning sensation Loss of balance Ringing in the ears	Nose/throat	Bloody nose Congestion Smell changes Runny nose Sore throat Hoarseness
Oral	Dry mouth Bleeding gums Mouth pain Tongue problems Taste changes Jaw pain Dentures (if yes, ask about fit, pain)	Respiratory	Cough Shortness of breath Wheezing Productive sputum Blood in sputum
Cardiovascular	Chest pain Palpitations Swelling of the legs Shortness of breath with exertion Sleeping with many pillows for better breathing Wakes up due to difficulty breathing Painful varicose veins	Gastrointestinal	Fecal incontinence Abdominal pain Constipation Diarrhea Blood in stools Excessive gas/bloating Painful swallowing Trouble swallowing Nausea Vomiting Heartburn

(continued)

5

Table 5.2 (continued)

Genitourinary	Leakage of urine Frequent nighttime urination Urinary frequency Urination urgency Painful urination Blood in urine Problems with erection Vaginal itching/dryness Spotting/discharge Painful intercourse Impotence	Breast	Nipple discharge Pain Breast mass
Musculoskeletal	Falls Fear of falling Neck pain Painful gait Back pain Joint pain or swelling Muscle pain Stiffness	Neurological	Memory loss Dizziness or lightheadedness Headaches Fainting Loss of consciousness Numbness or tingling of hands or feet Tremors Involuntary movements
Skin	Itching Rash Mass or swelling	Endocrine	Hot flashes Heat/cold intolerance Excessive thirst Excessive urination
Psychiatric	Depression Anxiety Sleep problems Irritability Visual hallucinations Hear voices Suicidal ideations Homicidal ideations Abusive relationship Alcoholism Substance abuse problems	Hematologic/lymphatic	Easy bruising Bleeding Swollen lymph nodes

5.3.1 Healthcare History

- You will encounter many adults with multiple chronic conditions that can in turn contribute to functional limitations. Being specific about the time course of onset and potential resolution of medical problems and functional impairments can help provide clues to how they may be related. For example, finding out that a patient's falls began shortly after they developed and started treatment for insomnia would be important information to help mitigate further fall risk.
- Because older patients often see multiple providers, it will be helpful to review a list of those providers with their contact information and reach out to these providers for additional information or discussion. A review of health maintenance and immunizations is also important.

5.3.2 Medications

- Special attention should be paid to review an older patient's medications, including over-the-counter and herbal supplements. Research has demonstrated that about one-third of adults aged 57–85 take at least five prescription medications, with 50% of older adults taking at least one medication that is not medically necessary [6].
- Also approximately 50% of older adults have reported taking an over-the-counter medication or herbal supplement [6]. This places our older adult patients at increased risk of adverse drug events that can lead to geriatric syndromes such as falls and delirium.

5.3.3 Functional Status

- The Activities of Daily Living (ADLs) and Instrumental Activities of Daily Living (IADLs) should be routinely explored to assess a patient's functional status.
- When discussing the ADLs and IADLs, it is important to determine which ones your patient can do independently, which they require assistance to perform, and which they are totally dependent on the help of others to perform.
- Some older adults will hesitate to answer questions about their function such as falls or difficulty bathing because of the implications these answers may have on their autonomy.

- The importance of the assessment of functional status in older adults cannot be overstated as it is a strong predictor of an older person's prognosis [7–9].
- Activities of Daily Living:
  - Bathing
  - Dressing
  - Toileting
  - Transferring
  - Continence
  - Feeding
- Instrumental Activities of Daily Living:
  - Managing finances
  - Medication management
  - Travel
  - Laundry
  - Housekeeping
  - Shopping
  - Cooking
  - Cleaning
  - Telephone use

5.3.4 Pain

- It is important to be specific when asking your older adult patients about pain and its relationship to physical function. The 2011 National Health and Aging Trends Study on prevalence and impact of pain among older adults found that older adults frequently reported many different sites of pain. Furthermore, the study found that pain in older adult patients was strongly associated with decreased physical function [10].
- We traditionally ask patients, "What is your pain on a scale from 0–10?" However, this may be difficult for an older adult patient with multiple different sites of pain to answer. A more thorough investigation of the sites of pain and exploration of the underlying causes is important in limiting functional impairment in your older adult patients. Please see ▶ Chap. 42 for further information on the assessment and treatment of pain in older adults.

5.3.5 Sexual Activity

- While obtaining your history, it is important to keep in mind that some older adults may feel uncomfortable disclosing certain information in front of their family or caregivers. Questions involving incontinence and sexual activity may be embarrassing to older adults.
- Given these concerns, it is important to ensure that you have time alone with your patient to discuss more sensitive concerns. Having family or caregivers leave during the physical exam can provide time alone with the patient. Time alone with the patient is also an important time to inquire about concerns for abuse or neglect.

5.3.6 Caregiver Burden

- Caregiver burden is very prevalent among persons caring for the geriatric population [11]. If your patient has a caregiver, be sure to explore any burden or stress he or she may be experiencing.
- Family members and caregivers may also appreciate time alone with you to express concerns they may be hesitant to discuss in the older patient's presence.

5.4 Physical Examination

5.4.1 General Assessment

- Careful observation of the older adult patient can provide particularly important information on functional status and possible limitations. This observation begins as soon as you see your patient and continues through your history and physical exam.
- Upon first meeting the patient, you may observe glasses and hearing aids that provide evidence for impaired special senses. Fall alert devices, assistive devices such as canes and walkers, or an older adult who requires assistance from another person can be clues to functional impairment.
- While conducting your history, noting the pace of speech, the fluency of speech and the coherence of the answers, as well as the patient's affect can provide clues to possible diagnoses of dementia, delirium, or depression.
- During your physical exam, taking notice of cachexia or obesity can provide important information about nutritional status. An older adult who is noted to be cachectic with generalized weakness, fatigue, motor slowing, and decreased muscle mass may also qualify as frail.
- Noticing poor personal hygiene, disheveled clothing, or strong odors such as urine can be clues to an older adult who is struggling with self-care or neglect.

5.4.2 Vitals

Temperature Older adult patients are often less able to mount a temperature response than the general population. For that reason, obtaining a baseline temperature is particularly important in older adults [11]. Fever in frail older adults is defined as a single oral temperature > 37.8 °C (>100 °F), persistent oral or tympanic membrane temperature ≥ 37.2 °C (99.0 °F), rectal temperature ≥ 37.5 °C (99.5 °F), or a rise in temperature of ≥1.1 °C (≥2 °F) above baseline temperature [12]. Fever as it is usually defined in adults is absent in 30 to 50 percent of frail, older adults, even in the setting of serious infections [11]. Hypothermia, or a core temperature below 35 °C (95 °F), is more common in older adults than the general population and can be indicative of the presence of sepsis, hypothyroidism, adrenal insufficiency, malnutrition, and hypoglycemia, among other causes [5]. These facts make it critically important to take a baseline temperature reading and follow the above definitions.

Heart rate Resting heart rate does not change with age. However, due to age-related changes in the cardiac conduction system, older adults are more likely than the general population to suffer from atrial arrhythmias such as atrial fibrillation or supraventricular tachycardia as well as an increase in premature ventricular beats and ventricular arrhythmias [13]. Using the radial artery to feel the pulse and measuring the heart rate can identify bradycardia, tachycardia, and irregularity, all of which could signify a serious medical issue or the side effect of a medication (e.g., cholinesterase inhibitors, albuterol). If you notice the following abnormalities in the pulse of your patients, you should consider the associated arrhythmias in your differential diagnosis.

- Tachycardia: sinus tachycardia, supraventricular tachycardia
- Bradycardia: sick sinus syndrome, second- or third-degree heart block
- Irregularly irregular: most likely atrial fibrillation, less likely multifocal atrial tachycardia, or frequent premature atrial or ventricular beats
- Regularly irregular: consistently dropped beats such as second-degree atrioventricular block or consistently added beats such as premature ventricular contractions

If the radial artery pulse is difficult to ascertain, using the apical heart rate may yield more accurate information about rate and regularity [5]. Any abnormalities detected in the pulse should be followed up with an EKG for further exploration of possible arrhythmias.

Blood pressure Careful monitoring of blood pressure in your older adult patients is extremely important. According to the CDC, 64% of men and 69% of women aged 65–74 and 66% of men and 78% of women aged 75 and older have hypertension [14]. Obtaining an accurate blood pressure is key to diagnosing and monitoring treatment effects. There are multiple considerations to keep in mind to ensure that you are obtaining an accurate blood pressure in your older adult patients. Once the patient is seated comfortably and with their arm relaxed and supported at the level of the heart:

- Ask about and look for any restrictions in which limb you can use
  - Lymphedema
  - Prior axillary lymph node dissections (i.e., breast cancer)
  - Vascular access for dialysis
  - Active infection/rash
  - Pain
- Ensure appropriate cuff size and position
  - The bottom edge of the cuff should be positioned approximately 1 inch above the antecubital fold
  - A cuff too small could overestimate blood pressure
  - Too large a cuff can underestimate blood pressure
- The hypertension seen with aging is often characterized by a significant increase in systolic blood pressure with no change, or even a decrease, in diastolic blood pressure creating a wide pulse pressure [15]. In older adults, it is especially important to ensure that there is no auscultatory gap. An auscultatory gap occurs when the Korotkoff sounds (the blood flow sounds you hear when taking a blood pressure with a sphygmomanometer over the brachial artery in the antecubital fossa) disappear temporarily and reappear again at a lower pressure. To ensure that you do not miss an auscultatory gap, inflate the cuff to at least 200 mm Hg and to continue to listen until a pressure of 50 mm Hg. If the auscultatory gap is missed, you may record the systolic blood pressure as lower than its true value, or the diastolic blood pressure as higher than its true value. The blood pressure should be measured in both arms at least once as long as there are no identified limb restrictions.
- Older adult patients are also more likely than the general population to have pseudohypertension. Pseudohypertension is an artificially elevated blood pressure level due to stiff peripheral arteries. Suspect pseudohypertension in patients with persistently elevated blood pressure who developed hypotensive symptoms on antihypertensive drug therapy [5]. In order to detect pseudohypertension, an Osler maneuver can be performed. The Osler maneuver is performed by palpating the radial or brachial artery, inflating the blood pressure cuff above systolic pressure and determining if the pulseless artery is palpable. If the pulseless artery is palpable, this is considered to be Osler positive and suggests that the true intra-arterial blood pressure reading may be lower than the blood pressure obtained by auscultation.
- Twenty percent of older adult patients and up to 50% of frail older adults in nursing homes have been found to have postural or orthostatic hypotension [5].
  - If your older adult patient is reporting dizziness or if you are considering starting antihypertensives or other medications that may contribute to postural hypotension, you should measure both blood pressure and pulse with the patient lying and standing.
  - Older adults have increased susceptibility to postural hypotension because reflex orthostatic mechanisms can be impaired due to age-related changes and medication use.
  - Low blood volume can also contribute to exaggerated postural changes in older adults.
  - Postural or orthostatic hypotension is defined as a drop in systolic blood pressure (SBP) of $\geq$20 mm Hg or diastolic blood pressure (DBP) $\geq$ 10 mm Hg when blood pressure is initially checked with the patient laying down and then within 3 minutes after standing up [5].
  - Orthostatic hypotension poses a significant concern for frail older adults where it has been associated with increased falls and syncope [16].

Respiratory rate Checking the respiratory rate provides you with an opportunity to learn much more than just the rate or respiration. The usual rate in adults is about 12 to 18 breaths per minute, and this does not change in normal aging [17]. While measuring the respiratory rate, you should also be observing the depth of breathing as well as noticing the respiratory effort. Signs of increased work of breathing include:

- Tachypnea (elevated respiratory rate)
- Activation of the accessory muscles in the neck including the sternocleidomastoid and scalene during inspiration
- Retractions in the supraclavicular fossa during inspiration
- Activation of the intercostal or abdominal muscles during expiration

This information can help you identify uncontrolled chronic medical conditions such as heart failure or pain, provide information on an acute illness such as sepsis or a metabolic disorder, or even point to a mental health disease such as anxiety.

Oxygen saturation A normal oxygen saturation level does not change with normal aging. Therefore, decreased oxygen saturation as measured by pulse oximetry can be a clue to a serious disease process in older adult patients. In one study of older adults evaluated in the emergency department, the most common causes of hypoxia were pneumonia, congestive heart failure, COPD, myocardial ischemia, sepsis, and bronchitis [18].

5.4.3 Height, Weight, and Nutrition

Height and weight Measure an older adult's weight and height at each visit. Weight can be measured on chair or bed scales for those unable to stand. If monitoring weight daily, for example, in a patient with congestive heart failure, weight should be checked on the same scale at the same time of day.

Body mass index The body mass index (BMI) is a measure of body fat that is calculated by dividing the weight of the person in kilograms by the square of the height in meters. In older adults, however, due to increased adiposity and decreased muscle mass, their BMI may poorly identify obesity [19]. Clinical guidelines have defined a person with a BMI between 18.5 and 24.9 as normal, of 25 to 29.9 as overweight, and of 30 and higher as obesity [20]. However, a large meta-analysis of 197,940 older adults demonstrated that mortality was lowest for elderly adults with a BMI between 24 and 30. Mortality was increased at both BMIs lower than 24 and higher than 30. Therefore, for older adults, an appropriate and safe BMI is higher than for the general population [21].

Nutrition Nutritional status is of special concern for older adults. Inappropriate food intake, poor oral health, social isolation, disability, chronic medical conditions, and medications all contribute to an increased risk of malnutrition in older adults [22, 23]. Good nutritional status is necessary for adequate functioning, energy, and a sense of well-being [24]. Older adults who suffer from malnutrition have been found to suffer from increased risk of infection, delay in recovery from illness, complications from procedures, and increased mortality [25]. Because of the increased risk of malnutrition and its complications, one simple tool that can be used for clinical assessment is the Mini Nutritional Assessment short form (▶ http://www.mna-elderly.com). It is a widely validated tool that includes six questions about food intake, weight loss, acute disease, function, cognition, and the body mass index [26–28].

5.4.4 Head

- It is important to visualize and palpate the head and skull of older adult patients for evidence of trauma, especially in cases of delirium or sudden changes in level of consciousness.
- An older adult presenting with temporal tenderness associated with jaw claudication and visual changes is concerning for a serious autoimmune condition called temporal arteritis.
- An increase in the head circumference with a prominent brow ridge and frontal bossing is indicative of Paget's disease.

5.4.5 Eyes

Age-related changes There are numerous age-related changes in the eye to be aware of. These include:

- Darkening of the skin around the orbits
- Loss of fat within the orbits causing eyes to appear sunken
- Crow's feet (wrinkling of the skin around the eye)
- Smaller pupil size
- Slowed pupillary light reflex
- Decreased tear production
- Decreased adaptation to the dark
- Increased thickness and opacity of the lens

Prior history Inquire about prior eye surgeries, particularly if pupils are asymmetric. Other more serious causes for unequal pupils are diabetes or central nervous system lesions. Pupillary diameter normally decreases with age and may react sluggishly to light and accommodation but should remain equal in size [29].

Structures Begin the examination of the eyes with the structures surrounding the eye. Xanthomas are fat deposits usually in the skin near the eyes that may be associated with elevated lipid levels. Ectropion (outward sagging of the lower lid exposing the inner lid) can contribute to drying of the eyes and increased risk of infection. Entropion, when the lower lid turns in, can cause eyelashes to brush against the cornea. Observe for discharge, ocular redness, conjunctival color, extraocular movements, hemorrhage, and protrusion.

Visual field abnormalities Visual field abnormalities can be caused by a variety of neurologic and ophthalmologic processes such as stroke or glaucoma that occur more commonly with advanced age. The confrontation test is a simple method to test for visual field abnormalities. While the tester sits facing the patient three feet away, the patient covers one eye. The tester covers his/her contralateral eye. The tester then holds his/her arms straight out to the sides while putting up certain number fingers. The patient looks straight ahead to the tester's nose and is asked to say the number of fingers the tester is holding up. The fingers should be positioned bilaterally and in both the upper and lower halves of the visual field to ensure that all four quadrants of the visual field are included.

Visual acuity Decreased visual acuity is common in older adults and can increase the risk of falls and delirium as well as diminish quality of life [30]. Use a Snellen chart to test for visual acuity for reading and distance, with and without glasses. ◻ Table 5.3 presents information on common age-related disorders of the eye that can contribute to vision loss in older adults.

5.4.6 Ears

Examination Begin the examination by inspecting the outer ear. Examine the pinnae for painless nodules, which could represent basal cell carcinomas, rheumatoid nodules, or even gouty tophi. As we age, common changes that occur include increased ear lobe length, hair growth in the canal, and accumulation of cerumen. Cerumen in the canal may be a significant cause of conductive hearing loss and is common in patients with hearing aids too. Look for inflammation of the ear canal and possible exudate caused my otitis externa. Otitis externa may be due to an allergic reaction, infection, or irritation due to hearing aids.

The normal tympanic membrane has a grayish or pink color and is translucent. A light reflex is seen upon shining light with the otoscope due to its conical shape. The tympanic membrane in older adults may appear thickened and less mobile, a condition called tympanosclerosis. This may result from scarring due to frequent or prolonged otitis media. You should also look for the presence of perforation and effusion, which may be seen in cases of allergy or upper respiratory tract infections.

Hearing assessment Most older adults experience some degree of hearing loss, and many older adults find that it negatively impacts quality of life. Older adults with cognitive impairment and hearing loss present an especially challenging situation as the combination may lead to social isolation and paranoia while making testing of mental status challenging.

Two easy to perform tests, the whispered voice test and the single question screening, "Do you have difficulty with your hearing?" were found by the USPSTF [31] to be effective screening for hearing loss. You can conduct the whispered voice test by standing two feet behind the seated patient so that your patient cannot read your lips. Ask the patient to cover the ear you are not testing with a finger. Exhale fully to ensure a quiet voice and whisper a series of three numbers and letters, such as 1-A-3. If the patient does not give the correct answer for the initial three numbers and letters, repeat a second series of three. The screening is positive for hearing loss if four out of the 6 total numbers and letters are incorrect.

◻ **Table 5.3** Common age-related eye disorders contributing to vision loss in older adults

Disorder	Description	Symptoms/findings
Macular degeneration	Degeneration of the macula (the region of the retina with the sharpest visual acuity)	Decreased visual acuity Preserved peripheral vision
Glaucoma	Elevation in intraocular pressure, >22 mm Hg	Loss of peripheral vision early progresses to blindness if untreated
Cataracts	Thickening and opacification of lens	Appears as an opaque/black area on the orange reflection from the retina on fundoscopic exam Blurred, decreased vision Poor night vision

5.4.7 Nose

Examination Use a bright light or otoscope to examine the nasal mucosa and palpate the sinuses for tenderness. After the age of 60, there can be a small, gradual loss of sense of smell [29].

Loss of smell If your patient reports a sudden or noticeable loss of smell, you should investigate further. Loss of smell can cause decrease appetite, which may contribute to malnutrition and can impact quality of life [32]. Possibly modifiable causes include allergies, medications, dental problems, and smoking.

5.4.8 Oral Cavity

Risk factors Older adults often have multiple risk factors that are associated with poor oral health, including being disabled, homebound, or institutionalized [33]. A thorough examination of the oral cavity is necessary particularly in those patients with dysphagia, weight loss, cough, oral pain, or smokers. Older adults who use systemic or inhaled steroids are at risk for oral fungal infections or ulcers.

Examination Fissures at the angles of the mouth, known as cheilosis, may be a sign of poor nutrition and vitamin deficiency. Dry mouth, or xerostomia, a common problem in patients taking multiple medications [34, 35], can lead to dental caries, cracked lips, mucositis, and a fissured tongue. Examine the lips for ulcerations and the oral mucosa for irregular lesions using a tongue blade to move the buccal mucosa away from the teeth. If dentures are present, remove them to look for areas of irritation and suspicious lesions. Older adults with poorly fitting dentures present with erythematous changes in the mucosa.

Oral cavity On the examination of the oral cavity, you may notice white patches or plaques on the mucous membranes that look as though they are painted on. Leukoplakia (premalignant condition), oral thrush (fungal infection), and oral lichen planus (chronic inflammatory condition of the mucous membranes) may have a similar appearance. Leukoplakia can't be scrapped off with a tongue blade and should be biopsied, as opposed to oral thrush. After inspecting the oral cavity, you should palpate for areas of induration. This is especially important if your patient has a history of tobacco or alcohol use. Ask the patient to stick their tongue out for proper inspection. Palpate the tongue by grabbing the tip of the tongue with a gauze and pulling it gently to the sides while palpating the oral mucosa with your other hand [5].

Tongue Note its symmetry and if any deviations (the twelfth cranial nerve). Look for fasciculations (spontaneous contractions), which can be suggestive of lower motor neuron disease or possibly alcohol withdrawal. You may also notice abnormal movements such as tardive dyskinesia (repetitive sticking out of tongue). Pay attention to the surface and note if the tongue is tender, red, and inflamed; this could be a sign of a vitamin deficiency such as vitamin B12 or iron. If the tongue appears hairy or black, this is usually an asymptomatic condition that occurs when a person is taking antibiotics that inhibit the normal oral flora and allow for fungal overgrowth.

Teeth After examination of the oral mucosa examine the teeth. Dental carries have a soft white, yellow, or brown appearance. Older adults with caries may complain of sensitivity to cold, heat, or even sweets. Periodontal disease is a major cause of tooth loss in older adults. About 17% of seniors age 65 and over have periodontal disease [36]. Periodontal disease involves inflammation and destruction of the structures that support the teeth [37]. Clues to periodontal disease include [5]:

- Bad breath
- Red, swollen gums
- Tender, bleeding gums
- Pain when chewing
- Loose teeth
- Tooth sensitivity
- Gums that have pulled away from the teeth
- Changes in the way the teeth align during the patient's bite
- Change in the fit of partial dentures

5.4.9 Cranial Nerves

While focusing on the head and face, many providers will also incorporate their cranial nerve examination. We discussed the decrease in sense of smell (CN I) as well as the changes that can occur with a more sluggish pupillary light reflex and decreased visual acuity (CN II) and decreased hearing (CN VIII) above. In addition to these changes, extraocular motion can also be impaired, with the most noticeable change occurring in vertical gaze (CN III, IV, VI) [29]. Testing for the remaining cranial nerves is typically not affected by age-related changes.

5.4.10 Neck

Structures Multiple structures in the neck can provide valuable information about the health of an older adult including the lymph nodes, trachea, thyroid, carotid arteries, and jugular veins. Palpate the lymph nodes in the anterior and posterior cervical chains as well as the supraclavicular fossa. You may recall that an enlarged lymph node in the left supraclavicular fossa known as Virchow's node is a hallmark sign of metastatic gastrointestinal cancer. After examination of the lymph nodes, inspect and palpate the trachea to ensure it is not deviated.

Thyroid examination A good physical exam is important in diagnosing thyroid disease in older adults as it often presents very subtly. Palpate the thyroid while standing both in front and behind the patient. Providing the patient with a small cup of water and asking them to swallow can enhance your ability to palpate the thyroid gland. When you palpate an enlarged thyroid gland, it is important to try to determine if there are discrete nodules present or if the gland is more diffusely enlarged. If the thyroid is enlarged, you may also feel a vascular thrill, and you can listen over the gland for the presence of a thyroid bruit.

Hypothyroidism may present with only depression or worsening cognition. Furthermore, the more subtle symptoms of hypothyroidism, such as dry skin, constipation, increased fatigue, and sleepiness, may be misinterpreted by patients and healthcare providers and attributed to age-related changes [5]. Hyperthyroidism may also present in an atypical manner in older adults such as with new-onset atrial fibrillation. It is less likely that your older adult patients will have exophthalmos or report restlessness or hyperactivity.

Carotid arteries The carotid arteries should be gently palpated, one at a time. Note if the pulsations are symmetric while considering the characteristics of the pulsations. Pulsus parvus et tardus, where the carotid upstroke is delayed, the peak plateaued, the amplitude diminished, and the downslope slowed, is the traditional finding of aortic stenosis. Aortic regurgitation, however, can present with a bounding or collapsing pulse where the upstroke of the pulsation is sharp and the downstroke falls rapidly. This type of bounding pulsation can also be seen in patients with hypertension or thyrotoxicosis.

After palpation, auscultate the carotid arteries with the bell of the stethoscope for the presence of bruits. Asymptomatic carotid bruits are not uncommon and, as one would expect, their presence increases with age. A large meta-analysis demonstrated that the prevalence of asymptomatic carotid bruit increases from 0.2% men and 0% women <50 years to as high as 7.5% men and women over 80 years [38]. Even though they may be asymptomatic, carotid bruits are important to note because they serve as a marker of generalized cardiovascular disease and have been associated with a long-term increase in both cerebrovascular and cardiac events [5]. It is important to keep in mind that radiation to the carotids from an aortic stenosis murmur can be confused with a carotid bruit due to turbulent flow within the carotids. The presence of a murmur consistent with aortic stenosis on cardiac auscultation can help you to distinguish between the two.

Jugular veins Examination of the jugular veins for distension can provide important information on the volume status of your older adult patients. Examination of the right internal jugular vein is preferred because it is more directly in line with the superior vena cava. It is important to look for the jugular venous pulsation while your patient is seated upright as elevated jugular venous pressures are often best seen with the patient in the upright position. At times, it can be difficult to distinguish the jugular venous from the carotid pulsations. ◘ Table 5.4 describes the ways these two pulsations may be differentiated.

◘ Table 5.4 Ways to distinguish jugular venous pulsations from carotid pulsations

	Venous pulsation	Carotid pulsation
Visualization	Double pulsation of the A and V waves visible, with strong downstroke (X descent)	Single, strong upstroke
Location best visualized	Slightly lateral, lower in the neck, supraclavicular region	Medial, higher in the neck, submandibular region
Palpation	Under normal circumstances not palpable (may be palpable with severe TR)	More easily palpable
Compression at the base of the neck	Compressible, pulsations will disappear	Not compressible, pulsations will continue
Change with respiration	Pressure decreases with inspiration	Should not change significantly with inspiration
Change with position	Will decrease with raising head, increase with lying flat, raising legs above heart	Should not change significantly with position changes

5.4.11 Heart

Atypical presentation As we age, the prevalence of cardiovascular disease increases. It is estimated that 43.7 million adults age 60 and older suffer from at least one type of cardiovascular disease [39]. As with other diseases we have discussed, older adults with cardiovascular disease may not present with the typical presentations seen in younger adults. For example, rather than complaining of chest pain, older adults with angina pectoris may report dyspnea, palpitations, or syncope with exertion.

A note on myocardial infarction Diagnosing myocardial infarction in older adults may require a high level of clinical suspicion. You should add myocardial infarction to your differential diagnosis whenever an older adult presents with symptoms of transient ischemic attack or stroke; nonspecific symptoms such as generalized weakness, fatigue, or confusion; or even epigastric pain nausea or vomiting. When an older adult does experience pain that may be more typical of myocardial infarction, they may attribute it to other medical conditions they have. Examples of this include jaw pain that may be attributed to arthritis or epigastric pain that may be attributed to peptic ulcer disease or hiatal hernia [40].

Examination Begin your examination by palpating the point of maximal impulse (PMI) located in the midclavicular line. Ask a patient to lean forward, or to lay in the left lateral decubitus position if you are unable to easily palpate the PMI. An older adult with a hypertrophied left ventricle may have a PMI that is laterally displaced and may be felt as more vigorous than normal. If your patient is experiencing right ventricular hypertrophy from causes such as chronic obstructive pulmonary disease and pulmonary hypertension, you may feel a right ventricular heave near the xiphoid process. The four valve areas described below should also be palpated for thrills using the ball of your hand.

- Aortic: right 2nd intercostal space
- Pulmonic: left 2nd and 3rd intercostal space
- Tricuspid: left 4th and 5th intercostal space near the lower left sternal border
- Mitral: left 5th intercostal space in the midclavicular line near the apex

Continue by listening throughout the precordium using the diaphragm of your stethoscope for the first and second heart sounds. Next, listen at the apex with the bell of your stethoscope for possible 3rd and 4th heart sounds (S_3 and S_4). S_4 can be a normal physical exam finding in older adults due to the decrease in ventricular compliance that occurs with aging. Though S_3, can be heard in healthy younger adults, it is almost always indicative of pathology in adults over the age of 40. Also known as a ventricular gallop, S_3 signifies increased filling pressures in the left ventricle. Causes of a pathologic S3 include:

- Heart failure (more likely heard in systolic than diastolic)
- Decreased myocardial contractility
- Coronary artery disease
- Aortic regurgitation
- Mitral regurgitation

Systolic murmurs can be heard very commonly in adults age 65 and older, although not all are indicative of a pathologic condition. It is estimated that more than one in ten adults age 65 and older suffer from moderate to severe valve disease [41]. Table 5.5 describes common murmurs heard during the physical examination of older adults.

Though some systolic murmurs such as aortic sclerosis may not be clinically significant, diastolic murmurs are always significant and require further investigation.

5.4.12 Lungs

Risk of pneumonia for older adults Pneumonia occurs four times more commonly in older adults than younger, and older adults with pneumonia are more likely than younger adults to require hospitalization and to die as a result of their pneumonia [42]. Because of this, it is important for you to have a high level of clinical suspicion and to be able to make the diagnosis and begin antimicrobial therapy early in the course of the infection in your older adult patients.

Inspection Previously, we discussed the importance of noticing the respiratory rate and observing for signs of increased work of breathing (see section on respiratory rate and oxygen saturation above). Continue now with inspection of the anteroposterior (AP) diameter of the chest. Normally the chest is wider than it is deep, with a normal ratio around 0.7. As we age, that normal ratio can increase to 0.9 [43].

A barrel chest, where the depth of the chest is greater than the width, may be observed in older adults with COPD and in older adults with kyphosis, which is a markedly pronounced curvature of the thoracic spine.

Percussion Follow your visualization with percussion of the lungs. In COPD percussion may sound hyperresonant (or higher in pitch than percussion over normal lung) because of trapping of gas leading to overinflation. Areas of dullness to percussion (lower pitch) suggest a consolidation, as you may find with a mass or pneumonia, or an effusion. Checking tactile fremitus by placing the soft area of your palm on the ulnar side of your hand on the patient's chest while the patient says 99 can help you distinguish between a consolidation and effusion.

- Fremitus is increased in the area overlying a consolidation.
- Fremitus in decreased in the area overlying an effusion.

Auscultation, as described below, can also help you to distinguish a consolidation from an effusion. Bronchial breath sounds may be auscultated over a consolidation. Breath sounds will be absent or diminished over an effusion

Auscultation After percussion and checking for tactile fremitus, you will proceed to auscultation of the lungs. When performing auscultation of breath sounds in an older adult patient, be careful to ensure that your patient does not begin to feel dizzy due to hyperventilation, as this can cause syncope.

Table 5.5 Common heart murmurs heard in older adults

Murmur	Common characteristics	Causes	Exam maneuvers
Aortic stenosis	Mid-systolic Harsh Crescendo-decrescendo	Calcific degeneration of the aortic valve	Best heard at the right second intercostal space Can radiate into the carotids or toward the apex S_2 is suggestive of it
Aortic sclerosis	Mid-systolic Harsh Crescendo-decrescendo	Thickening of the aortic valve without concurrent stenosis Common due to age-related changes in the aortic valve	Best heard at the right second intercostal space Doesn't affect the pulse pressure
Aortic regurgitation	Early diastolic Low intensity High pitched Blowing Decrescendo	Degenerative aortic valve disease Dilation of the aortic root/ascending aorta	Best heard at right second intercostal space Radiates to lower left sternal border or apex Enhanced by patient leaning forward, exhaling completely, and holding breath at end exhalation
Mitral regurgitation	Holosystolic Blowing	Mitral valve prolapse (myxomatous degeneration) Effects of ischemic heart disease on the mitral valve	Best heard at apex Radiates to left axilla

Table 5.6 Common normal and adventitious breath sounds

Sound	Quality	Physiology	Possible pathology
Vesicular breath sounds	Soft, low pitched, short expiratory phase	Normal breath sounds	
Bronchial breath sounds	Loud, high pitched, inspiration and expiration of nearly equal length	Normal over trachea but indicative of consolidation in peripheral lung fields	Pneumonia Mass
Rales or crackles	High pitched, discontinuous, crackling heard at middle to end of inspiration	Sounds of fluid or mucus in small airways	Congestive Heart Failure Pneumonia Atelectasis
Rhonchi	Low pitched, continuous, coarse, occur during both inspiration and expiration, may clear with cough	Sounds of fluid or mucus in larger airways	Pneumonia
Wheezes	High pitched, musical, continuous, most pronounced during expiration	Bronchospasm	Asthma COPD Pulmonary edema

- While listening to the anterior and posterior lung fields, pay close attention to the breath sounds you are hearing as they can provide valuable clues to underlying pathology. Table 5.6 reviews the breath sounds you should listen for.
- Keep in mind that rales may be heard in older adults even in the absence of congestive heart failure or pneumonia. They may indicate atelectasis, especially in older adult patients who are frail, debilitated, or confined to bed. If this is the case, they will usually clear when the patient takes a few deep breaths or coughs.

5.4.13 Musculoskeletal

Common disorders Musculoskeletal disorders can be of great significance for older adults as they may contribute to pain, falls, and issues with gait and balance that can negatively impact their quality of life. One such condition to keep in mind is lumbar spinal stenosis. Older adults with spinal stenosis will often present with complaints of back and leg pain that limit their ability to walk and may progress to lower extremity paresthesias. The pain is often relieved by sitting and leaning forward [44]. Conditions like polymyalgia rheumatica (PMR) require a high level of clinical suspicion to diagnose. PMR is the most commonly diagnosed rheumatic disease in older adults. The hallmarks are symmetrical abrupt-onset pain and stiffness of the muscles of the shoulder and pelvic girdles [45].

Examination The examination of the back and spine can be conducted in conjunction with the posterior pulmonary exam. As we discussed above, the presence of kyphosis should be noted, as should any scoliosis (lateral curvature of the spine). In an older adult with acute back pain and increased kyphosis, the spine should be palpated for point tenderness. The presence of point tenderness would increase your suspicion of vertebral compression fracture.

As you examine the muscle bulk, you may notice that older adults experience a loss of muscle mass as they age. Sarcopenia is the loss of lean muscle mass and strength that occurs with aging. There are thought to be many contributing causes including sedentary lifestyle and inflammation as well as endocrine and metabolic changes [46].

Range of motion Active range of motion of the joints should be tested, followed by passive range of motion if there is a significant limitation in active range. While examining range of motion, it is important to realize that range of motion also decreases with age. Osteoarthritis is a significant contributor to decreased range of motion in older adults. Studies have demonstrated that around 33% of adults age 65 and older have osteoarthritis in at least one joint [47]. A decreased range of external rotation at the hip can be an early indicator of osteoarthritis. The knees and hands are also frequently affected by osteoarthritis.

Joint deformities Joint examination may also reveal the presence of joint swelling and deformities. This can provide useful information to support diagnoses of osteoarthritis, rheumatoid arthritis, infection, and gout. The hands are a particularly important place to examine for joint deformities.

- Heberden's nodes are bony overgrowths of the distal interphalangeal (DIP) joints seen in osteoarthritis.
- The proximal interphalangeal (PIP) and metacarpophalangeal joints are commonly affected by rheumatoid arthritis.
- Rheumatoid arthritis can also cause ulnar deviation of the fingers.
- Swan neck deformities (extension of PIP and flexion of DIP joints) and boutonniere deformities (flexion of PIP and extension of DIP joints) are also seen in rheumatoid arthritis.

Contractures Contractures may be found in older adults with dementia or other neurologic conditions and occur secondary to muscle spasticity that results when there is a lack of joint motion. Contractures can cause significant limitations in functional ability as well as contribute to increased fall risk and be a source of pain for our older adult patients [48].

5.4.14 Peripheral Neurologic Examination

Age-related changes The nervous system is the site of many age-related changes in older adult patients. Recall from our discussion of the musculoskeletal system that muscle bulk and strength decrease with age. It is important to determine if the weakness is symmetric or if specific muscle groups are involved. Indicators of proximal muscle weakness include difficulty rising from a chair, which requires the hip muscles, or combing one's hair, which uses the muscles of the shoulder girdle. Distal muscle weakness can be detected if the patient has difficulty standing on her toes, which requires the use of the gastrocnemius and soleus muscles, or weakness in the intrinsic muscles of the hands. Determining patterns of muscle weakness can help diagnose the etiology of myopathies such as polymyositis (proximal) and inclusion body myositis (distal) [49].

Examination While conducting the musculoskeletal examination, many providers will also conduct the seated portions of the peripheral neurologic examination. We previously discussed the cranial nerve examination during our examination of the head and neck. For this portion, we will discuss the motor, sensory, and reflex examinations.

- Examination of the musculature of the older adult may also demonstrate increased muscle tone and rigidity. This may be seen in pathologic conditions such as Parkinson's but has also been noted in normal aging. This may be detected if passive range of motion of the patient's limb demonstrates increased involuntary rigidity [29].
- Age-related sensory changes include a decrease in vibratory sense, especially in the lower extremities. This is tested by placing a vibrating tuning fork on the pad of the patient's finger or toe. Proprioception, or position sense, tested by asking the patient to identify if their finger or toe is being moved up or down while their eyes are closed, can also be impaired in older adults. Light touch sensation, tested using a soft cotton-tipped applicator or piece of gauze, and sharp/pain sensation are often maintained [29]. However, because of the subjective nature of sensory testing, it can be difficult, or even impossible, in older adults with cognitive impairment or aphasia.
- Reflexes also diminish and may be lost as patient's age. This is especially noticeable at the Achilles tendon where by the age of 80 about one third of healthy people will not have Achilles tendon reflexes. While the Achilles tendon reflex is frequently lost, reflexes at the patella, biceps, and triceps are maintained though may be diminished [29].
- Peripheral neurologic examination may also reveal tremors in older adults with the prevalence of tremor reaching 10% in those 90 years of age and older [29]. Tremors that occur or worsen with activity are most commonly essential tremors and age-related tremors. Both are commonly observed in the hands, head, jaw, and forearms. In contrast, the tremors of Parkinson's disease usually occur at rest and rarely affects the head early in the course of the disease.

5.4.15 Skin and Nails

Age-related changes While you are conducting the above examinations, you should also be examining your patient's skin. The skin of your older adult patient is thinner and drier because of a loss of subcutaneous fat, sweat glands, and sebaceous glands [50]. Easy bruising and bleeding are common and are enhanced in many older adult patients who take aspirin or other blood thinners. Skin also loses elasticity as we age, which contributes to the wrinkling and creasing that occurs with age as well as a loss of skin turgor even in adults who are well hydrated [50].

Careful examination may also reveal some of the many lesions that occur with increased frequency as skin ages [51].

- Skin tags: benign, soft, fleshy growths, often on a pedicle.
- Solar lentigines: commonly known as age spots, sun spots, or liver spots; are hyperpigmented macular lesions commonly seen on the face, back of hands, arms
- Seborrheic keratoses: benign, raised, brown, sharply demarcated, waxy-appearing tan to brown plaques often seen on face, shoulders, chest.
- Actinic keratoses: premalignant, scaly, rough patches; can be pink, red, tan; seen most often in sun-exposed areas.
- Basal cell carcinomas: most frequently occurring of all cancers; raised, pearly, or shiny appearing; often pink or red; may ulcerate.
- Squamous cell carcinomas: erythematous plaques with scale on sun-exposed areas, may develop crusting, erosions, or ulcerations.
- Melanomas: look for the ABCDEs to distinguish possible melanoma lesions from benign growths.
  - Asymmetry
  - Borders: irregular, uneven, scalloped, notched
  - Color: presence of multiple colors within same lesion, including tan, brown, black, red, white, blue
  - Diameter: larger than ¼ inch or 6 mm
  - Evolving: changing over time

Elder abuse Signs of elder abuse may be missed by professionals due to lack of awareness and inadequate training on detecting abuse. The elderly may be reluctant to report abuse themselves because of fear of retaliation or lack of physical and/or cognitive ability to report or because they do not want to get the abuser in trouble. Elder abuse is fully covered in ► Chap. 23.

Pressure ulcers The skin should also be assessed for pressure ulcers, particularly in frail older adults or those with limited mobility.

- Pressure ulcers are staged as follows [52]:
  - In Stage 1 skin is intact and may be warm or tender. In lighter-skinned people, the area is reddened and doesn't blanch (lose color with finger pressure); in darker-skinned people, the area is not red but has a different color than the surrounding area.
  - In Stage 2 the skin is broken, and the area is tender and painful.
  - By Stage 3 the ulcer has extended into the subcutaneous tissue.
  - In Stage 4 muscle and bone can be seen.
  - Ulcers are considered unstageable if you are unable to see the bottom of the wound because it is covered by necrotic tissue or eschar.
- In deep tissue injury, the overlying skin is intact, but you may observe a non-blanching maroon or purple area, or a hemorrhagic-appearing bulla or vesicle. A thin eschar may develop over time and cover the deep tissue injury. In older adults with darker skin, the color change may be difficult to appreciate; however, you may feel an area of bogginess or firmness or note that the skin is a different temperature at a point of pressure such as the heels, occiput, or sacrum [50].
- Pressure ulcers and skin tears result in pain, disfigurement, decreased quality of life, increased healthcare costs, longer hospitalizations, and increased morbidity [53]. A pressure ulcer can develop over a short period of time (e.g., as a result of several hours of lying in place). Constant vigilance is required to prevent the development of pressure ulcers in institutionalized or hospitalized older adults [54]. Recurrent or extensive decubiti in older adults might signal abuse or neglect.

Nails The nails should also be examined while looking at the skin. The condition of an older adult's finger and toenails can provide information on his or her ability to care for oneself or suggest if they are being well cared for by others.

- Clubbing of the finger nails may be a clue to an underlying disorder resulting in chronic hypoxia such as chronic lung disease and lung carcinoma. A normal nail, when viewed from the side, forms an angle with the skin of the nail bed less than 180 degrees. Clubbing results when the angle is greater than normal and the finger has a "rounded" appearance [5].
- Onychomycosis, or dermatophyte infection of the nail, is common in older adults affecting 20% of people over the age of 60 [5]. This is the most common cause of thickening of the toenails and can make it difficult for older adults to care for their nails.

5.4.16 Supine Examination

After you have completed the seated examination, you may have the patient lie down for the supine examination. This is an important opportunity to consider the comfort of your older adult patient. Many older adults may be uncomfortable lying completely flat. In this case it can be beneficial to have a pillow present to support the head and upper back or to raise the head of the bed slightly. This is also an important time to ensure that you are using sheets and good draping technique to ensure comfort, warmth, and modesty. Uncover only the part of the body you wish to examine, and recover that portion when your exam is complete.

5.4.17 Breast

Age-related changes As adult women age, the breasts lose glandular tissue and fat, which makes the breasts smaller and less full. There is also a decrease in the elasticity of the connective tissue that contributes to the breasts sagging. These changes do, however, make it easier to detect masses.

Examination All four quadrants of the breast as well as the portion that extends upward into the axilla should be examined for masses, symmetry, and skin changes. The nipples should be examined for retraction and palpated in an attempt to express any discharge. While nipple retraction can be an age-related change, you should still be able to evert the nipple with gentle pressure. If you are unable to do so, this indicates that the retraction may be secondary to an underlying growth. It is also important in older adult patients with large breasts to examine the skin under the breasts for evidence of maceration or fungal infection.

The breasts of older adult males must also be examined. While most men have little to no palpable breast tissue, breast enlargement, or gynecomastia, can occur in situations where there is an increase in estrogen, a decrease in testosterone, or as a result of medication. Your differential for gynecomastia may include obesity, thyroid disease, testicular tumors, liver disease, bronchogenic carcinoma, and other types of cancer.

5.4.18 Abdominal

Age-related changes In older adults the abdominal exam can be more challenging and requires careful attention due atypical presentations [55]. For example, an acute abdomen may present with less severe pain, and guarding and rebound may be absent or less pronounced. While gathering the history, patients might not be able to localize well the area of discomfort and asking an accompanying caregiver will be necessary.

Observation Expose the abdomen, if possible, while the patient is lying flat. Note if the abdomen appears relax or tense. Pay attention to the skin coloration (e.g., jaundice), bruising, or rashes. Look for any scars, bulging (e.g., hernias), pulsations (e.g., aneurysms), distention, tubes, or any wounds.

Auscultation Take some time to auscultate all four quadrants. Hypoactive sounds may be a sign of intestinal obstruction, paralytic ileus, ischemia, or volvulus particularly in someone with severe changes in the bowel movements and nausea/vomiting. In addition to diarrhea (e.g., colitis) as a cause, patients with hyperactive bowel sounds may also have a bowel obstruction. Listen for bruits particularly over the aorta area, iliac, and femoral arteries. If a patient has a history of kidney transplant attempt to listen for the area where the graft is for bruits which could be due stenosis [56].

Percussion Percuss the abdomen for evaluation of distribution of gas. Sounds may range from tympanic to dull depending on the underlying problem. As an example, a patient with volvulus will have an area quite tympanic and a patient with an underlying solid mass will have dull sounds. Don't forget to percuss the costovertebral angles in the back to elicit tenderness in the flanks in someone you are concern for pyelonephritis (inflammation of the kidney). This could be incorporated as part of your lung or back exam to avoid repositioning the patient multiple times.

Palpation Palpate throughout the abdomen starting away from the area that has pain or discomfort. Warn your older patient before initiating the examination, particularly those with cognitive or visual impairment. Warm up your hands to avoid causing sudden contractions that can cause more pain or stress. Press down gently and slowly press more deeply otherwise, you may not reach any viscera or deeper structures. If you feel some resistance, attempt to distinguish voluntary guarding from involuntary. Some techniques that can reduce voluntary guarding and allow for better understanding of your findings are [5]:

- Palpate after asking the patient to exhale to relax the abdominal muscles.
- Ask the patient to mouth-breathe with the jaws wide open.

Atypical presentation Keep in mind the aforementioned about the atypical presentations in older adults during certain serious medical issues. However, if an older adult has evidence of guarding, rigidity, rebound tenderness, or percussion tenderness, that could be evidence of peritonitis (e.g., cholecystitis, bowel perforation). Also remember that mesenteric ischemia is a medical emergency and may present somewhat subtle in older adults. Older adults may present with vague abdominal pain, vomiting, and diarrhea, making the diagnosis quite challenging [57]. However, the hallmark is severely poorly localized abdominal pain with minimal physical findings [58]. The abdomen can remain soft with little tenderness.

Digital rectal examination While performing the abdominal exam, it might be easier to include the digital rectal exam (DRE) and genitourinary exam (discussed later on). Many times this part of the exam is left out by medical students and even physicians due to time constraints, level of discomfort, fear, or lack of proper training [59]. This often leads to invaluable information as older adults commonly suffer from fecal impaction, which can often be managed in the ambulatory setting. Also an enlarged prostate detected by DRE, with or without nodularities, can be the etiology of urinary retention causing significant lower abdominal pain. Other possible sources of pain identify during the rectal exam are hemorrhoids, fissures, fistulous tracts, or masses. Note any evidence of rectal bleeding and collect a stool sample to test for hemoccult blood if indicated.

5.4.19 Genitourinary

Age-related changes Older adults can experience symptoms that can be burdensome due physiologic changes or medical conditions. Commonly patients don't seek help for issues such as urinary incontinence due to embarrassment or reduced health expectations [60]. One of the most fundamental parts of the evaluation of the genitourinary anatomy is to directly ask the patient for any concerns they may have. Women experience vaginal changes due to the fall in estrogen levels. They can feel itchiness or burning which might be due to the vaginal mucosa becoming thinner, pale, and dry without much lubrication. The history should include questions about their level of sexual activity, preferences, and impact on satisfaction. Men should be asked about erectile dysfunction as they frequently won't bring it up.

Pelvic floor disorders Female patients that complain of a pressure or a bulging sensation when bearing down or voiding, particularly those who had vaginal deliveries or pelvic surgeries, most likely have a pelvic organ prolapse. Certain questions are helpful in the evaluation of women with pelvic floor disorders [61]:

- Urinary incontinence:
  - Do you ever leak urine?
  - Does the urine leakage happen with activities such as with a cough, sneeze, rising from a seater position, or running?
  - Does the urine leakage happen after a sudden strong urge to void? With rushing to the restroom?
- Overactive bladder:
  - How many times during the day do you urinate?
  - How many times during the night do you wake up just to urinate?
- Anorectal incontinence:
  - Do you have accidental bowel leakage?
- Pelvic organ prolapse:
  - Do you ever feel or see a bulge from the vagina?

Examination If the answers to these questions indicate any form of distress from your patient, evaluate further with a physical exam. Perform the examination with the woman's bladder empty. Observe for color, excoriations, soiling, discharge, or any deformities. Patients should be asked about any loss of sensation or sudden loss of continence. A simple technique to evaluate for incontinence is the cough test [62].

This test is performed with a full bladder, and by asking the patient to cough in the supine or lithotomy position. The test is positive if involuntary leakage is seen. A similar exam can be performed in a standing position if the patient is able to do so. Ask the patient to stand up on top of a large towel with feet apart. Instruct the patient to perform the Valsalva maneuver and cough. Observe for urine leakage and possible pelvic prolapse.

Similarly, men experienced hormone-related changes with androgen-dependent proliferation of prostate epithelial and stromal tissue [5]. Men with enlarged prostates and lower urinary tract symptoms will report dribbling, urinary hesitancy, and incomplete emptying. It's important to look at the medications list, especially if the change evolved rapidly after initiating a new medication as many medications can contribute to urinary retention.

5.4.20 Vascular

Examination When the patient is in the supine position, this is a good time to palpate the dorsalis pedis and posterior tibial pulses in the feet as well as to palpate and auscultate the femoral arteries. Auscultation of the femoral arteries may provide evidence of atherosclerotic disease if bruits are heard. The femoral area should also be palpated for evidence of lymphadenopathy.

Arterial insufficiency This is also a good time to examine the skin of the lower extremities for lesions as described above in the section on skin. While examining the skin of the lower extremities, it is important to be mindful of evidence of arterial insufficiency which include [63]:

- Laterally placed ulcers
- Loss of hair
- Atrophic, dry, shiny-appearing skin
- Delayed capillary refill when the toenails are pressed and released

Venous insufficiency may be manifested by the following [63]:

- Pigmented, medially placed ulcers
- Hyperpigmented skin
- Edema
- Presence of varicose veins

5.4.21 Gait and Balance

For older adults, falls are common, can cause significant morbidity, and can negatively impact quality of life [64]. Therefore, an assessment of gait and balance are an integral part of the physical examination. ▶ Chapter 26 provides additional information on screening and assessment of falls. Common easy to perform screening tests for gait and balance disorders include the following:

- Three-Stage Balance Test
  - Have patient stand with feet together side by side.
  - Next is semi-tandem with the heel of one foot positioned next to the arch of the other foot.
  - Third is full tandem with one foot in front of the other with the heel of the front foot touching the toes of the back foot.
  - If the patient is unable to maintain each position for 10 seconds he or she is at increased risk of falls.
- Romberg Test
  - Patient stands with feet together, arms at sides, eyes closed for 15 seconds.
  - Observe for sway and need to move feet to maintain position.
  - May indicate impaired proprioception, increase reliance on visual input to maintain balance, and decreased strength.
- Timed Up and Go Test
  - The patient starts seated in chair and is timed while standing up without using their arms, walking 3 meters, turning, walking back to chair, and sitting back down.
  - The patient may use whatever walking aid (i.e., cane, walker) they normally use.
  - Time cutoffs vary by the population studied, but generally between 12 and 15 seconds have been used in many study populations with those taking longer than that identified as high risk of falls [65].

5.4.22 Cognitive Assessment

A comprehensive assessment of an older adult patient should also include an assessment of cognition and function. Please see ▶ Chap. 20 for comprehensive information on assessing memory. Screening for depression and anxiety should also become a routine part of your history and physical when seeing older adult patients. ▶ Chapter 17 will discuss screening for depression in older adult patients.

5.5 Summary

Throughout this chapter, you have learned that the physical examination of the older adult patient can provide information that is vital to your ability to develop a differential and plan of care for your complex older adult patients. The knowledge of changes in the physical exam that occur as part of the normal aging process and abnormal findings that you will encounter commonly in your older adult patients will enable you to distinguish normal from abnormal and sick from well in this special population. You will now be able to go forward and use this information as part of your comprehensive geriatric assessment to devise plans of care that will allow your patients to maximize function and quality of life.

References

1. Kurrle S, Cameron I, Geeves R. A quick ward assessment of older patients by junior doctors. BMJ. 2015;350:h607.
2. Gravenstein S, Besdine RW. From Occam's razor to multimorbidity: geriatrics comes of age. Aging Clin Exp Res. 2008;20(3):179–80.
3. Kane RL, Shamliyan T, Talley K, Pacala J. The association between geriatric syndromes and survival. J Am Geriatr Soc. 2012;60(5): 896–904.
4. Elsawy B, Higgins KE. The geriatric assessment. Am Fam Physician. 2011;83(1):48–56.
5. Bickley L, Bates HR. Guide to physical examination and history taking. Philadelphia: Lippincott Raven; 2016.
6. Maher RL, Hanlon J, Hajjar ER. Clinical consequences of polypharmacy in elderly. Expert Opin Drug Saf. 2014;13(1):57–65.
7. Muscari A, Bianchi G, Forti P, Giovagnoli M, Magalotti D, Pandolfi P, et al. Physical activity and other determinants of survival in the oldest adults. J Am Geriatr Soc. 2017;65(2):402–6.
8. Huang CC, Lee JD, Yang DC, Shih HI, Sun CY, Chang CM. Associations between geriatric syndromes and mortality in Community-Dwelling Elderly: results of a National Longitudinal Study in Taiwan. J Am Med Dir Assoc. 2017;18(3):246–51.
9. Bahat G, Tufan F, Bahat Z, Tufan A, Aydin Y, Akpinar TS, et al. Observational cohort study on correlates of mortality in older community-dwelling outpatients: the value of functional assessment. Geriatr Gerontol Int. 2015;15(11):1219–26.
10. Patel KV, Guralnik JM, Dansie EJ, Turk DC. Prevalence and impact of pain among older adults in the United States: findings from the 2011 National Health and Aging Trends Study. Pain. 2013;154(12): 2649–57.
11. Yoshikawa TT, Norman DC. Geriatric infectious diseases: current concepts on diagnosis and management. J Am Geriatr Soc. 2017;65(3):631–41.
12. High KP, Bradley SF, Gravenstein S, Mehr DR, Quagliarello VJ, Richards C, et al. Clinical practice guideline for the evaluation of fever and infection in older adult residents of long-term care facilities: 2008 update by the Infectious Diseases Society of America. J Am Geriatr Soc. 2009;57(3):375–94.
13. Strait JB, Lakatta EG. Aging-associated cardiovascular changes and their relationship to heart failure. Heart Fail Clin. 2012;8(1):143–64.
14. High Blood Pressure Facts Centers for disease control and prevention2016 [updated November 30, 2016; cited 2017]. Available from: https://www.cdc.gov/bloodpressure/facts.htm.
15. Sun Z. Aging, arterial stiffness, and hypertension. Hypertension. 2015;65(2):252–6.
16. Tinetti M, Han L, Lee D, McAvay G, Peduzzi P, Gross C, et al. Antihypertensive medications and serious fall injuries in a nationally representative sample of older adults. JAMA Intern Med. 2014;174(4):588–95.
17. Williams M. The basic geriatric respiratory examination medscape2009 [January 27, 2018]. Available from: https://www.medscape.com/viewarticle/712242_7.
18. Mower WR, Myers G, Nicklin EL, Kearin KT, Baraff LJ, Sachs C. Pulse oximetry as a fifth vital sign in emergency geriatric assessment. Acad Emerg Med. 1998;5(9):858–65.
19. Batsis JA, Mackenzie TA, Bartels SJ, Sahakyan KR, Somers VK, Lopez-Jimenez F. Diagnostic accuracy of body mass index to identify obesity in older adults: NHANES 1999–2004. Int J Obes. 2016;40(5):761.
20. Han TS, Tajar A, Lean MEJ. Obesity and weight management in the elderly. Br Med Bull. 2011;97(1):169–96.
21. Winter JE, MacInnis RJ, Wattanapenpaiboon N, Nowson CA. BMI and all-cause mortality in older adults: a meta-analysis. Am J Clin Nutr. 2014;99(4):875–90.
22. Favaro-Moreira NC, Krausch-Hofmann S. Risk factors for malnutrition in older adults: a systematic review of the literature based on longitudinal data. 2016;7(3):507–22.
23. Burks CE, Jones CW, Braz VA, Swor RA, Richmond NL, Hwang KS, et al. Risk factors for malnutrition among older adults in the emergency department: a multicenter study. J Am Geriatr Soc. 2017;65(8):1741–7.
24. Ahmed T, Haboubi N. Assessment and management of nutrition in older people and its importance to health. Clin Interv Aging. 2010;5:207.
25. Starr KNP, McDonald SR, Bales CW. Nutritional vulnerability in older adults: a continuum of concerns. Curr Nutr Rep. 2015;4(2): 176–84.
26. Huhmann MB, Perez V, Alexander DD, Thomas DR. A self-completed nutrition screening tool for community-dwelling older adults with high reliability: a comparison study. J Nutr Health Aging. 2013;17(4):339–44.
27. Skipper A, Ferguson M, Thompson K, Castellanos VH, Porcari J. Nutrition screening tools: an analysis of the evidence. JPEN J Parenter Enteral Nutr. 2012;36(3):292–8.
28. Kaiser MJ, Bauer JM, Ramsch C, Uter W, Guigoz Y, Cederholm T, et al. Validation of the Mini Nutritional Assessment short-form (MNA-SF): a practical tool for identification of nutritional status. J Nutr Health Aging. 2009;13(9):782–8.
29. Schott JM. The neurology of ageing: what is normal? Pract Neurol. 2017;17(3):172–82.
30. Brown RL, Barrett AE. Visual impairment and quality of life among older adults: an examination of explanations for the relationship. J Gerontol B Psychol Sci Soc Sci. 2011;66B(3):364–73.
31. Moyer VA. Screening for cervical cancer: US Preventive Services Task Force recommendation statement. Ann Intern Med. 2012;156(12):880–91.
32. Takahashi P. Is loss of taste and smell normal with aging or could loss of taste and smell have other causes? Mayo Clinic webpage2014 [updated November 11, 2014; cited 2017]. Available from: http://www.mayoclinic.org/healthy-lifestyle/healthy-aging/expert-answers/loss-of-taste-and-smell/faq-20058455.
33. Friedman PK, Kaufman LB, Karpas SL. Oral health disparity in older adults. Dent Clin N Am. 2014;58(4):757–70.
34. Stein P, Aalboe J. Dental care in the frail older adult: special considerations and recommendations. J Calif Dent Assoc. 2015;43(7): 363–8.
35. Yellowitz JA, Schneiderman MT. Elder's oral health crisis. J Evid Based Dent Pract. 2014;14:191–200.
36. Research NIoDaC. Periodontal disease in seniors (Age 65 and Over) NIDCR2014 [updated March 07, 2014]. Available from: https://www.nidcr.nih.gov/DataStatistics/FindDataByTopic/GumDisease/PeriodontaldiseaseSeniors65over.htm.
37. Renvert S, Persson GR. Treatment of periodontal disease in older adults. Periodontol. 2016;72(1):108–19.
38. de Weerd M, Greving JP, Hedblad B, Lorenz MW, Mathiesen EB, O'Leary DH, et al. Prevalence of asymptomatic carotid artery stenosis in the general population: an individual participant data meta-analysis. Stroke. 2010;41(6):1294–7.
39. Association AH. Statistical fact sheet: older Americans and cardiovascular diseases 2016. [September, 25, 2017]. Available from: https://www.heart.org/idc/groups/heart-public/@wcm/@sop/@smd/documents/downloadable/ucm_483970.pdf.
40. Williams BCA, Landefeld CS, Ahalt C, Conant R, Chen H. Current diagnosis and treatment: geriatrics 2E: New York, NY: McGraw-Hill; 2014. p. 608.
41. d'Arcy JL, Coffey S, Loudon MA, Kennedy A, Pearson-Stuttard J, Birks J, et al. Large-scale community echocardiographic screening reveals a major burden of undiagnosed valvular heart disease in older people: the OxVALVE Population Cohort Study. Eur Heart J. 2016;37(47):3515–22.
42. Stupka JE, Mortensen EM, Anzueto A, Restrepo MI. Community-acquired pneumonia in elderly patients. Aging Health. 2009;5(6):763–74.
43. McGee SR. Evidence based physical diagnosis. 4th ed. Philadelphia: Elsevier; 2018.
44. Suri P, Rainville J, Kalichman L, Katz JN. Does this older adult with lower extremity pain have the clinical syndrome of lumbar spinal stenosis? JAMA. 2010;304(23):2628–36.

5

45. Patil P, Dasgupta B. Polymyalgia rheumatica in older adults. Aging Health. 2013;9(5):483–95.
46. Evans WJ. Sarcopenia should reflect the contribution of age-associated changes in skeletal muscle to risk of morbidity and mortality in elderly people. J Am Med Dir Assoc. 2015;16(7):546–7.
47. Neogi T. The epidemiology and impact of pain in osteoarthritis. Osteoarthr Cartil. 2013;21(9):1145–53.
48. Wagner LM, Clevenger C. Contractures in nursing home residents. J Am Med Dir Assoc. 2010;11(2):94–9.
49. Daroff RB, Jankovic J, Mazziotta JC, Pomeroy SL, Bradley WG. Daroff RB, Jankovic J, Mazziotta JC, Pomeroy SL, editors. Bradley's neurology in clinical practice. 7th ed. 1 online resource p.
50. Chang AL, Wong JW, Endo JO, Norman RA. Geriatric dermatology review: major changes in skin function in older patients and their contribution to common clinical challenges. J Am Med Dir Assoc. 2013;14(10):724–30.
51. Bolognia J, Jorizzo JL, Schaffer JV. Dermatology. 3rd ed. Philadelphia: Elsevier Saunders; 2012.
52. Bhattacharya S, Mishra R. Pressure ulcers: current understanding and newer modalities of treatment. Indian J Plast Surg. 2015; 48(1):4.
53. Gorecki C, Brown JM, Nelson EA, Briggs M, Schoonhoven L, Dealey C, et al. Impact of pressure ulcers on quality of life in older patients: a systematic review. J Am Geriatr Soc. 2009;57(7):1175–83.
54. Stansby G, Avital L, Jones K, Marsden G. Prevention and management of pressure ulcers in primary and secondary care: summary of NICE guidance. BMJ. 2014;348:g2592.
55. Ragsdale L, Southerland L. Acute abdominal pain in the older adult. Emerg Med Clin North Am. 2011;29(2):429–48.
56. Kaufman D. Assessment and management of the renal transplant patient 2013. URL: http://emedicine.medscape.com/article/429314-overview (Accessed 9 Aug 2013).
57. Kärkkäinen JM. Acute mesenteric ischemia in elderly patients. Expert Rev Gastroenterol Hepatol. 2016;10(9):985–8.
58. Ansari P. Acute mesenteric ischemia merck manual online2017 [updated January 2017; cited 2018]. Available from: www.merckmanuals.com/professional/gastrointestinal.../acute-mesenteric-ischemia.
59. Dabson AM, Magin PJ, Heading G, Pond D. Medical students' experiences learning intimate physical examination skills: a qualitative study. BMC Med Educ. 2014;14:39.
60. Chan L, Tse V. Multidisciplinary care of urinary incontinence a handbook for health professionals. London: Springer; 2013. Available from: http://BN7ZQ5YK2C.search.serialssolutions.com/?V=1.0&L=BN7ZQ5YK2C&S=JCs&C=TC0000796459&T=marc&tab=BOOKS.
61. Parker-Autry C, Tan J. Updates in the evaluation of older women with pelvic floor disorders. Curr Geriatr Rep. 2017;6(3):149–57.
62. Wood LN, Anger JT. Urinary incontinence in women. BMJ. 2014;349(15):4531–42.
63. Goldsmith LA, Fitzpatrick TB. Fitzpatrick's dermatology in general medicine. New York: McGraw-Hill Professional; 2012. Available from: http://BN7ZQ5YK2C.search.serialssolutions.com/?V=1.0&L=BN7ZQ5YK2C&S=JCs&C=TC0000746305&T=marc&tab=BOOKS.
64. Bergen G, Stevens MR, Burns ER. Falls and fall injuries among adults aged >/=65 years - United States, 2014. MMWR Morb Mortal Wkly Rep. 2016;65(37):993–8.
65. Herman T, Giladi N, Hausdorff JM. Properties of the 'timed up and go' test: more than meets the eye. Gerontology. 2011;57(3):203–10.

Testing in the Elderly

Michael Bogaisky

A. Chun (ed.), *Geriatric Practice*, https://doi.org/10.1007/978-3-030-19625-7_6

6

Case

A 78-year-old female is brought to the emergency room by ambulance after a fall on the street. A passerby helped her stand up and called 911 because she seemed confused. She does not know why she was brought to the ER and is unable to give a history of her fall. She reports feeling well and denies all somatic complaints on a thorough review of symptoms, including dizziness, chest pain, palpitations, headache, joint or muscle pains, dysuria, urinary frequency, pelvic pain, cough, dyspnea, or fever.

Her temperature is 100.1 °F, BP 106/54, pulse 94 bpm, respiratory rate 22 breaths/minute, oxygen saturation 93%, and weight 49 kg.

She is a thin, short female who appears slightly anxious and asks repeatedly when she can go home. You note slight breathlessness with speaking with no use of accessory muscles of respiration and lungs which are clear to auscultation. Cardiac exam reveals a regular rate with normal S1 and S2 with no murmurs, rugs, or gallops. She has an abrasion on her right forearm and right knee. Her left leg has 1+ pitting edema to the mid-shin with no redness, warmth, or calf tenderness. Mental status exam reveals that she is oriented to person; knows that she is in a hospital, although not which one; and knows the year but not the month or day of the week. Her speech is fluent and she responds promptly to questions. Her gait is wide-based with shortened stride length and slow gait speed.

Given her low-grade temperature, confusion, and fall, you are concerned that she has an infection of some type. Her tachypnea, borderline tachycardia, and borderline normal oxygen saturation make you concerned for a pulmonary infection. You decide to order a CBC, chemistry panel, urinalysis, urine culture, blood cultures, and a chest X-ray. Her unilateral leg swelling, along with the prior findings, raises concern for deep vein thrombosis with pulmonary embolism. Based on the simplified Geneva score, you calculate that she has low pretest probability of pulmonary embolism and decide to check her D-dimer level and an EKG.

To further evaluate her confusion, you also order a TSH.

Lab testing reveals:

Test	Value	Reference range	Unit
WBC	6.4	(4.8–10.8)	K/μL
Neutrophil %	68	(37–79)	%
BUN	30	(9–30)	mg/dL
Creatinine	1.2	(0.5–1.5)	mg/dL
eGFR	46	(>60)	mL/min/1.73 m^2
D-dimer	580	(<500)	μg/L
TSH	7.3	(0.4–4.8)	mIU/L
Free T4	1.2	(0.8–2.0)	ng/dL

Urinalysis is positive for leukocyte esterase with 40 WBCs on urine microscopy (reference range 0–3/HPF).

Her chest X-ray shows no infiltrates.

An EKG shows sinus rhythm with a rate of 96 beats/minute.

Based on these laboratory tests, you determine that she has delirium due to a urinary tract infection and plan to give her empiric ciprofloxacin 250 mg orally twice per day until her urine culture comes back. Because of her positive D-dimer test, you order a lower extremity duplex ultrasound and a CT angiogram of the chest to rule out a deep vein thrombosis with pulmonary embolism. You start enoxaparin 50 mg SQ every 12 hours as coverage until these tests can be performed. You are concerned that her elevated TSH and normal free T4 levels may represent subclinical hypothyroidism. You wonder if this might contribute to her confusion. You decide to discuss starting levothyroxine with your attending.

Laboratory data can play a significant role in the care of older adults and even more so in patients with dementia or altered mental status, such as in the case above, where the ability to obtain a history may be limited. Evaluation of laboratory data in older adults is complicated by a number of factors including lack of representation of older adults in populations sampled to determine the reference ranges for laboratory tests, misconceptions regarding the meaning of laboratory reference ranges, normal physiologic changes with aging which influence results of some tests, difficulty distinguishing normal changes with aging from pathologic changes, and the frequent presence of chronic conditions and use of medications which may alter test results.

Even in younger patients, clinicians sometimes struggle to determine whether a laboratory test indicates that a patient is "normal." What constitutes an abnormal result can shift depending on factors such as sex, age, and ethnicity as well as whether the intended purpose of a test is to screen for general health, diagnose a particular disease, manage a disease, follow up on a past result, or determine risk for developing a disease in the future [1, 2].

Starting from the 1960s to 1970s, laboratories shifted away from reporting "normal values" in favor of reporting "reference intervals" due to an increasing awareness that the term "normal" is hard to define clinically. Starting in the 1970s, international societies began to codify the criteria for creating reference intervals which are in widespread use today. Reference intervals for lab tests are determined by assembling a reference population, who are all given the test in question. Reference populations typically consist of "healthy" subjects, to avoid any confounding effects of ill-health on test results. They often are people with no chronic diseases who are on no medications [3].

Chronic disease, however, is the norm with aging. In 2008, 92% of older adults in the USA reported having one or more chronic diseases [4]. In 2010, 87% of US older adults reported using one or more prescription medications [5]. Sampling methods which enroll only subjects with no chronic conditions on no medications exclude the majority of older adults from determination of laboratory reference ranges. A study comparing reference intervals for lab tests generated from elderly nursing home residents to standard reference populations found that only 7% of the older subjects were free from chronic disease and would have been considered eligible for inclusion in a reference population under usual sampling criteria [6]. It has been argued that "healthy" senior reference subjects without any disease or medication use are so rare as to be unrepresentative of seniors as a whole [7]. In practice, because of the rarity of older adults who meet typical sampling criteria, most adult reference populations consist of subjects less than 60 years old [7].

Once a reference population is assembled, the range of values of the test in the sampled population is enumerated. The reference interval is most often determined from the range of values in which 95% of the population falls, designating the bottom 2.5% and upper 2.5% of values as outside of the reference range. Five percent of all results from what were considered to be "healthy" people thus fall outside of the reported reference range and are considered abnormal [3]. In practice, this approach can be useful for screening purposes, particularly if a value falls far outside the reference range. However, values falling near the upper or lower limit may be hard to interpret as they may truly be normal results [1].

For parameters which change with age, this approach can be particularly problematic. There is a risk for false negatives, and thus missed diagnoses, and a risk for false-positive results leading to inappropriate and burdensome interventions. For example, Surks and colleagues demonstrated, in cross-sectional studies of US and Israeli populations, that levels of thyroid-stimulating hormone (TSH) rise progressively with age among subjects with normal serum T4 levels. In the USA, the 97.5th percentile for TSH rises from 3.56 mIU/L in 20–29-year-olds to 7.49 mIU/L in those over the age of 80. Seventy percent of people who would traditionally be considered to have subclinical hypothyroidism via a typical single reference range for TSH for all ages were within a normal range using age-specific reference ranges [8]. The goal for treatment of hypothyroidism with levothyroxine is to achieve normalization of elevated TSH levels. Based on the above data, as well as evidence that the elderly have improved longevity with higher TSH levels and increased risk of harms with higher doses of levothyroxine, the American Thyroid Association, in its most recent guidelines for the treatment of hypothyroidism, recommended that the target TSH in older adults should be raised from the prior standard of 0.4–4.0 mIU/L to 4–6 mIU/L [9]. While TSH may rise, free T4 and T3 levels remain stable with aging [10].

An alternative approach from using reference ranges derived from healthy populations is to test patients with and without disease to try to determine a threshold level for a test beyond which the probability of a specific disease is high enough to prompt further clinical actions. These threshold levels have been called "clinical decision limits."

An example of a clinical decision limit is D-dimer testing for the diagnosis of venous thromboembolic disease (VTE). D-dimers are protein fragments produced by naturally occurring degradation of the fibrin component of blood clots. D-dimer levels rise with deep vein thrombosis or pulmonary embolism; however, they also rise in inflammatory conditions, malignancy, liver disease, trauma and with aging [11]. As a result, elevated D-dimer levels are a sensitive indicator of the presence of VTE but have poor specificity. Studies have shown that using a lower cutoff level increases the sensitivity of the test at the expense of poorer specificity. Raising the cutoff level improves specificity but lowers the sensitivity [12]. Because VTE is a potentially fatal condition, a clinical decision limit for D-dimer levels which maximizes sensitivity, and thus has poor test specificity, is thought to be optimal, minimizing the chance of missed diagnoses. D-dimer testing can be used to "rule out" VTE when negative and the pretest probability of VTE is considered low. Positive tests, because of their poor specificity, require further confirmatory tests [13].

However, inflammation is increasingly common with advancing age, leading to a rising prevalence of elevated D-dimer levels among older people without VTE. As a result, D-dimer testing becomes progressively less useful as a test to rule out VTE as age rises. In one study, using a standard clinical decision limit for D-dimer levels, D-dimer testing allowed for the exclusion of pulmonary embolism in 58% of people less than 40 years old, 26% of people aged 60–69, 17% of people aged 70–79, and only 5% of people aged 80 or above [14]. Recognition of this issue has led to suggestions that the clinical decision limit for D-dimer testing for VTE in older adults should be adjusted upward. In 2014, a clinical trial tested adjusting the clinical decision limit for D-dimer testing upward in older adults from the standard 500 μg/L cutoff to a cutoff determined by multiplying age by 10 in people aged 50 years and older. Use of the age-adjusted D-dimer decision limit increased the proportion of people aged 75 years old and older who could be safely ruled out for pulmonary embolism from 1 in 16 to 1 in 3.4 [15].

Aging also influences levels of other inflammatory markers. Westergren, who developed the method most commonly used to measure the erythrocyte sedimentation rate (ESR), reported a rise in ESR levels with aging [16]. Women have also been noted to have higher ESR levels than men. Miller used data from 27,000 subjects to develop a formula to estimate the upper limit for normal ESR with age as (age (in years) plus 10 if female) divided by 2 [17]. C-reactive protein levels have also been reported to increase with aging and to be higher in older adults with rheumatoid arthritis, potentially impacting judgments regarding success of anti-inflammatory treatment [18, 19]. Ferritin levels increase in healthy subjects with increasing age [20]. As a result, it has been proposed that the cutoff of ferritin levels for diagnosing iron deficiency should be increased from 25 to 50 ng/mL in the elderly [21].

The glomerular filtration rate (GFR) in the kidneys declines, on average, by 1 mL/min per year after age 40; however, 1/3 of adults showed no evidence of decline with age in a longitudinal study [22]. A decline in GFR leads to increased levels of serum creatinine. However, creatinine levels are proportional to muscle mass, which also declines universally with age [23]. As a result, creatinine levels can remain stable as renal function declines in older adults, making creatinine an unreliable indicator of renal function in the elderly. Equations have been developed to estimate the GFR. Many laboratories automatically report an estimated GFR, called an "eGFR," with every chemistry panel. The most commonly used equation in lab reports is the 4-variable version of the Modification of Diet in Renal Disease (MDRD) equation. The MDRD equation uses age, race, gender, and creatinine to estimate the GFR. However, this equation was derived in a population with no subjects over the age of 70 and does not contain a variable for weight, which would allow for adjustment for lower muscle mass with aging [24]. Some labs have begun to report eGFR using the newer CKD-EPI equation, a "super equation" which was derived by pooling the data from several large studies. The CKD-EPI equation also uses age, race, gender, and creatinine to estimate the GFR and does not include weight [25]. The Cockcroft-Gault equation, which uses age, weight, gender, and creatinine to estimate creatinine clearance, has been shown in one study to be a more accurate predictor of renal function in older adults than the MDRD equation and CKD-EPI equations [26]. Both the MDRD and CKD-EPI equations tend to give a higher estimate of kidney function in older adults than the Cockcroft-Gault equation, leading to increased risk for overdosing of drugs. Because the Cockcroft-Gault equation uses weight as a variable, it is not as amenable to automatic reporting of eGFR by labs as the MDRD or CKD-EPI equations and requires direct calculation by the practitioner.

The decline in GFR with aging is also accompanied by declines in renal tubular function. The reduced tubular function leads to reduced ability to compensate for sudden changes in water or electrolyte intake, which helps to account for the increased prevalence of hyper- and hyponatremia in the elderly. However, in a non-stress state, there is no change in baseline sodium, potassium, chloride, or calcium levels with aging [27]. There have been older reports of slightly decreased serum bicarbonate levels with aging reflecting a mild acidosis [28]. However, recent studies have not shown this. Some have suggested that the earlier findings may be due to specific Western dietary patterns with high animal protein intake, and thus higher dietary acid load, combined with greater problems excreting excess acid with aging, rather than from aging alone [29].

Phosphorus levels have been shown to decline with age, decreasing steadily in one cross-sectional study from a mean of 3.8 mg/dL in men in their 20s to 3.0 mg/dL in those 84 years of age and older. In women in the same study, phosphorus decreased from a mean of 3.7 mg/dL in their 20s to 3.4 in those 84 and older [30, 31]. There was no associated decrease in serum calcium levels. This may be related to a decline in tubular phosphate reabsorption with aging [30]. It has been suggested that the lower limit of normal for phosphorus in older adults should be 2.2 mg/dL rather than 2.5 [31].

Aging in the liver is associated with decreases in hepatic blood flow and liver volume [32]. Despite these changes, levels of liver chemistry tests such as aspartate aminotransferase and alkaline phosphatase do not change with age. There is a slight decline in albumin with age. In one longitudinal study of 3438 community-dwelling subjects aged 65–89, over a 5-year period there was a decline in albumin of 0.015 g/dL per year in men and 0.012 g/dL per year in women. Despite this decline, most older adults remained within the reference range. Using a threshold of 3.5 g/dL, only 2.4% of men and 1.5% of women had hypoalbuminemia [33].

Levels of alanine aminotransferase (ALT) have been reported to decline with age in both longitudinal [34] and cross-sectional analyses [35, 36], potentially peaking in the 40–50s in cross-sectional analyses and declining by 20% over 10 years of follow-up in the longitudinal study, from a mean of 20 to 16 IU/L. One study found that the decline in ALT levels with age led to decreased sensitivity of three commonly used tests for diagnosis of nonalcoholic fatty liver disease that rely on a rise in ALT levels in patients with the disease. The authors posited that age-specific reference ranges for ALT might need to be defined [37].

One population-based longitudinal cohort study reported that bilirubin increased slightly with age from a mean of 0.48 mg/dL at baseline in a population with a mean age of 66 years to 0.68 mg/dL after an average of 13 years of follow-up. The absolute bilirubin levels stayed within the typical reference range [38]. Two older, smaller cross-sectional studies did not find such an increase with age [39, 40].

Glucose levels tend to increase with age. Aging has been associated with an increase in central adiposity and decreased lean muscle mass, contributing to the development of insulin resistance, as well as impairments in pancreatic beta cell function, leading to decreased insulin secretion [41]. Fasting plasma glucose increases on average by 1–2 mg/dL per decade while 2-hour oral glucose tolerance test levels rise by 6 mg/dL per decade from the third to the eighth decade of life [41, 42]. These changes are associated with an increasing prevalence of impaired fasting glucose, impaired glucose tolerance, and diabetes mellitus with aging [43]. For example, the prevalence of diabetes mellitus in 2012 in the USA among those aged 20–44 years was 2.5%, 12.5% among those aged 45–64 years, and 21% in those aged 65–79 years [44]. There are studies suggesting a progressive increase in mortality associated with rising glucose levels in older adults [45].

Studies among middle-aged individuals have shown that risk for diabetes starts to rise in the high-normal range of fasting plasma glucose (90–99 mg/dL), challenging the concept of "normality" in glucose testing and suggesting that, rather than a discrete threshold, there may be a continuum of risk for diabetes [2].

Glycemic targets for treatment of diabetes mellitus are often expressed in terms of hemoglobin A1c (HbA1c) levels. HbA1c is formed by glycation, the nonenzymatic attachment of glucose to the hemoglobin in red blood cells (RBCs). HbA1c levels reflect the average blood glucose levels over the lifespan of RBCs (120 days on average). Diseases which alter the rate of production or destruction of RBCs can impact HbA1c levels, making them less representative of actual glucose levels. Conditions which lower the accuracy of HbA1c are more common in the elderly. Severe chronic kidney disease can increase HbA1c levels via lower erythropoietin levels, which lead to longer RBC lifespan and thus higher levels of HbA1c. Kidney disease can also increase glycation of RBCs through lipid peroxidation of hemoglobin. Anemia due to iron deficiency and vitamin B12 deficiency are associated with decreased erythropoiesis, leading to false elevation of HbA1c levels [46].

Average hemoglobin levels decrease slightly with aging. For example, in a cross-sectional study of the US adult population, the mean hemoglobin level decreased from 15.2 g/dL in Caucasian men aged 50–59 to 14.9 at age 60–69 and 14.7 at age 70–79 [47]. Anemia is also more common in the elderly. The prevalence of anemia in the US population aged 65 and over was estimated in one study as 11% [48]. The majority had mild anemia, with only 2.8% of women and 1.6% of men with hemoglobin <11 g/dL and only 0.9% of women and 0.5% of men below 10 g/dL. The prevalence of anemia rises with increasing age, to 20% of adults 85 and older [48].

Many diseases which lower hemoglobin levels are more common in the elderly, including nutritional deficiencies, chronic kidney disease, cancer, and chronic inflammatory states. Several studies investigating the epidemiology of anemia in the elderly have shown that no cause of anemia can be found in 1/3 of cases [48]. Authors have argued about whether there is a benign form of anemia and whether a proportion of the anemia seen in older adults is due to "aging" rather than disease [49]. Aging is associated with senescence of hematopoietic stem cells as well as a declining bone marrow cellularity [50]. Whether these changes alone are enough to explain declines in hemoglobin or if there are yet unknown pathological causes of anemia in the elderly is not clear.

Anemia has been associated with increased risk for functional decline and mortality even in analyses which have controlled for age, comorbidity, and specific causes of anemia [51–53]. Whether this association is causal or a result of underlying disease states associated with anemia is not clear.

Since 1968, anemia has most often been defined by criteria proposed by the World Health Organization (WHO) as hemoglobin <13 g/dL in men and <12 mg/dL in women. The validity of the WHO anemia criteria has been questioned in the elderly. The WHO criteria were developed largely from studies of nutritional deficiencies in anemia during pregnancy in women in developing countries. No elderly people were included in the studies used to create the WHO criteria. They also did not include people of African descent, a population with an increased prevalence of hemoglobinopathies [50, 52].

There is no clear consensus for alternate criteria. Other cutoffs for diagnosing anemia have been proposed based on data from population distributions for hemoglobin in the elderly. One study suggested slightly lower levels than the WHO criteria for African-Americans and the elderly and slightly higher levels for Caucasians [47]. Another study proposed that cutoffs should be lower in the frail elderly [50]. Other studies have looked at the association between hemoglobin levels and mortality to examine the validity of the WHO criteria. One study of US adults aged 65 and older proposed that the cutoffs for anemia should be slightly higher than the WHO criteria in Caucasian men and women (<13.4 and 12.4 g/dL) and significantly lower in African-American men and women (<12.3 and 11.3 g/dL) [51]. A similar study which used data from a nationally representative population in England found support for use of the WHO criteria [52].

There is a concern that if a component of the decline in hemoglobin commonly seen with aging is physiologic rather than pathologic, then the current diagnostic criteria may lead to overdiagnosis of anemia in the elderly and unnecessary testing. Proponents of maintaining the current diagnostic criteria fear missing significant disease.

In Western populations, the reference interval for the platelet count has been widely accepted as 150 to 400 or 450 × 10^3/μL. However, platelet counts have been shown to decline with age. There is also significant variation in platelet counts with gender and ethnic background [54]. A cross-sectional study of a nationally representative population in the USA showed that females had higher platelet counts than males and African-Americans had higher platelet counts than Caucasians. There was a decline in platelet counts in all of these groups with age. For example, in Caucasian males, the mean platelet count declined from 260 × 10^3/μL at age 17–19 to 242 at age 60–69 and 232 at age 70 and over. For Caucasian women, platelet counts declined from 300 × 10^3/μL at age 17–19 to 264 at age 60–69 and 254 at age 70 and over. On average, platelet counts declined 10 × 10^3/μL by age 60–69 from young adulthood levels and by 20 × 10^3/μL in those older than 70 years [55].

A population-based study of 40,987 subjects in Italy without malignancy, liver disease, or inherited thrombocytopenia also documented a decline in platelet count with age, as well as gender differences in adulthood, with male platelet counts lower than female, but no gender differences under age 15. The authors proposed both age- and gender-based reference intervals for platelet counts of 141–362 × 10^3/μL for men aged 15–64, 122–350 for men aged >64 years, 156–405 for women aged 15–64, and 140–379 for women aged >64 years [56]. No similar age or gender-based reference ranges have been proposed for other Western populations.

The mechanism for the decline in platelet counts with age is not clear. One theory is that there may be a survival advantage with lower platelet counts or, alternatively, it may be due to a reduction in hematopoietic function with age [55]. While the observed mean changes with age are small, they may have real impacts on the diagnosis of thrombocytopenia and thrombocytosis in the elderly.

The white blood cell (WBC) count and the WBC differential do not change with normal aging. Aging, however, is associated with declines in WBC function, part of an overall decline in humoral and cell-mediated immune function which has been called "immune senescence" [57]. A less robust immune response in the setting of infection can cloud recognition that an infection is taking place and delay diagnosis. Older adults may have bacteremia without a rise in WBCs [58]. Older adults are less likely to mount a fever in response to infection than younger adults [59]. Instead, nonspecific symptoms such as altered mental status, weakness, falls, urinary incontinence, and malaise may be the first signs of serious infection in older adults. However, noninfectious problems can also cause similar symptoms.

When in doubt, clinicians sometimes rely on culture results to determine if older patients with nonspecific symptoms have an infection; however blood and urine cultures can give false-positive results. As many as half of positive blood cultures are due to contaminants [60] and can lead to inappropriate antibiotic exposure and prolonged hospital length of stay [61]. Older women and men frequently have positive urine cultures without symptoms or signs of infection. This has been termed "asymptomatic bacteriuria." Asymptomatic bacteriuria is rarely seen in younger adults and becomes increasingly common at older ages. Asymptomatic bacteriuria is present in up to 20% of community-dwelling women over age 80 and 5–10% of men over age 80 as well as between 15% and 50% of nursing home residents [62].

Pyuria (presence of WBCs on urinalysis) is universally seen with asymptomatic bacteriuria. Presence of pyuria on urinalysis, the magnitude of pyuria, or the magnitude of the colony count seen on urine culture cannot be used to distinguish true infection from asymptomatic bacteriuria [63]. Studies have shown no benefits of treatment of asymptomatic bacteriuria [62]. Nevertheless, older adults with nonspecific symptoms of illness with positive urine cultures are often treated for urinary tract infections, exposing them needlessly to the potential for antibiotic-associated adverse drug effects as well as the potential harms from premature closure of the search for the true underlying diagnosis. Experts recommend that positive urine cultures should not be treated in older adults without specific signs of infection localizing to the urinary tract, such as dysuria, urinary frequency, urgency, suprapubic discomfort, or costovertebral angle tenderness [63] (▶ Box 6.1; ◘ Table 6.1).

Box 6.1 Laboratory tests which do not change with age

Free T4 and T3
Sodium
Chloride
Potassium
Bicarbonate
Calcium
Aspartate aminotransferase
Alkaline phosphatase
White blood cell count

◘ Table 6.1 Laboratory tests which change with age

Test	Change with aging	Clinical implication
TSH	The 97.5th percentile for TSH rises from 3.56 mIU/L in 20–29-year-olds to 7.49 mIU/L in those over the age of 80 [8]	The American Thyroid Association has stated that it may be appropriate for the target TSH in older adults treated for hypothryoidism to be raised from the prior standard of 0.4–4.0 mIU/L to 4–6 mIU/L [9]
Phosphorus	Decreases from a mean of 3.8 mg/dL in men in their 20s to 3.0 mg/dL in those 84 years of age and older. In women in the same study, phosphorus decreased from a mean of 3.7 mg/dL in their 20s to 3.4 in those 84 and older [30, 31]	It has been suggested that the lower limit of normal for phosphorus in older adults should be 2.2 mg/dL rather than 2.5 [31]
Erythrocyte sedimentation rate	Rises	The upper limit for normal ESR with age was estimated in one study as (age (in years) plus 10 if female) divided by 2 [17]
C-reactive protein	Rises	May impact diagnostic uses of this analyte as well as use in monitoring responses to therapeutics
D-dimer	Rises	An age-adjusted cut-off for D-dimer level (age × 10) has been clinically validated for use in adults above the age of 50 in diagnosis of pulmonary embolism [15]
Ferritin	Rises	Joosten proposed that the cutoff of ferritin levels for diagnosing iron deficiency should be increased from 25 to 50 ng/mL in the elderly [21]

Table 6.1 (continued)

Test	Change with aging	Clinical implication
Albumin	Slight decline	Unclear
Alanine aminotransferase	Declined by 20% over 10 years of follow-up in one longitudinal study, from a mean of 20 to 16 IU/L [34]	One study showed decreased sensitivity of tests for diagnosis of nonalcoholic fatty liver disease in the elderly [37]
Bilirubin	A slight increase shown in one longitudinal study [38] but two smaller cross-sectional studies did not show this [39, 40]	Unclear
Glucose	Fasting and postprandial levels rise	Increased prevalence of impaired fasting glucose, impaired glucose tolerance, and diabetes mellitus with aging [44]
Hemoglobin	Slight decline in mean hemoglobin with age	Anemia is more common in the elderly but the majority of older adults don't meet criteria for anemia. Alternate cutoffs for diagnosis of anemia in the elderly have been proposed but none have widespread acceptance
Platelets	Declines a small amount, on average in one study by 10×10^9/L by age 60–69 and 20×10^9/L in those older than 70 years [55]	Alternate reference ranges for age and gender have been proposed in Italy [56] but not in other populations
Urine culture	Increasing prevalence of asymptomatic bacteriuria present in up to 20% of community-dwelling women over age 80 and 5–10% of men over age 80 as well as between 15% and 50% of nursing home residents [62]	Increased risk of overdiagnosis of urinary tract infection in the elderly

Case Discussion

Our interpretation of the case changes once we consider age-related issues in laboratory test interpretation in older adults.

While the eGFR based on the MDRD equation reported by the lab is 46 mL/min/1.73 m^2, the patient's estimated Creatinine Clearance based on the Cockcroft-Gault equation is 29 mL/min. If we feel that she needs treatment for DVT or PE, the correct enoxaparin dose for her level of kidney function is 50 mg SQ once daily rather than 50 mg SQ every 12 hours. Treatment for a UTI with ciprofloxacin should be 250 mg every 18 hours rather than 250 mg every 12 hours.

However, we may no longer feel that she needs treatment for DVT or PE. While her D-dimer level of 580 μg/L is above the standard clinical decision limit of 500 μg/L, it is below her age-adjusted clinical decision limit of 780 μg/L. Combined with her low pretest probability of pulmonary embolism based on the simplified Geneva rule, it is reasonable to forego anticoagulation and further workup for PE.

While the patient has pyuria on her urinalysis, she has no localizing symptoms to suggest a urinary tract infection. The pyuria may represent asymptomatic bacteriuria. It may be prudent to withhold antibiotics.

The patient's TSH is in a normal range for a 78-year-old. Combined with the normal free T4 level, there is no evidence for subclinical hypothyroidism. Even if there was a concern for subclinical hypothyroidism, a recent trial found no evidence of benefit of treatment in older adults [64].

A call to her daughter reveals that she has dementia and appears to be at her baseline mental status. She has gait impairment with a history of falls but refuses to use an assistive device. The unilateral leg swelling is chronic and due to venous insufficiency.

Your interpretation of the abnormal clinical and laboratory findings is transformed with consideration of normal age-related changes in laboratory data and, equally importantly, with obtaining a more complete history. You start to make plans with her daughter for discharge home.

References

1. Ceriotti F, Henny J. "Are my laboratory results normal?" Considerations to be made concerning reference intervals and decision limits. EJIFCC. 2008;19(2):106–14.
2. Arky RA. Doctor, is my sugar normal? N Engl J Med. 2005;353:1511–3.
3. Ozarda Y. Reference intervals: current status, recent developments and future considerations. Biochem Med (Zagreb). 2016;26(1):5–16.
4. Hung WW, Ross JS, Boockvar KS, Siu AL. Recent trends in chronic disease, impairment and disability among older adults in the United States. BMC Geriatr. 2011;11:47.
5. Qato DM, Wilder J, Schumm LP, Gillet V, Alexander GC. Changes in prescription and over-the-counter medication and dietary supplement use among older adults in the United States, 2005 vs 2011. JAMA Intern Med. 2016;176(4):473–82.
6. Edvardsson M, Levander MS, Ernerudh J, Theodorsson E, Grodzinsky E. Clinical use of conventional reference intervals in the frail elderly. J Eval Clin Pract. 2015;21(2):229–35.

6

7. Risch M, Nydegger U, Risch L. SENIORLAB: a prospective observational study investigating laboratory parameters and their reference intervals in the elderly. Medicine (Baltimore). 2017;96(1):e5726.
8. Surks MI, Hollowell JG. Age-specific distribution of serum thyrotropin and antithyroid antibodies in the US population: implications for the prevalence of subclinical hypothyroidism. J Clin Endocrinol Metab. 2007;92(12):4575–82.
9. Jonklaas J, Bianco AC, Bauer AJ, Burman KD, Cappola AR, Celi FS, Cooper DS, Kim BW, Peeters RP, Rosenthal MS, Sawka AM, American Thyroid Association Task Force on Thyroid Hormone Replacement. Guidelines for the treatment of hypothyroidism: prepared by the American thyroid association task force on thyroid hormone replacement. Thyroid. 2014;24(12):1670–751.
10. Kim MI. Hypothyroidism in the elderly [Updated 2017 Mar 15]. In: De Groot LJ, Chrousos G, Dungan K, et al., editors. Endotext [Internet]. South Dartmouth: MDText.com, Inc.
11. Kabrhel C, Mark Courtney D, Camargo CA Jr, Plewa MC, Nordenholz KE, Moore CL, Richman PB, Smithline HA, Beam DM, Kline JA. Factors associated with positive D-dimer results in patients evaluated for pulmonary embolism. Acad Emerg Med. 2010;17(6):589–97.
12. Demers C, Ginsberg JS, Johnston M, Brill-Edwards P, Panju A. D-dimer and thrombin-antithrombin III complexes in patients with clinically suspected pulmonary embolism. Thromb Haemost. 1992;67(4):408–12.
13. Stein PD, Hull RD, Patel KC, Olson RE, Ghali WA, Brant R, Biel RK, Bharadia V, Kalra NK. D-dimer for the exclusion of acute venous thrombosis and pulmonary embolism: a systematic review. Ann Intern Med. 2004;140(8):589–602.
14. Righini M, Goehring C, Bounameaux H, Perrier A. Effects of age on the performance of common diagnostic tests for pulmonary embolism. Am J Med. 2000;109(5):357–61.
15. Righini M, Van Es J, Den Exter PL, et al. Age-adjusted D-dimer cutoff levels to rule out pulmonary embolism: the ADJUST-PE study. JAMA. 2014;311(11):1117–24.
16. Böttiger LE, Svedberg CA. Normal erythrocyte sedimentation rate and age. Br Med J. 1967;2:85–7.
17. Miller A, Green M, Robinson D. Simple rule for calculating normal erythrocyte sedimentation rate. Br Med J. 1983;286:266.
18. Puzianowska-Kuźnicka M, Owczarz M, Wieczorowska-Tobis K. Interleukin-6 and C-reactive protein, successful aging, and mortality: the PolSenior study. Immun Ageing. 2016;13:21.
19. Siemons L, Ten Klooster PM, Vonkeman HE, van Riel PL, Glas CA, van de Laar MA. How age and sex affect the erythrocyte sedimentation rate and C-reactive protein in early rheumatoid arthritis. BMC Musculoskelet Disord. 2014;15:368.
20. Casale G, Bonora C, Migliavacca A, Zurita IE, de Nicola P. Serum ferritin and ageing. Age Ageing. 1981;10(2):119–22.
21. Joosten E, Hiele M, Ghoos Y, Pelemans W, Boogaerts MA. Diagnosis of iron-deficiency anemia in a hospitalized geriatric population. Am J Med. 1991;90(5):653–4.
22. Lindeman RD, Tobin J, Shock NW. Longitudinal studies on the rate of decline in renal function with age. J Am Geriatr Soc. 1985;33(4): 278–85.
23. Goodpaster BH, Park SW, Harris TB, Kritchevsky SB, Nevitt M, Schwartz AV, Simonsick EM, Tylavsky FA, Visser M, Newman AB. The loss of skeletal muscle strength, mass, and quality in older adults: the health, aging and body composition study. J Gerontol A Biol Sci Med Sci. 2006;61(10):1059–64.
24. Levey AS, Bosch JP, Lewis JB, Greene T, Rogers N, Roth D, et al. A more accurate method to estimate glomerular filtration rate from serum creatinine: a new prediction equation. Ann Intern Med. 1999;130:461–70.
25. Levey AS, Stevens LA, Schmid CH, Zhang YL, Castro AF 3rd, Feldman HI, Kusek JW, Eggers P, Van Lente F, Greene T, Coresh J, CKD-EPI (Chronic Kidney Disease Epidemiology Collaboration). A new equation to estimate glomerular filtration rate. Ann Intern Med. 2009;150(9):604–12.
26. Dowling TC, Wang E-S, Ferrucci L, Sorkin JD. Glomerular filtration rate equations overestimate creatinine clearance in older individuals enrolled in the Baltimore Longitudinal Study on Aging (BLSA): impact on renal drug dosing. Pharmacotherapy. 2013;33(9):912–21.
27. Schlanger LE, Bailey JL, Sands JM. Electrolytes in the aging. Adv Chronic Kidney Dis. 2010;17(4):308–19.
28. Frassetto LA, Morris RCJ, Sebastian A. Effect of age on blood acid-base composition in adult humans: role of age-related renal functional decline. Am J Phys. 1996;271:F1114–22.
29. Amodu A, Abramowitz MK. Dietary acid, age, and serum bicarbonate levels among adults in the United States. Clin J Am Soc Nephrol. 2013;8(12):2034–42.
30. Cirillo M, Ciacci C, De Santo NG. Age, renal tubular phosphate reabsorption and serum phosphate levels in adults. N Engl J Med. 2008;359:864–6.
31. Lederer E, Nayak V. Disorders of fluid and electrolyte balance. In: Halter JB, Ouslander JG, Studenski S, editors. Hazzard's geriatric medicine and gerontology. New York: McGraw-Hill; 2017. p. 1330.
32. Kim H, Kisseleva T, Brenner DA. Aging and liver disease. Curr Opin Gastroenterol. 2015;31(3):184–91.
33. Gom I, Fukushima H, Shiraki M, et al. Relationship between serum albumin level and aging in community-dwelling self-supported elderly population. J Nutr Sci Vitaminol (Tokyo). 2007;53(1):37–42.
34. Dong MH, Bettencourt R, Brenner DA, Barrett-Connor E, Loomba R. Serum levels of alanine aminotransferase decrease with age in longitudinal analysis. Clin Gastroenterol Hepatol. 2012;10(3):285–90.
35. Elinav E, Ben-Dov IZ, Ackerman E, Kiderman A, Glikberg F, Shapira Y, Ackerman Z. Correlation between serum alanine aminotransferase activity and age: an inverted U curve pattern. Am J Gastroenterol. 2005;100(10):2201–4.
36. Le Couteur DG, Blyth FM, et al. The association of alanine transaminase with aging, frailty, and mortality. J Gerontol A Biol Sci Med Sci. 2010;65(7):712–7.
37. McPherson S, Hardy T, Dufour JF, Petta S, Romero-Gomez M, Allison M, Oliveira CP, Francque S, Van Gaal L, Schattenberg JM, Tiniakos D, Burt A, Bugianesi E, Ratziu V, Day CP, Anstee QM. Age as a confounding factor for the accurate non-invasive diagnosis of advanced NAFLD fibrosis. Am J Gastroenterol. 2017;112(5):740–51.
38. Boland BS, Dong MH, Bettencourt R, Barrett-Connor E, Loomba R. Association of serum bilirubin with aging and mortality. J Clin Exp Hepatol. 2014;4(1):1–7.
39. Rosenthal P, Pincus M, Fink D. Sex- and age-related differences in bilirubin concentrations in serum. Clin Chem. 1984;30(8):1380–2.
40. Tietz NW, Shuey DF, Wekstein DR. Laboratory values in fit aging individuals--sexagenarians through centenarians. Clin Chem. 1992;38(6):1167–85.
41. Chang AM, Halter JB. Aging and insulin secretion. Am J Physiol Endocrinol Metab. 2003;284(1):E7–12.
42. DeFronzo RA. Glucose intolerance and aging. Diabetes Care. 1981;4(4):493–501.
43. Meigs JB, Muller DC, Nathan DM, Blake DR, Andres R, Baltimore Longitudinal Study of Aging. The natural history of progression from normal glucose tolerance to type 2 diabetes in the Baltimore Longitudinal Study of Aging. Diabetes. 2003;52(6):1475–84.
44. Geiss LS, Wang J, Cheng YJ, Thompson TJ, Barker L, Li Y, Albright AL, Gregg EW. Prevalence and incidence trends for diagnosed diabetes among adults aged 20 to 79 years, United States, 1980–2012. JAMA. 2014;312(12):1218–26.
45. Palta P, Huang ES, Kalyani RR, Golden SH, Yeh HC. Hemoglobin A(1c) and mortality in older adults with and without diabetes: results from the National Health and Nutrition Examination Surveys (1988-2011). Diabetes Care. 2017;40(4):453–60.
46. O'Keeffe DT, Maraka S, Rizza RA. HbA1c in the evaluation of diabetes mellitus. JAMA. 2016;315(6):605–6.
47. Beutler E, Waalen J. The definition of anemia: what is the lower limit of normal of the blood hemoglobin concentration? Blood. 2006;107(5):1747–50.

48. Guralnik JM, Eisenstaedt RS, Ferrucci L, Klein HG, Woodman RC. Prevalence of anemia in persons 65 years and older in the United States: evidence for a high rate of unexplained anemia. Blood. 2004;104(8):2263–8.
49. Paltiel O, Clarfield AM. Anemia in elderly people: risk marker or risk factor? CMAJ. 2009;181(3–4):129–30.
50. Mahlknecht U, Kaiser S. Age-related changes in peripheral blood counts in humans. Exp Ther Med. 2010;1(6):1019–25.
51. Patel KV, Longo DL, Ershler WB, Yu B, Semba RD, Ferrucci L, Guralnik JM. Haemoglobin concentration and the risk of death in older adults: differences by race/ethnicity in the NHANES III follow-up. Br J Haematol. 2009;145(4):514–23.
52. Mindell J, Moody A, Ali A, Hirani V. Using longitudinal data from the health survey for England to resolve discrepancies in thresholds for haemoglobin in older adults. Br J Haematol. 2013;160(3):368–76.
53. Penninx BW, Guralnik JM, Onder G, Ferrucci L, Wallace RB, Pahor M. Anemia and decline in physical performance among older persons. Am J Med. 2003;115(2):104–10.
54. Balduini CL, Noris P. Platelet count and aging. Haematologica. 2014;99(6):953–5.
55. Segal JB, Moliterno AR. Platelet counts differ by sex, ethnicity, and age in the United States. Ann Epidemiol. 2006;16(2):123–30.
56. Biino G, Santimone I, Minelli C, Sorice R, Frongia B, Traglia M, Ulivi S, Di Castelnuovo A, Gögele M, Nutile T, Francavilla M, Sala C, Pirastu N, Cerletti C, Iacoviello L, Gasparini P, Toniolo D, Ciullo M, Pramstaller P, Pirastu M, de Gaetano G, Balduini CL. Age- and sex-related variations in platelet count in Italy: a proposal of reference ranges based on 40987 subjects' data. PLoS One. 2013;8(1):e54289.
57. Ponnappan S, Ponnappan U. Aging and immune function: molecular mechanisms to interventions. Antioxid Redox Signal. 2011;14(8):1551–85.
58. Fontanarosa PB, Kaeberlein FJ, Gerson LW, Thomson RB. Difficulty in predicting bacteremia in elderly emergency patients. Ann Emerg Med. 1992;21(7):842–8.
59. Gavazzi G, Krause KH. Ageing and infection. Lancet Infect Dis. 2002;2(11):659–66.
60. Coburn B, Morris AM, Tomlinson G, Detsky AS. Does this adult patient with suspected bacteremia require blood cultures? JAMA. 2012;308(5):502–11.
61. Bates DW, Goldman L, Lee TH. Contaminant blood cultures and resource utilization. The true consequences of false-positive results. JAMA. 1991;265(3):365–9.
62. Nicolle LE. Urinary tract infections in the older adult. Clin Geriatr Med. 2016;32(3):523–38.
63. Finucane TE. "Urinary tract infection": requiem for a heavyweight. J Am Geriatr Soc. 2017;65(8):1650–5.
64. Stott DJ, Rodondi N, Kearney PM, Ford I, Westendorp RGJ, Mooijaart SP, Sattar N, Aubert CE, Aujesky D, Bauer DC, Baumgartner C, Blum MR, Browne JP, Byrne S, Collet TH, Dekkers OM, den Elzen WPJ, Du Puy RS, Ellis G, Feller M, Floriani C, Hendry K, Hurley C, Jukema JW, Kean S, Kelly M, Krebs D, Langhorne P, McCarthy G, McCarthy V, McConnachie A, McDade M, Messow M, O'Flynn A, O'Riordan D, Poortvliet RKE, Quinn TJ, Russell A, Sinnott C, Smit JWA, Van Dorland HA, Walsh KA, Walsh EK, Watt T, Wilson R, Gussekloo J, TRUST Study Group. Thyroid hormone therapy for older adults with subclinical hypothyroidism. N Engl J Med. 2017;376(26):2534–44.

Differential Diagnoses in the Setting of Advanced Age and Multiple Conditions

Ayla Pelleg and Ravishankar Ramaswamy

A. Chun (ed.), *Geriatric Practice*, https://doi.org/10.1007/978-3-030-19625-7_7

7.1 Introduction

Ms. Adler is an 89-year-old female with a past medical history significant for hypertension, diabetes, mild cognitive impairment, and a history of a myocardial infarction 10 years ago who comes to the emergency department with her daughter after having an unwitnessed fall at home. Ms. Adler recalls taking her medications that morning and eating breakfast; she does not know if she lost consciousness and cannot recall if she felt dizzy or nauseous before falling. Her medications include aspirin, metoprolol, hydrochlorothiazide, metformin, and glargine insulin.

Ms. Adler is a patient commonly encountered in various medical settings. She has multiple medical problems, is on many medications, and had a sentinel event, a fall, which could lead to significant morbidity. Was Ms. Adler's fall due to her cognitive impairment, deconditioning, hypoglycemia, orthostatic hypotension, a cardiac arrhythmia, environmental factors like loose rugs on the floor, impaired vision, a combination of the above, or none of the above? When a patient comes to the ambulatory clinic, emergency department, or even seen at home and has a chief complaint, generating a differential diagnosis is the first step to a working diagnosis and plan of care.

This chapter will delve into the formulation of a differential diagnosis and how to approach differential diagnoses in geriatric patients and those with multiple medical conditions. Geriatric and multiple condition patients are similar in that they both have a pathophysiological milieu that is different from a healthy, young adult. Both are likely to be burdened by chronic medical conditions, which are treated with multiple medications and in many cases are likely to have a complex psychosocial situation that complicates diagnosis and management. For this chapter, the approach to differential diagnosis will be similar for these two groups of patients.

7.2 What Is a Differential Diagnosis?

A differential diagnosis begins when a patient presents with any symptom(s) or sign(s). It is a dynamic process based on information received that starts off broad and becomes narrower with more information provided. A diagnosis can help determine the underlying cause of a disease. Determining which diseases may be causing a symptom is a combination of information gathering from history taking, physical examination, laboratory and radiographic data, and obtaining collateral information from family members and caregivers.

Formulating a differential diagnosis is a key skill learned and perfected by medical professionals. Medical errors account for the third leading cause of death in the US [1]. When formulating differential diagnoses, 32% of medical errors were related to clinician assessment errors [2]. Given the increase in medical error and complexities of patients as they live longer, a differential diagnosis and how to approach older adults and multiple condition patients are crucial.

Coming up with a differential diagnosis requires clinical experience and knowledge as well as using intuition and analytical processes [3]. Medical professionals can be blinded from anchoring biases, previous experiences or pattern recognition, and inaccurate information that may result in medical error or misdiagnosis. Understanding how to interpret symptoms and signs as well as medical data including vital signs, laboratory values, and radiographic imaging is equally as important. When it comes to older adults and those with multiple conditions, presentations may be subtle and analytical data may have smaller differences, which will be further explained later in this chapter as well as in other chapters of this book.

7.3 How to Approach a Differential Diagnosis?

There is not one standardized method of teaching differential diagnoses to medical learners. There are many ways to approach a differential diagnosis, often dependent on the health profession and location of training. One approach entails taking a symptom and coming up with possible diagnoses based on organ systems. Common organ system categories include neurology, pulmonary, cardiovascular, gastrointestinal, renal/genitourinary, gynecology, hematology, infectious, endocrinology, or psychiatry. Within disease categories, there are various mnemonics that can be used to help remember possible diagnosis categories.

One strategy is a comprehensive system-based approach that goes after a certain Dr. Tom Prince who works at a Pediatric General Hospital (TOM G PRINCE MD PGH). This approach can be applied in the following way for a patient presenting with a cough.

- **T**rauma/**T**oxin/meds: Silicosis, asbestosis, trauma leading to pneumothorax, ACE inhibitors
- **O**ncologic/**O**phthalmologic: Lung cancer, bronchogenic cancer
- **M**SK/rheumatology/autoimmune: Sarcoidosis, lupus with pleuritis
- **G**astrointestinal: GERD, esophageal spasm, Zenker's diverticulum
- **P**ulmonary: Asthma, COPD, atelectasis, bronchiectasis
- **R**enal: N/A
- **I**nfectious: Pneumonia, upper respiratory infection, bronchitis, sinusitis, allergic rhinitis, TB, influenza
- **N**eurologic: Diaphragmatic spasms
- **C**ardiovascular: Congestive heart failure
- **E**ndocrine: N/A
- **M**etabolic/genetic: N/A
- **D**ermatologic: N/A
- **P**sychiatric: Tic disorder
- **G**U/**G**yn: N/A
- **H**eme: Pulmonary embolism

Table 7.1 Acronyms for differential diagnosis

Acronym	Medicine	I vindicate AIDS	A vitamin CDE
Categories	Metabolic/Medications Endocrine Degenerative Infection/Ischemia/Infarction Congenital Iatrogenic/Idiopathic Neoplastic Electrical *(neurological/psychiatric)*	Inflammatory Vascular Infectious Neoplastic Degenerative Idiopathic Congenital Autoimmune Trauma Endocrine/metabolic Allergic Iatrogenic Drugs Social	Acquired Vascular Inflammatory Trauma/Toxin Autoimmune Metabolic/Medication Infection Neoplastic Congenital Degenerative Endocrine/Electrical

Table 7.1 outlines other mnemonics for approaching a differential diagnosis. Besides an organ or systems-based approach, another way to approach a differential diagnosis is to look at illness onset whether it is acute or chronic. For a symptom like cough, the differential may include infections like bronchitis or pneumonia (*acute*) and malignancy (*chronic*). The time frame of a symptom can help narrow a differential diagnosis. Knowledge of the prevalence and population demographics will help with identifying which differentials are *more likely* or *common*. Furthermore, diseases that should *not be missed* such as a heart attack or stroke ought to be part of a differential diagnosis. The organization of differential diagnosis can be by severity of illness or most severe consequences if not identified.

As outlined in *Harrison's Principles of Internal Medicine*, some medical clinicians approach a differential diagnosis with pattern recognition through experience, memorization, and analytic reasoning via data collection and interpretation [4]. One must be cautious of not falling into heuristics, shortcuts, or simplifying decisions. More specifically, an "availability heuristic" can often occur, which is when a decision on a diagnosis is based on a recent patient case. That recent patient case may be an anomaly or may not be appropriate for a different patient. To help prevent this, a differential diagnosis approach should be broad, thoughtful, and systematic.

7.4 What Is Unique About Geriatric Patients?

Mr. Molina is a 78-year-old man who comes in for a routine visit to establish care with a new primary care doctor. He has no self-reported medical problems. He reports being able to do most of his activities of daily living (ADLs) independently. Recently, he has noticed that he gets short of breath when walking up the flights of stairs at the 63rd street subway station. He has even had to stop and rest when carrying a heavy bag. What is causing his shortness of breath?

In the US, a geriatric patient is a person above the age of 65 years. This can be considered an arbitrary designation or a matter of convenience as that is the age Americans become eligible for Medicare. Some experts think an age of 75 years is more likely to represent the impact of chronic conditions and changes with aging on health as well as the need for expert geriatric care. The 85+ age group is the fastest growing cohort in the US today and will require more attention from medical providers [5]. Age is a strong independent risk factor for many medical conditions. Older adults have higher prevalence for certain diseases and syndromes, including cognitive disorders (dementia and mild cognitive impairment), functional disabilities (from a stroke, Parkinson's disease, and arthritis), cardiovascular diseases, and cancer.

Homeostasis is the ability of the body to maintain equilibrium even in the presence of external stimuli. With aging, there are changes to most organs and a reduction in size and function, which diminish the "physiological reserve" needed to maintain homeostasis in times of stress (Fig. 7.1). Hence, it takes a lower dose of an insult, such as an infection or medication, to supersede the physiologic reserve of an older adult and manifest as clinical symptoms. The word "decompensation" is sometimes used to describe the inability of an organ (or an older adult) to compensate for acute overload from any form of stress. This *homeostenosis* or decompensation is thought to be gradual with time but can decline sharply with an acute illness. The age at which homeostenosis sets in or becomes clinically applicable can be different in every older adult; this age depends on their milieu of genetics, medical history, access to healthcare, and other social determinants. This may explain why as a geriatric healthcare provider, "If you have seen one 80-year old, you have seen ONE 80-year old!" This emphasizes the importance of looking beyond the chronological age of patients and assessing all medical problems and medically related complexities in a holistic manner.

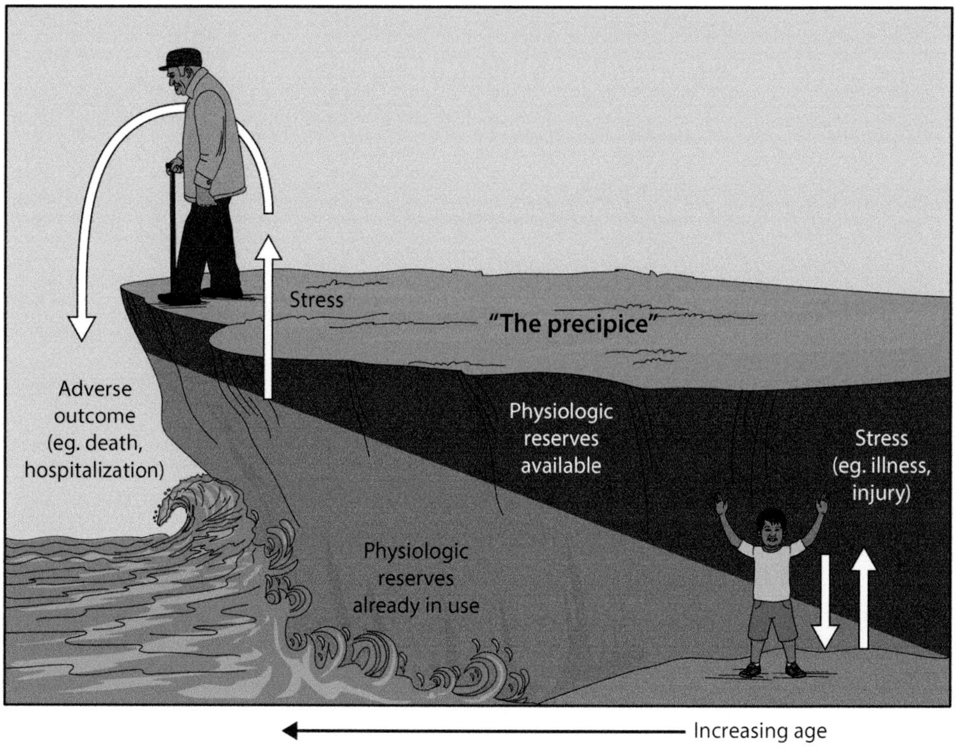

Fig. 7.1 Geriatrics and homeostenosis. (Based on information from Taffet [31])

7

In the above case of Mr. Molina with his shortness of breath, one could assume it is normal for physical exertional capacity to decline with aging. In the heart, normal aging brings about structural, histologic, molecular, and functional changes that contribute to this decreased physical tolerance. Some of these cardiac changes include: increased thickness of left ventricular wall, calcification of aortic and mitral valves, decrease in number of cardiomyocytes, decline in beta-adrenergic responsiveness, and a reduction in diastolic function and maximal heart rate [6]. Mr. Molina's cardiac changes with aging could cause his shortness of breath; however, other factors must be considered as well.

Age in itself can be considered another predisposing factor that increases vulnerability to poor outcomes when exposed to noxious stimuli (Fig. 7.2). The greater the baseline vulnerability, the lower the intensity of the precipitating insult needed to cause a devastating outcome like morbidity or mortality. Although age is an important predictor, practitioners should not forget to view a younger person with disabilities and/or multiple chronic conditions as being just as or more vulnerable compared to a healthy counterpart.

There are physiologic changes with aging that affect pharmacokinetics (what the body does to the drug) and pharmacodynamics (what the drug does to the body). These changes make drug interactions and adverse drug events (ADE) more likely and should be considered as part of the differential diagnosis in a geriatric patient. An older adult presenting with new onset fatigue could have, for example, anemia or cancer, but should also be suspected of having an amplified effect of a medication, such as metoprolol (a beta-blocker), that could have been initiated recently. In fact, several presentations of geriatric syndromes including dementia, delirium, depression, falls, urinary incontinence, and constipation can result from adverse drug events and inappropriate medication use [7]. The use of multiple or inappropriate medications or polypharmacy, which is common in older adults, can accentuate the likelihood of an ADE being the primary cause of a clinical presentation [8]. Appreciating this is vital because the majority of these ADE are considered preventable.

Single risk factors can lead to multiple disease states. One example of this is smoking and its correlation to cancers, heart disease, pulmonary disease, and vascular disease. It is worth emphasizing that in older adults, multiple etiologies or risk factors can be associated with a certain presentation of illness or disability. This is called a *multifactorial* causation. Not only are conditions with a multifactorial causation more challenging to identify and attribute; they are also more difficult to cure and palliate. Ms. Adler and her injurious fall described at the beginning of this chapter is an example of multifactorial causation. Her fall may be attributed to progressive cataracts, dehydration, inappropriate footwear, even worsening arthritis pain among others, or a combination of all factors. This multifactorial causation can cloud differential diagnoses and make presentations less straightforward.

Geriatric healthcare providers also need to look for what are often called *atypical presentations*. In reality, these presentations are not atypical, but can be common for older people who are ill. These presentations lack the usual signs and symptoms characterizing a particular condition or diagnosis often studied and validated in younger adults. For example, dyspnea and not chest pain is the most common presentation of myocardial infarction in older adults [9]. Fever, the cardinal feature of infection, is absent in 30–50% of frail, older adults, even in the setting of serious infections

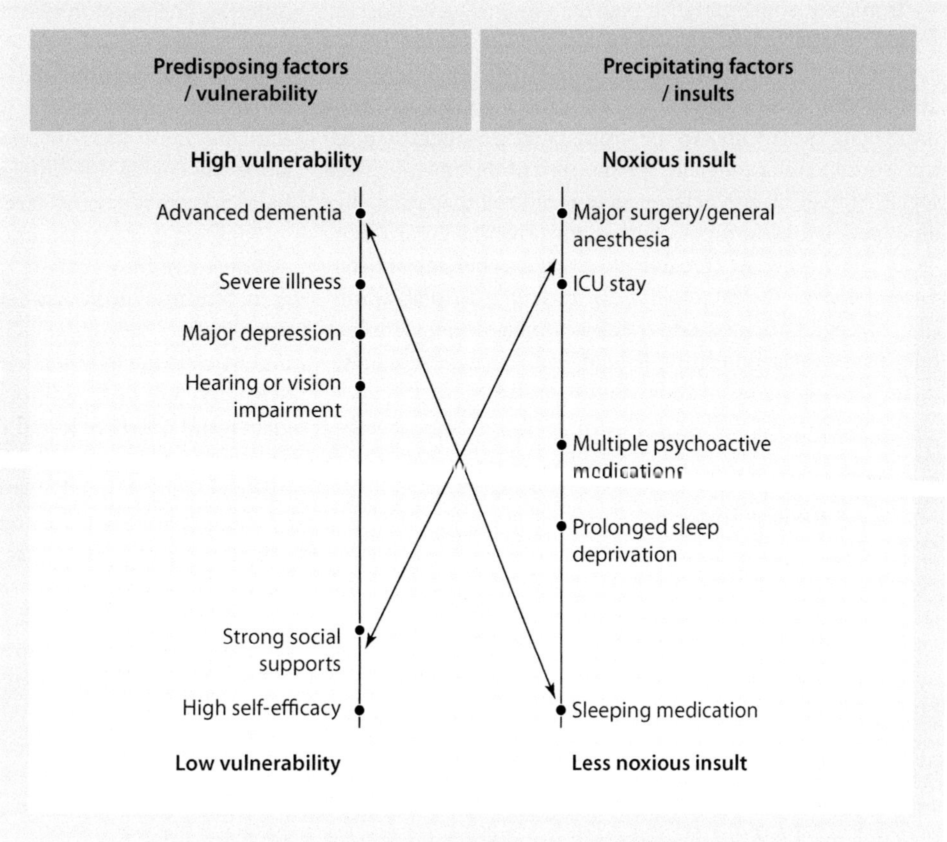

■ **Fig. 7.2** Vulnerability and insults in older adults. (Modified from Halter et al. [32])

like pneumonia or endocarditis [10, 11]. The blunted febrile response in older adults is due to changes in multiple systems including the immune system and thermoregulatory processes. These and other pathophysiologic changes of aging in organ systems also cause other vital signs (blood pressure, pulse, and respiratory rate) to not respond appropriately when stressed [12]. Changes can be subtle. Hence, practitioners in geriatrics may need a heightened awareness and look beyond the typical vital signs or single point measurements (like an elevated white blood cell count) to detect these atypical presentations.

Another important factor to consider is the heightened interrelationship of the biopsychosocial factors with somatic presentation of disease in older adults as compared to younger adults [13]. Incidence of psychological dysfunction like depression and apathy is higher. Moreover, social determinants like absence of spousal or family support, unemployment, limited health literacy, and food insecurity can greatly complicate a presentation in older adults. ■ Figure 7.3 depicts this concept wherein the functional status is influenced by not only the physical manifestation of disease but also by the psychological and socioeconomic factors. Consider, for example, an 84-year-old lady who presents with dizziness, near fainting, and inability to get out of the home in the past week. In addition to the plethora of differential diagnoses for a younger adult, medication nonadherence from not understanding medication instructions, an ADE from concurrent use of multiple neuropsychiatric medications, and progressive cognitive decline leading to reduced ability to cook and eat balanced meals are possible causes that must be included for an older adult. This highlights the importance of a holistic approach to data gathering, i.e., eliciting pertinent functional, psychological, and social history as part of the history of present illness [14].

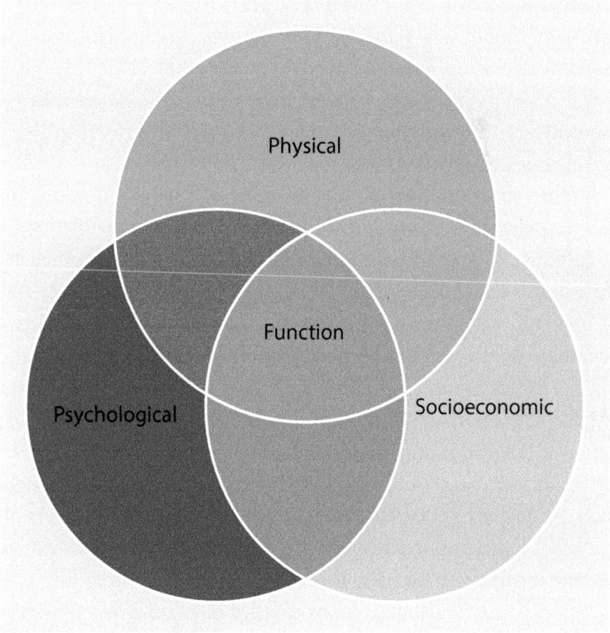

■ **Fig. 7.3** Holistic patient approach. (Modified from Kane et al. [33])

Ironically, some geriatric patients admitted to a hospital are also at risk for being labeled as a *social admission*. This is a patient in whom no acute medical issues are felt to be contributing; rather the patient's social circumstances are felt to be the driving cause. Often in these situations, a thoughtful medical workup is not pursued. It is important to remember that social admissions are heterogeneous and multifactorial (like other geriatric syndromes), with many potential contributing factors. Hence, while caregiver stress or another social determinant may be the causative factor in such a hospital admission, one must not miss a reversible or undiagnosed pathology [15]. Every social admission should be an invitation to investigate the underlying and contributing causes.

7.5 What Is Unique About Multiple Condition Patients?

When a patient is referred as having multiple conditions, the term multimorbidity may come to mind. Multimorbidity is when a patient has two or more chronic, degenerative, or terminal illnesses that are difficult to control and when combined together can provide serious side effects [16]. Patients with multimorbidity often have increased healthcare utilization, have decreased functionality, have increased pain and suffering, and often have shorter life expectancies. Identifying the etiology of a symptom and creating a differential diagnosis are challenging in multimorbidity due to the difficulty in correlating symptoms to a particular disease process. There are less linear relationships between disease pathology and symptoms when a patient has many diseases [17]. Like geriatric patients, multiple condition patients have atypical presentations and further complications from infections and interventions.

The American Geriatrics Society (AGS) created an expert panel providing recommendations on how to care for older adults with multimorbidity [18]. These guiding principles highlight the importance of asking patients their primary concerns, considering patient preferences and prognosis, evaluating interactions among treatments and conditions, and weighing benefits and harms when considering treatments. Multiple condition patients are likely to have a greater number of medications and healthcare providers and specialists involved in their care, thereby presenting similar challenges like a complex geriatric patient. A practical approach to multimorbid patients includes prioritization of medical issues, exploring patient's goals and preferences, and coordinating care with the healthcare team members (clinicians, pharmacists, social workers, and mental health providers) [19].

7.6 What Are Challenges in Creating a Differential Diagnosis?

The complexities described so far bring many challenges to coming up with differential diagnoses for geriatric and multiple condition patients. Based on pathophysiology and differing presentation symptoms, geriatric and multiple condition patients require closer attention given atypical presentations. This section will delve into various barriers, its detrimental impact on patients' health, and strategies to mitigate them. In most cases, being aware of these barriers alone will enable the clinician to draw a better set of differentials and provide better care.

Gathering information or history taking in a geriatric or multiple condition patient can be challenging for many reasons. Subtle or profound cognitive, mood, hearing, or visual impairments can impede efficient and accurate data gathering. Knowledge of baseline impairments among patients can help clinicians seek additional information from family, caregivers, and others involved with patient care. Patients should be encouraged to use their vision and hearing aids at each medical visit. A quick cognitive assessment like the clock-drawing or the Mini-Cog test can assess deficits in executive functioning and delayed recall.

It is not unusual for a geriatric healthcare provider to indulge in detective work to get the whole story, which is crucial for formulating an accurate differential diagnosis. When relevant, an extra step with a phone call to the pharmacist, the specialist physician, or the home care agency will clarify a key component of history. Further, in order to differentiate between baseline impairment and superimposed pathological change as the cause of the patient's presentation, the time frame of the presenting complaint is important. An older adult with worsening confusion over a few days should be evaluated for an infection and other causes of delirium, whereas someone with cognitive worsening over months to years likely has some form of progressive dementia.

Low health literacy is ubiquitous, but poorly recognized [20]. This can be particularly problematic in geriatric and multiple condition patients, who are likely to have multiple chronic problems, are prescribed multiple medications, follow with multiple specialists, and hence have to process and utilize a lot of medical information to take care of their health. This can lead to behaviors often inaccurately categorized as nonadherent. To improve the patient-physician interaction, a clinician should use *universal communication precautions* – minimal use of medical jargon, deliver information in small packets, and check for understanding using teach-back methods. *Ask Me 3*® is another strategy that empowers patients to be an advocate for themselves and relay complex information from one provider to another. It consists of three questions that patients should ask their provider at the end of the visit: *What is my main problem? What do I need to do? Why is it important for me to do this?* [21].

An under-evaluated component of history taking that is pertinent in older adults is the social history. Alcohol misuse by older adults is often overlooked, likely either due to physician biases about aging adults or due to attribution of symptoms and signs to other problems common in geriatric patients [22]. Relating back to the beginning of the chapter, think about Ms. Adler who presented with a fall. If she was not asked about alcohol use, peripheral sensory neuropathy secondary to chronic alcohol would not be part of the differential diagnosis. Many older adults continue to drink the same quantity of alcohol as they did when they were younger, without realizing that their body composition changes with aging, which makes them more likely to experience harmful effects of alcohol ("You do become a cheaper drunk with age."). Compounding that problem is the common occurrence of low or reduced drinking of water among older adults. We suggest the routine use of CAGE screening questions to look for alcohol use disorder in older adults that endorse drinking any amount of alcohol [23].

Also, clinicians may be inclined to avoid asking details of sexual activity in their geriatric patient, often from false assumptions, ageist beliefs, or personal discomfort in asking a sexual history. This is despite the fact that 25–50% of older adults continue to be sexually active [24]. Asking a sexual history and considering a sexually transmitted illness may be appropriate for a differential diagnosis. Approaching this sensitive (and possibly uncomfortable) topic with an open-ended question such as "Tell me about your sex life?" can be helpful before probing for more specific details.

Knowledge of a patient's religious practice and cultural background can influence history taking and the differential diagnosis [25]. For example, fasting rituals during Ramadan and Yom Kippur can lead to hypoglycemia and dehydration-related presentations. Psychiatric diagnoses can be challenging to explore in certain cultures that still stigmatize mental health disorders or consider depression and apathy to be a normal part of aging.

It cannot be stressed enough that a detailed medication history is one of the most crucial components of a geriatric patient history, especially those with multiple conditions and medications. Medication reconciliation, which is a several step process, includes confirming the medication indication, dose, frequency, and patient's compliance as well as understanding potential side effects from the medication [26]. Clinicians faced with challenging lists of medications should seek assistance from team members – pharmacists, nurses, and doctors – to reduce medication discrepancies. In today's electronic world, utilization of online resources and mobile applications to perform a drug interaction check at the bedside is feasible and highly recommended.

When performing the physical examination, clinicians should review the vital signs closely. As mentioned earlier in the chapter, older adults are less likely to mount a febrile response to infection or injury. Conversely, they are more likely to present with a lower temperature than normal; the use of reliable low-reading thermometers can accurately identify hypothermia. While older adults are at risk for strokes and heart attacks from chronic hypertension, they are uniquely predisposed to dangerous presentations from hypotension. If feasible, clinicians should attempt to get orthostatic vital signs for all patients. If not, a standing blood pressure alone can be helpful in identifying those at risk for orthostatic hypotension [27].

7.7 How to Approach Geriatric or Multiple Condition Patients?

At first glance, a differential diagnosis may be similar between young and older adults. However, age and disease complexity are important in determining what is most likely and what needs immediate versus deferred action. When drawing differential diagnoses in older adults and those with multiple conditions, one may be reminded of Hickam's dictum ("Patients can have as many diseases as they damn well please."), which supports the possibility of various disease processes contributing simultaneously to a patient presentation [28]. In contrast, the counter-strategy of Occam's razor (based on a principle of diagnostic parsimony) supports a single unified diagnosis to explain a multitude of symptoms, signs, and laboratory data. This paradigm in which clinical findings lead directly to a unifying diagnosis has been found true in fewer than half of older patients studied [29]. Similar to Hickam's dictum theory, older adults are likely to have multiple diagnoses that explain a clinical presentation. Thinking back about our patients, Ms. Adler who fell and Mr. Molina who had progressive shortness of breath, they both have multiple diagnoses and disease processes that can explain their clinical presentations, aligning with Hickam's dictum theory.

A comprehensive geriatric assessment that includes a detailed psychosocial and functional assessment along with geriatric-specific screenings for hearing, vision, depression, and cognitive impairment is ideal; however, it may not be practical in every clinical setting. Busy clinicians will need a strategy to quickly develop an age-appropriate differential to help provide patient-centered care. Learners and geriatric healthcare providers may want to utilize the following tools to ensure complete data gathering and appropriate hypothesis generation. These tools will also minimize biases that may lead to errors in clinical reasoning and premature closure when generating differential diagnoses.

Geriatric ROS At the conclusion of history taking, the Geriatric Review of Systems (ROS) can be utilized to further assess symptoms and systems, which are not only more common in older adults but also unlikely to be shared with the clinician unless specifically asked. The DEEP IN mnemonic is a helpful way to remember the components of the Geriatric ROS.

- **D** – *D*ementia, *D*epression, *D*riving, *D*rugs
- **E** – *E*yes (vision)
- **E** – *E*ars (hearing)
- **P** – *P*hysical Performance, *P*halls (for falls), *P*sychosocial
- **I** – *I*ncontinence (and constipation)
- **N** – *N*utrition

Positive findings in the Geriatric ROS will help formulate a more relevant differential diagnosis. For example, in the case of Ms. Adler who fell at home, the knowledge of worsening urinary incontinence will allow consideration of a urinary infection or a home hazard. An example of a home hazard may be lack of optimal lighting, causing a fall at home.

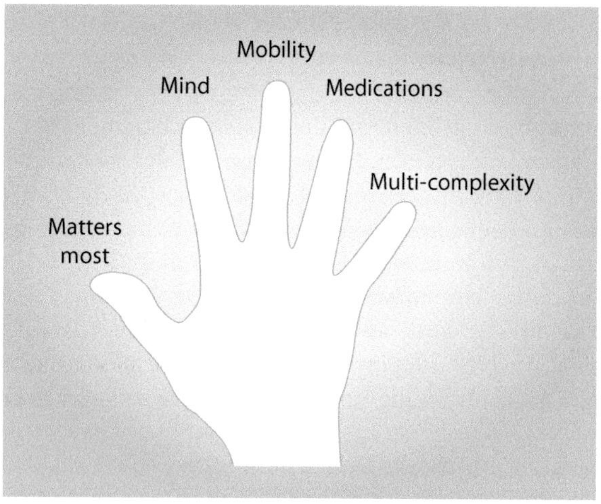

7

Fig. 7.4 Geriatric 5Ms. (Modified from Frank Molnar and Allen Huang, University of Ottawa Mary Tinetti, Yale University)

Geriatric 5Ms© Once data gathering is completed, the next step is to streamline obtained information and create a prioritized differential diagnosis list. Any of the strategies mentioned in ► Sect. 7.3 and Table 7.1 of this chapter can help with this process (acute/chronic, most likely/rare/not-to-be-missed, severity-based, etc.). In the case of older adults and those with multiple conditions, prioritizing a differential diagnosis can be further enhanced by the use of a *geriatric lens* in order to ensure inclusion of syndromes and issues that are more prominent in older adults. The Geriatric 5Ms depicted in Fig. 7.4 by the five fingers of the hand is a simplified communication framework to describe core competencies in Geriatrics in a manner that learners and clinicians can easily understand and remember [30]. It reminds clinicians to be cognizant of the disorders of the **m**ind, **m**obility, and **m**edications, to acknowledge the **m**ulti-complexity of many geriatric patient situations, and above all, to tailor the management based on what **m**atters most to that patient.

For example, by purposefully applying the Geriatric 5Ms to Ms. Adler's case, the following can be added to the differential diagnosis: progression of her mild cognitive impairment to dementia or depression (**m**ind), arthritis or age-related deconditioning (**m**obility), hypoglycemia or orthostatic hypotension from inappropriate use of one of her diabetes or hypertension medications (**m**edications), reduced dietary intake from a recent change in her social support (**m**ulti-complexity), and her preference for wearing socks in the home despite prior counseling to use flexible shoes for walking inside the home (**m**atters most).

In conclusion, providing high-quality patient-centered care begins with the development of an accurate and pertinent differential diagnosis. Tools like the Geriatric ROS and the Geriatric 5Ms offer a holistic and comprehensive approach to the differential diagnosis process for our geriatric and multiple condition patients.

Take-Home Messages

- Geriatric and multiple condition patients are similar in the complexity they present to the clinician. They are likely to have several chronic conditions, take multiple medications, and have a higher likelihood of psychosocial factors affecting their health.
- Being aware that clinical presentations of common conditions in this population can differ significantly from that in younger adults can reduce the risk of missed diagnoses, morbidity, and mortality.
- Reduction in physiologic reserve in most organ systems (homeostenosis) and pharmacokinetic and pharmacodynamic changes with aging predispose older adults to be more vulnerable to poor outcomes from exposure to precipitating stressors, including various medications.
- A detailed social history, with attention to substance use, sexual activity, cultural and religious practices, and caregiver stress can be crucial.
- Obtaining collateral information from family members and caregivers is often necessary and very helpful, particularly for patients with cognitive disorders or altered mental status.
- Geriatric and multiple condition patients are at higher risk for drug interactions and adverse drug events as the cause of the clinical presentation; hence, medication reconciliation should be prioritized.
- Using the Geriatric Review of Systems in the data gathering process and the Geriatric 5Ms (mind, mobility, medications, multi-complexity, matters most) in the differential diagnosis generation process can be a vital part of a systematic approach to older adults and those with multiple conditions.

References

1. Makary MA, Daniel M. Medical error-the third leading cause of death in the US. BMJ. 2016;353:i2139.
2. Schiff GD, Hasan O, Kim S, et al. Diagnostic error in medicine: analysis of 583 physician-reported errors. Arch Intern Med. 2009;169(20):1881–7.
3. Stern SD, Cifu AS, Altkorn D. Diagnostic process. In: Symptom to diagnosis: an evidence-based guide. 3rd ed. New York: McGraw-Hill; 2014.
4. Mark DB, Wong JB. Decision-making in clinical medicine. In: Kasper D, et al., editors. Harrison's principles of internal medicine. 19th ed. New York: McGraw-Hill; 2014.
5. He W, Goodkind D, Kowal P. U.S. Census Bureau, International population reports, P95/16-1, an aging world: 2015. Washington, DC: U.S. Government Publishing Office; 2016. Available from:

https://www.census.gov/content/dam/Census/library/publications/2016/demo/p95-16-1.pdf.
6. Arbab-Zadeh A, Dijk E, Prasad A, et al. Effect of aging and physical activity on left ventricular compliance. Circulation. 2004;110(13):1799–805.
7. Saraf AA, Petersen AW, Simmons SF, et al. Medications associated with geriatric syndromes and their prevalence in older hospitalized adults discharged to skilled nursing facilities. J Hosp Med. 2016;11(10):694–700.
8. Budnitz DS, Pollock DA, Weidenbach KN, et al. National surveillance of emergency department visits for outpatient adverse drug events. JAMA. 2006;296(15):1858–66.
9. Carro A, Kaski JC. Myocardial infarction in the elderly. Aging Dis. 2011;2(2):116–37.
10. Henschke PJ. Infections in the elderly. Med J Aust. 1993;158(12):830–4.
11. Musgrave T, Verghese A. Clinical features of pneumonia in the elderly. Semin Respir Infect. 1990;5(4):269–75.
12. Chester JG, Rudolph JL. Vital signs in older patients: age-related changes. J Am Med Dir Assoc. 2011;12(5):337–43.
13. Mooijaart SP, Broekhuizen K, Trompet S, et al. Evidence-based medicine in older patients: how can we do better? Neth J Med. 2015;73(5):211–8.
14. Kane RL, Ouslander JG, Resnick B, Malone ML. Evaluating the geriatric patient. In: Essentials of clinical geriatrics. 8th ed. New York: McGraw-Hill; 2013.
15. Oliver D. "Acopia" and "social admission" are not diagnoses: why older people deserve better. J R Soc Med. 2008;101(4):168–74.
16. Wallace E, Salisbury C, Guthrie B, et al. Managing patients with multimorbidity in primary care. BMJ. 2015;350:h176.
17. Halter JB, Ouslander JG, Studenski S, High KP, Asthana S, Supiano MA, Ritchie CS. Evaluation, management, and decision-making. In: Hazzard's geriatric medicine and gerontology. 7th ed. New York: McGraw-Hill; 2016.
18. American Geriatrics Society Expert Panel on the Care of Older Adults with Multimorbidity. Guiding principles for the care of older adults with multimorbidity: an approach for clinicians. J Am Geriatr Soc. 2012;60(10):E1–E25.
19. Ramaswamy R. Complex care: treating an older patient with multiple comorbidities. Am Fam Physician. 2014;89(5):392–4.
20. Paasche-Orlow M. Caring for patients with limited health literacy: a 76-year-old man with multiple medical problems. JAMA. 2011;306(10):1122–9.
21. Institute for Healthcare Improvement [Internet]. Ask me three: good questions for your health. Cambridge: National Patient Safety Foundation. 2016. Available from: http://www.npsf.org/page/askme3.
22. Graham K. Identifying and measuring alcohol abuse among the elderly: serious problems with existing instrumentation. J Stud Alcohol. 1986;47(4):322–6.
23. Steinweg DL, Worth H. Alcoholism: the keys to the CAGE. Am J Med. 1993;94(5):520–3.
24. Ni Lochlainn M, Kenny RA. Sexual activity and aging. J Am Med Dir Assoc. 2013;14(8):565–72.
25. Gopalkrishnan N, Babacan H. Cultural diversity and mental health. Australas Psychiatry. 2015;23(6 Suppl):6–8.
26. American Medical Association [Internet]. The physician's role in medication reconciliation: issues, strategies and safety principles. 2007. Available from: https://bcpsqc.ca/documents/2012/09/AMA-The-physician%E2%80%99s-role-in-Medication-Reconciliation.pdf.
27. Conti RC. Blood pressure measurement: sitting and standing? Clin Cardiol. 2008;31(9):395–6.
28. Mani N, Slevin N, Hudson A. What three wise men have to say about diagnosis. BMJ. 2011;343:d7769.
29. Fried LP, Storer DJ, King DE, Lodder F. Diagnosis of illness presentation in the elderly. J Am Geriatr Soc. 1991;39(2):117–23.
30. Tinetti M, Huang A, Molnar F. The geriatrics 5M's: a new way of communicating what we do. J Am Geriatr Soc. 2017;65(9):2115.
31. Taffet GE. Physiology of aging. In: Cassel CK, Leipzig RM, Cohen HJ, et al., editors. Geriatric medicine: an evidence-based approach. 4th ed. New York: Springer; 2003.
32. Halter JB, Ouslander JG, Tinetti ME, Studenski S, High KP, Asthana S. Hazzard's geriatric medicine and gerontology. 6th ed. New York: McGraw-Hill Companies; 2009.
33. Kane RL, Ouslander JG, Abrass IB, Resnick B. Essentials of clinical geriatrics. 7th ed. New York: McGraw Hill Companies; 2013.

Common Acute Illness

Noelle Marie Javier, Martine Sanon, and Sara Suleman

A. Chun (ed.), *Geriatric Practice*, https://doi.org/10.1007/978-3-030-19625-7_8

8.1 Sepsis in the Older Adult

8.1.1 Introduction

Sepsis is a serious universal health problem that if left untreated will lead to high morbidity and mortality. Older adults have a high susceptibility to developing sepsis in part related to the natural consequence of immunosenescence. The two most common causes of sepsis in the older adults are pneumonia and urinary tract infections (UTIs). Multiple medical problems further add to the severity of sepsis and subsequent organ dysfunction. It is important to recognize that older adults present atypically when infected which could lead to delays in early medical management. These symptoms include generalized body weakness, anorexia, and confusion. The cornerstone of successful management of sepsis requires early intervention with source identification, pathogen speciation, risk factor modification, and appropriate antimicrobial therapy administration.

Case Presentation

GC is an 88-year-old female residing in a high-rise building who was transferred to the hospital for worsening mental status. She has a past medical history pertinent for neurocognitive impairment, hypertension, mild COPD, osteoporosis, type 2 diabetes mellitus on insulin, and osteoarthritis. Upon arrival at the emergency room, she was found to have a respiratory rate of 24, blood pressure of 140/70 mmHg, temperature of 100.4F, and white blood cell count of 17,000 cells/microLiter. Her chest radiograph revealed a non-specific lower lobe infiltrate. Per her home health aide, she might have aspirated after she was given a food supplement shortly after dinner and after she was found to have been coughing incessantly. She was then started on intravenous ceftriaxone and azithromycin. A few hours into her stay, she developed hypotension requiring intravenous fluids. Blood cultures revealed gram positive cocci in clusters. She was empirically treated with vancomycin. Her daughter arrives and requests the provider to give her a medical update.

8

8.1.2 Discussion

Sepsis continues to be a serious universal health problem associated with high morbidity and mortality despite improvements in approach to diagnosis and treatment [1]. Older adults are at particularly increased susceptibility to developing sepsis. Pneumonia accounts for 50% of all cases of sepsis [2].

Sepsis is defined as a clinical syndrome of systemic inflammation related to its response to an infection. On the other hand, bacteremia denotes the presence of bacteria in the blood [3]. Although not every patient with bacteremia has sepsis, the syndrome is under-recognized in patients with bacteremia especially among older patients who may not exhibit the common manifestations of the systemic inflammatory response syndrome. ◘ Table 8.1 shows the definition and continuum from inflammation to infection [3].

◘ Table 8.1 Definitions of sepsis, bacteremia, and related disorders[a]

Disorder	Definition
Infection	A pathologic process caused by the invasion of normally sterile tissue or fluid or body cavity by pathogenic or potentially pathogenic microorganisms
Bacteremia	Presence of bacteria in the blood
SIRS	The systemic inflammatory response to a variety of clinical insults exhibited by at least two of the following: (1) temperature >38 °C or <36 °C, (2) heart rate >90 beats/min, (3) respiratory rate >20 breaths/min with a $PaCO_2 < 32$ mm Hg, and (4) WBC > 12,000/mm^3 or <4000/mm^3 or >10% immature (band) forms
Sepsis	SIRS and documented or suspected infection
Severe sepsis	Sepsis complicated by organ dysfunction
Septic shock	Sepsis complicated by hypotension (ie, SBP < 90 mm Hg or MAP < 60 mm Hg) despite adequate fluid resuscitation

Abbreviations: MAP mean arterial pressure, *SBP* systolic blood pressure, *SIRS* systemic inflammatory response syndrome, *WBC* white blood cells

[a]American College of Chest Physicians/Society of Critical Care Medicine Consensus Conference definitions [1]

8.1.2.1 Risk Factors

There are well-known risk factors for sepsis that relate to an older adult's predisposition to infection and to the likelihood of progression to organ dysfunction. Non-modifiable risk factors include age, gender, and ethnicity. There is a higher prevalence of developing sepsis in the very young and the very old patients. It also appears that there is a male predilection and African- American propensity for its development. A study by Martin et al. in 2006 concluded that compared to younger patients, geriatric patients aged 65 years and above had 13 times more risk of developing sepsis with a twofold risk of death from sepsis. For those who survived, they were more likely to be functionally debilitated requiring skilled nursing and rehabilitation after hospitalization. Another well-known risk factor for developing sepsis is a compromised immune system that stems from immunosenescence as a function of aging. This pertains to a dysregulated immune function that is a direct result of a reduced number of T lymphocytes associated with a consequent decreased ability to mount an appropriate response to new pathogens [4]. This puts them at higher risk for more severe infections and/or relapses and recurrences. Further compounding this picture is the high likelihood that an older adult has multiple concurrent chronic conditions such as heart disease, cancer, and other progressive organ-specific diseases. The Centers for Disease Control (CDC) estimates that 80% of older adults have at least one chronic condition and 50% have two chronic conditions [5]. The consequences of having these chronic conditions include recurrent hospitalizations that may require procedural manipulation leading to an even heightened predisposition to sepsis. It is well-supported that multiple comorbidities are associated with higher severity of sepsis and subsequent organ dysfunction [6, 7]. As previously mentioned, procedural manipulation for an organic pathology may not be uncommon. The presence of invasive devices such as Foley catheters and intravenous lines are potential sources for infection. In fact, up to 25% of hospitalized patients have Foley catheters whereas over 90% of patients in the intensive care units have a Foley in place for strict monitoring of urine output [8]. Among patients older than 65 years, the genitourinary system was the most common site of sepsis.

8.1.2.2 Geriatric Considerations

Infections in the older adult may occur atypically as far as clinical manifestations are concerned [9]. The implication therefore leads to diagnostic and therapeutic delays leading to significant morbidity and mortality. Conversely, clinicians may overprescribe antimicrobial therapy in relation to a fear that any form of atypical clinical manifestation may be indicative of an infection putting people at risk for developing superimposed infection with Clostridium difficile, adverse drug reactions, and antimicrobial therapy resistance.

The 2016 Surviving Sepsis Campaign includes guidelines for pediatric patients and adult patients without clear distinction for the special population, i.e., older adults. Keeping in mind that there are age-related changes to the way patients respond to infection, there arises the challenge of ambiguity in clinical presentation. Often times, the older adults present without localized features typical of sepsis [10]. This paucity of symptomatology could lead to older adult patients progressing more rapidly to severe sepsis or septic shock with severe cardiovascular dysfunction [11]. Elderly patients typically suffer from one or more chronic conditions in addition to recurrent hospitalizations thereby depleting an already impaired physiologic response to critical illness; hence there is a call to action to identify sepsis signs and symptoms early on so that timely and appropriate interventions could be put into place [12].

Flaherty and Zwicker looked into the atypical presentation of illness in an older adult patient [13]. They further categorized atypical presentation into *vague* presentation, *altered* presentation, and *non-presentation* or under-reporting of illness. *Vague* presentation pertains to symptoms that are considered non-specific. Examples include changes in behavior, functional decline, falls, confusion, anorexia, malaise, generalized weakness, and urinary incontinence [14]. The 2013 study by Wester looked at a large sample ($n = 700$) of patients with bacteremia. They found that the older adult patients presented with atypical symptoms notably confusion, falls, malaise, incontinence, and immobility [6]. Only about 20% of patients with altered mentation are thought to be an atypical symptom of acute illness. Agitation and withdrawal behavior are sometimes the sole presentation of acute sepsis in older adults. Further complicating this scenario is the fact that older patients may present with altered mentation even in diseases that are not of infectious origin. This deters early diagnosis and management of acute illness. The *altered* presentation of atypical illness pertains to signs and symptoms that are otherwise well-known to a younger cohort of patients but not the elderly. The presence of fever and leukocytosis are oftentimes blunted. A systematic review by Lu in 2010 found that older patients aged 60 and above have body temperatures that are considered lower than normal [15]. This is possibly attributed to age-related changes in vasomotor function, skeletal muscle response, and temperature perception. Hence, with sepsis, hypothermia is a more ominous sign of sepsis rather than hyperpyrexia. This is further supported by the fact that there is evidence showing hypothermia as an independent predictor of mortality for elderly patients with sepsis. As far as leukocytosis goes, about 60% of patients will present with this diagnostic finding when serious infection is present [16]. The last form of atypical presentation is *non-presentation* of acute illness. This refers to conditions and symptomatology that are considered by older adult patients as "part of normal aging." These tend to go under-noticed and under-reported. Some examples include progressive hearing loss, stiffness of muscles, and dental problems. The presentation of sepsis is therefore challenging as older adult patients could dismiss new symptomatology that may be considered as normal and will have learned to cope with them. It is therefore necessary to have a good grasp of normal age-related changes in aging as well as the atypical forms of presentation for early diagnosis and intervention. A comprehensive evaluation with emphasis on nuances and subtleties of symptoms is mandatory.

8.1.2.3 Pathophysiology

The susceptibility to developing infections in the older adult relates to the changes in the immune system as part of the normal process of aging. Adaptive immunity is significantly impaired such that cell-mediated and humoral immunity responses are diminished [17, 18]. As cytokine and chemokine signaling are altered with advancing age, higher levels of pro-inflammatory cytokines such as tumor necrosis factor alpha and interleukin-6 are implicated in sepsis. These in turn lead to leukocytic activation, leukocyte-vascular endothelium adhesion, and endothelial dysfunction [19]. There is also a component of a prothrombotic state in sepsis possibly related to tissue factor expression from activated immune cells that subsequently leads to the clotting factor-associated microvascular thrombosis, capillary blood flow damage, and reduced blood perfusion [20].

8.1.2.4 Disease Management

The cornerstone of successful management of sepsis requires early intervention with source identification, pathogen speciation, risk factor modification, and antimicrobial therapy administration. In some cases, surgical management might be warranted such as drainage of an abscess and removal of infected surgical devices in vivo. Empiric antibiotic therapy with broad-spectrum coverage should be started as soon as sepsis is suspected (within the first hour) while continuing to pursue an investigation of the possible source(s). For the older adult patient, it is important to take note of the unique aspects of drug dosing, drug level monitoring, and adverse drug effects in relation to altered pharmacokinetics [21]. All patients with severe sepsis and septic shock should receive aggressive fluid resuscitation without delay. For the geriatric population, it is also important to monitor for the risk of fluid overload leading to respiratory symptoms though the risk of under-resuscitation is more likely than over-resuscitation due to the increase capacitance of the vasculature as a result of sepsis. In patients with septic shock and therefore unresponsive to fluids, use of vasopressive agents such as norepinephrine or dopamine may be indicated. Vasopressin may be utilized as an adjunct to catecholamines for refractory shock [22]. In very specific instances, there might be a role for hydrocortisone supplementation though may sound counter-intuitive due to the effect of steroids on an already impaired immune system [23]. Additional supportive measures that may be utilized in severely ill patients include periodic blood transfusions and low tidal volume mechanical ventilation (<6 mL/kg predicted body weight) [24].

The severity of sepsis correlates directly with higher mortality rates. This is probably the most important prognostic marker. However, there are other variables that are independent predictors of mortality such as older age, severe preexisting illnesses, and a gram positive infection. There are some studies that showed that older patients with bacteremia have a higher risk for death [25]. Octogenarians and older were 2.4 times more likely to die in the hospital compared to a much younger cohort of geriatric patients [26]. Moreover for patients who survive sepsis, there are an observed functional decline and impaired quality of life [27].

Case Conclusion

GC was subsequently transferred to the medical floor where she was continued on the previous antibiotics. Final speciation of the blood culture revealed staphylococcus epidermidis. Since this was believed to be a colonizer, vancomycin was discontinued. She had another episode of relative hypotension and required at least a liter of fluids. Her blood pressure improved. Further workup did not reveal any urinary tract infection. Subsequent days showed a decreasing trend in the white blood cell count. Her antibiotics were continued for 5 days. During her hospitalization, she started to perk up and slowly advanced her diet to a more regular one while also continuing inpatient physical therapy. She was discharged to a skilled nursing facility in stable condition and with further need for rehabilitation.

8.2 Pneumonia in the Elderly

8.2.1 Introduction

With the rising population of older adults 65 years and above, there is a corresponding higher risk for acquiring infection such as pneumonia due to altered immune system as a function of aging. Furthermore, concurrent medical conditions and functional disability are associated with increased risk for serious infection. The clinical presentation of pneumonia in the older adult is insidious, non-specific, and atypical. It is therefore important to start empiric antimicrobial therapy while awaiting results of diagnostic tests. Hospitalization is oftentimes necessary. Early targeted management will help prevent worsening of infection leading up to severe sepsis and septic shock. Unfortunately, patients with severe pneumonia have the worst prognosis overall.

Case Presentation

GC is an 88-year-old female who was recently treated in the hospital for pneumonia and with a known medical history of neurocognitive impairment, hypertension, diabetes, osteoporosis, type 2 diabetes mellitus on insulin, mild COPD, and osteoarthritis presented to the clinic with malaise and weakness. On further workup she was observed to have a high white blood cell count of 18,000 cells/microliter. Her chest radiograph was notable for an infiltrate. She was initially prescribed an oral antibiotic however before taking her first dose, she fell getting up a flight of stairs. Her husband called 911 and was subsequently brought to the ED. Her blood pressure was 90/60 mmHg. Her baseline blood pressure reading is in the 130s mmHg. She was immediately started on IVF with good response and started on broad spectrum antibiotics. There was no fracture of her lower extremities.

8.2.2 Discussion

There is an increasing number of older adults in America. By 2030, it is projected that about 20% of the population (71 million) belong to the geriatric age group. It is a noticeable trend in the patient population across care settings from hospitals to nursing homes [28]. Older adults are especially vulnerable to pneumococcal pneumonia and hence active vaccination is strongly encouraged by healthcare providers. It is important for medical providers to recognize that multiple chronic medical conditions and functional disability are associated with an increased risk for serious infection [29]. Moreover, medical management is oftentimes delayed because of atypical presentations such as weakness and confusion; paucity of classic clinical cues such as fever; and the masking of symptoms related to competing acute medical illnesses in the background of age-related changes to the immune system known as immunosenescence.

8.2.2.1 Risk Factors

A number of risk factors may be associated with the development of infection such as pneumonia to include malnutrition, alcoholism, urinary incontinence, and institutionalization. The mortality of pneumonia in older adults is approximately three to five times that of younger adults, but the rate is profoundly influenced by comorbidity which confers a relative risk of 4.1. Comorbidity is defined as cancer, collagen vascular disease, or advanced liver disease. Other independent risk factors for mortality upon hospital admission include functional disability, old-old age (>85 years old), hypotension (systolic <90 mmHg), tachycardia (>110 beats per minute), and serum creatinine level of >1.5 mg/Dl [30].

8.2.2.2 Geriatric Considerations

In this population, the presentation of pneumonia is insidious. Non-specific and atypical symptoms may herald the onset of the clinical manifestations of pneumonia. Acute confusion, malaise, and weakness may be the initial manifestations. The classic symptoms of fever, cough, chest pain, and rigors may not necessarily be present. The atypical manifestation poses a challenge in the early detection and subsequent intervention for pneumonia resulting in further complications such as severe sepsis.

8.2.2.3 Pathophysiology

Typical community-acquired bacterial pathogens include *Streptococcus pneumoniae, Haemophilus influenzae, Moraxella catarrhalis, Legionella* species, *Mycoplasma pneumoniae, Chlamydia pneumoniae*, and *Staphylococcus aureus*. Common nosocomial pathogens include *Klebsiella pneumoniae, Escherichia coli*, and *Pseudomonas* species. When patients get admitted to the ICU for other medical reasons, they are especially susceptible to developing pneumonia. An intubated patient is a classic example.

Ventilator-associated pneumonia (VAP) is a specific type of pneumonia defined as a pulmonary infection arising in greater than or equal to 48 hours after endotracheal intubation with no evidence of pneumonia at the time of intubation or the diagnosis of a new pulmonary infection if the initial admission to the ICU was for pneumonia [31]. In a prospective cohort study of 27 European ICUs by Blot et al., VAP for older patients intubated for at least 2 days did not occur more frequently among the elderly, but the associated mortality in these patients was higher. *Enterobacteriaceae, E. coli*, and *Klebsiella* species were the prevalent microorganisms associated with VAP [32].

8.2.2.4 Disease Management and Overall Impact

Antimicrobial therapy is necessary in treating pneumonia irrespective of severity. However parenteral antibiotics are required for patients with severe pneumonia. The speciation of microorganisms and antibiotic nomograms will assist in the selection of the appropriate antibiotics. Hospitalization is often necessary for older adults especially when other associated factors previously mentioned as well as potential complications exist such as empyema, sepsis, endocarditis, and meningitis among others. Prognosis in relation to disease trajectory is worse for older adult patients with severe pneumonia. Additionally, when this happens, oftentimes patients will require a higher level of monitoring such as the intensive care unit setting.

The study by Blot also confirmed that older age, diabetes mellitus, septic shock, and infection with a high-risk pathogen are important predictors for mortality in this population. These predictors are not the same for older patients residing in nursing homes and presenting with lower respiratory tract infections. A nested cohort study by Carusone et al. in 2007 identified that the severity of pneumonia and its radiographic confirmation conferred greater risk for hospitalization and mortality [33]. In two separate studies looking at outcomes implicating the role of functional status on the morbidity and mortality risk, Torres' study showed that functional status was an independent risk factor for short- and long-term mortality in hospitalized patients with community acquired pneumonia (CAP), whereas CAP severity influenced functional decline [34]. Mody's prospective cohort study on the other hand concluded that older adults who were functionally independent before admission were more likely to present with less severe pneumonia and a shorter length of stay [35]. Therefore, assessment of physical function before and during hospitalization should be an integral part of the comprehensive clinical evaluation in all older adults with pneumonia. This information is helpful in re-evaluating pneumonia severity scores which do not typically include functional status as a parameter to take into consideration.

Case Conclusion

GC was subsequently admitted to the hospital again and completed the course of antibiotics for 5 days. She started feeling better although she reported that on the third day of admission, she developed episodes of diarrhea which improved spontaneously. She is back to her usual happy self. Initial recommendation was for subacute rehabilitation. However, she herself felt well enough to continue physical therapy at home especially since she has a home health aide 12 hours a day. Her daughter agreed with this plan. She was advised close follow-up in the clinic within a week post-discharge.

8.3 Coronary Artery Disease (CAD)/ Acute Coronary Syndrome (ACS)

8.3.1 Introduction

Advanced age is a known risk factor for the development of coronary artery disease (CAD) by virtue of the cumulative effects of the normal aging process and presence of cardiovascular risk factors such as hypertension, obesity, and diabetes mellitus. It is considered an independent predictor of poor outcomes following an acute coronary syndrome. Age-associated physiological changes and the presence of chronic co-morbidities such as heart failure, diabetes mellitus (DM), renal disease, and anemia often account for variations in the clinical presentation of ACS in older adults. It is important to have a high index of suspicion for ACS along with the appreciation of its context. This is needed in assessing elders to achieve timely diagnosis and appropriate treatment.

Case Presentation

GC is an 88-year-old female residing independently in a high-rise building who was visiting her grandchildren in the northeast when she complained of fatigue, dyspnea, and nausea. She has a past medical history pertinent for neurocognitive impairment, hypertension, osteoporosis, type 2 diabetes mellitus on insulin, mild COPD, and osteoarthritis. She initially thought that this had something to do with the food that she had eaten and the numerous activities she had with her grandchildren. Her symptoms continued to persist. She was not eating or drinking as much. Her daughter who had checked in on her encouraged her mother to seek help. In the ED, she was found to have a blood pressure of 160/70 mmHg. Her normal is around 130s mmHg. She had a heart rate of 87 and respiratory rate of 20. She was not febrile. Her blood sugar was 180 mg/dL. Her last food intake was supper the night of her ED visit. Initial electrocardiogram was non-diagnostic. It showed old Q waves in the inferior leads. She had a mild heart attack in the past as per her. Her urinalysis was not indicative of any infection. Her chest radiograph did not show any infiltrate. GC is concerned that she might have yet again another bout of pneumonia. She was hospitalized twice in the last 6 months for this. Blood work was done. While awaiting her test results, she was given a dose of aspirin and nitroglycerin with some relief of her dyspnea and nausea.

Case Discussion

Advanced age is a well-known risk factor for coronary artery disease (CAD) and an independent predictor of poor outcomes following an acute coronary syndrome (ACS). Cardiovascular disease remains the leading cause of death in adults over the age of 65. The rising prevalence of cardiovascular disease with advancing age may be attributed to the cumulative effects of the normal aging process and cardiovascular risk factors, which also increase with age. It is estimated that about 60% of hospital admissions for ACS (which includes unstable angina and acute myocardial infarction) occur in this age group [36].

8.3.1.1 Risk Factors

Advanced age has been independently associated with increased mortality in both ST elevation MI (STEMI) and non-ST elevation MI (NSTEMI). Mortality is at least three-fold higher in patients over 85 years old compared to those under the age of 65. Each 10-year increase in age has been shown to be associated with a 75% increase in hospital mortality. The risk continues 30 days to 1 year after hospitalization, with mortality rates of 15% for older adults 75–85 years old and 25% for adults older than 85 years [37]. Other well-known risk factors include a history of smoking, hypertension, obesity, renal disease, and diabetes mellitus.

8.3.1.2 Geriatric Considerations

Older adults with acute coronary syndrome often have an atypical presentation of cardiac symptoms that can cause delays in care and impact patient outcomes. They are less likely to present with the typical ischemic chest pain often described as "pressure-like" quality, sub-sternal, radiating to jaw, neck or left shoulder. Chest pain is less frequent, and patients are more likely to describe dyspnea on exertion or fatigue. As a result of this atypical presentation, older patients who present to the emergency department with ACS and a chief complaint other than chest pain are often misdiagnosed and undertreated and have higher in-hospital mortality rates than adults aged younger than 65 years with chest pain [38]. Age-associated physiological changes and the presence of chronic co-morbidities such as heart failure, diabetes mellitus (DM), renal disease, and anemia often account for variations in the clinical presentation of ACS in older adults. It is important to have a high index of suspicion for ACS along with the appreciation of its context. This is needed in assessing elders to achieve timely diagnosis and appropriate treatment [39].

As previously mentioned, chest pain may be absent, and dyspnea or acute shortness of breath is often the presenting symptom of acute MI in the elderly. Other vague symptoms such as confusion, dizziness, syncope, or gastrointestinal complaints such as nausea and vomiting can be described. The symptoms may also be less likely to be induced by physical exertion. Rather, these are often precipitated by hemodynamic stressors such as an acute illness, infection or dehydration [40]. Older adults tend to have non-diagnostic electrocardiograms (ECG) due to baseline changes such as left ventricular hypertrophy (LVH), left bundle branch block (LBBB), paced rhythm, prior MI-related EKG findings, and electrolyte abnormalities. Normal cardiac changes with aging include premature ventricular contractions (PVCs) with age, first degree atrioventricular (AV) block, left atrial dilatation (LAD), and less likely to have ST segment elevation (STE) changes.

The combination of an atypical presentation, vague symptoms with physical exam findings, and non-diagnostic EKGs often leads to a delayed presentation in an acute care setting and consequently delays workup and management. It is also important to note that the differential diagnoses for acute MI in the elderly is broad and includes other cardiovascular conditions as well as a number of pulmonary, gastrointestinal, musculoskeletal, or neurological disorders. Major cardiovascular conditions include unstable angina, aortic dissection, pericarditis, and acute pulmonary edema. It is important to consider pulmonary disorders such as pneumonia, pulmonary embolism, and pleural effusion; gastrointestinal diseases such as esophagitis, reflux esophagitis, peptic ulcer disease, pancreatitis, and cholelithiasis; musculoskeletal conditions such as costochondritis and muscular strain; and psychiatric issues such as anxiety and hyperventilation syndrome [41].

8.3.1.3 Pathophysiology

The mechanism implicated in the development of atherosclerosis includes the complex interplay of numerous factors to include oxidative stress, mitochondrial function, genetics, lipid metabolism, extracellular matrix, coagulation and hemostasis, inflammation, and endothelial homeostasis. All of these play important roles in vascular aging per se. The signaling factors can contribute to both age-related macrovascular and microvascular remodeling leading to myocardial dysfunction and ischemia.

8.3.1.4 Disease Management and Overall Impact

While age is an important and well-known determinant of outcomes for patients with acute coronary syndromes (ACS), there still tends to be a disproportionately lower use of cardiovascular medications and invasive treatment even among elderly patients with ACS who would potentially stand to benefit [42]. Many clinical trials continue to exclude patients on the basis of age, which often leads to limited data to guide the care of older adults. As a result, there is uncertainty about benefits and risks particularly with newer medications or invasive treatments and in the setting of advanced age or complex health status. The clinical decision making for older patients can be challenging in this heterogeneous population. It is imperative to take into consideration not only the relative risk and benefit of treatments or interventions, but also conditions unique to older patients such as geriatric syndromes of polypharmacy and frailty, cognitive impairment, physical function, independence, support system, and quality of life that influence treatment goals and outcomes. Treatment decisions in both the inpatient and outpatient setting should be individualized and informed by patient's preference and health status [43].

It is critical that all medical providers involved in the care of older adults in a clinical setting appreciate the fact that the older the patient, the more likely he or she will have an atypical presentation of ACS, including NSTEMI or STEMI [44]. Myocardial infarctions often occur without chest pain in patients with advanced age. As previously mentioned, history and physical exam findings may be unrevealing, and EKG interpretation may differ. It is important to consider other possible angina equivalent in order to prevent delays in care and workup as these may impact management decisions and clinical outcomes. Frontline providers such as emergency nurses are often the first healthcare providers to assess and triage older adults for ACS and initiate life-saving evidence-based protocols such as aspirin or oxygen. Emergency providers including physicians, nurses, physician assistants, and nurse practitioners must be knowledgeable and vigilant in their assessment of ACS and identifying red flags in this high-risk population. Patients presenting with atypical symptoms are less likely to receive an aspirin, thrombolytic therapy, or percutaneous coronary intervention (PCI). These delays in time to treatment modalities place older adults with ACS at risk for higher mortality. Early recognition of symptoms suggestive of ACS by the emergency care team can improve patient outcomes. Nurses and physician extenders need to have a good understanding of the different symptoms in older adults and incorporate questions about how they normally function to include the subtleties in changes and atypical presentations. Using these strategies, the inter-professional care team of emergency nurses, physicians, physician assistants, and social workers can increase the likelihood of early recognition of ACS, reducing treatment delays and improving hospital mortality rates [37].

Family and Caregiver Role and Educational Resources

All patients and/or their families and caregivers should have an understanding of their disease process especially those at high risk for cardiovascular disease. In this heterogeneous population of older adults, the role of family and caregivers can vary based on the patient's acute presentation, diagnosis, management, and baseline cognitive and functional status. Therefore, it is important to have an individualized approach when it comes to post-acute management, care transitions, and follow-up plans.

Clear information about the patient's diet, changes in medications, post-procedural care, and follow-up appointments should be reviewed and documented in the discharge instructions. All the patient's medications should be reconciled at the time of discharge with the medication list from admission. It is important to educate both patient and caregiver about the symptoms of coronary artery disease to include recurrent ischemia, complications from the disease and current treatments, and the urgency to report such symptoms to avert further ischemic damage [45, 46].

Community Resources

It is extremely important that a careful and comprehensive transition plan is provided at the time of hospital discharge for older adults admitted with ACS. The patients' risk-stratification, medications, and interventions initiated in the acute hospital setting may impact important medical decisions in other areas [47].

Outpatient follow-up arrangements should be made prior to discharge with the primary care physician and a cardiologist. It is important to gather resources with the help of discharge planners, social workers, pharmacists, consultants if needed to manage co-morbidities, nutritionists, cardiac rehabilitation personnel, and nursing personnel in every care setting. Safe transitions of care among the different settings of the ACS patient are a vital component of optimizing treatment in both inpatient and outpatient settings.

Case Conclusion

GC underwent further workup in the emergency department. She presented with high troponin levels. Her serial electrocardiographic readings did not show any ST segment elevation. By this time, she was already started on aspirin and as needed morphine and nitroglycerin. She was given atorvastatin in addition to the above medications. At home she was on maintenance losartan and metoprolol. Both were continued for as long as her blood pressure readings could tolerate. She was managed medically with close monitoring by the cardiology team. While in the hospital, she was seen by a nutritionist regarding her diabetic diet and by the physical therapist who worked with the cardiologist regarding the most appropriate bedside cardiac rehabilitation exercises. After a few days in the hospital, a decision was made to continue her rehabilitation in a subacute facility.

8.4 COPD in the Elderly

8.4.1 Introduction

Chronic obstructive pulmonary disease (COPD) is a prevalent disease in the elderly that is associated with high morbidity and mortality. It is a major public health challenge. Older adults are at high risk for developing COPD given age-related pulmonary changes in function and cumulative effects of exposure to risk factors over time. The systemic manifestations along with the presence of common medical problems cause significant symptom burden that affects overall quality of life. The main goals of COPD management include reduction of symptoms, frequency, and severity of exacerbations and a decreased risk of hospitalizations. Smoking cessation should be encouraged and supported at every encounter. COPD treatment in the elderly requires a comprehensive inter-professional approach to the optimal prevention and management of exacerbations and progression.

Case Presentation

GC is an 88 year-old female with a past medical history of hypertension, CAD, type 2 diabetes on insulin, osteoporosis, COPD, and osteoarthritis who started to develop progressive shortness of breath and intermittent cough while recuperating in a subacute rehabilitation facility. Her cough is productive with whitish sputum that is worse in the morning. She has a long-standing history of smoking one pack per day since age 40. She did not report of any fever, chills, chest pain, nausea, vomiting, abdominal pain, constipation, and diarrhea. Vital signs included normal temperature 97.9 °C, normotensive at 135/85 mmHg, respirations 18 per minute, and heart rate of 85 beats per minute. Focused physical exam findings revealed non-labored breathing, clear lung fields with prolonged expiratory phase, decreased breath sounds at the bases, and faint wheezing on expiration bilaterally. Her heart sounds showed regular rate and rhythm and normal S1 and S2 with strong peripheral pulses. There were no JVD and peripheral edema. Chest radiograph demonstrated hyper-inflated lungs and normal heart and mediastinum without any evidence of pleural effusion, consolidation, or pneumothorax.

Laboratory markers were notable for WBC 5000 per microliter, hemoglobin of 14 grams per deciliter, and platelets of 400,000 cells per microliter. The basic metabolic panel and renal function tests were within normal range. Previous spirometry testing a few days ago showed forced vital capacity (FVC) 75%, forced expiratory volume in 1 second (FEV1) 60% and post-bronchodilator FVC 85%-FEV1 65%. The primary team, patient, and the daughter have all been in communication with each other regarding the plan to either manage her in the skilled facility or transfer her to the emergency department. GC verbalized that she has been in and out of the hospital over the last 6 months and would prefer to remain in the current setting.

8.4.2 Discussion

Chronic obstructive pulmonary disease (COPD) is a debilitating chronic condition that is associated with high morbidity and mortality globally [48]. It is estimated that 3.2 million people died of COPD in 2015. This is an 11.6% increase compared to the 1990s. In the United States, COPD is prevalent in more than 14% of adult population older than 65 years old [49]. It is the third leading cause of death in over 150,000 older Americans. Both the death rate and prevalence of COPD increase with age[l]. COPD is half as prevalent as asthma but has eight times more common deaths than asthma. Its high prevalence and chronicity is associated with substantial economic and social burden with a direct relationship between the severity of the disease and cost of care including workplace and home productivity [50]. Burden of obstructive disease impacts an elderly person's physical, psychological, and social function thereby decreasing overall quality of life [51].

8.4.2.1 Risk Factors

An aging lung is vulnerable to respiratory infections, e.g., pneumonia, which contribute greatly to the onset and progression of COPD. Smoking, whether active or second-hand exposure, is the single biggest risk factor leading to chronic lung inflammation. Exposure to noxious particles from outdoor pollution, occupational exposure (e.g., organic and inorganic dusts and chemicals and fumes), and biomass fuels (smoke from cooking and heating homes with open fires) in poorly ventilated dwellings are important risk factors for developing chronic airflow limitation [52]. Other risk factors that may contribute to developing COPD are genetics (alpha-1-antitrypsin deficiency), congenital lung abnormalities, bronchial hyper-reactivity, and low socioeconomic status [51, 53].

8.4.2.2 Geriatric Considerations

Chronic obstructive pulmonary disease (COPD) is a complex disease that puts older persons at high risk due to age-related pulmonary changes and cumulative effect of exposure to noxious stimuli over the years.[liv] Structural changes that occur are chest wall rigidity and poor compliance due to kyphoscoliosis, calcification of intercostal cartilage, or arthritis of the costovertebral joints. There are loss of elastic recoil and a decrease in respiratory muscle (diaphragm and intercostal muscles) strength due to sarcopenia and muscle atrophy [53]. Changes at the level of the connective tissue lead to parenchymal change and destruction. The tracheobronchial tree diameter narrows and alveolar ducts enlarge leading to homogenous airspace enlargement but decreased alveolar surface area for gaseous exchange. This is commonly described as *senile emphysema* as it can be found in non-smokers and mimics smoking-induced COPD.[li] Age-related lung changes cause airflow limitation, air trapping, hyperinflation, decline in minute ventilation, and increased ventilation-perfusion mismatch. On spirometry, these changes are reflected as decreased forced vital capacity (FVC) and forced expiratory volume in 1 second (FEV_1) of 25–30 mL/year in non-smokers and approximately 60–70 mL/year in smokers ≥65 years old, increase in residual volume (RV), and functional residual capacity (FRC) [50, 54]. Further PaO_2 decreases will cause more hypoxia that in turn increases the normal Alveolar-arterial (A-a) gradient. They are at risk for aspiration-related infections due to loss of airway protection or swallowing abnormalities, decreased pulmonary capillary density, and increased mucous plugging. In addition, reduced peripheral chemosensitivity to carbon dioxide (CO2) can lead to altered ventilatory response to hypercapnia and a decline in innate and adaptive cell and humoral-mediated immunity. Collectively, complex changes of an aging lung predispose them to respiratory infections increasing morbidity and mortality in older adults [53]. Patients typically present with a combination of signs and symptoms of chronic bronchitis, emphysema, and reactive airway disease. Symptoms include chronic progressive cough and shortness of breath with colorless sputum that vary day to day and often present earlier than airflow limitation. Intermittent wheezing and chest tightness can also be present. Dyspnea, occurring late in life, is a cardinal symptom of COPD and can cause significant disability and anxiety due to air hunger. COPD diagnosis should be suspected in a patient with chronic and progressive symptoms of shortness of breath, cough, and/or sputum production with a history of exposure to risk factors, e.g., smoking. COPD is under-diagnosed in the elderly. Older adults are less likely to seek attention as they consider dyspnea a normal part of the aging process. Physicians underestimate symptom severity due to less prominent tachycardia or pulsus paradoxus during COPD exacerbations [54].

8.4.2.3 Pathophysiology

Global Initiative for Chronic Obstructive Lung Disease (GOLD) defines COPD as a common preventable and treatable disease. It is characterized by persistent airflow limitation that is usually progressive and associated with an enhanced chronic inflammatory response in the airways and the lungs to noxious particles or gases. COPD is a syndrome that is comprised of inflammatory chronic bronchitis (CB), bronchiectasis, emphysema, and reversible airways disease [53, 54].

To diagnose COPD, obtain a thorough medical history including exposure to risk factors, pattern of symptom development, past medical history (including any lung abnormalities, hospitalizations for respiratory disorders, other co-morbidities), family history for chronic respiratory diseases, impact of disease on the patient's life, and social and family support available to the patient [55].

COPD symptoms like cough, sputum production, and/or shortness of breath are not specific and can occur in other chronic illnesses. Objective testing with spirometry helps establish diagnosis and severity of airway limitation using the GOLD criteria. Spirometry is reproducible and easily performed in an office setting. A ratio of FEV1/FVC < 0.70 post-bronchodilator therapy is diagnostic for persistent airflow limitation and thus of COPD. Repeated measures on two separate occasions can be used to confirm obstruction defect. The reduced ratio of FEV1/FVC fails to distinguish between age-related airflow limitation and COPD-related airflow obstruction thus over-diagnosing and mistreating COPD in older adults. Hence, it is recommended to consider using FEV1/FVC score z score < −1.64 (defining the lower limit of normal at the fifth percentile of the normal distribution). This is associated with respiratory symptoms, impaired mobility, frailty status, COPD hospitalizations, and mortality [56]. It is important to correlate spirometric measurements with symptoms and risk factors. Additional pulmonary testing can include measuring lung volumes, performing a 6-minute walk test, and diffusion lung capacity of carbon monoxide (DLCO). Patients with an FEV1 < 50% should get evaluated with arterial blood gas (ABG) testing to screen for hypoxia and hypercapnia. Although the physical exam is part of the assessment, it is rarely diagnostic and lacks sensitivity. Elderly patients are limited in performing spirometry due to lack of coordination and cognitive impairment. Only

70% of community-dwelling adults can perform spirometry assessments [51]. The Mini Mental State Exam (MMSE) can be used quickly to exclude adults with cognitive dysfunction. The differential diagnosis to be considered in COPD management includes congestive heart failure (CHF), asthma, bronchiectasis, vocal cord dysfunction, respiratory tract tumors, and other chronic pulmonary disorders. Elderly patients with COPD should be assessed for concomitant chronic diseases. Age-related pulmonary function changes coupled with COPD burden has a multi-factorial impact on the older adult in the areas of nutrition, cognition, and physical function. Having COPD increases the risk of other diseases, e.g., cardiovascular disease, osteoporosis, anxiety, depression, diabetes mellitus, and lung cancer. Comorbidities have an independent influence on mortality and hospitalization. Patients with COPD requiring long-term oxygen therapy are more likely to die of acute on chronic respiratory failure. Once COPD diagnosis is established, the next step in management would be to perform an evaluation of the level of airflow obstruction, its impact on patients' health status, and risk of future exacerbations. These assessments will allow physicians to individualize treatment plans. Spirometry will assess airflow limitation and categorize severity into GOLD 1 through 4. Refer to ◘ Table 8.2 for GOLD classification of severity. Patients' symptoms should be objectively measured with tools such as the COPD Assessment Test (CAT) (8 domain scale ranked 0 through 5 in each domain that goes from 0 through 40 in which a score of more than 10 represents significant symptoms), Modified British Medical Research Council (mMRC) Questionnaire (scale where patients self-report breathlessness from 0 through 4), and the COPD Control Questionnaire (CCQ). COPD exacerbations refer to acute worsening of respiratory symptoms requiring additional therapies. It is important to know how often a patient is treated for flare-ups with antibiotics and/or corticosteroids. Exacerbations are classified as mild, moderate, and severe. *Mild* exacerbations are treated with short-acting bronchodilators (SABDs) only. *Moderate* exacerbations are treated with SABDs plus antibiotics and/or oral corticosteroids. *Severe* exacerbations require hospitalizations. The latter can be associated with acute respiratory failure and poor prognosis with a high likelihood of mortality. A history of more than two exacerbations per year is a good predictor of the risk for future exacerbations.[li]

◘ Table 8.2 Grading of Severity of airflow limitation in COPD (Based on post-bronchodilator FEV1) Based on GOLD guidelines 2018

In patients with $FEV_1/FVC < 0.70$:		
GOLD 1:	Mild	$FEV_1 \geq 80\%$ predicted
GOLD 2:	Moderate	$50\% \leq FEV_1 < 80\%$ predicted
GOLD 3:	Severe	$30\% \leq FEV_1 < 50\%$ predicted
GOLD 4:	Very severe	$FEV_1 < 30\%$ predicted

Definition of abbreviation: COPD chronic obstructive pulmonary disease, *GOLD* Global Initiative for Chronic Obstructive Lung Disease

8.4.2.4 Disease Management and Overall Impact

COPD management should be focused on reducing symptoms, risk of future exacerbations, and further lung injury. GOLD recommends categorizing patients using the ABCD tool when assessing symptom burden, risk of future exacerbations, and GOLD severity on an ongoing basis. Refer to ◘ Fig. 8.1 for the refined ABCD assessment tool. The first domain is to determine how breathless a patient is using either the COPD Assessment Test (CAT) or mMRC test. If the mMRC is 0 to 1 or the CAT < 10, the patient falls in category A or C. If the mMRC ≥2 or the CAT ≥ 10, then the patient falls into category B or D. Next, assess the COPD risk in two domains using the GOLD classification and history of exacerbations. GOLD severity 1 or 2 and 0 to 1 exacerbations fall under category A and B. Likewise GOLD severity 3 or 4 with ≥2 exacerbations falls under category C and D. When assessing the risk, choose the highest risk according to GOLD grade or exacerbation history.

Pharmacotherapy in COPD management is similar to that of a younger patient. Older patients are often excluded from clinical trials due to advanced age and the presence of multiple co-morbidities. The goal of COPD management is to reduce symptoms, reduce frequency and severity of exacerbations, and improve exercise tolerance in patients. COPD treatments should be based according to individual assessment of symptoms, severity and exacerbation risks then categorized into categories A through D. Refer to ◘ Table 8.3 for pharmacologic treatment approach for COPD. Most common classes of medications used to treat include bronchodilators (beta-2-agonists and anti-muscarinics), combination bronchodilator therapy, corticosteroids (inhaled and oral), methylxanthines (e.g., theophylline), phosphodiesterase-4 inhibitors (roflumilast), and antibiotics (macrolides). Most common short-acting beta-2-agonist (SABA) used is albuterol; long-acting beta-2-agonist (LABA) is formoterol; short-acting anti-muscarinic (SAMA) is ipratropium; and long-acting anti-muscarinic (LAMA) agent is tiotropium. Other pharmacologic treatments used for COPD include alpha-1-antitrypsin augmentation therapy, antitussives, and vasodilators [52].

Inhaler drugs should be individualized based on patient access, cost, and most importantly patient's ability to use the inhaler. Proper inhaler technique is of high relevance and cannot be over-emphasized. Techniques should be demonstrated and confirmed using the *teach-back* approach at every visit to ensure adherence and correct use of the inhaler. Although COPD is not a curable disease, clinical trials have demonstrated mortality benefits with non-pharmacologic therapies such as smoking cessation. Efforts should be made to identify and reduce exposure to risk factors. Cigarette smoking is common and easily identifiable. Smoking cessation is the most important therapeutic intervention to

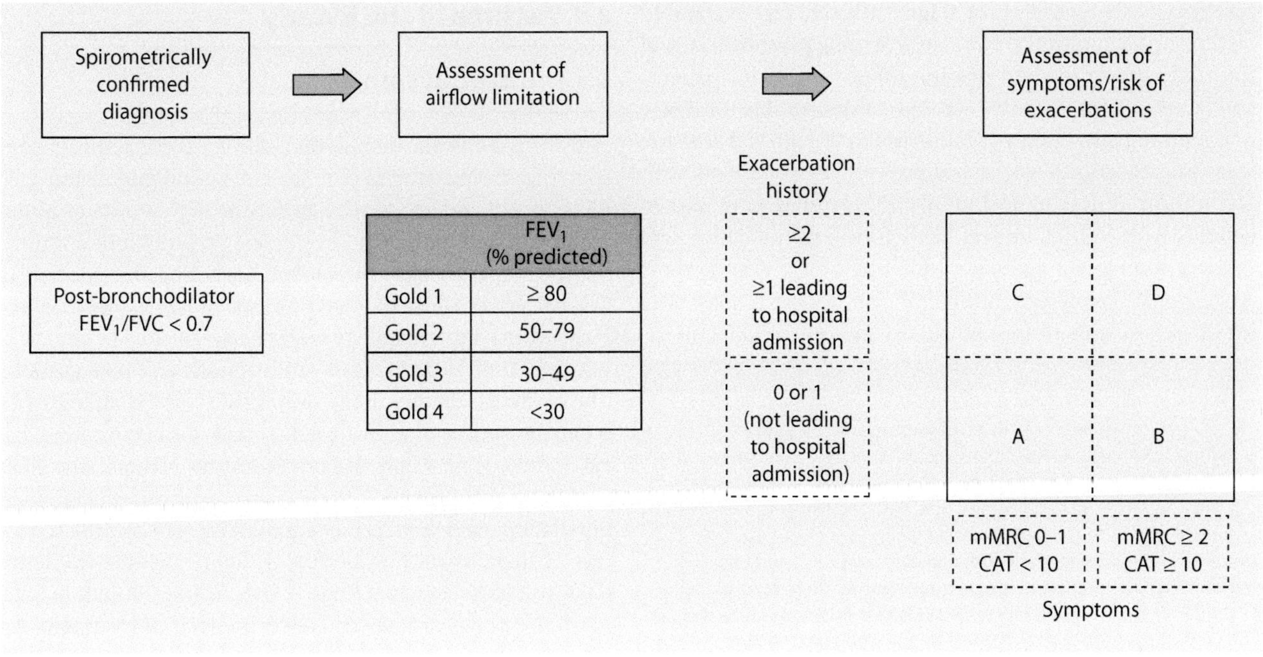

Fig. 8.1 The refined ABCD assessment tool

Table 8.3 Pharmacologic treatment for COPD (table recreated based on GOLD 2018 guidelines). LABA = long-acting beta-2-agonist. LAMA = long-acting antimuscarinic agent. ICS = inhaled corticosteroid [51, 56]

Patient category	FEV 1 predicted	Exacerbation history	Symptoms	Suggested therapy
A	GOLD 1 mild FEV1 ≥ 80%	0–1 per year	Few: mMRC 0–1 CAT < 10	Bronchodilators prn (short- or long-acting)
B	GOLD 2 moderate FEV1 50–79%		Significant: mMRC ≥ 2 CAT > 10	LABA *or* LAMA *or* LABA + LAMA
C	GOLD 3 severe FEV1 30–49%	≥2 per year or ≥1 leading to hospitalization	Few: mMRC 0–1 CAT < 10	LAMA *or* LABA + LAMA or *or* LABA + ICS
D	GOLD 4 very severe FEV1 < 30%		Significant: mMRC ≥ 2 CAT > 10	LAMA + LABA or LABA + ICS or LABA + LAMA + ICS Consider: Roflumilast (if FEV1 < 50% and chronic bronchitis) or macrolide (in former smokers)

improve healthcare and reduce mortality. Therefore, individuals who smoke should be encouraged and supported in quitting efforts. Mortality benefit is also seen with long-term oxygen therapy in hypoxic patients, non-invasive ventilation, and lung volume reduction surgery (LVRS) in certain populations. In addition, patients should regularly participate in physical activity to avoid physical deconditioning which can worsen chronic dyspnea. Patients with high symptom burden (belonging to Groups B, C, D) should partake in pulmonary rehabilitation for improvement in symptoms and quality of life. Annual influenza [57] and pneumococcal polysaccharide vaccines (PCV 13 and PPSV 23) should be given to all patients with COPD especially those with severe COPD and cardiac disease as they decrease incidence of lower respiratory tract infections. Overall, healthcare professionals should offer education and coach patients to adapt behaviors that will help manage the disease.

COPD is a highly symptomatic disease that can significantly worsen physical, social, and emotional function. Symptoms of the disease include dyspnea, fatigue, cough, weight loss, lung infections, and concurrent mental health considerations such as anxiety, insomnia, depression, and social isolation. With ongoing COPD management, providers should either incorporate or refer patients to palliative care specialists regardless of stage. Palliative care is focused on reducing symptoms while also providing psychosocial and spiritual support for best possible quality of life for patients and families [58]. Palliative care specialists are able to engage in communication and education with patients and families regarding prognosis, goals, and preferences in patients with life-limiting illness to include COPD. Studies have shown patients with COPD are less likely to receive palliative care services compared to patients with lung cancer despite similar end-of-life symptom burden [59, 60].

Case Conclusion

GC was immediately given nebulizations with albuterol and ipratropium with a maintenance plan of every 6 hours of treatment. She was placed on oxygen via nasal cannula which provided relief to her dyspnea. She was empirically started on azithromycin to reduce severity of illness and hospitalization. She was continued on her inhaled corticosteroids and had received a prior dose of intravenous solumedrol to control the inflammation. She stayed in the skilled facility. Hospitalization was averted. She was extremely happy with this decision although she also knew that if her condition changed, she would have to be transferred to the hospital.

8

8.5 Asthma in the Elderly

8.5.1 Introduction

Asthma is a chronic disease that affects people across the age spectrum from young to old. The older adult population aged 65 years old and above account for the highest rate of hospitalizations and mortality. The clinical presentation of asthma varies in the geriatric population including the concept of normal aging when the symptom of breathlessness occurs. Hence, the symptomatology might be overlooked by clinicians which in turn leads to a delay in diagnosis and management. The challenge also lies in the overlap of symptomatology with other diseases such as heart failure and obstructive lung disease. There is no single diagnostic test for asthma. The goals of asthma management are the same as in the general adult population, namely, to achieve good symptom control; reduce risk of impairment and decline in lung function; minimize risks of future exacerbations, fixed airflow limitation; and minimize polypharmacy and adverse effects of treatment. An interdisciplinary approach and education of caregivers on how to administer medications are critical to a successful adherence to the care plan for optimal control of asthma symptoms.

Case Presentation

GC is an 88-year-old female with a past medical history of mild cognitive impairment, hypertension, coronary artery disease, GERD, type 2 diabetes, osteoarthritis, osteoporosis, and mild COPD who presented to her primary care provider with 8 weeks of cough and shortness of breath. These symptoms were preceded by an upper respiratory tract infection (cough, sore throat, nasal congestion, malaise, and subjective fevers). After the resolution of her URI, she then developed a non-productive cough with periods of shortness of breath both at rest and with activity. Her shortness of breath and cough have also awakened her from sleep numerous times in the past month. Though she lives alone and is quite independent, she has a home health aide for about 12 hours four times per week. She had a 5–10 pack-year smoking history in her 20s. On her lung exam she was found to have non-labored breathing with a prolonged expiratory phase and faint wheezing bilaterally. Chest x-ray was unremarkable for any acute pulmonic process. The patient recounted that when she was in her 20s, she had recurrent hospitalizations for wheezing requiring steroids and inhalers. There were no prior episodes of intubation. In the clinic, she was given a nebulization treatment with albuterol and ipratropium. She insisted to finish the treatment so she can avoid going into the hospital again.

8.5.2 Discussion

Asthma is one of the most common chronic diseases worldwide. Traditionally, it is considered a disease of childhood and adolescents. However, its prevalence among US adults age 65 years and older is 6.6% as compared to 6–8% in younger adults [61]. The older adult population account for the highest rate of asthma hospitalizations [62] with more than 50% of fatalities annually in this age group resulting in high hospital and medication costs [63]. As the aging population is expected to rapidly increase up to 86 million by year 2050, the number of older adults with asthma will continue to rise thus having a great impact from a global healthcare perspective [64].

8.5.2.1 Risk Factors

Age and genetics are the two biggest risk factors for the development of asthma. In addition to classic asthma triggers, cold temperatures, environmental allergens, or irritants, asthma in the elderly (AIE) can also be triggered by medications (aspirin, non-steroidal anti-inflammatory, ACE inhibitors, or beta-blockers) which are commonly used in this population. AIE can be divided in two categories. The first category, *early-onset asthma*, includes adults who develop classic asthma symptoms in childhood or early adulthood with persistence later in life. The second category, *late-onset asthma*, includes adults who develop asthma at an advanced age [54, 65]. Diagnosing the latter is challenging as it is less common with marked heterogeneity in presentation as compared to classic early-onset asthma and the presence of other chronic conditions such as COPD that can mimic asthma. This makes the differential diagnosis of asthma in the elderly patients longer as compared to younger asthmatics.

8.5.2.2 Geriatric Considerations

As with any chronic illness, there are challenges to diagnosis and management of asthma in the elderly. Symptoms are often overlooked by physicians and patients as patients perceive breathlessness as normal part of aging, physical deconditioning, age-related lung function decline, and chronic airway remodeling (increase chest wall stiffness, decreased respiratory muscle, and elastic recoil), low reversibility potentially leading to fixed airflow obstruction, absence of atopy/allergy symptoms, and less reporting of nocturnal symptoms [54]. A spectrum of phenotypic expressions, age-related lung changes, lifetime accumulation of insults by environmental factors, and co-existence of other co-morbidities in the older population makes asthma an under-reported, overlooked, under-diagnosed, misdiagnosed, and thus undertreated medical condition. Failure to appropriately diagnose, treat, and manage asthma leads to increased symptom burden and poor psychological and physical quality of life [64]. Thus, special consideration and additional strategies need to be incorporated when managing asthma in older adults. Despite the difference in presentation, asthma is treated with the same principles as in all ages.

8.5.2.3 Pathophysiology

Asthma is a heterogeneous disease characterized by chronic airway inflammation and episodic symptoms varying in intensity such as wheezing, shortness of breath, and chest tightness along with airflow obstruction and bronchial hyper-responsiveness [54].

8.5.2.4 Disease Management and Overall Impact

There is no single diagnostic test for asthma. To establish diagnosis of asthma, a clinician should determine that symptoms of airflow obstruction or airway hyper-responsiveness are present and that airway obstruction is at least partially reversible. A clinician must get a detailed history, perform a physical exam, and test to confirm expiratory flow limitation. History of variable respiratory symptoms includes wheezing, shortness of breath, cough, and chest tightness varying in time and intensity. These symptoms tend to worsen at night or early morning upon waking up. They are triggered by exercise, cold air, laughter, and exposure to allergens. They are often preceded by or worsen with upper respiratory infections. As asthma symptoms are very non-specific and can overlap with other chronic conditions, alternative diagnoses must be excluded. Asthma can have symptoms that can mimic other respiratory conditions such as recurrent respiratory infections, COPD, post-infectious tussive syndrome, rhinosinusitis cardiovascular causes, GERD, vocal cord dysfunction, medication-related cough, post-nasal drip, or airway obstruction by malignancy. Among patients with longstanding smoking history of greater than 20 pack-years, one may need to consider asthma-COPD overlap as a diagnosis. Alternative diagnoses must be ruled out before confirming asthma. The symptomatology of asthma determines the category of asthma, i.e., intermittent versus persistent. Mild intermittent asthma presents with occasional symptoms of cough, wheezing, or shortness of breath during the week and nocturnal symptoms during the month. Persistent asthma is further stratified into mild, moderate, or severe. This requires more frequent symptoms during the week, nights, and need for bronchodilator therapies. Spirometry, peak expiratory flow, or response to short-acting bronchodilators will help isolate symptoms with respiratory etiology. Initial spirometry testing must be performed to obtain baseline readings and to confirm that the forced expiratory volume in 1 second (FEV_1) and FEV_1/FVC are low. FEV_1/FVC is normally >0.75–0.80 in adults. A positive bronchodilator test (BD) needs to be performed to detect if airflow obstruction is partially reversible. An increase in FEV_1 of more than 12% and >200 ml from baseline 10–15 minutes after 200–400 mcg albuterol or equivalent administered signifies a positive response. To obtain better test results, hold patients BD medication short-acting beta-blocker (SABA) ≥4 hours and long-acting beta-blocker (LABA) ≥15 hours. There are barriers to the elderly performing effective pulmonary function testing (PFT). Clinicians have difficulty interpreting these results due to age-related pulmonary changes. Kyphoscoliosis, decreasing chest wall compliance, degenerative arthritic changes seen along the costovertebral joints, calcification of the costal cartilages, sarcopenia causing intercostal muscle atrophy, a 25% reduction in diaphragmatic strength, sensory deficits, and impaired coordination make it challenging to perform forced expiratory maneuvers efficiently with a decrease in FEV1. Connective tissue changes of the alveolar sacs and airway remodeling contribute to fixed obstruction. Pulmonary function tests (PFTs) may easily be mistaken for COPD, age-related physiological changes with decreases in FVC and PaO_2, increased residual volume (RV), increased functional residual capacity (FRC), and coexistence of asthma-COPD overlap (ACO) are some of the reasons why it is challenging for clinicians to interpret PFT's [66]. There are a 25–30 mL/year decline in FVC and FEV_1 among non-smokers and a 60–70 mL/year among smokers with an overall decrease in the FEV_1/FVC ratio in adults ≥65 years old. As such PFTs' role in diagnosing asthma in elderly patients is limited. The reversibility of BD response is less pronounced in the elderly patients. The methacholine challenge test is used less often because of more frequent contraindications especially in patients with cardiovascular disease.

There is lack of evidence-based guidelines for the treatment of asthma in the elderly population as older patients are often excluded from clinical trials. The treatment guidelines are adopted from studies conducted on a much younger cohort [63]. The first step before initiating therapy includes a preliminary assessment asthma severity (see ◘ Fig. 8.2). Based on this, one is then able to follow the stepwise approach to achieve asthma control (refer to ◘ Fig. 8.3) [54].

Long-term use of inhaled corticosteroids (ICS) is the cornerstone of asthma management in the elderly population. Long-acting B-blockers (LABA) can be added as adjunctive therapy when low-to-moderate dose ICS is not helpful. The goals of asthma management are the same as the younger adults, i.e., to achieve good symptom control; reduce risk of impairment and decline in lung function; minimize risks of future exacerbations, fixed airflow limitation; and minimize polypharmacy and adverse effects of treatment. It is essential to periodically monitor treatment progression and

Classifying asthma severity youths ≥ 12 years of age and adults

- Classifying severity for patients who are not currently taking long-term control medications.

Components of severity		Classification of asthma severity (Youths ≥12 years of age and adults)			
		Impairment	Persistent		
			Mild	Moderate	Severe
Impairment Normal FEV_1/FVC: 8–19 yr 85% 20–39 yr 80% 40–59 yr 75% 60–80 yr 70%	Symptoms	≤2 days/week	>2 days/week but not daily	Daily	Throughout the day
	Nighttime awakenings	≤2x/month	3–4x/month	**>1x/week but** not nightly	Often 7x/week
	Short-acting $beta_2$-agonist use for symptom control (not prevention of EIB)	≤2 days/week	**>2 days/week** but not **>lx/day**	Daily	Several times per day
	Interference with normal activity	None	Minor limitation	Some limitation	Extremely limited
	Lung function	• Normal FEV_1 between exacerbations • FEV_1 **>80%** predicted • FEV_1 /FVC normal	• FEV_1 ≥80% predicted • FEV_1/FVC normal	• FEV_1 **<60%** but <80% predicted • FEV_1 /FVC reduced 5%	• FEV_1 **<60%** predicted • FEV_1 /FVC reduced **>5%**
Risk	Exacerbations requiring oral systemic corticosteroids	0–1/year (see note)	≥2/year (see note) →		
		← Consider severity and interval since last exacerbation. Frequency and severity may fluctuate over time for patients in any severity category. →			
		Relative annual risk of exacerbations may be related to FEV			

- Level of severity is determined by assessment of both impairment and risk. Assess impairment domain by patient's/caregiver's recall of previous 2–4 weeks and spirometry. Assign severity to the most severe category in which any feature occurs.

- At present, there are inadequate data to correspond frequencies of exacerbations with different levels of asthma severity. In general, more frequent and intense exacerbations (e.g., requiring urgent, unscheduled care, hospitalization, or ICU admission) indicate greater underlying disease severity. For treatment purposes, patients who had ≥2 exacerbations requiring oral systemic corticosteroids in the past year may be considered the same as patients who have persistent asthma, even in the absence of impairment levels consistent with persistent asthma.

Fig. 8.2 Assessing asthma severity. (Modified from US Department of Health and Human Services. National Heart, Lung, and Blood Institute. National Asthma Education and Prevention Program. Expert Panel Report 3: Guidelines for the Diagnosis and Management of Asthma. August 28, 2007)

adjust therapy accordingly. This can be done either through symptom-based monitoring or using a peak flow meter. The Asthma Control Test or Asthma Control Questionnaires are useful tools to monitor adults. However, its use can be limited to elderly patients with visual and cognitive impairment [65]. In the elderly, the management of chronic symptoms (e.g., coughing, breathlessness during day or night, or after exertion) should be used to guide a treatment regimen

Stepwise approach for managing asthma in youths ≥ 12 years of age and adults

Intermittent asthma	**Persistent asthma: daily medication** Consult with asthma specialist if step 4 care or higher is required. Consider consultation at step 3.				
Step 1	**Step 2**	**Step 3**	**Step 4**	**Step 5**	**Step 6**
Preferred:	***Preferred:***	***Preferred:***	***Preferred:***	***Preferred:***	***Preferred:***
SABA PRN	Low-dose ICS	Low-dose ICS + LABA OR Medium-dose ICS	Medium-dose ICS + LABA	High-dose ICS + LABA	High-dose ICS + LABA + oral corticosteroid
	Alternative: Cromolyn, LTRA, Nedocromil, or Theophylline	***Alternative:*** Low-dose ICS + either LTRA, Theophylline, or Zileuton	***Alternative:*** Medium-dose ICS + either LTRA, Theophylline, or Zileuton	AND Consider Omalizumab for patients who have allergies	AND Consider Omalizumab for patients who have allergies

Step up if needed (first, check adherence, environmental control, and comorbid conditions)

Assess control

Step down if possible (and asthma is well controlled at least 3 months)

Each step: Patient education, environmental control, and management of comorbidities.

Steps 2–4: Consider subcutaneous allergen immunotherapy for patients who have allergic asthma (see notes).

Quick-Relief Medication for All Patients

- SABA as needed for symptoms. Intensity of treatment depends on severity of symptoms: up to 3 treatments at 20-minute intervals as needed. Short course of oral systemic corticosteroids may be needed.
- Use of SABA >2days a week for symptom relief (not prevention of EIB) generally indicates inadequate control and the need to step up treatment.

Key: **Alphabetical order is used when more than one treatment option is listed within either preferred or alternative therapy.** EIB, exercise-induced bronchospasm; ICS, inhaled corticosteroid; LABA, long-acting inhaled beta$_2$-agonist; LTRA, leukotriene receptor antagonist; SABA, inhaled short-acting beta$_2$-agonist

Fig. 8.3 Stepwise approach to achieving asthma control. (Modified from US Department of Health and Human Services. National Heart, Lung, and Blood Institute. National Asthma Education and Prevention Program. Expert Panel Report 3: Guidelines for the Diagnosis and Management of Asthma. August 28, 2007)

that requires infrequent use of (≤2 days a week and ≤2 nights a month) of SABA for quick symptom relief. There should be none or minimal interruptions in carrying out daily activities while also maintaining a near normal pulmonary function. Clinicians should be working very closely with the patients and their families to meet their asthma management expectations. Furthermore, therapy plans should target the reduction of the risk of recurrent asthma exacerbations, minimizing the need for ED visits and hospitalizations. Elderly patients are frequently admitted for asthma exacerbations as they have reduced β2 responsiveness to BD therapy in the ED as compared to younger adults [65]. Chronic co-morbidities are very common in older patients and should be given careful attention when treating asthmatic patients. This is very important as multiple co-morbidities mean increased number of medications with net effect of polypharmacy and multiple drug interactions. This has an effect on patient's asthma symptoms and medication adherence. Higher doses and chronic use of ICS can lead to skin thinning, risk of easy bruising, and oral thrush. A patient with coronary artery disease is on non-selective B-blockers (e.g., carvedilol and labetalol). In theory B-blockers can potentially worsen asthma symptoms. It is imperative that the medication list be reviewed, simplified, and oftentimes discontinued appropriately. However, asthma is not a contraindication to selective B-blockers. Medication adherences should be monitored in patients with depression and dementia and in those who are unable to afford prescription therapies due to multiple co-payments for drugs need for other co-morbidities. An interdisciplinary approach involving family members, caregivers, and social workers should be taken when creating individualized treatment plans for patients. This will ensure optimum medication adherence. Despite the limited clinical data on the adverse effects of asthma medication on the elderly, we know that this population has an increased risk of adverse events due to age-related pharmacodynamic and pharmacokinetic changes [54]. Hence it is important to be vigilant in monitoring B2-mediated hypokalemia, narrow angle glaucoma, prostatic hyperplasia, or bladder neck obstruction especially among patients taking long-acting anti-muscarinic agents. On rare occasions there are some patients who are started on theophylline therapy to manage asthma symptoms. Theophylline has a very narrow therapeutic index; therefore blood levels need to be monitored closely. Special consideration should be given to the choice of inhaler device recommended in this age group. Providers should directly observe patients' inhaler techniques to ensure accuracy and adequacy of the inhaler. The patient knows how to use the device correctly by checking their technique. Before stepping-up treatment plans, observe the patient to make sure they are using the inhaler correctly. Poor technique means poor asthma symptom control. Other limitations to device use in the elderly include the need for coordination and manual dexterity to use capsule-based inhaler versus metered-dose inhalers (MDI). Inhaler devices also require an inspiratory flow which can be compromised with increasing age. A spacer device can be very helpful in patients who are unable to generate a deep inhalation technique or coordinate the use of an MDI. A spacer also allows more medications to be delivered to the lungs and decrease oropharyngeal deposition. Nebulizers are another alternative option to deliver inhalation medications albeit it also requires medication preparation, regular maintenance of the machine, portability, and limited number of medications available in nebulizer form. Despite the alternatives, a patient with cognitive impairment and dementia will still not be able to correctly use any of these devices [66]. An interdisciplinary approach and education of caregivers on how to administer medication are crucial to ensure medication adherence and control of asthma symptoms [67].

8

Case Conclusion

GC was subsequently diagnosed to have an overlap diagnosis of asthmatic bronchitis/COPD. She was treated with nebulizations, inhaled corticosteroids, and oxygen therapy for her COPD. Her peak flow rate was monitored well. She was advised to keep a diary of her symptoms diurnally and nocturnally. It was made clear that she needed to get her annual flu vaccine. Since she had previous hospitalizations for pneumonia exacerbating her COPD, she was also started on maintenance azithromycin. She was advised to stay away from triggers such as pollens and strong scents. She was subsequently sent home with close follow-up with her pulmonologist in a week's time.

8.6 Acute Kidney Injury (AKI) in the Elderly

8.6.1 Introduction

Acute kidney injury (AKI) is a sudden deterioration in kidney function leading to an accumulation of nitrogenous waste products that are normally cleared by the kidney. These changes occur over a period of time and affect the body's normal physiologic homeostasis. Elderly patients are more susceptible to AKI due to the presence of multiple co-morbidities, impaired ability to recover from disease, and a consequential decline in overall renal function with advancing age. Mortality rates in elderly patients with multi-organ failure and AKI can be as high as 50%. AKI in the elderly is associated with short- and long-term morbidity and mortality. AKI outcomes in older patients affect their overall quality of life. When possible, all preventative measures should be taken to prevent AKI. The treatment of AKI is non-specific which includes hydration and avoidance of nephrotoxic agents. Occasionally, AKI treatment will require renal replacement therapy (RRT). Dialysis in the elderly should be individualized and initiated in a shared decision-making process.

Case Presentation

GC is an 88-year-old female with a history of mild chronic obstructive pulmonary disease (COPD), hypertension, coronary artery disease, gastroesophageal reflux disease (GERD), type 2 diabetes, cognitive impairment, osteoporosis, and osteoarthritis who presented to the emergency room from home with acute onset of confusion. Her daughter, who lives nearby, stated that her mother was recently treated for asthmatic bronchitis. She was maintained on azithromycin to prevent recurrent hospitalizations. She subsequently developed loose bowel movements and could not keep up with fluid losses. She lost her appetite and was not drinking fluids. There is no history of recent travel. She was also taking intermittent doses of naproxen for crampy abdominal pain. In the emergency room her vitals included a temperature of 39 °C, normotensive 135/85 mmHg, respiratory rate 18 breaths per minute, and heart rate 102 beats per minute. Focused physical exam findings revealed slightly labored breathing, with prolonged expiratory phase and wheezing bilaterally. She had tachycardia. There was no jugular venous distention or peripheral edema. Chest radiograph demonstrated hyper-inflated lungs with a questionable infiltrate. Her initial labs showed elevated blood urea nitrogen at 35 mg per deciliter and creatinine at 2.5 mg per deciliter with a baseline of 1.2. She had a mildly elevated potassium at 5.5 millimoles per liter.

8.6.2 Discussion

Acute kidney injury (AKI) previously known as acute renal failure (ARF) is a sudden deterioration in kidney function leading to an accumulation of nitrogenous waste products that are normally cleared by the kidney. These changes occur over a period of hours to days and affect the body's normal physiologic homeostasis. The incidence of AKI is rising among all ages particularly the elderly above the age of 65 [68]. It is estimated that AKI occurs in up to 7% of hospitalized patients and 30% of patients in the intensive care unit (ICU) [69]. The mortality rate among hospitalized elderly patients above the age of 65 years old is high [70]. AKI is not limited to a hospital setting and can occur among community dwelling adults. Elderly patients are more susceptible to AKI due to the presence of multiple co-morbidities, impaired ability to recover from the disease, and a consequential decline in overall renal function with advancing age. Mortality rates in elderly patients with multi-organ failure and AKI can be as high as 50% [71]. Many patients who survive the acute event are left with decreased glomerular filtration rate (GFR) and chronic kidney disease (CKD) that can eventually progress to end-stage renal disease (ESRD) [71]. Per US Renal Data System (USRDS) national census on patients receiving renal replacement therapy, it is estimated that there is at least a 40% increase in adults 75 years or older getting dialysis. Epidemiological studies have shown that even mild reversible AKI has important clinical outcomes including the risk of death [72].

8.6.2.1 Risk Factors

Ongoing age-dependent functional and structural changes in a kidney lead to a loss in renal mass and reserve. In an event of an insult, a normal functioning kidney can compensate and adapt to maintain homeostasis and GFR. However, a kidney of an older adult is less likely able to do so because of decreased renal reserve and presence of other co-morbid conditions (e.g., diabetes, hypertension) and pre-existing renal vascular diseases in this age group. In addition, elderly patients are often taking multiple medications (often nephrotoxic) and are subject to more invasive procedures requiring radiocontrast agents. The cumulative insults over time put a kidney of an elderly person vulnerable to developing AKI. AKI in the elderly is associated with significant morbidity and mortality [71–73].

8.6.2.2 Geriatric Considerations

All older adults experience age-related structural changes in the kidney resulting in spontaneous progressive decline in renal function over a period of time [74]. Age-related structural changes include thickening of the basement membrane, mesangial expansion, and focal glomerulosclerosis. Functional changes include an average of 10% decrease in renal blood flow per decade. Where normal blood flow in a healthy kidney is 1200 mL/min/1.73 m^2, by the ninth decade the flow decreases to 300 mL/min/1.73 m^2. There is an average of 8 mL/min per decade decline in GFR after age 40. Kidney function is measured through levels of serum creatinine. Creatinine is metabolized in the muscle and excreted in the urine. The decline in muscle mass with aging, regardless of etiology, results in a decrease in serum creatinine. Normal serum creatinine in a frail older adult, obese, or an amputated patient can be misleading. Hence, GFR is widely accepted as the best overall marker for kidney function. It is difficult to measure GFR directly, so it is estimated. GFR is used to dose medications that are cleared by the kidneys. The steady functional decline in renal blood flow, GFR, and serum creatinine combined impair the ability of the kidney to excrete salt or water load. These changes pose an increased risk for acute kidney injury. An aging kidney, despite being able to maintain homeostasis, is vulnerable to physiologic stress and insults due to its limited reserve [72].

8.6.2.3 Pathophysiology

Acute kidney injury (AKI) is defined as a sudden loss of kidney function resulting in low urine output, an acute elevation of serum creatinine (SCr), and blood urea nitrogen (BUN). Serum creatinine is an important indicator of kidney health. It is a byproduct of muscle metabolism and is mainly excreted by the kidney with some secretion at the level of the kidney tubules. Hence the levels of serum creatinine vary with age, muscle mass, volume of distribution, and hydration status. Therefore, a frail older adult with a decreased muscle mass will have low to normal serum creatinine levels. A higher serum creatinine for this patient, despite it seemingly appearing normal, might mislead a provider for diagnosing AKI. Hence, GFR measurement is helpful for diagnoses and appropriate medication dosing [73, 74]. Per KDIGO (Kidney Disease: Improving Global Outcomes), a patient is diagnosed with AKI if they have an increase in SCr by $\geq$0.3 mg/dl ($\geq$26.5 μmol/l) within 48 hours or SCr $\geq$ 1.5 times the baseline creatinine or decrease in urine output <0.5 ml/kg/h over at least 6 hours [73]. These abrupt changes are usually reversible. It is possible to have AKI without injury to the renal parenchyma. Hence AKI is a clinical diagnosis rather than a structural one. Severity of AKI can range from asymptomatic and transient to rapidly progressive causing plasma electrolyte imbalances and ineffective volume regulation [69]. The etiologies of AKI in the elderly population is not any different from those in the general populations. They can be classified into prerenal, intrarenal, and postrenal. *Prerenal* etiology accounts for about one-third of the causes of AKI. The injury occurs due to hypoperfusion of the kidney in the setting of volume depletion, low cardiac output, or medication effects. Intravascular volume depletion in an elderly patient can be due to dehydration secondary to vomiting, diarrhea, active bleeding, and medications such as diuretics. For example, a nursing resident who is bedridden and has diarrhea is unable to compensate for oral intake and usually presents with dehydration, hypernatremia, and an AKI [69, 75].

A variety of disorders can cause *intrarenal* AKI which can further be subdivided depending on the part of the kidney that is affected, i.e., glomerulus, vasculature, tubules, or the interstitium.

- Glomerulonephritis is the inflammation of the glomerulus. Disorders affecting the glomerulus present with dysmorphic red blood cells, red blood cell casts, and proteinuria on urinalysis. The most common causes of glomerulonephritis in the elderly include anti-neutrophil cytoplasmic antibody, p-ANCA-associated diseases, or positive anti-myeloperoxidase (MPO) antibody. Examples of p-ANCA-associated diseases are rheumatoid arthritis and microscopic polyangiitis.
- Vasculature: Renal artery obstruction, atheroembolism (post-procedure cholesterol emboli), or large vessel vasculitis can cause AKI. Most older adults have

simultaneous co-morbid disease and are on multiple medications that can impair the normal circulatory system, e.g., angiotensin-converting enzyme inhibitors, angiotensin receptor blockers, or nonsteroidal anti-inflammatory drugs. These medications have an effect on decreasing the GFR especially in states with decreased renal perfusion (e.g., sepsis, heart failure, dehydration, etc.) and thus increase further risk of AKI.
- Acute tubular necrosis (ATN): Renal tubules are lined by epithelial cells that can be damaged by nephrotoxic or ischemic causes. Nephrotoxic causes are medications such as aminoglycosides or chemotherapy drugs and radiocontrast dyes. Ischemic causes of ATN include sepsis and prolonged volume depletion that can lead to tubular injury.
- Acute interstitial nephritis (AIN) is caused by an allergic reaction to a medication. One can appreciate white blood cells and eosinophils in the urine. However, this finding lacks sensitivity and specificity.

Post-renal etiologies of AKI can vary from diseases causing anatomical obstruction to medications (e.g., anti-cholinergic) causing neurogenic bladder. In older males, the possible causes include prostate disease (e.g., benign prostatic hypertrophy or BPH or prostate carcinoma), urethral stricture, and ureter and bladder obstruction. In females, pelvic malignancies are commonly seen to cause post-renal obstruction [77]. Elderly patients with AKI commonly require a urethral catheterization to relieve obstruction.

8.6.2.4 Disease Management and Overall Impact

With any disease, workup should include a thorough history and physical examination, current medication review, and documentation of recent procedures with or without contrast dye. Further history should be obtained specific to investigate any pre-renal, intrinsic, or post-renal etiologies. A detailed history must include any changes in urine output, color, and/or symptoms during urination. When patients present with post-renal AKI, a urinary catheterization can be both diagnostic and therapeutic. Further diagnostic testing includes imaging of the kidney, ureter, and bladder (KUB) to look for any signs of obstruction. Additional testing for urine includes urinalysis and urine electrolytes. A simple urinalysis can provide clues such as dysmorphic red blood cells or red blood cell casts that can be present in glomerulonephritis. Urine electrolyte measurement can help calculate the fractional excretion of sodium (FE_{Na}). Fractional excretion of urea (FEUrea) is calculated when patients are on diuretics. A calculated $FE_{Na} < 1\%$ or FEUrea < 40% indicates that the etiology of AKI is likely pre-renal [8]. If patient has rapidly progressive renal failure or the etiology of AKI is unknown, renal biopsies can also be done. However, detailed discussions should be held with patient and families to discuss the risks and benefits of the procedure [74].

Kidney Disease Improving Global Outcomes (KDIGO) outlines the stages and criteria for diagnosing of acute kidney injury (AKI) [75]:
- Stage 1: 1.5–2 times baseline or ≥0.3 mg/dL (≥26.5 mmol/L) increase in the serum creatinine or urine output <0.5 mL/kg per hour for 6–12 hours
- Stage 2: 2–3 times baseline increase in the serum creatinine or urine output <0.5 mL/kg per hour for ≥12 hours
- Stage 3: >3 times baseline increase in the serum creatinine, increase in serum creatinine to ≥4.0 mg/dL (≥354 mmol/L), urine output of <0.3 mL/kg per hour for ≥24 hours, or anuria for ≥12 hours, or on renal replacement therapy (RRT)

Patients with AKI have variable illness trajectory. Patients may either recover fully, require permanent renal replacement therapy (RRT), partially recover and be left with CKD, or may die of the acute illness. There are no specific therapies for AKI treatment. No matter the etiology, treatment is aimed to keep renal injury to a minimum and restore kidney function to maintain the normal physiologic homeostasis. This involves treating any electrolyte imbalances, acid base disturbances, volume overload, and uremic symptoms. If supportive therapy is not successful, then patients are started on renal replacement therapy (RRT). RRT in a younger patient has been shown to be well-tolerated due to less medical co-morbidities and increased renal reserve. In older people with multiple co-morbidities, RRT is an aggressive therapy that is poorly tolerated and confers a worse prognosis. Hence the decision to start or withdraw dialysis in elderly patients should involve a shared decision-making process and integrate one's life expectancy and individual goals. Advance care planning can assist in identifying individual goals and hope for physical and cognitive recovery. Goals of care should be discussed in advance to include risks and benefits of hemodialysis therapy [76]. Since there are no specific therapeutic options available to treat AKI, it is important to prevent renal injury from happening as it is associated with greater morbidity and mortality. Older patients are susceptible to renal injury due to decreased renal reserve, age-related decline in GFR, or CKD caused by the multiple renal injuries during the course of their lifetime (e.g., diabetes, hypertension). Hence, it is important to take measures to prevent AKI by minimizing exposure where possible to nephrotoxins (e.g., nonsteroidal anti-inflammatory agents, aminoglycosides, iodinated contrast, etc.) and to properly dose medications. There are situations where AKI may not be preventable. It is important in situations like these to maintain euvolemia and avoid hypotension [77].

Case Conclusion

GC was admitted to the hospital for acute kidney injury likely related to dehydration from diarrhea and use of naproxen. She was given intravenous fluids. Her medications were dosed appropriately based on her renal function. Nephrotoxic agents were avoided. The kidney specialists were involved in her care given her history of hypertension and diabetes. Furthermore, the offending antibiotic was discontinued. She did not test positive for Clostridium difficile diarrhea. After a couple of doses of loperamide, her bowel movements firmed up. She was finally able to drink some more fluids and slowly restarted her meals. Repeat chest radiograph did not reveal any infiltrate. She was not treated for any infection at this time.

Additionally, she was advised to get out of bed and sit on the chair when she can to avoid further deconditioning.

8.7 Dizziness

8.7.1 Introduction

Dizziness is a common complaint for the aging population with a prevalence of 30% in people aged over 60 years and increasing to 50% in the very old (older than 85 years). Dizziness can be caused by a number of benign or serious conditions, making the diagnosis more complex. In evaluating older adults with dizziness, it is important to understand how the patient describes their symptoms and confirm if the symptoms were continuous or episodic. Compared to their younger counterparts, dizziness in older people is not only more common but also more persistent, and can be more debilitating. The approach to therapy is multi-factorial that must take into account the multiple and varied causes with targeted interventions. It is important to balance both pharmacologic and non-pharmacologic therapies.

Case Presentation

GC is an 88-year-old female with mild cognitive impairment, mild COPD, osteoporosis, type 2 diabetes on insulin, osteoarthritis, and GERD who is being treated in the hospital for acute kidney injury believed to be related to her previous episodes of diarrhea and use of naproxen. She was being managed with IV fluids and advised to get out of bed to chair. Physical therapy was called in the next day to evaluate her. Upon standing, she felt light-headed and a bit nauseated. Orthostatic blood pressure readings were checked. Her sitting blood pressure was 140/90 while her standing blood pressure was 110/70 with a heart rate of 103 beats per minute. She could not complete her walking exercises and was advised to sit down. Further physical therapy was postponed for the following day. In the meanwhile, her daughter visits her at night and managed to assist her mother to go to the bathroom to void. Again, the change in position prompted GC to hold on to her daughter. She had expressed light-headedness and nausea. The daughter summons the nurse for assistance.

8.7.2 Discussion

Dizziness is a common complaint for the aging population with a prevalence of 30% in people aged over 60 years, and increasing to 50% in the very old (older than 85 years) [78]. Dizziness can be caused by a number of benign or serious conditions, making diagnosis more complex. In older adults, the differential diagnoses for dizziness can be broad, and even the most common causes of dizziness may manifest differently.

8.7.2.1 Risk Factors

The common risk factors that cause dizziness in the older adult population include balance symptoms and difficulties with gait stability that exponentially increases with age. Medications are a common contributor to dizziness and ataxia as elderly patients are often on multiple drugs, which place them at high risk for these side effects [79].

8.7.2.2 Geriatric Considerations

In evaluating older adults with dizziness, it is important to understand how the patient describes their symptoms and confirm if the symptoms are continuous or episodic. Many older adults will use vague terms such as light-headed, unsteady, or dizzy to describe similar sensations. The causes of dizziness can be categorized into otologic (vertigo), central (disequilibrium), medical (presyncope), and psychogenic (light-headedness) etiologies. It is important to review the terminology which can distinguish the various etiologies:

- Vertigo: sensation that the room is spinning or tilting.
- Disequilibrium: sense of imbalance that usually involves the trunk or legs without sensation of the head moving.
- Faintness or light-headedness may be a precursor to syncope or presyncope which can be life-threatening.

Compared to their younger cohorts, dizziness in older people is not only more common but also more persistent, and can be more debilitating. It has more causes and less likely due to a psychological reason. In 20–40% of dizzy patients in primary care, the underlying cause remains unknown [80]. Approximately half of all older adults complain of symptoms which fall in two or more categories. The patient history can generally classify dizziness into one of four categories described above. The main causes of vertigo are benign paroxysmal positional vertigo, Meniere's disease, vestibular neuritis, and labyrinthitis. Many medications can cause presyncope, and regimens should be assessed in patients with this type of dizziness. Especially in older adults with polypharmacy, dizziness is often cited as an adverse drug event. A thorough history assessing cardiac and neurologic symptoms can identify life-threatening diagnosis. Vascular events, tumors, Parkinson's disease, and diabetic neuropathy should be considered with the diagnosis of disequilibrium. Psychiatric disorders, such as depression, anxiety, and hyperventilation syndrome, can cause vague light-headedness (◘ Tables 8.4 and 8.5).

8

8.7.2.3 Pathophysiology

Presbystasis is the term used to describe the loss of vestibular and balance functions associated with aging. Dizziness can be viewed as a multi-factorial geriatric syndrome involving many different symptoms and derived from many different sensory, neurologic, cardiovascular, and other systems. The underlying causes of dizziness in older adults can often fall into one of three broad categories including normal age-related decline in the acuity of the sensory and motor pathways, i.e., loss of hair cells in labyrinth; pathological changes in aging, where older adults are more susceptible to age-related changes with time; and finally a number of environmental and lifestyle factors (e.g., polypharmacy) [80].

There are a number of age-related physiological changes that contribute to the symptom of dizziness in the elderly. Age-related degeneration of different neural structures affects balance, including the vestibular receptors, central vestibular neurons, cerebellum, and visual and proprioceptive pathways. The number of hair cells in the vestibular organs and

◘ Table 8.5 Drugs that can cause ataxia (Hain/ Ramaswamy) [81]

Anticonvulsants	(e.g., phenytoin, carbamazepine)
Antihypertensive medications and drugs with hypotension as side effects	Adrenergic blockers (e.g., propranolol, terazosin) Diuretics (e.g., furosemide) Vasodilators (e.g., isosorbide, nifedipine) Tricyclic antidepressants (e.g., nortriptyline) Phenothiazines (e.g., chlorpromazine) Dopamine agonists (e.g., L-dopa/carbidopa)
Ototoxic drugs and vestibular suppressants Some of the mycin antibiotics	(e.g., gentamicin)
Psychotropic agents	Sedatives (e.g., barbiturates and benzodiazepines) Drugs with Parkinsonism as side effects (e.g., phenothiazines) Drugs with anticholinergic side effects (e.g., amitriptyline)
Miscellaneous drugs	Cimetidine

◘ Table 8.4 Causes of dizziness in the elderly (Hain and Ramaswamy) [81]

Otologic (vertigo-peripheral)	Central (disequilibrium)	Medical (presyncope)	Psychogenic (light-headedness)
BPPV	Vascular events involving the cerebellum and brainstem	Hypotension (orthostasis)	Anxiety disorders
Meniere's syndrome	Vertebrobasilar migraine	Cardiac event (includes occult cardiac arrhythmias and acute myocardial infarctions)	Panic attacks
Vestibular neuritis	Seizures	Infection	Somatization syndrome
Bilateral vestibular paresis (often secondary to ototoxic medications)	Parkinson's disease (due to postural instability and orthostatic hypotension due to dysautonomia exacerbated by dopaminergic agents)	Low blood glucose	Malingering
Labyrinthitis	Diabetic neuropathy	Medications	Agoraphobia
	Tumor		Depression
	Infection: Brain abscess Meningitis		Hyperventilation syndrome

the number of fibers in the superior and inferior vestibular nerves decrease with age [82], all of which can impair vestibular pathways. The proprioceptive system also undergoes several changes with age which impact postural stability, vibration and tactile stimuli, and position and directional movements. Age-related changes to visual system including decline in depth perception, visual acuity, and decline in motor system, strength, and function all contribute to the symptom of dizziness and imbalance and have been shown to have a strong association with falls in this population. The presence of dizziness in the elderly is a strong predictor of accidental falls and injuries. It is estimated that about 30% of adults older than 65 will fall at least once a year, and about 50% will fall again. This number increases with advanced age. Falls are the leading cause of accidental death in people older than 65 years and represent the number one reason for hospital admission for non-fatal falls in this population [82]. Fall-related injuries can lead to mobility restrictions, loss of independence, and unwanted care transitions to skilled nursing facilities.

8.7.2.4 Disease Management and Overall Impact

Dizziness accounts for an estimated 5 percent of primary care clinic visits and is also one of the most common presentations for older adults in the emergency department. The differential diagnoses of dizziness can be narrowed with easy-to-perform physical examination tests, including evaluation for nystagmus, the Dix-Hallpike maneuver, and orthostatic blood pressure testing. The diagnosis is largely based on a constellation of clinical features obtained with careful history taking and bedside examinations. Laboratory testing and radiography play a little role in diagnosis. A final diagnosis is not obtained in about 20 percent of cases. The differential diagnosis of acute dizziness can be challenging as dizziness itself can be a manifestation of conditions varying from life-threatening disorders to normal physiologic responses. The evaluation of dizziness relies on a thorough history and physical exam which can often guide subsequent cardiac, neurologic, or other lab and diagnostic studies. Most causes of vertigo are benign and self-limiting, while cardiovascular causes can be life-threatening [83]. Vestibular disease and medications are noted to be the most common cause of dizziness in the primary care setting, while cardiovascular disease is considered to be the most common cause of dizziness in the acute care setting. For patients who present with syncope (loss of consciousness due to decreased blood flow to the brain) or presyncope, it is important to include a thorough cardiac history inquiring about chest pain and palpitations that can be caused by dysrhythmias or myocardial ischemia. Vasovagal (neurocardiogenic) syncope can occur under emotional stress, fear, pain, or injury and results from an overstimulation of the sympathetic nervous system resulting in peripheral vasodilatation and bradycardia which in turn causes hypotension. This often occurs with vomiting, urinating, or coughing. Postural hypotension may also cause dizziness. Many medications prescribed for hypertension, atrial fibrillation, and other cardiac diseases can lead to postural hypotension. Other causes of postural hypotension in the acute care setting include dehydration, sepsis, and gastrointestinal bleeding leading to volume loss [85]. These patients often present with alterations in vital signs, electrocardiographic findings, or changes in medications that can guide further workup. Treatment of vertigo includes the Epley maneuver (canalith repositioning) and vestibular rehabilitation for benign paroxysmal positional vertigo, intra-tympanic dexamethasone or gentamicin for Meniere's disease, and steroids for vestibular neuritis. Orthostatic hypotension that causes presyncope can be treated with alpha agonists, mineralocorticoids, or lifestyle changes. Disequilibrium and lightheadedness can be alleviated by treating the underlying cause [85]. Particular attention should be paid to potentially life-threatening disorders as a cause of acute dizziness or vertigo. Certain bedside physical exam findings which can detect central vestibular signs, such as direction-changing nystagmus, and skew deviation in patients are more sensitive than brain imaging in detecting stroke presenting with acute isolated dizziness/vertigo. Isolated positional vertigo is almost always caused by BPPV and can readily be treated with canalith repositioning maneuvers once the involved semicircular canal is determined. Even with developments in imaging technology, the diagnosis of acute dizziness/vertigo largely relies on bedside examination [84]. While it is important to distinguish between the various etiologies of dizziness, in many patients, a clear etiology may not be determined. Medications such as anti-vertiginous drugs, anti-histamines, or vasodilators are known to give temporary relief, but the literature suggests the counterproductive effects of these drugs can limit their use [85]. Treatment with medications must be used with greater caution in older adults as they may be more sensitive to side effects. Vestibular physical therapy is often helpful and should be utilized in many situations [85]. For older patients who suffer with continuous dizziness, a referral to an inter-professional rehabilitation team which treats dizziness and vestibular disorders can be an effective option. Team members typically include a nurse, physician, and specialists such as audiologist, physical therapist, occupational therapist, and a research scientist. This multidisciplinary approach, involving a group of professionals with varying expertise is effective in the treatment of vestibular and balance disorders. Vestibular rehabilitation therapy (VRT) deals with the management of vertiginous patient by alleviating the symptoms and increasing the threshold to vertigo. Activities of daily living (ADLs) are also a part of the therapy which eases their performance in function with the symptoms.

The role of rehabilitation in the management of vertigo is limited to a very specific group of conditions. An occupational therapist who is a part of the multidisciplinary team treating the vertiginous patient, with the knowledge of physiology and therapeutic benefit of vestibular rehabilitation can widen the rehabilitation spectrum for various diseases producing vertigo and dysequilibrium, to resolve or minimize these symptoms.

Other key resources for successful management of dizziness and vertigo include family members and caregivers who play an integral role in supporting patients with dizziness. They are often needed to collaborate history and clinical presentation and provide information about medication changes, prodromal symptoms, etc. They also play a significant role in VRT to ensure that the treatment modalities are incorporated to daily activities to ensure safety and wellness. The efficient management and resolution of disabling symptoms depends on diagnostic and rehabilitative planning which requires a multidisciplinary team approach comprising of not only the clinical team of neuro-otologists, rehabilitation therapists, psychiatrists, and medical social workers but also the patient and their family members and caregivers who can continue the education and support the patient needs as they rehabilitate. This often takes patience and time to aid recovery from vertigo and dysequilibrium [85]. As previously mentioned, the presence of dizziness in the elderly is a strong predictor of falls, which is the leading cause of accidental death in people older than 65 years. Family members and caregivers play an integral role in identifying patients risks for falls, and providing the support and assistance they need to mitigate the risk of traumatic and debilitating falls [86]. Resources such as the Fall precautions: STEADI guide can be a useful tool to educate patients and caregivers [87].

Case Conclusion

GC was given more fluids to ensure that she had adequate hydration. Medications that would further lower her blood pressure were ceased for now. She was given exercises to properly maneuver from bed to chair. She continued her physical therapy on a daily basis with much improvement in walking speed and stance. She did not fall. Her daughter was very pleased with her progress. She was subsequently discharged to home with recommendations for ongoing home physical therapy.

8.8 Urinary Tract Infection

8.8.1 Introduction

Urinary tract infections (UTI) are common in both community-dwelling and long-term care older adult residents. Women appear to be more affected than men. Although UTI is one of the most commonly reported infections in older adults, its definition varies across the literature. It is further challenged by the atypical nature of symptomatology in this population. Given that the risk of harm in delaying UTI treatment in clinically stable patients is low, the risk-benefit balance favors a more meticulous approach to diagnoses and antibiotic prescription.

Case Presentation

GC is an 88-year-old female with a past medical history of mild cognitive impairment, mild COPD, osteoporosis, type 2 diabetes, CAD, osteoarthritis, and hypertension who was seen in the clinic today complaining of urinary frequency alternating with hesitancy. She did not report of any fever or chills. However, over the last few days she complained of malaise. At one point, she almost fell walking to the bathroom. She had been feeling not quite her usual self. On physical examination, she did not have any suprapubic and abdominal tenderness. A spot urinalysis was done. This tested positive for leukocyte esterase and negative for nitrite. Furthermore, she had some white blood cells in the urine. She was empirically treated with Bactrim DS 1 tab oral BID. As per her, this is not her first UTI episode. She had had a couple over the last few months.

8.8.2 Discussion

Urinary tract infections (UTI) are common in both community-dwelling and long-term care older adult residents. It is the second most common infection diagnosed in the acute hospital setting and accounts for almost 5% of all emergency department visits by adults aged 65 years and older in the USA [88, 89]. It is responsible for an estimated 7 million office visits [90]. Its approximate prevalence in long-term care facilities is close to 30% to 40% of all healthcare-associated infections [91, 92]. Women appear to be more affected than men [93]. The risk factors for women might be associated with postmenopausal state, worsening incontinence, debility, and alteration of the vaginal milieu in relation to greater exposure to antimicrobial therapy. Although UTI is one of the most commonly reported infections in older adults, its definition varies across the literature. It is further challenged by the atypical nature of symptomatology in the older adult population. Given that the risk of harm in delaying UTI treatment in clinically stable patients is low, the risk-benefit balance favors a more meticulous approach to diagnoses and antibiotic prescription.

8.8.2.1 Risk Factors

There are multiple predisposing risk factors including but are not limited to the following that can lead to the development of UTI in the older adult [94]:

1. Increasing age
2. Increasing rates of urinary retention and incontinence
3. Immunosenescence
4. Anatomic abnormalities such as BPH
5. Uncontrolled diabetes mellitus
6. Long-term medical institutionalization
7. Prolonged immobility
8. Autonomic dysfunction from other neurologic diseases
9. Medications such as sodium-glucose cotransporter 2- inhibitors
10. Vaginal atrophy
11. Sexual intercourse
12. Presence of urinary instrumentation, e.g., catheterization

UTI in the Community-Dwelling Older Adult

Disease Management and Overall Impact

In general, UTI in the community-dwelling older adult population requires the presence of localized genitourinary symptoms, pyuria, and a positive urine culture. The symptoms most commonly reported include dysuria with or without frequency, urgency, suprapubic pain, and hematuria. Atypical symptoms that may manifest include lower abdominal pain, back pain, constipation, fatigue, falls, confusion or acute change in mental status, lack of appetite, and incontinence among others. It is imperative that providers recognize these variations in clinical presentation so that appropriate goal-directed prevention and treatment strategies may be utilized. Diagnosis requires at the very least a urinary dipstick to assess for the presence of leukocyte esterase or nitrite and concurrent urinalysis to look for pyuria. The confirmatory test is urine culture to look for bacteriuria and evaluate for antibiotic susceptibilities. The most frequent pathogen for UTI in this population is Escherichia coli. Other common microbes in descending prevalence include Proteus spp, Klebsiella spp, and Enterococcus spp. A study by Little and colleagues examined the impact of several management strategies on the use of antibiotics for cases of uncomplicated UTI [95]. The investigators found no differences in symptom duration, severity of frequency of symptoms, or severity of unwell symptoms between the antibiotic management of strategies. For most women who present with nonspecific symptoms, a trial of hydration is reasonable while awaiting completion of a diagnostic workup. This will delay use of antibiotics thereby decreasing unnecessary exposure. The study by Knottnerus et al. supports this management [96]. More than half of the women in this study who delayed antibiotic initiation reported improvement of their symptoms. A major key point is that none of these women who delayed antibiotics developed complications of untreated UTI such as pyelonephritis. When deciding to use antibiotics, it is essential to choose the appropriate agent based on efficacy, dosing, and duration of treatment while minimizing unwanted side effects and inappropriate resistance. For treatment of uncomplicated UTI, the Infectious Disease Society of America (IDSA) and European Society for Microbiology and Infectious Diseases propose the use of nitrofurantoin monohydrate/macrocrystals at 100 mg twice daily dosing for a 5 day duration or the TMP/SMX 1160/800 mg, 1 double strength twice daily for 3 days [97]. Another option is fosfomycin at a single dose of 3 grams though efficacy is inferior to the first two. It is important to note that these same medications may be used for men; however the therapy is typically extended to 1–2 weeks. Further studies need to be done to ascertain the optimal length of UTI treatment in older men.

UTI in Long-Term Care

Disease Management and Overall Impact

Older adults who reside in long-term facilities are at increased risk of developing UTI. Some risk factors that are implicated include physical disability, neurocognitive disorders such as dementia and Parkinson's disease, and the prevalent use of urinary catheters either as temporizing measures to assist in voiding or as a function of an organic pathology such as severe BPH, post-op status, neoplasia, autonomic dysfunction, etc. Eriksson et al. found a link when a history of UTI in the preceding year was tied to the occurrence of vertebral fractures, multi-infarct dementia, and stroke [98]. In 2012, the Society for Healthcare Epidemiology of America (SHEA) updated the surveillance definitions of infections in long-term care facilities. The McGeer criteria were revised as follows [99]:

1. At least one of the following: acute dysuria; pain, swelling, or tenderness of the testes, epididymis, or prostate; or fever or leukocytosis. And at least one of the following localizing urinary tract sub-criteria (e.g., costovertebral angle tenderness or pain, hematuria, new or marked increase in incontinence) or in the absence of fever or leukocytosis, two or more of the localizing urinary sub-criteria (such as suprapubic pain, gross hematuria, new or marked incontinence/urgency/frequency)
2. One of the following microbiological sub-criteria (at least 10^5 cfu/mL of no more than two species of microbes in a voided urine sample or at least 10^2 of any number of microbes in a specimen collected by straight catheter)

The diagnostic workup is similar to the previous older adult population. A urinalysis and urine dipstick should be obtained. If pyuria is present or the dipstick is positive for leukocyte esterase and nitrite, a urine culture should be obtained to evaluate for the presence of bacteriuria and to document antibiotic susceptibility. It is important to highlight that the absence of both nitrite and leukocyte esterase confers a 100% negative predictive value for the diagnosis of UTI in this population. Urine culture alone is often not helpful in evaluating diffuse non-specific symptoms in older long-term care residents and should not be routinely performed in asymptomatic patients. As far as pathogens are concerned, the microbes mirror the frequency of pathogens for UTI in the community. *E.coli* accounts for the majority followed by *Proteus*, *Klebsiella*, and *Enterococcus* spp. The latter along with *Staphylococcus aureus* account for 4.5% and 4.1% of cases, respectively. The antibiotic management for UTI in this population is similar to community dwellers in that TMP/SMX and nitrofurantoin are acceptable first-line options. Though cautious use of nitrofurantoin in patients with renal insufficiency is warranted, it also has been shown to have overall lower rates of resistance compared to TMP/SMX and fluoroquinolones. One caveat on the use of nitrofurantoin should underscore that *Proteus* species-positive patients may have intrinsic resistance to this antibiotic. In 2001, the SHEA recommended a 7 day course of antibiotics for women with lower level UTI, while simple cystitis may be given for 3 to 5 days. In general, the optimal duration of antibiotics in institutionalized patients has not been well-studied.

8.8.2.2 Geriatric Considerations

Older adults may not necessarily present with symptoms typical of UTI as in the younger adult population owing in large part to immunosenescence and homeostenosis. The first phenomenon describes the alteration in the host response to varying stimuli including infectious and inflammatory markers. The second phenomenon is the altered physiologic coping response when the reserves of the older adult diminish over time. These signs and symptoms include but are not limited to the following:

1. Change in behavior or mental status, e.g., lethargy, confusion/delirium, etc.
2. Changes in physical strength such as body weakness, malaise, etc.
3. Changes in appetite and weight, i.e., weight loss, anorexia
4. Possibly a history of falls (deemed controversial)

A prospective study by Rowe in 2013 looked at the association of suspected UTIs in five nursing homes with history of falls [100]. The authors concluded that there was no association between the two in spite of the fact that a history of falls is often considered a reason to test a nursing home resident for UTI.

8.8.2.3 Pathophysiology

The development of UTI begins with the colonization of the urogenital tract by pathogens from the fecal flora subsequently leading up to their ascension via the urethra and into the bladder, ureter, and kidneys. Bacterial adhesion to the uroepithelium is therefore a critical step in the pathogenesis of UTIs. Furthermore, when a patient is bacteremic related to sepsis, there is a tendency to have bacterial seeding into the kidneys, ureter, and bladder. Persistent urinary dysbiosis could compromise host defenses and lead to recurrent UTIs.

8.8.2.4 Disease Management and Overall Impact

Asymptomatic Bacteriuria in the Older Adult

Asymptomatic bacteriuria is defined as the presence of bacteria in the urine with or without pyuria in the absence of clinical symptoms indicating UTI. A study on long-term care by Nicolle et al. showed a prevalence of 25–50% of adult residents with bacteriuria at any given time [101]. After adjusting for concurrent medical problems, those with ASB did not have higher rates of mortality. Furthermore, antimicrobial therapy for ASB did not reduce the rates of complications and may in fact increase the risk for a subsequent symptomatic UTI. The current guidelines from the Infectious Diseases Society of America recommend treating ASB in a certain population, i.e., pregnant women and patients undergoing urologic procedures that will likely result in some type of mucosal injury (◘ Fig. 8.4).

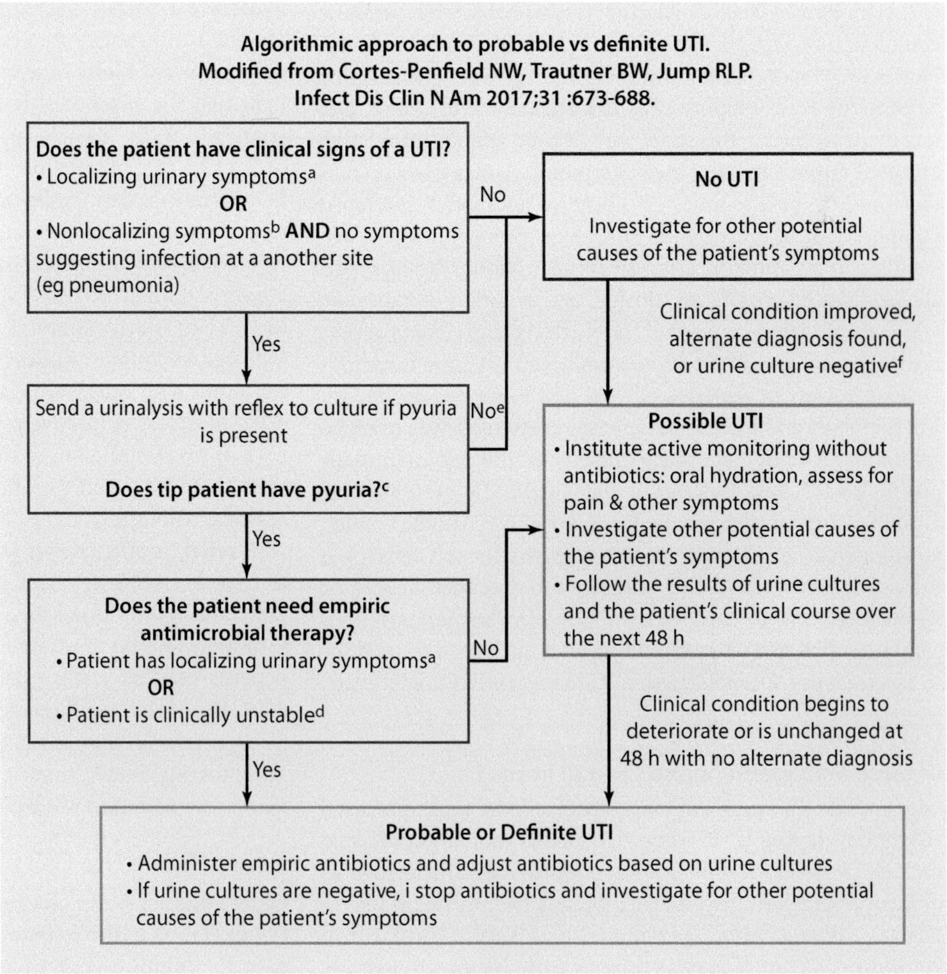
Algorithmic approach to probable vs definite UTI.
Modified from Cortes-Penfield NW, Trautner BW, Jump RLP.
Infect Dis Clin N Am 2017;31 :673-688.
Does the patient have clinical signs of a UTI?
• Localizing urinary symptoms[a]
OR
• Nonlocalizing symptoms[b] AND no symptoms suggesting infection at a another site (eg pneumonia)
No
No UTI
Investigate for other potential causes of the patient's symptoms
Yes
Clinical condition improved, alternate diagnosis found, or urine culture negative[f]
Send a urinalysis with reflex to culture if pyuria is present
Does tip patient have pyuria?[c]
No[e]
Possible UTI
• Institute active monitoring without antibiotics: oral hydration, assess for pain & other symptoms
• Investigate other potential causes of the patient's symptoms
• Follow the results of urine cultures and the patient's clinical course over the next 48 h
Yes
Does the patient need empiric antimicrobial therapy?
• Patient has localizing urinary symptoms[a]
OR
• Patient is clinically unstable[d]
No
Clinical condition begins to deteriorate or is unchanged at 48 h with no alternate diagnosis
Yes
Probable or Definite UTI
• Administer empiric antibiotics and adjust antibiotics based on urine cultures
• If urine cultures are negative, i stop antibiotics and investigate for other potential causes of the patient's symptoms

◘ **Fig. 8.4** Algorithmic approach to probable vs definite UTI. (Modified from Cortes-Penfield et al. [94])

Preventative Management

It is highly important to counsel patients, families, and their caregivers that UTI is a preventable disease. Specific considerations that are worth mentioning include but not limited to the following:

1. Avoidance of urinary tract instrumentation
2. Optimal control of blood sugar
3. Increased hydration
4. Improvement in mobility
5. Overuse of unwarranted antibiotic therapy leading to medication resistance

Case Conclusion

GC completed her course of oral antibiotics. She was advised to drink plenty of fluids to include cranberry juice. She was feeling much better and appeared to have been back to her baseline function. Both she and her daughter who lives with her are pleased with the progress she had made.

References

1. Rhodes A, Evans L, Levy M, et al. Surviving sepsis campaign: international guidelines for management of severe sepsis and septic shock: 2016. Crit Care Med. 2017;45(3):486–552.
2. Centers for Disease Control and Prevention. The state of aging and health in America 2013. Atlanta: Centers for Disease Control and Prevention, US Department of Health and Human Services; 2013.
3. Girard TD, Wesley EE. Bacteremia and Sepsis in older adults. Clin Geriatr Med. 2007;23:633–47.
4. Martin GS, Mannino DM, Moss M. The effect of age on the development and outcome of adult sepsis. Crit Care Med. 2006;34(1):15–21.
5. Centers for Disease Control and Prevention. Healthy Aging at a glance 2011. https://www.cdc.gov/chronicdisease/resources/publications/aag/healthy-aging.htm. Accessed January 11, 2018.
6. Wester AL, Dunlop O, Melby KK, Dahle UR, Wylier TB. Age-related differences in symptoms, diagnosis, and prognosis of bacteremia. BMC Infect Dis. 2013;13:346.
7. Nasa P, Juneja D, Singh O. Severe sepsis and septic shock in the elderly: an overview. World J Crit Care Med. 2012;1(1):3–30.
8. Laupland KB, Bagshaw SM, Gregson DB, Kirkpatrick AW, Ross T, Church DL. Intensive care unit-acquired urinary tract infections in a regional critical care system. J Crit Care. 2005;9(2):R60–5.
9. Norman DC. Clinical features of infections in older adults. Clin Geriatr Med. 2016;32:433–41.
10. Green JE, Ariathianto Y, Wong SM, Aboltins C, Lim K. Clinical and inflammatory response to blood-stream infections in octogenarians. BMC Geriatr. 2014;14(1):55.
11. De Gaudio AR, Rinaldi S, Chelazzi C, Borracci T. Pathophysiology of sepsis in the elderly: clinical impact and therapeutic considerations. Curr Drug Targets. 2009;10(1):60–70.
12. Umberger R, Callen B, Brown ML. Severe sepsis in older adults. Crit Care Nurs Q. 2015;38(3):259–70.
13. Flaherty E, Zwicker D. Atypical presentation. BMJ. 2005;330:773–4.
14. Rajagopalan S, Yoshikawa TT. Antimicrobial therapy in the elderly. Med Clin North Am. 2001;85(1):133–47.
15. Lu SH, Leasure AR, Dai YT. A systematic review of body temperature variations in older people. J Clin Nurs. 2010;1(2):4–16.
16. Mouton CP, Pierce B, Espino DV. Common infections in older adults. Am Fam Physician. 2001;63(2):257–69.
17. Fry TJ, Mackall CL. Current concepts of thymic aging. Semin Immunopathol. 2002;24(1):7–22.
18. Weksler ME, Goodhardt M, Szabo P. The effect of age on B cell development and humoral immunity. Semin Immunopathol. 2002;24(1):35–52.
19. Wheeler AP, Bernard GR. Treating patients with severe sepsis. N Engl J Med. 1999;340(3):207–14.
20. Opal SM, Esmom CT. Bench-to-bedside review: functional relationships between coagulation and the innate immune response and their respective roles in the pathogenesis of sepsis. Crit Care. 2003;7(1):23–38.
21. Williamson J. Principles of antibiotic use in older adults. Clin Geriatr Med. 2007;23(3):481.
22. Russell JA, Walley KR, Singer J, et al. A randomized controlled trial of low dose vasopressin versus norephinephrine infusion in patients who have septic shock. Am J Respir Crit Care Med. 2007;175:A508.
23. Sprung CL, Annane D, Briegel J, et al. Corticosteroid therapy of septic shock. Am J Respir Crit Care Med. 2007;175:A507.
24. The Acute Respiratory Distress Syndrome Network. Ventilation with lower tidal volumes as compared with traditional tidal volumes for acute lung injury and the acute respiratory distress syndrome. N Engl J Med. 2000;342(18):1301–8.
25. Jensen AG, Wachmann CH, Espersen F, et al. Treatment and outcome of Staphylococcus aureus bacteremia: a prospective study of 278 cases. Arch Intern Med. 2002;162(1):25–32.
26. Brun-Buisson C, Doyon F, Carlet J. Bacteremia and severe sepsis in adults: a multicenter prospective survey in ICU's and wards of 24 hospitals. French Bacteremia-Sepsis Study Group. Am J Respir Crit Care Med. 1996;154(3):617–24.
27. Chassagne P, Perol MB, Doucet J, et al. Is presentation of bacteremia in the elderly the same as in younger patients? Am J Med. 1996;100(1):65–70.
28. Goldrick BA. Infection in the older adult. Am J Nurs. 2005;105(6):31–4.
29. Moran D. Infections in the elderly. Top Emerg Med. 2003;25(2):174–81.
30. Conte HA, Chen Y, Mehal W, et al. A prognostic rule for elderly patients admitted with community acquired pneumonia. Am J Med. 1999;106(1):20–8.
31. Gavazz G, Krause KH. Ageing and infection. Lancet Infect Dis. 2002;2:659–66.
32. Blot S, Koulenti D, Dimopoulos G, Martin C, Komnos C, et al. Prevalence, risk factors, and mortality for ventilator-associated pneumonia in middle-aged, old, and very old critically ill patients. Crit Care Med. 2014;42(3):601–9.
33. Carusone SB, Walter SD, Brazil K, Loeb MB. Pneumonia and lower respiratory infections in nursing home residents: predictors of hospitalization and mortality. J Am Geriatr Soc. 2007;55:414–9.
34. Torres OH, Munoz J, Ruiz D, Ris J, Gich I, et al. Outcome predictors of pneumonia in elderly patients: importance of functional assessment. J Am Geriatr Soc. 2004;52(10):1603–9.
35. Mody L, Sun R, Bradley SF. Assessment of pneumonia in older adults: effect of functional status. J Am Geriatr Soc. 2006;54(7):1062–7.
36. Dai X, Busby-Whitehead J, Alexander KP. Acute coronary syndrome in the older adults. J Geriatr Cardiol. 2016;13(2):101–8.
37. Gillis N, Arslanian-Engoren C, Struble L. Acute coronary syndromes in older adults: a review of literature. J Emerg Nurs. 2014;40(3):270–5.
38. Samaras N, Chevalley T, Samaras D, Gold G. Older patients in the emergency department: a review. Ann Emerg Med. 2010;56(3):261–9.
39. Canto JG, Rogers WJ, Goldberg RJ, Peterson ED, Wenger NK, et al. Association of age and sex with myocardial infarction symptom presentation and in-hospital mortality. JAMA. 2012;307(8):813–22.
40. El-Menyar A, Zubaid M, Sulaiman K, et al. Atypical presentation of acute coronary syndrome: a significant independent predictor of in-hospital mortality. J Cardiol. 2011;57(2):165–71.
41. Brieger D, Eagle K, Goodman S, et al. Acute coronary syndromes without chest pain, an under-diagnosed and under-treated high-risk group: insights from the Global Registry of Acute Coronary Events. Chest. 2004;126(2):461–9.

42. Hwang S, Ryan C, Zerwic J. The influence of age on acute myocardial infarction symptoms and patient delay in seeking treatment. Prog Cardiovasc Nurs. 2006;21(1):20–7.
43. Chan PS, Spertus JA, Nallamothu BK. Long-term outcomes in Elderly Survivors of In-Hospital Cardiac arrest. N Engl J Med. 2013;368(11):1019–26.
44. Alexander K, Newby L, Cannon C, et al. Acute coronary care in the elderly, part I: non-ST segment elevation acute coronary syndromes: a scientific statement for healthcare professionals from the American Heart Association Council on Clinical Cardiology: in collaboration with the Society of Geriatric Cardiology. Circulation. 2007;115(19):2349–569.
45. The American Heart Association Online Educational Resource http://www.heart.org/HEARTORG/Conditions/HeartAttack/Heart-Attack-Tools-and-Resources_UCM_002043_Article.jsp#.WhSYzOOWzct.
46. https://www.hospitalmedicine.org/Web/Quality_Innovation/Implementaton_Toolkit/ACS/Reliable_Interventions/patient_education.aspx.
47. https://www.hospitalmedicine.org/Web/Quality_Innovation/Implementation_Toolkit/ACS/Reliable_Interventions/discharge_transitions.asp.
48. Soriano JB, Abajobir AA, Abate KH, Abera SF, Agrawal A, Ahmed MB, et al. Global, regional, and national deaths, prevalence, disability-adjusted life years, and years lived with disability for chronic obstructive pulmonary disease and asthma, 1990–2015: a systematic analysis for the Global Burden of Disease Study 2015. Lancet Respir Med. 2017;5(9):691–706.
49. Gooneratne NS, Patel NP, Corcoran A. Chronic obstructive pulmonary disease diagnosis and management in older adults. J Am Geriatr Soc. 2010;58(6):1153–62.
50. Global Initiative for Obstructive Lung Disease (GOLD). Global Strategy for the Diagnosis, Management, and Prevention of Chronic Obstructive Pulmonary Disease http://goldcopd.org/wp-content/uploads/2017/11/GOLD-2018-v6.0-FINAL-revised-20-Nov_WMS.pdf. Published 2018. Accessed 14 Jan 2018.
51. Renwick DS, Connolly MJ. Impact of obstructive airways disease on quality of life in older adults. Thorax. 1996;51(5):520–5.
52. Albertson TE, Louie S, Chan AL. The diagnosis and treatment of elderly patients with acute exacerbation of chronic obstructive pulmonary disease and chronic bronchitis. J Am Geriatr Soc. 2010;58(3):570–9.
53. Fragoso C, Akgün KM, Jeffery SM, Kapo JM, Possick JD, Rochester CL, Lee PJ. Chronic obstructive pulmonary disease. In: Halter JB, Ouslander JG, Studenski S, High KP, Asthana S, Supiano MA, Ritchie C, editors. Hazzard's geriatric medicine and gerontology. 7th ed. New York: McGraw-Hill Education; 2017. Retrieved from http://accessmedicine.mhmedical.com/content.aspx?bookid=1923&sectionid=144525549. Last accessed 28 Dec 2017.
54. Akgün MK, Pisani M. Pulmonology. In: Medina-Walpole A, Pacala JT, Potter JF, editors. Geriatrics review syllabus: a core curriculum in geriatric medicine, vol. 1-Book Section. 9th ed. New York: American Geriatrics Society; 2016. Retrieved from https://geriatricscareonline.org/FullText/B023/B023_VOL001_PART001_SEC006_CH047?parent_product_id=B023_VOL001_PART001_SEC006.
55. Vaz Fragoso CA, Gill TM. Defining chronic obstructive pulmonary disease in an aging population: defining chronic obstructive pulmonary disease. J Am Geriatr Soc. 2010;58(11):2224–6.
56. Health United States Report, Centers for Disease Control and Prevention. Table 20. https://www.cdc.gov/nchs/data/hus/hus16.pdf. Published 2016. Accessed 10 Jan 2018.
57. Huang CL, Nguyen PA, Kuo P, Iqbal U, Hsu YHE, Jian WS. Influenza vaccination and reduction in risk of ischemic heart disease among chronic obstructive pulmonary elderly. Comput Methods Prog Biomed. 2013;111(2):507–11.
58. American Academy of Hospice and Palliative Medicine Center to Advance Palliative Care Hospice and Palliative Nurses Association Last Acts Partnership National Hospice and Palliative Care Organization. National consensus project for quality palliative care: clinical practice guidelines for quality palliative care, executive summary. J Palliat Med. 2004;7(5):611–27. https://doi.org/10.1089/jpm.2004.7.611.
59. Au DH, Udris EM, Fihn SD, McDonell MB, Curtis JR. Differences in health care utilization at the end of life among patients with chronic obstructive pulmonary disease and patients with lung cancer. Arch Intern Med. 2006;166(3):326–31.
60. Goodridge D, Lawson J, Duggleby W, Marciniuk D, Rennie D, Stang M. Health care utilization of patients with chronic obstructive pulmonary disease and lung cancer in the last 12 months of life. Respir Med. 2008;102(6):885–91.
61. Centers for Disease Control and Prevention. Most recent asthma data. https://www.cdc.gov/asthma/most_recent_data.htm. 2016. Updated June 7, 2017. Accessed 5 Jan 2018.
62. Skloot GS, Busse PJ, Braman SS, Kovacs EJ, Dixon AE, Vaz Fragoso CA. An official American Thoracic Society workshop report: evaluation and management of asthma in the elderly. Ann Am Thorac Soc. 2016;13(11):2064–77.
63. Global Initiative for Asthma. Global Strategy for Asthma Management and Prevention http://ginasthma.org/2017-gina-report-global-strategy-for-asthma-management-and-prevention/. 2017. Accessed 5 Jan 2018.
64. Hanania NA, King MJ, Braman SS, Saltoun C, Wise RA, Enright P. Asthma in the elderly: current understanding and future research needs: a report of a National Institute on Aging (NIA) Workshop. J Allergy Clin Immunol. 2011;128(3 Suppl):S4–S24.
65. National Asthma Education and Prevention Program: Expert panel report III: Guidelines for the diagnosis and management of asthma. Bethesda, MD: National Heart, Lung, and Blood Institute, 2007. (NIH publication no. 07–4051) https://www.ncbi.nlm.nih.gov/books/NBK7232/pdf/Bookshelf_NBK7232.pdf. Accessed on 1 Jan 2018.
66. Chotirmall SH, Watts M, Branagan P, Donegan CF, Moore A, McElvaney NG. Diagnosis and management of asthma in older adults: diagnosis and management of asthma in older adults. J Am Geriatr Soc. 2009;57(5):901–9.
67. Shanker S, Rojas M, Caufield C. Aging of the respiratory system. In: Halter JB, Ouslander JG, Studenski S, High KP, Asthana S, Supiano MA, Ritchie C, editors. Hazzard's geriatric medicine and gerontology, vol. 1–Book, Section. 7th ed. New York, NY: McGraw-Hill Education; 2017. Retrieved from accessmedicine.mhmedical.com/content.aspx?aid=1136594252.
68. Khaled A, Paul P. Acute kidney injury in elderly. Clin Geriatr Med. 2009;25(3):331–58.
69. Waikar SS, Bonventre JV. Acute kidney injury. In: Kasper D, Fauci A, Hauser S, Longo D, Jameson J, Loscalzo J, editors. Harrison's principles of internal medicine. 19th ed. New York: McGraw-Hill; 2014.. http://accessmedicine.mhmedical.com.eresources.mssm.edu/content.aspx?bookid=1130&sectionid=79746409. Accessed 28 Dec 2017.
70. Santacruz F, Barreto S, Mayor MM, Cabrera W, Breuer N. Mortality in elderly patients with acute renal failure. Ren Fail. 1996;18(4):601–5.
71. Gong Y, Zhang F, Feng D, Gu Y. Elderly patients with acute kidney injury (AKI): clinical features and risk factors for mortality. Arch Gerontol Geriatr. 2011;54:47–51.
72. Wiggins J, Patel S. Aging of the kidney. In: Halter JB, Ouslander JGS, Studenski S, High KP, Asthana S, Supiano MA, Ritchie C, editors. Hazzard's geriatric medicine and gerontology. 7th ed. New York: McGraw-Hill Education; 2017. Retrieved from http://accessmedicine.mhmedical.com/content.aspx?bookid=1923&sectionid=144525549.Accessed December 28, 2017.
73. Kidney Disease Improving Global Outcomes (KDIGO 2012) http://www.kdigo.org/clinical_practice_guidelines/pdf/CKD/KDIGO_2012_CKD_GL.pdf. 2013. Accessed 14 Jan 2018.
74. Pascual J, Llano F, Ortuno J. The elderly patient with acute renal failure. J Am Soc Nephrol. 1995;6(2):144–53.
75. Rosner MH. Acute kidney injury in the elderly. Clin Geriatr Med. 2013;29(3):565–78.

76. Anderson S, Eldadah B, Halter JB, Hazzard WR, Himmelfarb J, Horne FM, High KP. Acute kidney injury in older adults. J Am Soc Nephrol. 2011;22(1):28–38, 8–38.
77. Bitzer M. Renal disease. In: Halter JB, Ouslander JO, Studenski S, High KP, Asthana S, Supiano MA, Ritchie C, editors. Hazzard's geriatric medicine and gerontology 2017. 7th ed. New York: McGraw-Hill Education; 2017. Retrieved from http://accessmedicine.mhmedical.com/content.aspx?bookid=1923&sectionid=144525549. Accessed 28 Dec 2017.
78. Barin K, Dodson EE. Dizziness in the elderly. Otolaryngol Clin N Am. 2011;44(2):437–54.
79. Davis LE. Dizziness in elderly men. J Am Geriatr Soc. 1994;42(11):1184–8.
80. Post RE, Dickerson LM. Dizziness: a diagnostic approach. Am Fam Physician. 2010;82(4):361–9.
81. Hain TC, Ramaswamy T. Dizziness in the elderly. http://projects.galter.northwestern.edu/geriatrics/chapters/dizziness.cfm.
82. Fernández L, Breinbauer HA, Delano PH. Vertigo and Dizziness in the elderly. Front Neurol. 2015;6:144.
83. Ehrich MA, Meldon SW, Ma J, Woolard R. "Dizziness, weakness, vertigo" Geriatric emergency medicine: American College of Emergency Physicians (ACP). McGraw Hill; 2004.
84. Jung I, Kim JS. Approach to dizziness in the emergency department. Clin Exp Emerg Med. 2015;2(2):75–88.
85. Konnur MK. Vertigo and vestibular rehabilitation. J Postgrad Med. 2000;46(3):222–3.
86. Maarsingh OR, Dros J, Schellevis FG, van Weert HC, et al. Causes of persistent dizziness in elderly patients in primary care. Ann Fam Med. 2010;8(3):196–205.
87. https://www.cdc.gov/steadi/pdf/preventing_falls_in_older_patients_provider_pocket_guide_2015-04-a.pdf last accessed: May 9, 2018.
88. Nicolle LE, Bradley S, Colgan R, et al. Infectious Diseases Society of America guidelines for the diagnosis and treatment of asymptomatic bacteriuria in adults. Clin Infect Dis. 2005;40(5):643–54.
89. Curns AT, Holman RC, Sejvar JJ, et al. Infectious disease hospitalizations among older adults in the United States from 1990 through 2003. Arch Intern Med. 2005;165(21):2514–20.
90. Ruben FL, Dearwarter SR, Norden CW, et al. Clinical infections in the non-institutionalized geriatric age group: methods utilized and incidence of infections, the Pittsburgh good health study. Am J Epidemiol. 1995;141(2):145–57.
91. Tsan L, Langberg R, Davis C, et al. Nursing home-associated infections in the Department of Veterans Affairs community living centers. Am J Infect Control. 2010;38(6):461–6.
92. Cotter M, Donlon S, Roche F, et al. Healthcare-associated infection in Irish long-term care facilities: results from the first National Prevalence Study. J Hosp Infect. 2012;80(3):212–6.
93. Jackson SL, Boyko EJ, Scholes D, et al. Predictors of urinary tract infection after menopause: a prospective study. Am J Med. 2004;117(2):903–11.
94. Cortes-Penfield NW, Trautner BW, Jump RL. Urinary tract infection and asymptomatic bacteriuria in older adults. Infect Dis Clin N Am. 2017;31:673–88.
95. Little P, Moore MV, Turner S, et al. Effectiveness of five different approaches in management of urinary tract infection: randomized controlled trial. BMJ. 2010;340:c199.
96. Knottnerus BJ, Geerlings SE, Moll Van Charante EP, et al. Women with symptoms of uncomplicated urinary tract infection are often willing to delay antibiotic treatment: a prospective cohort study. BMC Fam Pract. 2013;14:71.
97. Grover ML, Bracamonte JD, Kanodia AK, et al. Urinary tract infection in women over the age of 65: is age alone a marker of complication? J Am Board Fam Med. 2009;22(3):266–71.
98. Eriksson I, Gustafson Y, Fagerstrom L, et al. Prevalence and factors associated with urinary tract infections (UTIs) in very old women. Arch Gerontol Geriatr. 2010;50(2):132–5.
99. Finucane TE. "Urinary tract infection" – requiem for a heavyweight. J Am Geriatr Soc. 2017;65:1650–5.
100. Rowe T, Towle V, Van Ness PH, et al. Lack of positive association between falls and bacteriuria plus pyuria in older nursing home residents. Infect Control Hosp Epidemiol. 2007;28(7):889–91.
101. Nicolle LE, SHEA Long Term Care Committee. Urinary tract infections in long-term care facilities. Infect Control Hosp Epidemiol. 2001;22(3):167–75.

Multi-morbidity (Multiple Conditions)

Contents

Patient-Centered Care for Persons with Multiple Conditions

Michelle Martinchek and Katherine Thompson

A. Chun (ed.), *Geriatric Practice*, https://doi.org/10.1007/978-3-030-19625-7_9

What is the optimal patient-centered approach to care for this patient with multiple conditions? How might that look different from following all of the clinical practice guidelines recommendations designed for her individual conditions?

Multimorbidity is when multiple chronic conditions exist within a single patient. These conditions can be physical (cancer, congestive heart failure, osteoarthritis), mental (depression, dementia, substance abuse), or both. As a provider, it is crucial to develop an approach to caring for multimorbid patients, as this is a steadily increasing population with complex care needs. Patients with multimorbidity account for a significant percentage of health care spending in the United States. These patients have higher health-care utilization [1] and are at increased risk for poorer quality of life and earlier death than age matched counterparts without multimorbidity [2].

Patient-centered care, sometimes also referred to as "person-centered care," means that individuals' values and preferences are elicited and, once expressed, guide all aspects of care, supporting realistic health and life goals [3]. Patient-centered care is important for all patients but particularly important for persons with multiple conditions for a number of reasons. Often, both the potential harms and potential benefits of treatment options are less clear for multimorbid patients, and patient preferences become even more paramount in decision-making. Additionally, aggressive management of risk factors to prevent future disease can impose a large treatment burden with unclear benefits. Multimorbid patients often have a wider variety of health-care experiences which may shape a wide variety of goals and preferences for care. Multimorbid patients may also have different resources and different limitations to care than healthier patients. All conditions and treatments must be considered in the larger context of the patient's overall disease burden and functional status.

In recognition of the growing population of multimorbid patients and the need for a focus on patient-centered care in this population, health-care providers have sought to develop rational approaches to guide care for multimorbid patients. It is important to note that an increasingly multimorbid population is a worldwide phenomenon and many international organizations have developed similar guidelines and recommendations to review data and best practices for multimorbid patients. The National Institute for Health and Care Excellence (NICE) in the United Kingdom and the World Health Organization are two such examples [4, 5]. Each of these organizations attempts to outline key principles and challenges for clinicians to provide rational, patient-centered care to multimorbid patients. Here, the Guiding Principles for the Care of Older Adults with Multimorbidity: An Approach for Clinicians [6] will be reviewed. These guiding principles were developed by the American Geriatrics Society Expert Panel on the Care of Older Adults with Multimorbidity. Using expertise in the field, and a structured review of the literature, the panel developed these principles to help guide clinicians as well as inform researchers and policy-makers. These principles provide an excellent framework for providers making medical decisions with multimorbid patients.

Case

Mrs. T is a 79-year-old woman presenting for a routine health visit. She has a history of coronary artery disease, peripheral vascular disease, osteoporosis, osteoarthritis of the knees, and depression. Since her last visit, she has had two falls. After both falls, she was able to get up on her own and believes she "just tripped." She is very worried she will break a hip and lose her independence and states "I would rather be dead than live in a nursing home." She prefers not to take prescription medications if possible and is currently only taking a daily multivitamin and occasional acetaminophen for pain. She is widowed and lives alone in her own apartment but has a daughter that checks in on her and brings her groceries once a week. She is a former smoker but does not currently smoke. She drinks alcohol, about three drinks per day. She has very limited financial resources. She is independent in all activities of daily living and instrumental activities of daily living except for shopping. She does not have a car and her daughter takes her out to run errands as needed, but she also occasionally uses public transportation. She can walk about ½ block before getting leg pain.

Physical Exam

Vital signs: 145/87 76 Ht 5′5″ Wt 112lbs

Thin, pleasant, well-groomed, no acute distress. She has a somewhat flat affect, but is interactive and appropriate. Orientation intact, mental status exam unremarkable. Heart is regular rate and rhythm. Diminished but palpable pulses in her feet. Lungs are clear. There is a large healing bruise over the L hip, no tenderness to palpation. There is mild joint line tenderness over both knee joints with some bony overgrowth, no joint effusions.

9.1 Guiding Principle 1: Elicit and Incorporate Patient Preferences into Medical Decision-Making for Older Adults with Multimorbidity [6]

Beginning the medical decision-making process with an assessment of a patient's health-care goals and preferences is an essential starting point in providing patient-centered care to multimorbid patients. The majority of medical decisions carry with them a range of possible diagnostic or therapeutic options with different potential harms or benefits. This is particularly true for patients with multimorbidity where both potential harms and potential benefits may be less clear. Multimorbid older adult patients may vary widely in their health-care goals and preferences. Many place high value on retaining function and independence [7]. Others may value preserving quantity of remaining life, preventing specific disease processes, avoiding specific symptoms, or maintaining specific functional roles (being a caregiver, etc.). Patients may have different levels of willingness or ability to participate in the needed "work" required for specific treatment options (take medications, attend clinician visits, undergo procedures, pay for treatment, diet or exercise, etc.) [8]. However, assessing these goals and preferences may help both optimize adherence to a care plan and ensure that all involved providers are aligning treatments around the patient's main goals [9]. It is also important to note that the term "patient preferences" may expand to include family, caregivers, or others if cognitive impairment is present or if the patient chooses to include others in the medical decision-making process.

Case Practice for Guiding Principle 1: Elicit Patient Preferences

In the above case, Ms. T states she would "rather be dead than live in a nursing home." She also prefers not to take prescription medicines if possible.

When weighing patient goals and preferences for this patient, does one goal take precedence over another? For instance, if medical treatment for osteoporosis might minimize the patient's risk of hip fracture and functional independence, would she consider taking a medication? How would you explain the risks and benefits of a bisphosphonate to this patient in terms of her goals and preferences?

9.2 Guiding Principle 2: Recognizing the Limitations of the Evidence Base, Interpret and Apply the Medical Literature Specifically to Older Adults with Multimorbidity [6]

Incorporating evidence from the medical literature to guide care decisions is foundational to the practice of medicine; however, there are several limitations to applying this approach in multimorbid patients. Recognizing and accounting for these limitations is imperative to providing patient-centered care for multimorbid patients. First, clinical trials often enroll patients who only have the specific disease process under study without other chronic conditions or who are relatively healthier or younger. It may be difficult to apply results of these studies to patients who are older or multimorbid as they may be more likely to experience harms or burdens of treatment or be subject to medication interactions or side effects. Second, it is important to evaluate the outcomes assessed for any study. Surrogate outcomes such as improvement in laboratory test results may carry little meaning for a patient and have little impact on their health. Studies of interventions that affect "patient-important" outcomes—those that align with a patient's individual goals and preferences—are more likely to have positive impact on a patient's health. Examples of patient-important outcomes may include prevention of a specific disease process (stroke, heart attack) or improvement in quality of life, physical functioning, or ability to be independent. Third, when reviewing evidence behind a treatment decision, it is important to consider both the potential benefits and harms. Often, potential benefits are described in more detail than potential harms. Additionally, for multimorbid patients, treatment of one disease process may exacerbate or interact with another disease process. It is important to assess whether or not the potential for unintended effects or interactions on other conditions was studied or reported on.

Case Practice for Guiding Principle 2: Interpreting the Evidence

What evidence exists for medications or interventions to prevent fractures in osteoporosis? What are the benefits vs. harms of various options? For example, what are the possible harms of treating Ms. T with an oral bisphosphonate? What are the benefits? Are potential interactions with other disease processes described in the literature?

9.3 Guiding Principle 3: Frame Clinical Management Decisions Within the Context of Risks, Burdens, Benefits, and Prognosis (e.g., Remaining Life Expectancy, Functional Status, Quality of Life) for Older Adults with Multimorbidity [6]

A person's prognosis should help to inform, but not necessarily dictate, care decisions. Prognosis may be considered in terms of estimated remaining life expectancy, but also in the context of development of specific disease states, functional dependence, etc. Prognosis can be difficult to estimate and even more difficult to discuss with patients. Using prognostic tools can help clinicians estimate prognosis, although they still often provide only a rough guide. Use of life table data [10] or an aggregator of mortality indices such as can be found on ► eprognosis.ucsf.edu [11] can help clinicians more accurately estimate prognosis and may prove especially useful in differentiating between short-term (within the next year), medium-range (within the next 5 years), and long-term (beyond 5 years) clinical decisions [6]. For instance, in diabetes decision-making, a patient with a remaining life expectancy of less than 1 year may opt for a hemoglobin A1c target in the 8–9 range to avoid short-term risks of hypoglycemic episodes, while a patient with a remaining life expectancy of more than 5 years may opt for a lower hemoglobin A1c target to avoid possible consequences of longer-term hyperglycemia. Discussing prognosis with patients can be difficult. A recent study examining communication preferences of older adults about screening tests found that specific wording of life expectancy was important [12]. Many felt the language of "you may not live long enough to benefit from this test" was unnecessarily harsh compared with the more positive messaging of "this test would not help you live longer."

Case Practice for Guiding Principle 3: Estimating Prognosis

Use life table data [10] to estimate Ms. T's remaining life expectancy. Use a prognosis calculator such as can be found on ► eprognosis.ucsf.edu to estimate Ms. T's 1-, 5-, or 10-year mortality risk. How does this impact your care plan? How would you discuss this information with Ms. T?

Case Practice for Guiding Principle 4: Complexity and Feasibility

What plan will Ms. T be willing/able to adhere to? What factors may affect her adherence? What non-pharmacologic options are available? Would patient education be beneficial? If so, regarding what?

9.4 Guiding Principle 4: Consider Treatment Complexity and Feasibility When Making Clinical Management Decisions for Older Adults with Multimorbidity [6]

Treatment complexity is common and can lead to adverse effects in multimorbid patients. For instance, following the clinical practice guidelines for treatment of a hypothetical patient with osteoporosis, osteoarthritis, type 2 diabetes, hypertension, and COPD—five of the most commonly billed Medicare diagnoses—results in a treatment regimen that may include twelve different medications delivered at five time points through the day with multiple potential drug-drug and drug-disease interactions [13]. The cost of this regimen may be hundreds of dollars a month or even more. It is easy to see how complex treatment regimens put patients at higher risk of nonadherence, adverse reactions, and decreased quality of life [14]. When deciding on a treatment regimen in a multimorbid patient, clinical feasibility and individual preferences should inform choices about treatment. Factors such as financial and insurance resources, cognitive impairment, caregiver involvement, potential side effects, health literacy and health beliefs, and desired outcomes all may impact feasibility of a medical plan. Some patients may be able to manage more complex treatment regimens than others based on their support system, cognitive ability, financial situation, or health-care goals. A discussion of such factors between patient and provider in the context of deciding on a feasible treatment regimen may lead to improved adherence [6]. Additionally, some evidence exists that chronic disease self-management programs may improve health status measures [15]. Care transitions are times when patients are at high risk for increased treatment complexity but also provide opportunities to review regimens with patients, reduce polypharmacy, and enhance feasibility.

9.5 Guiding Principle 5: Use Strategies for Choosing Therapies That Optimize Benefit, Minimize Harm, and Enhance Quality of Life for Older Adults with Multimorbidity [6]

For multimorbid patients, optimizing care plans usually involves prioritization of treatments and interventions based on maximizing benefit, minimizing harms, and enhancing quality of life. Patients with multimorbidity have a higher likelihood of experiencing adverse drug reactions [16] and drug-drug or drug-disease interactions [17]. Prescription of all potentially clinically indicated drugs in a patient with multimorbidity may result in burdensome treatment complexity, non-adherence, and adverse drug reactions [13]. Thus, the most essential drugs and interventions to enable a patient to meet their stated goals and still be clinically feasible must be sought. Identifying treatments that may be potentially inappropriate is a good first step, and several tools are available to assist clinicians in this process (see Approach to Polypharmacy, below). An inter-professional team approach may also help to optimize care plans and minimize polypharmacy in multimorbid patients. For instance, a diabetes educator may help provide patient education on diet and exercise to help improve blood sugar control without medication changes. A pharmacist may perform a structured medication review using an evidence-based tool to minimize polypharmacy. A physical therapist may work with a patient with osteoarthritis to improve mobility and decrease pain. Any changes made to optimize a patient's treatment plan should be made in a stepwise fashion, so results of individual changes can be monitored before the next change is made.

Case Practice for Guiding Principle 5: Optimizing Treatment Plan

Would you recommend pharmacologic treatment of osteoporosis to minimize Ms. T's fracture risk? Why or why not? What factors might influence this decision? What non-pharmacologic treatments will be part of your plan? What interventions might help promote adherence? What are the downsides and the upsides to your plan for this patient? How will you communicate that to this patient?

The above Guiding Principles for the Care of Older Adults with Multimorbidity [6] provide a framework to assist clinicians in providing patient-centered care to older adults with multiple chronic conditions. Individualizing care to account for a patient's own goals, chronic conditions, needs, and resources is paramount. In addition, a number of specific care models have been developed to help meet the needs of multimorbid patients.

9.6 Care Models for Persons with Multiple Conditions

Persons with multiple conditions often have unique care needs, and numerous care models have been developed to more fully address these needs. These care models occur in different care settings, such as in the community, home, outpatient clinic, hospital, or post-acute and long-term care settings. Many of these care models were designed to care for older adults, who often have multiple medical conditions. Some of these care models span across multiple settings or specifically address transitions between care settings. Individuals may be served by these care models for variable lengths of time. Care is often provided by interprofessional teams. These care models are designed to provide high-quality, safe, cost-effective care to patients with complex needs and aim to improve outcomes compared to traditional care models. Some examples of these care models will be reviewed to illustrate the innovation underway in the care for persons with multiple conditions.

9

9.7 Care Across Settings

There has been increasing focus in recent years on person-centered care, in which individuals' needs, values, and preferences are determined and guide all aspects of their health care. Person-centered care focuses on individual functional abilities and goals and re-defines quality and value. It recognizes that people may have needs not only related to chronic medical problems and functional limitations but also to challenges in the physical environment and need for social support [18]. Several care models utilize these person-centered care tenets, including Geriatric Resources for Assessment and Care of Elders (GRACE) and Program for All-Inclusive Care for the Elderly (PACE).

The GRACE model is designed to support older adults and their primary care physicians [19, 20]. It includes a support team that does an initial comprehensive geriatric assessment of the patient in the home and then meets with a larger interdisciplinary team to develop an individualized care plan, which is then discussed with the PCP and modified as appropriate. This model provides ongoing collaboration and coordination with providers across multiple sites of care. Meanwhile, PACE is a community-based model designed to serve frail, high-risk elderly adults. In order to qualify, individuals must be at least 55 years old, meet criteria for nursing home eligibility, and live in a defined area where the PACE program is available [21]. Participants are largely dual eligible for Medicare and Medicaid. Once enrolled, participants received individualized care designed by an interdisciplinary team, which includes services ranging from primary and specialty care to acute care and nursing care, which are mostly provided at a day center, where complex medical, social, and therapy services are provided. It has been shown to reduce hospitalization and readmission rates in participants [22].

9.8 Outpatient Care

There are several models in the outpatient care setting that are designed to accommodate individuals with multiple medical conditions. The traditional model of office-based primary care includes a primary care physician who manages most of the medical conditions, with input from specialist consultants as needed. Another model of care for complex older patients includes either a consultative or co-management model in which a geriatrician provides recommendations for evaluation and management for older adults with multiple chronic conditions. This model generally utilizes a comprehensive geriatric assessment (CGA), which is a multidisciplinary evaluation of key domains that may impact an older adult's health and the creation of management plans for the issues discovered during the assessment [23]. Finally, another example of a primary care model specifically for patients with multiple chronic conditions is called guided care, in which a trained guided care nurse works closely with patients and physicians to provide coordinated, patient-centered care [24]. In addition to primary care, models exist for the care of patients with specific medical conditions. For example, collaborative care models have been developed for the care of patients with dementia [25].

Given that a high proportion of health-care costs are attributed to individuals with multiple chronic conditions, these patients—particularly the sickest—have been the focus of intensive primary care programs. One model to deliver primary care is the patient-centered medical home (PCMH), which is a delivery model where care is coordinated through the primary care physician, with the aim to have a centralized setting that develops a partnership between patients and physicians. The goal is integrated and coordinated care with a focus on quality. Recent programs modeled on the PCMH have focused on delivery of care to the sickest, highest-cost patients which are often referred to as "High-Intensity Primary Care" programs or "Ambulatory Intensive Care Units." These may either be primary care replacement (home or clinic based) or augmentation of primary care [26]. Home-based primary care often includes interprofessional care teams that meet regularly and after-hours support [27]. Outside of formalized care models, it is important to note that a significant amount of care often occurs within a patient's home. This may include a combination of home nursing services; physical, occupational, or speech therapists; paid and unpaid caregivers and homemakers; and additional services provided by community organizations and local, state, and federal agencies.

9.9 Acute Care Models

Admission to an acute care hospital is often a high-risk period for older adults and persons with multiple conditions due to the risk of functional decline. Many inpatient care models are designed to try to prevent this decline in acutely ill patients. One care model aims to circumvent this potential for decline by not admitting patients to a traditional hospital in the first place. The hospital at home program has been utilized to avoid hospitalization completely, allow for early discharge from the hospital, or provide terminal care hospital at home. Admission avoidance hospital at home may achieve either similar or improved clinical outcomes and patient and caregiver satisfaction as traditional inpatient hospitalization with decreased costs [28, 29]. These programs have recruited patients with a number of different clinical conditions and provide hospital level care including nursing and physician care as well as diagnostic and therapeutic services.

9.10 Emergency Department

Older adults make up a high percentage of emergency room care, with an increasing number of visits. Older adults are more likely to be triaged to higher levels of urgency and spend more time in the ED and utilize more resources compared to younger adults, speaking to the diagnostic and therapeutic challenges in caring for older adults with multiple conditions [30]. Recently, "Geriatric Emergency Department Guidelines" were created as a framework for the creation of Emergency Departments that are friendly to older adults [31]. These guidelines include physical recommendations to improve care, recommendations for a robust interdisciplinary team, screening tools for geriatric patients, information on the appropriate management of geriatric syndromes, and a recommendation to provide access to palliative care and end-of-life care for medically complex patients in the geriatric ED [31].

9.11 Inpatient Hospitalization

Once patients are admitted to an acute inpatient hospital, there are several well-known programs designed to improve the quality of care for older adults with multiple conditions. The acute care for elders (ACE) model was originally conceptualized to prevent the decline in functionality and poor outcomes such as increased dependency that can occur during the hospitalization of older adults [32]. Important components included patient-centered care, frequent medical review, early rehabilitation and discharge planning, a prepared environment specific for older adults, and regular meetings and input from interdisciplinary teams [32]. These models have been found to be associated with both patient and systems level outcomes such as fewer falls, less delirium, less functional decline, shorter length of stay, decreased institutionalization with more discharges home, and lower costs [32].

Other acute care programs have been designed to target specific outcomes. One example is the Hospital Elder Life Program, which was designed to prevent delirium in hospitalized older adults. This program screens older adults for specific delirium risk factors and provides targeted interventions for these risk factors implemented by an interdisciplinary team and is unique in incorporating trained volunteers [33]. It has shown favorable outcomes including preventing cognitive and functional decline in hospitalized older adults and has been replicated and implemented in many different settings.

Many care models include input and participation from nurses, but the Nurses Improving Care for Healthsystem Elders (NICHE) program is unique in that it is both a nursing education and consultation program designed to improve care in health-care organizations [34]. Other care models target specific conditions. For example, co-management programs, where the care of patients is shared between teams of providers from different specialties, are commonly used for geriatric patients with hip fracture [35]. Finally, inpatient consultative models are often utilized in the care of older adults admitted to the hospital. These models may include consultation by a geriatrician or a more formalized CGA [23].

9.12 Transitions of Care

Periods of care transitions are particularly vulnerable periods for adults with multiple medical conditions. During these care transitions, patients may have changes in medications, need for follow-up of treatment or diagnostic studies, specialized care instructions, and new or unmet care needs. Thus, several care models have been developed to improve the quality of these care transitions. These transitions may occur from the hospital to home, from the hospital to post-acute or long-term care, and from nursing facilities to home. Many of these transitional care models include some or all of the Joint Commission's seven foundations of safe and effective transitions of care to home [36], outlined in ▶ Box 9.1. These models are designed to reduce the risk of hospital readmissions and unnecessary costs in vulnerable patients. Examples of evidence-based transition of care models from hospital to home are listed in ◘ Table 9.1. Similar care models have also been developed for other care transitions, including those from a skilled nursing facility (SNF) to home. These models are promising, although further work is ongoing [37]. Best practice recommendations for transitioning patients from a SNF to home focus on identification of the primary care physician (PCP) and timely follow-up after SNF discharge, appropriate transmission of information and needed follow-up to the PCP and outpatient team, and patient follow-up to address any questions and ensure receipt of crucial services and appropriate medication reconciliation [38].

Box 9.1 Foundations of safe and effective transitions of care to home identified by the Joint Commission [36]

- Leadership support
- Multidisciplinary collaboration
- Early identification of patients/clients at risk
- Transitional planning
- Medication management
- Patient and family action/engagement
- Transfer of information

Table 9.1 Evidence-based transitions of care models from hospital to home

Program	Brief description
Project RED [48]	A bundle consisting of 12 discharge components including both patient education and discharge planning, medication reconciliation, and discharge instructions, which are designed to reduce re-hospitalizations
Care Transitions Program [49]	Provides specific tools to patients with complex care needs and their caregivers as well as support from a transition coach. Goal to learn self-management skills to aid in transition from hospital to home
Transitional Care Model [50]	Nurse-led intervention that targets older adults at risk for poor outcomes as they move across health-care settings and see different clinicians
Better Outcomes for Older Adults Through Safe Transitions (BOOST) [51]	Initiative to improve transitions and reduce readmissions for hospitals across the United States through a toolkit, mentoring from experts, and ongoing evaluation and quality improvement

9

9.13 Post-acute Care and Long-Term Care

Skilled nursing facilities, also known as nursing homes, are sites of care for patients both in the post-acute care setting and there for long-term care. Patients at these facilities for post-acute care often have sub-acute rehabilitation needs or are there for skilled nursing services. Other patients, particularly those who need significant assistance with activities of daily living, may live at the facility for long-term care. The heterogeneity of patients who often have multiple chronic conditions poses challenges for successful care implementation in this setting. One well-known example of a care model in skilled nursing facilities is a program titled Interventions to Reduce Acute Care Transfers (INTERACT). This is a quality improvement program that focuses on the identification, evaluation, and management of acute changes in condition of nursing home residents. It also includes information on communication, documentation, and decision support tools for management. Additionally, it places emphasis on advanced care planning, hospice, and palliative care in patients with end-stage illness [39, 40].

9.14 Palliative Care Models

Once patients with multiple medical conditions become seriously ill, community-based palliative care may best meet the needs of these individuals and their families. These models aim to provide support outside of the hospital setting and can be delivered in many different settings including home and long-term care settings. Palliative care focuses on symptom management and quality of life and is often enacted by a multidisciplinary team. Once patients are nearing the end of life and choose to forgo further active treatment to focus on symptom management, transition to hospice services may be appropriate. Patients must meet criteria for hospice based on disease severity, and appropriateness is determined by the hospice team. Hospice care is also provided by a multidisciplinary team and can occur in many care settings including at home, a nursing home, or inpatient hospice unit.

Advanced care planning plays an important role in each stage of care. Advanced care planning is multifaceted and aims to discuss and understand a patient's wishes and values so they can be applied in different situations. Many states now employ tools for documentation for advanced care planning, such as Physician Orders for Life-Sustaining Treatment (POLST), which are transferrable across multiple care settings [41]. Common topics included in POLST tools are listed in ▶ Box 9.2.

Box 9.2 Common areas covered in Physician Orders for Life Sustaining Treatment (POLST) tools, which vary by state

- Cardiopulmonary resuscitation (CPR)
- Medical interventions
- Medically administered nutrition
- Advanced directive information – includes information on health-care power of attorney and living will

9.15 Shared Decision-Making

Throughout different settings of care, shared decision-making is a crucial component of care for adults with multiple medical conditions. Often, these decisions are complex and the evidence base to support these decisions may be limited as patients with multi-morbidity are often underrepresented in randomized controlled trials. Additionally, the benefit to harm tradeoffs of diagnostic or therapeutic options may differ in adults with many medical conditions, who may already take multiple medications, be more susceptible to side effects, or have a limited life expectancy. In many situations, there is no clear best choice for how to proceed. The shared decision-making process recognizes this and focuses on reaching shared decisions through conversations and communication between the clinician and patients that is enhanced by the clinical expertise of the physician, available medical evidence, and the patient's expertise on their own experiences, goals, and preferences [42]. After the patient and clinician share information, the goal of shared decision-making is to build consensus and agree on a treatment option [43]. While many patients prefer to be involved in medical decision-making, they may have vastly different preferences on the level of information they want and components that are important during the decision-making process [44]. Decision aids are designed to help support people during this process of weighing the benefits and harms of treatment options and have overall been successful in doing so [44]. There are a variety of decision aids available for specific health issues. These are often educational tools that provide information for patients on various medical decisions, for example, whether to undergo screening for colorectal or prostate cancer. Other tools may provide a framework for providers to utilize in shared decision-making or provide useful information to be introduced during the process, such as calculations of prognosis or life expectancy.

9.16 Approach to Polypharmacy

In patients with multiple medical conditions, common decisions revolve around whether to stop or start new medications. Patients with multiple medical conditions often are prescribed an increasing number of medications and are at risk for polypharmacy. There are many definitions for polypharmacy that revolve around a specific number of medications, but one particularly useful definition for clinical practice is the use of more medications than are clinically indicated [45]. Polypharmacy increases the risk of drug-related adverse events. Additionally, there are several barriers to taking a medication regimen correctly. These range from financial costs, physical barriers (e.g., the ability to twist off a medication cap or correctly inject insulin), health literacy, the burden of time to take multiple medications, and intact cognition to remember to take medications on a set schedule. Simplifying medication regimens is often an important step in improving the quality of care and daily life for patients with multiple conditions.

The first step in addressing polypharmacy is identifying which medications an individual is taking. Individuals with multiple medical conditions may be prescribed medications from multiple specialty providers or pharmacies. One of the most effective methods to ensure the medication list is complete is to have patients bring in all medications they have from all prescribers and pharmacies, in addition to all over-the-counter medications and vitamins. Then, the clinician can review each medication with the patient to compile a thorough medication list.

Once a medication list is defined, efforts can be made to ensure the appropriateness of the medication list. This includes identifying any possible drug side effects and weighing the risks versus the potential benefits of each medication. This process should take into account a patient's own goals and values. It is helpful to ensure the medication list is appropriate for the medical conditions identified and does not include unnecessary medications or omit medications that may be helpful. It is also useful to know the patient's life expectancy in assessing potential benefits of treatment. There are several decision tools available to assist clinicians in ensuring the appropriateness of a medication list, many of which were specifically designed to be used with older adults. A few examples of these tools are listed in ◘ Table 9.2. There are also tools available to help providers and patients in shared decision-making for specific conditions. For example, in deciding whether or not to start anticoagulation for atrial fibrillation to try to decrease stroke risk, it may be useful to calculate the patient's risk of stroke using the CHAD2VASC score and compare it to the patient's risk of bleeding with the HASBLED score [46, 47]. These risk scores can be used to provide information on available evidence for use in the shared decision-making process, which is an important component of care for patients with multiple medical conditions.

◘ **Table 9.2** Examples of tools used to assist providers in assuring the appropriateness of medication lists in patients with multiple medical conditions

Tool	Brief description
Beer's criteria [52]	Guidelines for safely prescribing medications for older adults. Includes potentially inappropriate medication use in older adults, potentially inappropriate medications due to drug-disease or drug-syndrome interactions or due to drug-drug interactions, potentially inappropriate medications to be used with caution in older adults, and medications that should be avoided or have their dose reduced with varying levels of kidney function
START [53]	List of medications to consider starting among certain patients who meet indications
STOPP [54]	List of medications to consider stopping in older adults because the risks may outweigh the benefits
Anticholinergic risk scale [55]	Rates the anticholinergic properties of medications. Drugs that are anticholinergic may cause significant side effects in older adults particularly, such as worsening cognition or sedation, increased fall risk, constipation, dry mouth, visual changes, urinary retention, and others

References

1. Lehnert T, Heider D, Leicht H, et al. Review: health care utilization and costs of elderly persons with multiple chronic conditions. Med Care Res Rev. 2011;68(4):387–420.
2. Boyd CM, Fortin M. Future of multimorbidity research: how should understanding of multimorbidity inform health system design? Public Health Rev. 2010;32:451–74.
3. Person-Centered Care. A definition and essential elements. American Geriatrics Society Expert Panel on person-centered care. J Am Geriatr Soc. 2016;64(1):15–8.
4. Multimorbidity: assessment, prioritisation and management of care for people with commonly occurring multimorbidity. National Guideline Centre (UK). London: National Institute for Health and Care Excellence (UK); 2016.
5. Multimorbidity: technical series on Safer Primary Care. Geneva: World Health Organization; 2016. Licence: CC BY-NC-SA 3.0 IGO.
6. Guiding principles for the care of older adults with multimorbidity: an approach for clinicians: American Geriatrics Society Expert Panel on the care of older adults with multimorbidity. J Am Geriatr Soc. 2012;60(10):E1–E25.

7. Fried T, Tinetti M, Agostini J, Iannone L, Towle V. Health outcome prioritization to Elicit preferences of older persons with multiple health conditions. Patient Educ Couns. 2011;83(2):278–82.
8. Tinetti ME, Naik AD, Dodson JA. Moving from disease-centered to patient goals-directed care for patients with multiple chronic conditions: patient value-based care. JAMA Cardiol. 2016;1(1):9–10.
9. Naik AD, Dyer CB, Kunik ME, McCullough LB. Patient autonomy for the management of chronic conditions: a 2-component reconceptualization. Am J Bioeth. 2009;9(2):23–30.
10. Walter LC, Covinsky KE. Cancer screening in elderly patients: a framework for individualized decision making. JAMA. 2001;285(21):2750–6.
11. ePrognosis. Available from: https://eprognosis.ucsf.edu, Accessed 23 Feb 2018.
12. Schoenborn NL, Lee K, Pollack CE, Armacost K, Dy SM, Bridges JFP, Xue QL, Wolff AC, Boyd C. Older Adults' views and communication preferences about cancer screening cessation. JAMA Intern Med. 2017;177(8):1121–8.
13. Boyd CM, Darer J, Boult C, Fried LP, Boult L, Wu AW. Clinical practice guidelines and quality of care for older patients with multiple comorbid diseases: implications for pay for performance. JAMA. 2005;294(6):716–24.
14. George J, Vuong T, Bailey MJ, et al. Medication regimen complexity and adherence in patients at risk of medication misadventure. J Pharm Pract Res. 2006;36:99–102.
15. Franek J. Self-management support interventions for persons with chronic disease: an evidence-based analysis. Ont Health Technol Assess Ser. 2013;13(9):1–60. eCollection 2013.
16. Alhawassi TM, Krass I, Bajorek BV, Pont LG. A systematic review of the prevalence and risk factors for adverse drug reactions in the elderly in the acute care setting. Clin Interv Aging. 2014;9:2079–86.
17. Nobili A, Pasina L, Tettamanti M, Lucca U, Riva E, Marzona I, et al. Potentially severe drug interactions in elderly outpatients: results of an observational study of an administrative prescription database. J Clin Pharm Ther. 2009;34:377–86.
18. Westphal EC, Alkema G, Seidel R, Chernof B. How to get better care with lower costs? See the person, not the patient. J Am Geriatr Soc. 2016;64(1):19–21.
19. Counsell SR, Callahan CM, Buttar AB, Clark DO, Frank KI. Geriatric Resources for Assessment and Care of Elders (GRACE): a new model of primary care for low-income seniors. J Am Geriatr Soc. 2006;54(7):1136–41.
20. Counsell SR, Callahan CM, Clark DO, Tu W, Buttar AB, Stump TE, et al. Geriatric care management for low-income seniors: a randomized controlled trial. JAMA. 2007;298(22):2623–33.
21. Eng C, Pedulla J, Eleazer GP, McCann R, Fox N. Program of All-inclusive Care for the Elderly (PACE): an innovative model of integrated geriatric care and financing. J Am Geriatr Soc. 1997;45(2):223–32.
22. Segelman M, Szydlowski J, Kinosian B, McNabney M, Raziano DB, Eng C, et al. Hospitalizations in the program of all-inclusive care for the elderly. J Am Geriatr Soc. 2014;62(2):320–4.
23. Pilotto A, Cella A, Daragjati J, Veronese N, Musacchio C, Mello AM, et al. Three decades of comprehensive geriatric assessment: evidence coming from different healthcare settings and specific clinical conditions. J Am Med Dir Assoc. 2017;18(2):192.e1–.e11.
24. Guided Care [Available from: http://www.guidedcare.org.
25. Galvin JE, Valois L, Zweig Y. Collaborative transdisciplinary team approach for dementia care. Neurodegener Dis Manag. 2014; 4(6):455–69.
26. Edwards ST, Peterson K, Chan B, Anderson J, Helfand M. Effectiveness of intensive primary care interventions: a systematic review. J Gen Intern Med. 2017;32(12):1377–86.
27. Stall N, Nowaczynski M, Sinha SK. Systematic review of outcomes from home-based primary care programs for homebound older adults. J Am Geriatr Soc. 2014;62(12):2243–51.
28. Shepperd S, Iliffe S, Doll HA, Clarke MJ, Kalra L, Wilson AD, et al. Admission avoidance hospital at home. Cochrane Database Syst Rev. 2016;9:CD007491.
29. Conley J, O'Brien CW, Leff BA, Bolen S, Zulman D. Alternative strategies to inpatient hospitalization for acute medical conditions: a systematic review. JAMA Intern Med. 2016;176(11):1693–702.
30. Kahn JH, Magauran BG, Olshaker JS, Shankar KN. Current trends in geriatric emergency medicine. Emerg Med Clin North Am. 2016;34(3):435–52.
31. Physicians ACoE, Society AG, Association EN, Medicine SfAE, Force GEDGT. Geriatric emergency department guidelines. Ann Emerg Med. 2014;63(5):e7–25.
32. Fox MT, Persaud M, Maimets I, O'Brien K, Brooks D, Tregunno D, et al. Effectiveness of acute geriatric unit care using acute care for elders components: a systematic review and meta-analysis. J Am Geriatr Soc. 2012;60(12):2237–45.
33. Inouye SK, Bogardus ST, Baker DI, Leo-Summers L, Cooney LM. The Hospital Elder Life Program: a model of care to prevent cognitive and functional decline in older hospitalized patients. Hospital Elder Life Program. J Am Geriatr Soc. 2000;48(12):1697–706.
34. Capezuti E, Boltz M, Cline D, Dickson VV, Rosenberg MC, Wagner L, et al. Nurses Improving Care for Healthsystem Elders - a model for optimising the geriatric nursing practice environment. J Clin Nurs. 2012;21(21–22):3117–25.
35. Chen P, Hung WW. Geriatric orthopedic co-management of older adults with hip fracture: an emerging standard. Ann Transl Med. 2015;3(16):224.
36. Labson MC. Adapting the joint commission's seven foundations of safe and effective transitions of care to home. Home Healthc Now. 2015;33(3):142–6.
37. Toles M, Colón-Emeric C, Asafu-Adjei J, Moreton E, Hanson LC. Transitional care of older adults in skilled nursing facilities: a systematic review. Geriatr Nurs. 2016;37(4):296–301.
38. Lindquist LA, Miller RK, Saltsman WS, Carnahan J, Rowe TA, Arbaje AI, et al. SGIM-AMDA-AGS consensus best practice recommendations for transitioning patients' healthcare from skilled nursing facilities to the community. J Gen Intern Med. 2017;32(2):199–203.
39. Kane RL, Huckfeldt P, Tappen R, Engstrom G, Rojido C, Newman D, et al. Effects of an intervention to reduce hospitalizations from nursing homes: a randomized implementation trial of the INTERACT program. JAMA Intern Med. 2017;177(9):1257–64.
40. Ouslander JG, Bonner A, Herndon L, Shutes J. The Interventions to Reduce Acute Care Transfers (INTERACT) quality improvement program: an overview for medical directors and primary care clinicians in long term care. J Am Med Dir Assoc. 2014;15(3):162–70.
41. Struck BD, Brown EA, Madison S. Advance care planning in the outpatient geriatric medicine setting. Prim Care. 2017;44(3):511–8.
42. Sepucha KR, Simmons LH, Barry MJ, Edgman-Levitan S, Licurse AM, Chaguturu SK. Ten years, forty decision aids, and thousands of patient uses: shared decision making at Massachusetts General Hospital. Health Aff (Millwood). 2016;35(4):630–6.
43. Levine DM, Landon BE, Linder JA. Trends in patient-perceived shared decision making among adults in the United States, 2002-2014. Ann Fam Med. 2017;15(6):552–6.
44. van Weert JC, van Munster BC, Sanders R, Spijker R, Hooft L, Jansen J. Decision aids to help older people make health decisions: a systematic review and meta-analysis. BMC Med Inform Decis Mak. 2016;16:45.
45. Riker GI, Setter SM. Polypharmacy in older adults at home: what it is and what to do about it--implications for home healthcare and hospice. Home Healthc Nurse. 2012;30(8):474–85; quiz 86-7.
46. Lip GY, Nieuwlaat R, Pisters R, Lane DA, Crijns HJ. Refining clinical risk stratification for predicting stroke and thromboembolism in atrial fibrillation using a novel risk factor-based approach: the euro heart survey on atrial fibrillation. Chest. 2010;137(2):263–72.
47. Pisters R, Lane DA, Nieuwlaat R, de Vos CB, Crijns HJ, Lip GY. A novel user-friendly score (HAS-BLED) to assess 1-year risk of major bleeding in patients with atrial fibrillation: the Euro Heart Survey. Chest. 2010;138(5):1093–100.
48. Project Red [Available from: http://www.bu.edu/fammed/projectred/index.html.

49. Coleman EA, Parry C, Chalmers S, Min SJ. The care transitions intervention: results of a randomized controlled trial. Arch Intern Med. 2006;166(17):1822–8.
50. Hirschman KB, Shaid E, McCauley K, Pauly MV, Naylor MD. Continuity of care: the transitional care model. Online J Issues Nurs. 2015;20(3):1.
51. Hansen LO, Greenwald JL, Budnitz T, Howell E, Halasyamani L, Maynard G, et al. Project BOOST: effectiveness of a multihospital effort to reduce rehospitalization. J Hosp Med. 2013;8(8):421–7.
52. American Geriatrics Society 2019 Updated AGS Beers Criteria® for potentially inappropriate medication use in older adults. J Am Geriatr Soc. 2019;67: 674–94. https://doi.org/10.1111/jgs.15767.
53. Barry PJ, Gallagher P, Ryan C, O'mahony D. START (screening tool to alert doctors to the right treatment)--an evidence-based screening tool to detect prescribing omissions in elderly patients. Age Ageing. 2007;36(6):632–8.
54. Gallagher P, Ryan C, Byrne S, Kennedy J, O'Mahony D. STOPP (Screening Tool of Older Person's Prescriptions) and START (Screening Tool to Alert doctors to Right Treatment). Consensus validation. Int J Clin Pharmacol Ther. 2008;46(2):72–83.
55. Rudolph JL, Salow MJ, Angelini MC, McGlinchey RE. The anticholinergic risk scale and anticholinergic adverse effects in older persons. Arch Intern Med. 2008;168(5):508–13.

Geriatric Preoperative Evaluation of the Older Adult

Stephanie Le, Nami Safai Haeri, and Allen D. Andrade

A. Chun (ed.), *Geriatric Practice*, https://doi.org/10.1007/978-3-030-19625-7_10

Clinical Scenario

Ms. MN is an 89-year-old active older adult with obstructive jaundice and a surgically resectable mass in the head of her pancreas. She lives alone and is independently mobile, cognitively intact, and socially active. She has a history of hypertension and diet-controlled diabetes. She is independent with activities of daily living (ADLS) and instrumental activities of daily living (IADLS). She is able to walk two blocks without pause but has not really had the need to climb stairs and is unsure if she will have difficulty climbing them. On examination she is jaundiced and appears exhausted but comfortable. Her cardiac, pulmonary, abdominal, neurologic, and musculoskeletal exams are unremarkable. She takes less than 20 seconds on the timed up and go test which suggests good mobility. On admission, an electrocardiogram showed no acute changes. 2D ECHO, nuclear stress test, and chest x-ray were unremarkable. A complete blood count showed a mild normocytic anemia. A comprehensive metabolic panel demonstrated an obstructive pattern on the hepatic panel. A goal of care conversation was subsequently conducted with the patient and her family to discuss surgical resection of the mass. Given the patient's age and recent poor health, she was deemed to be at increased risk of post-operative complications and a prolonged, complicated post-surgical recovery period. The patient recognized that without the potentially curative surgical procedure, her life expectancy would be limited. Given her self-reported good quality of life, she felt that attempting the procedure, even if it led to further morbidity or death, was more acceptable to her than following a conservative approach. Although the medical and surgical teams and the patient's family expressed concerns regarding proceeding with surgery, they all acknowledged the patients view point and the goals of care she outlined. After finding no medical contraindications to surgery, the patient proceeded to have a pancreaticoduodenectomy.

10

10.1 Background

The geriatric preoperative assessment includes risk factor assessment with a focus on risk reduction of potential complications in the medical, social, functional, and neuropsychological domains. Recent comparative trials confirm that older adults who participate in a geriatric preoperative assessment have fewer complications, shorter hospitalizations, more frequent discharge to home, and fewer readmissions than a comparison group [1]. The geriatrician's role in a preoperative assessment goes beyond pre-procedure medical optimization by including additional plans for how to preserve the older adult's function, cognition, and social well-being. The geriatrician can prepare patients on what to expect during the post-operative recovery period, lay the groundwork for patients through transition planning, and explain settings for rehabilitation, short-stay skilled nursing facilities, or long-term acute care hospitals. Geriatric preoperative assessments also take into consideration the impact of aging on older adult's ability to tolerate surgery. The patient's ability to tolerate surgery rests not on the patient's physiologic reserve but also on environmental factors such as urgency of the surgery, nutrition, and social support. We have divided this chapter into a medical assessment organized around major relevant organ systems followed by functional, social, and psychological assessments relevant to a geriatric preoperative evaluation.

10.2 Medical Assessment

10.2.1 Cardiovascular System

An older adult's cardiovascular system has a reduced ability to compensate for stress. Changes in cardiac conduction also increase the risk of arrhythmia. Older patients are more prone to having perioperative cardiac adverse events [2]. We recommend calculating the revised cardiac risk index (RCRI), which is designed to predict post-operative complications such as myocardial infarction, pulmonary edema, ventricular fibrillation or cardiac arrest, and complete heart block. In patients with low risk by the RCRI, no further testing is indicated. In higher-risk patients, we recommend pursuing further cardiovascular testing if it will change clinical management [3]. An alternative to the RCRI is the American College of Surgeons National Surgical Quality Improvement Program (NSQIP) score which was designed to determine risk factors associated with intraoperative and post-operative myocardial infarction or cardiac arrest [4]. Routine 12-lead electrocardiogram testing is not recommended for everyone. Obtain an electrocardiogram only in patients with coronary heart disease, heart failure, significant arrhythmia, peripheral arterial disease, cerebrovascular disease, shortness of breath, or other significant structural heart disease, except in those undergoing low-risk surgeries. A 12-lead electrocardiogram may be considered in other asymptomatic patients who are undergoing higher-risk surgeries. Pursue an echocardiogram in patients with shortness of breath of unknown origin or any patient with previously documented left ventricular dysfunction with no assessment within the past year [3]. In patients with elevated cardiac risk and moderate or good functional capacity (more than 4 metabolic equivalent of task (MET)), no further testing is recommended. Examples of activities with METs greater than 4 include climbing a flight of stairs, walking up a hill, and walking on level ground at 4 mph [3].

In patients with elevated cardiac risk and unknown or poor functional capacity – less than 4 METs – pharmacologic stress testing is recommended if the results will change management [3]. Twenty-four-hour ambulatory monitoring is indicated primarily for patients with syncope or significant bradycardia or tachycardia if not previously evaluated. Preoperative angiography is recommended in patients with proven myocardial ischemia and unstable chest pain (Canadian Cardiovascular Society Class III–IV) despite adequate medical therapy who require non-urgent, non-cardiac surgery. In patients with intermediate or high cardiovascular risk, a referral to a cardiologist for further evaluation may be indicated.

Heart failure (HF) The initial step in preoperative evaluation of patient with heart failure is assessment of functional status, symptoms and signs of heart failure, and comorbidities that may exacerbate the heart failure. In general, patients with a heart failure who are asymptomatic at the time of surgery should continue their current medical regimen. Patients with symptomatic heart failure should be medically optimized prior to surgery unless the surgery is emergent. Natriuretic peptides should be assessed as routine preoperative evaluation in patients with known cardiac dysfunction. In patients with arrhythmias, we recommend continuing oral antiarrhythmic drugs before surgery. Patients with permanent pacemaker (PPM)/automated implantable cardioverter-defibrillator (AICD) should undergo interrogation of the device prior to surgery [5].

Valvular heart disease In symptomatic patients with aortic stenosis, consider aortic valve replacement before non-cardiac surgery. Asymptomatic patients with aortic stenosis can proceed with elective surgeries. In asymptomatic patients with mitral stenosis if systolic pulmonary artery pressure is <50 mmHg and valve area is >1.5 cm^2, non-cardiac surgery can be performed. In symptomatic patients with mitral stenosis or in patients with systolic pulmonary artery pressure >50 mmHg, correct the mitral stenosis before non-cardiac surgery. In aortic or mitral regurgitation, non-cardiac surgery can be performed safely in asymptomatic patients. If a patient is symptomatic or has LV dysfunction, consider valve replacement [5]. New techniques and technology in minimally invasive surgery have broadened the eligibility of patients for various valve repairs and replacement. Transcatheter aortic valve replacement (TAVR) is an alternative for patients unable to undergo open heart surgery [6].

Prosthetic heart valves All mechanical valves require anticoagulation. When patients on anticoagulants are planned to have a surgical procedure with a high risk of bleeding, it may be necessary to stop their usual anticoagulant to reduce bleeding risk during the perioperative period. In patients with certain high-risk conditions, substituting an alternative anticoagulant with a short half-life while a patient's usual anticoagulant is held (a process known as "bridging") is recommended to minimize the risk of thrombotic events. Usually heparin or enoxaparin is used as a bridging agent. Of note, patients on direct-acting oral anticoagulants (DOACs) may not need to bridge since they have shorter half-lives and the duration that the patient is off of them is shorter. Bridging is indicated in patients with mechanical aortic valve plus additional clotting risk (atrial fibrillation, previous VTE, systolic heart failure with EF <30%, multiple mechanical valves, other hypercoagulable condition), older mechanical valve, and mechanical mitral or tricuspid valve (■ Table 10.1).

■ **Table 10.1** Anticoagulation bridging therapy

Condition	When bridging is recommended
Atrial fibrillation	For patients with a CHADS2VASC > ≥5 *or* stroke within the last 3 months
Mechanical aortic valve	If additional stroke risk exists
Mechanical mitral valve	Always in major procedures where holding anticoagulation is necessary
DVT/PE	Occurred within the last 3 months prior to surgery
Thromboembolic stroke	Occurred within the last 3 months prior to surgery
Coronary stents	Recently placed – within 3 months prior to surgery

Resuming anticoagulation: Resumption of anticoagulation may vary depending on whether hemostasis has been achieved. Discussion with the surgeon performing the procedure is necessary to determine a safe time to resume anticoagulation. Generally, warfarin may be resumed within 24 hours of the procedure. Short-acting anticoagulants for post-operative bridging can be resumed after 24 hours, or later if there is higher risk.

Atrial fibrillation Anticoagulation bridging is beneficial if the patient has had a stroke within the past 6 months or if their CHADS2VASC score is ≥5 [7].

Guidelines for surgical delay after coronary revascularization Surgery should be delayed if possible after revascularization with coronary stenting. Ideally, anti-platelet agents (P2Y12 receptor inhibitors such as clopidogrel) should be continued, although the risks of bleeding vs. in-stent thrombosis must be weighed. If P2Y12 inhibitors must be discontinued, aspirin should be continued. Patients with high cardiac risk should be initiated on appropriate high-intensity statins [8].

Hypertension Anesthesia can lead to an increase in blood pressure in normotensive individuals. When hypertension is discovered in a preoperative evaluation, testing for target organ damage is recommended. In patients with blood pressure of 180/110 mmHg and above, the potential benefits of delaying surgery to optimize pharmacological therapy should be weighed against the risk of delaying the procedure. There is no clear evidence favoring one mode of antihypertensive therapy over another. There is no recommendation on whether diuretics should be discontinued prior to surgery. Beta blockers should be continued in the perioperative period and continued throughout the hospital stay. In patients with intermediate to high risk, it may be even reasonable to begin perioperative beta blockers; however, we do not recommend initiation of beta blocker on the day of surgery. Hold angiotensin-converting enzyme inhibitors/receptor blockers for a period of 24 hours prior to surgery except in those with heart failure or with inadequately treated hypertension that cannot be improved before surgery [3].

Peripheral arterial disease When assessing an older adult for possible revascularization, functional status is among the most important things to consider. Revascularization is a high-risk surgery; thus, medical optimization and careful candidate selection is crucial for successful outcomes. Surgery is most likely to be beneficial to older adults as a means to preserve ambulation and independence. Studies have some good outcomes after revascularization both for chronic and critical limb ischemia, with upward of 70% of patients returning to live at home post-procedure [9].

10.2.2 Pulmonary System

Increasing age is an independent risk factor for post-operative pulmonary complications. Older adults develop an impaired ability to cough effectively over time (decreased respiratory muscle strength, increase chest wall stiffness), decreased mucociliary clearance, and greater ventilation-perfusion mismatch leading to an increased risk of pneumonia and hypoxia in the post-operative period [10]. Studies have shown a twofold risk for patients aged 60–69 and threefold for aged 70–79 for pulmonary complications. However, age may not be the strongest predictor of pulmonary complication. The type of surgery has been shown in one study to be a greater predictive factor. Proximity to the diaphragm and thoracic cavity increases pulmonary risk. This is thought to be due to pain, splinting, and inability to take deep breaths. Neurosurgery, neck surgery, aortic surgery, and other vascular surgeries also carry higher pulmonary risk [11]. Age ≥ 70 was only slightly higher risk than renal dysfunction, low albumin, and poor functional status. The American College of Physicians identifies the following risk factors to identify patients who require pulmonary evaluation: chronic obstructive pulmonary disease, age older than 60 years, American Society of Anesthesiologists (ASA) class II or greater, functionally dependent, and congestive heart failure. No specific models exist to predict pulmonary risk in older adults. A sample of commonly used risk assessment models for the general population is discussed below. While not aimed at older adults exclusively, these models can help guide discussion regarding the risk of post-operative complication, especially the possibility of longer-term intubation and tracheostomy which are important topics to explore with patients and families during the preoperative assessment. ARISCAT risk index [12] predicts the risk of any post-operative pulmonary complications, including respiratory infection, respiratory failure, bronchospasm, atelectasis, pleural effusion, pneumothorax, or aspiration pneumonitis. Arozullah respiratory failure index [13] predicts the likelihood of remaining on the ventilator 48 hours after surgery. Gupta calculator [14] predicts the likelihood of post-operative respiratory failure, definite specifically as the inability to come off a ventilator after 48 hours. The literature is not specific to geriatric patients; however, the following are reasonable guidelines to determine which patients may benefit from pulmonary function tests: those undergoing lung resection, coronary artery bypass grafting, pre-existing asthma or chronic obstructive pulmonary disease, and likely undiagnosed obstructive airway diseases. Routine chest x-ray is not recommended as part of a preoperative assessment for low-risk patients. Older adults are automatically considered at high risk by most assessment standards. Additionally, they have a higher prevalence of abnormal chest x-ray findings [15]. However, the clinical significance of abnormal chest x-ray is very low. A meta-analysis by Archer et al. demonstrated that abnormal chest x-ray that changed management occurred in only 0.1% of cases. Additionally, only 1.4% of these abnormal findings were "unexpected," meaning they would not have been predicted by history and exam [16]. A low serum albumin (<3.0) is correlated with a high likelihood of post-operative pulmonary complication. Nutrition status and other chronic diseases in older adults (cirrhosis, heart failure) may predispose to low albumin states. Elevated BUN increases risk of post-operative respiratory failure, though it is not as strong a predictor as albumin [17]. *Common conditions that affect pulmonary outcomes:* Functional status is a key component of a comprehensive geriatric assessment and has a significant impact on post-operative pulmonary complications. Partial dependence has 1.65 odds ratio of pulmonary complication; total dependence has 2.51 odds ratio of pulmonary complication; being categorized as ASA class II or higher is linked to increased risk of pulmonary complication and has an odds ratio of 4.8. Patients with cognitive impairment, prior stroke, gastroesophageal reflux disease, diabetes, dry mouth, and poor dentition are at increased risk for post-operative pneumonia. Smoking increases the incidence of pulmonary complications. Limited data exists on smoking cessation preoperatively, and no data is specific for older populations. In younger adults, smoking cessation more than 8 weeks prior to surgery has the greatest risk reduction. Chronic obstructive pulmonary disease increases risk of post-operative pulmonary complication, with an odds ratio of 1.79. Asthma has not been linked to increased pulmonary complication. Congestive heart failure significantly increases pulmonary complications, with an odds ratio of 2.93 [11]. *Venothrombolism:* The issue of anticoagulation in older adults is challenging. The benefit in terms of stroke prevention or treatment of deep vein thrombosis/pulmonary embolism must be weighed against the risk of bleeding. Several bleeding risk scores exist, including the HEMORR2HAGES risk index, HAS-BLED risk score, ATRIA, and OBRI. The HAS-BLED score has been shown to best predict clinically relevant bleeding, particularly intracranial hemorrhage [18]. Falls are a problem in older adults and often are cited as the reason for withholding anticoagulation. Subsequently we may be undertreating older adults. Evidence shows that patients with moderate to high risk of stroke still benefit from anticoagulation, even if they are at a high fall risk [19]. While bleeding is a concern in older adults, rates of major bleeding have been found to be relatively low. A large study of 1500 patient found 2.4 major bleeding events for every 1000 patient-months. Insufficient education about bleeding risk and polypharmacy were the greatest risk factors for bleeding [20]. Stroke risk increases with age; therefore, there is increased benefit of oral anticoagulation with age. However, anti-platelets have been found to have decreased benefit for stroke prevention with age [21]. *Warfarin:* If there are 24 hours or more until surgery, give vitamin K to reverse the effect of warfarin [22]. There is no benefit to lower international normalized ratio (INR) goals with warfarin for preventing ischemic stroke in older adults. Tightly controlled INR with warfarin decreases risk of intracranial hemorrhage. The advantage of warfarin is that it is reversible but the disadvantage is the need for frequent monitoring. Direct-acting oral anticoagulants (DOACs) have a lower rate of intracranial hemorrhage than warfarin. *Dabigatran:* RE-LY trial found that at the 110 mg dose, dabigatran was noninferior to warfarin for stroke prevention but had a lower rate of bleeding [23]. Currently dabigatran is the only DOAC with an approved reversal agent: idarucizumab. *Rivaroxaban:* ROCKET-AF demonstrates non-inferiority to warfarin for stroke prevention. There were similar rates of bleeding but lower overall rates of intracranial hemorrhage [24]. *Apixaban:* ARISTOTLE trial showed that apixaban is superior to warfarin for stroke prevention, results in less bleeding, and has improved mortality [25]. Oral anticoagulants and antiplatelets are generally held prior to elective surgery. Discussion with the surgeon is necessary to determine which anticoagulants need to be held. Additional consultation with cardiology or hematology may be necessary in high-risk patients. For patients on anticoagulation receiving implantable cardiac defibrillator/pacemaker placement, continuing anticoagulation with warfarin has shown decreased rates of pocket hematoma than when bridging with heparin [26]. Known venous thromboembolism (VTE): The highest risk of recurrence of VTE is within 3 months of the event. Elective surgery should be delayed if possible to avoid this period [27].

VTE prophylaxis VTE prophylaxis should be used in patients with higher risk for DVT. Older adults have an increased risk of DVT. Other factors are prior DVT, malignancy, infection/inflammation, and stroke. Those who are immobile post-operative also are at increased risk and should have prophylaxis. Hip replacements carry a higher risk for DVT, as do abdominal/pelvic surgery in those with cancer [28].

10.2.3 Gastroenterology System

10.2.3.1 Liver Disease

Liver disease incurs a higher operative risk, even in younger patients. While there are surgical risk-prediction models for patients with cirrhosis and end-stage liver disease, including the Child-Pugh score and the MELD [29], neither of these were studied in older adults. *Coagulopathy in liver disease:* Valuating INR is reasonable to assess coagulopathy. Improvement in nutrition status may be beneficial in correcting INR. *Hepatic encephalopathy:* Hepatic encephalopathy predicts a poorer prognosis in patients with liver disease. Post-operatively, hepatic encephalopathy should be considered as a cause of altered mental status in cirrhotic patients. *Inflammatory bowel disease (IBD):* discussion with a gastroenterologist in patients with IBD is recommended prior to surgery, particularly if there is active disease or use of immune-modulating treatments. *Constipation:* Older adults are at risk of constipation in the post-operative setting for multiple reasons. The use of opiates for post-operative pain is a common cause, as is relative immobility. A good bowel regimen should include a motility-stimulating agent such as senna or a bisacodyl suppository. Docusate is generally ineffective for post-operative constipation in older adults. *Enteral feeding:* Temporary enteral feeding may be required post-operatively depending on the type of surgery and post-operative complications. The need for enteral feeding should be discussed with patients and families prior to surgery, with care to distinguish between temporary and long-term enteral feeding. For patients with advanced dementia, enteral feeding has not been shown to improve nutrition status or prolong survival nor does it decrease aspiration risk [30].

10.2.4 Renal System

Loss of kidney function with age increases acute kidney injury and renal failure risk. Changes in renal physiology also increase sensitivity to hypotension and increase the risk of acute kidney injury [31]. Renal function declines with age due to a multitude of physiologic changes. These changes also predispose to a higher risk of acute kidney injury and greater incidence of chronic kidney disease [32]. Similarly, the physiologic stresses created by surgery and anesthesia may be magnified. Patients with chronic kidney disease have at least doubled the likelihood of cardiovascular events and death after surgery as those with normal renal function [33]. The incidence of acute kidney injury after surgery is high. After cardiac surgery the rate can be up to 25% [34]. Additionally, a systemic review and meta-analysis found that those with acute kidney injury had a substantially increased risk of developing chronic kidney disease or end-stage renal disease, with a hazard ratio of 8.8 [35]. *Dialysis:* There is a higher post-operative mortality in hemodialysis patients [36]. A nephrologist should be involved in the preoperative screening process for any dialysis patients. A new dialysis requirement post-operatively is a poor prognostic factor. Older adults ≥75 years of age have a high 3-month mortality after starting dialysis, even in non-emergent settings [37]. Prior to any major surgery with a risk for AKI or renal failure, a thorough discussion of the risks and benefits of dialysis should be initiated with patients and their families/healthcare proxies. While there is no specific evidence to support this practice, it is generally recommended to hold diuretics on the day of surgery due to the theoretical risk for intraoperative hypotension [38].

Angiotensin-converting enzyme inhibitor/receptor blockers can be discontinued the evening before surgery, possibly 24 hours up to surgery. Increased incidence of intraoperative hypotension was found in patients who continued their angiotensin-converting enzyme inhibitor/receptor blockers on the morning of surgery [39]. Non-steroidal anti-inflammatory drugs: Discontinue prior to surgery to reduce acute kidney injury.

Dose adjustment and glomerular filtration rate (GFR) calculation Medications should always be dose-adjusted based upon renal function. The Crockoft-Gault formula, while widely used for calculation of creatinine clearance, should be used with caution in older adults as it is inaccurate and underestimates GFR (National Institute of Diabetes and Digestive and Kidney Diseases – NIDDK). Two alternatives being studied for calculating GFR are Chronic Kidney Disease Epidemiology Collaboration (CKD-EPI) and Modification of Diet in Renal Disease (MDRD) study. CKD-EPI may be more accurate for GFR calculations for patients ≥65 years old. Discussion with a pharmacist is recommended if there is concern about renal impairment. It should be noted that the Crockoft-Gault formula is used in studies that validate medications for approval with the FDA.

10.2.5 Endocrine System

Diabetes Preoperative glucose levels of >200 mg/dL has been found to be associated with deep wound infections [40]. For elective procedures, check HbA1C or have a glucometer diary, and if poorly controlled, surgery should be postponed. The American Diabetes Association (ADA) has endorsed a target glucose range of 80–180 mg/dL for the perioperative period. Patients on insulin should receive half their usual dose of intermediate-acting NPH insulin dose or full doses of a long-acting or pump basal insulin. Monitor blood glucose every 4–6 hours while NPO and correct with short-acting insulin if needed [41]. Basal insulin analogs and pump can be continued preoperatively and on the day of the surgery [42]. Oral hypoglycemic drugs or non-insulin injectable agents can be continued until the morning of surgery. They can be reinstated as soon as the patient is eating well. Consider cancelling non-emergent surgeries in patients with metabolic abnormalities (diabetic ketoacidosis, hyperosmolar hyperglycemia state) or blood glucose level above 400–500 mg/dL [43]. *Thyroid disease:* Myxedema coma is a potential risk in older adults with moderate to severe hypothyroidism undergoing surgery. If surgery is non-urgent, consider postponing until a euthyroid state is achieved. Patients with subclinical hypothyroidism may proceed with either urgent or elective surgeries. In severe hypothyroidism (myxedema coma; clinical symptoms such as altered mentation, pericardial effusion, or heart failure; or very low levels of T4), surgery should be postponed until hypothyroidism has been treated. If surgery is emergent, then start treating the patient as soon as the diagnosis is made [44]. Hyperthyroidism can result in thyroid storm with surgical stress. Treat hyperthyroidism before elective surgery. If surgery cannot be postponed, then initiate treatment as soon as possible. Hyperthyroid patients who require urgent surgery should be evaluated for possible cardiopulmonary disease such as arrhythmia, ischemia, and heart failure [45]. Thyroid medications (levothyroxine, propylthiouracil, etc.) should be continued in the perioperative period.

Adrenal insufficiency Adrenal insufficiency puts the patient at increased risk for perioperative cardiovascular collapse. Steroids at dose equivalent or greater to prednisone >20 mg/day for ≥3 weeks are considered to have iatrogenic suppression of the HPA axis and require stress dose steroids in the perioperative period. Consider adrenal insufficiency in patients on lower doses (5–20 mg/day) as well, and it is reasonable to give empiric corticosteroid coverage. Given the risk of stress-dose steroids (hyperglycemia, mania/psychosis, delirium), it is reasonable to perform testing to rule out adrenal insufficiency in those on lower doses to avoid unnecessary glucocorticoid use.

Morbid obesity Obstructive sleep apnea (OSA) and metabolic syndrome should be evaluated preoperatively. Perioperative continuous positive airway pressure in patients with OSA is recommended to decrease the chance for some of the post-operative pulmonary complications, such as atelectasis, pneumonia, and reintubation [46].

Nutrition Check for dietary preferences or restrictions to ensure an appropriate diet is ordered. Identify if the patient is having difficulty with loose fitting dentures or dental issues that need further evaluation, and assess if there are any signs of aspiration (coughing with eating, trouble swallowing). Record patient's weight, perform a brief nutritional assessment such as the mini nutritional assessment tool, and check for use of any supplements or vitamins [47].

Surgical mortality is higher in malnourished patients. Albumin has been traditionally used as a marker of poor nutrition, although this practice has become controversial. Regardless, there is a correlation between low albumin and poor surgical outcomes, including increased length of stay. Weight loss of ≥10% within 6 months prior to surgery is also a predictor of negative post-operative outcomes [47]. Older adults should undergo daily evaluation of their ability to take in adequate nutrition and risk of aspiration. Initiate dietary consultation and/or formal swallowing assessment if indicated. Patients who use dentures should have them easily available. Vision should also be assessed, as this can impair the ability to eat, and a patient's glasses should be easily accessible if needed. Patients should have an elevated head of bed and be sitting upright while eating and for 1 hour after completion of eating. Enteral feeding has to be started as early as possible [48].

10.3 Anesthesia

An anesthesia plan should be carefully tailored to each older adult undergoing surgery. This should include a prophylactic bowel regimen [49]. Scheduled acetaminophen is an appropriate first-line treatment option. In cases with contraindication to acetaminophen or if acetaminophen is insufficient to achieve pain control, then patients may require low-dose opiates or may benefit from local or regional pain management techniques [50]. Most studies examining elective surgery suggest no difference in post-operative delirium when regional and general anesthesia are compared [51]. Epidural anesthesia may provide benefits over general anesthesia in an older adult, including decreasing atelectasis, allowing for earlier extubation and reducing the length of ICU stays [52]. Post-anesthesia, slower recovery of psychomotor and neurocognitive function may be observed in older adults compared to younger populations, with cognition sometimes taking months to recover [53].

Review medications and evaluate for potential discontinuation of nonessential ones in the perioperative period. Inappropriate medication use in older patients before cancer surgery has been associated with increased incidence of postoperative delirium [54]. Consider potential for withdrawal, progression of disease with interruption of drug, and interactions with anesthetic agents as well [55]. For example medications such as rivastigmine or donepezil that are commonly prescribed for patients with dementia are associated with a prolonged effect of the anesthetic succinylcholine or the interaction between SSRI antidepressants with some of the serotonergic medications administered in the perioperative period may lead into serotonin syndrome. We also need to keep in mind that sometimes clinical depression or acute psychosis may develop following acute withdrawal of regular antidepressants or benzodiazepines. Always check for herbs or over-the-counter medication use. For example, ginkgo biloba may increase risk for bleeding during the surgery or Kava may increase sedative effect of anesthesia [56].

10.4 Psychological Assessment

Decision-making capacity The assessment of decision-making capacity generally is comprised of the ability of a patient to communicate a choice, understand health information, and appreciate the medical consequences of decisions and reasons about treatment options. Keep in mind that capacity is situation dependent. Patients with cognitive impairment may still retain the capacity to make certain decisions. In patients who do not have the capacity to make decisions, it is important to identify an alternate decision-maker. One such person may be the patient-appointed healthcare proxy. If no healthcare proxy has been appointed, next of kin and surrogacy laws generally determine the legal decision-maker. If no surrogates exist, then it may be necessary to seek legal guardianship [57].

Mental illness – schizophrenia This encompasses a wide spectrum of disease. Some individuals will still retain capacity to make decisions. *Depression:* This can affect decision-making capacity and can interfere with recovery from surgery. Depression should be screened for and treated appropriately prior to surgery. Antidepressants should be continued during the perioperative period. Stopping the antidepressant during the preoperative period may cause withdrawal (discontinuation syndrome). Symptoms of withdrawal include nausea, abdominal pain, diarrhea, affective symptoms, and insomnia [58]. Lithium: Kidney injury and changes in renal function can affect lithium levels during the preoperative period, risking lithium toxicity. Monitor renal function closely and adjust lithium doses as needed. Antipsychotics should be continued through the perioperative period. It should be noted that tramadol can interact with antipsychotics, SSRIs, and TCAs and lower the seizure threshold. Additionally, neuroleptic malignant syndrome and serotonin syndrome should be considered on the differential for altered mental status and fever for patients taking antidepressants or antipsychotics. *Substance abuse:* All patients should be screened for substance abuse prior to surgery. Withdrawal from alcohol may be deadly. While withdrawal from cocaine or heroin may not be fatal, it can be a cause of delirium post-operatively. Screening for prescription drug abuse is also important. Tobacco cessation should be recommended and a referral for treatment offered. *Preoperative cognitive status/dementia:* It is important to establish a baseline cognitive status on all patients undergoing surgery. Older adults should be screened for possible dementia or mild cognitive impairment. Two commonly used screening tools for dementia are the Folstein Mini Mental Status Exam (MMSE) and the Montreal Cognitive Assessment (MOCA). The MMSE and other screening tests are generally 70–90% sensitive and 80–90% specific for dementia [59].

Post-anesthesia cognitive dysfunction A large study of 1200 patients over the age of 60 found that about 25% had post-operative cognitive dysfunction. This generally improved, with only 10% reporting continued cognitive dysfunction after 3 months. However, about 1% of those patients had not returned to baseline after 2 years [60]. This phenomenon highlights the importance of baseline cognitive assessments, as well as establishing healthcare proxies and advanced directives. *Seizure:* Anesthesia and metabolic disturbances around surgery can cause seizures. Tramadol can interact with antipsychotics, SSRIs, and TCAs and lower the seizure threshold.

Cerebrovascular disease Patients at high risk of stroke should be medically optimized, controlling blood pressure, hyperlipidemia, diabetes, and hypo-/hyperthyroidism. Specialist referral would be appropriate if a patient has had a recent stroke. While there is some data on preoperative screening for carotid stenosis, there is no data to support this specifically in older adults. Symptomatic carotid stenosis (previous TIA or stroke) should be treated.

Post-operative delirium prevention Studies on pharmacologic therapy for delirium prevention and treatment are limited, with small studies and inconclusive data. Antipsychotics such as haloperidol and seroquel are commonly employed for treatment of agitation in delirium. There is no conclusive data on effectiveness or the superiority of one drug over another. Conservative measures for delirium prevention should be initiated in all older adults post-operatively. These include reducing tethers (lines, catheters, restraints), early mobilization, frequent reorientation, maintaining proper day/night cycles (ideally have the patient's bed near a window with the shades open), managing constipation, managing pain, ensuring proper vision and hearing devices are available if needed, and avoiding medications that cause or worsen delirium such as sedatives, anticholinergics, and antihistamines. While opiates may contribute to delirium, their use should be balanced against appropriate pain control (inadequate pain control can also cause delirium).

Antiepileptics These should be continued preoperatively, and levels monitored if indicated. Renal function should be closely monitored and medications dose-adjusted as appropriate.

Parkinson's medications These should be continued preoperatively. Stopping medications for Parkinson's disease can cause withdrawal or a flare of symptoms [61].

10.5 Functional Assessment

An assessment of an older adult's functional ability plays an important role in relation to post-surgical complications as well as transition planning options to a location other than a patient's home due to increased personal care needs. The preoperative period offers a unique period to assess and document baseline functional status and intervene through physical therapy, post-operative transition planning to subacute or acute rehabilitation or consideration for home physical therapy services. There is an increased interest in preoperative optimization via structure exercise programs with both aerobic and resistance exercise. Rehabilitation prior to surgery has not yet been sufficiently studied. Improving functional ability prior to surgery is appealing, as studies have shown in cancer patients that the inability to perform activities of daily living (ADLs) and instrumental activities of daily living (IADLs) is correlated with increased morbidity, mortality, and increased length of stay. We recommend documenting any history of falls in the past year, sensory impairments (hearing, vision, or swallowing), gait and mobility limitations, adaptive equipment needs (canes, walkers, wheelchair), and an assessment of ADLs, IADLs, and performance status during the preoperative evaluation [62]. Preoperative functional assessments such as the "Timed Up and Go" screening tool have shown to predict outcomes in elderly cancer patients as well as post-orthopedic surgery [63]. Patients who require more than 15 seconds to complete the Timed Up and Go test are at increased risk of falls. A significant change in functional status from baseline in a patient with preserved functional ability will influence transition planning to acute or subacute rehabilitation due to rehabilitation potential for return to baseline functional status.

Frailty This is the age-related decline in physiologic reserve and reduced ability to handle stressors. Frailty is a predictor of negative post-operative outcomes such as morbidity, mortality, increased length of stay, and discharge to facility. Frailty is common in older adults. There are multiple frailty assessment tools that include unintentional weight loss, generalized weakness, poor energy and endurance, low physical activity, and slow gait. The choice of frailty assessment instruments needs to be individualized based on evaluation time constraints and availability of objective measurement such as grip strength assessments or gait speed [64].

10.6 Social Assessment

Preoperative assessments should include current home address, type of abode if the patient lives in a private residence (i.e., elevator- or stair-accessible apartment), single-family home, assisted living, or long-term care facility, need to climb stairs in the home, and need for wheelchair access. Alternative living arrangements need to be explored if the patient is unable to safely function at home or has insufficient social supports or resources to meet their skilled (registered nurse) or unskilled needs (home health aide) during the post-operative recovery period. Identification of family members, formal and informal caretakers, health insurance information, prior use of Medicare rehabilitation days, ability to pay for private home health aides, or a private hire geriatric care manager to coordinate care are useful for post-surgical transition planning. Information on current services such as meals on wheels or certified home healthcare agency (CHHA) services is important to identify to resume or modify such services post-operatively. Working with interdisciplinary team members including social workers and case managers is highly valuable for navigating these assessments. *Advanced care planning and goals of care:* Geriatricians have an opportunity to ensure that the intended surgical procedure and anticipated outcome is in line with the patient's overall goals of care. This ensures that healthcare providers best meet patient expectations during the post-surgical recovery period and beyond. Delirium, prolonged or unexpected intubation, or other unexpected events leading to an inability to make decisions can lead to significant stress and conflict if appropriate preparations are not made. Ensure a clear alternate decision-maker has been designated (healthcare proxy, surrogate, guardian), and encourage patients to make their wishes known to this person prior to the operation. Advance care planning is the process which allows patient to voice the care they would want to receive if they were unable to communicate. Advance directives such as a living will are the documentation of what patient's value, their beliefs, and treatment preferences. The process includes the opportunity to appoint a healthcare agent/proxy or identify surrogates/next of kin to allow for these individuals to participate in a discussion preoperatively. Non-emergent surgeries in particular offer an opportunity to explore what patient's value and ensure that anticipated surgical outcomes are in line with the patient's goals of care.

Case Conclusion

Ms. MN had a complicated post-operative course where she needed to be surgically re-explored for an anastomotic leak which was repaired. She developed post-operative delirium and renal failure requiring dialysis and needed prolonged mechanical ventilation and hemodynamic support in an intensive care unit. She ultimately died just over a month following the procedure due to ongoing multiorgan failure. The geriatric team met with the family to provide support and debrief following the patient's death. The patient's family, while grieving, recognized that the patient understood the surgical risks involved and was grateful that we honored her informed decision to pursue the surgery despite the risks and subsequent negative outcome.

References

1. McDonald SR, Heflin MT, Whitson HE, Dalton TO, Lidsky ME, Liu P, et al. Association of integrated care coordination with postsurgical outcomes in high-risk older adults: the Perioperative Optimization of Senior Health (POSH) initiative. JAMA Surg. 2018;153(5):454.
2. Halter J, Ouslander J, Tinetti M, Studenski S, High K, Asthana S. Hazzard's geriatric medicine and gerontology: New York: McGraw-Hill Prof Med/Tech; 2009.
3. Fleisher LA, Fleischmann KE, Auerbach AD, Barnason SA, Beckman JA, Bozkurt B, et al. 2014 ACC/AHA guideline on perioperative cardiovascular evaluation and management of patients undergoing noncardiac surgery. Circulation. 2014:CIR. 0000000000000106.
4. Gupta PK, Gupta H, Sundaram A, Kaushik M, Fang X, Miller WJ, et al. Development and validation of a risk calculator for prediction of cardiac risk after surgery. Circulation. 2011; https://doi.org/10.1161/CIRCULATIONAHA.110.015701.
5. Baumgartner H, Falk V, Bax JJ, De Bonis M, Hamm C, Holm PJ, et al. 2017 ESC/EACTS guidelines for the management of valvular heart disease. Eur Heart J. 2017;38(36):2739–91.
6. Thyregod HGH, Steinbrüchel DA, Ihlemann N, Nissen H, Kjeldsen BJ, Petursson P, et al. Transcatheter versus surgical aortic valve replacement in patients with severe aortic valve stenosis: 1-year results from the all-comers NOTION randomized clinical trial. J Am Coll Cardiol. 2015;65(20):2184–94.
7. Douketis JD, Spyropoulos AC, Kaatz S, Becker RC, Caprini JA, Dunn AS, et al. Perioperative bridging anticoagulation in patients with atrial fibrillation. N Engl J Med. 2015;373(9):823–33.
8. Levine GN, Bates ER, Bittl JA, Brindis RG, Fihn SD, Fleisher LA, et al. ACC/AHA guideline focused update on duration of dual antiplatelet therapy in patients with coronary artery disease: a report of the American College of Cardiology/American Heart Association Task Force on Clinical Practice Guidelines: an update of the 2011 ACCF/AHA/SCAI guideline for percutaneous coronary intervention, 2011 ACCF/AHA guideline for coronary artery bypass graft surgery, 2012 ACC/AHA/ACP/AATS/PCNA/SCAI/STS guideline for the diagnosis and management of patients with stable ischemic heart disease, 2013 ACCF/AHA guideline for the management of ST-elevation myocardial infarction, 2014 AHA/ACC guideline for the management of patients with non–ST-elevation acute coronary syndromes, and 2014 ACC/AHA guideline on perioperative cardiovascular evaluation and management of patients undergoing noncardiac surgery. Circulation. 2016;134(10):e123–e55.
9. Chakos A, Wilson-Smith A, Arora S, Nguyen TC, Dhoble A, Tarantini G, et al. Long term outcomes of transcatheter aortic valve implantation (TAVI): a systematic review of 5-year survival and beyond. Ann Cardiothorac Surg. 2017;6(5):432.
10. Enright PL, Kronmal RA, Manolio TA, Schenker MB, Hyatt RE. Respiratory muscle strength in the elderly. Correlates and reference values. Cardiovascular Health Study Research Group. Am J Respir Crit Care Med. 1994;149(2):430–8.
11. Qaseem A, Snow V, Fitterman N, Hornbake ER, Lawrence VA, Smetana GW, et al. Risk assessment for and strategies to reduce perioperative pulmonary complications for patients undergoing noncardiothoracic surgery: a guideline from the American College of Physicians Reducing Perioperative Pulmonary Complications in Noncardiothoracic Surgery. Ann Intern Med. 2006;144(8):575–80.
12. Canet J, Gallart L, Gomar C, Paluzie G, Valles J, Castillo J, et al. Prediction of postoperative pulmonary complications in a population-based surgical cohort. Anesthesiology. 2010;113(6):1338–50.
13. Arozullah AM, Daley J, Henderson WG, Khuri SF, Program NVASQI. Multifactorial risk index for predicting postoperative respiratory failure in men after major noncardiac surgery. Ann Surg. 2000;232(2):242.
14. Goldman L, Caldera DL, Nussbaum SR, Southwick FS, Krogstad D, Murray B, et al. Multifactorial index of cardiac risk in noncardiac surgical procedures. N Engl J Med. 1977;297(16):845–50.
15. Rucker L, Frye EB, Staten MA. Usefulness of screening chest roentgenograms in preoperative patients. JAMA. 1983;250(23):3209–11.
16. Archer C, Levy AR, McGregor M. Value of routine preoperative chest x-rays: a meta-analysis. Can J Anaesth. 1993;40(11):1022–7.
17. Smetana GW, Lawrence VA, Cornell JE. Preoperative pulmonary risk stratification for noncardiothoracic surgery: systematic review for the American College of Physicians Preoperative Pulmonary Risk Stratification for Noncardiothoracic Surgery. Ann Intern Med. 2006;144(8):581–95.
18. Apostolakis S, Lane DA, Guo Y, Buller H, Lip GY. Performance of the HEMORR2HAGES, ATRIA, and HAS-BLED bleeding risk–prediction scores in nonwarfarin anticoagulated atrial fibrillation patients. J Am Coll Cardiol. 2013;61(3):386–7.
19. Gage BF, Birman-Deych E, Kerzner R, Radford MJ, Nilasena DS, Rich MW. Incidence of intracranial hemorrhage in patients with atrial fibrillation who are prone to fall. Am J Med. 2005;118(6):612–7.
20. Kagansky N, Knobler H, Rimon E, Ozer Z, Levy S. Safety of anticoagulation therapy in well-informed older patients. Arch Intern Med. 2004;164(18):2044–50.
21. Mant J, Hobbs FR, Fletcher K, Roalfe A, Fitzmaurice D, Lip GY, et al. Warfarin versus aspirin for stroke prevention in an elderly community population with atrial fibrillation (the Birmingham Atrial Fibrillation Treatment of the Aged Study, BAFTA): a randomised controlled trial. Lancet. 2007;370(9586):493–503.
22. Goldstein JN, Refaai MA, Milling TJ, Lewis B, Goldberg-Alberts R, Hug BA, et al. Four-factor prothrombin complex concentrate versus plasma for rapid vitamin K antagonist reversal in patients needing urgent surgical or invasive interventions: a phase 3b, open-label, non-inferiority, randomised trial. Lancet. 2015;385(9982):2077–87.
23. Connolly SJ, Ezekowitz MD, Yusuf S, Eikelboom J, Oldgren J, Parekh A, et al. Dabigatran versus warfarin in patients with atrial fibrillation. N Engl J Med. 2009;361(12):1139–51.
24. Patel MR, Mahaffey KW, Garg J, Pan G, Singer DE, Hacke W, et al. Rivaroxaban versus warfarin in nonvalvular atrial fibrillation. N Engl J Med. 2011;365(10):883–91.
25. Granger CB, Alexander JH, McMurray JJ, Lopes RD, Hylek EM, Hanna M, et al. Apixaban versus warfarin in patients with atrial fibrillation. N Engl J Med. 2011;365(11):981–92.

26. Birnie DH, Healey JS, Wells GA, Verma A, Tang AS, Krahn AD, et al. Pacemaker or defibrillator surgery without interruption of anticoagulation. N Engl J Med. 2013;368(22):2084–93.
27. Douketis JD. Perioperative anticoagulation management in patients who are receiving oral anticoagulant therapy: a practical guide for clinicians. Thromb Res. 2002;108(1):3–13.
28. Arnesen H, Dahl O, Aspelin T, Seljeflot I, Kierulf P, Lyberg T. Sustained prothrombotic profile after hip replacement surgery: the influence of prolonged prophylaxis with dalteparin. J Thromb Haemost. 2003;1(5):971–5.
29. Ziser A, Plevak DJ, Wiesner RH, Rakela J, Offord KP, Brown DL. Morbidity and mortality in cirrhotic patients undergoing anesthesia and surgery. Anesthesiology. 1999;90(1):42–53.
30. Lan S-H, Lu L-C, Yen Y-Y, Hsieh Y-P, Chen J-C, Wu W, et al. Tube feeding among elder in long-term care facilities: a systematic review and meta-analysis. J Nutr Health Aging. 2017;21(1):31–7.
31. Nyengaard J, Bendtsen T. Glomerular number and size in relation to age, kidney weight, and body surface in normal man. Anat Rec. 1992;232(2):194–201.
32. Weinstein JR, Anderson S. The aging kidney: physiological changes. Adv Chronic Kidney Dis. 2010;17(4):302–7.
33. Mathew A, Devereaux P, O'hare A, Tonelli M, Thiessen-Philbrook H, Nevis I, et al. Chronic kidney disease and postoperative mortality: a systematic review and meta-analysis. Kidney Int. 2008;73(9):1069–81.
34. Bastin AJ, Ostermann M, Slack AJ, Diller G-P, Finney SJ, Evans TW. Acute kidney injury after cardiac surgery according to risk/injury/failure/loss/end-stage, acute kidney injury network, and kidney disease: improving global outcomes classifications. J Crit Care. 2013;28(4):389–96.
35. Coca SG, Singanamala S, Parikh CR. Chronic kidney disease after acute kidney injury: a systematic review and meta-analysis. Kidney Int. 2012;81(5):442–8.
36. Rahmanian PB, Adams DH, Castillo JG, Vassalotti J, Filsoufi F. Early and late outcome of cardiac surgery in dialysis-dependent patients: single-center experience with 245 consecutive patients. J Thorac Cardiovasc Surg. 2008;135(4):915–22.
37. Couchoud CG, Beuscart J-BR, Aldigier J-C, Brunet PJ, Moranne OP. Development of a risk stratification algorithm to improve patient-centered care and decision making for incident elderly patients with end-stage renal disease. Kidney Int. 2015;88(5):1178–86.
38. Khan NA, Campbell NR, Frost SD, Gilbert K, Michota FA, Usmani A, et al. Risk of intraoperative hypotension with loop diuretics: a randomized controlled trial. Am J Med. 2010;123(11):1059. e1–8.
39. Coriat P, Richer C, Douraki T, Gomez C, Hendricks K, Giudicelli J-F, et al. Influence of chronic angiotensin-converting enzyme inhibition on anesthetic induction. Anesthesiology. 1994;81(2):299–307.
40. Trick WE, Scheckler WE, Tokars JI, Jones KC, Reppen ML, Smith EM, et al. Modifiable risk factors associated with deep sternal site infection after coronary artery bypass grafting. J Thorac Cardiovasc Surg. 2000;119(1):108–14.
41. Association AD. 14. Diabetes Care in the Hospital: standards of medical care in diabetes—2018. Diabetes Care. 2018;41(Supplement 1):S144–S51.
42. Clement S, Braithwaite SS, Magee MF, Ahmann A, Smith EP, Schafer RG, et al. Management of diabetes and hyperglycemia in hospitals. Diabetes Care. 2004;27(2):553–91.
43. Sudhakaran S, Surani SR. Guidelines for perioperative management of the diabetic patient. Surg Res Pract. 2015;2015:284063.
44. Bennett-Guerrero E, Kramer DC, Schwinn DA. Effect of chronic and acute thyroid hormone reduction on perioperative outcome. Anesth Analg. 1997;85(1):30–6.
45. Langley RW, Burch HB. Perioperative management of the thyrotoxic patient. Endocrinol Metab Clin N Am. 2003;32(2):519–34.
46. Böhmer AB, Wappler F. Preoperative evaluation and preparation of the morbidly obese patient. Curr Opin Anesthesiol. 2017;30(1):126–32.
47. Cohendy R, Rubenstein L, Eledjam J. Preoperative nutritional evaluation of elderly patients. Aging Clin Exp Res. 2001;13(4):293–7.
48. Mohanty S, Rosenthal RA, Russell MM, Neuman MD, Ko CY, Esnaola NF. Optimal perioperative management of the geriatric patient: a best practices guideline from the American College of Surgeons NSQIP and the American Geriatrics Society. J Am Coll Surg. 2016;222(5):930–47.
49. Colburn JL, Mohanty S, Burton JR. Surgical guidelines for perioperative management of older adults: what geriatricians need to know. J Am Geriatr Soc. 2017;65:1339.
50. Chin RP-H, Ho C-H, Cheung LP-C. Scheduled analgesic regimen improves rehabilitation after hip fracture surgery. Clin Orthop Relat Res. 2013;471(7):2349–60.
51. Bryson GL, Wyand A. Evidence-based clinical update: general anesthesia and the risk of delirium and postoperative cognitive dysfunction. Can J Anesth. 2006;53(7):669.
52. Rigg JR, Jamrozik K, Myles PS, Silbert BS, Peyton PJ, Parsons RW, et al. Epidural anaesthesia and analgesia and outcome of major surgery: a randomised trial. Lancet. 2002;359(9314):1276–82.
53. Shinozaki M, Usui Y, Yamaguchi S, Okuda Y, Kitajima T. Recovery of psychomotor function after propofol sedation is prolonged in the elderly. Can J Anesth. 2002;49(9):927–31.
54. Jeong YM, Lee E, Kim K-I, Chung JE, Park HI, Lee BK, et al. Association of pre-operative medication use with post-operative delirium in surgical oncology patients receiving comprehensive geriatric assessment. BMC Geriatr. 2016;16(1):134.
55. Chow WB, Rosenthal RA, Merkow RP, Ko CY, Esnaola NF. Optimal preoperative assessment of the geriatric surgical patient: a best practices guideline from the American College of Surgeons National Surgical Quality Improvement Program and the American Geriatrics Society. J Am Coll Surg. 20120;215(4):453–66.
56. Kennedy J, Van Rij A, Spears G, Pettigrew R, Tucker I. Polypharmacy in a general surgical unit and consequences of drug withdrawal. Br J Clin Pharmacol. 2000;49(4):353–62.
57. Appelbaum PS. Assessment of patients' competence to consent to treatment. N Engl J Med. 2007;357(18):1834–40.
58. Attri JP, Bala N, Chatrath V. Psychiatric patient and anaesthesia. Indian J Anaesth. 2012;56(1):8.
59. Tsoi KK, Chan JY, Hirai HW, Wong SY, Kwok TC. Cognitive tests to detect dementia: a systematic review and meta-analysis. JAMA Intern Med. 2015;175(9):1450–8.
60. Fines DP, Severn AM. Anaesthesia and cognitive disturbance in the elderly. Continuing education in Anaesthesia. Crit Care Pain. 2006;6(1):37–40.
61. Onofrj M, Thomas A. Acute akinesia in Parkinson disease. Neurology. 2005;64(7):1162–9.
62. Audisio RA. Shall we operate? Preoperative assessment in elderly cancer patients (PACE) can help A SIOG surgical task force prospective study. Crit Rev Oncol Hematol. 2008;65:156.
63. Huisman MG, Van Leeuwen BL, Ugolini G, Montroni I, Spiliotis J, Stabilini C, et al. "Timed up & go": a screening tool for predicting 30-day morbidity in onco-geriatric surgical patients? A multicenter cohort study. PLoS One. 2014;9(1):e0086863.
64. Beggs T, Sepehri A, Szwajcer A, Tangri N, Arora RC. Frailty and perioperative outcomes: a narrative review. Can J Anaesth/Journal canadien d'anesthésie. 2015;62(2):143–57.

Common Chronic Conditions

Erika Diaz Narvaez, Komal D'Souza, and Veronica Rivera

A. Chun (ed.), *Geriatric Practice*, https://doi.org/10.1007/978-3-030-19625-7_11

11.1 Introduction

One of the cornerstones of excellent geriatric care is caring for older adults with multiple chronic conditions or "multimorbidity." More than 50 percent of older adults have three or more chronic conditions. The combinations and severity of these chronic conditions can have varying cumulative effects on each individual [1].

Multimorbidity has significant impact and increases risk of death, institutionalization, increased utilization of healthcare resources, decreased quality of life, and higher rates of adverse effects of treatment or interventions. Unfortunately, older adults with multimorbidity are also commonly excluded from clinical trials and observational studies. Almost all existing guidelines have single-disease focus and do not take into consideration comorbid illness. There are also no clear approaches to decision-making and clinical management of older adults with multimorbidity. In 2012, the American Geriatrics Society Clinical Practice and Models of Care Committee created "Guiding Principles for the Care of Older Adults with Multimorbidity" as a framework for the management of multimorbidity.

The guiding principles developed involve conducting a complete review of a care plan for persons with multimorbidity, reviewing the current medical conditions and interventions, considering patient preferences, reviewing relevant evidence for significant outcomes, assessing prognosis, evaluating interactions within and among treatments and conditions, reexamining benefits and harms of the treatment plan, and lastly communicating and deciding for or against an intervention or treatment. They also suggest reassessing over time to evaluate benefit, feasibility, adherence, and alignment with patient preferences [1].

More than 50 percent of older adults have three or more chronic conditions. It is not uncommon to encounter an older adult with the following profile: 85-year-old with history of dementia, coronary artery disease, aortic stenosis s/p aortic valve replacement, hypertension, hyperlipidemia, type 2 diabetes mellitus, chronic kidney disease stage III, gastroesophageal reflux disease, constipation with recurrent small bowel obstruction, and urinary incontinence. A patient such as this one requires a great deal of thoughtful assessment and review of each chronic condition as well as careful consideration of how each condition may affect the other coexisting conditions.

11.2 Part I: Cardiovascular Disease

Cardiovascular disease is perhaps the most common disease found in older adults with multimorbidity: it is listed as the underlying cause of death for about 1 out of every 3 deaths in the United States. About 2200 Americans die of cardiovascular disease each day. In 2010, the estimated global cost of cardiovascular disease was $863 billion, estimated to rise to $1044 billion by 2030. Given the importance of cardiovascular disease, this section will cover coronary artery disease, hypertension, and atrial fibrillation.

11.2.1 Coronary Artery Disease

Coronary artery disease (CAD) is the leading cause of death attributable to cardiovascular disease in the United States, accounting for 45% of the deaths. The American Heart Association's (AHA's) Heart Disease and Stroke 2012 update shows that more than >16 million American adults have CAD, with a prevalence exceeding 80% in those >80 years of age [3]. The estimated annual incidence of myocardial infarction (MI) in the United States is 580,000 for new attacks and 210,000 for recurrent attacks. The average age at the first MI is 65.3 years for males and 71.8 years for females. Coronary artery disease and myocardial infarction were 2 of the 10 most expensive hospital principal discharge diagnoses, costing $10.4 billion and $11.5 billion respectively.

Coronary artery disease is an umbrella term that includes stable ischemic heart disease (SIHD) and acute coronary syndrome (ACS) including unstable angina, non-ST-elevation myocardial infarction (NSTEMI), and ST-elevation myocardial infarction (STEMI). For the purpose of this chapter on common chronic conditions, we will focus on SIDH. Risk factors for CAD are age, male sex, obesity or metabolic syndrome, smoking, hyperlipidemia, known CAD, diabetes mellitus, hypertension, physical inactivity, and family history of premature ischemic heart disease (i.e., onset in a father, brother, or son before age 55 or in a mother, sister, or daughter before age 65). A history of cerebrovascular or peripheral artery disease (PAD) also increases the likelihood of ischemic heart disease.

The patient presenting with angina must be categorized as having stable angina or acute coronary syndrome (ACS). Patients presenting with any suspicion for ACS should be transferred promptly to an emergency department for evaluation and treatment [5]. The presentation of acute coronary syndrome (ACS) in the elderly is complicated and varied, given the physiological and structural cardiovascular changes of aging [2] and the presence of comorbidities such as diabetes and hypertension. The typical presentation for ACS is the presence of acute chest, epigastric, neck, jaw, or arm pain or discomfort or pressure without an apparent non-cardiac source [6]. Classic chest pain is reported only by one third of patients older than 85. Given the limited amount of activity in this population, the classic activity-related pain onset might not be present [2], but although the presentation of ACS may be painless, it is often symptomatic.

SIHD refers to patients with known or suspected SIHD who have no recent or acute changes in their current symptoms, suggesting that no active thrombotic process is underway [4]. SIHD stems from thrombotic and/or atherosclerotic obstruction of coronary arteries, the risk of which grows with age. The incidence of SIHD is expected to increase greatly as the population of older adults expands over the next few decades.

Diagnostic studies for SIHD can be conducted in an outpatient setting. These should include the standard 12-lead electrocardiogram (ECG) and standard exercise ECG in patients with an intermediate pretest probability of CHD who have an interpretable ECG and are able to exercise. For patients with an uninterpretable ECG, the exam should include exercise stress with nuclear myocardial perfusion imaging (MPI) or echocardiography, looking for worsening wall motion abnormalities and changes in global left ventricular function during or immediately after stress. For patients with an intermediate pretest probability, cardiac/coronary computed tomography angiography (CCTA) might be reasonable as it can define the coronary anatomy and help to plan further therapy for patients at high risk of mortality. If the patient is at low or intermediate risk for mortality, therapeutic decisions should be directed toward improving symptoms and function. Angiography is performed to differentiate high-risk from low-risk patients. Those who are determined to be at low or intermediate risk with no persisting symptoms should be started on evidence-based medical therapy and should defer revascularization, as it does not improve survival nor adverse cardiac events [5].

Guideline-Directed Medical Therapy (GDMT) includes many antianginal medications such as beta blockers, calcium channel blockers, long-acting nitrates, and newer agents such as ranolazine, which have similar antianginal efficacy and acceptable safety and side effect profile. Beta blockers, which have been shown to improve survival in patients after myocardial infarction and in patients with hypertension, are considered first-line therapy. If beta blockers are contraindicated, calcium channel blockers or long-acting nitrates should be prescribed for symptom relief or in cases when the initial treatment with beta blockers alone is unsuccessful. Sublingual nitroglycerin or nitroglycerin spray is recommended for immediate relief of angina [5].

Treatment also includes lifestyle modifications, including dietary changes and smoking cessation. Furthermore, treatment should include management of lipids, hypertension, and diabetes mellitus. Aspirin 75 to 162 mg daily should be continued indefinitely in the absence of contraindications and ACE inhibitors should be prescribed in all patients with SIHD who also have hypertension, diabetes mellitus, LVEF 40% or less, or CKD, unless contraindicated.

If symptoms are relieved with medical therapy, that treatment should be continued without proceeding to revascularization. If symptoms persist, a discussion with the patient needs to explain the risks and benefits of percutaneous coronary intervention or coronary artery bypass surgery and to elicit their goals of care.

11.2.2 Hypertension

According to the AHA Heart Disease and Stroke Statistics 2017, about 85.7 million, or 34%, of American adults have high blood pressure [3]. In the United States, hypertension accounted for more cardiovascular disease (CV) deaths than any other modifiable CV risk factor and was second only to cigarette smoking as a preventable cause of death [13]. MESA (Multi-Ethnic Study of Atherosclerosis) found that for adults 45 years of age without hypertension, the 40-year risk of developing hypertension was 93% for African-American, 92% for Hispanic, 86% for white, and 84% for Chinese adults [12]. In the Framingham Heart Study, approximately 90% of adults free of hypertension at age 55 or 65 years developed hypertension during their lifetimes [17]. Because of its extremely high prevalence in older adults, hypertension is a leading cause of preventable morbidity and mortality. It is also under-recognized as a major contributor to premature disability and institutionalization.

Studies have demonstrated graded associations between higher systolic blood pressure (SBP) and diastolic blood pressure (DBP) and increased CVD risk. Although the relative risk of incident CVD associated with higher SBP and DBP is smaller at older ages, the corresponding high BP-related increase in absolute risk is larger given the higher absolute risk of CVD at an older age [11]. Isolated systolic hypertension is the predominant form of hypertension in older adults, and it has been demonstrated that lowering BP in isolated systolic hypertension (defined as SBP ≥160 mm Hg with variable DBP ≤90, ≤95, or ≤110 mm Hg) is effective in reducing the risk of fatal and nonfatal stroke, cardiovascular events, and death [19].

An age-associated increase in arterial vascular stiffness has been demonstrated, this may be due to alterations in vessel structure such as increase in smooth muscle cell size and number, increase in medial collagen deposition, and decrease in elastin content. Given the fact that stroke volume does not change with age, the change in arterial compliance may account for the age-associated increase in SBP [11] (◘ Table 11.1).

Patients with hypertension often have other CVD risk factors. Modifiable risk factors include current cigarette smoking, diabetes mellitus, dyslipidemia, obesity, physical inactivity, excess intake of alcohol, and unhealthy diet, such as excess intake of sodium and insufficient intake of potassium, calcium, magnesium, protein, especially from vegetables, fiber, and fish fats. Fixed risk factors are known to be CKD, family history of HTN, increased age, low socioeconomic and educational status, male sex, and obstructive sleep apnea.

A thorough medical history should focus on questions that might help to identify target organ damage and possible secondary causes of hypertension, as well as to assist in planning an effective treatment regimen. In the case of older patients, treatment goals and risk tolerance should also be

◘ Table 11.1 The new BP categories according to the 2017 Hypertension Guidelines JNC 8

	SBP	DBP
Normal	<120 mm Hg	<80 mm Hg
Elevated	120–129 mm Hg	<80 mm Hg
Hypertension stage 1	130–139 mm Hg	80–89 mm Hg
Hypertension stage 2	SBP ≥140 mm Hg	≥90 mm Hg

elicited, and an assessment of multiple chronic conditions, frailty, and prognosis should be performed. This should include consideration of the time required to see benefit from intervention, which may not be realized for some individuals. Medical history questions should focus on the pattern of BP measurements and changes over time, the patient's dietary habits, physical activity, alcohol consumption, and tobacco use, as well as on any recent lifestyle changes, including meals away from home. It is also important to know if the patient has family history of hypertension and to inquire into possible occurrence of symptoms that indicate a secondary cause such as the ones listed below, which may warrant further testing:

- Pheochromocytoma: BP lability, episodic pallor, and dizziness
- Cushing's syndrome: Central obesity, facial rounding, easy bruisability
- Hypokalemia from primary aldosteronism or secondary aldosteronism due to renovascular disease: Muscle cramps, weakness
- Hyperthyroidism: Weight loss, palpitations, heat intolerance
- Renal disease: Edema, fatigue, frequent urination
- Residual hypertension associated with coarctation: History of coarctation repair
- Obstructive sleep apnea: Snoring, hypersomnolence

A thorough physical exam needs to be performed, starting with BP measurement. Though the process is relatively easy, errors are common. The correct method for measuring BP is to have the patient sit quietly for 5 minutes before a reading is taken, support the limb used to measure BP, ensure the BP cuff is at heart level, use the correct cuff size, and, for auscultatory readings, and deflate the cuff slowly [15]. The timing of BP measurements in relation to ingestion of the patient's antihypertensive medication should be standardized. Change in BP from seated to standing position should be measured to detect orthostatic hypotension (a decline >20 mm Hg in SBP or >10 mm Hg in DBP after 1 minute is abnormal) [19].

Because individual BP measurements tend to vary, a single reading is inadequate for clinical decision-making. An average of 2 to 3 BP measurements obtained on 2 to 3 separate occasions will minimize random error and will provide a more accurate basis for estimation of BP. It is important to note that there can be inconsistencies between office and out-of-office BPs. Masked hypertension, or masked HTN, manifests as lower BP in a medical environment than at home. White-coat hypertension, or elevated blood pressure reading in a medical environment, averages approximately 13% and as high as 35% in some hypertensive populations [16]. Ambulatory BP monitoring is recommended in both cases. Another option is to use automated oscillometric devices in the office, since they provide an opportunity to obtain repeated measurements without a provider present, thereby minimizing the potential for a white-coat effect. Out-of-office BP readings are recommended either by self-monitoring or by ambulatory monitoring. If self-monitoring is used, it is important to ensure that the BP measurement device used has been validated [19]. Lastly, the physical examination should also include an assessment of hypertension-related target organ damage.

In any new diagnosis of hypertension, testing is required to facilitate CV risk factor profiling, to establish a baseline for medication use, and to screen for secondary causes of hypertension. The recommended tests are fasting blood glucose; complete blood count; lipid profile; complete metabolic panel to assess serum creatinine with eGFR, serum sodium, potassium, and calcium; thyroid-stimulating hormone; urinalysis; and electrocardiogram. Optional testing includes an echocardiogram, test for uric acid, and a test to determine urinary albumin to creatinine ratio [19]. Monitoring of serum sodium and potassium levels is helpful during diuretic or renin-angiotensin system blocker titration, as are serum creatinine and urinary albumin as markers of CKD progression.

It is also necessary to look for signs of secondary hypertension. Such signs include new-onset or uncontrolled hypertension in adults; drug-resistant/induced hypertension; abrupt onset of hypertension; onset of hypertension at <30 years of age or onset of diastolic hypertension in older adults (age ≥ 65 years-old); exacerbation of previously controlled hypertension; disproportionate target organ damage for degree of hypertension; accelerated/malignant hypertension; and unprovoked or excessive hypokalemia. If there is any suspicion of secondary hypertension, a screen is required and, with a positive screening test, a referral to a clinician with specific expertise in this area [19].

Treatment of hypertension in older patients is complicated given the high comorbidity burden and associated conditions, such as frailty and dementia. For these reasons, eliciting the goals of care and conducting a thorough assessment that may offer insight into prognosis is important, as is the consideration of time required to see benefit from intervention. For example, patients with prevalent and frequent falls, advanced cognitive impairment, and multiple comorbidities may be at risk of adverse outcomes with intensive BP lowering, especially when they require multiple BP-lowering medications. Older persons in this category typically reside in nursing homes and assisting living facilities, are unable to live independently in the community, and have not been represented in RCTs. Older persons may present with neurogenic orthostatic hypotension associated with supine hypertension. This is particularly common in Parkinson's disease and other neurodegenerative disorders.

Several RCTs have demonstrated the safety of more intensive treatment for hypertension. Both HYVET (Hypertension in the Very Elderly Trial) and SPRINT included community-dwelling frail older adults, and both trials were stopped early for benefit. In SPRINT, the benefit was for an SBP goal of <120 mm Hg. BP-lowering therapy is one of the few interventions shown to reduce CVD morbidity and mortality risk in frail older adults and does not increase the risk of orthostatic hypotension or the risk of injurious falls [18].

The BP target for ambulatory community-dwelling older adults should be ≤130/80 mm Hg, based on the fact that most of this population have an Atherosclerotic Cardiovascular Disease (ASCVD) risk score ≥10% and history of CVD (CHD, stroke, or HF). According to the National Health and Nutrition Examination Survey (NHANES) 2011–2014 data set, the actual number is 88% for adults ≥65 years old; 100% for adults ≥75 years of age have an ASCVD risk score ≥10% and history of CVD. For older adults (≥65 years of age) with hypertension and a high burden of comorbidity and limited life expectancy, clinical judgment, patient preference, and a team-based approach to assess risk/benefit are reasonable for decisions about the intensity of BP-lowering and choice of antihypertensive drugs.

Nonpharmacologic therapy is the preferred therapy for adults with elevated BP and an appropriate first-line therapy for adults with stage 1 hypertension who have an estimated 10-year ASCVD risk of <10%. Adherence to and impact of nonpharmacologic therapy should be assessed within 3 to 6 months. Such therapy includes weight loss if the patient is obese; heart-healthy diet, such as the DASH (Dietary Approaches to Stop Hypertension) diet that is a diet rich in fruits, vegetables, whole grains, and low-fat dairy products, with reduced content of saturated and total fat; and increased physical activity with a structured exercise program at least 90–150 min/week. If the patient currently consumes alcohol, they should be advised to drink no more than 2 drinks per day. A three-month trial may be given, and if BP shows no improvement medications should be started.

Initiation of antihypertensive therapy with 2 agents should be undertaken cautiously in older persons, with careful monitoring for orthostatic hypotension and history of falls. BP-lowering medications are recommended for patients with an average SBP of 130 mm Hg or higher or an average DBP of 80 mm Hg or higher, given the fact that for individuals older than age 79, the 10-year ASCVD risk is generally >10%. If the patient is <79 years but >65, has no history of CVD, and has an estimated 10-year ASCVD risk <10%, treatment should be started if the SBP is 140 mm Hg or higher or a DBP is 90 mm Hg or higher.

Adults with stage 2 hypertension should be evaluated by or referred to a primary care provider within 1 month of the initial diagnosis and start a combination of nonpharmacologic and antihypertensive drug therapy (with two agents of different classes), with a repeat BP evaluation in 1 month. For adults with a very high average BP (e.g., SBP ≥ 180 mm Hg or DBP ≥ 110 mm Hg), an evaluation should be followed by prompt antihypertensive drug treatment.

For initiation of antihypertensive drug therapy, first-line agents include thiazide diuretics, calcium channel blockers (CCBs), and angiotensin-converting enzyme inhibitors (ACE-I) or angiotensin II receptor blockers (ARBs) [19]. ACE-I or ARBs together are not recommended because the combination can be harmful. Therapy can then be individualized for each patient based on their coexisting conditions. For patients with stable angina and hypertension, GDMT beta blockers should be started, with ACE inhibitors or ARBs as first-line therapy, with the addition of other drugs (such as dihydropyridine CCBs, thiazide diuretics, and/or mineralocorticoid receptor antagonists) as needed to control hypertension. If the patient has angina, dihydropyridine CCBs or beta blockers can be used. If a patient has heart failure with preserved ejection fraction and symptoms of volume overload, they should be started on diuretics. If the patient has persistent hypertension after management of volume overload, the patient should be prescribed an ACE-I or ARB and beta blockers. For patients with chronic kidney disease (stage 3 or higher or stage 1 or 2 with albuminuria), treatment with an ACE-I or ARB is indicated. ACE-Is or ARBs may also be considered in the presence of albuminuria for patients with concomitant diabetes mellitus. For patients with atrial fibrillation (AF), treatment of hypertension with an ARB can be useful for prevention of recurrence of AF. Lastly, in asymptomatic aortic stenosis, start low-dose antihypertensive, and then gradually titrate upward as needed [19].

11.2.3 Atrial Fibrillation

Atrial fibrillation (AF), the most common sustained cardiac rhythm disturbance, has increasing prevalence with age. The estimate of the current prevalence of AF in the United States is around 2.3 million and is expected to increase to 5.6 million by 2050. AF occurs in almost 9% of the population > 80 years of age. The lifetime risks for AF are 1 in 6 even in the absence of predisposing cardiac conditions [10].

AF is associated with systemic thromboembolism, gradual worsening of ventricular function, the subsequent development of heart failure, and increased mortality. In patients 80–89 years old, 36% of strokes occur in those with AF. The annual risk of stroke for octogenarians with AF is in the range of 3–8% per year, depending on associated stroke risk factors.

AF is a supraventricular tachyarrhythmia characterized by uncoordinated atrial activation with consequent deterioration of atrial mechanical function. It is seen on the electrocardiogram (ECG) as the absence of P waves or the replacement of P waves by rapid oscillations or fibrillatory waves. This is associated with an irregular, frequently rapid ventricular response when atrioventricular (AV) conduction is intact [9].

Predisposing factors for AF are varied and include familial AF, congenital heart disease, neurogenic secondary to subarachnoid hemorrhage or strokes; post cardiac, pulmonary, or esophageal surgeries; primary or metastatic disease in or adjacent to the atrial wall; changes in autonomic tone (increased parasympathetic or sympathetic activity); endocrine disorders like hyperthyroidism and pheochromocytoma; inflammatory or infiltrative atrial disease including age-induced atrial fibrotic changes; atrial ischemia secondary to coronary artery; elevated atrial pressure secondary to systemic hypertension, ventricular hypertrophy, pulmonary hypertension, valve disease, myocardial disease with systolic or diastolic dysfunction; and electrophysiological abnormalities like enhanced automaticity or conduction abnormalities. Drug and alcohol use, as well as caffeine intake, are also considered predisposing factors.

Table 11.2 Classification of Atrial Fibrillation

Classification of atrial fibrillation (AF) [9]	
Recurrent AF	2 or more episodes
Paroxysmal AF	Arrhythmia terminates spontaneously
Persistent AF	Sustained beyond 7 days, requiring electrical or pharmacological termination, also includes cases of long-standing AF (e.g., greater than 1 year)
Permanent AF	Cardioversion has failed or has not been attempted because it is futile

Over time, the pattern of AF may be defined in terms of the number, frequency, and duration of episodes; mode of onset; triggers; and response to therapy, but these features may be impossible to discern when AF is first encountered (Table 11.2).

AF may present with palpitations, chest pain, dyspnea, fatigue, lightheadedness, syncope, exacerbation of HF, hemodynamic alterations, and thromboembolic complications. It can also be asymptomatic or have symptoms only during paroxysmal AF, making it difficult to identify the exact onset [9]. Once AF has become more permanent, the palpitations and other symptoms may decrease, especially in older patients. The irregularity and rate of ventricular response, underlying functional status, duration of AF, and individual patient factors may also affect the symptom presentation.

A thorough medical history should focus on characterizing the pattern of the arrhythmia (paroxysmal or persistent); predisposing and associated factors to try to elucidate its cause (see predisposing factors above), especially underlying heart disease or other reversible conditions, such as hyperthyroidism; symptoms and their tolerability; and history of prior management, including response to any pharmacological treatments. Questions should elicit details about the first symptomatic attack or date of discovery of AF; its frequency and duration; triggers, including alcohol, caffeine, exercise, and emotional stress; and modes of termination [9]. Take into account that vagally mediated AF may occur during sleep or after a large meal and is more likely to arise during a period of rest followed by a period of stress. In addition, try to discern whether the patient has noticed a decline in activity over time, especially when there is no other obvious explanation that is helpful for management decisions.

During the physical examination, key findings include irregular pulse, irregular heart sounds, irregular jugular venous pulsations, and variation in the intensity of the first heart sound. The exam may also reveal associated valvular heart disease or signs of heart failure.

A single outpatient visit can usually include both the workup of a patient with AF and the initiation of therapy. The basic workup includes electrocardiogram (ECG) documentation by at least a single-lead recording during the arrhythmia; identifying rhythm to verify AF; noting signs of LV hypertrophy; documenting P-wave duration and morphology or fibrillatory waves; looking for preexcitation, bundle-branch block, signs of prior MI; and measuring the R-R, QRS, and QT intervals. A portable ECG recording tool may help establish the diagnosis in cases of paroxysmal AF. A transthoracic echocardiogram may be performed to look for valvular heart disease and to assess chamber size and function, and signs of pulmonary hypertension or pericardial disease. Blood tests of thyroid, renal, and hepatic function should be conducted to look for reversible causes [9].

Management of older adult patients with AF involves two broad areas: symptom control and stroke risk reduction [7]. First and foremost, rate control strategy is sufficient to manage symptoms. Rate control, in which ventricular rate is controlled with no commitment to restore or maintain sinus rhythm, is the preferred strategy over rhythm control [7]. The second objective is prevention of thromboembolism.

Management also depends on several factors. These include type and duration of AF; severity and type of symptoms; associated cardiovascular disease, since symptoms may more likely progress; and patient age, medical conditions, functional status and goals of care with considerations of how permanent AF is likely to affect the patient in the future. In two big clinical trials (RACE and AFFIRM), it was shown that patients who could tolerate rate-controlled AF had outcomes similar to those randomized to rhythm control. Drugs and ablation are effective for both rate and rhythm control. For rhythm control, drugs are typically the first choice, and left atrial ablation is a second-line choice, especially in patients with symptomatic lone AF. In special circumstances, surgery may be the preferred option. Regardless of the approach, the need for anticoagulation is based on stroke risk and not on whether sinus rhythm is maintained.

For patients with symptomatic AF lasting many weeks, initial therapy may be anticoagulation and rate control, while the long-term goal is to restore sinus rhythm. When cardioversion is contemplated and the duration of AF is unknown or exceeds 48 hours, patients who do not require long-term anticoagulation may benefit from short-term anticoagulation. If rate control offers inadequate symptomatic relief, restoration of sinus rhythm becomes a clear long-term goal. Early cardioversion may be necessary if AF causes hypotension or worsening HF, making the establishment of sinus rhythm a combined short- and long-term therapeutic goal.

For rate control in patients with persistent or permanent AF, current guidelines recommend using pharmacological agents, that is, beta blocker or nondihydropyridine calcium channel antagonists. In the acute setting, in the absence of preexcitation, intravenous administration of beta blockers (esmolol, metoprolol, or propranolol) or nondihydropyridine calcium channel antagonists (verapamil, diltiazem) is recommended to slow the ventricular response to AF, and hypotension or heart failure (HF). Digoxin or amiodarone is recommended to control the heart rate in patients with AF and HF. When pharmacological therapy is insufficient or associated with side effects, it is reasonable to use ablation of the AV node or accessory pathway to control heart rate. Intravenous procainamide, disopyramide, ibutilide, or amiodarone may be considered for hemodynamically stable patients with AF involving conduction over an accessory pathway [9].

To prevent thromboembolism, guidelines recommend antithrombotic therapy to prevent thromboembolism for all patients with AF, except those with lone AF or contraindications [9]. AF is associated with five times the risk of stroke and is the cause of 25% of strokes in older adults [7]. The most recent American College of Cardiology/AHA guidelines recommend anticoagulation in individuals with CHA2DS2-VASc score of 2 or greater. However, despite the high risk of stroke, older age is associated with greater risk of bleeding complications including intracranial hemorrhage, gastrointestinal hemorrhage, and traumatic bleeding secondary to falls and this often causes a dilemma for clinicians. Two risk scoring instruments CHA2DS2-VASc, for stroke risk, and HAS-BLED, for bleeding risk, are often used to assist in clinical decision-making [8].

The selection of the antithrombotic agent should be based upon the absolute risks of stroke and bleeding and the relative risk and benefit for a given patient [9]. For patients without mechanical heart valves at high risk of stroke or with more than 1 moderate risk factor, chronic oral anticoagulant therapy with warfarin, a vitamin K antagonist, is recommended in a dose adjusted to achieve the target intensity international normalized ratio (INR) of 2.0 to 3.0, unless contraindicated. INR should be determined at least weekly during initiation of therapy and monthly when anticoagulation is stable [9]. Newer direct-acting oral anticoagulants (such as apixiban, dabigatran, and rivaroxaban) are associated with lower rates of all-cause mortality, hemorrhagic stroke, ischemic stroke, and major bleeding compared to warfarin. They also have the benefit of requiring less monitoring. Of note, dabigatran and rivaroxaban must be dose-adjusted for individuals with renal insufficiency [7].

Aspirin is recommended as an alternative to vitamin K antagonists in low-risk patients or in those with contraindications to oral anticoagulation; however it is less effective in stroke prevention in patients over 75 years of age. In older adults who are unable to have long-term anticoagulation, percutaneous left atrial appendage occlusion devices might be an alternative option; however there is still limited data in this area.

11.3 Part II: Renal Disease

11.3.1 Chronic Kidney Disease

Chronic kidney disease (CKD) is defined as functional (albuminuria, abnormal urine sediment, tubular dysfunction) or structural (detected by imaging, histologic abnormalities, prior kidney transplant) abnormalities of the kidney that last 3 months or more, with or without glomerular filtration rate (GFR) <60 ml/min/1.73 m^2. It is also defined by GFR of <60 mL/min/1.73 m^2 for ≥3 months, with or without kidney damage [20]. Overall prevalence of CKD (stages 1–5) in the US adult general population was 14.8% in 2011–2014; individuals of age 60 years experience the highest prevalence of CKD, and the prevalence in this group has been shown to increase [22].

Table 11.3 Chronic Kidney Disease (CKD) categories

eGFR categories		
G1	Normal or high	>90 ml/min/1.73 m^2
G2	Mildly decreased	60–89 ml/min/1.73 m^2
G3a	Mildly to moderately decreased	45–59 ml/min/1.73 m^2
G3b	Moderately to severely decreased	30–44 ml/min/1.73 m^2
G4	Severely decreased	15–29 ml/min/1.73 m^2
G5	Kidney Failure	<15 ml/min/1.73 m^2
Albuminuria categories		
A1	Normal to mildly increased	<30 mg/g
A2	Moderately increased	30–300 mg/g
A3	Severely increased	>300 mg/g

CKD staging is done by the Kidney Disease Improving Global Outcomes (KDIGO) group staging system, which is based on estimated glomerular filtration rate (eGFR) and albuminuria. These categories are combined for risk stratification. For example, Gi+A1 is a low-risk normal patient, but G5 A3 is very high-risk for adverse outcomes. For risk stratification of CKD, it is important to know the following: cause of CKD; GFR category; albuminuria category; and other risk factors and comorbid conditions [20] (Table 11.3).

The most common etiologies for CKD are diabetic nephropathy HTN and glomerulonephritis. Other causes of CKD are autoimmune diseases, systemic infections, urinary tract infections, urinary stones, obstruction of lower urinary tract, and drug toxicity. Other risk factors include older age, family history of CKD, reduction in kidney mass, low birth weight, US racial or ethnic minority status, and low income or educational level [22].

Patients are usually asymptomatic until the eGFR is very low. Once they reach CKD stage V level, the patient may experience fatigue, SOB, hypertension, LE edema, and other signs of fluid overload. If the patient develops overt kidney failure, they may experience symptoms of uremia which may include AMS, anorexia, nausea, vomiting, fatigue, and serositis [21].

A thorough history is needed to assess risk factors such as diabetes, hypertension, vascular disease, any causes of prerenal azotemia such as heart failure or intravascular volume depletion, contrast dye exposures, NSAID use, benign prostatic hypertrophy, and prior use of nephrotoxic medications. Any past personal or family history of kidney disease or urologic abnormalities, such as polycystic kidney disease or hereditary nephritis, needs to be identified. It is also important to ask about symptoms such as urinary symptoms, redness, decreased energy, impairment in thinking clearly, anorexia, insomnia, pruritus, nocturnal muscle cramps, edema of extremities, or puffiness around the eyes in the morning.

The cause of CKD may be assigned based on the presence or absence of systemic disease and the location within the kidney of observed or presumed pathologic-anatomic findings. The clinical context includes personal and family history, social and environmental factors, medications, a physical examination, laboratory measures, imaging, and pathologic diagnosis to determine the causes of kidney disease [20]. Initial assessment should be done with serum creatinine and a GFR estimating equation. If the patient is identified with low GFR, proteinuria can be measured either as albumin-creatinine ratio (ACR), protein-creatinine ratio (PCR), or dipstick.

Other important tests to order are CBC, LFTs, phosphorus, PTH, cholesterol, ESR, and serum protein electrophoresis. If the patient has CKD G3a, measure phosphate, PTH, and alkaline phosphatase; if elevated, vitamin D needs to be checked [20]. Renal ultrasound can be done to check for tumors, infiltrative disease, cystic disease, small kidneys are suggestive of CKD, and to check for cyst stones, masses, and hydronephrosis. MRA, CT, CTA, or duplex Doppler ultrasound can be used to exclude renal artery stenosis. Renal biopsy is needed in select cases only.

Screen for anemia with CBC when clinically indicated for GFR categories G1–G2, at least annually for GFR categories G3a–G3b, and at least twice a year for GFR categories G4–G5. Serum levels of calcium, phosphate, PTH, and alkaline phosphatase should be measured at least once in patients in GFR categories G3b–G5 to document baseline values. In this patient's routine bone mineral density, test results may be misleading. Phosphate concentrations should be maintained in the normal range. Optimal PTH level is unknown, but if high or abnormal, patients should be evaluated for hyperphosphatemia, hypocalcemia, and vitamin D deficiency [20].

In people identified as having kidney disease, repeat testing (eGFR and albuminuria) should be scheduled based on stage, previous values, and clinical context, but should be done at least annually—more often for higher risk of progression or if decisions need to be made. People without kidney disease may have repeat evaluations every year or more frequently [20].

Treatment of CKD is guided toward slowing the progression of kidney failure. In older patients, treatment should consider age, comorbidities, other therapies, and adverse effects such as orthostatic hypotension. Target BP is systolic of ≤130 mm Hg and diastolic ≤80 mm Hg. Diabetes control should be improved and target hemoglobin A1c (HbA1c) should be 7.0%. High protein intake should be avoided. Vitamin D should only be prescribed if deficiency present, not to suppress elevated PTH. And bisphosphonates should be avoided in GFR categories G4–G5. If serum bicarbonate level is <22 mmol/l, supplementation with oral bicarbonate is suggested unless contraindicated to maintain serum bicarbonate within normal range [20].

All patients with CKD are at risk for cardiovascular disease. The level of care offered to patients with CKD in case they have ischemic heart disease or heart failure should be the same as if offered to those without CKD. GFR should be taken into account when dosing drugs. If patients with GFR categories G3a-G5 have a temporary increased risk for acute kidney injury (AKI), all potentially nephrotoxic and renally excreted agents should be held. These agents may include RAS blockers, diuretics, NSAIDs, metformin, lithium, and digoxin. Patients with CKD should also avoid using herbal remedies and should seek medical advice prior to using over-the-counter medications or nutritional supplements [20].

Patients should be referred to a nephrologist if they have AKI or abrupt sustained fall in GFR, if they are GFR categories G4–G5, and if they have a consistent finding of albuminuria, progression of CKD as defined above, unexplained urinary red cell casts, CKD and refractory hypertension (on 4+ antihypertensives), recurrent or extensive nephrolithiasis, hereditary kidney disease, or persistent electrolytes abnormalities [20].

For patients with progressive CKD with risk of kidney failure within 1 year at 10–20% should be referred for renal replacement therapy (RRT) planning. Dialysis should be initiated when symptoms or signs attributable to kidney failure are present (such as serositis, acid-base or electrolytes abnormalities, or pruritus), inability to control volume status or blood pressure, cognitive impairment, or deterioration in nutritional status. This usually occurs with GFR raging between 5 and 10 ml/min/1.73 m^2. Renal transplantation should be considered when the GFR is <20 ml/min/1.73 m^2, and there is evidence of progressive and irreversible CKD over the past 6–12 months [20].

11.4 Part III: Gastroenterological Disorders

11.4.1 Dysphagia

Dysphagia is the sensation of difficulty passing food or liquid from the mouth to the stomach. It is most commonly a consequence of other diseases, such as gastrointestinal or neurologic disorders, and is thus more common in multimorbid older adults. Dysphagia was found in approximately 22% of community-dwelling older adults with the prevalence increasing to 30% in hospitalized older adults and 68% in older adults in long-term care settings [26–28].

The normal process of swallowing is a complex combination of voluntary and involuntary neurologic and muscular processes that are traditionally separated into oral, pharyngeal, and esophageal processes [23]. Normal aging can cause neurologic and muscular changes that can slow the swallowing mechanism, and these changes have been reported in asymptomatic older adults without dysphagia [23]. Normal changes associated with swallowing in older adults have been referred to as presbyphagia [25]. Although presbyphagia can be expected in older adults, dysphagia is not expected in healthy older adults. When dysphagia is reported in older adults, further investigation should be conducted for underlying etiology and treatment.

Dysphagia can be classified by its anatomical origin: oropharyngeal or esophageal [23]. Oropharyngeal dysphagia is also known as transfer dysphagia, as it refers to difficulty transferring oral contents from the hypopharynx to the esophagus [24]. Esophageal dysphagia refers to difficulty in passing contents from the esophagus to the stomach [24]. Both oropharyngeal and esophageal dysphagia can be further classified into structural disorders and motor disorders of the central nervous systems, peripheral nervous system, or myopathies (◘ Figs. 11.1 and 11.2). The differential diagnosis for etiology of dysphagia is vast; history, physical exam, and diagnostic testing may help to diagnose and treat the etiology of the disease.

The evaluation of dysphagia begins with a careful history. A detailed past medical history, including any neurologic or gastrointestinal disorders which may predispose to symptoms, should be elicited.

Medications may affect normal swallowing as well. Medications or chemotherapy may cause neuromuscular dysfunction or xerostomia, which may impair swallowing [23]. Also, pill-induced esophagitis may lead to swallowing difficulties. Common medications associated with pill-induced esophagitis include tetracycline, potassium chloride, nonsteroidal anti-inflammatory drugs, quinidine, and alendronate [23].

Furthermore, tobacco and alcohol use are risk factors for the development of malignancies that may manifest as dysphagia. Associated symptoms, such as weight loss, blood loss, progressive symptoms, symptoms causing awakening at night, and odynophagia are all 'alarm' symptoms that merit a prompt workup [24].

Symptoms associated with oropharyngeal dysphagia include drooling, cough with eating, and aspiration which may manifest as pneumonitis or pneumonia [24]. Oropharyngeal dysphagia may occur immediately after consuming food or drink, and patients may find it difficult to initiate a swallow [23]. Common symptoms of esophageal dysphagia include reflux and chest pain and these symptoms may occur a few seconds after consuming food or drink [23, 24]. Also, the sensation of dysphagia below the suprasternal notch reliably correlates to esophageal dysphagia [24]. However, patients with esophageal dysphagia may localize their symptoms to the lower neck; thus the localization of symptoms may not always correlate the anatomical etiology [24]. Physical exam signs such as oral masses, cervical adenopathy, and any abnormality on neurological exam may also help in diagnosing the etiology of dysphagia [23].

There are several diagnostic tests that can be used to evaluate dysphagia. The most common tests are barium radiography, videofluoroscopic swallowing study (VFSS or commonly known as modified barium swallow), fiberoptic endoscopic evaluation of swallowing (FEES), upper endoscopy, and

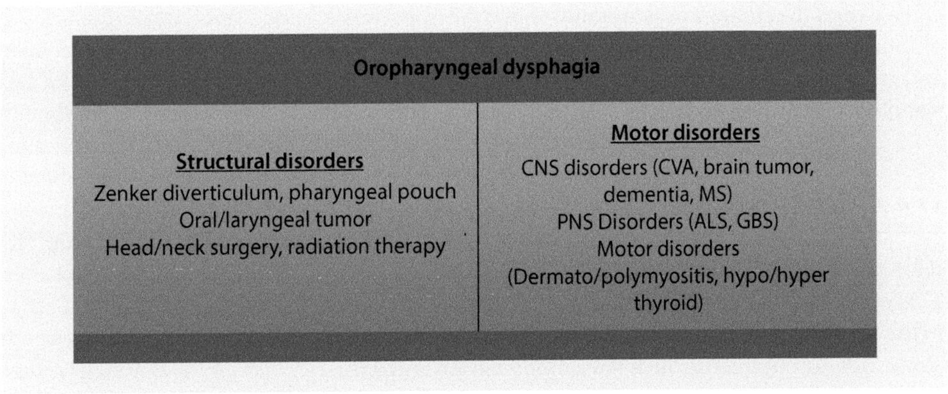

◘ **Fig. 11.1** Etiologies of oropharyngeal dysphagia. (Adapted from Aslam et al. [23])

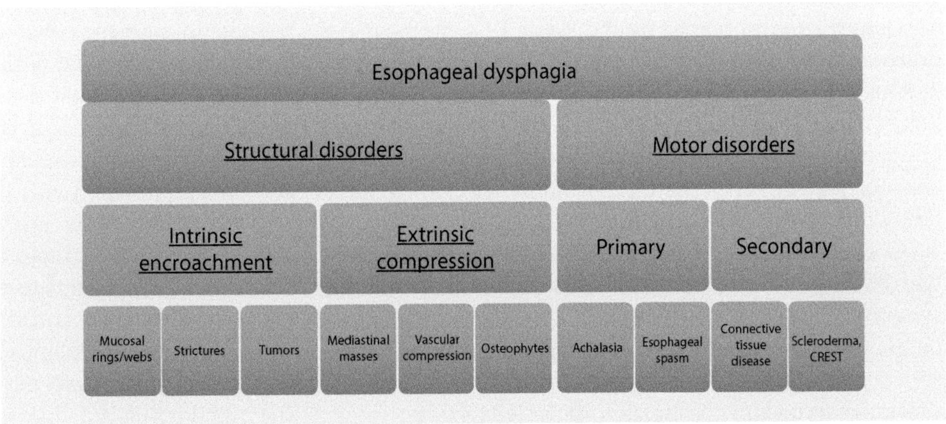

◘ **Fig. 11.2** Etiologies of esophageal dysphagia. (Adapted from Aslam et al. [23])

esophageal manometry [23]. Upon suspicion of oropharyngeal dysphagia, modified barium swallow is often the first diagnostic test ordered. This test can then be used to guide the FEES evaluation, which has the advantage of being able to be done at bedside or within a long-term care setting [23]. For esophageal dysphagia, upper endoscopy is commonly performed to evaluate for structural and motor disorders [23]. Modified barium swallow may also provide the diagnosis for some structural disorders, such as strictures, and motor disorders such as achalasia [23]. Esophageal manometry can provide the diagnosis for motor disorders such as achalasia or esophageal spasm when prior endoscopy is unrevealing [23].

Treatment of the underlying etiology of dysphagia may lead to significant relief. Treatment of common disorders such as gastrointestinal reflux disorder (GERD) or removal of potentially offending medications may lead to significant relief of symptoms [24]. Procedures such as dilatation, surgery, chemotherapy, or radiation may relieve mechanical obstruction from structural disorders [23]. Furthermore, swallowing therapy may ease symptoms by teaching compensatory mechanisms for dysphagia. Techniques such as chin tuck and head rotation have been found to decrease aspiration events [25]. The consistency of the food and liquids in the diet may also be modified based on the results of the swallowing evaluation [25].

Dysphagia may be a symptom of localized benign pathology or herald malignancy or systemic disease. Given the broad differential for dysphagia, careful history and physical exam with subsequent diagnostic measures should be undertaken to find the etiology of symptoms. Given the importance of food and liquid intake related to quality of life, diagnosis and treatment should be pursued to attempt to relieve the symptoms of dysphagia.

11.4.2 Constipation

It is estimated that chronic constipation can affect from 2% to 27% of the population [33]. The annual cost of constipation in the United States is more than $800 million in medications alone, not accounting for hospitalizations related to constipation. For nursing home residents, the prevalence of constipation reaches as high as 50%, and 75% of nursing home residents use a daily laxative therapy.

Constipation is defined by the Rome III Criteria as the presence of at least two of the following symptoms in at least 25% of defecations: straining during defecation, passage of lumpy or hard stool, sensation of incomplete evacuation, use of manual maneuvers to facilitate defecation (digital evacuation or support of pelvic floor), and/or fewer than three bowel movements per week [32].

Constipation can be classified as acute, chronic and secondary, or functional. Chronic constipation is defined as symptoms present for at least three months with symptom onset at least six months prior to diagnosis. Functional constipation is a diagnosis of exclusion after excluding all the causes for secondary constipation (▫ Table 11.4).

▫ Table 11.4 Causes of secondary constipation

Mechanical causes	Obstruction due to cancer, strictures, rectocele, sigmoidocele, compression from pelvic or abdominal process
Pelvic floor dysfunction	Secondary to poor toilet habits, painful defecation, obstetric or back injury, and brain-gut dysfunction.
Metabolic causes	Diabetes, hypothyroidism, hypercalcemia, hypokalemia, heavy metal poisoning
Neurological disease	Parkinson's, multisystem atrophy, multiple sclerosis, Shy-Drager syndrome
Medications	Opioids, anticholinergics, NSAIDs, antihypertensives (CCB, BB, diuretics), iron supplements

Functional constipation in relation with aging may be due to normal age-related changes such as reduced number of intrinsic cholinergic neurons that cause decreased bolus constriction, inefficient peristalsis, and delayed transit [29]. It also may be secondary to reduced water intake since older adults lack thirst. Older adults may have reduced rectal sensation that may lead to stool impaction; and sarcopenia of aging may lead to weak abdominal muscles, decreasing the intraabdominal pressure during straining.

When taking an initial history, it is important to ask about patient's perception of normal bowel habits, defecation frequency, and onset and duration of symptoms like straining, stool incontinence, need for digital manipulation of stool, rectal pain or bleeding, weight loss, abdominal pain, or bloating. Patient may be asked to characterize stool in terms of color, size, and volume; here, the Bristol Stool Scale may be useful [31]. Alarm symptoms include new onset constipation, rectal bleeding, anemia, weight loss, history of abdominal or pelvic malignancy, abdominal surgery, and severe/intractable constipation. These warrant further workup to identify systemic disease or neoplasia. Recurring problems of a long duration that are poorly relieved with dietary measures or laxatives suggest a functional colorectal disorder.

A physical exam should be performed to look for signs of systemic disease like Parkinson's disease, prior stroke, hypothyroidism, or diabetes. Abdominal examination should be conducted, evaluating for distention, masses and bowel sounds. In women, pelvic examination may be warranted to rule out an internal prolapse or rectocele. Perineal exam and rectal exam should also be performed. Rectal exam may reveal fecal impaction. It is important to remember that a digital rectal exam is reliable in detecting normal, but not abnormal, sphincter tone [30].

Diagnostic studies are reserved for patients that have alarm signs and symptoms as described above. Initial workup includes complete cell blood count, basic metabolic panel, calcium level, and thyroid function tests to look for secondary causes. Colonoscopy is indicated in all patients over age 50 who have not undergone screening colonoscopy. Abdominal CT may be done if there are concerns for masses. Colonic transit or pelvic floor function studies are considered only with severe, intractable constipation with no secondary cause. Manometry and balloon expulsion tests can help identify the presence of dyssynergic defecation but are considered only if they will affect management decisions. Defecography or pelvic magnetic resonance imaging is indicated if the results of anal manometry or balloon expulsion tests are equivocal, or if there is a clinical suspicion of a structural rectal abnormality [30].

The goal of treatment of constipation in adults is to improve quality of life by relieving symptoms and restoring normal bowel habits. Initial treatment should include nonpharmacologic measures. Behavioral modifications that support regular bowel habits include scheduling toileting around the same time every day, instruction on the best sitting position for defecation, avoiding distractions while defecating, and utilizing the gastrocolic reflex 15–20 min prior to defecation. Also, patients may need to increase their activity 30–60 min after a meal. Dietary modifications should also promote an increase in dietary fiber from fruits and vegetables, combination of soluble and insoluble fiber, and adequate water intake. It is also imperative to thoroughly review medication lists and remove any that may cause constipation as side effect, if possible.

If nonpharmacologic measures fail to relieve symptoms, laxatives may be needed and include the following categories. First, fiber supplements include soluble fibers (such as psyllium and methylcellulose) and insoluble fibers (bran, flax seed, and rye). Soluble fibers are better tolerated. Next, surfactant laxatives or stool softeners such as docusate sodium are used for mild intermittent constipation. They are well tolerated but are not very effective for older adults.

Osmotic laxatives, which work by having an osmotic effect in the intestines, are an excellent choice and include agents such as magnesium hydroxide, lactulose, sorbitol, and polyethylene glycol. In addition to osmotic laxatives, stimulant laxatives such as senna and bisacodyl can also be added. Lastly, prosecretory agents lubiprostone, a chloride channel activator, and linaclotide, a guanylate cyclase-C activator, can be used when constipation has failed all other therapies. Tap-water enemas are also indicated for severe cases [30].

11.4.3 Fecal Incontinence

Fecal incontinence is defined as the involuntary loss of either flatus, mucous, liquid stool, or solid stool. Fecal incontinence is the second most common cause of institutionalization, and as a result, it greatly affects quality of life. According to the National Health and Nutrition Examination Survey (NHANES), the prevalence of fecal incontinence is 8.3% in non-institutionalized adults, and it is similar in men and women, and it increases with age, so it can be 15.3% in participants aged 70 years and older [36].

In older adults, aging is associated with thickening of internal anal sphincter and thinning of the external anal sphincter. These changes result in decreased anal squeeze pressures, reduced rectal capacity, and decreased sensation to rectal distention [34]. Risk factors for fecal incontinence include urinary incontinence, watery stools, more than 21 bowel movements per week, obesity, pelvic surgery, obstetric trauma, anorectal surgery, and sedentary lifestyle. Chronic illnesses including stroke and dementia are also predisposing factors.

When taking a history, it is important to ask about fecal incontinence, as patients are less likely to volunteer this information due to fear or embarrassment. It should be asked as part of the geriatric review of systems, and it is also important to ask if the incontinence is flatus, liquid stool, and/or solid stool. Other historical features should include duration of symptoms, frequency, urgency, time of day, dietary relationships, relation to exertional activities, dyschezia, time to evacuation, frequency of bowel movements, and rectal bleeding. Questions must be geared to exclude pseudo-incontinence, which is soiling, frequency, and urgency, likely secondary to leakage or drainage from prolapsed mucosa, hemorrhoidal disease, or inflamed rectal mucosa as observed with gastroenteritis, inflammatory bowel disease, or irritable bowel syndrome. In pseudo-incontinence there is an intact sphincter mechanism [35].

History must also include associated comorbidities, medications, number of pregnancies and deliveries, perineal injuries and/or trauma, and perineal or colorectal procedures. Lastly, it is very important to ask about the impact that fecal incontinence has on the patient's quality of life.

A complete physical exam including abdominal exam is important. Inspect the patient in left lateral decubitus looking for prior scars, hygiene, hemorrhoids, prolapses, and fistulae. In females, vaginal examination is necessary. Rectal examination will be looking for sensory deficits by eliciting the anal wink, looking for impacted stool, laxity of perineal body, and masses. Valsalva maneuver is to be performed during rectal exam to evaluate the resting and squeeze pressures.

If additional workup is warranted, diagnostic studies may include electromyography (EMG) and pudendal nerve terminal motor latency (PNTML) to identify neurologic or sensory deficits of anorectal function; anorectal manometry to assess sphincter function, rectal sensation, and compliance; anoscopy to inspect for hemorrhoids, fistulae, or mucosal inflammation; colonoscopy to evaluate the entire colon if concern for neoplasm or irritable bowel disease; and endoanal ultrasound to identify sphincter defects [35].

For the management of fecal incontinence, nonpharmacologic measures should also be the first-line treatment. Dietary modifications to increase fiber intake gradually are recommended. A food diary helps identify possible triggers of fecal incontinence, including lactose in lactose-intolerant patients, caffeine, alcohol, fruit juices, and certain vegetables (beans, broccoli, cauliflower) that can decrease colonic transit time and predispose to fecal incontinence. Behavioral modifications should promote scheduled toileting aimed at having a daily complete bowel movement at a scheduled time and prevent overflow incontinence due to impaction or constipation. Also, anal hygiene is an important aspect of the management, as it may prevent pruritus ani and excoriations. Other treatment options include physical therapy with biofeedback and pelvic floor exercises.

Pharmacologic interventions may also be indicated. For example, a bowel regimen with supplemental fiber can be used to normalize stool consistency. Antidiarrheal medications, to increase colon transit time and to help solidify stool, include loperamide, diphenoxylate and codeine. Lastly, stool softeners and laxatives may prevent fecal impaction or constipation, therefore preventing overflow diarrhea if this is occurring [35].

Other treatment options include surgical sphincter repair if there is a disrupted anal sphincter. There are also artificial bowel sphincters. Sacral nerve stimulation (SNS) is a less invasive method, however, has unclear benefit. Another option is sphincter submucosal injection of bulking agents such as polytetrafluoroethylene, autologous fat, glutaraldehyde crosslinked collagen, carbon beads, silicone biomaterial, and stabilized nonanimal hyaluronic acid with dextranomer. Finally, a colostomy may allow stool to be collected via a stoma bag in a relatively controlled fashion and does not require sphincter control [35].

11.5 Part IV: Endocrine Disorders

11.5.1 Thyroid Disorders

Common chronic conditions in older adults often include thyroid disorder. In this section, we will focus on hypothyroidism and hyperthyroidism.

11.5.1.1 Hypothyroidism

The prevalence estimated for hypothyroidism for older adults ranges from 0.5% to 5% for clear hypothyroid disease and is estimated at 5–10% for subclinical hypothyroidism [38]. The most common causes are autoimmune, following treatment for hyperthyroidism, pituitary, or hypothalamic disorders, or medications.

Symptoms of hypothyroidism for older adults maybe be atypical. Clinical features of hypothyroidism, such as dry skin, constipation, weakness, anemia, hyponatremia, and gait disturbances, can often be mistaken for other diseases in older adults. Because of this, and because of the insidious onset of symptoms, most cases of hypothyroidism are not confirmed with a clinical exam but rather with laboratory screening [38].

For diagnostic testing, thyroid-stimulating hormone (TSH) testing remains the most sensitive test to detect primary thyroid disorders. However, although the mechanism is not exactly clear, there is evidence to suggest that serum TSH changes in older adults above the traditional reference range. Therefore, it is important to consider that changes in serum TSH may be more physiologic in older adults rather than reflective of actual disease. It has also been studied and documented that serum T3 levels decrease with aging while serum T4 remains unaffected [37]. Also, the presence of serious acute or chronic nonthyroid-related illness can also affect thyroid function tests in the short-term period. Thyroid function tests should be repeated for confirmation in the stable outpatient setting. The presence of true hypothyroid illness can be confirmed by a consistently increased TSH and decreased free T4 [38].

Treatment for subclinical hypothyroid with a TSH of between 5 and 10, normal free T4, and no symptoms is controversial. Most agree that it is indicated to treat if TSH is above 10. Also, the presence of high-titer antithyroid peroxidase antibodies suggestive of Hashimoto's disease is associated with eventual over-hypothyroidism [38]. It is important that levothyroxine be given on an empty stomach and to wait 1 hour before eating to avoid reduced absorption related to food and other medications, especially vitamins like calcium and iron. Starting dose is 25–50 mcg and can increase by 12–25 mcg intervals every 6 weeks with repeat TSH testing (Reuben, [39, 43]). It is also important to note that with patients who have severe cardiac disease, it is sometimes advisable to start replacement at even lower doses, to avoid exacerbation of cardiac symptoms such as angina [38]. Thyroid hormone replacement also decreases with aging due to decreased clearance rate.

11.5.1.2 Hyperthyroidism

The prevalence of hyperthyroidism is 0.5–2.3% of older adults, and 15–25% of all cases of thyrotoxicosis are in adults over 60 years of age. The etiology of hyperthyroidism in most cases is Graves' disease, but toxic multinodular goiters and adenomas are more common in older adults. Medications such as amiodarone in particular may also cause hyperthyroidism.

Older adults are less likely to present with the clinical features, including heat intolerance, tremor, nervousness, or goiter, but may rather present with weight loss, dyspnea, heart failure, or atrial fibrillation. Workup predominantly includes laboratory evaluation. If the TSH is low and free T4 is normal, it is recommended to repeat labs in 6 weeks. If TSH is still low, check free T3 and T4. If the TSH remains low, but the free T3 and T4 are normal, then this is subclinical hyperthyroidism. If the TSH is low and T3 or T4 are elevated, it is recommended to check radioactive iodine uptake. If there is thyroid nodularity, checking a thyroid scan is recommended.

Subclinical hyperthyroidism is defined as low TSH with normal range free T4 and free T3. About 1–5% of patients with subclinical hyperthyroidism progress to overt hyperthyroidism [37]. Treatment of hyperthyroidism should be considered in older adults with TSH <0.1mIU/L due to Graves or thyroid nodular disease. There is insufficient evidence to treat patients with TSH between 0.1 and 0.45mIU/L, unless the patient also presents with underlying cardiovascular disease or low bone mineral density. Radioactive iodine therapy is the treatment of choice for older adults with hyperthyroidism due to Graves' disease or toxic nodular thyroid disease. Surgery and medications are also options. β-blocking agents can be used to help symptoms of tachycardia, tremor, and anxiety.

11.5.2 Diabetes Mellitus

Diabetes mellitus is a highly prevalent chronic condition for older adults: about 25% of people over the age of 65 have diabetes, and about 50% of older adults have prediabetes. Older adults with diabetes have higher rates of complications such as functional decline, premature death, and coexisting illnesses such as hypertension and coronary artery disease. Older adults with diabetes are also at higher risk for geriatric syndromes such as polypharmacy, cognitive impairment, urinary incontinence, and falls [41].

Diabetes is a group of metabolic diseases characterized by hyperglycemia due to deficiencies in insulin secretion, insulin action, or both. Type 1 diabetes is an autoimmune disease where pancreatic beta cells are destroyed and lead to an absolute deficiency of insulin secretion. Type 2 diabetes is a progressive disorder that is due to insulin resistance and inadequate insulin secretory response. The classic clinical features of diabetes include polyuria, polydipsia, or polyphagia; however, these may be absent in older adults. Older adults may present with dehydration, confusion, incontinence, and diabetes complications such as neuropathy or nephropathy [40]. Most often, patients are asymptomatic, and diagnosis is based on routine laboratory evaluation similar to younger patients (hemoglobin A1C and plasma glucose levels). It's important to remember that hemoglobin A1C level may not be as accurate in older patients with conditions such as anemia, recent blood transfusions, treatment with erythropoietin, or chronic kidney disease [40].

The treatment goals for older adults with diabetes should be tailored to individual patients based on their functional capacity and life expectancy. This table, adopted from the American Diabetes Association, classifies patients into three categories: healthy (few coexisting chronic illnesses, intact functional and cognitive status); complex/intermediate (multiple existing chronic illnesses or 2+IADL impairments or mild to moderate cognitive impairment); and very complex/poor health (LTC facility or end-stage chronic illnesses or moderate to severe cognitive impairment or 2+ADL dependencies) (Table 11.5).

There are limited long-term studies illustrating the benefits of tight glycemic, blood pressure, and lipid control in healthy older adults. However, patients who are expected to have longer life expectancy and may benefit from this management should be offered management similar to younger patients. Patients who have complex medical comorbidities are less likely to benefit from tight glycemic control with the goal of reducing microvascular complications but rather are at higher risk of hypoglycemia and its complications. The glycemic goals, however, at least be sufficient to avoid complications such as dehydration, poor wound healing, and hyperglycemic hyperosmolar coma.

Treatment for diabetes includes both nonpharmacologic and pharmacologic options. Nonpharmacologic treatment includes lifestyle changes such as exercise and alcohol and smoking cessation, as well as nutrition advice. There are many classes of medications used to control diabetes. The following table will review the available classes of diabetes medications and special considerations for older adults. Also, in general the cost of medications can become another factor, given the amount of polypharmacy in older adults (Table 11.6).

In addition to antihyperglycemia treatment, if it is appropriate, based on function and goals of care, it is important to consider these other treatments for older adults with diabetes as endorsed by the American Geriatrics Society [42]. Aspirin therapy is recommended for all older adults who have diabetes and cardiovascular disease, unless contraindicated. Older adults with diabetes should also have controlled hypertension with a goal of <140/90 unless they are in the category of very poor health and limited life expectancy. For older adults with DM, evidence clearly supports lipid management for patients with diabetes and under 75yo. For those over 75yo, consider overall health status first. It is also important to refer diabetic patients for routine eye and feet care, at least annually. Nephropathy screening with annual screening for albuminuria should also be conducted.

Patients with diabetes are also at higher risk for depression. It is recommended to screen for depression during initial treatment period and if there is decline in clinical status. Also, it is important to consider screening for neurocognitive disorders. Persons with diabetes have higher incidence of all-cause dementia. Furthermore, the presence of cognitive impairment complicates patients' ability to manage their diabetes, including glucose monitoring and adjustment of medications, especially insulin. Lastly, as with all good geriatric care, attention to syndromes such as polypharmacy, urinary incontinence, pain, and falls is essential.

Table 11.5 Diabetes stratification based on complexity of illness

Patient health	A1C goal	Fasting glucose or postprandial	Bedtime glucose	BP goal	Lipid treatment
Healthy	<7.5	90–130	90–150	<140/80	Statin
Complex/intermediate	<8.0	90–150	100–180	<140/80	Statin
Very complex/poor health	8.5–9.0	100–180	110–200	<150/90	Consider statin

Table adopted from ADA, Diabetes Care [41]

Table 11.6 Pharmacologic options for diabetes management

Class and agent	Considerations
Biguanides Metformin	Works by decreasing hepatic glucose production Contraindicated if eGFR is <30 and not recommended if GFR is 30–45 Hold before contrast studies Caution in patients with impaired hepatic function or congestive heart failure due to increased risk of lactic acidosis May cause weight loss Gastrointestinal side effects of nausea or diarrhea are common
Second-generation sulfonylureas Glimepiride Glipizide Glyburide	Works by increasing insulin secretion Can cause hypoglycemia and weight gain. Must be used with caution Shorter duration glipizide is preferred sulfonylurea. Glyburide is not advised for older adults Use of clarithromycin, levofloxacin, ciprofloxacin, trimethoprim-sulfamethoxazole, and metronidazole are associated with increased risk of hypoglycemia
α-Glucosidase inhibitors Acarbose	Works by slowing down intestinal glucose digestion and absorption Main side effect is gastrointestinal (flatulence)
DPP-4 enzyme inhibitors Linagliptin (Tradjenta) Sitagliptin (Januvia)	Works by increasing insulin secretion and decreasing glucagon secretion Few side effects and minimal hypoglycemia
Meglitinides Nateglinide (Starlix) Repaglinide (Prandin)	Works by increasing insulin secretion. Can cause hypoglycemia and weight gain Avoid nateglinide in renal dysfunction
Thiazolidinoediones Pioglitazone (Actos) Rosiglitazone (Avandia)	Works by increasing insulin sensitivity Increases risk of heart failure. Avoid in class III or IV heart failure Monitor LFTs. Avoid if there is clinical evidence of liver disease
SGLT2 (sodium-glucose transporter 2) inhibitors Canagliflozin (Invokana) Dapagliflozin (Farxiga) Empagliflozin (Jardiance)	Work by decreasing glucose reabsorption from the kidney May cause ketoacidosis, acute kidney injury, urinary tract infections, increased LDL, and fracture risk Avoid in patients with renal impairment
GLP-1 receptor agonists Dulaglutide (Trulicity) Exanatide (Byetta) Liraglutide (Victoza)	Work by activating GLP-1 receptors and increasing insulin secretion Hypoglycemia common if combined with sulfonylurea or insulin Risks include acute pancreatitis or medullary thyroid cancer May be associated with vomiting, diarrhea, or nausea
Amylin analogue Pramlintide (Symlin)	Nausea common Risk of hypoglycemia when used with insulin
Insulin therapy	Requires patient or caregiver to have good visual or motor skills and cognitive ability Once-daily basal insulin preferable option, if possible, over multiple daily injections which is more complex to manage

11

11.5.3 Osteoporosis

Osteoporosis is a systemic condition that is characterized by low bone mass that increases the risk of bone fracture. According to the National Health and Nutrition Examination Survey (NHANES), from 2005 to 2010, 16.2% of all US adults had osteoporosis of the lumbar spine or femur neck [45]. It is even more common in females and all adults over the age of 80 [45]. As the population ages, the burden of osteoporosis will continue to climb higher.

Other important risk factors include weight, height, previous fracture, glucocorticoid use and tobacco and alcohol intake [46]. Given the importance of age and female sex as risk factors for osteoporosis, the US Preventive Services Task Force (USPSTF) recommends that all women over the age of 65 should be screened for osteoporosis [48]. Furthermore, younger postmenopausal women should also be considered for screening. The USPTF has recommended that women between the ages of 50 and 65 be evaluated using the FRAX (▶ https://www.shef.ac.uk/FRAX) tool to determine the need for osteoporosis screening [48]. A woman aged 50–65 with a FRAX score of 9.3%, which is an equivalent score of a 65-year-old white woman without other risk factors, should undergo osteoporosis screening [48].

Osteoporosis screening is typically conducted using the dual energy x-ray absorptiometry (DEXA) scan. The DEXA scan measures bone mineral density at the hip and lumbar spine [44]. The DEXA scan reports bone density as T scores for adults over the age of 50. Per the World Health Organization, adults with a T score less than or equal to

15. Pickering TG, Hall JE, Appel LJ, et al. Recommendations for blood pressure measurement in humans and experimental animals: part 1: blood pressure measurement in humans: a statement for professionals from the Subcommittee of Professional and Public Education of the American Heart Association Council on High Blood Pressure Research. Circulation. 2005;111:697–716.
16. Pickering TG, James GD, Boddie C, et al. How common is white coat hypertension? JAMA. 1988;259:225–8.
17. Vasan RS, Beiser A, Seshadri S, et al. Residual lifetime risk for developing hypertension in middle-aged women and men: the Framingham Heart Study. JAMA. 2002;287:1003–10.
18. Weiss J, et al. Intensive blood pressure treatment in adults aged 60 and older. Ann Intern Med. 2017;166:419–29.
19. Whelton PK, et al. 2017 ACC/AHA/AAPA/ABC/ACPM/AGS/APhA/ASH/ASPC/NMA/PCNA guideline for the prevention, detection, evaluation, and management of high blood pressure in adults: a report of the American College of Cardiology/American Heart Association Task Force on Clinical Practice Guidelines. Hypertension. 2017.

Chronic Kidney Disease

20. Kidney Disease: Improving Global Outcomes (KDIGO) CKD Work Group. KDIGO 2012 clinical practice guideline for the evaluation and management of chronic kidney disease. Kidney Int Suppl. 2013;3:1–150.
21. Munikrishnappa D. Chronic kidney disease (CKD) in the elderly–a geriatrician's perspective. Aging Male. 2007;10(3):113–37.
22. US Renal Data System: USRDS 2017 annual data report: Volume I - CKD in the United States 2017.

Dysphagia

23. Aslam M, et al. Dysphagia in the elderly. Gastroenterol Hepatol. 2013;9(12):784–95.
24. Geriatrics Review Syllabus, 7th edn. Chapter 29: Dysphagia.
25. Humbert IA, et al. Dysphagia in the elderly. Phys Med Rehabil Clin N Am. 2008;19:853–66.
26. Layne KA, et al. Using the Fleming Index of Dysphagia to establish prevalence. Dysphagia. 1989;4(1):39–42.
27. Lindgren S, et al. Prevalence of swallowing complaints and clinical findings among 50–79-year-old men and women in an urban population. Dysphagia. 1991;6(4):187–92.
28. Steele CM, et al. Mealtime difficulties in a home for the aged: not just dysphagia. Dysphagia. 1997;12(1):43–50.

Constipation

29. Bernard CE, Gibbons SJ, Gomez-Pinilla PJ, et al. Effect of age on the enteric nervous system of the human colon. Neurogastroenterol Motil. 2009;21:746–e46.
30. Dharmarajan. In: Pitchumoni CS, Dharmarajan TS, editors. Geriatric gastroenterology: Springer; 2012.
31. Lindberg G, et al. World Gastroenterology Organisation global guideline: constipation A global perspective. J Clin Gastroenterol. 2011;45(6):483:483–7.
32. Longstreth GF, Thompson WG, Chey WD, et al. Functional bowel disorders. Gastroenterology. 2006;130:1480–91.
33. Pinto Sanchez MI, Bercik P. Epidemiology and burden of chronic constipation. Can J Gastroenterol. 2011;25(Suppl B):11B–5B.

Fecal Incontinence

34. Papachrysostomou M, Pye SD, Wild SR, et al. Significance of the thickness of the anal sphincters with age and its relevance in faecal incontinence. Scand J Gastroenterol. 1994;29:710–4.
35. Sanjiv K. In: Pitchumoni CS, Dharmarajan TS, editor troenterology: Springer; 2012. p. 533–339.
36. Whitehead WE, Borrud L, Goode PS, et al. Feca in US adults: epidemiology and risk factors. Ga 2009;137:512–7.

Thyroid

37. Visser WE, et al. Thyroid disorders in older adults. En Clin N Am. 2013;42(2):287–303.
38. Geriatrics Review Syllabus, 7th edn. Chapter 59: metabolic disorders.
39. Geriatrics at Your Fingertips. 2017. Chapter endocri

Diabetes Mellitus

40. Lipska KJ, et al. Polypharmacy in the aging patie glycemic control in older adults with Type 2 c 2016;315(10):1034–45.
41. American Diabetes Association. Older adults: medical care in diabetes. 2018. Diabetes Care. 20 S119–25.
42. American Geriatrics Society Expert Panel on Care with Diabetes Mellitus, Moreno G, Mangione CM, berg E. Guidelines abstracted from the American G Guidelines for Improving the Care of Older Adu tes Mellitus: 2013 update. J Am Geriatr Soc. 201 https://doi.org/10.1111/jgs.12514.
43. Geriatrics at Your Fingertips. 2017. Chapter endocri

Osteoporosis

44. Ensrud KE, Crandall CJ. In the clinic: osteoporosis. 2017;166:ITC 17–32.
45. Looker AC, Frenk SM. Percentage of adults aged 6 osteoporosis or low bone mass at the femur neck United States, 2005–2010. Atlanta: Centers for I National Centers for Health Statistics; 2015.
46. O'Connor KM. Evaluation and treatment of osteop North Am. 2016;100:807–26.
47. Pavone V, Testa G, Giardina SMC, Vescio A, Re G. Pharmacologic therapy of osteoporosis: a sys review of literature. Front Pharmacol [Interne 2017 December 13]. 8. Available from: https://c fphar.2017.00803.
48. US Preventative Services Task Force. Screening f U.S. Preventive Services Task Force Recommenda Annals of Internal Medicine March 2011 Volume 15

Osteoarthritis

49. Barbour KE, Helmick CG, Boring M, Brady TJ. Vital s of doctor-diagnosed arthritis and arthritis-attri limitation—United States, 2013–2015. Morb M 2017;66:246–53.
50. Gelber AC, Cotton D, Rao JK, Taichman D, William osteoarthritis. Ann Intern Med. 2014;161:ITC1 1–16
51. Lespasio MJ, Piuzzi NS, Husni ME, Muschler GF, G MA. Knee osteoarthritis: a primer [Internet]. Perr 2017 November 18]. 21. Available from: https:// TPP/16-183
52. Taylor N. Nonsurgical management of osteoarthr the older adult. Clin Geriatr Med. 2017;33:41–51.

−2.5 has osteoporosis, a T score between −1.0 and −2.5 is osteopenia and greater than −1.0 is normal [44]. There are no evidence-based guidelines for re-screening patients with osteopenia; however, repeat DEXA should be done for these patients given their risk of developing osteoporosis. Osteoporosis can also be diagnosed from a fragility fracture, which is a fracture occurring in the absence of major trauma [46]. Treatment should also be considered in postmenopausal women with osteopenia, and a 10-year probability of hip fracture is 3% or greater, or risk of major osteoporotic fracture (hip, shoulder, wrist) is greater than or equal to 20% per the FRAX calculator [46].

All older adults should be counseled on preventive measures to maintain good musculoskeletal health. Important preventive measures for musculoskeletal health include maintaining a normal body weight, exercise, and adequate intake of calcium and vitamin D [44]. It is important that Vitamin D deficiency be treated prior to initiating other treatment for osteoporosis [47].

The goal of pharmacologic treatment for osteoporosis is to increase bone mass by increasing bone formation and/or decreasing bone resorption. Bisphosphonates are first-line treatment for osteoporosis, and these medications work by decreasing bone resorption [47]. The most commonly used bisphosphonates are oral medications that are taken on a daily or weekly basis. There are also intravenous formulations that can be given for patients who do not tolerate oral preparations [44]. It is important to note that bisphosphonates are contraindicated in patients with severe renal impairment, a glomerular filtration rate (GFR) less than 30–35 mL/min [47]. Rare but important adverse effects that have been associated with bisphosphonates include osteonecrosis of the jaw and atypical femur fractures. Bisphosphonate therapy may need to be suspended prior to invasive dental procedures [46]. Also, it has been proposed that patients on bisphosphonates be placed on a drug holiday after 5 years of medication use depending on their risk of fracture off of the medication [46].

Other pharmacologic treatments include selective estrogen receptor modulators, parathyroid hormone analogues, and monoclonal antibody treatments which are options for patients who cannot tolerate bisphosphonates. Teriparatide or recombinant human 1–34 parathyroid hormone works by increasing bone remodeling [46]. Teriparatide has been shown to significantly reduce vertebral and non-vertebral fractures, but data has not shown efficacy in reducing hip fractures [46]. Denosumab is a monoclonal antibody that works by decreasing osteoclast formation [46]. It has been shown to reduce osteoporotic fracture risk at all sites.

11.6 Part V: Musculoskeletal Disorders

Musculoskeletal disorders are very common in older adults. Given the high overall prevalence of these conditions, they are often present in patients with multimorbidity. Certain risk factors that are common to many musculoskeletal conditions—such as age, gender, and weight—are also risk factors for other diseases commonly found in multimorbid patients, such as cardiovascular and endocrine conditions. In this section, we will focus on one commonly occurring conditions in multimorbid patients—osteoarthritis.

11.6.1 Osteoarthritis

The burden of osteoarthritis in older adults in the United States is extremely high. According to the National Health Information Survey, approximately 22 million adults in the United States older than 65 have arthritis [49]. This represents nearly half of the older adults living in the United States. Furthermore, with the projected aging of the American population, the burden of osteoarthritis will certainly climb higher.

The major risk factors for osteoarthritis include age, family history, ethnicity, and female sex. The most important modifiable risk factor for osteoarthritis is obesity [51]. It has also been shown that patients with comorbid conditions of heart disease and diabetes are more likely to have osteoarthritis compared to those without these conditions [49].

Diagnosis of osteoarthritis can be made by history and physical exam with radiologic confirmation if needed [50]. Common symptoms of osteoarthritis include joint stiffness and pain [50]. Signs on exam include tenderness along the joint line, bony enlargement, and crepitus with movement of joint [50]. Common radiologic findings include joint space narrowing and osteophyte formation [50]. Although osteoarthritis is a very common etiology of joint pain, a differential diagnosis for joint pain should be considered. Other potential etiologies for joint pain include other forms of arthritis (gouty arthritis, rheumatoid arthritis, septic arthritis), calcium pyrophosphate dihydrate deposition disease, osteonecrosis, and Paget's disease of the bone [51]. If there is clinical suspicion for these conditions, appropriate diagnostic workup should be undertaken (▫ Table 11.7).

Management of osteoarthritis includes both pharmacologic and nonpharmacologic measures. All patients should be counseled on lifestyle changes including weight loss [51]. Other nonpharmacologic measures that may be considered include physical therapy, orthotics, and other supportive or assistive devices [50]. Physical therapy and braces and devices should be tailored to the patient and joint by trained providers [50].

Given that older adults are often multimorbid and given the potential side effects associated with certain analgesics, pharmacologic therapy for osteoarthritis should be chosen judiciously. The favorable outcome versus side effect profile of topical nonsteroidal anti-inflammatory drugs (NSAIDs) merits these agents as first choice for pharmacologic therapy of osteoarthritis [52]. The American College of Rheumatology strongly recommends topical NSAIDs over oral NSAIDs for treatment of osteoarthritis [52]. If the patient and joint (typically larger joints like the knee and shoulder) are amenable to joint injections, these injections should be considered to reduce pill burden and potential side effects from systemic

Table 11.7 Common differential diagnoses of OA

Condition	Distinguishing features
Rheumatoid arthritis	Inflammatory signs (fatigue, prolonged stiffness), rarely involves distal interphalangeal joints. Elevated inflammatory markers. Rheumatoid factor and anticyclic citrullinated peptide antibody may be positive
Gouty arthritis	Acute episode of mono- or polyarticular arthritis with erythema and possible edema. Monosodium urate crystals seen on synovial fluid. Tophi may be present
Calcium pyrophosphate deposition disease (CPPD)	Chondrocalcinosis seen on radiographs. CPPD crystals seen on synovial fluid
Septic arthritis	Acute episode of monoarthritis with warmth, erythema, and edema
Polymyalgia rheumatica	Proximal muscle (shoulder, upper arms, hips, thighs, neck) pain and stiffness. Negative radiographs. Elevated inflammatory markers

therapy [52]. The most commonly administered joint injections are glucocorticoid joint injections although several other types of injections are available [52]. Other types of joint injections include hyaluronic acid and protein-rich plasma injections. However, evidence studying the effectiveness of these injections has had varying results [50].

If oral pharmacologic therapy is indicated, acetaminophen at a dose of 2–3 grams daily should be the first-line therapy [52]. NSAIDs can be used on an intermittent basis but patients should be cautioned on the risks of NSAID use [52]. Potential adverse effects of NSAIDs include increased risk of GI bleeding and renal toxicity. Opioids and opioid receptor agonists can be used judiciously if all other pharmacologic therapies are ineffective [52]. Finally, if the patient is a candidate for joint replacement surgery, they should be referred to a surgeon for further discussion of surgical options [51]. If a patient is referred for joint replacement surgery there are potential risks especially in older, multimorbid patients. Perioperative factors to consider include the risks of anesthesia and postoperative analgesics, postoperative delirium, and the potential need for rehab placement after surgery.

11.7 Conclusion

While we have reviewed the evidence-based approach for many of the most common chronic conditions for older adults in this chapter, there are still many other chronic conditions that unfortunately plague our older patients. It is important for clinicians to approach each older patient while considering the multiple problems that may be coexisting. It is also imperative to address an older adult's preferences and goals as well as prognosis and existence of other geriatric syndromes such as dementia or falls.

References

Introduction

1. American Geriatrics Society Expert Pa Adults with Multimorbidity. J Am E1–E25.

Coronary Artery Disease

2. Loengard AU. In: Soriano R, et al., e peripheral arterial diseases in fundame case-based approach. New York: Spring
3. Benjamin EJ, et al., on behalf of the A Statistics Committee and Stroke Statisti ease and stroke statistics—2017 updat can Heart Association. [published onlin 2017]. Circulation. 2017;135:e146.
4. Dai X, et al. Stable ischemic heart disea atr Cardiol. 2016;13(2):109–14.
5. Fihn SD, et al. 2012 ACCF/AHA/ACP/A line for the diagnosis and manageme ischemic heart disease: a report of th diology Foundation/American Heart Practice Guidelines, and the American (ican Association for Thoracic Surgery, Nurses Association, Society for Cardic Interventions, and Society of Thoracic S 2012;60:2564–603.
6. Luepker RV, et al. Case Definitions for Ac in Epidemiology and Clinical Research the AHA Council on Epidemiology and Committee; World Heart Federation Cc Prevention; the European Society of Ca Epidemiology and Prevention; Centers vention; and the National Heart, Lung, tion. 2003;108:2543–9.

Atrial Fibrillation

7. Desai Y, et al. Management of atrial fib Am Geriatr Soc. 2017;65(1):185–93.
8. Edholm K, Ragle N, Rondina M. Antit atrial fibrillation in the elderly. Med 417–30.
9. Fuster V, et al. ACC/AHA/ESC guidelin patients with atrial fibrillation: executi American College of Cardiology/Amer Force on Practice Guidelines and the ology Committee for Practice Guidelir (Committee to Develop Guidelines for t with Atrial Fibrillation). Circulation. 200
10. Kannel WB, Benjamin EJ. Current perce of atrial fibrillation. Cardiol Clin. 2009;2

Hypertension

11. Apoeso. In: Soriano R, et al., editors. Hy of geriatric medicine a case-based ap 2007.
12. Carson AP, Howard G, Burke GL, et al. tension incidence among middle-aged ethnic study of atherosclerosis. Hypert
13. Danaei G, Ding EL, Mozaffarian D, et al death in the United States: comparativ lifestyle, and metabolic risk factors. PLo
14. Lewington S, Clarke R, Qizilbash N, et a usual blood pressure to vascular morta vidual data for one million adults in 61 2002;360:1903–13.

Geriatric Considerations in Common Surgical Conditions

Adora Tricia V. Santos and Steven Y. Chao

A. Chun (ed.), *Geriatric Practice*, https://doi.org/10.1007/978-3-030-19625-7_12

12.1 Introduction

It is estimated that by the year 2030, about 20% of Americans will be older than 65, while one out of four elderly individuals will be older than 85 years of age. Twenty-one percent of those over age 60 will undergo surgery and anesthesia as compared with only 12% of those aged 45 to 60 years. Despite the higher numbers of elderly patients having surgery, mortality and morbidity rates have been declining. Older age appears to have assumed less influence as a determinant of adverse outcomes, as perioperative care has improved. A better understanding of the associated risk factors leading to perioperative complications may help providers to further lower the risk and is discussed in more detail in ▶ Chap. 10—Geriatric Preoperative Evaluation of the Older Adult. This chapter will describe some of the most common surgeries completed in older adults.

12.2 Breast Cancer

With the aging population in the United States, there has been an increase in the prevalence of breast cancer in the geriatric population. In fact, following skin cancer, it is the most common cancer and second most common cause of cancer-related deaths. Risk factors for the development of breast cancer are well established and are attributed to almost half of the reported cases. A much smaller percentage of breast cancers can be attributed to genetic mutations, such as BRCA1 and BRCA2.

12.2.1 Surgical Considerations

Currently, the main surgical treatment options for breast cancer include the modified radical mastectomy (MRM) and breast-conserving therapy (BCT). Which type of surgery is appropriate to recommend for the patient is dependent both on the stage of cancer and patient preference. For cancers that are not amenable to breast-conserving therapy (i.e., T3 tumors or multifocal tumors), a modified radical mastectomy is indicated. The modified radical mastectomy involves removal of the breast, including the pectoralis fascia. Multiple studies have shown that a patient's age should not preclude the surgeon from offering the MRM when appropriate, as operative mortalities have been reported to be between 0.2% and 4.5% [1].

In the early stages of breast cancer, BCT is considered to be an appropriate treatment in patients of all ages, with strong evidence to support that BCT is as effective in creating a disease-free state as MRM in the appropriate patient population. Contraindications to BCT can be found in ▶ Box 12.1. BCT in the elderly provides a better quality of life, and several studies have shown that at 10 years follow-up, there is a lower rate of recurrence in those >55 years old [1]. It is important to note that patients who undergo BCT with postoperative radiation will have a significant reduction in local recurrence at 5 and 15 years [1]. In the geriatric population, postoperative radiation is well tolerated and is in fact better tolerated in those >65 years of age than those in the younger populations.

Previously, the standard of care for patients with sentinel node-positive breast cancer was that they required an axillary lymph node dissection (ALND), which is the excision of all of the level I and level II axillary lymph nodes. However, in 2010, the ACS Oncology Group published their randomized trial, the Z11 trial, which analyzed the safety of performing solely a sentinel lymph node biopsy (SLNB) for patients with T1 or T2 N0 M0 breast cancer undergoing breast-conserving therapy [2]. They concluded that there was no significant difference in 5-year recurrence rates between the two groups [2].

Box 12.1 Contraindications to Breast-Conserving Therapy

1. 2+ primary tumors in different breast quadrants
2. Diffuse malignant-appearing microcalcifications
3. Prior therapeutic irradiation
4. Positive margins despite multiple attempts at BCT

12.2.2 Hormone Therapy

The benefit of the use of hormone therapy is determined by the ER and PR hormone receptor status of the cancer. In the postmenopausal state, in ER/PR-positive patients, current guidelines recommend the use of an aromatase inhibitor along with a selective estrogen receptor modulator, such as anastrozole or tamoxifen, respectively, with the addition of trastuzumab in HER-2 positive disease [3].

12.2.3 OncotypeDx

While ER/PR/HER-2 positivity helps determine the use of hormone therapy, the OncotypeDx genomic assay is now being used to determine whether the addition of systemic chemotherapy will significantly affect a patient's 5-year risk of recurrence [4]. This gene assay is applied to those with early-stage ER+, node-negative cancers. A patient receives a score between 0 and 100 and, from this result, can be placed into low-, intermediate-, and high-risk groups of recurrence. A score <10 has been shown to have a 5-year disease-free survival of 93.8% and an overall survival of 98% with adjuvant endocrine therapy alone, without the use of systemic chemotherapy [5]. Studies have shown that those in the high-risk group (recurrence score >25) would benefit the most from systemic chemotherapy. Further studies are needed at this time to determine the benefit of systemic chemotherapy in addition to hormonal therapy in those with scores of 11–25.

12.2.4 Breast Cancer Staging

Traditionally, breast cancer staging was based on anatomic characteristics of the primary tumor, using the TNM system, similar to other cancer staging systems. However, in 2018, the American Joint Committee for Cancer (AJCC) has incorporated the use of tumor genetics into its staging system for breast cancers [6]. A tumor's genetics, including ER/PR/HER-2 positivity, has played an important role in determining a patient's treatment plan, as described above. However, a tumor's genetics have not yet been used in classifying patients into prognostic stage groups and help determine which patients better benefit from systemic chemotherapy. With the new staging system, a patient's prognosis is determined not just by tumor size, presence of positive nodes, and distant metastasis. The new AJCC guidelines now incorporate ER/PR/HER-2 positivity, as well as OncotypeDx® scores into the staging system.

12.3 Prostate Cancer

Prostate cancer is the second leading cause of death from cancer in men, the most significant risk factor being age [7]. Most patients with prostate cancer are asymptomatic, and the presence of symptoms suggests advanced disease at presentation. According to the National Comprehensive Cancer Network recommendations, there is no current recommendation age for when to start and stop screening; however, there are several recommendations for screening methods and time intervals. In patients who elect to partake in an early detection program, the recommendation is for baseline PSA (prostate-specific antigen) levels as well as a baseline digital rectal examination. However, the use of PSA levels is controversial. In fact, the US Preventive Services Task Force recommends against the routine use of obtaining PSA levels as a screening method for prostate cancer. These recommendations are based on the fact that multiple studies have not showed a reduction in overall mortality in patients who were routinely screened for prostate cancer [8].

12.3.1 Staging

The American Joint Cancer Committee has defined a TNM staging system as seen in ◘ Table 12.1 [9].

12.3.2 Biopsy

Transrectal ultrasound is a minimally invasive method used to detect prostate cancer [7]. A biopsy needle is used to take multiple biopsies of the prostate, which has shown improved cancer detection as well as the ability to provide information on the staging of cancer.

12.3.3 Surgical Considerations

A radical prostatectomy is the surgical treatment of choice for prostate cancer and can be performed through open techniques, either through a lower midline incision or perineal

◘ **Table 12.1** Prostate cancer TNM classification

TX	Primary tumor cannot be assessed		NX	Regional lymph nodes not assessed	MX	Distant metastasis cannot be assessed	
T0	No evidence of primary tumor		N0	No regional lymph node metastasis	M0	No distant metastasis	
T1	Clinically unapparent tumor neither palpable nor visible by imaging		N1	Metastasis in regional lymph nodes	M1	Distant metastasis	
	1a	Histologic finding <5% of tissue				1a	Non-regional lymph nodes
	1b	Histologic finding >5% of tissue				1b	Bones
	1c	Tumor identified by needle biopsy				1c	Other site with or without bone disease
T2	Tumor confined within prostate						
T3	Tumor extends through prostate capsule						
T4	Tumor is fixed or invades adjacent structures other than seminal vesicles						
Staging							
I	T1a		N0		M0		
II	T1–2		N0		M0		
III	T3		N0		M0		
IV	T4		N0		M0		
	Any T		N1		M0		
	Any T		Any N		M1		

incision [7]. Advances in technology have allowed for this procedure to be now predominantly performed laparoscopically and robotically.

12.4 Upper Gastrointestinal Disorders

12.4.1 Esophageal Cancer

Esophageal cancer is prevalent both in the United States and worldwide, with squamous cell carcinoma being more common worldwide and adenocarcinoma being more common in the United States [9]. These types of cancers typically manifest late and in the elderly population, with a 5-year survival of 15–25% [10].

Esophageal adenocarcinoma arises from Barrett's esophagus in the setting of gastroesophageal reflux disease (GERD); however, smoking and obesity are also strong risk factors for the development of adenocarcinoma [9]. Chronic GERD can lead to metaplastic changes, so endoscopic biopsies should be taken to evaluate for these changes that may degenerate into cancer. While there are no set guidelines for screening for esophageal cancer, several studies have recommended that patients with dysphagia and chronic GERD symptoms should be screened [9–11]. Once the diagnosis of esophageal cancer has been made, there are several treatment options, whose indications will depend on the stage of the cancer on discovery. Complete staging should be performed with endoscopic ultrasound to determine the depth of invasion and local nodal involvement, and PET/CT should be added for larger lesions to evaluate for metastatic lesions [9]. Therapeutic options can range from endoscopic ablation to esophagectomy, which will depend on the stage of the lesion [9].

12.4.2 Peptic Ulcer Disease

Peptic ulcer disease originates from mucosal damage that leads to ulceration of the stomach lining and is most commonly caused by *H. pylori* infection and NSAID use [12]. *H. pylori* has also been found to be the most common cause of gastritis, as well as for mucosa-associated lymphoid tissue (MALT) lymphoma [12].

Upper endoscopy can be used to visually diagnose peptic ulcer disease, while also having the advantage of the ability to take tissue samples to biopsy for *H. pylori*, as well as cancer [12]. However, endoscopic biopsies are not required to identify *H. pylori*. Less invasive methods include an immunoassay looking for IgG antibodies, a urea breath test, and stool antigen studies. It is important to be aware that the sensitivity is affected by the recent use of proton pump inhibitors, so these medications should be held for 2 weeks prior to test administration [12].

Once the diagnosis of peptic ulcer disease is made, treatment is directed at decreasing the acidic environment of the stomach, improving the mucosal barrier, and eradication of *H. pylori*, as well as avoidance of medications that lead to gastritis such as NSAIDs. The use of antacids, H2 receptor blockers, and PPIs can help decrease the acidic environment of the stomach. Sucralfate is a therapeutic option that likely helps with improving the mucosal barrier of the stomach, allowing for a layer of protection to the stomach lining against the acidic environment of the stomach [11]. In peptic ulcer disease caused by *H. pylori*, treatment is directed at the eradication of the bacteria and acid suppression [12]. Triple therapy for the eradication of *H. pylori* includes the use of PPI, amoxicillin and clarithromycin, or metronidazole in the penicillin-allergic patients for 2 weeks. In those whose treatment fails with triple therapy, quadruple therapy is initiated by the addition of bismuth.

12.4.3 MALT Lymphoma

MALT lymphoma is a type of lymphoma that involves mucosa-associated lymphoid tissue, usually originating from the stomach. Since MALT lymphoma is strongly associated with *H. pylori* infections, treatment is directed toward the eradication of the bacteria as described above [12]. Treatment usually leads to complete remission of MALT lymphoma, however, follow-up endoscopy 2 months after completion of therapy is necessary to evaluate and confirm response to treatment [12].

12.4.4 Gastric Cancer

Gastric cancer is a common cause of cancer and cancer death in the United States, with a peak incidence in the elderly population in the seventh decade of life [12]. There are multiple environmental and genetic risk factors to take into consideration when suspecting gastric cancer, which can be seen in ◘ Table 12.2.

◘ **Table 12.2** Risk factors for gastric cancer

Nutritional	Environmental	Social	Medical	Others
Low fat/protein	Poor food preparation	Low socioeconomic class	Prior gastric surgery	Male gender
Salted meat/fish	Lack of refrigeration		*H. pylori* infection	
High nitrates	Poor drinking water		Gastric atrophy and gastritis	
High complex carbohydrates	Smoking		Adenomatous polyps	

Symptoms of gastric cancer are usually nonspecific but may include epigastric pain not relieved with eating, early satiety, and weight loss [12]. Diagnosis is made with endoscopy and endoscopic ultrasound, and can be both diagnostic and therapeutic, by allowing for biopsies, and in the case of obstructing or bleeding lesions, stent placement and hemostasis can be achieved. Once the diagnosis of gastric cancer is made, staging should be completed, and treatment should be tailored based on completion (◘ Table 12.3) [13]. Endoscopic ultrasound is used to determine the depth of tumor invasion

◘ Table 12.3 Gastric cancer TNM classification [13]

Tx		Primary tumor cannot be assessed	NX		Regional lymph nodes cannot be assessed	M0	No distant metastasis
T0		No evidence of primary tumor	N0		No regional lymph node metastasis	M1	Distant metastasis
Tis		Carcinoma in situ	N1		Metastasis in 1–2 regional lymph nodes		
T1		Tumor invades lamina propria, muscularis mucosa, or submucosa	N2		Metastasis in 3–6 regional lymph nodes		
	1a	Invades lamina propria/muscularis mucosa	N3		Metastasis in >7 lymph nodes		
	1b	Invades submucosa					
T2		Invades muscularis propria		3a	Metastasis in 7–15 lymph nodes		
				3b	Metastasis in >16 lymph nodes		
T3		Penetrates subserosal tissue, no invasion of viscera					
T4		Invades serosa or adjacent structures					
	4a	Invades serosa					
	4b	Invades adjacent structures					

Staging			
0	Tis	N0	M0
1A	T1	N1	M0
1B	T2	N0	M0
	T1	N1	M0
IIA	T3	N0	M0
	T2	N1	M0
	T1	N2	M0
IIB	T4a	N0	M0
	T3	N1	M0
	T2	N2	M0
	T1	N3	M0
IIIA	T4a	N1	M0
	T3	N2	M0
	T2	N3	M0
IIIB	T4b	N0–N1	M0
	T4a	N2	M0
	T3	N3	M0
IIIC	T4b	N2	M0
	T4b	N3	M0
	T4b	N3	M0
IV	Any T	Any N	M1

and regional nodal involvement. The addition of a CT of the chest, abdomen, and pelvis will complete the staging of gastric cancer in order to assess for distant disease. Once the staging is completed, surgical therapy is determined based on final staging as well as the location of the primary cancer on the stomach. According to the National Comprehensive Cancer Network recommendations, neoadjuvant and adjuvant chemoradiation is also considered based on the location, stage, and biology of gastric cancer.

After surgical treatment, recurrences most often occur within the first 3 years postoperatively, and therefore, patients should be screened more closely in this time period; however, at this time there is no definitive evidence for screening intervals and duration [12].

12.5 Hernias

Hernias become more common in the geriatric population as a result of the weakening of the abdominal wall and comorbidities that increase abdominal pressure, like COPD [14]. However, when considering hernia repair in the geriatric patient, one must consider the morbidity and mortality associated with hernia repair in this particular population. These risks include wound infection, wound hematoma, mesh infection, bleeding, respiratory disease, and ischemic heart disease. This is particularly true in the setting of emergency repair which has a higher chance of postoperative morbidity. Hernia complications requiring emergent intervention would include incarceration or strangulation.

12.5.1 Surgical Considerations

Hernia repairs, both inguinal and ventral, are typically repaired either open or laparoscopically. There has been much debate regarding which method is safer and more effective in the geriatric population. A recent review of the literature showed low complication rates for both methods even in the aging patient with a decreased time back to work and lower rates of residual chronic pain postoperatively in the laparoscopic group [15].

12.6 Colorectal Disease

12.6.1 Diverticular Disease

Diverticular disease is one of the most common disease processes in developed countries, and the incidence increases greatly in the geriatric population [16]. Acute inflammation of colonic diverticula, as seen in diverticulitis, can often be managed with nonoperative therapy of bowel rest and antibiotics; however, there are instances in which surgical management is required, which is often associated with significant morbidity.

Table 12.4 Hinchey classification of perforated diverticulitis [18]

I	Pericolonic or mesenteric abscess
II	Pelvic abscess
III	Purulent peritonitis
IV	Feculent peritonitis

In the setting of acute diverticulitis, management will be dependent on the patient clinical picture, and patients can be divided into uncomplicated and complicated diverticulitis. Patients with significant tenderness on exam, who meet SIRS criteria, should be managed with bowel rest and IV antibiotics [17]. Patients should be referred for colonoscopy approximately 6–8 weeks after clinical symptoms have resolved, to screen for neoplasm which may also present like diverticulitis. The American Society of Colon and Rectal Surgeons now recommend that elective colectomy after an episode of uncomplicated diverticulitis is not required and should be considered following a recovery from an episode of complicated diverticulitis. However, the decision for surgery should be individualized to each patient [17].

Complicated diverticulitis is associated with abscess or fistula and may require more aggressive management. Table 12.4 lists the Hinchey classification for perforated diverticulitis and can aid the surgeon in determining management [18]. Stage I and II are often managed with IV antibiotics. In the event of a well-formed abscess and appropriate access, a percutaneous drainage is an option. On the other hand, stage III and IV often warrant emergent surgical exploration, particularly if the patient meets sepsis criteria. Operative management can vary from laparoscopy or laparotomy with colon resection with or without anastomosis, depending on the extent of peritonitis and patient clinical status.

12.6.2 Colorectal Cancer

Colorectal cancer is one of the most common types of cancers worldwide. The risk of colorectal cancer is directly related to age with the median age of diagnosis being 67. Timing and frequency of screening for colon cancer should be tailored to each individual patient. According to the American Cancer Society, in average-risk patients, those with no personal or family history of colorectal cancer, screening should begin at age 45. In patients with at least one first-degree relative with colorectal cancer at any age, screening colonoscopies should begin at age 40, or 10 years prior to the earliest age of diagnosis of the family member. Recommendations for endoscopic resection and frequency of repeat colonoscopies are dependent on what is found on initial screening colonoscopy.

The staging of colorectal cancer is based on a TNM staging system (Table 12.5) [19]. Evaluation for the metastatic disease includes CT chest, abdomen, and pelvis. Carcinoembryonic antigen (CEA) levels are also obtained

Table 12.5 Colorectal cancer TNM classification [19]

TX	Primary tumor cannot be assessed	NX		Regional nodes cannot be assessed	M0		No distant metastasis
T0	No evidence of primary tumor	N0		No regional metastasis	M1	a	Metastasis confined to one organ
T1	Tumor invades submucosa	N1	a	Metastasis in 1 regional lymph node		b	Metastasis to more than one organ
T2	Tumor invades muscularis propria		b	Metastasis in 2–3 regional lymph nodes			
T3	Tumor invades through muscularis propria		c	Metastasis to regional tissues			
T4a	Tumor penetrates through peritoneum	N2	a	Metastasis to 4–6 regional lymph nodes			
T4b	Tumor invades other organs		b	Metastasis to 7+ regional lymph nodes			
Colon cancer staging							
0	Tis			N0	M0		
1	T1			N0	M0		
	T2			N0	M0		
IIA	T3			N0	M0		
IIB	T4a			N0	M0		
IIC	T4B			N0	M0		
IIIA	T1–T2			N1/N1c	M0		
	T1			N2a	M0		
IIIB	T3–T4a			N1/N1c	M0		
	T2–T3			N2a	M0		
	T1–T2			N2b	M0		
IIIC	T4a			N2a	M0		
	T3–T4a			N2b	M0		
	T4b			N1–N2	M0		
IVA	Any T			Any N	M1a		
IVB	Any T			Any N	M1b		

and used in the postoperative period for surveillance for possible recurrent disease.

The workup for rectal cancer is similar to that of colon cancer. It is particularly important to determine the distance of the tumor to the anal sphincters, as this distance will determine surgical management [19]. A completion colonoscopy should also be performed in these patients to look for synchronous colonic lesions. The main difference between colon cancer and rectal cancer is the use of neoadjuvant chemotherapy, in addition to surgery and adjuvant therapy. The use of neoadjuvant therapy is recommended by the NCCN for stage II and higher stages of rectal cancers. Neoadjuvant therapy in these patients has been shown to be of benefit for several reasons. The main advantage includes the downstaging of tumors and better local control, which can change the operative management of the tumor and increase chances for sphincter preservation [20, 21].

Postoperatively, follow-up of patients with colorectal cancer is dependent on the stage of colon cancer. Those with stage I and II colon cancer may be followed with repeat colonoscopy within a year postoperatively and then every 5 years if no new polyps are detected [17]. CEA levels should be obtained every 3 months for the first 2 years, regardless of preoperative CEA level. If CEA levels are noted to rise, a metastatic workup is mandated. In stage I and II colorectal cancer, routine adjuvant chemotherapy is not recommended. Neoadjuvant as well as adjuvant chemotherapy may be of benefit in stage IV colon cancer in order to aid in the resectability of the cancer.

The treatment plan for colorectal cancer can be both different and difficult for geriatric patients. Successful treatment includes a multidisciplinary approach that includes surgeons, oncologists, radiation oncologists, anesthesiologists, gastroenterologists, pathologists, and radiologists. Geriatric patients should have their algorithms individualized based on their own age, comorbidities, functional status, advance directives, frailty, and social situations. More fit patients should be treated like younger patients in terms of an aggressive approach. However, this aggressive approach may not be appropriate for older and more frail patients due to high risk of mortality and morbidity. In the case of rectal cancer, after complete treatment with surgery, radiation, and chemotherapy, the patient may develop permanent bowel habit changes and incontinence or permanent ostomy leading to significant quality-of-life dysfunction. All of these risks must be thoroughly discussed with the patient with a possibility of the change of treatment plans as well as palliation [22].

12.7 Biliary Disease

12.7.1 Acute Calculous Cholecystitis and Choledocholithiasis

The management of acute cholecystitis can be managed operatively and nonoperatively, which can be decided based on surgeon preference and clinical condition of the patient. In acute cholecystitis, while the primary cause is obstruction of the cystic duct, it is associated with a superimposed infectious process, so the treatment is IV antibiotics along with prompt cholecystectomy. However, in the elderly population, particularly those with severe comorbidities that are considered to be a prohibitively high operative risk, a percutaneous cholecystostomy tube can be placed to drain the gallbladder of infected bile [23]. Biliary drainage allows for time to allow the inflammation to resolve, as well as medical optimization prior to interval cholecystectomy.

12.7.2 Acute Cholangitis

Acute cholangitis is an infection of the biliary tree caused by an obstruction of the biliary duct system [23]. Acute cholangitis presents with fever, jaundice, and right upper quadrant abdominal pain (Charcot's triad). The triad becomes Reynold's pentad in the setting of altered mental status and hypotension. Stable patients with cholangitis can quickly decompensate to septic shock and require immediate diagnosis and treatment with fluid resuscitation and broad-spectrum antibiotics. Definitive decompression of the biliary tree as well as drainage of infected bile should be performed promptly. This can be performed endoscopically, percutaneously, or operatively, dependent on the resources available to the institution.

Endoscopic treatment allows for definitive management by relieving the obstruction, whether by removing the obstructing stone or stent placement across an external obstruction [23]. However, percutaneous drainage, during which a drain is placed into the common bile duct, only allows for decompression of the biliary tree above the site of obstruction but does not relieve the obstruction in the duct. Operative management consists of common bile duct exploration with the placement of a T-tube for biliary drainage.

12.7.3 Biliary Pancreatitis

Obstruction of the common bile duct from a stone can cause inflammation to the pancreas from the increased pressure in the ducts proximal to the obstruction. Endoscopic ultrasound along with ERCP allows for diagnosis and treatment, as it allows for stone removal with or without stent placement to prevent future obstructions [23]. Once the pancreatitis has resolved, which can be determined by clinical resolution of abdominal pain, cholecystectomy is warranted to remove the source of gallstones that may cause a recurrence of biliary pancreatitis, preferably prior to discharge.

12.7.4 Surgical Considerations

It is known that the elderly patient population who undergo surgery for treatment of biliary disease in an emergent setting have higher mortality rates than their younger counterparts [24]. However, the morbidity and mortality rates are lower if the patient is allowed to recover from their acute illness and surgery is performed on an elective basis. Therefore, it is important that the surgeon takes these facts into consideration when treating acute biliary disease in the elderly. In the setting of choledocholithiasis, the use of ERCP in an emergent setting has been found to be safe and effective and will allow the patient to undergo medical optimization before elective surgery. In the case where the risks of nonoperative management of cholecystitis strongly outweigh the risk of emergent surgical management, percutaneous cholecystostomy has been found to allow for clinical improvement with >85% rates of clinical improvement, allowing for the patient to undergo cholecystectomy once the acute process has resolved [25].

12.8 Trauma

In the aging population in the United States, it is prudent for the surgeon to be aware of certain considerations that need to be taken when it comes to trauma in the geriatric patient. Trauma is the fifth most common cause of death in the elderly patients, with the most common cause of death resulting from falls [26]. Advanced age is known to be a risk factor for poor outcomes in trauma patients. This increased risk is due to multiple factors, including preexisting medical conditions, medications, and altered baseline mental status.

12.8.1 Initial Evaluation

The American College of Surgeons recommends following the same initial evaluation as any other trauma patient, with a few special considerations. The elderly trauma patient often has multiple comorbidities which put them at risk for more complications and poorer outcomes than the younger patient [27]. These comorbidities may preclude the trauma patient to nontraumatic events that could complicate their hospital stay, such as acute coronary syndrome, hypovolemia, pneumonia, acute renal failure, cerebrovascular accident, and syncope.

In addition to making the elderly patient more susceptible to nontraumatic events, patients with multiple comorbidities often take multiple medications, and it is important to consider polypharmacy as a cause of their traumatic injury. This patient population also is often on anticoagulation medications, which puts these patients at higher risk of bleeding events that may be devastating. It has been shown that having a rapid anticoagulation reversal protocol in place will lead to better outcomes in the injured patient [28]. Warfarin has multiple modes of reversal, including vitamin K and plasma; however, there are newer prothrombin complex concentrates that contain factors that rapidly reverse the effect of warfarin. On the other hand, patients who are taking direct Xa inhibitors, or direct thrombin inhibitors such as rivaroxaban and dabigatran, do not have rapid means of reversal and must be taken into consideration during initial assessment and management of the geriatric trauma patient.

When taking into consideration a trauma patient's medications, it is also important to be aware of medication side effects that may mask concerning signs or symptoms. For example, a patient who is on a beta-blockade for blood pressure control or atrial fibrillation may not show initial signs of acute blood loss, such as tachycardia, until a significant amount of blood has been lost.

It is crucial that the surgeon not overlook the potential for injuries in the elderly population, as relatively low-risk mechanisms may lead to a devastating injury. The ACS recommends the liberal use of CT scanning to rule out occult injuries [28]. This population is more susceptible to injuries due to physiologic changes related to age. For example, cerebrovascular injury is more common in the elderly due to cerebral atrophy, and fractures are more common despite low-risk mechanisms due to increased bone fragility [26].

Finally, much like in pediatric patients, it is important to be aware of the possibility of non-accidental traumas in the elderly, particularly those who live with relatives or are institutionalized [26].

12.8.2 Post-trauma Care

Taking care of a geriatric patient who sustains traumatic injuries that require hospitalization needs careful assessments and prompt development of treatment and follow-up plans. Historically, the Frailty Index has been used to predict a patient's disposition, whether it be home, short-term rehabilitation, or acute rehabilitation, and should be calculated early in order to aid in timely disposition once the patient has met discharge criteria [29].

When treating the geriatric trauma patient, it is also important to take into consideration any medications being prescribed to the patient, whether it be pain medications, antiarrhythmic agents, diuretics, or antibiotics. The ACS recommends following Beers Criteria [30] when taking into consideration medications being prescribed to patients during their hospital stay in order to prevent further complications in the already fragile patient population.

12.9 Conclusion

Surgery is common in older adults, but older age appears to have assumed less influence as a determinant of adverse outcome as perioperative care has improved. Despite the higher numbers of elderly patients having surgery, mortality and morbidity rates have been declining. As surgery becomes more common, it is important to have knowledge of common conditions and their potential surgical management options to optimize care for older adults.

References

1. Kalogerakos K, Sofoudis C, Koumousidis A, Tzonis P, Maniou I. Breast cancer surgery in the elderly women: a review. OA Women's Health. 2014;2(1):3.
2. Giuliano AE, McCall L, Beitsch P, et al. Locoregional recurrence after sentinel lymph node dissection with or without axillary dissection in patients with sentinel lymph node metastases: the American College of Surgeons Oncology Group Z0011 randomized trial. Ann Surg. 2010;252(3):426–33.
3. Puhalla S, Bhattacharya S, Davidson NE. Hormonal therapy in breast cancer: a model disease for the personalization of cancer care. Mol Oncol. 2012;6(2):222–36.
4. McVeigh TP, Hughes LM, Miller N, et al. The impact of Oncotype DX testing on breast cancer management and chemotherapy prescribing patterns in a tertiary referral centre. Eur J Cancer. 2014;50(16):2763–70.
5. Sparano JA, Gray RJ, Makower DF, et al. Prospective validation of a 21-gene expression assay in breast cancer. N Engl J Med. 2015;373(21):2005–14.
6. Giuliano AE, Connolly JL, Edge SB, et al. Breast cancer – major changes in the American Joint Committee on Cancer eighth edition cancer staging manual. CA Cancer J Clin. 2017;67(4):290–303.
7. Presti JC. Urology. In: Surgery: basic science and clinical evidence. 2nd ed. New York: Springer; 2008. p. 2175–96.
8. Moyer VA. Screening for prostate cancer: U.S. preventive services task force recommendation statement. Ann Intern Med. 2012;157:120–34.
9. Spicer JD, Dhupar R, Kim JY, Sepesi B, Hofstetter W. Esophagus. In: Sabiston textbook of surgery: the biological basis of modern surgical practice. 20th ed. Philadelphia: Elsevier; 2016. p. 1013–64.
10. Arnal MJ, Arenas AF, Arbeloa AL. Esophageal cancer: risk factors, screening and endoscopic treatment in western and eastern countries. World J Gastroenterol. 2015;21(26):7933–43.
11. Wang YK, Hsu WH, Wang SS, Lu CY, Kuo FC, Su YC. Current pharmacological management of gastroesophageal reflux disease. Gastroenterol Res Pract. 2013;2013:1–12.
12. Teitelbaum EN, Hungness ES, Mahvi DM. Stomach. In: Sabiston textbook of surgery: the biological basis of modern surgical practice. 20th ed. Philadelphia: Elsevier; 2016. p. 1188–236.
13. Ajani JA, Barthel JS, Bekaii-Saab T, et al. NCCN guidelines for gastric cancer. J Natl Compr Cancer Netw. 2010;8:378–409.

14. Compagna R, Rossi R, Fappiano F, et al. Emergency groin hernia repair: implications in elderly. BMC Surg. 2013;13(S29):19–22.
15. Bates AT, Divino C. Laparoscopic surgery in the elderly: a review of the literature. Aging Dis. 2015;6(2):149–55.
16. Comparato G, Pilotto A, Franze A, Franceschi M, DiMario F. Diverticular disease in the elderly. Dig Dis. 2007;25:151–9.
17. Feingold D, Steele SR, Lee S, et al. Practice parameters for the treatment of sigmoid diverticulitis. Dis Colon Rectum. 2014;57(3): 284–94.
18. Hinchey EJ, Schaal PG, Richard GK. Treatment of perforated diverticular disease of the colon. Adv Surg. 1978;12:85–109.
19. Mahmoud NN, Bleier JI, Aarons CB, Paulson EC, Shanmugan S, Colon FRD. Rectum. In: Sabiston textbook of surgery. 20th ed. Philadelphia: Elsevier; 2016. p. 1312–93.
20. Messersmith WA. NCCN guidelines for colorectal cancer. J Natl Compr Canc Netw. 2017;15(5S):699–702.
21. Li Y, Wang J, Ma X, et al. A review of neoadjuvant chemoradiotherapy for locally advanced rectal cancer. Int J Biol Sci. 2016;12(8): 1022–31.
22. Millan M, Merino S, et al. Treatment of colorectal cancer in the elderly. World J Gastrointest Oncol. 2015;7(10):204–20.
23. Jackson PG, Evans SR. Biliary system. In: Sabiston textbook of surgery. 20th ed. Philadelphia: Elsevier; 2016. p. 1482–519.
24. Siegel JH, Kasmin FE. Biliary tract diseases in the elderly: management and outcomes. Gut. 1997;41(4):433–5.
25. Zarour S, Imam A, Kouniavsky G, Zbar A, Mavor E. Percutaneous cholecystostomy in the management of high-risk patients presenting with acute cholecystitis: timing and outcome at a single institution. Am J Surg. 2017;214(3):456–61.
26. Yeo H, Indes J, Rosenthal RA. Surgery in the geriatric patient. In: Sabiston textbook of surgery. 20th ed. Philadelphia: Elsevier; 2016. p. 327–59.
27. Victorino GP, Chang TJ, Pal JD. Trauma in the elderly patient. Arch Surg. 2003;138(10):1093–8.
28. ACS TQIP Geriatric Trauma Management Guidelines. https://www.facs.org/~/media/files/quality%20programs/trauma/tqip/geriatric%20guide%20tqip.ashx. Accessed 11/1/2018.
29. Joseph B, Pandit V, Zangbar B, et al. Validating trauma-specific frailty index for geriatric trauma patients: a prospective analysis. J Am Coll Surg. 2014;219(1):10–7.
30. American Geriatrics Society 2015 Beers Criteria Update Expert Panel. American Geriatrics Society 2015 updated Beers Criteria for potentially inappropriate medication use in older adults. J Am Geriatr Soc. 2015;63:2227–46.

Medication Management (MEDICATIONS)

Contents

Prescription Selection and Dosing

Sharon See

A. Chun (ed.), *Geriatric Practice*, https://doi.org/10.1007/978-3-030-19625-7_13

13.1 Introduction

Most medical school education is based on disease-oriented evidence (DOE). This is evidence that includes information about pathophysiology, pharmacology, and prognosis [1]. It often requires memorization of a vast amount of content knowledge and facts. Pharmacology is the science of drugs including their origin, composition, pharmacokinetics, therapeutic use, and toxicology [2]. This includes medication class, mechanisms of action, indications, and side effects. This basic science education is important to providing the basis for critical thinking, and it is essential to understand diseases in order to diagnose, prevent, or treat. However, by itself, it is not sufficient for patient care in clinical practice. As medical students enter their clinical experiences after building their medical database, contact with patients requires a deeper knowledge of the medications they will soon be empowered to prescribe. This requires knowledge of patient-oriented evidence that matters (POEMs) and clinical application of drugs (pharmacotherapy) [1].

Patient-oriented evidence differs from disease-oriented evidence in that it evaluates the effectiveness of treatments in a way that patients will understand and care about. Knowing the difference between POEMs and DOEs can help clinicians with decision-making at the bedside and help them keep up with the literature. [◘ Table 13.1] [2–4] Consider the following scenario: You are looking at two different studies on a new hypertensive agent called LOWERSBP. Study 1 is a randomized controlled trial comparing LOWERSBP to placebo and showed that LOWERSBP lowers blood pressure by 5 mm Hg more than placebo, which only lowered blood pressure by 2 mm Hg. Study 2 is a randomized controlled trial comparing LOWERSBP to placebo and showed that LOWERSBP decreased the risk of stroke statistically significantly more than placebo. Which study reports an outcome that patients and clinicians care about? While a patient understands conceptually that she takes her blood pressure medicine to lower her numbers, it may matter more that it will prevent her from developing a stroke which may make her unable to talk, work and may change her lifestyle dramatically. Using this patient-oriented evidence can help patients understand the importance of their treatments in a relatable, relevant manner.

Pharmacotherapy is the treatment of disease through the use of drugs and differs from pharmacology in that it focuses on the patient-oriented evidence-based application of medication use for disease state management. This chapter will introduce the reader to a pathway to rational prescribing practices with a focus on special considerations unique to older adults as well as utilizing disease state knowledge, patient-oriented evidence and pharmacotherapy to help guide decision-making.

13.2 Polypharmacy

There is no consensus on the definition of polypharmacy but it is agreed that it can lead to negative consequences including increased costs, adverse events, medication nonadherence, decline in functional status, falls, and cognitive impairment [5]. In 2010–2011, 87% of adults aged 62–85 were taking prescription medication. Thirty-six percent of older adults were on more than five prescription medications, and 67% of older adults were on five or more medications and supplements. The most common drugs prescribed for older adults included antihyperlipidemics, antihypertensives, anticoagulants, and analgesics [6]. In a Veteran population, patients on more than five medications were associated with having adverse drug events (ADE) adjusted OR 2.85, 95% CI (1.03–7.85), and those on more than nine medications were four times more likely to develop an ADE (adjusted OR 3.90, 95% CI [1.43–10.61] [7]. A CDC study reported that 24% of emergency department hospitalizations were for adverse events with 46% attributed to adults older than 65 years of age. Approximately two-thirds of the adverse events in these older adults were due to opioids, diabetes medications, and anticoagulants [8]. Drug interactions are another consequence of polypharmacy. In a study of over 2000 older adults in the community aged 63–85 years old, in 2010–2011, 15% were prescribed drug combinations that could potentially cause a major drug-drug interaction. This was almost two times higher than in 2005–2006 [6].

Polypharmacy is commonly associated with inappropriate prescribing. While polypharmacy is often detrimental to older adults, sometimes it is necessary. For example, a patient with reduced ejection fraction heart failure (HFrEF) will

◘ **Table 13.1** Patient-oriented evidence that matters (POEMs) vs disease-oriented evidence (DOE) [3, 4]

Example	Disease-oriented evidence (DOE)	Patient-oriented evidence (POE)	Comment
Beta blockers in HFrEF	Blocks the neurohormonal surge associated with HFrEF; negative inotropes and chronotropes	Reduce morbidity and mortality	POE agrees with DOE
Antiarrhythmics (encainide/flecainide)	Decrease PVCs on ECG in patients with LVH after a myocardial infarction	Increased mortality	POE contradicts DOE

HFrEF Heart failure with reduced ejection fraction, *PVC* Premature ventricular contractions, *ECG* Electrocardiogram, *LVH* Left ventricular hypertrophy

13

need to be on at least four medications according to evidence-based guidelines [9]. A patient may have multiple conditions that warrant medications for each problem. The goal of every clinician should be to identify polypharmacy in older adults and have the skills to assess the appropriateness of medications, identify and avoid prescribing cascades and seek opportunities to deprescribe, reduce frequencies, eliminate duplication of therapies, and/or switch to combination medications if available. Deprescribing is the process by which clinicians discontinue medications after careful consideration of risks versus benefits and patient goals and values [10]. Medications with no clear indication such as a proton pump inhibitor in a patient without peptic ulcer disease or GERD would be good candidates for deprescribing. Other appropriate situations for deprescribing include discontinuing drugs where the time to benefit may go beyond the life expectancy of a patient. If a patient is expected to die within 6 months, it may be reasonable to discontinue a statin since its time to benefit to prevent a cardiovascular event is 5 years [11].

There are several common medications that are often inappropriately prescribed in older adults. This includes sedative hypnotics, anticholinergic drugs, benzodiazepines, first-generation antihistamines, and anticoagulants. Older adults are prone to medication errors due to unique pharmacokinetics and pharmacodynamic changes. The Beers criteria provide a list of potentially harmful drugs in older adults and, if prescribed, must be used with caution [12]. The recommendations in this guideline seek to decrease or avoid potential adverse events, aid in drug selection, and be used in research studies to evaluate medication use in older adults. This guideline also provides recommendations for renal dosing for commonly used medications as well as drug combinations that can lead to clinically important drug-drug interactions.

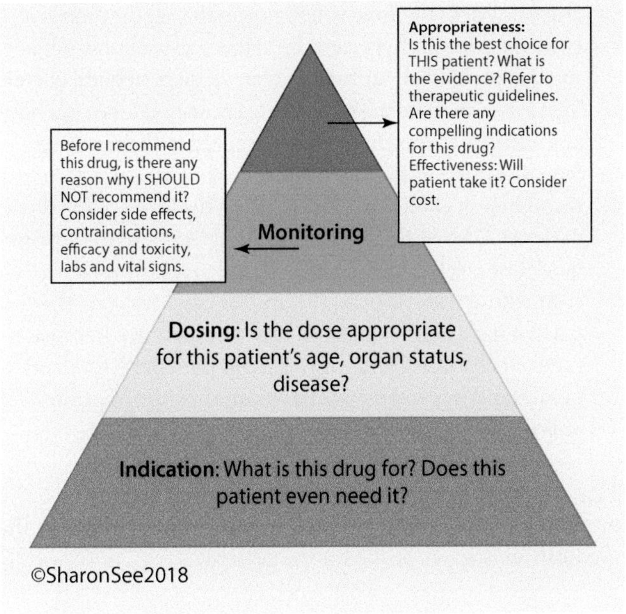

■ **Fig. 13.1** Hierarchy of Medication Evaluation

13.3 Principles of Prescribing

Good prescribing practices can help to avoid polypharmacy and the negative consequences that accompany it. The Hierarchy of Medication Evaluation (HME) is an algorithm that the author (SS) created and uses to assess patient medications (■ Fig. 13.1) This pyramid resembles Bloom's taxonomy where lower order thinking resides at the base of the pyramid and more critical thinking is at the peak. (■ Fig. 13.2) [13] In the same way, HME begins with the most basic content at the bottom of the pyramid. Throughout medical training, the medical student must work his way up from content and memorization toward truly understanding and determining the appropriateness of his medication selection. This HME can be applied to assess current medications or aid in rational prescribing decision-making. Each step is described below:

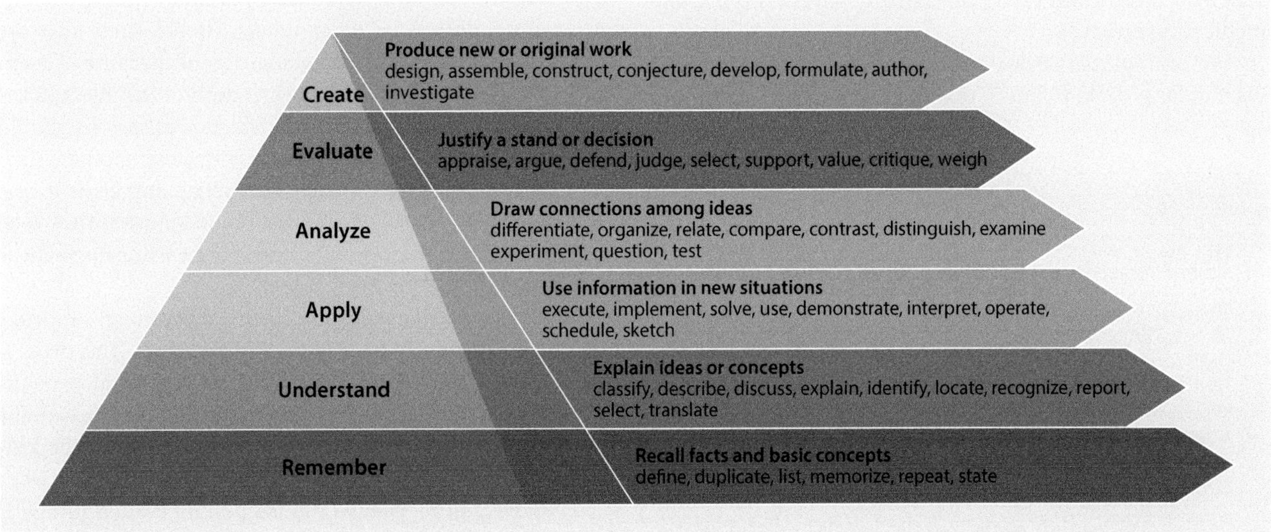

■ **Fig. 13.2** Revised Blooms Taxonomy. (Modified from [13])

13.3.1 Hierarchy of Medication Evaluation

- Step 1: Indication – What is the drug for? This step is the most basic skill of medication evaluation and requires content knowledge. Is there a matching indication for the drug being considered? If not, perhaps the patient does not need it.
- Step 2: Dosing – Is this drug dose appropriate for this patient's renal or hepatic function? Older adults have reduced renal and hepatic function, and as a result, many medications need their doses adjusted because they cannot be cleared.
- Step 3: Monitoring – Before prescribing this medication, is there any reason why you SHOULD NOT recommend it? Who should *not* get this drug? Asking this negative question will help the prescriber consider contraindications to the drug and come to a quick conclusion about going forward with the prescription. Another important question to ask in this step is, "How will you know if the drug is working?" "How will you know if the medication is causing toxicities?" Here you need to know monitoring parameters for efficacy and toxicity (◘ Table 13.2) [14–16]. If the drug you are considering is the beta-blocker metoprolol, then you know its efficacy parameter is blood pressure and its toxicity parameter is heart rate (bradycardia).
- Step 4: Appropriateness – This is the step that requires higher level thinking. Once you have passed each previous step, it is time to consider the evidence. Is this the best choice for this patient according to evidence-based medicine and guidelines? What is the effectiveness of this drug in this patient? (◘ Table 13.2) [14–16]. Will the patient take it? Consider frequency, dosage form, and cost.

13

As the prescriber proceeds up the HME, he/she should stop at each step and ask the relevant questions for that step before moving on. A prescriber may halt his decision to prescribe a medication at any point in the pyramid. In turn, this HME may help avoid unnecessary prescribing, adverse events, and medication errors.

For example, an 80-year-old man comes to clinic and has been taking amlodipine 5 mg daily for hypertension for 1 year. His blood pressure is 135/88 mmHg. His past medical history includes HFrEF, asthma, and osteoarthritis. This patient has normal renal function. He just moved to town and is seeing you for the first time for a physical. Let's use the HME to determine whether this medication is a rational, best choice for this patient's hypertension.

- Step 1: Indication – Amlodipine is a dihydropyridine calcium channel blocker which is indicated for hypertension. Proceed to the next step.
- Step 2: Dosing – Amlodipine 5 mg daily is an appropriate hypertensive dose and does not require to be adjusted in this patient. Proceed to the next step.
- Step 3: Monitoring – Is there any reason why this patient should *not* be on this medication? This requires you to know the contraindications and adverse effect of this drug. Does this person have any allergies to this medication? We also want to know, how will I know if this medication is efficacious for his hypertension? How will we know if it's causing problems? Amlodipine can cause peripheral edema. This is not an issue in this patient. The patient does not have any allergies to this medication. Proceed to the next step.
- Step 4: Appropriateness – According to best practice and standards of care, is amlodipine the best choice for this patient? According to the 2017 ACC/AHA hypertension guidelines, selection of antihypertensives is based on compelling indications [17]. In this case, because the patient has HFrEF, an ACEI is the best choice because it reduces mortality and morbidity in patients with heart failure and hypertension. Based on this information, amlodipine is not the best choice for this patient.

This example demonstrates that a positive response to the questions posed in Steps 1–3 does not necessarily mean the medication is appropriate for the patient.

◘ Table 13.2 Efficacy versus effectiveness [14, 15, 16]

Efficacy	Effectiveness
These types of trials may are done in "ideal" settings	These types of trials are conducted in "real world" settings
Exubera (inhaled insulin) was shown in studies to lower HbA1c in Type 2 diabetes Efficacy: Good	Patients did not like Exubera because the inhaler was too big and bulky and expensive compared to subcutaneous insulin Effectiveness: Bad

HbA1c Hemoglobin A_{1c}

13.4 Renal and Hepatic Considerations

As mentioned earlier, renal function declines with age which affects drug dosing in older adults. Medications that are renally eliminated require dose adjustments because of accumulation which may lead to exaggeration of the effect of the primary medication and/or toxic effects. Prescribers should also be aware that medications with active metabolites (such as glyburide) will accumulate with renal impairment and lead to toxicities. Prescribers must reconcile what they read in drug dosing references and understand why dosing adjustments are required for medications.

Two common reasons for dose adjustment of drugs include: 1. The drug is renally eliminated. 2. The drug is metabolized by the liver. Medication management depends on what happens if the drug is not adjusted. If the reason for dose adjustment is because a drug is eliminated by the kidneys and the patient has renal failure, then the prescriber needs to determine what would happen if he did nothing. If the consequence of drug accumulation leads to a minor side effect such as sedation, perhaps the dose can be reduced. If the result of drug accumulation leads to a severe adverse effect such as renal tubular necrosis, then the decision would be to discontinue the drug and seek alternatives. Prescribers must be familiar with the toxicities of the medications they prescribe to help them make prescribing decisions.

13.4.1 Renal Considerations

Glomerular filtration rate (GFR) indicates how well the nephrons of the kidney are filtering. Serum creatinine is a by-product of muscle metabolism and is cleared by glomerular filtration. Creatinine clearance (CrCl) is not synonymous with GFR [18]. Serum creatinine is a filtration marker that can best determine GFR. Daily creatinine production declines with age [19]. Calculating CrCl using various equations can estimate GFR. The Cockcroft-Gault (CG) equation is the pharmaceutical industry standard for pharmacokinetic drug dosing studies [20]; however, there is growing support for alternate, more accurate ways to determine GFR using the Modification of Diet in Renal Disease (MDRD) study equation. The Cockcroft-Gault equation is based on two basic assumptions: 1. serum creatinine is at steady state and 2. weight, age, and gender reflect normal muscle mass. (Fig. 13.3) [19, 21] Because muscle produces creatinine, changes in muscle mass can affect creatinine production. Oftentimes, renal function in older adults is deemed normal because of attention paid solely to serum creatinine which is often below 1 mg/dL. A normal or low serum creatinine is misleading however, because this is attributed to lower lean body mass in older adults rather than normal renal function. To avoid missing true renal impairment, it is important to calculate CrCl rather than focusing solely on serum creatinine. In older adults, some clinicians round up the creatinine to 1 mg/dL when the actual creatinine is less than 1 mg/dL to compensate for overestimating CrCl although this can lead to underestimating CrCl and potentially underdosing of medication [18, 19]. The CG calculation is an estimate of CrCl and clinical judgment should be used to determine which method of calculation to use (rounding creatinine to 1 mg/dl or using actual creatinine). It is reasonable to calculate both and then determine which one is more plausible. For example, the CrCl of an 88 year old, 70 kg with Cr of 0.5 mg/dl = 101 ml/min vs Cr 1 mg/dl = 51 ml/min. Which is more plausible in an 88 year old? The MDRD equation estimates GFR using body surface area and race and is purported to be a more accurate measure of CrCl compared to 24-hour urine collection and Cockcroft-Gault equation. The MDRD equation is less accurate when GFR > 60 mL/min/1.73 m2 and more useful when GFR < 60 mL/min/1.73 m2 assuming average body size and muscle mass. For a majority of patients, there is not a significant difference in drug dosing adjustments using either Cockcroft-Gault or MDRD equation [22]. Table 13.3 provides a list of common medications that require renal dose adjustments [23].

$$\text{CrCl (ml/min)} = \frac{(140\text{-age}) \times \text{IBW (kg) (0.85 if female)}}{72 \times \text{Cr (mg/dL)}}$$

CrCl = Creatinine clearance
IBW = Ideal body weight
Cr = Serum creatinine

Fig. 13.3 Cockgroft-Gault Equation. (Modified from [21])

Table 13.3 Common medications that require dose reduction in CKD [23]

Class	Examples
ACEI	Lisinopril, enalapril
BB	Atenolol
Diuretics	Hydrochlorothiazide (avoid when CrCl <30 ml/min)
Oral diabetes agents	Glyburide (avoid), metformin
Antimicrobials	Ampicillin/sulbactam, TMP/SMX, fluoroquinolones, nitrofurantoin, carbapenems
HMG Co-A Reductase Inhibitors	Pravastatin, rosuvastatin, simvastatin
Other	Allopurinol, H2 blockers, gabapentin

CKD Chronic kidney disease, *ACEI* Ace inhibitors, *BB* Beta-blockers, *TMP/SMX* trimethoprim-sulfamethoxazole

Case 1

Scenario 1: An 88-year-old woman comes to the pharmacy for her glyburide prescription. You look up the drug in your drug reference and realize that it should not be used in patients with CrCl <60 ml/min. She has a CrCl of 20 ml/min.

Question: Why should it not be used with CrCl <60 ml/min?

Answer: Glyburide has an active metabolite that is 50% eliminated renally and has an extremely long half-life of 10 hours. The active metabolite would accumulate resulting in toxicity, in this case hypoglycemia.

Scenario 2: The pharmacy only has glyburide in stock and the closest pharmacy is 3 hours away in the next town.

Question: Should the pharmacist send the patient to the nearest pharmacy which is 3 hours away to get an alternative medication like glipizide (which does not have an active metabolite and is not renally cleared) or can she suggest to the provider to reduce the dose?

Answer: In this situation, the pharmacist can recommend to reduce the dose rather than inconvenience the patient.

Case 2

Scenario 1: The drug monograph for metformin says: Do not give if CrCl <30 ml/min.

Question: Why?

Answer: It's excreted 90% as unchanged drug in the urine. So, it will accumulate and cause toxicity, in this case lactic acidosis.

Scenario 2: The drug monograph also says: Do not give if the patient has uncontrolled reduced ejection fraction.

Question: Why?

Answer: With heart failure, there is decreased perfusion to the entire body including the kidneys. If there is reduced perfusion, the drug will not be renally eliminated and would accumulate and thus increase the risk of lactic acidosis.

In both scenarios, renal impairment causes the accumulation of the drug which will lead to toxicities of that drug. Its dosing parameters are based on the fact that it is 90% renally eliminated. Metformin itself does not cause renal failure. It requires dose adjustments because it is an elimination issue.

13.4.2 Hepatic Considerations

Older adults have a reduced ability to metabolize medications due to smaller livers and decreased liver blood flow. This can result in an increase of bioavailability of some medications leading to adverse effects. Liver impairment such as cirrhosis can also affect the metabolism and clearance of medications via several mechanisms. Drugs can accumulate due to decreased hepatic clearance and have increased bioavailability or fail to be metabolized to active or inactive metabolites due to the reduction of first-pass metabolism and hepatic enzyme activity. Patients with liver disease also have decreased protein binding which prevents certain medications from being distributed throughout the body resulting in a lower volume of distribution and ultimately may require higher loading doses [24]. Liver disease can also cause a renal failure which can lead to the decreased renal elimination of drugs resulting in toxicities.

13

A reduction of first-pass metabolism and hepatic metabolic enzymes can result in higher bioavailability of certain medications. Specifically, Phase I reactions (hydrolysis, oxidation and reduction) decline with in older adults, however Phase II reactions (conjugation) are preserved [18, 25]. Drugs that undergo Phase I biotransformation are metabolized by cytochrome P450 enzymes putting elderly patients at risk for CYP 450 drug interactions.

Unlike in renal disease where the calculation of CrCl using the Cockcroft-Gault equation can be useful for drug dosing, there is no equivalent measurement to determine how hepatic disease can alter a drug's pharmacokinetic or pharmacodynamic parameters. The FDA requires a pharmacokinetic study of a drug in a patient with liver disease only if the absorbed drug is >20% is hepatically metabolized or cleared or < 20% if it has a narrow therapeutic index. This parameter limits the number of medications with these PK studies [26]. The tool that is used to aid with drug dosing in liver disease is the Child Pugh Scoring Tool. This is a scoring system that utilizes five criteria to determine the severity of liver disease. They include bilirubin, ascites, albumin, prothrombin time or INR, presence of encephalopathy. Each item is scored and totaled. Liver disease severity is classified Mild: Grade A < 7 points, moderate: Grade B 7–9 points, or severe: Grade C 10–15 points (Table 13.4) [18, 27]. Medication package inserts include Child Pugh Scoring to aid in dose adjustments in hepatic disease for applicable drugs.

Table 13.4 Child-Pugh Scoring [27]

Test/symptom	Score 1 point	Score 2 points	Score 3 points
Total bilirubin (mg/dL)	<2.0	2.0–3.0	>3.0
Serum albumin (g/dL)	>3.5	2.8–3.5	<2.8
Prothrombin time (seconds prolonged over control)	<4	4–6	>6
Ascites	Absent	Slight	Moderate
Hepatic encephalopathy	None	Moderate	Severe

Scenario: A 78-year-old woman is admitted to the hospital for alcohol withdrawal. You activate your hospital's alcohol withdrawal protocol which gives the option of starting a diazepam or lorazepam pathway.

Question: Which benzodiazepine should you choose for this patient?

Answer: Diazepam undergoes Phase I metabolism and has a long half-life (60–72 hours) and is metabolized to an active metabolize desmethyldiazepam which has a half-life of 152–174 hours. On the other hand, lorazepam undergoes Phase II metabolism and is rapidly conjugated to an inactive metabolite. Because older adults have reduced Phase I metabolism and intact Phase II metabolism, lorazepam would be the optimal benzodiazepine to choose in this scenario. Other benzodiazepines that undergo Phase II metabolism include oxazepam and temazepam.

13.5 Conclusion

Rational prescribing in older adults requires thoughtful decision-making with the aid of tools such as the Hierarchy of Medication Evaluation which focuses on important questions at each step. As prescribers progress through the HME, attention focuses on assessing the appropriateness of medications and requires prescribers to consider contraindications or side effects. Basic disease state knowledge along with patient-oriented evidence is necessary to answer this question. Prescribers must consider the consequences of polypharmacy and pay close attention to the renal and hepatic function of older adults.

References

1. Slawson DC, Shaughnessy AF, Bennett JH. Becoming a medical information master: feeling good about not knowing everything. J Fam Pract. 1994;38(5):505–13.
2. Introduction. In: Trevor AJ, Katzung BG, Kruidering-Hall M, editors. Katzung & Trevor's pharmacology: examination & board review, 11th ed. New York: McGraw-Hill; 2015 http://accesspharmacy.mhmedical.com.jerome.stjohns.edu:81/content.aspx?bookid=1568&sectionid=95700839. Accessed 13 Jan 2018.
3. Sackner-Bernstein JD, Mancini DM. Rationale for treatment of patients with chronic heart failure with adrenergic blockade. JAMA. 1995;274:1462.
4. Echt DS, Liebson PR, Mitchell LB, Peters RW, Obias-Manno D, Barker AH, et al. Mortality and morbidity in patients receiving encainide, flecainide, or placebo. The Cardiac Arrhythmia Suppression Trial. N Engl J Med. 1991;324(12):781–8.
5. Maher RL, Hanlon JT, Hajjar ER. Clinical consequences of polypharmacy in elderly. Expert Opin Drug Saf. 2014;13(1):57.
6. Qato DM, Wilder J, Schumm LP, Gillet V, Alexander GC. Changes in prescription and over-the-counter medication and dietary supplement use among older adults in the United States, 2005 vs 2011. JAMA Intern Med. 2016;176(4):473–82.
7. Marcum ZA, Amuan ME, Hanlon JT, Aspinall SL, Handler SM, Ruby CM, et al. Prevalence of unplanned hospitalizations caused by adverse drug reactions among older veterans. J Am Geriatr Soc. 2012;60(1):34–41.
8. Koronkowski MJ, Semla TP, Schmader KE, Hanlon JT. Recent literature update on medication risk in older adults, 2015-2016. J Am Geriatr Soc. 2017;65(7):1401–5.
9. Yancy CW, Jessup M, Bozkurt B, Butler J, Casey DE Jr, Drazner MH, et al. American College of Cardiology Foundation; American Heart Association Task Force on Practice Guidelines. 2013 ACCF/AHA guideline for the management of heart failure: a report of the American College of Cardiology Foundation/American Heart Association Task Force on Practice Guidelines. J Am Coll Cardiol. 2013;62(16):e147–239. https://doi.org/10.1016/j.jacc.2013.05.019. Epub 2013 Jun 5. PubMed PMID: 23747642.
10. Scott IA, Hilmer SN, Reeve E, Potter K, Le Couteur D, Rigby D, et al. Reducing inappropriate polypharmacy: the process of deprescribing. JAMA Intern Med. 2015;175(5):827–34.
11. Heart Protection Study Collaborative Group. MRC/BHF Heart Protection Study of cholesterol lowering with simvastatin in 20,536 high-risk individuals: a randomised placebo-controlled trial. Lancet. 2002;360(9326):7–22.
12. The American Geriatrics Society 2015 Beers Criteria Update Expert Panel. American Geriatrics Society 2015 updated Beers Criteria for potentially inappropriate medication use in older adults. J Am Geriatr Soc. 2015;63(11):2227–46.
13. Blooms Taxonomy Graphic. Vanderbilt University Center for Teaching and Learning. [cited 2018 Jan 13. Available from: https://cft.vanderbilt.edu/guides-sub-pages/blooms-taxonomy/.
14. Singal AG, Higgins PD, Waljee AK. A primer on effectiveness and efficacy trials. Clin Transl Gastroenterol. 2014;5:e45. https://doi.org/10.1038/ctg.2013.13. PubMed PMID: 24384867; PubMed Central PMCID: PMC3912314.
15. Profit L. Exubera® (inhaled insulin): an evidence-based review of its effectiveness in the management of diabetes. Core Evid. 2005;1(2):89–101.
16. Heinemann L. The failure of Exubera: are we beating a dead horse? J Diabetes Sci Technol (Online). 2008;2(3):518–29.
17. 2017 ACC/AHA/AAPA/ABC/ACPM/AGS/APhA/ASH/ASPC/NMA/PCNA Guideline for the prevention, detection, evaluation, and management of high blood pressure in adults: a report of the American College of Cardiology/American Heart Association Task Force on Clinical Practice Guidelines. J Am Coll Cardiol 2017;Nov 13:[Epub ahead of print].
18. Bauer LA, editor. Drug dosing in special populations: renal and hepatic disease, Dialysis, heart failure, obesity, and drug interactions. In: Applied clinical pharmacokinetics. 3rd ed. New York: McGraw-Hill; http://accesspharmacy.mhmedical.com.jerome.stjohns.edu:81/content.aspx?bookid=1374&sectionid=74719619. Accessed 13 Jan 2018.
19. Winter ME. Basic clinical pharmacokinetics. 4th ed. Philadelphia: Lippincott Williams & Wilkins; 2004.
20. Food and Drug Administration. Guidance for industry: pharmacokinetics in patients with impaired renal function — study design, data analysis, and impact on dosing and labeling. Rockville: U.S. Department of Health and Human Services; 1998.
21. Cockcroft DW, Gault MH. Prediction of creatinine clearance from serum creatinine. Nephron. 1976;16:31–41.
22. FAQ GFR Estimates, National Kidney Foundation. Accessed 12/15/17 www.kidney.org.
23. Munar MY, Singh H. Drug dosing adjustments in patients with chronic kidney disease. Am Fam Physician. 2007;75(10):1487–96. Review. PubMed PMID: 17555141.
24. Hajjar ER, Gray SL, Slattum PW Jr, Hersh LR, Naples JG, Hanlon JT. Geriatrics. In: DiPiro JT, Talbert RL, Yee GC, Matzke GR, Wells BG, Posey L, editors. Pharmacotherapy: a pathophysiologic approach. 10th ed. New York: McGraw-Hill; http://accesspharmacy.mhmedical.com.jerome.stjohns.edu:81/content.aspx?bookid=1861&sectionid=146077984. Accessed 13 Jan 2018.
25. Guidance for industry pharmacokinetics in patients with impaired hepatic function: study design, data analysis, and impact on dosing and labeling. Rockville: U.S. Department of Health and Human Services; 2003.
26. Verbeeck R, Horsmans Y. Effect of hepatic insufficiency on pharmacokinetics and drug dosing. Pharm World Sci. 1998;20:183. https://doi.org/10.1023/A:1008656930082.
27. Pugh RN, Murray-Lyon IM, Dawson JL, Pietroni MC, Williams R. Transection of the oesophagus for bleeding oesophageal varices. Br J Surg. 1973;60(8):646–9.

High-Risk Prescriptions for Aging Patients

Khusbu Patel

A. Chun (ed.), *Geriatric Practice*, https://doi.org/10.1007/978-3-030-19625-7_14

14.1 Competency

Identify medications, including anticholinergic, psychoactive, anticoagulant, analgesic, hypoglycemic, and cardiovascular drugs that should be avoided or used with caution in older adults, and explain the potential problems associated with each.

Case

HPI

A 70-year-old female presents to your practice for a follow-up visit with the primary care provider. The patient reports a recent fall last week in the restroom after getting up in the middle of the night to urinate. She denies any injuries or any other falls in the past but does admit to feeling dizzy and confused at night several times a week.

Past Medical History

- Diabetes
- Hypertension
- Atrial fibrillation, persistent
- Chronic kidney disease (stage 3b, GFR 30–44 ml/min)
- Osteoarthritis
- Urinary incontinence
- Insomnia
- Dementia

Allergies

- No known allergies

Social History

- Nonsmoker, occasional social drinks (1–2 times/year)

Review of Systems

- Eyes: Denies vision changes and eye pain
- Ears/Nose/Throat: Denies runny nose, sinus pain, ear pain, tinnitus, or pain with swallowing
- Respiratory: No wheezing or asthma
- GI: Denies nausea, vomiting, diarrhea, or abdominal pain. Occasional constipation
- GU: Positive for incomplete voiding and some difficulty initiating urination
- MSK: Osteoarthritis of both knees
- Neuro: Complains of confusion. No headaches, numbness, or tingling
- Psychiatric: Denies depression, anxiety, or changes in mood

Physical Exam

- General: Well appearing, no distress. Recent fall with no injuries
- BP, 132/80 mmHg (sitting), 128/74 mmHg (standing); RR, 24 bpm; HR, 54 beats/min; T, 98 °F
- Wt, 132 lb; Ht, 64 inches
- HEENT: PERRL. Moist mucous membranes. No acute visual changes, allergies, hearing loss, sore throat, or neck stiffness
- Lymph Nodes: No lymphadenopathy
- Lungs: No wheezes or rhonchi heard
- Cardiac: Normal S_1 S_2 heart sounds without murmur/gallop/rub. No S3,S4
- Extremities: No cyanosis, clubbing, or edema
- Abdomen: Soft, non-tender, not distended
- GI: Positive bowel sounds and denies abdominal pain or constipation
- Neurologic: Unsteadiness in gait and dizziness. Denies numbness or tingling

Medications

- Zolpidem: 10 mg daily
- Glyburide: 10 mg daily
- Ibuprofen: 800 mg TID
- Donepezil: 5 mg daily
- Apixaban: 5 mg daily
- Metoprolol ER: 50 mg daily
- Lisinopril: 20 mg daily
- Atorvastatin: 40 mg daily

Laboratory Values (at Last Visit)

- Estimated Glomerular Filtration Rate: 39.4 ml/min/1.73m^2
- Hemoglobin A1c: 6.9%

Test	Results	Reference interval
Sodium	140	137–145 mmol/L
Potassium	4.5	3.5–5.1 mmol/L
Chloride	102	98–107 mmol/L
CO2	27	19–27 mmol/L
BUN	17	7–26 mmol/L
Creatinine	1.4	0.5–0.95 mg/dL
Glucose	102	75–100 mg/dL
AGAP	11	5–17
Calcium	10	8.8–10.3 mg/dL

14.2 Background

Potentially inappropriate or high-risk medications in geriatric patients can generally be defined as drugs that cause more harm than benefit and lead to poor outcomes. Changes in pharmacokinetics (absorption, distribution, metabolism, and elimination) and pharmacodynamics (the effect of the drug on the body) with ageing may lead to increased sensitivity or unpredictable side effects of drugs. This is complicated by the fact that many disease-based guidelines do not offer recommendations for older adults due to the lack of studies or data in this population, which is especially common in people over the age of 80 years [1]. In order to make treatment decisions, evidence is often extrapolated from younger populations, and the value of a treatment option is placed on clinical judgment. Examples of patient factors that should be considered when deciding to initiate a new drug therapy include comorbidities, drug interactions, and renal function of the patient. The following chapter will review types and categories of high-risk medications and tools to mitigate potential adverse effects.

14.3 Potentially Inappropriate Medications (PIMs)

The American Geriatric Society (AGS) Beers Criteria is a well-known evidence-based guide for identifying medications that should be avoided or used with caution in all geriatric patients [2]. In the last iteration of the Beers Criteria, the AGS panel stratified medication recommendations based on drug-disease interactions, drug interactions, and anticholinergic potential. Medications are considered to have a drug-disease interaction when a drug or drug class can exacerbate a preexisting disease (e.g., nonsteroidal anti-inflammatory drug (NSAID) use in heart failure). Drugs included in Beers Criteria can apply to multiple settings; therefore, it is often used as a reference to determine quality metrics by insurers or institutions.

Another common tool is the Screening Tool of Older Persons' potentially inappropriate Prescriptions (STOPP)/Screening Tool to Alert doctors to Right Treatment (START) criteria. The STOPP component of the tool identifies potentially inappropriate prescribing, whereas the START recommendations describe medications to initiate based on comorbidities (e.g., laxatives in patients receiving opioids) [3, 4]. The STOPP/START and Beers Criteria are independent of each other but should be used collectively to assess medication appropriateness and adverse drug events [5]. It is important to note that both of the aforementioned tools along with other available guides capture complex concepts as concise information; therefore, the recommendations are not considered to be contraindications. Patient factors and the strength of evidence supporting the guidance should be reviewed in order to ultimately determine if a medication change should be made [6]. Furthermore, Beers Criteria has direct application within the United States, but the explicit recommendations may vary between tools that have more on an international presence [3, 7, 8]. Nevertheless, all of the available guidelines or tools to identify high-risk medications should be used in a complementary fashion [9].

14.4 Special Considerations for Older Adults

The acronym *STEPS* is a mnemonic aid that can be used to identify medication appropriateness, safety, tolerability, efficacy, price, and simplicity [10] (◘ Fig. 14.1). A general rule to follow is to "start low, and go slow" especially with medications that have an unpredictable dose response or side effect. Below we review various classes of high-risk medications with examples from the chapter patient case.

14.4.1 Psychoactive

Medications that affect the central nervous system may have anticholinergic properties, increase risk of falls or delirium, or lead to other poor outcomes [2]. As an example, benzodiazepine and nonbenzodiazepine hypnotics have been associated with the aforementioned adverse events with minimal improvement in sleep latency and duration [11]. Alternatives in the chapter case after a taper of the nonbenzodiazepine hypnotic, zolpidem, include sleep hygiene and trial of safer treatment alternatives for insomnia [12]. Antipsychotics (first- and second-generation) are another group of medications to avoid unless the patient has bipolar disease or schizophrenia and should not be used as a chem-

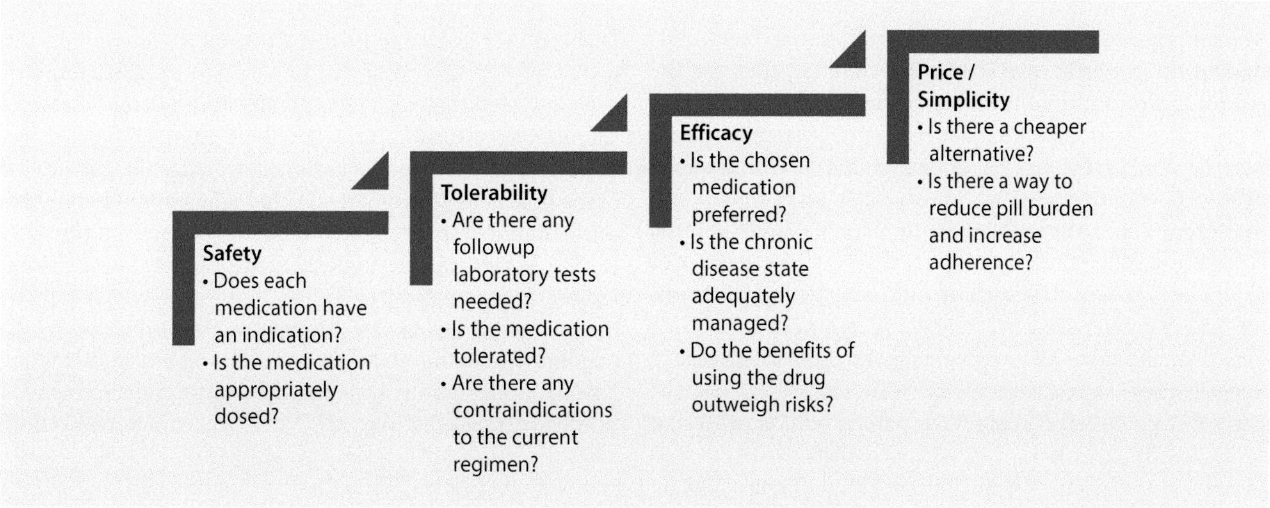

◘ **Fig. 14.1** Taking the right *STEPS* to evaluate medication appropriateness for high-risk medications

ical restraint in patients with behavioral problems; however, second-generation antipsychotics can be used in patients where other modalities have failed or if the patient is a harm to himself/herself or others [13]. Other types of psychoactive medications to avoid in older adults include tricyclic antidepressants (TCAs) and barbiturates as safer treatment options are available.

14.4.2 Cardiovascular

Management of hypertension or other cardiovascular conditions should involve medications with relatively lower rates of orthostatic hypotension and bradycardia. This includes avoiding peripheral alpha-1 blockers (e.g., doxazosin) and central alpha blockers (e.g., clonidine) as first-line agents for the management of blood pressure. Safer alternatives to treat benign hypertension include thiazides, calcium channel blockers, angiotensin-converting enzyme inhibitors (ACEI), or angiotensin II receptor blockers (ARBs). Counseling patients to rise slowly out of bed and to maintain adequate hydration are some nonpharmacological strategies to reduce risk of orthostatic hypotension. In addition, dosing diuretics in the morning to avoid nighttime ambulation may help reduce the risk of falls. The Beers Criteria lists several medications to use with caution in atrial fibrillation (e.g., amiodarone and digoxin) as beta-blockers or nondihydropyridine calcium channel blockers are safer alternatives [2]. In the chapter patient case, a beta-blocker and direct oral anticoagulants (DOACs) are used for the management of atrial fibrillation. No issues exist with the regimen; however, close attention should be placed on renal dosing requirements for DOACs. In addition, concurrent use of medications that increase the risk of bleeding (e.g., ibuprofen) should be avoided with both warfarin and DOACs [14].

14.4.3 Analgesic

Several types of pain medications should be used with caution in the geriatric population. NSAIDs can increase the risk of gastrointestinal bleeding or peptic ulcer disease in high-risk groups including older adults, systemic steroid use, or concurrent use of anticoagulants or antiplatelet drugs [2]. Gastroprotective agents such as proton pump inhibitors can reduce the risk in patients with chronic NSAID use, albeit these agents have their own consequences [15]. Certain NSAIDS, such as indomethacin and ketorolac, have a greater risk of central nervous system (CNS) side effects or bleeding risk, respectively. In the patient case, a drug-disease interaction exists with ibuprofen, as the patient is potentially taking it for pain several times a day. Part of the care planning should include adding other treatment modalities, such as acetaminophen or topical agents, since the patient has chronic kidney disease and concomitant anticoagulant use [16, 17]. Other analgesic medications, such as opioids, should be used with caution due to the risk of falls, confusion, and addiction. In a situation where opioids are used to manage nonmalignant pain, the agent should be initiated at the lowest dose and titrated based on response [18]. A bowel regimen should be considered at the same time for constipation with an opioid [4, 19]. Skeletal muscle relaxants, often used for lower back pain, should also be limited to the lowest dose and for acute treatment [2, 20].

14.4.4 Anticholinergic

Medications with anticholinergic potential may potentiate the risk of falls, delirium, and cognitive impairment [21]. In addition, there may be a positive correlation between the cumulative anticholinergic medication use and dementia risk [22]. Polypharmacy often defined as the use of multiple medications to treat the same or coexisting diseases may increase this risk. In the chapter patient case, donepezil, an acetylcholinesterase inhibitor for dementia, is used. This medication is known to exacerbate symptoms of urinary incontinence with minimal improvement in dementia [23, 24]. The plan can include discontinuation of donepezil and considering an antimuscarinic agent, which may improve urgency associated with urinary incontinence [2]. There are multiple published tools that can aid in identifying risk with anticholinergic medications [25–28]. Examples of medication classes that are considered with high anticholinergic potential include first-generation antihistamines, skeletal muscle relaxants, tricyclic antidepressants, antimuscarinics, and antispasmodics [2] (◘ Table 14.1).

14.4.5 Hypoglycemic

Diabetes A1c goals can be less stringent in older adults due to risk of hypoglycemia and impaired autonomic response with low blood glucose [20, 29, 30]. Sliding scale insulin, a set number of insulin units based on pre-meal glucose values, should be avoided regardless of whether the patient is at home or at a nursing facility due to higher risk of hypoglycemia without improvement in hyperglycemia management [2, 31]. When considering oral medication options, chronic kidney disease may play an important role in which diabetes medications are used. For example, metformin is not recommended when the eGFR is less than 30 mL/min/1.73m^2. Dosing modifications are needed for most of diabetes medications in renal disease [32]. Often, there are medications within a drug class that are comparatively better than others due to either how the drug is metabolized, half-life, or side effect profile. The sulfonylurea, glyburide, is used in the chapter case, which has a longer duration of action and active metabolites compared to other agents in its class such as glipizide and glimepiride. Therefore, glyburide is listed specifically on Beers Criteria as an agent to avoid as it is more likely to cause hypoglycemia [2].

Table 14.1 Medications associated with moderate to high anticholinergic properties

Class	Examples of medications[a]	Common alternative suggestions[b]
Antiarrhythmic	Disopyramide	*Rate control*: nondihydropyridine CCB (e.g., diltiazem) or beta-blocker
Antidepressant	TCAs (amitriptyline has relatively more anticholinergic potential), paroxetine	*Depression*: SSRI (note that paroxetine has the most anticholinergic effects in the class), SNRI, bupropion, mirtazapine *Neuropathic pain*: SNRI, gabapentin, pregabalin, capsaicin topical, lidocaine patch
Antiemetic	Prochlorperazine, promethazine	*Nausea/vomiting*: prochlorperazine may not be an issue if used short term or ondansetron
Antihistamines	Chlorpheniramine, diphenhydramine, meclizine, hydroxyzine	*Acute allergic conditions*: diphenhydramine has relatively more anticholinergic potential but can be used for acute treatment of allergic conditions *Chronic allergic conditions*: second-generation antihistamine (e.g., cetirizine, fexofenadine, loratadine) or intranasal corticosteroids (for allergic rhinitis)
Antimuscarinic	Darifenacin, fesoterodine, oxybutynin, solifenacin, tolterodine, trospium	*Urinary incontinence*: topical preparations are thought to be less anticholinergic (i.e., oxybutynin patch)
Antiparkinsonian	Benztropine, trihexyphenidyl	*Parkinson's disease*: levodopa/carbidopa dosed based on timing of daily activities
Antipsychotic	Chlorpromazine, clozapine, loxapine, olanzapine, perphenazine	*Psychiatric condition*: use agents with less anticholinergic properties if possible *Behavior changes with dementia*: if nonpharmacological approaches have failed and patient has psychosis or is a danger to self or others, low-dose nonanticholinergic agent (e.g., risperidone, quetiapine) for shortest duration possible
Antispasmotics	Dicyclomine, hyoscyamine, scopolamine	*Motion sickness*: nonpharmacological options (pressure band or ginger) *Gastrointestinal*: loperamide
Skeletal muscle relaxants	Cyclobenzaprine	*Acute mild or moderate pain*: acetaminophen, NSAIDs if no heart failure or eGFR>30 mL/min *Spasticity*: baclofen or tizanidine may be safer options

Adapted from [a]American Geriatrics Society 2015 Beers Criteria Update Expert Panel [2]; [b]Hanlon et al. [26]
Abbreviations: *SSRI* selective serotonin reuptake inhibitor, *SNRI* selective norepinephrine reuptake inhibitor, *TCA* tricyclic antidepressants, *CCB* calcium channel blocker

Case Discussion

Due to the risk of falls and adverse drug events seen in older adults, an accurate and complete medication review should be performed on a regular basis and when any medication changes are made. In the chapter patient case, the patient presents after feeling confused and dizzy at night and a recent fall, which adds need to perform a medication review.

Table 14.2 provides a summary of PIMs and strategies to address them. Although not reviewed in this chapter, considerations of underprescribing like using low-dose aspirin for primary prevention or immunizations should also be reviewed [4].

Table 14.2 Summary of potentially inappropriate medications in the chapter case

Medication	PIM	Rationale based on Beers Criteria[a]	Clinical application strategies
Zolpidem	Yes	Risk of delirium, falls fractures; increased emergency department visits and hospitalizations; motor vehicle crashes; minimal improvement in sleep latency and duration	Taper and discontinue; consider melatonin or nonpharmacological interventions such as sleep hygiene. In general, limit to less than 3 CNS active medications[a]
Glyburide	Yes	Higher risk of severe prolonged hypoglycemia in older adults	Discontinue agent, and consider patient-specific HbA1c goal before adding shorter-acting sulfonylurea (e.g., glipizide or glimepiride) or other diabetes medication based on medication and medical history
Ibuprofen	Yes	Risk of bleeding with concomitant anticoagulant use	Limit use of NSAIDs; consider use of acetaminophen or topical products (e.g., topical NSAIDs, capsaicin, or lidocaine) and nonpharmacological modalities
Donepezil	Yes	Increased risk of orthostatic hypotension or bradycardia	Review cumulative anticholinergic effect of all medications; consider discontinuation due to risk of falls and exacerbation of urinary incontinence
Apixaban	No	Appropriate use: anticoagulation for atrial fibrillation	Avoid apixaban if CrCl <25 ml/min. Monitor for changes in renal function as needed
Metoprolol	No	Appropriate use: rate control in atrial fibrillation	Monitor heart rate when changing dose
Lisinopril	No	Appropriate use: hypertension and kidney protection	Monitor renal function and basic metabolic panel based on renal function.
Atorvastatin	No	Appropriate use: cardiovascular risk reduction	No need for routine monitoring unless patient has myopathy

Abbreviations: *CNS* central nervous system, *HbA1c* hemoglobin A1c, *NSAIDs* nonsteroidal anti-inflammatory drugs, *PIM* potentially inappropriate medications

[a]American Geriatrics Society 2015 Beers Criteria Update Expert Panel [2]

14

14.5 Interprofessional Care

The provision of safe medication practices involves an interdisciplinary approach to care. Person-centered care means to use an individual's values and preferences to drive all aspects of care while supporting realistic health and life goals [33]. According to the American Geriatrics Society (AGS), person-centered care is more comprehensive than patient-centered care as the latter mainly implies clinical or medical needs [33]. The members of an interdisciplinary team may depend on the care setting, but high-risk medications should be evaluated when there is a change in health status or goals. The healthcare providers completing the medication reconciliation can include a nurse, pharmacist, or physician depending on the institution but often involves a multidisciplinary approach. The family or caregivers play an important role in management of medications and can provide valuable input and guidance. For example, if the patient needs insulin, education should be provided for administration and monitoring to the patient and/or caregivers depending on the functional status of the patient. Aside from injectable medications, another example where a caregiver plays an important role is when there are multiple medication changes after a heart failure admission [34]. Overall, a team approach should be emphasized to manage underlying conditions by using safe and simple regimens and nonpharmacological options. Use of high-risk medications should be limited to short durations in situations where benefit outweighs risk.

14.6 Hospital Versus Outpatient Care

The type of high-risk medications may be different when comparing community-dwelling, inpatient, and nursing home patients; however, transitions of care is an integral time where reviewing medication changes is key to reducing adverse events. In the hospital setting, this means starting the discharge planning shortly after hospital admission so that coordination can be seamless between healthcare providers, caregivers, and family members [35, 36]. If the patient is transitioned to a nursing facility or home, a fall risk assessment should also include medication review. An available tool from the Agency of Healthcare Research and Quality (AHRQ) stratifies fall risk on a point value based on the medication class with analgesics, antipsychotics, anticonvulsants, and benzodiazepines having the highest risk [37]. Although this tool is not comprehensive for all medications, medications listed with a medium risk of falls include antihypertensive, cardiac drugs, antiarrhythmic, and antidepressants. Since the described tool is mostly for medications, it should be used for other guides to assess fall risk [38, 39].

Key Learning Pearls

- Tools such as the Beer's Criteria can be used to identify potentially inappropriate medications.
- Medications that are safe in younger adults may not be appropriate in older adults due to age-related physiological changes or lack of studies.
- Multiple classes of medications have anticholinergic side effects; however, the decision to add an agent for a condition should be based on the cumulative effect of all of the anticholinergic medications prescribed to the patient, the efficacy of the medication, and the potential side effects.
- A medication reconciliation or "pruning" of the medication list should be a constant process during outpatient visits, hospital admissions, and transitions of care.

References

1. Herrera AP, Snipes SA, King DW, Torres-Vigil I, Goldberg DS, Weinberg AD. Disparate inclusion of older adults in clinical trials: priorities and opportunities for policy and practice change. Am J Public Health. 2010;100(Suppl 1):S105–12.
2. American Geriatrics Society 2015 Beers Criteria Update Expert Panel. American Geriatrics Society 2015 updated Beers Criteria for potentially inappropriate medication use in older adults. J Am Geriatr Soc. 2015;63(11):2227–46.
3. Gallagher P, Ryan C, Byrne S, Kennedy J, O'Mahony D. STOPP (Screening Tool of Older Person's Prescriptions) and START (Screening Tool to Alert doctors to Right Treatment). Consensus validation. Int J Clin Pharmacol Ther. 2008;46(2):72–83.
4. Mahony DO, Sullivan DO, Byrne S, Connor MNO, Ryan C, Gallagher P. Corrigendum: STOPP/START criteria for potentially inappropriate prescribing in older people: version 2. Age Ageing. 2018; 47(3):489.
5. Barenholtz Levy H, Marcus EL. Potentially inappropriate medications in older adults: why the revised criteria matter. Ann Pharmacother. 2016;50(7):599–603.
6. Steinman MA, Beizer JL, DuBeau CE, Laird RD, Lundebjerg NE, Mulhausen P. How to use the American Geriatrics Society 2015 Beers Criteria-a guide for patients, clinicians, health systems, and payors. J Am Geriatr Soc. 2015;63(12):e1–7.
7. Renom-Guiteras A, Meyer G, Thürmann PA. The EU(7)-PIM list: a list of potentially inappropriate medications for older people consented by experts from seven European countries. Eur J Clin Pharmacol. 2015;71(7):861–75.
8. Holt S, Schmiedl S, Thürmann PA. Potentially inappropriate medications in the elderly: the PRISCUS list. Dtsch Arztebl Int. 2010;107(31–32):543–51.
9. Brown JD, Hutchison LC, Martin BC. Comparing the tools to identify potentially inappropriate medications in the elderly and future research directions. J Gerontol Geriatr Res. 2016;5(4):1.
10. Pegler S, Underhill J. Evaluating the safety and effectiveness of new drugs. Am Fam Physician. 2010;82(1):53–7.
11. Schroeck JL, Ford J, Conway EL, Kurtzhalts KE, Gee ME, Vollmer KA, et al. Review of safety and efficacy of sleep medicines in older adults. Clin Ther. 2016;38(11):2340–72.
12. Bloom HG, Ahmed I, Alessi CA, Ancoli-Israel S, Buysse DJ, Kryger MH, et al. Evidence-based recommendations for the assessment and management of sleep disorders in older persons. J Am Geriatr Soc. 2009;57(5):761–89.
13. Reus VI, Fochtmann LJ, Eyler AE, Hilty DM, Horvitz-Lennon M, Jibson MD, et al. The American Psychiatric Association practice guideline on the use of antipsychotics to treat agitation or psychosis in patients with dementia. Am J Psychiatry. 2016;173(5):543–6
14. January CT, Wann LS, Alpert JS, Calkins H, Cigarroa JE, Cleveland JC, et al. 2014 AHA/ACC/HRS guideline for the management of patients with atrial fibrillation: executive summary: a report of the American College of Cardiology/American Heart Association Task Force on practice guidelines and the Heart Rhythm Society. Circulation. 2014;130(23):2071–104.
15. Safety of long-term PPI use. JAMA. 2017;318(12):1177–8.
16. American Geriatrics Society. Pharmacological management of persistent pain in older persons. J Am Geriatr Soc. 2009;57(8):1331–46.
17. Pham PC, Khaing K, Sievers TM, Pham PM, Miller JM, Pham SV, et al. 2017 update on pain management in patients with chronic kidney disease. Clin Kidney J. 2017;10(5):688–97.
18. Dowell D, Haegerich TM, Chou RCDC. Guideline for prescribing opioids for chronic pain--United States, 2016. JAMA. 2016;315(15):1624–45.
19. Mounsey A, Raleigh M, Wilson A. Management of constipation in older adults. Am Fam Physician. 2015;92(6):500–4.
20. Spence MM, Shin PJ, Lee EA, Gibbs NE. Risk of injury associated with skeletal muscle relaxant use in older adults. Ann Pharmacother. 2013;47(7–8):993–8.
21. Salahudeen MS, Hilmer SN, Nishtala PS. Comparison of anticholinergic risk scales and associations with adverse health outcomes in older people. J Am Geriatr Soc. 2015;63(1):85–90.
22. Gray SL, Anderson ML, Dublin S, Hanlon JT, Hubbard R, Walker R, et al. Cumulative use of strong anticholinergics and incident dementia: a prospective cohort study. JAMA Intern Med. 2015;175(3):401–7.
23. Gill SS, Mamdani M, Naglie G, Streiner DL, Bronskill SE, Kopp A, et al. A prescribing cascade involving cholinesterase inhibitors and anticholinergic drugs. Arch Intern Med. 2005;165(7):808–13.
24. Siegler EL, Reidenberg M. Treatment of urinary incontinence with anticholinergics in patients taking cholinesterase inhibitors for dementia. Clin Pharmacol Ther. 2004;75(5):484–8.
25. Carnahan RM, Lund BC, Perry PJ, Pollock BG, Culp KR. The Anticholinergic Drug Scale as a measure of drug-related anticholinergic burden: associations with serum anticholinergic activity. J Clin Pharmacol. 2006;46(12):1481–6.
26. Hanlon JT, Semla TP, Schmader KE. Alternative medications for medications in the use of high-risk medications in the elderly and potentially harmful drug-disease interactions in the elderly quality measures. J Am Geriatr Soc. 2015;63(12):e8–e18.
27. Kouladjian L, Gnjidic D, Chen TF, Mangoni AA, Hilmer SN. Drug Burden Index in older adults: theoretical and practical issues. Clin Interv Aging. 2014;9:1503–15.
28. Rudolph JL, Salow MJ, Angelini MC, McGlinchey RE. The anticholinergic risk scale and anticholinergic adverse effects in older persons. Arch Intern Med. 2008;168(5):508–13.
29. Moreno G, Mangione CM, Kimbro L, Vaisberg E, Mellitus AG. Guidelines abstracted from the American Geriatrics Society guidelines for improving the care of older adults with diabetes mellitus: 2013 update. J Am Geriatr Soc. 2013;61(11):2020–6.

30. American Diabetes Association. 11. Older adults. Diabetes Care. 2018;41(Suppl 1):S119–S25.
31. Munshi MN, Florez H, Huang ES, Kalyani RR, Mupanomunda M, Pandya N, et al. Management of diabetes in long-term care and skilled nursing facilities: a position statement of the American Diabetes Association. Diabetes Care. 2016;39(2):308–18.
32. American Diabetes Association. 8. Pharmacologic approaches to glycemic treatment. Diabetes Care. 2018;41(Suppl 1):S73–85.
33. American Geriatrics Society. Person-centered care: a definition and essential elements. J Am Geriatr Soc. 2016;64(1):15–8.
34. Díez-Villanueva P, Alfonso F. Heart failure in the elderly. J Geriatr Cardiol. 2016;13(2):115–7.
35. Panel on Prevention of Falls in Older Persons AeGSaBGS. Summary of the updated American Geriatrics Society/British Geriatrics Society clinical practice guideline for prevention of falls in older persons. J Am Geriatr Soc. 2011;59(1):148–57.
36. Labson MC. Adapting the joint commission's seven foundations of safe and effective transitions of care to home. Home Healthc Now. 2015;33(3):142–6.
37. Agency for Healthcare Quality and Safety. Tool 3I: medication fall risk score and evaluation tools. Rockville: Agency for Healthcare Quality and Safety; 2013.
38. Moyer VA, Force USPST. Prevention of falls in community-dwelling older adults: U.S. Preventive Services Task Force recommendation statement. Ann Intern Med. 2012;157(3):197–8.
39. Ganz D, Huang C, Saliba D, et al. Preventing falls in hospitals: a toolkit for improving quality of care. Rockville: Agency for Healthcare Research and Quality; 2013. Available at: https://www.ahrq.gov/professionals/systems/hospital/fallpxtoolkit/index.html. Accessed 10 June 2018.

Dietary Botanicals and Supplements

Alan Remde and Raymond Teets

A. Chun (ed.), *Geriatric Practice*, https://doi.org/10.1007/978-3-030-19625-7_15

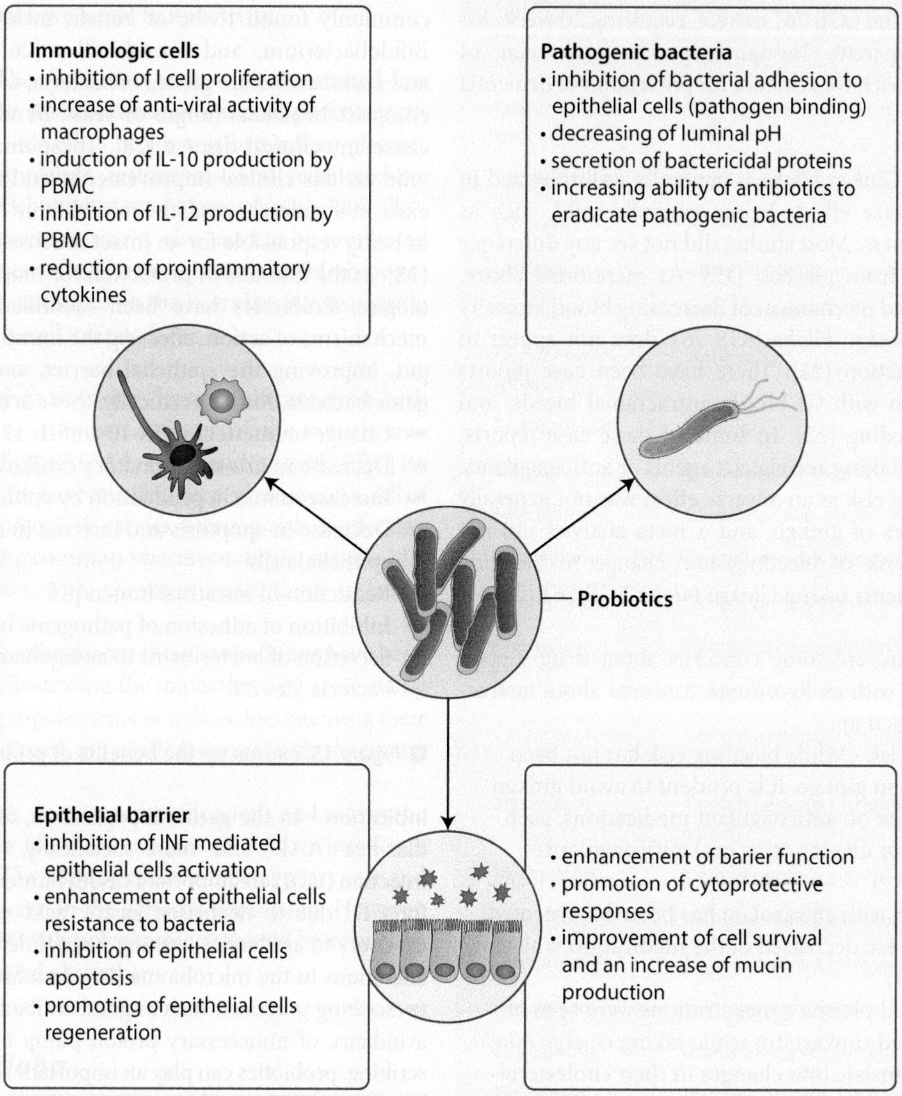
Immunologic cells
• inhibition of I cell proliferation
• increase of anti-viral activity of macrophages
• induction of IL-10 production by PBMC
• inhibition of IL-12 production by PBMC
• reduction of proinflammatory cytokines
Pathogenic bacteria
• inhibition of bacterial adhesion to epithelial cells (pathogen binding)
• decreasing of luminal pH
• secretion of bactericidal proteins
• increasing ability of antibiotics to eradicate pathogenic bacteria
Probiotics
Epithelial barrier
• inhibition of INF mediated epithelial cells activation
• enhancement of epithelial cells resistance to bacteria
• inhibition of epithelial cells apoptosis
• promoting of epithelial cells regeneration
• enhancement of barier function
• promotion of cytoprotective responses
• improvement of cell survival and an increase of mucin production

Fig. 15.3 Probiotic mechanism of action graphic. (Modified from Dylag et al. [26])

and *Lactobacillus acidophilus*. The probiotics need to be started within 2 days of initiation of antibiotics and continued for 21 days [30]. Administer the probiotics separately (>2 hours) from the antibiotics, to diminish any untoward effects of the antibiotic on the probiotic [33]. Lastly, the daily dose should be at or above a threshold of 10–20 billion colony forming units, which can be taken together or divided up twice a day.

Adverse effects The side effect profile for probiotics is generally benign – an Agency for Healthcare Research and Quality (AHRQ) study evaluated the available literature for adverse effects and found none requiring hospitalization [34]. The recent Cochrane review identified common mild side effects being equivalent to the controls and included abdominal cramping, nausea, soft stools, flatulence, and taste disturbance [31]. Contraindications for probiotics are minimal: avoid use in patients with central lines especially if immunosuppressed and also in patients who have severe pancreatitis – outcomes for patients with severe pancreatitis may worsen when given probiotics [35].

Summary *Clostridium difficile* infection is an illness that elders are at particular risk, especially when hospitalized and receiving antibiotics. Probiotics, specifically *Saccharomyces boulardii* and two *Lactobacillus* genera provide beneficial prevention for CDI. The risk profile appears low, with minimal adverse effects and very few known drug-supplement interactions.

15.5 Glucosamine and Chondroitin Sulfate

Background Glucosamine sulfate is a normal constituent of glycosaminoglycans in cartilage matrix and synovial fluid. It is believed to support the cartilage by stimulating chondrocytes and synovial cells while inhibiting cytokines that increase inflammation via creation of COX-2. There is speculation that the sulfate moiety provides clinical benefit in the synovial fluid by strengthening cartilage and aiding glycosaminoglycan synthesis, implying that non-sulfated glucosamine forms may not be as effective; however, this is unproven. Chondroitin is a glycosaminoglycan that appears to inhibit cartilage degradation by blocking leukocyte elastase and increasing creation of hyaluronic acid. Chondroitin is usually made from bovine trachea. Glucosamine and chondroitin (GC and CS) are often used together and have often been evaluated together in studies, however their bioavailability and therefore efficacy may be improved when taken separately. Other supplements combined with GC/ and/or CS in practice and studies include methylsulfonylmethane (MSM), curcumin [36, 37], boswellia, quercetin [37], and others.

Indications Efficacy of GC/CS for the treatment of osteoarthritis (OA) is controversial, with some studies showing benefit and others no benefit, however this may be a reflection of poor bioavailability of some forms [38–41]. (Natural Medicines database, accessed 9/5/2019, lists Glucosamine sulfate as '*Likely effective*', and Chondroitin sulfate as '*Possibly effective*'). Pharmaceutical grade crystalline Glucosamine sufate, e.g. Dona brand or combination products like InvigoFlex distributed by WynnPharm (with or without Chondroitin sulfate) has the best clinical evidence, and therefore may be the preferred formulation. See: Differentiation of patented crystalline glucosamine sulfate from other glucosamine preparations will optimize osteoarthritis treatment [42]. Some major trials do suggest improvement in joint narrowing in patients with OA [43], while its ability to reduce pain in studies has been mixed [44, 45].

Doses/practical considerations Use pharmaceutical grade Glucosamine sulfate such as Dona brand. New evidence suggests that taking Glucosamine sufate and Chondroitin sulfate separately, e.g. 10–12 hours apart, may enhance their bioavailability, as opposed to the common GS/CS combinations often promoted. A "fair trial" to assess benefits in a patient with OA might be 3 months.

Adverse effects GC/CS is generally tolerated well but may occasionally cause GI upset or more rare side effects. Various theoretical concerns, such as that glucosamine might raise blood pressure or blood sugar, have not been an issue in clinical studies or experience (Natural Medicines database, accessed 9/5/19).

Contraindications/cautions Theoretical concerns that chondroitin may interfere with cell adhesion and increase prostate cancer progression, as well as a theoretical and remote concern of prion disease from diseased cow trachea, have not been demonstrated in clinical trials; nevertheless, it may be prudent to avoid chondroitin in men with prostate cancer. In addition, due to possible slight increase in eye pressure on glucosamine, patients with severe glaucoma should avoid it or have their eye pressure closely monitored (Natural Medicines database, accessed 9/5/19).

Interactions Monitor PT/INR levels in patients on warfarin and GC/GS. Other interactions are minor or theoretical (Natural Medicines database, accessed 9/5/2019).

Summary Glucosamine sulfate and chondroitin sulfate can be used safely in geriatric patients with osteoarthritis and may provide some benefit. At dosages of 1500 mg and 1200 mg daily, respectively, taken apart, the geriatric patient may be able to achieve some pain control and reduce progression of OA. This improved pain control may allow for less use of medications such as nonsteroidal anti-inflammatory drugs (NSAIDs), which carry some risk for elderly patients.

15.6 Vitamin D

Background Vitamin D (calciferol) is the name for a family of hormones/vitamins that have central roles in calcium/bone metabolism as well as modulating immune, cellular differentiation and myriad other functions. Vitamin D metabolic systems are found in virtually all organs and tissues, implying its central role in health. Typically, about 80% comes from photosynthesis, induced by direct sunlight on bare skin (however, this effect does not significantly occur through windows, sunscreen, or clothes), with the remaining 20% coming from diet [46]. Because it is a fat-soluble hormone, we can deposit it in our body's "fat depot bank" during the warmer months to be released as needed during the "vitamin D winter." This ability to store vitamin D allows us to survive at more polar latitudes and likely was a main evolutionary driver of paler skin during our species' migration out of our ancestral African home, where our normal skin color is darker to protect against damage from intense solar radiation [47]. As with most hormones, the cholecalciferol formed in the skin or absorbed from food is a pre-hormone; the body will activate this as needed in the liver and kidneys and locally in different tissues as needed to serve its functions. See ◻ Fig. 15.4 for a description of metabolism and effects of vitamin D [48, 49]. Vitamin D assessment and supplementation is often mis-interpreted and mis-applied. Generally speaking, there is little evidence that supplementing in patients who are not deficient has any clinical benefit, therefore limit supplementation to those who are clearly deficient as measured by a validated 25 (OH) Vit. D lab value. Like most nutrients, there is likely a range of of adequate levels in different individuals, e.g. a level of 15 ng/ml may be adequate for one person and mildly deficient for another. The RDA is set to cover 97.5% of the population based on present understanding of the role of Vit. D in the body, which is likely in its infancy, especially as relates to non-musculoskeletal functions of Vit. D. When to test for Vit. D deficiency is highly controversial. Routine screening is clearly not indicated, but whether to test for (and then treat if deficient) patients with various chronic diseases associated with Vit. D deficiency (causality usually unproven) is unclear. Since most chronic diseases, such as cardiovascular, metabolic, depressive, autoimmune disorders, etc. often are highly multi-factorial, it is unlikely that correcting Vit. D deficiciency per se will have a marked effect in most

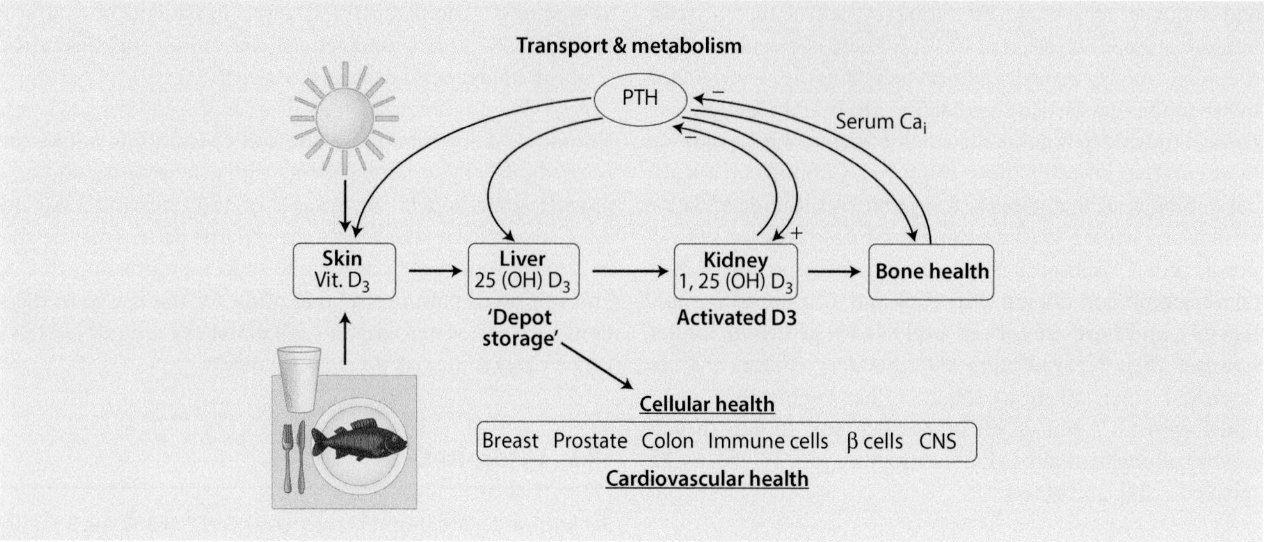

Fig. 15.4 Vitamin D graphic

cases. This is reflected in numerous randomized controlled trials with often mixed or conflicting results. But this does not imply that one should not treat clear Vitamin D deficiency, just that one should not view it as a magic bullet.

Indications Vitamin D should be given as supplementation to prevent and correct vitamin D deficiency when natural sources are difficult or impractical to obtain because of lifestyle or medical issues. Correcting deficiency is especially important if geriatric patients are suffering from disorders likely related to vitamin D deficiency such as osteoporosis and frequent unexplained falls, though it is unclear if Vitamin D supplementation by itself is effective at reducing these disorders. Vitamin D deficiency is considered the most common nutritional deficiency worldwide, probably due to indoor living styles with avoidance of sun exposure (note that *excess* sun exposure definitely is bad for the skin, including increasing risk of skin cancer). Technically, skin photosynthesis of vitamin D is optimized at 1/4 the minimal erythema (slight pinking of skin) sun exposure dose for one's skin phototype. For example, 15 minutes per day would be needed for light skin, while 45 minutes per day would be needed for very dark skin/day. This sensible dose does not appear to significantly increase skin cancer. Main dietary sources are fortified foods such as milk and fish liver oils.

15

Monitoring Avoid routine screening or supplementation for Vitamin D deficiency in community dwelling patients, as there is no convincing evidence of benefit in this setting. Screen for vitamin D deficiency in those at high risk, such as insufficient sun exposure, and in diseases associated with vitamin D deficiency. Such individuals include patients with the following conditions:

- Osteoporosis or osteopenia
- Frequent unexplained falls
- Severe chronic kidney disease
- Hyperparathyroidism
- Malabsorption syndromes such as after bariatric surgery
- Ingestion of medications that interfere with vitamin D

Most vitamin D deficiency is asymptomatic, though if severe can present with myalgias and osteomalacia-/osteoporosis-related symptoms in adults. Lab definitions of deficiency are somewhat variable depending on method used but are generally as follows:

- Vitamin D insufficiency (low-normal levels): 20–29 ng/ml (50–73 nmol/L). This category is controversial and considered normal by some authorities. There is little evidence that treatment or maintenance supplementation in response to a level is this range has any clinically meaningful benefit it most clinical situations. Levels in this range in the fall season (when the patient should be Vt. D replete from a warm season's worth of sunlight and is about to enter the 'Vitamin D winter' in which they cannot photosynthesize Vit. D from the sun at temperate latitudes) could be supplemented to allow a buffer zone of Vit. D stores. If the patient likely will get some sun, levels in the spring (when the patient has used up their 'Vitamin D stores') at this level may not need treatment.
- Mild deficiency: 12–19 ng/mL (30–49 nmol/L). This range may be sufficient in some individuals, but since it is not practically posible to be clear if this is sufficient or not for a given individual, treating and then putting on a maintenance dose if still at risk for Vit. D deficiency is considered reasonable by many authorities to ensure has adequate stores.
- Moderate deficiency: 5–11 ng/mL (12.5–29 nmol/L). Treat all patients, then likely put on a maintenance dose.
- Severe deficiency: <5 ng/mL (12.5 nmol/L). Treat all patients, then put on a maintenance dose.

Routine lab vitamin D screening or monitoring is not needed but can be done if concern that patient is not correcting a deficiency or is having health issues suspected to be worsened by vitamin D deficiency, such as osteoporosis, frequent falls, and others. There is extensive literature showing associations between vitamin D deficiency and many chronic diseases (causality yet unproven), including cardiovascular disease, cancer, autoimmune diseases, worsening of various infectious diseases such as HIV and TB, asthma, hypertension, cognitive decline, depression, and many others [49].

Dose/practical considerations For prevention of vitamin D deficiency in adults at risk of deficiency, a practical dose of 1000 units/day of vitamin D3 (cholecalciferol), taken with healthy fat in a meal, is usually sufficient. This dose, while moderately above the RDA, takes into account human inconsistency in pill taking and variations in absorption, and is in the safe range. 2–3 times or occasionally even higher doses may be needed in malabsorption syndromes, morbid obesity and drug-induced Vt. D deficiencies. To treat vitamin D deficiency generally requires 50,000 units orally per week of vitamin D for 8 weeks or more, depending on the level of deficiency. As an alternative, cholecalciferol (vitamin D3) at 5000 units orally per day can be given, again for 8 weeks. If the original cause of the deficiency is likely to continue, once repletion is completed, supplement with a maintenance dose (e.g., 1000 units/daily) indefinitely is important to prevent relapse of the deficiency.

Vitamin D deficiency treatment in severe liver or kidney disease requires special considerations such as using the hydroxylated forms to compensate for the loss of natural hydroxylation in the liver and kidney.

Adverse effects Vitamin D when properly prescribed is very safe. Avoid excess doses in patients with a risk of hypercalcemia. Except in special situations, avoid excess maintenance doses above the upper tolerable limit of 4000 units/day or artificially raising the serum level above 40–60 ng/mL with supplementation.

Interactions Various medications can interfere with vitamin D absorption or metabolism and thus may require monitoring of levels and supplementation. Such medications include some anticonvulsant, anti-tuberculosis, and HIV drugs.

Summary Vitamin D is clinically relevant in the geriatric population given risks of osteoporosis, frequent falls, and related fractures as well as possible deficiencies when homebound or institutionalized. Patients at risk should be evaluated for deficiency and corrected to normal levels with oral vitamin D supplementation.

15.7 S-Adenosylmethionine (SAMe)

Background SAMe is a natural substance involved in methyl donation that is synthesized in and supports the liver, supports neurotransmitter metabolism, and may be helpful in two common problems in the elderly: depression and arthritis. There are mixed studies on antidepressant effects [50, 51, 52], Adjunctive S-adenosylmethionine (SAMe) in treating non-remittent major depressive disorder: An 8-week double-blind, randomized, controlled trial. SAMe appears to have analgesic and anti-inflammatory properties equivalent to NSAIDs, but with less side effects. It may stimulate cartilage growth helpful for joint support (preliminary evidence), with studies showing benefit for osteoarthritis of the knee, hip, hand, and spine (moderate evidence, Natural Medicines database SAMe, accessed 9/5/19).

Indications SAMe has evidence for use in three disparate clinical conditions:

1. Osteoarthritis
2. Possibly for Depression can be used as an alternative or adjunct to conventional antidepressant medications
3. Possibly as an adjunct in liver disease [53], and also in fibromyalgia [54], though the evidence is less strong than for the above two conditions

Important note For supplements not derived from plants, being cognizant of how processing occurs is still important. Here there are parallels with pharmaceuticals, where a single molecule is relevant, ensuring that such active principle is bioavailable and in correct formulation. For instance, SAMe is sensitive to heat, moisture, and stomach acid, so only use enteric-coated tablets in blister packs. In addition, SAMe products have stabilizing compounds such as tosylates, so only ~1/2 of the total ingredients of a pill are actual SAMe – it's important to verify that any formulation is delivering the actual amount of active SAMe intended. Like herbal supplements, ConsumerLab.com can be a guide on high-quality and least expensive brands. SAMe is utilized in the body with cofactors folate, B12, and B6, so consider supplementing these if there is concern of low nutritional status (ConsumerLab.com, SAMe, accessed 8/18/19).

Dose/practical considerations Doses shown to be effective, reflective of the actual SAMe component, (which can be higher than what is often listed on the bottle) for osteoarthritis are 800–1200 mg as a total daily dose, divided two to three times per day; and for depression 400–1600 mg/day, in divided doses. Again, these doses should be reflective of the actual active SAMe component taken orally, which can be higher than what is often listed on the bottle. For fibromyalgia, 800 mg/day may be helpful. It can take a few weeks for SAMe to reach its full effect, and so the provider can "front-load" the dose for quicker effect but then might increase the chance of side effects. Thus the recommendation in the elderly is to start low and gradually titrate up the dose.

Adverse effects SAMe side effects are generally minimal but at higher doses can be associated with GI upset, headache, and agitation. Counseling patients to avoid taking it in evening can help mitigate any insomnia risk. SAMe has not been found to cause weight gain or sexual dysfunction (Natural Medicines database, accessed 8/18/19).

Contraindications As SAMe may have an antidepressant effect, it should not be used in elders with bipolar disorder, as it could trigger a manic phase.

Interactions SAMe does interact with a few medications. Levodopa (L-dopa) used in Parkinson's disease treatment may deplete brain SAMe levels; thus, supplementation may improve depression in Parkinson's disease. SAMe might however decrease L-dopa effectiveness. Serotonin syndrome when combined with selective serotonin reuptake inhibitors (SSRIs) and other anti-depressants appears rare, but it is prudent to not use SAMe in patients taking monoamine oxidase inhibitors (MAOIs) (Natural Medicines database, accessed 9/5/19).

15.8 Turmeric/Curcumin

Background *Curcuma longa* is a culinary herb that, when standardized to the curcumin content, has been found to have anti-inflammatory and antioxidant properties. When turmeric is ingested in cooking, curcumin content is less, and so effects described below are in the context of more processed turmeric [55–58]. In this botanical, curcumin is believed to be the main active principle, and so here curcumin will be used when talking about medicinal benefits; turmeric is the plant from which it is derived.

Indications Curcumin has been shown to be beneficial in various conditions affecting the geriatric population. Curcumin in multiple small randomized controlled trials (mid-level evidence) demonstrates efficacy in knee osteoarthritis with preliminary evidence of benefit in other sites (e.g., hand, hip) and other forms of arthritis such as rheumatoid arthritis [57]. Benefit has been found for curcumin alone or when taken with other dietary supplements such as boswellia, glucosamine, etc. [36, 59–71]. In addition to the pain relief benefit found in arthritis, there is preliminary data that curcumin may have other beneficial effects, such as in:

15

- Improving the hyperlipidemia profile [58, 72]
- Decreasing progression of pre-diabetes to diabetes mellitus type 2 (DM2) [73]
- Preliminary evidence that curcumin benefits a multitude of other inflammatory conditions [58, 74, 75]

Dose/practical considerations A typical dose for the 95% curcumin standardized extract for arthritis is 500 mg three times a day. The supplement should be taken with healthy fat and black pepper (ConsumerLab.com accessed 9/5/2019) – this improves the bioavailability. Use of high bioavailable curcumin is important, since little is absorbed from the GI tract otherwise. Curcumin products complexed with piperine (the active enhancer in black pepper) are also on the market. These complexed products have better bioavailability, and so dose would be lower [55–57].

Contraindications/cautions Turmeric/curcumin generally is well tolerated. Caution the patient about theoretical increased risk of bleeding with curcumin if on anti-platelet drugs and anti-coagulants such as DOACs or warfarin, though antiplatelet agents such as aspirin probably don't need to be avoided. Patients with a history of active biliary colic should also avoid curcumin, as it can stimulate gallbladder contraction. While there is some evidence that curcumn appears to protect the liver, for example in non-alcoholic fatthy liver disease (NAFLD), there are uncommon reports of elevated liver enzymes and very rarely auto-immune hepatitis that possibly could have been due to the botanical. In addition, turmeric has small amounts of oxalates which theoretically could exacerbate risk of stone formation in patients with a history of calcium oxalate kidney stones (ConsumerLabs.com and Natural Medicines database accessed 9/5/2019).

Interactions Avoid the use of curcumin with critical drugs metabolized by the P450 3A system such as tacrolimus. Theoretically curcumin could bind iron, so monitor iron levels in those deficient or with marginal stores and take curcumin at a different time than iron supplements. Piperine extract (BioPerine) theoretically could alter some drug levels, so if it is part of the curcumin complex, take curcumin at different times from pharmaceuticals. Lastly, as mentioned above, curcumin may provide a mild hypoglycemic effect when patients are already on diabetic medications. Diabetics who opt to take this supplement should have their glucose levels closely monitored (Natural Medicines database accessed 9/5/19).

Summary Turmeric/curcumin may offer elderly patients a well-tolerated means of decreasing arthritis pain, with a safe side effect profile. It also has an intriguing anti-inflammatory profile that plays a role both in pain benefit and broader anti-inflammatory conditions. However, bioavailability can be limited without the correctly processed product, and caution should be taken with patients who are on polypharmacy.

15.9 Coenzyme Q10 (CoQ10)

Background CoQ10 is an essential cofactor in the human mitochondrial electron transport pathway that generates cellular ATP. It acts as a powerful lipid-soluble antioxidant to reduce free radical damage from this energy production. It is endogenously synthesized via the mevalonate pathway (which is blocked by statin drugs) and can also be obtained from the diet in small amounts from fish, organ meats, and wheat germ. CoQ10 is in virtually all cells, with especially high concentrations in the heart. CoQ10 levels are highest during the first 20 years of life and decline with age, so deficiency is relatively common in the elderly. Statins may aggravate this deficiency, and CoQ10 serum levels can be assessed for deficiency. It may be used with other nutrients such as selenium (Se) and other antioxidant vitamins, omega-3 fatty acids, ribose, carnitine, and taurine to support the "energy chain," especially in heart function [76–80].

Indications Ingestion of CoQ10 is helpful to prevent or correct deficiency. Its safety and freedom from drug interactions make it useful in many conditions suffered by the elderly:

- Cardiovascular disease: typically 50–200 mg per day. Preliminary to mid-level evidence supports the following benefits:
  - Coronary artery disease (CAD) – improved function and reduced cardiac events [81], reduced cardiovascular mortality in elderly with CoQ10 and selenium [82], and better lipid goals with nutraceuticals containing CoQ10 [83]. Of note, evidence is conflicting in the use of CoQ10 in prevention of statin-induced myopathy. A typical dose used in this context is 50–200 mg per day [84, 85].
  - Congestive heart failure (CHF) – mainly positive results in later trials. The Q-SYMBIO trial demonstrated improved key CHF endpoints including lower mortality, using CoQ10 100 mg TID for 2 years [86]. Other studies largely support the use in CHF, whether in preserved or reduced ejection fraction subtype [87–89].
  - CoQ10 may also decrease atrial fibrillation in heart failure [90] and may improve blood pressure in hypertensive patients, the latter through a possible related anti-inflammatory and vascular function [91].
- There is some suggestion that CoQ10 can be helpful in neurodegenerative diseases such as in Parkinson's disease. Mild cognitive impairment possibly may be improved in Parkinson's disease, as an example [92]. Doses in this context appear to be higher, at anywhere from 300 mg up to 2400 mg per day [93].
- Hospital-free days and maintenance of healthcare quality of life in elderly with CoQ10 and selenium (Se) [94].
- DM – 100–200 mg per day modestly decreases A1C (mixed evidence).
- Preliminary evidence of benefit of CoQ10 alone or with other supplements such as selenium (Se) for many other medical problems such as metabolic syndrome and hyperlipidemia [95–98], diabetic retinopathy [99, 100], skin aging [101, 102], nonalcoholic fatty liver disease (NAFLD) [103], chronic fatigue [104, 105], cancer-related fatigue [106] and depression (in MS patients [107]), oxidative stress in hemolysis patients [108], and migraines [109].

Dose/practical considerations As a lipid-soluble supplement, bioavailability of CoQ10 can vary among supplement products. Softgel or chewables have better bioavailability than tablets. Doses for heart failure are typically 200–600 mg/day. It is worth noting that, on average, the monthly cost for 100 mg per day is approximately $30 and for 1200 mg per day of CoQ10 is approximately $300. As such it is important to discuss cost with patients.

Adverse effects CoQ10 is very well tolerated and has minimal adverse effects. There is a theoretical risk that it can decrease PT/INR on warfarin, so this should be monitored [110]. In addition, as mentioned above, CoQ10 can mildly lower blood pressure and blood sugar – monitoring may be prudent.

Contraindications/cautions No specific contraindications have been identified in the geriatric population.

Interactions No clinically significant interactions known. As mentioned above, CoQ10 can slightly lower blood sugar and BP, so monitor with medications used for these purposes.

Summary CoQ10 may be useful for elderly with heart disease, statin-induced myopathy, and possibly neurodegenerative and some other disorders. It is a more expensive supplement, and so counseling about cost is prudent with patients.

15.10 Magnesium (Mg)

Background As a mineral, magnesium is present and available in many whole food sources; however, these food sources are not present in a more processed diet. That is, magnesium ingestion may be low in patients who are not ingesting much of the following whole foods: legumes, nuts, dark leafy greens, halibut, unprocessed grains, and fortified cereals, meat, and dairy.

Indications Magnesium supplementation is indicated for the prevention or correction of magnesium deficiency, which is common [111, 112]. As stated above, many Americans including especially the elderly consume less than the RDA of about 320 (Females) – 420 (Males) mg/day, mainly due to a lack of eating the whole foods rich in magnesium. In addition, there are select groups at risk for Mg deficiency, and these include patients with the following conditions [112]:

- Regular alcohol use (esp. spirits), predisposing to stroke, sarcopenia, cardiomyopathy, steatohepatitis, and cirrhosis. Even moderate alcohol use promotes magnesiuresis.
- GI disorders: malabsorption, chronic diarrhea, inflammatory conditions, short bowel syndrome, and intestinal resection.
- Elderly (especially hospitalized): due to decreased GI magnesium absorption, increases in urinary excretion, use of certain medications (e.g., diuretics, proton-pump inhibitors (PPIs)), and poor dietary intake, elders are at risk of low total magnesium levels.
- Diabetes mellitus: approximately 33% of diabetes have low Mg intake, which is significant, since hypomagnesemia impairs glucose handling [113].

It's important to have a high suspicion for Mg deficiency in any of the above clinical settings, especially if serum values are low or low normal or if there is unexplained/persistent low potassium (which is found in ~40% of low Mg cases) or low calcium, phosphorus, or sodium serum levels. Expected beneficial effects of correcting Mg deficiency include [112]:

- Cardiovascular: May lower BP modestly and may reduce risk of stroke and atrial fibrillation and may improve prognosis in CHF and MI. Improves risk of digitalis toxicity/side effects.
- Metabolic: Adequate Mg intake is associated with improved metabolic syndrome, diabetes mellitus control, and HDL levels.
- Musculoskeletal: Adequate Mg is associated with improved bone density and is required for proper vitamin D function.
- Renal: Correcting Mg deficiency likely lowers risk of calcium oxalate nephrolithiasis. Chronic low Mg is associated with kidney disease [114].

Dose/practical considerations All nutrients ideally should be gained from whole foods; however, if need to supplement Mg, it is best to take magnesium in divided doses, since gut absorption is slow and most of a high single daily dose will be wasted leading to osmotic diarrhea. Avoid prolonged supplementation that exceeds the upper tolerable limit (UL) of 360 mg/day unless in special clinical situations. Various Mg salts are roughly equivalent, but magnesium citrate in a slow absorbed formulation has reasonably good bioavailability. Severe hypomagnesemia would require IV $MgSO_4$ and is outside the scope of this chapter.

Adverse effects Excess doses of Mg can lead to osmotic diarrhea, since the body can only absorb a small amount at a time. Magnesium needs to be given cautiously in patients with chronic kidney disease (CKD).

Contraindications/cautions Mg appears safe if sensibly dosed to correct deficiency; however, because both low and high serum Mg levels are associated with increased hospital mortality [115, 116], supplement with magnesium only if suspecting deficiency, and follow levels to make sure they are not excessive. Advanced CKD impairs excretion of Mg – use caution in dosing and monitor levels if CKD stages 4 or 5.

15

Interactions Medication classes that can lead to Mg loss or impaired function include diuretics and PPIs (though the Mg impairment effect of PPIs may not be that clinically significant) [117, 118].

Summary Magnesium deficiency is common but often missed. In addition, common medical conditions and medications used in the elderly put them at risk for lower magnesium levels. Correcting Mg deficiency is important for health, especially relating to healthy cardiovascular, neuromuscular, and metabolic function. However excess Mg may also be hazardous and should be avoided.

15.11 Summary

Supplements, like all therapeutics, need to be used based on solid evidence, careful selection, and thorough communication and have a legitimate place in the proper treatment of elderly patients. A shared decision-making approach with open dialog helps elderly patients make the best decision around supplement use, and proper documentation of supplement use in the medical record enhances surveillance for potential side effects and botanical/pharmaceutical interactions, thus optimizing benefit/risk ratio.

References

1. FDA US. Dietary supplements: what you need to know [updated 11/29/179/13/18]. Available from: https://www.fda.gov/Food/DietarySupplements/UsingDietarySupplements/ucm109760.htm.
2. Gahche JJ, Bailey RL, Potischman N, Dwyer JT. Dietary supplement use was very high among older adults in the United States in 2011–2014. J Nutr. 2017;147(10):1968–76.
3. Consumerlab.com. [1/10/18]. Available from: https://www.consumerlab.com.
4. Pharmacopeia US. Dietary Supplements Verification Program. Available from: http://www.usp.org/verification-services/dietary-supplements-verification-program.
5. NSF. Dietary Supplements GMP Registration. Available from: http://www.nsf.org/services/by-industry/dietary-supplements/dietary-supplements-gmp-registration.
6. Farahani MS, Bahramsoltani R, Farzaei MH, Abdollahi M, Rahimi R. Plant-derived natural medicines for the management of depression: an overview of mechanisms of action. Rev Neurosci. 2015;26(3):305–21.
7. Concerto C, Boo H, Hu C, Sandilya P, Krish A, Chusid E, et al. Hypericum perforatum extract modulates cortical plasticity in humans. Psychopharmacology. 2018;235(1):145–53.
8. Linde K, Berner MM, Kriston L. St John's wort for major depression. Cochrane Database Syst Rev. 2008;(4):CD000448.
9. Varteresian T, Lavretsky H. Natural products and supplements for geriatric depression and cognitive disorders: an evaluation of the research. Curr Psychiatry Rep. 2014;16(8):456.
10. Kasper S. Phytopharmaceutical treatment of anxiety, depression, and dementia in the elderly: evidence from randomized, controlled clinical trials. Wien Med Wochenschr. 2015;165(11-12):-217–28.
11. Kasper S, Gastpar M, Muller WE, Volz HP, Dienel A, Kieser M, et al. Efficacy of St. John's wort extract WS 5570 in acute treatment of mild depression: a reanalysis of data from controlled clinical trials. Eur Arch Psychiatry Clin Neurosci. 2008;258(1):59–63.
12. Shi S, Klotz U. Drug interactions with herbal medicines. Clin Pharmacokinet. 2012;51(2):77–104.
13. Knüppel L, Linde K. Adverse effects of St. John's Wort: a systematic review. J Clin Psychiatry. 2004.
14. Council AAB. [Updated 8/12/19]. Available from: http://cms.herbalgram.org/herbclip/149/review42254.html. This is a monograph on Gingko biloba published by the American Botanical Council.
15. Weinmann S, Roll S, Schwarzbach C, Vauth C, Willich SN. Effects of Ginkgo biloba in dementia: systematic review and meta-analysis. BMC Geriatr. 2010;10:14.
16. von Gunten A, Schlaefke S, Uberla K. Efficacy of Ginkgo biloba extract EGb 761((R)) in dementia with behavioural and psychological symptoms: a systematic review. World J Biol Psychiatry. 2016;17(8):622–33.
17. Gauthier S, Schlaefke S. Efficacy and tolerability of Ginkgo biloba extract EGb 761(R) in dementia: a systematic review and meta-analysis of randomized placebo-controlled trials. Clin Interv Aging. 2014;9:2065–77.
18. Tan J, Peng H. Clinical analysis of Ginkgo biloba injection combined with traditional therapy in treatment of explosive deafness. Zhonghua Lao Dong Wei Sheng Zhi Ye Bing Za Zhi. 2015;33(4):279–81.

19. Savaskan E, Mueller H, Hoerr R, von Gunten A, Gauthier S. Treatment effects of Ginkgo biloba extract EGb 761® on the spectrum of behavioral and psychological symptoms of dementia: meta-analysis of randomized controlled trials. Int Psychogeriatr. 2017: 30(3):285–293.
20. Birks J, Evans JG. Ginkgo biloba for cognitive impairment and dementia. Cochrane Database Syst Rev. 2009;(1):CD003120.
21. Butler M, Nelson VA, Davila H, Ratner E, Fink HA, Hemmy LS, et al. Over-the-counter supplement interventions to prevent cognitive decline, mild cognitive impairment, and clinical Alzheimer-type dementia: a systematic review. Ann Intern Med. 2018;168(1):52–62.
22. Kellermann AJ, Kloft C. Is there a risk of bleeding associated with standardized Ginkgo biloba extract therapy? A systematic review and meta-analysis. Pharmacotherapy. 2011;31(5):490–502.
23. Markowitz JS, Donovan JL, Lindsay DeVane C, Sipkes L, Chavin KD. Multiple-dose administration of Ginkgo biloba did not affect cytochrome P-450 2D6 or 3A4 activity in normal volunteers. J Clin Psychopharmacol. 2003;23(6):576–81.
24. Guo CX, Pei Q, Yin JY, Peng XD, Zhou BT, Zhao YC, et al. Effects of Ginkgo biloba extracts on pharmacokinetics and efficacy of atorvastatin based on plasma indices. Xenobiotica. 2012;42(8):784–90.
25. Dai LL, Fan L, Wu HZ, Tan ZR, Chen Y, Peng XD, et al. Assessment of a pharmacokinetic and pharmacodynamic interaction between simvastatin and Ginkgo biloba extracts in healthy subjects. Xenobiotica. 2013;43(10):862–7.
26. Dylag K, Hubalewska-Mazgaj M, Surmiak M, Szmyd J, Brzozowski T. Probiotics in the mechanism of protection against gut inflammation and therapy of gastrointestinal disorders. Curr Pharm Des. 2014;20(7):1149–55.
27. Zhang YJ, Li S, Gan RY, Zhou T, Xu DP, Li HB. Impacts of gut bacteria on human health and diseases. Int J Mol Sci. 2015;16(4):7493–519.
28. Esposito S, Rigante D, Principi N. Do children's upper respiratory tract infections benefit from probiotics? BMC Infect Dis. 2014;14:194.
29. Donskey CJ. Clostridium difficile in older adults. Infect Dis Clin N Am. 2017;31(4):743–56.
30. Shen NT, Leff JA, Schneider Y, Crawford CV, Maw A, Bosworth B, et al. Cost-effectiveness analysis of probiotic use to prevent Clostridium difficile infection in hospitalized adults receiving antibiotics. Open Forum Infect Dis. 2017;4(3):ofx148.
31. Goldenberg JZ, Yap C, Lytvyn L, Lo CK, Beardsley J, Mertz D, et al. Probiotics for the prevention of Clostridium difficile-associated diarrhea in adults and children. Cochrane Database Syst Rev. 2017;(12):CD006095.
32. Hempel S, Newberry SJ, Maher AR, Wang Z, Miles JN, Shanman R, et al. Probiotics for the prevention and treatment of antibiotic-associated diarrhea: a systematic review and meta-analysis. JAMA. 2012;307(18):1959–69.
33. Hauser G, Salkic N, Vukelic K, JajacKnez A, Stimac D. Probiotics for standard triple Helicobacter pylori eradication: a randomized, double-blind, placebo-controlled trial. Medicine (Baltimore). 2015;94(17):e685.
34. Hempel S, Newberry S, Ruelaz A, Wang Z, Miles JN, Suttorp MJ, et al. Safety of probiotics used to reduce risk and prevent or treat disease. Evid Rep Technol Assess. 2011;200:1–645.
35. Besselink MG, van Santvoort HC, van der Heijden GJ, Buskens E, Gooszen HG, Dutch Acute Pancreatitis Study G. New randomized trial of probiotics in pancreatitis needed? Caution advised. Langenbeck's Arch Surg. 2009;394(1):191–2; author reply 3–4.
36. Sterzi S, Giordani L, Morrone M, Lena E, Magrone G, Scarpini C, et al. The efficacy and safety of a combination of glucosamine hydrochloride, chondroitin sulfate and bio-curcumin with exercise in the treatment of knee osteoarthritis: a randomized, double-blind, placebo-controlled study. Eur J Phys Rehabil Med. 2016;52(3):321–30.
37. Kanzaki N, Saito K, Maeda A, Kitagawa Y, Kiso Y, Watanabe K, et al. Effect of a dietary supplement containing glucosamine hydrochloride, chondroitin sulfate and quercetin glycosides on symptomatic knee osteoarthritis: a randomized, double-blind, placebo-controlled study. J Sci Food Agric. 2012;92(4):862–9.
38. Runhaar J, Rozendaal RM, van Middelkoop M, Bijlsma HJW, Doherty M, Dziedzic KS, et al. Subgroup analyses of the effectiveness of oral glucosamine for knee and hip osteoarthritis: a systematic review and individual patient data meta-analysis from the OA trial bank. Ann Rheum Dis. 2017;76(11):1862–9.
39. Harrison-Munoz S, Rojas-Briones V, Irarrazaval S. Is glucosamine effective for osteoarthritis? Medwave. 2017;17(Suppl1):e6867.
40. Roman-Blas JA, Castaneda S, Sanchez-Pernaute O, Largo R, Herrero-Beaumont G, Group CGCTS. Combined treatment with chondroitin sulfate and glucosamine sulfate shows no superiority over placebo for reduction of joint pain and functional impairment in patients with knee osteoarthritis: a six-month multicenter, randomized, double-blind, placebo-controlled clinical trial. Arthritis Rheumatol. 2017;69(1):77–85.
41. Selvan T, Rajiah K, Nainar MS, Mathew EM. A clinical study on glucosamine sulfate versus combination of glucosamine sulfate and NSAIDs in mild to moderate knee osteoarthritis. Sci World J. 2012;2012:902676.
42. Saengnipanthkul S, Waikakul S, Rojanasthien S, Totemchokchyakarn K, Srinkapaibulaya A, Cheh Chin T, Mai Hong N, Bruyere O, Cooper C, Reginster JY, Lwin M. International Journal of Rheumatic Diseases. 2019;22(3):376–385.
43. Fransen M, Agaliotis M, Nairn L, Votrubec M, Bridgett L, Su S, et al. Glucosamine and chondroitin for knee osteoarthritis: a double-blind randomised placebo-controlled clinical trial evaluating single and combination regimens. Ann Rheum Dis. 2015;74(5):851–8.
44. National Center for Complimentary and Alternative Medicine, National Institutes of Health. The NIH glucosamine/chondroitin arthritis intervention trial (GAIT). J Pain Palliat Care Pharmacother. 2008;22(1):39–43.
45. Reginster JY, Neuprez A, Lecart MP, Sarlet N, Bruyere O. Role of glucosamine in the treatment for osteoarthritis. Rheumatol Int. 2012;32(10):2959–67.
46. Holick MF. Vitamin D deficiency. N Engl J Med. 2007;357(3):266–81.
47. Tremezaygues L, Sticherling M, Pfohler C, Friedrich M, Meineke V, Seifert M, et al. Cutaneous photosynthesis of vitamin D: an evolutionary highly-conserved endocrine system that protects against environmental hazards including UV-radiation and microbial infections. Anticancer Res. 2006;26(4A):2743–8.
48. Pludowski P, Karczmarewicz E, Bayer M, Carter G, Chlebna-Sokol D, Czech-Kowalska J, et al. Practical guidelines for the supplementation of vitamin D and the treatment of deficits in Central Europe – recommended vitamin D intakes in the general population and groups at risk of vitamin D deficiency. Endokrynol Pol. 2013;64(4):319–27.
49. Institute of Medicine (US) Committee to Review Dietary Reference Intakes for Vitamin D and Calcium; Ross AC, Taylor CL, Yaktine AL, Del Valle HB, editors. Dietary Reference Intakes for Calcium and Vitamin D. Washington (DC): National Academies Press (US); 2011.
50. Galizia I, Oldani L, Macritchie K, Amari E, Dougall D, Jones TN, et al. S-adenosyl methionine (SAMe) for depression in adults. Cochrane Database Syst Rev. 2016;(10):CD011286.
51. Sharma A, Gerbarg P, Bottiglieri T, Massoumi L, Carpenter LL, Lavretsky H, et al. S-Adenosylmethionine (SAMe) for neuropsychiatric disorders: a clinician-oriented review of research. J Clin Psychiatry. 2017;78(6):e656–e67.
52. Sarris J; Byrne GJ; Bousman C; Stough C; Murphy J; MacDonald P; Adams L; Nazareth S; Oliver G; Cribb L; Savage K; Menon R; Chamoli S; Berk M; Ng C; Mischoulon D. European Neuropsychopharmacology. 2018;28(10):1126–1136.
53. Guo T, Chang L, Xiao Y, Liu Q. S-adenosyl-L-methionine for the treatment of chronic liver disease: a systematic review and meta-analysis. PLoS One. 2015;10(3):e0122124.
54. Jacobsen S, Danneskiold-Samsoe B, Andersen RB. Oral S-adenosylmethionine in primary fibromyalgia. Double-blind clinical evaluation. Scand J Rheumatol. 1991;20(4):294–302.
55. Shehzad A, Qureshi M, Anwar MN, Lee YS. Multifunctional curcumin mediate multitherapeutic effects. J Food Sci. 2017;82(9):2006–15.

56. Akuri MC, Barbalho SM, Val RM, Guiguer EL. Reflections about osteoarthritis and Curcuma longa. Pharmacogn Rev. 2017;11(21):8–12.
57. Amalraj A, Varma K, Jacob J, Divya C, Kunnumakkara AB, Stohs SJ, et al. A novel highly bioavailable curcumin formulation improves symptoms and diagnostic indicators in rheumatoid arthritis patients: a randomized, double-blind, placebo-controlled, two-dose, three-arm, and parallel-group study. J Med Food. 2017;20(10):1022–30.
58. Hewlings SJ, Kalman DS. Curcumin: a review of its' effects on human health. Foods. 2017;6(10):92.
59. Perkins K, Sahy W, Beckett RD. Efficacy of curcuma for treatment of osteoarthritis. J Evid Based Complementary Altern Med. 2017;22(1):156–65.
60. Liu X, Machado GC, Eyles JP, Ravi V, Hunter DJ. Dietary supplements for treating osteoarthritis: a systematic review and meta-analysis. Br J Sports Med. 2018;52:167–75.
61. Daily JW, Yang M, Park S. Efficacy of turmeric extracts and curcumin for alleviating the symptoms of joint arthritis: a systematic review and meta-analysis of randomized clinical trials. J Med Food. 2016;19(8):717–29.
62. Ross SM. Turmeric (Curcuma longa): effects of Curcuma longa extracts compared with ibuprofen for reduction of pain and functional improvement in patients with knee osteoarthritis. Holist Nurs Pract. 2016;30(3):183–6.
63. Belcaro G, Cesarone MR, Dugall M, Pellegrini L, Ledda A, Grossi MG, et al. Efficacy and safety of Meriva(R), a curcumin-phosphatidylcholine complex, during extended administration in osteoarthritis patients. Altern Med Rev. 2010;15(4):337–44.
64. Kuptniratsaikul V, Dajpratham P, Taechaarpornkul W, Buntragulpoontawee M, Lukkanapichonchut P, Chootip C, et al. Efficacy and safety of Curcuma domestica extracts compared with ibuprofen in patients with knee osteoarthritis: a multicenter study. Clin Interv Aging. 2014;9:451–8.
65. Pinsornsak P, Niempoog S. The efficacy of Curcuma Longa L. extract as an adjuvant therapy in primary knee osteoarthritis: a randomized control trial. J Med Assoc Thail. 2012;95(Suppl 1):S51–8.
66. Nakagawa Y, Mukai S, Yamada S, Matsuoka M, Tarumi E, Hashimoto T, et al. Short-term effects of highly-bioavailable curcumin for treating knee osteoarthritis: a randomized, double-blind, placebo-controlled prospective study. J Orthop Sci. 2014;19(6):933–9.
67. Kuptniratsaikul V, Thanakhumtorn S, Chinswangwatanakul P, Wattanamongkonsil L, Thamlikitkul V. Efficacy and safety of Curcuma domestica extracts in patients with knee osteoarthritis. J Altern Complement Med. 2009;15(8):891–7.
68. Chandran B, Goel A. A randomized, pilot study to assess the efficacy and safety of curcumin in patients with active rheumatoid arthritis. Phytother Res. 2012;26(11):1719–25.
69. Panahi Y, Rahimnia AR, Sharafi M, Alishiri G, Saburi A, Sahebkar A. Curcuminoid treatment for knee osteoarthritis: a randomized double-blind placebo-controlled trial. Phytother Res. 2014;28(11):1625–31.
70. Rahimnia AR, Panahi Y, Alishiri G, Sharafi M, Sahebkar A. Impact of supplementation with curcuminoids on systemic inflammation in patients with knee osteoarthritis: findings from a randomized double-blind placebo-controlled trial. Drug Res (Stuttg). 2015; 65(10):521–5.
71. Henrotin Y, Priem F, Mobasheri A. Curcumin: a new paradigm and therapeutic opportunity for the treatment of osteoarthritis: curcumin for osteoarthritis management. Springerplus. 2013;2(1):56.
72. Conrozier T, Mathieu P, Bonjean M, Marc JF, Renevier JL, Balblanc JC. A complex of three natural anti-inflammatory agents provides relief of osteoarthritis pain. Altern Ther Health Med. 2014;20(Suppl 1):32–7.
73. Chuengsamarn S, Rattanamongkolgul S, Luechapudiporn R, Phisalaphong C, Jirawatnotai S. Curcumin extract for prevention of type 2 diabetes. Diabetes Care. 2012;35(11):2121–7.
74. Ghosh S, Banerjee S, Sil PC. The beneficial role of curcumin on inflammation, diabetes and neurodegenerative disease: a recent update. Food Chem Toxicol. 2015;83:111–24.
75. Chuengsamarn S, Rattanamongkolgul S, Phonrat B, Tungtrongchitr R, Jirawatnotai S. Reduction of atherogenic risk in patients with type 2 diabetes by curcuminoid extract: a randomized controlled trial. J Nutr Biochem. 2014;25(2):144–50.
76. Gasiorowski A, Dutkiewicz J. Comprehensive rehabilitation in chronic heart failure. Ann Agric Environ Med. 2013;20(3):606–12.
77. Lee JH, Jarreau T, Prasad A, Lavie C, O'Keefe J, Ventura H. Nutritional assessment in heart failure patients. Congest Heart Fail. 2011;17(4):199–203.
78. Allard ML, Jeejeebhoy KN, Sole MJ. The management of conditioned nutritional requirements in heart failure. Heart Fail Rev. 2006;11(1):75–82.
79. Witte KK, Nikitin NP, Parker AC, von Haehling S, Volk HD, Anker SD, et al. The effect of micronutrient supplementation on quality-of-life and left ventricular function in elderly patients with chronic heart failure. Eur Heart J. 2005;26(21):2238–44.
80. Sole MJ, Jeejeebhoy KN. Conditioned nutritional requirements: therapeutic relevance to heart failure. Herz. 2002;27(2):174–8.
81. Aslanabadi N, Safaie N, Asgharzadeh Y, Houshmand F, Ghaffari S, Garjani A, et al. The randomized clinical trial of coenzyme Q10 for the prevention of periprocedural myocardial injury following elective percutaneous coronary intervention. Cardiovasc Ther. 2016;34(4):254–60.
82. Alehagen U, Alexander J, Aaseth J. Supplementation with selenium and coenzyme Q10 reduces cardiovascular mortality in elderly with low selenium status. A secondary analysis of a randomised clinical trial. PLoS One. 2016;11(7):e0157541.
83. Marazzi G, Pelliccia F, Campolongo G, Quattrino S, Cacciotti L, Volterrani M, et al. Usefulness of nutraceuticals (Armolipid Plus) versus ezetimibe and combination in statin-intolerant patients with dyslipidemia with coronary heart disease. Am J Cardiol. 2015;116(12):1798–801.
84. Okello E, Jiang X, Mohamed S, Zhao Q, Wang T. Combined statin/coenzyme Q10 as adjunctive treatment of chronic heart failure. Med Hypotheses. 2009;73(3):306–8.
85. Taylor BA, Lorson L, White CM, Thompson PD. A randomized trial of coenzyme Q10 in patients with confirmed statin myopathy. Atherosclerosis. 2015;238(2):329–35.
86. Mortensen SA, Rosenfeldt F, Kumar A, Dolliner P, Filipiak KJ, Pella D, et al. The effect of coenzyme Q10 on morbidity and mortality in chronic heart failure: results from Q-SYMBIO: a randomized double-blind trial. JACC Heart Fail. 2014;2(6):641–9.
87. Oleck S, Ventura HO. Coenzyme Q10 and utility in heart failure: just another supplement? Curr Heart Fail Rep. 2016;13(4):190–5.
88. Jankowski J, Korzeniowska K, Cieslewicz A, Jablecka A. Coenzyme Q10 – a new player in the treatment of heart failure? Pharmacol Rep. 2016;68(5):1015–9.
89. Fotino AD, Thompson-Paul AM, Bazzano LA. Effect of coenzyme Q(1)(0) supplementation on heart failure: a meta-analysis. Am J Clin Nutr. 2013;97(2):268–75.
90. Zhao Q, Kebbati AH, Zhang Y, Tang Y, Okello E, Huang C. Effect of coenzyme Q10 on the incidence of atrial fibrillation in patients with heart failure. J Investig Med. 2015;63(5):735–9.
91. Bagheri Nesami N, Mozaffari-Khosravi H, Najarzadeh A, Salehifar E. The effect of coenzyme Q10 supplementation on pro-inflammatory factors and adiponectin in mildly hypertensive patients: a randomized, double-blind, placebo-controlled trial. Int J Vitam Nutr Res. 2015;85(3–4):156–64.
92. Li Z, Wang P, Yu Z, Cong Y, Sun H, Zhang J, et al. The effect of creatine and coenzyme q10 combination therapy on mild cognitive impairment in Parkinson's disease. Eur Neurol. 2015;73(3–4):205–11.
93. Yoritaka A, Kawajiri S, Yamamoto Y, Nakahara T, Ando M, Hashimoto K, et al. Randomized, double-blind, placebo-controlled pilot trial of reduced coenzyme Q10 for Parkinson's disease. Parkinsonism Relat Disord. 2015;21(8):911–6.
94. Johansson P, Dahlstrom O, Dahlstrom U, Alehagen U. Improved health-related quality of life, and more days out of hospital with supplementation with selenium and coenzyme Q10 combined. results from a double blind, placebo-controlled prospective study. J Nutr Health Aging. 2015;19(9):870–7.

95. Cicero AF, Morbini M, Rosticci M, D'Addato S, Grandi E, Borghi C. Middle-term dietary supplementation with red yeast rice plus coenzyme Q10 improves lipid pattern, endothelial reactivity and arterial stiffness in moderately hypercholesterolemic subjects. Ann Nutr Metab. 2016;68(3):213–9.
96. Marazzi G, Campolongo G, Pelliccia F, Quattrino S, Vitale C, Cacciotti L, et al. Comparison of low-dose statin versus low-dose statin + Armolipid Plus in high-intensity statin-intolerant patients with a previous coronary event and percutaneous coronary intervention (ADHERENCE Trial). Am J Cardiol. 2017;120(6):893–7.
97. Raygan F, Rezavandi Z, Dadkhah Tehrani S, Farrokhian A, Asemi Z. The effects of coenzyme Q10 administration on glucose homeostasis parameters, lipid profiles, biomarkers of inflammation and oxidative stress in patients with metabolic syndrome. Eur J Nutr. 2016;55(8):2357–64.
98. Cicero AF, Colletti A, Fogacci F, Bove M, Rosticci M, Borghi C. Effects of a combined nutraceutical on lipid pattern, glucose metabolism and inflammatory parameters in moderately hypercholesterolemic subjects: a double blind, cross over, randomized clinical trial. High Blood Press Cardiovasc Prev. 2017;24(1):13–8.
99. Rodriguez-Carrizalez AD, Castellanos-Gonzalez JA, Martinez-Romero EC, Miller-Arrevillaga G, Pacheco-Moises FP, Roman-Pintos LM, et al. The effect of ubiquinone and combined antioxidant therapy on oxidative stress markers in non-proliferative diabetic retinopathy: a phase IIa, randomized, double-blind, and placebo-controlled study. Redox Rep. 2016;21(4):155–63.
100. Domanico D, Fragiotta S, Cutini A, Carnevale C, Zompatori L, Vingolo EM. Circulating levels of reactive oxygen species in patients with nonproliferative diabetic retinopathy and the influence of antioxidant supplementation: 6-month follow-up. Indian J Ophthalmol. 2015;63(1):9–14.
101. Zmitek K, Pogacnik T, Mervic L, Zmitek J, Pravst I. The effect of dietary intake of coenzyme Q10 on skin parameters and condition: results of a randomised, placebo-controlled, double-blind study. Biofactors. 2017;43(1):132–40.
102. Di Cerbo A, Laurino C, Palmieri B, Iannitti T. A dietary supplement improves facial photoaging and skin sebum, hydration and tonicity modulating serum fibronectin, neutrophil elastase 2, hyaluronic acid and carbonylated proteins. J Photochem Photobiol B. 2015;144:94–103.
103. Farsi F, Mohammadshahi M, Alavinejad P, Rezazadeh A, Zarei M, Engali KA. Functions of coenzyme Q10 supplementation on liver enzymes, markers of systemic inflammation, and adipokines in patients affected by nonalcoholic fatty liver disease: a double-blind, placebo-controlled, randomized clinical trial. J Am Coll Nutr. 2016;35(4):346–53.
104. Fukuda S, Nojima J, Kajimoto O, Yamaguti K, Nakatomi Y, Kuratsune H, et al. Ubiquinol-10 supplementation improves autonomic nervous function and cognitive function in chronic fatigue syndrome. Biofactors. 2016;42(4):431–40.
105. Castro-Marrero J, Cordero MD, Segundo MJ, Saez-Francas N, Calvo N, Roman-Malo L, et al. Does oral coenzyme Q10 plus NADH supplementation improve fatigue and biochemical parameters in chronic fatigue syndrome? Antioxid Redox Signal. 2015;22(8):679–85.
106. Iwase S, Kawaguchi T, Yotsumoto D, Doi T, Miyara K, Odagiri H, et al. Efficacy and safety of an amino acid jelly containing coenzyme Q10 and L-carnitine in controlling fatigue in breast cancer patients receiving chemotherapy: a multi-institutional, randomized, exploratory trial (JORTC-CAM01). Support Care Cancer. 2016;24(2):637–46.
107. Sanoobar M, Dehghan P, Khalili M, Azimi A, Seifar F. Coenzyme Q10 as a treatment for fatigue and depression in multiple sclerosis patients: a double blind randomized clinical trial. Nutr Neurosci. 2016;19(3):138–43.
108. Yeung CK, Billings FT, Claessens AJ, Roshanravan B, Linke L, Sundell MB, et al. Coenzyme Q10 dose-escalation study in hemodialysis patients: safety, tolerability, and effect on oxidative stress. BMC Nephrol. 2015;16:183.
109. Gaul C, Diener HC, Danesch U, Migravent Study G. Improvement of migraine symptoms with a proprietary supplement containing riboflavin, magnesium and Q10: a randomized, placebo-controlled, double-blind, multicenter trial. J Headache Pain. 2015;16:516.
110. Engelsen Engelsen reference: Engelsen J, Nielsen JD, Winther K. Effect of coenzyme Q10 and Ginkgo biloba on warfarin dosage in stable, long-term warfarin treated outpatients. A randomised, double blind, placebo-crossover trial. Thromb Haemost. 2002; 87(6):1075–6.
111. Bertinato J, Wang KC, Hayward S. Serum Magnesium Concentrations in the Canadian Population and Associations with Diabetes, Glycemic Regulation, and Insulin Resistance. Nutrients. 2017;9(3). pii: E296
112. Ross AC. Modern nutrition in health and disease. Philadelphia: Wolters Kluwer Health/Lippincott Williams & Wilkins; 2014.
113. Shardha AK, Vaswani AS, Faraz A, Alam MT, Kumar P. Frequency and risk factors associated with hypomagnesaemia in hypokalemic type-2 diabetic patients. J Coll Physicians Surg Pak. 2014;24(11):830–5.
114. Tin A, Grams ME, Maruthur NM, Astor BC, Couper D, Mosley TH, et al. Results from the Atherosclerosis Risk in Communities study suggest that low serum magnesium is associated with incident kidney disease. Kidney Int. 2015;87(4):820–7.
115. Cheungpasitporn W, Thongprayoon C, Mao MA, Srivali N, Ungprasert P, Varothai N, et al. Hypomagnesaemia linked to depression: a systematic review and meta-analysis. Intern Med J. 2015;45(4):436–40.
116. Haider DG, Lindner G, Ahmad SS, Sauter T, Wolzt M, Leichtle AB, et al. Hypermagnesemia is a strong independent risk factor for mortality in critically ill patients: results from a cross-sectional study. Eur J Intern Med. 2015;26(7):504–7.
117. Sharara AI, Chalhoub JM, Hammoud N, Harb AH, Sarkis FS, Hamadeh G. Low prevalence of hypomagnesemia in long-term recipients of proton pump inhibitors in a managed care cohort. Clin Gastroenterol Hepatol. 2016;14(2):317–21.
118. Luk CP, Parsons R, Lee YP, Hughes JD. Proton pump inhibitor-associated hypomagnesemia: what do FDA data tell us? Ann Pharmacother. 2013;47(6):773–80.

Understanding the Medication List and Addressing Polypharmacy in Older Adults

Daniel Z. Mansour, Kriti Sharma, and Nicole J. Brandt

A. Chun (ed.), *Geriatric Practice*, https://doi.org/10.1007/978-3-030-19625-7_16

Key Points

At the end of this book chapter, the learner should be able to:

- Define polypharmacy and the implications on caring for older adults.
- Identify at least two negative consequences of polypharmacy.
- Describe how polypharmacy impacts a patient's healthcare goals.
- List at least three tactics to address polypharmacy.

Case Study

JC is a widowed 78-year-old Asian male who is seen in the office by pharmacist/physician team for a follow-up treatment of hypertension and diabetes. Mr. JC lives alone and a home aid comes to his home to clean and cook. Current medical problem list includes chronic obstructive pulmonary disease (COPD), atrial fibrillation, left ventricular heart failure (LVHF) (Ejection Fracture (EF) = 34%), osteoarthritis (OA), and history of falls last of which was in the prior week. Body weight = 89 lbs, blood pressure (BP) = 170/95, heart rate (HR) = 85, pain = 7/10, HbA1C = 13% (2 months ago), fasting blood glucose (FBG) = 210 mg/dl (2 months ago), creatinine clearance (CrCl) = 29 ml/min (2 months ago).

16.1 Background and Epidemiology

It is estimated that 66% of adults aged >65 years in the United States take five or more medications [1, 2], and over 25% are prescribed ten or more medications [3]. As many as 50% of adverse drug events (ADEs) are due to the use of medications in older adults [4]. In recent years, the incidence of polypharmacy increased from an estimated 8.2% in 1999–2000 to 15% in 2011–2012 [5]. Organizations such as the Food and Drug Administration (FDA) have reported a high number of medication-related errors among older adults including overdosing, omitting, confusing medication with one another, drug-drug interactions, food-drug interactions, and wrong route of administration.

If medication-related problems were ranked as a disease, ADEs would be the fifth leading cause of death in the United States [6]. Thankfully, ADEs are one of the most preventable causative factors leading to hospital admission [7]. These data are of particular importance among older adults because of the increased medication burden in relation to their disease states and how they process medications compared to younger adults. In clinical practice, daily regimens consisting of tens of medications is not uncommon [8] and result in office visits involving polypharmacy which will be discussed [9].

Many older adults believe that "a pill will fix what ails them." The prescriber, more often than not, may feel pressured to "prescribe something" [10]. It is estimated that 80% of older adults have at least one chronic disease, and 68% have at least two [11], therefore, taking medications became the modality of choice in managing many of these chronic diseases compared to the invasive nature of surgery [12–14].

There are no national guidelines to treat polypharmacy [15], hence, implementing measures to prevent/manage polypharmacy on a case-by-case basis is common practice [16, 17]. Furthermore, 25% of older adults do not report to their healthcare providers the herbs and supplements they are taking at the provider's office. This is mostly because healthcare providers do not ask and because patients do not think their healthcare providers need to know [18]. Therefore, the need to educate and train healthcare providers who will work with older adults is needed to address polypharmacy and minimize adverse drug events [19].

Case (Continued)

When inspecting JC's medication vials, the following constitutes his medication list:

No.	Medication	Sig	Last date filled on vial	Prescriber
1	Metformin	500 mg PO BID	2 weeks prior to the appointment, takes PRN	Johannes, DO
2	Glucovance®	5/500 PO BID	17 days prior to appointment	Johannes, DO
3	Lisinopril	20 mg PO BID	57 days prior	Graham, MD
4	Aspirin	325 mg PO Q day	Unknown	Johannes, DO
5	Atenolol	50 mg PO Q day	57 days prior	Graham, MD
6	Omeprazole	40 mg PO Q day	Last fill date was 76 days ago filled for a 30 day supply	Stanley, MD
7	Ibuprofen	800 mg PO BID	Empty vial; patient states he has been told by community pharmacist it was too soon. Patient buys ibuprofen over the counter (OTC) and states taking 4 tablets as needed	Tree, PA
8	Albuterol Metered Dose Inhaler (MDI)	2 puffs PO Q 4 hours PRN	Patient states he uses 2 puffs when needed and has used more than one inhaler in the last month	Washington, CRNP

9	Advair® (fluticasone/ salmeterol 250 mcg/50mcg powder)	PO BID	6 months prior to appointment	Washington, CRNP
10	Furosemide	80 mg PO Q day	17 days prior to appointment	Graham, MD
11	Lidocaine 4% patches		Patient states he is applying up to 3 patches per day	Love, PA
12	Senna	2 tablets PO PRN		Noel, PharmD
13	Miralax®	1 tablespoonful PO BID		Love, PA
14	Ipratropium/albuterol nebulizer solution		Patient states he uses 7 boxes per month, last refill date was 17 days prior to appointment, and there was only one box presented at appointment	Tree, PA

Additionally, he had the following that he is using inconsistently: St. John's wort, omega-3, multivitamin, and Super Bio-Curcumin given to him by a friend.

16.1.1 Definition of Polypharmacy

While polypharmacy can be defined in terms of quantity of medications, as taking more than five regular prescribed medicines, it can also be defined qualitatively as the taking of multiple medications by a patient in whom the benefits are exceeded by the clinical and/or financial costs [20]. It can also be defined as prescribing, dispensing or administering medications beyond the clinical need of any given patient [21, 22] or despite no longer being clinically indicated [23]. Hence, assessing the number of medications can only serve as a starting point in evaluating a patient with *inappropriate* polypharmacy [24], with a more person-centered approach and questioning whether or how to adjust patients' medication regimens is warranted [25].

16.1.2 Factors that Lead to Polypharmacy

The most common risk factor for developing inappropriate polypharmacy is patient's sociodemographics and medical conditions [26]. Furthermore, polypharmacy can be complicated by the patient stockpiling their medications, sharing them with others or by various self-treatment approaches [1]. This can be seen with JC's case where he is not only prescribed multiple medications but he is self-treating and others are providing additional recommendations (e.g., a friend).

Moreover, in an attempt to increase patient's adherence, many pharmacy systems place their patients on "auto-refill." This may be problematic if the medication has been discontinued or dose changed due to hospitalization or a transition of care.

Multiple providers for the same patient can contribute to duplicative therapy or possibly to a prescribing cascade. The prescribing cascade, where one drug is prescribed to mask the adverse drug reaction of another is an increasingly common problem in medical practice and it constitutes a warning about irrational use of medicines that puts health at risk and increases treatment costs if it is not taken into account [27]. Examples of a prescribing cascade are shown in ◘ Table 16.1.

◘ Table 16.1 Examples of prescribing cascades [31, 32]

Initial drug therapy	Adverse drug event	Subsequent drug therapy
Antipsychotics	Extrapyramidal signs and symptoms	Antiparkinsonian therapy (e.g., carbidopa/levodopa)
Cholinesterase inhibitors	Urinary incontinence	Anticholinergics (e.g., oxybutynin)
Thiazide diuretics	Hyperuricemia	Gout treatment (e.g., allopurinol)
NSAIDs	Increased blood pressure	Antihypertensives (e.g., amlodipine)

Additionally, direct to consumer advertising (DTCA) can harm patient-physician relationship [28] and may contribute to the overuse of medications. Studies suggest that DTCA allows a patient to open up a conversation on prescribing with their physician and leads to more requests for advertised medications despite the physicians' reluctance [29]. Many patients are encouraged through DTCA to demand a prescription for a new medication, which could subsequently lead to unwanted polypharmacy and increased healthcare costs [29, 30].

16.2 Impact of Inappropriate Polypharmacy in Older Adults

Older adults who are nonpolypharmacy users perceived their health status to be better than did polypharmacy users [33]. This may be due to the fact that polypharmacy has been associated with a higher incidence of frailty, slower walk, and complex movement with evidence of a dose-response relationship [34] and that medical comorbidities are only partly explained [35]. Polypharmacy coupled with an increasing older adult population [7, 17] has led to many negative outcomes including but not limited to diminished medication-adherence [36]; increased adverse drug reactions [37]; increased risk of cognitive impairment [38]; increased risk of falls [39]; increased incidence of drug-drug, drug-food, drug-gene, and drug disease interactions [5, 17]; increased risk of overdosing [40]; increased out-of-pocket medication costs [18]; lower health-related quality of life scores among adults in the United States [41]; and unnecessary hospitalizations [42] which will be described further below.

16.2.1 Medication Nonadherence

The likelihood of nonadherence rises with the number of medications prescribed in older adults [43]. It is estimated that approximately 23% of new admissions to skilled nursing facilities are due to medication nonadherence [23]. Cost of medications may lead to the patient's nonadherence and therefore compounds the problem to increased direct and indirect costs of treatment [44]. One way to combat nonadherence is the implementation of protocols to automate the prescription of indicated discharge therapies and, hence, the potential to dramatically reduce nonadherence following discharge [45]. However, medications can only be beneficial when the patient actually takes them; that is why it is imperative that the healthcare team not only assesses adherence but also for health literacy. Medication adherence is strongly linked to the health literacy of the patient [46] and his/her psychological status [47]. Poor adherence to medication regimens can lead to disease progression, poor symptom control, hospital admissions, and even death.

16.2.2 Drug Interactions with Other Drugs, Food, Genes, and Diseases

With every medication added to an older adult regimen, the risk for drug-drug and drug-disease interactions increases exponentially [1]. In one study, almost half of the older adult participants were at risk for a potential drug-drug interaction, with approximately one-third having a potential interaction between their medications, herbs and/or nutritional supplements [1]. The following is a list of clinically significant drug-drug interactions [48]:

1. A combination of two or more of the following drugs resulting in renal dysfunction, electrolyte disorders, hypotension, inadequately treated hypertension or fluid retention: renin-angiotensin system inhibitors + diuretics + NSAIDs.
2. A combination of two or more of the following drugs resulting in bradycardia or hypotension: β-adrenocepter antagonists + digoxin + diuretics + calcium channel blockers + renin-angiotensin system inhibitors.
3. A combination of the following drugs resulting in inadequately controlled obstructive pulmonary symptoms: β-adrenocepter antagonists and β-sympathomimetics.
4. A combination of two or more of the following drugs resulting in inadequately controlled diabetes mellitus: antihyperglycemics + β-adrenocepter antagonists + diuretics + antipsychotics + corticosteroids + antibacterials.
5. A combination of two or more of the following drugs resulting in sedation or inadequately treated depression: antidepressants, antipsychotics + benzodiazepines + antiepileptics + opioids.
6. A combination of two or more of the following drugs resulting in anemia or bleeding complications: NSAIDs + salicylates + selective serotonin reuptake inhibitors; NSAIDs + corticosteroids + coumarins; coumarins + antimicrobials.
7. A combination of two or more of the following drugs resulting in inadequately treated hypothyroidism: iron supplements and bisphosphonates + thyroxine (levothyroxine sodium).
8. A combination of two or more of the following drugs resulting in constipation: iron supplements + antipsychotics + calcium channel antagonists + opioids.
9. A combination of the following drugs resulting in inadequately treated gout: gout medication + diuretics.
10. A combination of two or more of the following drugs resulting in hypercalcemia: thiazide diuretics + calcium + activated vitamin D (calcitriol).

16.2.3 Adverse Drug Events (ADEs)

As many as 50% of ADEs are due to the use of medications in older adults [4]. Consequently, polypharmacy can become one of the most preventable causative factors leading to hospital admissions [16]. In fact, ADEs were responsible for 6% of admissions to an acute geriatric unit, but over 75% of these admissions were considered avoidable when polypharmacy was an associated risk factor [49]. ADEs may be sub-classified into Type A or Type B reactions. Type A reactions relate to the mechanism of action and are seen if drug interactions cause an increase in the plasma levels of a medication, for example, bleeding on warfarin. Type B reactions are generally unpredictable, for instance, anaphylaxis or Stevens-Johnson syndrome. The risk of ADEs is 15% with two medications, and increases to 58% with five medications and 82% with over seven medications [50].

16.2.4 Rising Medication Costs

Polypharmacy contributes to healthcare costs to both the patient and the healthcare system. A retrospective cohort study identified an increased risk of taking a potentially inappropriate medication and an increased risk of outpatient visits, and hospitalization with an approximate 30% increase in medical costs in relation to polypharmacy [51]. Another study conducted in Sweden suggests that patients taking 5 or more medications faced a 6.2% rise in prescription drug expenditure and those taking 10 or more medications faced a 7.3% rise [26].

Case (Continued)

Based on JC's clinical scenario, do you think he may be exhibiting a prescribing cascade? Below will provide guidance to address polypharmacy and meet the improved medication use and safety.

16.3 Tactics to Address Polypharmacy

Primun non nocere, first do no harm, is the oldest precept in medicine. This principle is especially important in inappropriate polypharmacy, as increasing the number of drugs prescribed can increase the likelihood of adverse events [52]. Polypharmacy is common and is a known problem, but unfortunately, that does not tell us what to do about it [18]. Ideally, prevention of unnecessary polypharmacy should be the goal of the clinician, and the following approaches may help.

16.3.1 Medication Reconciliation

During transitions in care, medication discrepancies in older adults are commonly seen when they move from an institution to a local health setting or get discharged. These need to be addressed through structured medical reconciliation. Medication reconciliation may have a positive ripple effect on the patient-centered care delivery system [33] and is a tactic in managing the "medication list." A comprehensive list of medications should include all prescription medications, herbals, vitamins, nutritional (dietary) supplements (nutraceuticals), over-the-counter medications, vaccines, diagnostic and contrast agents, topicals, radioactive medications, parenteral nutrition, and intravenous solutions [53]. The purpose of medication reconciliation is to identify and resolve discrepancies—it is a process of comparing the medications a patient is taking (and should be taking) with newly ordered or prescribed medications. The comparison helps identify and tackle any duplications, omissions, and interactions. The medication name, dose, frequency, route, and purpose are some of the details used by clinician to reconcile the medication list.

It is a reasonable request to ask the patient to bring in all of their medications that they are currently taking or may have present at home to obtain a complete inventory. Then an assessment of whether that medication is clinically appropriate should be conducted by a qualified provider and reviewed with the patient. Pharmacists have distinct expertise that can contribute to team knowledge and competence in managing older patients with polypharmacy and multiple chronic conditions [54]. Many studies favor pharmacists providing medication and therapeutic management, patient education, and provider education to improve clinical outcomes and prescribing patterns [55] (▶ Box 16.1).

Box 16.1 Stepwise Assessment of Medication Appropriateness [56]

1. Is there an indication for the drug?
2. Is the medication effective for the condition?
3. Is the dosage correct?
4. Are the directions correct? Are they practical?
5. Are there any clinically significant drug-drug interactions?
6. Are there any clinically significant drug-disease interactions?
7. Is there unnecessary duplication with other drugs?
8. Is the duration of therapy acceptable?
9. Is this drug the least expensive alternative compared with others of equal effectiveness?

16.3.2 Shared Decision-Making

Collaborating with and engaging the patient, as key partners in maintaining their medication list, can help close the gap between what the clinician thinks their patient is taking and what they are actually taking [18]. Shared decision-making is a process in which clinicians and patients work together to clarify treatment, management, or self-management goals, sharing information about options and preferred outcomes with the aim of reaching mutual agreement on the best course of action [57]. Incorporating the likelihood of benefits and harms and patient preferences about treatment and treatment burden can lead to optimal collective decisions when exemplary communication skills are utilized [58]. One way to manage polypharmacy based on patient desires is to ask the patient about his/her treatment priorities and goals. Listing a patient's problems along with the treatments for that problem and his/her values and goals (which may differ from medical treatment) and then ordering them in priority can improve medication management [23].

16.3.3 Patient and Caregiver Engagement and Education

Not only is it imperative to develop the patient's goals of care with respect to medications; it is critical to ascertain the patient's and/or caregiver's knowledge on medications being prescribed [59–64]. Medicines that come with specific instructions on whether they need to be taken before or after a meal and also which foods should be avoided or are contraindicated should be pointed out carefully and the instructions must be mentioned legibly [61]. Other relevant information include dose, medication mode of action in simplified terms, possible side effects to monitor, and other specific instructions when necessary [59, 60, 62, 63]. It is helpful to provide reminder tools such as charts or schedules, also mentioning the time of next medication review as a part of the medication list [65–68].

16.3.4 Interprofessional Team Care

Interprofessional education is when students from two or more professions learn about, from and with each other to enable effective collaboration and improve health outcomes, while Interprofessional collaborative practice is when multiple health workers from different professional backgrounds work together with patients, families, careers, and communities to deliver the highest quality of care [69]. With the update spearheaded by the Interprofessional Education Collaborative (IPEC) in 2016, clinical institutions have a golden opportunity to implement its core competencies. Domains including teamwork and team-based practices, communication practices, roles and responsibilities, and values and ethics seem to influence, either directly or indirectly, patient's outcomes. Clinicians should work in concert hopefully minimizing potentially harmful drug and/or disease-state problems and preventing avoidable health-related sequelae [70]. One study demonstrated that consequences of polypharmacy could be avoided by case discussions in interprofessional team meetings, in which the presence of a dedicated clinic pharmacist is crucial [71]. Furthermore, pharmacist-led clinics addressing comprehensive medication reviews were associated with a statistically significant reduction in the number of medication-related problems [17, 72].

16.3.5 Deprescribing

16

Deprescribing is described as an art and has been defined as the process of identifying and discontinuing drugs that could potentially harm rather than benefit a patient. More specifically, it is the process of withdrawal of an inappropriate medication, supervised by a healthcare professional with the goal of managing polypharmacy and improving outcomes. The EMPOWER randomized controlled study suggests to use the same venues, i.e., television, radios, and computer screens to provide education [73] about the consequences of the overuse of medications. Deprescribing should be considered in all older adults on an individual basis which can achieve an optimal medication regimen [23].

Several tools (◘ Table 16.2) were identified to help with deprescribing such as the TRIMmethod for deprescribing [74]. The American Geriatrics Society Beers Criteria and the STOPP and START Criteria have been extensively used by various healthcare systems and providers to address potentially inappropriate prescribing. Furthermore, polydeprescribing has been associated with improved clinical outcomes, in comparison with outcomes of older people who adhere to all clinical guidelines and take all medications conventionally [75].

Case (Continued)

There are several issues with JC's case that could be addressed but will focus on just two:

1. Polypharmacy is evident through the number of medications. Omeprazole probably offsets the potential adverse drug reaction of ibuprofen. It appears that ibuprofen is being used beyond the recommended dose (in the setting of low creatinine clearance), which may be contributing to uncontrolled blood pressure (prescribing cascade).
2. Nonadherence is evident by the length of time since the last fill and one contributing factor is perhaps the number of prescribers providing care with potentially little or no communication amongst each other.

16.3.6 Pharmacogenomics

Pharmacogenetic testing is the study of how inter-individual variations in the DNA sequence of specific genes affect drug responses [76]. The current "fixed-dose strategy" approach in medicine often yields much inter-individual variation in drug response [76]. Pharmacogenetic testing has emerged as a promising approach toward optimizing a person-centered medication regimen, and a thorough understanding of a patient's individualized status of metabolizing medications via the cytochrome P450 enzyme system, e.g., CYP 3A4,

◘ Table 16.2 Tools for deprescribing

Tool	How it can help with deprescribing	Reference/website
AGS Beers criteria	To identify potentially inappropriate medication use in the elderly	▶ http://www.sigot.org/allegato_docs/1057_Beers-Criteria.pdf
STOPP and START criteria	Screening tool of older people's prescriptions/screening tool to alert to right treatment	▶ https://academic.oup.com/ageing/article/44/2/213/2812233
TRIM (tool to reduce inappropriate medication)	An automated online tool that extracts information on medications and chronic illness from EHR and has data entry options for chart review and patient assessment. It uses algorithms to identify reconciliations needs and inappropriate medications	▶ https://onlinelibrary.wiley.com/doi/epdf/10.1111/jgs.15042

CYP 2D6, etc., may lead to a more precise treatment approach [8]. More specifically, questions such as a patient's higher sensitivity to warfarin or predisposition to various drug interactions [8], statins' pharmacokinetics and pharmacodynamics in connection with their safe and effective use in older adults [77] may be answered. Hence, significant cost savings could result from reductions in polypharmacy as well as from fewer provider encounters and hospitalizations for exacerbations of underlying illness and because of adverse drug reactions [78].

Although not standard of care, genetic testing and assessment are widely used to determine the best antidepressant especially in patients who have failed a trial of antidepressants. In one study, 1167 outpatients with moderate to very severe treatment-resistant depression for whom at least one antidepressant medication had failed were divided into treatment groups. In the guided arm (n = 560), clinicians used genetic testing results to guide treatment decisions, while in the nonguided arm (n = 607), clinicians prescribed medication as they normally would without the benefit of genetic testing. The primary assessment was the Hamilton Depression scale (HAM-D17). Patients were assessed at baseline and at 4, 8, 12, and 24 weeks. Symptom improvement, response, and remission continued to improve by time in the guided arm, in which its patients were prescribed congruent antidepressants compared to patients in the non-guided arm, who were prescribed noncongruent antidepressants [79]. Despite the study's limitations, genetic testing and congruent prescribing have the potential to achieve optimal quality use of medicines, and to improve the efficacy and safety of medications resulting in more precision medicine [76].

16.4 Conclusion

This chapter highlights the implications that polypharmacy has on medication-related problems such as inappropriate prescribing, adverse drug events, and nonadherence which are still common among older adults [80]. Multiple tactics can be taken by the interprofessional team to maintain a dynamic medication list as well as engage and empower the patient. Ongoing communication as well as utilization of tools to facilitate the process will be needed to minimize unwanted polypharmacy.

Case (Closure)

Mr. JC is a typical example of an older adult who presents with multiple comorbidities, polypharmacy, and nonadherence. To achieve optimum outcomes for this patient, it will take an interprofessional team to work not only on stabilizing the patient's conditions clinically, but to empower him in every step of the treatment plan to take charge of his well-being. As mentioned before, medications exert their optimum effects and can only be beneficial when the patient actually takes them.

References

1. Loya AM, González-Stuart A, Rivera JO. Prevalence of polypharmacy, polyherbacy, nutritional supplement use and potential product interactions among older adults living on the United States-Mexico border. Drugs Aging. 2009;26:423–36.
2. Kim J, Parish AL. Polypharmacy and medication management in older adults. Nurs Clin. 2017;52:457–68.
3. Muscedere J, Kim P, Aitken P, Gaucher M, Osborn R, Farrell B, Holroyd-Leduc J, Mallery L, Siu H, Downar J. Proceedings of the Canadian frailty network summit: medication optimization for frail older Canadians, Toronto, Monday April 24, 2017. Can Geriatr J. 2017;20:253.
4. Gurwitz JH, Field TS, Harrold LR, Rothschild J, Debellis K, Seger AC, Cadoret C, Fish LS, Garber L, Kelleher M. Incidence and preventability of adverse drug events among older persons in the ambulatory setting. JAMA. 2003;289:1107–16.
5. Kantor ED, Rehm CD, Haas JS, Chan AT, Giovannucci EL. Trends in prescription drug use among adults in the United States from 1999–2012. JAMA. 2015;314:1818–30.
6. Fick DM, Cooper JW, Wade WE, Waller JL, Maclean JR, Beers MH. Updating the Beers criteria for potentially inappropriate medication use in older adults: results of a US consensus panel of experts. Arch Intern Med. 2003;163:2716–24.
7. Abe T, Tamiya N, Kitahara T, Hasegawa Y, Tokuda Y. Polypharmacy as a risk factor for hospital admission among elderly using emergency transport. BMC Health Serv Res. 2014;14:P2.
8. Finkelstein J, Friedman C, Hripcsak G, Cabrera M. Potential utility of precision medicine for older adults with polypharmacy: a case series study. Pharmgenomics Pers Med. 2016;9:31.
9. Aparasu RR, Mort JR, Brandt H. Polypharmacy trends in office visits by the elderly in the United States, 1990 and 2000. Res Soc Adm Pharm. 2005;1:446–59.
10. Woo TM, Robinson MV. Pharmacotherapeutics for advanced practice nurse prescribers. Philadelphia: F.A. Davis Company; 2015.
11. National Council on Aging. Healthy aging facts. 2016. https://www.ncoa.org/news/resources-for-reporters/get-the-facts/healthy-aging-facts/. Accessed 12 Jan 2018.
12. Yoo JC, Lim TK, Kim DH, Koh K-H. Comparison between the patients with surgery and without surgery after recommendation of surgical repair for symptomatic rotator cuff tear. J Orthop Sci. 2018;23:64–9.
13. Darrow JJ. Explaining the absence of surgical procedure regulation. Cornell J Law Public Policy. 2017;27:189–206.
14. Ferrailo DM, Veitz-Keenan A. No clinical quantifiable benefits between non-surgical and surgical endodontic treatment. Evid Based Dent. 2017;18:75.
15. Benetos A, Rossignol P, Cherubini A, Joly L, Grodzicki T, Rajkumar C, Strandberg TE, Petrovic M. Polypharmacy in the aging patient: management of hypertension in octogenarians. JAMA. 2015;314:170–80.
16. Abe T, Tamiya N, Kitahara T, Tokuda Y. Polypharmacy as a risk factor for hospital admission among ambulance-transported old-old patients. Acute Med Surg. 2016;3:107–13.
17. Yasu T, Koinuma M, Hayashi D, Horii T, Yashiro Y, Furuya J, Saitoh M, Seki R, Shirota M, Abe K. Association between polypharmacy and clinical ward pharmacy services in hospitals in Tokyo. Geriatr Gerontol Int. 2018;18:187–8.
18. Steinman MA. Polypharmacy—time to get beyond numbers. JAMA Intern Med. 2016;176:482–3.
19. Lyons BP, Dunson-Strane T, Sherman FT. The joys of caring for older adults: training practitioners to empower older adults. J Community Health. 2014;39:464–70.
20. Stefanacci RG, Khan T. Can managed care manage polypharmacy? Clin Geriatr Med. 2017;33:241–55.
21. Montamat SC, Cusack B. Overcoming problems with polypharmacy and drug misuse in the elderly. Clin Geriatr Med. 1992;8:143–58.

22. Gnjidic D, Hilmer SN, Blyth FM, Naganathan V, Waite L, Seibel MJ, McLachlan AJ, Cumming RG, Handelsman DJ, Le Couteur DG. Polypharmacy cutoff and outcomes: five or more medicines were used to identify community-dwelling older men at risk of different adverse outcomes. J Clin Epidemiol. 2012;65:989–95.
23. Brandt NJ. Optimizing medication use through deprescribing: tactics for this approach. J Gerontol Nurs. 2016;42:10–4.
24. Scott IA, Hilmer SN, Reeve E, Potter K, Le Couteur D, Rigby D, Gnjidic D, Del Mar CB, Roughead EE, Page A. Reducing inappropriate polypharmacy: the process of deprescribing. JAMA Intern Med. 2015;175:827–34.
25. Graham J. End-of-life medications draw more attention, greater scrutiny. JAMA. 2015;313:231–3.
26. Hovstadius B, Petersson G. Factors leading to excessive polypharmacy. Clin Geriatr Med. 2012;28:159–72.
27. Ponte ML, Wachs L, Wachs A, Serra HA. Prescribing cascade: a proposed new way to evaluate it. Med (B Aires). 2017;77:13–6.
28. Bailey TA, Fenney M. Perceptions of direct-to-consumer advertising and the older adult population. Consult Pharm J Am Soc Consult Pharm. 2016;31:215–20.
29. Mintzes B, Barer ML, Kravitz RL, Bassett K, Lexchin J, Kazanjian A, Evans RG, Pan R, Marion SA. How does direct-to-consumer advertising (DTCA) affect prescribing? A survey in primary care environments with and without legal DTCA. Can Med Assoc J. 2003;169:405–12.
30. Datti B, Carter MW. The effect of direct-to-consumer advertising on prescription drug use by older adults. Drugs Aging. 2006;23:71–81.
31. Rochon PA, Gurwitz JH. Optimising drug treatment for elderly people: the prescribing cascade. BMJ. 1997;315:1096–9.
32. Gill SS, Mamdani M, Naglie G, Streiner DL, Bronskill SE, Kopp A, Shulman KI, Lee PE, Rochon PA. A prescribing cascade involving cholinesterase inhibitors and anticholinergic drugs. Arch Intern Med. 2005;165:808–13.
33. Rasu R, Agbor-Bawa W, Rianon N. Impact of polypharmacy on seniors' self-perceived health status. South Med J. 2017;110: 540–5.
34. Veronese N, Stubbs B, Noale M, Solmi M, Pilotto A, Vaona A, Demurtas J, Mueller C, Huntley J, Crepaldi G. Polypharmacy is associated with higher frailty risk in older people: an 8-year longitudinal cohort study. J Am Med Dir Assoc. 2017;18:624–8.
35. George C, Verghese J. Polypharmacy and gait performance in community-dwelling older adults. J Am Geriatr Soc. 2017;65:2082–7.
36. Kvarnström K, Airaksinen M, Liira H. Barriers and facilitators to medication adherence: a qualitative study with general practitioners. BMJ Open. 2018;8:e015332.
37. Abe J, Umetsu R, Uranishi H, Suzuki H, Nishibata Y, Kato Y, Ueda N, Sasaoka S, Hatahira H, Motooka Y. Analysis of polypharmacy effects in older patients using Japanese Adverse Drug Event Report database. PLoS One. 2017;12:e0190102.
38. Harrison SL, O'Donnell LK, Bradley CE, Milte R, Dyer SM, Gnanamanickam ES, Liu E, Hilmer SN, Crotty M. Associations between the drug burden index, potentially inappropriate medications and quality of life in residential aged care. Drugs & Aging. 2018;35(1):83–91.
39. Ziere G, Dieleman JP, Hofman A, Pols HAP, Van Der Cammen TJM, Stricker BH. Polypharmacy and falls in the middle age and elderly population. Br J Clin Pharmacol. 2006;61:218–23.
40. von Lueder TG, Atar D. Comorbidities and polypharmacy. Heart Fail Clin. 2014;10:367–72.
41. Montiel-Luque A, Núñez-Montenegro AJ, Martín-Aurioles E, Canca-Sánchez JC, Toro-Toro MC, González-Correa JA, Polipresact Research Group. Medication-related factors associated with health-related quality of life in patients older than 65 years with polypharmacy. PLoS One. 2017;12:e0171320.
42. Strehblow C, Smeikal M, Fasching P. Polypharmacy and excessive polypharmacy in octogenarians and older acutely hospitalized patients polypharmazie und exzessive Polypharmazie bei akut hospitalisierten hochbetagten Patienten. Wien Klin Wochenschr. 2014;126:195–200.
43. Social Care Institute of Excellence. Research briefing 15: helping older people to take prescribed meditation in their home: what works? 2005. Published August 2005. Available from: https://www.scie.org.uk/publications/briefings/briefing15/.
44. Zaprutko T, Kopciuch D, Kus K, Merks P, Nowicka M, Augustyniak I, Nowakowska E. Affordability of medicines in the European Union. PLoS One. 2017;12:e0172753.
45. Brieger DB, Chow C, Gullick J, Hyun K, D'souza M, Briffa T, Concordance Investigators. Improving patient adherence to secondary prevention medications 6 months after an acute coronary syndrome: observational cohort study. Intern Med J. 2018;48:541–9.
46. Lee C, Lee K, Yu H, et al. Adverse events with sustained-release donepezil in Alzheimer disease. J Clin Psychopharmacol. 2017;37:401–4.
47. Hennein R, Hwang S, Au R, Levy D, Muntner P, Fox CS, Ma J. Barriers to medication adherence and links to cardiovascular disease risk factor control: the Framingham Heart Study. Intern Med J. 2018;48:414–21.
48. Tulner LR, Frankfort SV, Gijsen GJPT, van Campen JPCM, Koks CHW, Beijnen JH. Drug-drug interactions in a geriatric outpatient cohort. Drugs Aging. 2008;25:343–55.
49. Cabré M, Elias L, Garcia M, Palomera E, Serra-Prat M. Avoidable hospitalizations due to adverse drug reactions in an acute geriatric unit. Analysis of 3,292 patients. Med Clin (Barc). 2018;150:209–14.
50. Masoodi NA. Polypharmacy: to err is human, to correct divine. Br J Med Pract. 2008;1:6–9.
51. Akazawa M, Imai H, Igarashi A, Tsutani K. Potentially inappropriate medication use in elderly Japanese patients. Am J Geriatr Pharmacother. 2010;8:146–60.
52. Isidoro-García M, Sánchez-Martín A, García-Berrocal B, Román-Curto C. Primun non nocere, polypharmacy and pharmacogenetics. Pharmacogenomics. 2015;16:1903–5.
53. National Patient Safety Goals. 2005. http://www.jointcommission.org/PatientSafety/NationalPatientSafetyGoals/05_npsgs.htm. Accessed 12 Jan 2018.
54. Lee JK, Slack MK, Martin J, Ehrman C, Chisholm-Burns M. Geriatric patient care by US pharmacists in healthcare teams: systematic review and meta-analyses. J Am Geriatr Soc. 2013;61:1119–27.
55. Nkansah N, Mostovetsky O, Yu C, Chheng T, Beney J, Bond CM, Bero L. Effect of outpatient pharmacists' non-dispensing roles on patient outcomes and prescribing patterns. Cochrane Database Syst Rev. 2010;(7):CD000336.
56. Hanlon JT, Schmader KE, Samsa GP, Weinberger M, Uttech KM, Lewis IK, Cohen HJ, Feussner JR. A method for assessing drug therapy appropriateness. J Clin Epidemiol. 1992;45:1045–51.
57. Elwyn G, Dehlendorf C, Epstein RM, Marrin K, White J, Frosch DL. Shared decision making and motivational interviewing: achieving patient-centered care across the spectrum of health care problems. Ann Fam Med. 2014;12:270–5.
58. Lipska KJ, Krumholz H, Soones T, Lee SJ. Polypharmacy in the aging patient: a review of glycemic control in older adults with type 2 diabetes. JAMA. 2016;315:1034–45.
59. Nikolaus T, Kruse W, Bach M, Specht-Leible N, Oster P, Schlierf G. Elderly patients' problems with medication. Eur J Clin Pharmacol. 1996;49:255–9.
60. Barat I, Andreasen F, Damsgaard EMS. Drug therapy in the elderly: what doctors believe and patients actually do. Br J Clin Pharmacol. 2001;51:615–22.
61. Spiers MV, Kutzik DM, Lamar M. Variation in medication understanding among the elderly. Am J Health Syst Pharm. 2004;61:373–9.
62. Fineman B, DeFelice C. A study of medication compliance. Home Healthc Nurse. 1992;10:26–9.
63. Blenkiron P. The elderly and their medication: understanding and compliance in a family practice. Postgrad Med J. 1996;72: 671–6.
64. Cline CMJ, Björck-Linné AK, Israelsson BYA, Willenheimer RB, Erhardt LR. Non-compliance and knowledge of prescribed medication in elderly patients with heart failure. Eur J Heart Fail. 1999;1:145–9.

65. Lourens H, Woodward MC. Impact of a medication card on compliance in older people. Australas J Ageing. 1994;13:72–6.
66. Coleman EA, Smith JD, Frank JC, Min S, Parry C, Kramer AM. Preparing patients and caregivers to participate in care delivered across settings: the Care Transitions Intervention. J Am Geriatr Soc. 2004;52:1817–25.
67. Raynor DK, Booth TG, Blenkinsopp A. Effects of computer generated reminder charts on patients' compliance with drug regimens. BMJ. 1993;306:1158–61.
68. Goodyer LI, Miskelly F, Milligan P. Does encouraging good compli ance improve patients' clinical condition in heart failure? Br J Clin Pract. 1995;49:173–6.
69. World Health Organization. Framework for action on interprofessional education and collaborative practice. Geneva: WHO; 2010.
70. Patel R, Zhu L, Sohal D, Lenkova E, Koshki N, Woelfel J, Ranson C, Valle-Oseguera CS, Rogan EL. Use of 2015 Beers criteria medications by older medicare beneficiaries. Consult Pharm. 2018;33:48–54.
71. Maher RL, Hanlon J, Hajjar ER. Clinical consequences of polypharmacy in elderly. Expert Opin Drug Saf. 2014;13:57–65.
72. Kiel WJ, Phillips SW. Impact of pharmacist-conducted comprehensive medication reviews for older adult patients to reduce medication related problems. Pharmacy. 2017;6:2.
73. Tannenbaum C, Martin P, Tamblyn R, Benedetti A, Ahmed S. Reduction of inappropriate benzodiazepine prescriptions among older adults through direct patient education: the EMPOWER cluster randomized trial. JAMA Intern Med. 2014;174:890–8.
74. Niehoff KM, Rajeevan N, Charpentier PA, Miller PL, Goldstein MK, Fried TR. Development of the tool to reduce inappropriate medications (TRIM): a clinical decision support system to improve medication prescribing for older adults. Pharmacother J Hum Pharmacol Drug Ther. 2016;36:694–701.
75. Garfinkel D. Poly-de-prescribing to treat polypharmacy: efficacy and safety. Ther Adv Drug Saf. 2018;9:25–4. 32042098617736192.
76. Zhou S-F, Ming Di Y, Chan E, Du Y-M, Chow VD-W, Xue CC, Lai X, Wang J-C, Li CG, Tian M. Clinical pharmacogenetics and potential application in personalized medicine. Curr Drug Metab. 2008;9:738–84.
77. Gelissen IC, McLachlan AJ. The pharmacogenomics of statins. Pharmacol Res. 2014;88:99–106.
78. Rusnak JM, Kisabeth RM, Herbert DP, McNeil DM. Pharmacogenomics: a clinician's primer on emerging technologies for improved patient care. Mayo Clin Proc: Elsevier. 2001;76:299–309.
79. Brooks M. Genetic test identifies best antidepressant. Medscape Medical News. 2018.
80. Hanlon JT, Semla TP, Schmader KE. Medication misadventures in older adults: literature from 2013. J Am Geriatr Soc. 2014;62:1950–3.

Cognitive and Behavioral Disorders (MENTATION)

Contents

Depression in Older Adults: Principles of Diagnosis and Management

Elizabeth Mann, Gregory A. Hinrichsen, and Shahla Baharlou

A. Chun (ed.), *Geriatric Practice*, https://doi.org/10.1007/978-3-030-19625-7_17

Case

Ms. Martinez is an 84-year-old woman with well-controlled hypertension, diabetes with diabetic neuropathy, and stage III chronic kidney disease who has been under your care for the past 4 years. Typically, she comes to your office alone. Today, her daughter is with her. Her daughter tells you she is worried that her mom does not seem to have any energy or motivation anymore. She has not left the house in a month. Ms. Martinez denies depressed mood or anhedonia. However, she admits to lack of energy, decreased appetite, and difficulty sleeping for the past 2 months. She had a three pound weight loss since her last visit. Her review of systems, physical exam, and laboratory studies are normal.

17.1 Background

Depression is a common condition in patients of all ages. There is a misconception that depression is a normal part of aging. In fact, major depression affects only 5–10% of community-dwelling older adults [1]. Older adults are more likely to experience loss and bereavement, chronic illness, and functional impairment than younger adults. However, not all older adults who face these challenges become depressed, and older adults can suffer from depression in their absence.

It is important to determine whether patients with chronic illness also have depression because concomitant depression may lead to worse health outcomes. Patients with both depression and chronic illness have higher rates of healthcare utilization than those with chronic illness without depression [2].

Depression may present differently in older adults. Compared to younger adults, depressed older adults are less likely to report affective or mood-related symptoms and are more likely to present with cognitive changes including dementia, making a diagnosis of depression more challenging [3].

Diagnosing and treating late-life depression are important because untreated depression has been associated with a variety of serious adverse health outcomes including disability, diminished quality of life, and increased mortality [4].

This chapter will provide an overview of the symptoms, screening and diagnostic criteria, and evidence-based treatment options for community-dwelling older adults with depression.

17.2 Pathophysiology

Research into the pathophysiology of depression is an evolving field. Several neurobiologic systems have been implicated. Depression likely develops as a result of a complex interaction of these systems. Much research has shown that depression may be due to insufficient activity of serotonin and norepinephrine [5]. This research has formed the basis for some of the mainstays of pharmacologic depression management.

Disruption to the hypothalamic pituitary adrenal axis and alterations in cortisol levels have also been implicated in the pathophysiology of depression [5]. Inappropriately high cortisol levels in response to stress may be particularly relevant to the development of depression among older adults [6].

Endothelial pathology may also be associated with depression. Postmortem exams of older patients who suffered from depression have showed deep white matter changes, especially in the prefrontal cortex [7].

17.3 Clinical Features

17.3.1 Risk Factors

There are genetic and social factors that place patients of all ages at increased risk of developing depression. Some of the risk factors for depression in older adults specifically include medical illness, bereavement, sleep disturbances, disability, history of depression, and female gender [8].

17.3.2 Suicide in Older Adults

Suicide rates in late life are higher than at any point in life. While depression is less common in men compared with women, older males, notably white males over 85, have the highest rate of suicide of all age groups. Depression, health problems, life stresses, lack of social connectedness, and characterological rigidity are risk factors for suicide in later life [9]. There is a relationship between severity of depression and completed suicide [10]. Identification of major depression thus provides an important opportunity for both treatment of depression and prevention of late-life suicide.

17.3.3 Diagnosis

Depression is diagnosed by clinical assessment. A psychiatric evaluation is not required for the diagnosis of depression, and primary care providers commonly diagnose depression. The American Psychiatric Association's *Diagnostic and Statistical Manual of Mental Disorders, Fifth Edition* (DSM-5) describes the various depressive disorders and outlines diagnostic criteria [11]. ► Box 17.1 outlines the DSM-5 diagnostic criteria for major depressive disorder.

Some medical conditions can have symptoms that mimic the symptoms of depression. Patients should be asked a full review of systems and undergo physical exam and, in many cases, laboratory testing, to exclude other medical causes.

Box 17.1 DSM-5 Criteria for Major Depressive Disorder[a]

Depressed mood most of the day, nearly every day

Markedly diminished interest or pleasure in all, or almost all, activities most of the day, nearly every day

Significant weight loss when not dieting or weight gain or decrease or increase in appetite nearly every day

Insomnia or hypersomnia nearly every day

Psychomotor agitation or retardation nearly every day, observable by others

Fatigue or loss of energy nearly every day

Feelings of worthlessness or excessive or inappropriate guilt, nearly every day

Diminished ability to think, make decisions, or concentrate, nearly every day

Recurrent thoughts of death, recurrent suicidal ideation, or a suicide attempt

[a]Patients must report five or more symptoms during a 2-week period, and this must represent a change from prior functioning. One of these symptoms must be depressed mood or loss of interest or pleasure in most or all activities.

17.3.4 Diagnostic Challenges

It is estimated that fewer than 20% of cases of depression in older adults are detected [12]. There are a variety of reasons for this. In contrast to younger patients, older patients with depression are less likely to report depressed mood [3]. The presence of either anhedonia or depressed mood is required for a diagnosis of depression based on DSM-5 criteria [11]. Thus, providers who focus primarily on an older adult's report of depressed mood might overlook a diagnosable depression.

A diagnosis of depression may also be missed in patients suffering from chronic disease who have symptoms overlapping with those of depression. Multimorbidity, the presence of two or more chronic diseases, is more common in older adults. Many chronic health conditions common in older adults, including dementia, arthritis, malignancy, heart disease, Parkinson's disease, stroke, and thyroid disorders, have symptoms that can mimic depression. Patients with one or more of these conditions may suffer from fatigue, slowed movements, cognitive dysfunction, or sleep disorders. Distinguishing these health-related symptoms from the symptoms of depression can be challenging. While these symptoms may be present in nondepressed individuals, patients with the above chronic conditions have an increased risk of developing depression [2].

Older adults may exhibit some symptoms of depression that are less common in younger patients. For example, older patients might present with memory problems, social withdrawal, and irritability [3]. They are also more likely to have depression-related delusions or hallucinations than younger patients. It is vital that clinicians inquire about feelings of hopelessness, as these have been associated with suicidal ideation in older adults [3].

Given that older adults are likely to face loss of friends and family, bereavement is common in this population. The DSM-5 no longer excludes those experiencing bereavement in the diagnosis of major depression [11]. This is a change from prior editions, meant to capture more patients who might benefit from treatment.

Assessment of depression in older adults with cognitive impairment presents particular challenges since patients may not be able to accurately report changes in mood, behavior, and thinking that are characteristics of depression. Caregivers are often an important source of information, and they should be asked about whether they have noticed mood and behavioral changes.

17.3.5 Screening for Depression

The United States Preventive Services Task Force (USPSTF) recommends screening the general adult population for depression. The guidelines state "Screening should be implemented with adequate systems in place to ensure accurate diagnosis, effective treatment and appropriate follow-up" (Grade B) [13].

The Patient Health Questionnaire 2 (PHQ-2) is a brief, validated depression screening tool. It asks just two questions: "During the past month, have you been bothered by feeling down, depressed or hopeless?" and "During the past month, have you been bothered by little interest or pleasure in doing things?" Patients who answer "yes" to either or both questions screen positive for depression. The PHQ-2 can be administered by nonclinicians, making it useful for population-based screening. It has been validated in the older adult population, with a sensitivity of 100% and a specificity of 77% for detecting major depression as defined by DSM criteria [14].

The Geriatric Depression Scale (GDS) and the Patient Health Questionnaire 9 (PHQ-9) are more comprehensive screening instruments. The GDS has 30, 15, and 5 item versions. The GDS-15 and -5 are most commonly used in clinical practice. Both versions have been validated in patients over the age of 65 years, and the five-question version has a sensitivity of 97% and a specificity of 85% in detecting major depressive disorder compared to evaluation by a geropsychiatric specialist [15].

The PHQ-9 is a nine-question tool. It can be self-administered, it overlaps with the DSM criteria for major depressive disorder, inquiries about suicidality and impact on functioning, and it provides scores that indicate the severity of depression, ranging from mild to severe. The PHQ-9 is also available in several languages. In a validation study in older adults, a score of 8 or more had a sensitivity of 77% and a specificity of 83% for diagnosing major depression compared to evaluation by a geropsychiatric specialist [16] (▫ Table 17.1).

Table 17.1 Key general management consideration for depression in older adults

Factors to consider when planning treatment:
- Severity of symptoms or signs
- Possibility of grief
- History of depression and prior responses to treatment
- Concurrent comorbidities
- Cognitive impairment
- Patient treatment preferences
- Available psychosocial support
- Current medications
- Healthcare provider and local mental health resources (e.g., CoCMs)

Severity	PHQ-9	Treatment options	Monitor
1. Mild	5–9	Psychotherapy	Depressive symptoms and response to treatment including serial PHQ-9s.
2. Moderate	10–19	Psychotherapy +/–Antidepressants	Adherence and possible side effects to medications.
3. Severe	≥20	Psychiatry referral (antidepressants +/– psychotherapy +/– ECT)	Periodic serum sodium if on SSRIs or SNRIs

Medications to avoid:
- Tricyclic antidepressants (TCAs) due to anticholinergic effects
- Paroxetine unless patient has significant symptoms of anxiety due to drug interactions
- High dose of duloxetine or venlafaxine due to anticholinergic effects

Consider referral to psychiatrist:
- Severe depression (PHQ-9 ≥20)
- Psychotic symptoms (urgent)
- Suicidal or homicidal ideation (urgent)
- Comorbid substance use
- Significant comorbid anxiety
- Symptoms suspicious for bipolar disorder
- Lack of resources or uncomfortable managing the case
- Patients with history of psychotic depression or treatment with ECT

The gold standard for diagnosing depression remains clinical assessment. A comprehensive clinical assessment is indicated if a patient scores high on one of the above screening tests.

17.4 Treatment

Both pharmacologic and psychotherapeutic therapies have been shown to be effective in the treatment of depression in older adults [17]. Most older adults seek treatment for depression from their primary care provider. However, providing comprehensive depression care can be challenging in the busy primary care setting. Collaborative care models (CoCMs) provide an opportunity for primary care providers to optimize depression care.

17.4.1 Psychotherapeutic Interventions

Nonpharmacologic treatments for depression may be used in combination with or in place of pharmacologic therapy. Cognitive behavioral therapy, behavioral therapy, brief psychodynamic psychotherapy, problem-solving therapy, reminiscence therapy, and interpersonal psychotherapy have all been found effective for the treatment of depression in older patients [18]. Of note, very old patients, members of minority groups, and those with dementia have often been excluded from or underrepresented in clinical trials. Patients with dementia should not necessarily be excluded from psychotherapy; however, clinicians must judge whether the patient has enough cognitive capacity to engage and retain information from session to session. Another challenge to receiving psychotherapy is that patients may find it difficult to find a mental health professional with substantive training and experience with older adults.

17.4.2 Pharmacologic Therapies

The American Psychiatric Association (APA) recommends starting treatment with a selective serotonin reuptake inhibitor (SSRI), serotonin-norepinephrine reuptake inhibitor (SNRI), mirtazapine, or bupropion, depending on a patient's symptoms, clinical features, preferences, and prior treatment experiences [19].

SSRIs and SNRIs are generally well tolerated. Several SSRIs have been shown to be safe and effective in the older adult population, including citalopram, escitalopram, paroxetine, fluvoxamine, and sertraline. A 2012 meta-analysis of 51 double-blind RCTs found no significant difference in effectiveness among the above SSRIs [20].

Several SNRIs also have established efficacy in older adult populations, including venlafaxine and duloxetine; these should be prescribed at a lower dose than in younger patients [21]. Mirtazapine and trazodone, both serotonin modulators, have shown benefit in depression and also treat insomnia. Additionally, mirtazapine can increase appetite [22]. If a patient is struggling with weight loss and insomnia, low-dose mirtazapine might be considered as initial therapy or in combination with a low-dose SSRI. Bupropion, a dopamine and norepinephrine reuptake inhibitor, has more limited evidence among older adults but did show equivalent efficacy to paroxetine in one randomized controlled trial [23]. This can be an alternative in patients who do not tolerate serotonergic medications or have hyponatremia from SSRIs or SNRIs. Bupropion is contraindicated in patients with history of seizure [24].

The starting dose of antidepressants should be lower in older adults than in younger adults. The lower initial dose is intended to adjust for the alterations in drug serum concentrations, metabolism, and clearance that are seen in normal aging [19]. We recommend starting at about half of the dose used in younger age groups. Patients should be assessed for side effects after about 2 or 3 weeks; if they are tolerating the medication, the dose may be increased with the goal of reaching the recommended dose within several weeks [19]. Serum sodium should be monitored intermittently for those on SSRIs or SNRIs because of the risk of hyponatremia.

Evidence for when to switch to a new antidepressant or add an augmenting agent is limited in older adults. "Stepping-up" treatment by adding an augmenting agent such as bupropion or mirtazapine or starting psychotherapy should be considered if a patient has not yet achieved remission despite taking a therapeutic dose of an initial antidepressant for a sufficient period of time. In the STAR∗D trial, 50% of patients achieved remission after two treatment "steps" [25]. In this study, patients with more severe depression, additional psychiatric diagnoses, or multimorbidity were more likely to require more treatment steps. We recognize that stepping up treatment might be outside the scope of practice for some primary care providers. Psychiatry consultation would be advisable for patients with refractory symptoms, suicidality, or psychosis.

When starting any new medication in an older patient, physicians should consult the Beers Criteria for Potentially Inappropriate Medication Use in Older Adults. Antidepressants on this list include bupropion (lowers seizure threshold), tricyclic antidepressants (associated with a variety of significant adverse effects including constipation, delirium, and syncope), and SSRIs and SNRIs (monitor for hyponatremia, use care in patients with history of falls; paroxetine can have anticholinergic side effects) [24]. Medications listed on the Beers Criteria should not necessarily be avoided in older adults; rather, this list serves as a guide for providers seeking to choose the most appropriate treatment for each individual patient.

◘ Table 17.2 details some of those most commonly prescribed antidepressants.

◘ Table 17.2 Commonly prescribed antidepressants

Class of drug	Medication	Half-life	Dosage (mg/day)	Most common side effects	Precautions	Most useful
A. Antidepressants						
Tricyclic antidepressant	Desipramine	14.3–24.7	10–100	Anticholinergic side effects	Anticholinergic side effects	History of seizure Sedation desirable
Tricyclic antidepressant	Nortriptyline	15–39	10–100	Anticholinergic side effects	Anticholinergic side effects	History of seizure Sedation not desirable
SSRIs	Citalopram	33–37	20–40	Hyponatremia, headache, nausea, dizziness	Dose adjustment in severe renal impairment QTC prolongation with high dose	
SSRIs	Escitalopram	22–32	10–20	Hyponatremia, headache, nausea		Coexisting anxiety and depression
SSRIs	Fluoxetine	4–6 days	10–60	Hyponatremia, loss of appetite, nausea	Multiple drug-drug interactions due to P450 and CYP2D6 metabolism Risk of withdrawal if abruptly stopped	

(continued)

Table 17.2 (continued)

Class of drug	Medication	Half-life	Dosage (mg/day)	Most common side effects	Precautions	Most useful
SSRIs	Paroxetine	15–22	25–75	Diaphoresis, loss of appetite, nausea, hyponatremia	Multiple drug-drug interactions due to P450 and CYP2D6 metabolism Risk of withdrawal if abruptly stopped	
SSRIs	Sertraline	22–32	25–200	Hyponatremia	Dose adjust in liver impairment	
SNRIs	Duloxetine	11–16	30–90	Diaphoresis, nausea, diarrhea, dizziness	Avoid in liver failure Dose adjust in renal impairment	Coexisting anxiety and depression Coexisting neuropathic pain
SNRIs	Venlafaxine	3–7	37.5–375	Hypertension (much less with extended release form), dizziness, nausea.	Dose adjust in liver and renal impairment risk of withdrawal if abruptly stopped	Coexisting anxiety and depression
Others	Bupropion	12–30	100–450	Headache, insomnia	Dose adjust in liver and renal impairment	Weakly inhibits the neuronal uptake of dopamine, therefore preferred in patients with Parkinson's disease
Others	Mirtazapine	25–40	7.5–45	Increased appetite, weight gain, somnolence	Increase dose slowly in liver and renal impairment (CrCl <40 ml/min)	Poor appetite Insomnia
B. Stimulants						
Psycho-stimulants	Methylphenidate	3–5	10–30 in divided dose, typically 8 am and 12 pm	Tachyarrhythmia, decreased in appetite	Tolerance and dependence are possible	Adjuvant to antidepressant when rapid onset of action is required Limited life expectancy
Psycho-stimulants	Modafinil	15	100–400	Headache, nausea, insomnia	Decrease dose to 50% in severe hepatic failure Less potential for tolerance and dependence than methylphenidate	Adjuvant to antidepressant when rapid onset of action is required Limited life

17

Case Continued

Ms. Martinez scores a 16 on the PHQ-9. You explain that her depression is very likely causing her recent symptoms, and you both agree to start her on sertraline 25 mg daily. You also refer her to a psychotherapist. She will return for a follow-up appointment in 3 weeks.

17.4.3 Electroconvulsive Therapy

Electroconvulsive therapy is an effective treatment in older adults for the same indications as younger patients, and it is generally safe [26]. Recent randomized trials support the effectiveness of electroconvulsive therapy (ECT) both for acute treatment of depression and maintenance of remission in depressed older adults [27, 28]. The APA recommends considering ECT as first-line treatment in patients who suffer from severe depression with catatonia, refusal of food, psychotic features, severe treatment refractory depression, and active suicidal behavior [19].

Although there are no absolute contraindications for ECT, the following conditions may be associated with substantially increased risk [29, 30]:

- Unstable or severe cardiovascular conditions such as recent myocardial infarction, poorly compensated congestive heart failure, and severe valvular cardiac disease.
- Aneurysm or vascular malformation that might be susceptible to rupture with increased blood pressure.
- Increased intracranial pressure as may occur with some brain tumors or other space-occupying cerebral lesions including subdural hematoma, intracranial arachnoid cysts, normal pressure hydrocephalus, and recent cerebral infarction.
- Pulmonary conditions such as severe chronic obstructive pulmonary disease, asthma, or pneumonia.
- Metabolic abnormality (hypo- or hyperkalemia).
- High risk for anesthesia.

17.4.4 Collaborative Care Models (CoCMs)

Although depression in older adults can be successfully treated with medication or psychotherapy, many older adults don't receive adequate treatment in the primary care setting. This is not simply due to providers' lack of knowledge or comfort in treating depression. Interventions that focus on educating clinicians about depression have not been shown to help providers improve depression care in their practices [31]. In contrast, introducing collaborative depression care into primary care practices can lead to improvements in depression symptoms and quality of life [32].

Collaborative care models (CoCMs) have several components, central of which is the depression care manager (DCM). Often a licensed social worker or nurse case manager, the DCM is supervised by the patient's primary care provider. The DCM educates patients about depression as an illness, evaluates the severity of patients' depression and response to treatment on an ongoing basis, monitors adherence to treatment, provides psychosocial interventions, and coordinates care with primary providers. The CoCM team also includes a supervising psychiatrist and the patient. The model follows five main principles: patient-centered team care, population-based care, measurement-based treatment to target, evidence-based care, and accountable care [33].

A number of collaborative care models have been developed and studied in the older adult population. Improving Mood – Promoting Access to Collaborative Treatment (IMPACT) and Program to Encourage Active, Rewarding Lives for Seniors (PEARLS) are the best studied and most commonly implemented programs [33, 34]. IMPACT was originally designed for older adults in primary care. Several meta-analyses have documented that IMPACT and other collaborative care interventions are effective for both older and younger patients. Challenges to implementation of the model include reluctance of some patients to enroll or remain enrolled, in-person attendance of collaborative care visits for medically frail, lack of insurance coverage, and organizational barriers to establishing and sustaining collaborative care [35].

In the IMPACT program, a DCM is imbedded within the primary care clinic. The DCM assists with the initial assessment of patients, provides depression education, encourages patients to become active in their depression treatment, and coordinates care with the patient's primary care provider. DCMs provide Problem-Solving Treatment (PST), a brief (6–8 weeks) form of psychotherapy. The treatment team meets weekly to discuss patient's progress. Treatment response is monitored with biweekly PHQ-9s. Those who are not improving with medications or PST are seen by the psychiatrist for a consultation. In collaboration with the patient, the DCM develops a relapse prevention plan. The IMPACT model was studied in a 2002 randomized controlled trial with older adults published in *JAMA*. Patients in the intervention group had better adherence to medications and psychotherapeutic treatments, higher satisfaction with their care, and greater improvements in their depression compared with controls [32].

In the PEARLS program, a DCM provides eight in-home counseling sessions and three to six follow-up phone calls. The DCM uses PST and is supervised by a psychiatrist. Unlike IMPACT, which targets patients with moderate to severe depression, patients with mild depression can be enrolled in PEARLS. Progress is tracked using the PHQ-9. In a randomized controlled trial, older patients in the PEARLS intervention had a 50% reduction in depressive symptoms at 12 months. They were more likely to achieve complete remission and had greater improvements in quality of life and well-being compared to those receiving usual depression care [34].

The effectiveness of these CoCMs for behavioral health interventions is now recognized by CMS: CMS has recently announced that since January 2017, these services are billable through Medicare. Now is an opportune time for practices and institutions to consider incorporating these effective programs into their primary care practices.

17.4.5 Consider Referral to Psychiatrist

- Severe depression (PHQ-9 ≥20)
- Psychotic symptoms (urgent)
- Suicidal or homicidal ideation (urgent)
- Comorbid substance use
- Significant comorbid anxiety
- Symptoms suspicious for bipolar disorder
- Lack of resources or uncomfortable managing the case
- Patients with history of psychotic depression or treatment with ECT

Case Conclusion

Ms. Martinez returns to your office with her daughter for her scheduled follow-up appointment. She has been leaving the house more to attend weekly therapy appointments and to shop for groceries and attend church. She has not noticed any side effects to the sertraline you prescribed. She scores an 11 on the PHQ-9. Her appetite has not improved much and she is still having difficulty sleeping. Her serum sodium is normal. You prescribe mirtazapine 7.5 mg at bedtime for these symptoms and increased sertraline to 50 mg daily. You schedule another follow-up appointment in 4 weeks.

Take-Home Points

- Depression is not a normal part of aging.
- Prevalence of depression in community-dwelling older adults is 5–10%.
- The USPSTF recommends screening for depression. There are multiple validated screening tools.
- Older patients are at increased risk of suicide and should be screened for suicidality.
- Clinical assessment is the gold standard for diagnosing depression.
- Several nonpharmacologic and pharmacologic treatments have been studied and are effective in older adults.
- Electroconvulsive therapy is an effective treatment in older adults for the same indications as younger patients, and it is generally safe.

17.5 Conclusion

Depression is not part of normal aging, but for those older adults who are depressed, it is underdiagnosed and undertreated. Depression in older adults is a significant clinical and public health issue because of its potential impact on health and quality of life. Depression can be effectively diagnosed and treated in older patients. In primary care settings, treatment is best provided using a stepwise, comprehensive, team-based approach. CoCMs are an effective and financially viable option for improving depression care in the primary care setting.

References

1. Blazer DG. Depression in late life: a review and commentary. J Gerontol A Biol Sci Med Sci. 2003;58(3):249–65.
2. Chapman DP, Perry GS, Strine TW. The vital link between chronic disease and depressive disorders. Prev Chronic Dis. 2005;2(1):A14.
3. Gallo JJ, Rabins PV. Depression without sadness: alternative presentations of depression in late life. Am Fam Physician. 1999;60(3):820.
4. Schulz R, Beach SR, Ives DG, et al. Association between depression and mortality in older adults: the cardiovascular health study. Arch Intern Med. 2000;160(12):1761–8.
5. Belmaker RH, Agam G. Major depressive disorder. N Engl J Med. 2008;358(1):55–68.
6. Burke HM, Davis MC, Otte C, et al. Depression and cortisol responses to psychological stress: a meta-analysis. Psychoneuroendocrinology. 2005;30(9):846–56.
7. Tham MW, Woon PS, Sum MY, et al. White matter abnormalities in major depression: evidence from post-mortem, neuroimaging and genetic studies. J Affect Disord. 2011;132(1–2):26–36.
8. Cole MG, Dendukuri N. Risk factors for depression among elderly community subjects: a systematic review and meta-analysis. Am J Psychiatry. 2003;160(6):1147–56.
9. Conwell Y, Van Orden K, Caine ED. Suicide in older adults. Psychiatr Clin N Am. 2011;34(2):451–68.
10. Conwell Y, Lyness JM, Duberstein P, et al. Completed suicide among older patients in primary care practices: a controlled study. J Am Geriatr Soc. 2000;48(1):23–9.
11. American Psychiatric Association. Diagnostic and statistical manual of mental disorders: DSM-5. Washington, DC: American Psychiatric Association; 2013.
12. Unützer J, Patrick DL, Diehr P, et al. Quality adjusted life years in older adults with depressive symptoms and chronic medical disorders. Int Psychogeriatr. 2000;12(1):15–33.
13. Siu AL, and the USPSTF. Screening for depression in adults: US preventive services task force recommendation statement. JAMA. 2016;315(4):380–7.
14. Li C, Friedman B, Conwell Y, et al. Validity of the Patient Health Questionnaire 2 (PHQ-2) in identifying major depression in older people. J Am Geriatr Soc. 2007;55(4):596.
15. Hoyl MT, Alessi CA, Harker JO, et al. Development and testing of a five-item version of the geriatric depression scale. J Am Geriatr Soc. 1999;47(7):873.
16. Phelan E, Williams B, Meeker K, et al. A study of the diagnostic accuracy of the PHQ-9 in primary care elderly. BMC Fam Pract. 2010;11:63.
17. Pinquart M, Duberstein PR, Lyness JM. Treatments for later-life depressive conditions: a meta-analytic comparison of pharmacotherapy and psychotherapy. Am J Psychiatry. 2006;163(9):1493–501.
18. Scogin F, Welsh D, Hanson A, et al. Evidence-based psychotherapies for depression in older adults. Clin Psychol: Sci Pract. 2005;12(3):222–37.
19. American Psychiatric Association. Practice guideline for the treatment of patients with major depressive disorder. 2010. https://www.psychiatry.org/psychiatrists/practice/clinical-practice-guidelines. Accessed 24 Aug 2018.
20. Kok RM, Nolen WA, Heeren TJ. Efficacy of treatment in older depressed patients: a systematic review and meta-analysis of double-blind randomized controlled trials with antidepressants. J Affect Disord. 2012;141(2–3):103–15.
21. Weise BS. Geriatric depression: the use of antidepressants in the elderly. B C Med J. 2011;53(7):341–7.
22. Anttila SA, Leinonen EV. A review of the pharmacological and clinical profile of mirtazapine. CNS Drug Rev. 2001;7(3):249.
23. Weihs KL, Settle EC Jr, Batey SR, et al. Bupropion sustained release versus paroxetine for the treatment of depression in the elderly. J Clin Psychiatry. 2000;61(3):196–202.
24. American Geriatrics Society 2015 Beers Criteria Update Expert Panel. American Geriatrics Society 2015 updated Beers criteria for potentially inappropriate medication use in older adults. J Am Geriatr Soc. 2015;63(11):2227–46.
25. Rush AJ, Trivedi MH, Wisniewski SR, et al. Acute and longer-term outcomes in depressed outpatients requiring one or several treatment steps: a STAR*D report. Am J Psychiatry. 2006;163(11):1905–17.
26. Kellner CH, Hussain MM, Knapp RG, et al. Right unilateral ultrabrief pulse ECT in geriatric depression: phase 1 of the PRIDE study. Am J Psychiatry. 2016;173(11):1101–9.

27. O'Connor MK, Knapp R, Hussain M, et al. The influence of age on the response of major depression to electroconvulsive therapy: a CORE report. Am J Geriatr Psychiatry. 2001;9(4):382–90.
28. Kellner CH, Hussain MM, Knapp RG, et al. A novel strategy for continuation ECT in geriatric depression: phase 2 of the PRIDE study. Am J Psychiatry. 2016;173(11):1110–8.
29. Weiner RD. Chapter 3. In: The practice of electroconvulsive therapy: recommendations for treatment, training and privileging. 2nd ed. Washington, DC: American Psychiatric Publishing; 2001. p. 27–30.
30. Weiner RD, Krystal AD. Chapter 27: Electroconvulsive therapy. In: The American Psychiatric Publishing textbook of geriatric psychiatry. 4th ed. Arlington: American Psychiatric Publishing; 2009.
31. Callahan CM. Quality improvement research on late life depression in primary care. Med Care. 2001;39(8):772–84.
32. Unützer J, Katon W, Callahan CM, et al. Collaborative care management of late-life depression in the primary care setting: a randomized controlled trial. JAMA. 2002;288(22):2836–45.
33. AIMS Center, University of Washington Psychiatry and Behavioral Sciences. https://aims.uw.edu/collaborative-care/principles-collaborative-care. Accessed 5 Sept 2017.
34. Ciechanowski P, Wagner E, Schmaling K, et al. Community-integrated home-based depression treatment in older adults: a randomized controlled trial. JAMA. 2004;291(13):1569–77.
35. Thota AB, Sipe TA, Byard GJ, et al. Collaborative care to improve the management of depressive disorders: a community guide systematic review and meta-analysis. Am J Prev Med. 2012;42(5):525–38.

Behavioral and Psychiatric Symptoms in Dementia (BPSD)

Amy S. Aloysi and Eileen H. Callahan

A. Chun (ed.), *Geriatric Practice*, https://doi.org/10.1007/978-3-030-19625-7_18

18.1 Competency

1. Formulate a differential diagnosis and implement an evaluation in a patient who exhibits behavioral and psychiatric symptoms of dementia.
2. Develop a synergistic nonpharmacologic and pharmacologic management plan for a patient with behavioral and psychiatric symptoms of dementia.

Case

Mr. N is a 76-year-old married right-handed musician who was referred by his geriatrician for cognitive assessment. The patient was initially seen by a neurologist at age 72 for evaluation of a 3-year history of difficulty reading musical scores. MRI at that time showed mild microvascular ischemic disease and an old left thalamic infarction. His cognitive symptoms have progressed over time to include short-term memory impairment, word-finding difficulties, and dyspraxias including difficulty using the remote control and inability to write out checks. He also has a history of mild depressive spells throughout his life, never formally treated, but currently was experiencing depressed mood, lack of interest and motivation, poor sleep, extreme fatigue, and anxiety spells. He is in psychotherapy with a geriatric psychologist.

His voice has changed over the past 3 years, and he is undergoing speech therapy for moderate to severe dysphonia and dysarthria. Additional symptoms include a history of violent dream enactment starting 20 years ago, which has been gradually lessening. He has had recurrent well-formed visual hallucinations for the past 7 years. These have included formed components and less formed components (e.g. spots and patterns) amusing dogs and cats, spots and patterns on things with insight into their unreality. Over the past 5 years, he has had progressive gait impairment currently requiring walker. He has had a slight hand tremor.

Past medical history included esophageal cancer (resected 2000), spinal stenosis post decompression, vocal cord dysfunction, prostate cancer, hypertension, hyperlipidemia, deep venous thrombosis, and gastroesophageal reflux disease (GERD).

Medications include mirabegron for bladder dysfunction, nebivolol and amlodipine for hypertension, omeprazole for GERD, rivaroxaban for deep venous thrombosis (DVT), MVI, B12, and vitamin D. He has no known allergies. **Family medical history** there is no family history of dementia, psychiatric illness, movement disorders, however one sister died of a stroke and both parents suffered from cardiac disease.

On **examination**, the patient was a pleasant elderly African American male who presents with his girlfriend. He has a slight episode tremor of his hands. He has psychomotor slowing, and drools from the corner of his mouth. Speech is dysphonic, soft. Mood is described as depressed, affect is congruent. Thought process is linear and goal directed. Thought content does not reveal any delusionality or suicidal thoughts. Recurrent well-formed visual hallucinations as described, which do not distress him. Posture is forward-bent. Gait is wide-based, with short steps. Current MMSE is 28/30 (patient missing 2 items on a 3-item recall task). He is fully oriented with grossly intact attention and concentration. Insight and judgment are fair.

18.2 Background

Behavioral and psychological symptoms in dementia (BPSD) are common and ultimately affect the majority of patients with dementia at some point in their illness course. BPSD can involve complexly layered components including multidomain cognitive impairment, affective instability (depression, anxiety/agitation), neurovegetative dysregulation (e.g., sleep and appetite disturbance), and behavioral dyscontrol. BPSD are costly to society, personally taxing on families/caregivers, and a major contributor to institutional placement. We review the subtypes of dementias and behavioral disturbances that are commonly associated with each syndrome at various stages of disease. Optimal BPSD management typically requires a comprehensive and synergistic approach, including both behavioral and neuropsychopharmacologic strategies (latter reviewed in ▶ Chap. 21) carefully tailored to the individual patient, taking account of all comorbidities and their underlying pathogeneses. With targeted treatment, an integrated multidisciplinary approach offers the potential for optimizing patient functionality, quality of life, comfort, caregiver stress reduction, risk management (prevent serious consequences of BPSD), and overall prognosis.

18

18.2.1 Diagnostic Classification

Dementia diagnostic classification has been undergoing progressive renovation as etiologic understanding evolves, especially regarding socio-emotional neuroscience relevant to BPSD (see ◘ Fig. 18.1). This has driven transformation from clinical/top-down nosology to molecular and functional neuroanatomic pathologic/bottom-up classification schemes. This refinement has especially impacted classification of primary neurodegenerative disorders (e.g., parkinsonian-plus syndromes). It is therefore helpful to briefly summarize current dementia classification, as shown in ◘ Table 18.1, to facilitate case-based learning.

18.3 Diagnostic Approach

18.3.1 General Principles

- Although this chapter's focus is BPSD management, because optimal BPSD treatment requires a comprehensive and coordinated approach across neural/neuropsychiatric systems, we briefly summarize dementia diagnostic principles.

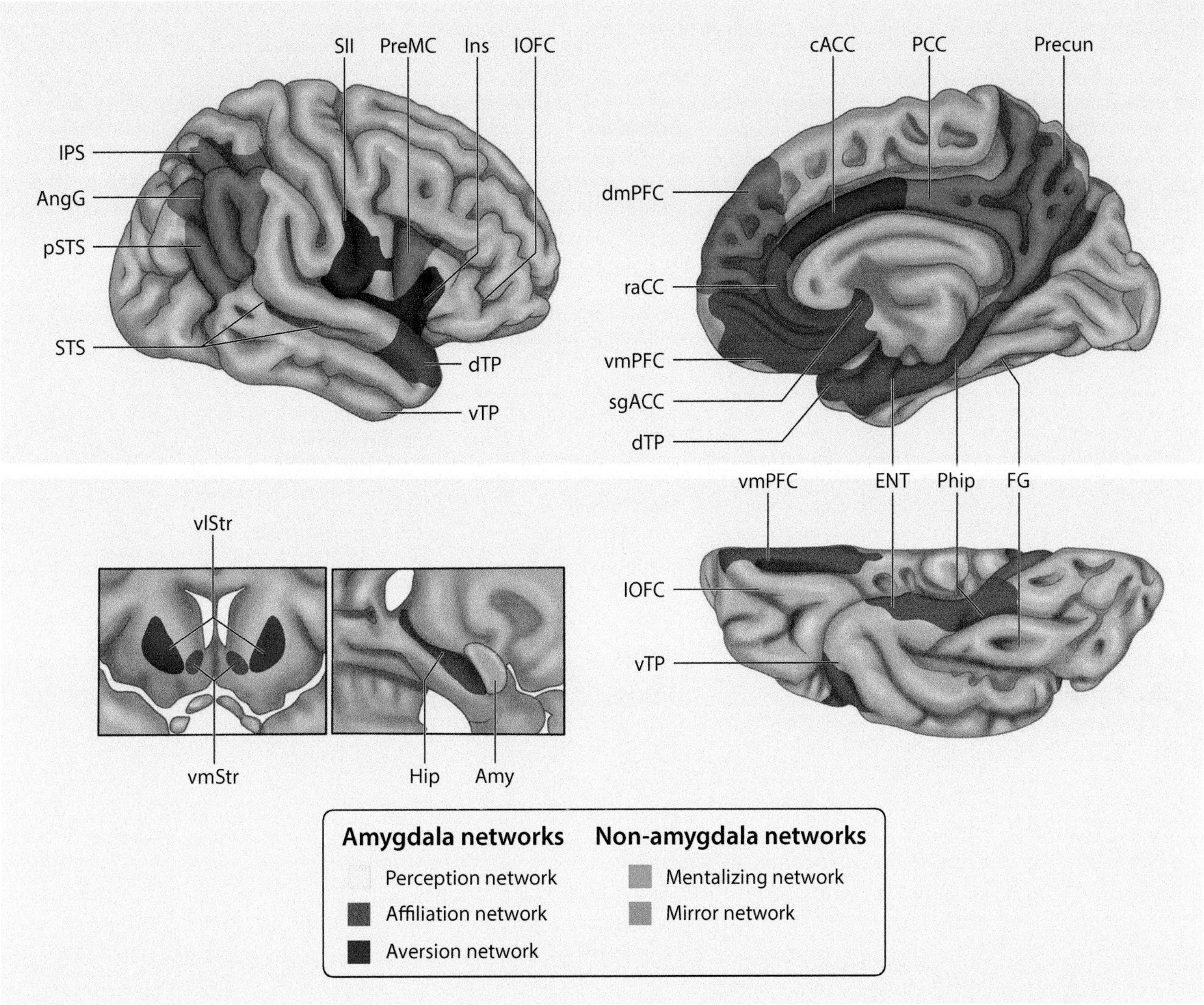

Fig. 18.1 Functional neuroanatomy of social behavior (from AAN-Continuum). (Adapted with permission from Dickerson [43])

- Observe the patient's behavior and interactions in a nondirected manner and formulate hypotheses for more specific testing. Because dementia syndromes often have overlapping clinical features, with multifactorial etiologies (e.g., PD-D, as shown in Fig. 18.2), it is important to just simply and accurately describe observed pathology without prematurely imposing diagnostic categories before attempting to formulate unifying and comprehensive diagnoses [43].
- Thorough history acquisition is essential for establishing BPSD profile, and a detailed multisystem review can narrow differential diagnosis by facilitating etiologic pattern recognition. BPSD can be an explicit complaint (i.e., when obvious to the patient, e.g., as in an expressive language disorder), a concern reported by informants but for which the patient is unaware (e.g., compartmental dysregulation in the context of (FTD)), or occult to patient and even family but incidentally detected on history-acquisition or examination (e.g., a more complex dyspraxia, like driving impairment). An intermediate permutation is when a BPSD issue is identified but mischaracterized (e.g., the abulia or disinhibition of FTD interpreted as depression or mania, respectively). The potentially nuanced, or even covert, nature of nonmemory dysfunction underscores the need to be vigilant for such impairments, and the need to interview a reliable informant when feasible. Be systematic and hierarchical in determining the basis for any BPSD in order to avoid falsely identifying a higher-order abnormality (such as dyspraxia) when the dysfunction is actually due to a lower-order defect (e.g., inattention or paresis). A complex functional deficit can only be correctly attributed when the intactness of simpler functions upon which it depends is confirmed [43].
- Be comprehensive: Disorders which produce BPSD are often complexly layered neuropsychiatric spectrum processes – i.e., they do not observe historical [classification] boundaries among cognitive, motor, and mood disorders. Consequently, comprehensive multineural system assessment is required to adequately capture data crucial for diagnostic precision [43].
- Adapt the method of cognitive examination and assessment to the setting. A variety of standardized assessment

Table 18.1 Dementia classification by neuropathology

Molecular/ histo-neuropathology	Clinical syndrome		Clinical features		
			Behavioral	Motor/autonomic	Posture/gait
Tauopathies (tau)	*Fronto-temporal dementia (FTD)*	*FTD-Tau (Pick's Disease)*	Dysexecutive −/+ primary progressive aphasia	Atypical	Atypical/ late-occurring
		FTDP-17	Dysexecutive	Parkinsonism	Parkinsonian
	Corticobasal ganglionic degeneration (CBGD)		Dysexecutive dysphasic asymmetric dyspraxia alien limb	Asymmetric parkinsonism Akinesia Rigidity Dystonia Myoclonus Frontal release signs Asymmetric Babinski sign	Postural instability
	Progressive supranuclear palsy (PSP)		Dysexecutive	Supranuclear ophthalmoplegia (especially vertical EOM palsy) Eyelid Dysfunction Dysarthria Dysphagia	Postural instability Frequent falls
Mixed amyloidopathies/tauopathies	*Alzheimer's Disease (AD)*		Dysmnesic	Atypical	Late-appearing
	Chronic traumatic encephalopathy (CTE)		Variable	Variable	Variable
Synucleinopathies (α-synuclein)	*Parkinson's disease dementia (PD-D)*		Dysexecutive	Parkinsonism (asymmetric)	Parkinsonian
	dementia with Lewy bodies (DLB)		Dysexecutive Visual hallucinations Consciousness fluctuations REM behavioral disorder	Parkinsonism	Prominent gait impairment
	Multisystem atrophy (MSA)	*MSA-P (striato-nigral degeneration)*	Dysexecutive	Parkinsonism	Parkinsonism
		MSA-A (Shy-Drager)	Dysexecutive	Variable parkinsonism Prominent dysautonomia	Variable gait dysfunction
		MSA-C (olivo-ponto-cerebellar degeneration)	Dysexecutive	Prominent cerebellar dysfunction	Cerebellar gait dysfunction
Huntington	*Huntington's disease (HD)*		Dysexecutive Dysinhibition Affective dysregulation	Chorieform movements	Progressive dysfunction
Prion/spongiform	*Creutzfeldt-Jacob disease (CJD)*	Sporadic/ iatrogenic	Global cognitive dysfunction	Mixed UMN and extrapyramidal signs	Dyspraxic and motor dysfunction-related
		Variant	Global cognitive dysfunction	Mixed UMN and extrapyramidal signs	Dyspraxic and motor dysfunction-related
		Familial *(Gerstmann–Sträussler–Scheinker)*	Progressive global dementia Mood dysregulation Thought content disturbance (psychosis)	Characterized by pyramidal, cerebellar, and parkinsonian features	Dyspraxic and motor dysfunction-related

Table 18.1 (continued)

Molecular/ histo-neuropathology	Clinical syndrome		Clinical features		
			Behavioral	Motor/autonomic	Posture/gait
Cerebrovascular	*Ischemic*	*Microvascular*	Bradyphrenia	Bradykinesia	Variable
		Thrombo-embolic	Variable	Variable	Variable
	Hemorrhagic	*Microangio-pathic*	Variable	Variable	Variable
		Lobar	Variable	Variable	Variable
Ventricular fluid dynamics	*Normal pressure hydrocephalus (NPH)*		Dysexecutive Depression	Secondary parkinsonism Urinary dyscontrol	Secondary parkinsonism Gait apraxia

Adapted from Goldstein [44]

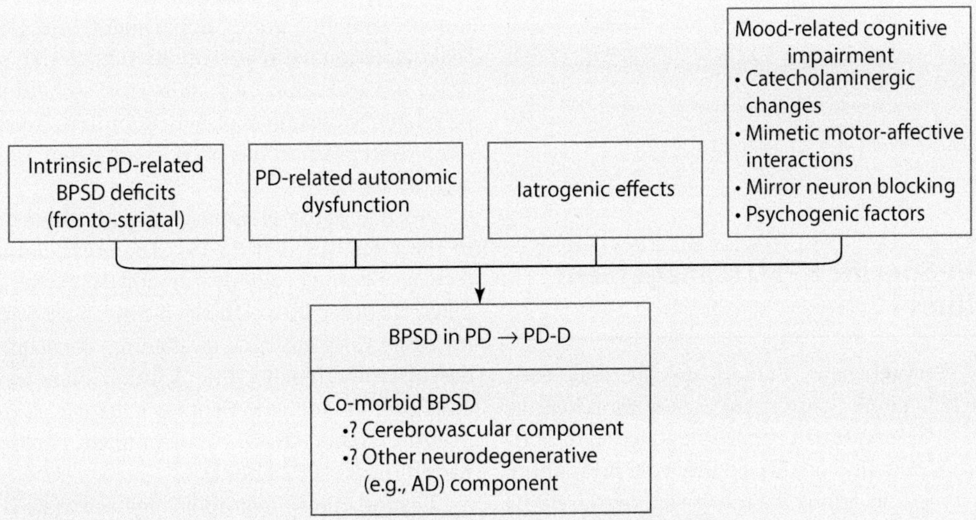

Fig. 18.2 Complexly layered BPSD components in PD-D. (Adapted from Aloysi and Aron [45])

inventories exist to facilitate efficient screening; the most widely used are the Folstein Mini-Mental Status Examination (MMSE) [1] and Montreal Cognitive Assessment (MoCA) [2]. Commercially available computerized neuropsychological screening instruments are available to extend the bedside or office evaluation [43].

- Consider formal neuropsychological testing: standardized and normed protocols represent the gold standard for characterizing current neurocognitive profile, thereby informing precise diagnosis and establishing a quantitative baseline for tracking [43].

18.3.2 Neurobehavioral Examination

A comprehensive hierarchical neurobehavioral domain-based examination is summarized in Fig. 18.3.

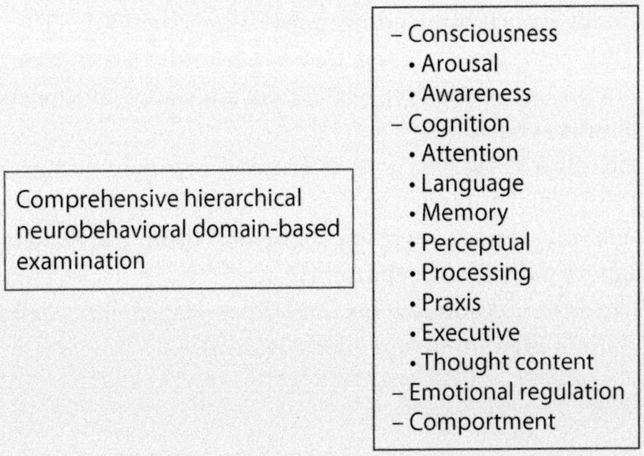

Fig. 18.3 Hierarchical neurobehavioral domain approach to BPSD assessment

18.3.3 Neurodiagnostics (◘ Table 18.2)

◘ **Table 18.2** BPSD neurodiagnostics

Brain imaging	Structural	CT	
		MRI	
	Functional	Perfusion	SPECT
		Metabolic	FDG-PET
	Molecular	DAT-SPECT	
		Amyloid PET	
Blood tests	Hematologic screens		
	Metabolic screens		
	Vitamin levels		
	Endocrine assays		
	Toxicity screens		
	Neurodegenerative genetic analyses		
CSF testing	CSF chemical, viral, and prion markers		
	CSF neurodegenerative markers		
Electrophysiologic	Electroencephalography (EEG)		

18.4 Domain-Specific BPSD Management Guidelines

The goal of a comprehensive domain-specific diagnostic assessment is to help guide a correspondingly comprehensive and synergistic BPSD treatment, since integrated care optimizes patient functionality, quality of life, risk prevention, and prognosis, as well as family/caregiver well-being. BPSD management can be further optimized by adhering to a correspondingly hierarchical strategy, with detailed attention to the choreography of treatment components.

While dementias are customarily typified by their associated cognitive deficits, targeting BPSD is a fundamental management priority, including optimizing cognition. That is, "gluing" a patient back together behaviorally is *foundational* to ambitiously and comprehensively managing all aspects of dementia syndromes.

RE-SEAM (◘ Fig. 18.4) is a useful acronym summarizing the initial approach to BPSD management for a patient, and family, "coming apart at the seams" from the escalating weight of a dementia syndrome.

The overarching strategy of BPSD management is defined by patient ***regulation*** and family ***education.***

BPSD management strategy
and therapeutic targets

R : regulate
E : educate
-
S : sleep
E : energy
A : appetite, agitation
M : mood

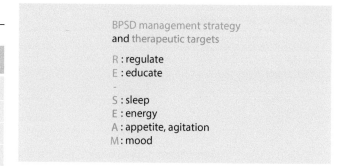

◘ **Fig. 18.4** RE-SEAM acronym summarizing initial approach to BPSD management

18.5 Sleep

Sleep regulation is foundational to optimal daytime cognitive proficiency, mood stabilization, motor function, and overall behavioral functionality. Sleep dysregulation can be correspondingly associated with cognitive impairment, mood instability, motor impairment, and global behavioral maladaptation, with potentially substantial impact on quality of life and safety (e.g., falls risk). In addition, sleep may be related to clearance of A-Beta protein from the brain, and sleep dysregulation has been investigated as a risk factor for AD [3].

Normal aging is associated with characteristic changes in the circadian rhythm [4]. The most common sleep pattern developing in elderly individuals is advanced sleep-wake phase disorder in which sleep-onset is in early evening followed by early morning awakening, consequently impairing daytime functionality [4]. Another common sleep pattern emerging in elderly patients is irregular sleep-wake rhythm disorder characterized by incomplete patches of sleep and wakefulness over 24 hours.

Beyond these common age-associated sleep pattern changes, select sleep disorders develop with increased predominance in older patient populations. Rapid eye movement (REM)-related behavioral disorder (RBD) is a distinct parasomnia which can be associated with, and can often be an important early harbinger (sometimes by decades) of, select neurodegenerative disorders, including Parkinson's disease and parkinsonian spectrum dementias. It is characterized by loss of muscle atony during REM sleep and resultant dream enactment [5]. Bed partners may notice fighting, shouting, or falling out of bed at night, and it can result in injury.

Sleep apnea is a sleep-respiratory disorder which can develop in older patients. Central and obstructive variants exist. Snoring and respiratory rate variation (including episodic gasping), often reported by bed partners, are common signs. Because sleep agents can worsen sleep apnea (e.g., via central respiratory suppression), if clinical suspicion warrants, it is crucial to identify and manage this syndrome *before* initiating any neuropsychopharmacologic intervention.

Characterizing sleep dysregulation sufficient for initiating targeted treatment can routinely be achieved by means of a detailed history acquisition, including obtaining collateral data from bed partners and/or caregivers. When clinical circumstances raise concern for a primary parasomnia and/or respiratory sleep disorder, more definitive diagnosis via a diagnostic nocturnal polysomnogram (NPSG) is indicated. For example, NPSG is essential for diagnosing and precisely managing (e.g., via CPAP titration) sleep apnea.

Management of sleep disorders begins with counseling. Patients and caregivers should be educated regarding sleep hygiene. This includes establishing set bedtime and wake times, securing a comfortable sleep environment, removal of sleep-dysregulating stimuli, and limiting caffeine amount and timing.

Given the potentially deleterious impact of sleep dysregulation on global functionality, quality of life, and risk management (e.g., driving safety, falls prevention), if sleep dysregulation and associated daytime wakefulness disturbance persist despite sleep hygiene optimization, targeted treatment is indicated.

Only select geriatric sleep disorders have solid evidence-based practice guidelines for treatment. Advanced sleep-wake phase disorder can be addressed with bright light therapy in the evening. Melatonin is a gentle first-line option to regulate circadian rhythm disorders [6]. RBD treatment can start with melatonin but often requires clonazepam [5]. Despite the frequency and severity of sleep disorders in dementia, there remains little evidence-basis for guiding their management [6]. Nevertheless, since sleep-wake cycle disturbances can be highly disruptive to patient and family, judicious use of sleep-facilitating agents may be required.

One strategy to follow when designing management of a geriatric sleep disorder is to identify any other aspects of patient neurovegetative function which might also require targeting, that is, to aim for achieving neuropsychopharmacologic synergy. For example, a geriatric patient with both initial insomnia and decreased appetite can be treated synergistically via mirtazapine. Or a patient with a pain syndrome with nocturnal predominance (e.g., neuropathy, osteoarthritis, spondylosis, etc.) can be treated with bedtime-only gabapentin or pregabalin.

Trazodone has acquired widespread application to sleep disorders in a variety of fragile patient populations, including dementia patients [7]. Newer agents such as the melatonin receptor agonist ramelteon are also options [8]. Insomnia-specific agents such as the non-benzodiazepine GABA-agonists (zolpidem, eszopiclone, zaleplon), also known as Z-drugs) can be helpful and reasonably safe when deployed with adequate precision and monitoring [9].

18.6 Energy

Fatigue and subjective energy-related symptomatology are commonly associated with dementia syndromes.

For example, apathy may be the most common neuropsychiatric feature of Alzheimer's disease but is often overlooked [10]. Energy anomalies can be either intrinsic to the primary dementia etiology or common comorbid syndromes.

Detection and management of fatigue-associated disorders commonly comorbid to dementia is essential, including screening for B12 deficiency, hypothyroidism, and anemia. Idiopathic fatigue and/or psychomotor retardation can be specifically targeted with CNS activating agents. A graduated algorithm including bupropion, amantadine, primary wakefulness agents (e.g., modafinil, armodafinil), and primary CNS stimulants (methylphenidate, amphetamine, and their derivatives) can all be considered in the management approach of fatigue [11]. Cholinesterase inhibitors such as donepezil, galantamine, and rivastigmine can also have activating effects [11].

If the need to advance to a primary CNS stimulant trial is reached, cardiology clearance, while not an official practice guideline, is wise to confirm absence of cardiac contraindications to ensure safety. Because of its relative safety, including absence of significant impact on seizure threshold a primary CNS stimulant trial is typically initiated with low-dose immediate-release methylphenidate to facilitate dosing precision [11]. Once a satisfactory titration is achieved, conversion to a once-daily long-acting formulation can be considered.

18.7 Appetite

Appetite is one of the key neurovegetative functions, and nutritional status is important to help maintain adequate neurological and psychiatric function. Vitamin deficiencies such as thiamine, vitamin B12, folic acid, as well as micronutrient deficiencies have been associated with neuropsychiatric syndromes. Some common causes of poor appetite are loss of sense of smell, mood disorders, medical conditions and some medications. Poor oral intake may also be associated with paranoid delusions that food is being poisoned, apraxia, inadequate caretaking, or dysphagia. A medical evaluation should be performed, the cause of the change in eating habits should be ascertained, and the problem addressed appropriately. The majority of patients with Alzheimer's disease, up to 80%, will suffer from an eating or swallowing disturbance [12], often in the later stages of the disease. Some patients require an evaluation with a speech pathologist and may include a formal swallowing evaluation. Treatment options may include nutritional supplements, additional caregiver assistance, creating a pleasant social milieu, providing familiar, favorite foods, or treating underlying medical or psychiatric conditions [13].

In addition to under-eating, overeating may develop in the setting of neurologic disease, particular in frontotemporal lobar dementia in which one of the early signs can be a change in dietary preferences or overeating [14]. Environmental measures to ensure access to appropriate quantities of nutritious food and restricting the compulsive eating is important. A case report describes the use of low dose topiramate to control abnormal eating and drinking behaviors in FTD [15]. Kluver-Bucy syndrome, characterized by hyperorality, placidity, hypermetamorphosis, dietary changes, and changes in sexual behavior and visual agnosia, may emerge due to injury, vascular insults, or degeneration of the temporal lobes [16].

18.8 Agitation and/or Psychosis

Agitation, in contrast to many other types of BPSD, is intrinsically defined by a patient's outwardly defined features. Agitation can be among the most challenging BPSD components to manage.

The initial approach to dementia-related agitation should be nonpharmacological, including caregiver education, milieu management, and identifying any underlying cause of the behavior, such as pain, under-/overstimulation, and constipation [17]. Additional behavioral interventions include environmental modification, caregiver skill development, activity engagement, music therapy, exercise, aromatherapy, light therapy, etc.

Neuropsychopharmacologic management is reserved for agitation-related behaviors which represent risk to the patient and/or others and are unresponsive to other means of control. Multiple psychotropic classes can be employed to target agitation. Agent selection typically involves a methodically graduated approach guided by specific agitation features, synergistic targeting of other BPSD components, and side effect vulnerability profile.

- **Antidepressants**

Antidepressants can be used to target impulsivity, and can be particularly helpful for behavioral disturbances in FTD. The CitAD study examined the effects of citalopram for agitation in AD; results suggest that citalopram can be effective in reducing agitation and caregiver distress, with improvement in the clinical global impressions of change in 40% of the citalopram group compared to 26% of the placebo arm. Maximum dosage has been revised to 20 mg due to risk of adverse cardiac effects, including QT interval prolongation [18]. Cognitive adverse effects were also noted [18]. Trazodone is a weak antidepressant but has a gentle sedating effect (hence its common application in geriatric sleep regulation) which can be helpful for ameliorating agitation.

- **Anticonvulsants**

There is limited evidence for use of anticonvulsants for agitation [19]. However, a graduated approach can start with gabapentin and culminate with valproate; latter can be an especially effective agent for agitation refractory to other interventions.

- **Primary Anxiolytics**

Buspirone is an atypical primary anxiolytic which can sometimes ameliorate agitation. Benzodiazepines are generally not recommended in the elderly, and are associated with cognitive impairment, delirium, and fall-related trauma [9]. However, like all psychotropics, when dementia-related agitation both (a) represents unacceptable risk to patient/others, and (b) is refractory to all other interventions, strategic benzodiazepine use with an intermediate half-life agent like lorazepam can be considered.

- **Neuroleptics**

American Psychiatric Association (APA) guidelines (2016) [20] provide recommendations on the use of antipsychotics in management of dementia-related agitation and/or psychosis (DRAP). Despite risk, neuroleptics retain utility in select circumstances when DRAP (a) represents unacceptable danger to patient/others; (b) treatment has the potential to relieve patient distress and/or caregiver burden; and (c) behavior is refractory to all other interventions.

Antipsychotics are classified as first generation (typical) or second generation (atypical). First generation neuroleptics, such as haloperidol are predominantly dopamine (D2) receptor blockers and carry more risk of extrapyramidal side effects (EPS), including parkinsonism, tremor, gait disturbance, and tardive dyskinesia. Second-generation neuroleptics include olanzapine, risperidone, quetiapine, and aripiprazole. These agents block D2-receptors but also have complex effects on multiple other transmitter systems including serotonin receptors (5HT2A). These agents generally carry less EPS risk.

APA guidelines do not specify particular neuroleptics but do indicate that haloperidol, outside of its role in the treatment of delirium, should *not* be first line treatment for nonemergent use in BPSD. Otherwise, choice of neuroleptic should be guided by phenomenology profile and available evidence base. The CATIE-AD (Clinical Antipsychotic Trials of Intervention Effectiveness–Alzheimer's Disease) Study (2008) [21] demonstrated greater efficacy of risperidone or olanzapine over quetiapine. Despite the common challenge of noncompliance complicating BPSD-related agitation, use of long-acting injectable depot agents is not recommended in the absence of a co-occurring chronic primary psychotic disorder.

Neuroleptics carry significant risks of adverse effects. In fact, neuroleptics are "black-boxed" for use in DRAP. All first and second generation antipsychotics carry a black-box warning for increased risk of mortality. Atypical antipsychotics were first implicated in 2005 when the FDA black box warning was issued based on meta-analyses revealing that 15 of 17 placebo-controlled studies showed increased mortality risk of 1.6–1.7 due to cardiac and infectious causes in elderly patients with BPSD who were treated with olanzapine, risperidone, aripiprazole, or quetiapine [22]. Mortality risk with typical agents can be up to 37% higher than with atypicals [23]. This risk appears to be cumulative and persists with ongoing treatment [24]. The DART-AD (Dementia Antipsychotic withdRrawal Trial – Alzheimer's disease) study showed increased risks of mortality associated with antipsychotics [25]. Both first- and second-generation (risperidone) neuroleptics were studied up to 3 years. Reduced survival was found in the neuroleptic-treated group relative to the placebo-treated group at 12-month endpoint (70% vs. 77%), as well as at 36-month follow-up (30% vs. 59%) [25]. While individual risks carried by specific neuroleptics remains ill-defined, one study comparing the relative mortality risk of four different agents over 180 days found morbidity risk with haloperidol to be greatest, followed by risperidone, olanzapine, and quetiapine [26].

Antipsychotics can also have cognitive side effects, ranging from subtle dysexecutive features to abulia and unacceptable sedation [27], mediated through anticholinergic and/or antidopaminergic mechanisms [28]. These effects, in combination with potential orthostatic hypotensive vulnerability, can significantly increase falls risk.

Before initiating a neuroleptic for DRAP, a careful assessment of risks and benefits of antipsychotic treatment must be made, taking into consideration severity, dangerousness, and distress caused by DRAP to the patient and impact on others/milieu. Use of a quantitative measure for monitoring is recommended. The Neuropsychiatric Inventory (NPI) is a useful rating scale for this purpose [29]. A discussion should be held with the patient and family/health care proxy before starting an antipsychotic. Starting dose should always be low, and then gently titrated to minimal effective dosage to control symptoms. Tolerability and risks should be continually reviewed.

When there is absence of response after a reasonably adequate trial by dosage and duration (e.g., 4 weeks), the neuroleptic should be gradually discontinued. If there is a positive response, a joint patient/family discussion should be held regarding risks/benefits of continued treatment relative to goals of care. APA guidelines recommend that when BPSD symptoms do respond to antipsychotics, and there are no prior failed attempts at discontinuation, attempt should be made to taper and withdraw the medication within 4 months [20]. However, relapse risk may be high: for a group of patients with AD and psychosis or agitation-aggression who responded to risperidone and maintained on treatment for 16 weeks, subsequent randomization to placebo led to relapse rate of 48% over the next 16 weeks while only 15% of those maintained on medication showed re-emergence of symptoms [30]. In contrast, a Cochrane review [31] concluded that some patients may be able to tolerate antipsychotic discontinuation, especially if DRAP signs are less severe.

Pimavanserin is a novel agent recently approved solely for Parkinson's disease-related psychosis [32]. Despite its novel pharmacology, pimavanserin is "black-boxed" for non-PD DRAP. Nevertheless, given the common parkinsonian dementia management challenge of simultaneous need for levodopa-based motoric optimization *and* parkinsonian cognitive dysfunction (including psychosis) exacerbated by levodopa, pimavanserin offers an innovative means for balancing these commonly conflicting management demands.

An increasingly available and potentially promisingly innovative DRAP treatment option is medical marijuana. This is commonly formulated as an oral oil combination of tetrahydrocannabinol (THC) and cannabidiol (CBD) in variable proportions depending on indications. Currently, 10 out of 24 states that license medical marijuana include dementia as one of the qualifying conditions [33]. Several studies of THC for agitation in dementia have demonstrated safety [34, 35], while one study showed that cannabis oil containing THC can significantly reduce delusions, agitation/aggression, irritability, apathy, insomnia, and caregiver distress as measured by the NPI [29]. Further studies are needed to inform development of evidence-based practice guidelines.

18.9 Mood

Mood disorders are commonly associated with dementias. They can be an independent comorbid process or intrinsic feature of the dementia etiology (e.g., as in Parkinson's disease dementia PD-D). Affective phenomenology occurring within the context of a dementia can be quite protean. Regardless of mechanism, affective symptomatology can significantly contribute to cognitive impairment (e.g., pseudo dementia). For example, ◘ Fig. 18.5 shows fMR images demonstrating differences in neuronal activation in attentional (cingulate) and memory (hippocampus) substrates when contrasting depressed patients with matched normal control subjects while performing a cognitive task [36]. Given the potential for mood disorders to exacerbate cognitive/behavioral dysfunction, and their tendency to be responsive to treatment, management of dementia-associated mood disorders should be given high priority.

Presentation of dementia-associated depression (DAD) can vary significantly. Mild depression can manifest as gradual failure-to-thrive complicated by malnutrition, dehydration and weight loss, while severe cases may appear as the rapid deterioration and loss of function atypical of the underlying dementia disease course.

Treatment of depression in dementia parallels that in nondemented elderly, including such principles as avoiding anticholinergic agents, initiating treatment at a low dose and gradually titrating to therapeutic effect, and monitoring closely for potential side effects.

While evidence base remains variable, DAD is generally treatable and should be aggressively targeted. Selective serotonin reuptake inhibitors (SSRIs) such as sertraline, citalopram, and escitalopram are typically first-line options. If an SSRI is ineffective, a Serotonin and Norepinephrine reuptake inhibitor (SNRI) such as venlafaxine or desvenlafaxine may be tried. Bupropion can be particularly helpful for psychomotorically slowed depression and can synergistically enhance executive functioning. Should depression be severe and fail to respond to treatment with oral agents, have psychotic features, and/or is associated with catatonia, electroconvulsive therapy (ECT) may be indicated [37].

Pseudobulbar affect, also known as pathologic laughing or crying (PLC), involves affective dysregulation

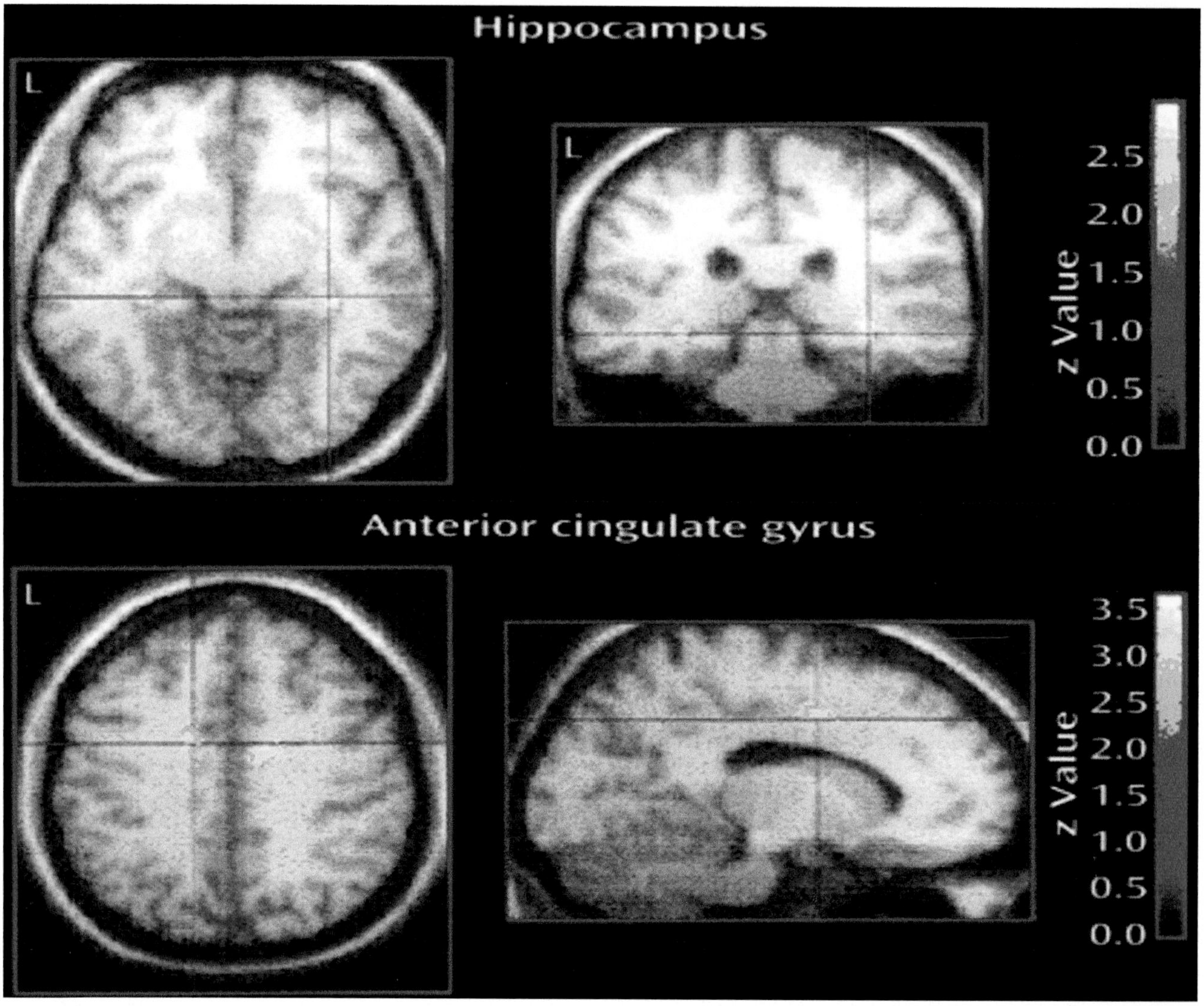

Fig. 18.5 Neural substrates of depression-associated cognitive impairment. (Reprinted with permission from American Journal of Psychiatry – De Asis et al. [36])

disconnected from context. Such seeming emotional "incontinence" is most commonly associated with neurologic syndromes including stroke, amyotrophic lateral sclerosis (ALS), multiple sclerosis (MS), and parkinsonian spectrum disorders [38]. A "catastrophic reaction" characterized by intense behavioral dysregulation triggered by anger or hostility represents a similar failure of regulatory control, often linked to underlying damage to frontal, parietal, cerebellar, and brainstem regions [38, 39]. Treatment options include the relatively new combination agent dextromethorphan/quinidine (Nudexta®), tricyclic antidepressants (TCAs), and SSRIs [38].

Late-onset mania in general is often associated with vascular disease or other neurological disorders [40].

A variety of dementia types can be associated with disinhibition, impulsivity, hyperactivity, and other manic-like symptoms. Frontotemporal lobar dementia (FTD) can be more likely to present with a manic syndrome [41]. Treatment can include anticonvulsant mood stabilizers (e.g., valproic acid), lithium, and/or atypical antipsychotics.

18.10 Management Infrastructure Design

18.10.1 Multidisciplinary Care Team

By its very multineural system nature, and common multimedical system comorbidities, BPSD management necessarily requires a multidisciplinary approach. Team components can be distinguished between "core" and "syndrome-specific":

- Core Team:
  - Geriatric psychiatry
  - Neuropsychiatry
  - Cognitive/behavioral neurology
  - Geriatrics
  - Neuropsychology
  - Social work/care manager
- Syndrome-specific
  - Movement disorder neurology
  - Vascular neurology
  - Sleep disorders
  - Cardiologist

- Neuro-urology
- Pain management
- Physical therapy
- Occupational therapy
- Speech and swallow therapy
- Visiting nurse services

Since management of one neural system commonly impacts another neural system (e.g., optimizing motor function in PD via use of dopaminergic agents routinely impacts cognitive/affective/behavioral function), integrated, synergistic management coordination is critical. To meet this challenge, one team member should be recognized as "quarterback," overseeing care to ensure multidisciplinary management is efficiently optimized and maximally aligned with explicit goals of care.

Outpatient dementia management is enhanced by dementia care coordination services; this can delay transition from home to a facility. The Maximizing INDependence at home trial (MIND), a model in which nonclinical community workers trained and supervised by geriatric clinicians provided home-based dementia care coordination, resulted in fewer unmet needs, delayed placement, and improved self-reported quality of life [42].

18.10.2 Environment/Milieu Management

Optimizing a dementia patient's home milieu can substantially ameliorate BPSD symptomatology.

This typically includes:

- Maximizing daytime light exposure to reduce sundowning vulnerability.
- Maintaining constancy of physical configuration.
- Maintaining staffing constancy.
- Optimizing daytime structured activity engagement.

18.10.3 Home Services

Visiting nursing agencies frequently have a behavioral specialty branch to provide in-home psychiatric services. This can be a valuable resource for patients who might not be able to travel to an outpatient practice setting, in addition to providing a data-rich window on patient status within their home environment via home safety, nutritional resource, home hygiene, falls risks, and other important assessments. Physical therapy, speech therapy, and occupational therapy services are often available for home provision. Within those rare circumstances in which (a) there exists grounds for concern regarding serious BPSD-related patient safety risk, and (b) intervention required to secure safety is obstructed by patient noncompliance and/or family opposition, consideration should be given for reporting situation to relevant local adult protective service agencies.

18.10.4 Community Resources

Structured Daily Activity/Quality-of-Life Enrichment A structured daily activity schedule customized to patient's interests, intellectual capacity, physical capacity, and compartmental regulatory capacity can be important for both managing BPSD symptomatology and patient course overall. Agencies and local volunteer programs can provide visiting companions which can facilitate patient engagement in structured activities and relieve family/caregiver burden. Adult day programs can provide a substantial structure for socialization and orientation. Local cultural institutions often have programs tailored toward patrons with dementia-related BPSD.

Family/Caregiver Support Educational Resources: The Alzheimer's Association is a well-established organization founded in 1980. It has an educational website, holds seminars in the community, and has BPSD-tailored patient programs.

18.10.4.1 Outpatient Versus Hospital Management

Most behavioral disturbances can be managed within an outpatient setting. However, when behavior endangers the safety of the patient and/or others, hospitalization may be warranted either to a medical unit or a geriatric psychiatry unit. All patients with an acute behavioral change, including patients with known BPSD, warrant an adequate medical evaluation on presentation to the emergency department in order to ensure identification of conditions which could cause a delirium (e.g., urinary tract infection, electrolyte disturbance, dehydration, vitamin deficiency, pneumonia, etc.), targeted treatment of which has the potential to restore baseline behavioral regulation and enable prompt return to current living configuration.

18.10.4.2 Indications for Living Configuration Change

It is important for the care team to educate family/caregivers regarding relevant criteria for determining optimal living configuration for patients with BPSD. As symptomatology evolves with dementia, it is also important to periodically check-in for any changes in patient status to ensure that current living configuration remains both safe and quality-of-life optimized. Costs and benefits regarding a living configuration change over time with dementia progression, thereby potentially changing their net balance regarding a particular configuration (see ◘ Fig. 18.6). Living configuration options which gradually progress from supervision to cueing to full assistance are summarized in ◘ Table 18.3.

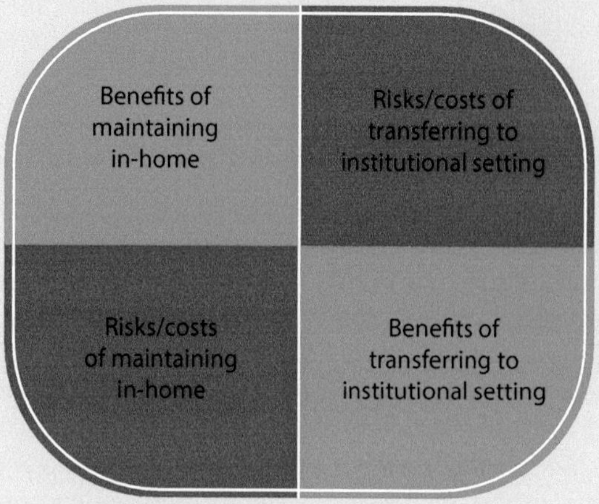

Fig. 18.6 Criteria for determining safety and optimization of living configuration for patients with BPSD

Table 18.3 Graduated living configuration options for patients with BPSD

Level/type of need	Living configuration
Socialization	Home with family/caregiver facilitation
ADL supervision	Home with caregiver supervision Assisted living
ADL assistance	Home with caregiver assistance Assisted living with caregiver assistance
ADL performance	Home with caregiver ADL support Assisted living with ADL support
Nursing care need	dementia unit of skilled nursing facility (SNF)

Case Conclusion

The case of Mr. N describes a patient with a cluster of cognitive, affective, perceptual, behavioral, and motoric symptoms which fit the syndrome of dementia with Lewy Bodies (DLB). His additional evaluation might include a sleep study to diagnose REM behavioral disturbance, and rule out sleep apnea due to large body habitus and excessive daytime fatigue. Neuropsychological testing would be helpful to clarify the cognitive dysfunction profile to inform optimal current management, prognosis, and establish quantitative benchmark for tracking. Treatment strategies might include an activating antidepressant such as bupropion for mood, energy, motivation, and executive function; a cholinesterase inhibitor such as donepezil, galantamine, or rivastigmine for cognition; and counseling him on sleep hygiene.

References

1. Folstein MF, Folstein SE, McHugh PR. "Mini-mental state": a practical method for grading the cognitive state of patients for the clinician. J Psychiatr Res [Internet]. 1975 [cited 2018 Feb 3];12(3):189–98. Available from: http://www.ncbi.nlm.nih.gov/pubmed/1202204.
2. Nasreddine ZS, Phillips NA, Bédirian V, Charbonneau S, Whitehead V, Collin I, et al. The Montreal Cognitive Assessment, MoCA: a brief screening tool for mild cognitive impairment. J Am Geriatr Soc [Internet]. 2005 [cited 2018 Feb 3];53(4):695–9. Available from: http://doi.wiley.com/10.1111/j.1532-5415.2005.53221.x.
3. Spira AP, Gottesman RF. Sleep disturbance: an emerging opportunity for Alzheimer's disease prevention? Int Psychogeriatr [Internet]. 2017 [cited 2017 Nov 26];29(4):529–31. Available from: https://www.cambridge.org/core/product/identifier/S1041610216002131/type/journal_article.
4. Pavlova M. Circadian rhythm sleep-wake disorders. Contin Lifelong Learn Neurol [Internet]. 2017 [cited 2017 Nov 26];23(4, Sleep Neurology):1051–63. Available from: http://www.ncbi.nlm.nih.gov/pubmed/28777176.
5. Bassetti CL, Bargiotas P. REM sleep behavior disorder. Front Neurol Neurosci [Internet]. 2018 [cited 2017 Nov 26];41:104–16. Available from: http://www.ncbi.nlm.nih.gov/pubmed/29145189.
6. Kinnunen KM, Vikhanova A, Livingston G. The management of sleep disorders in dementia. Curr Opin Psychiatry [Internet]. 2017 [cited 2017 Nov 26];30(6):491–7. Available from: http://www.ncbi.nlm.nih.gov/pubmed/28858007.
7. McCleery J, Cohen DA, Sharpley AL. Pharmacotherapies for sleep disturbances in dementia. Cochrane Database Syst Rev [Internet]. 2016 [cited 2018 Feb 3];11:CD009178. Available from: http://www.ncbi.nlm.nih.gov/pubmed/27851868.
8. Pinkhasov A, James SA, Fazzari M, Singh D, Lam S. Role of Ramelteon in reduction of as-needed antipsychotics in elderly patients with delirium in a general hospital setting. Clin Drug Investig [Internet]. 2017 [cited 2017 Dec 9];37(12):1137–41. Available from: http://www.ncbi.nlm.nih.gov/pubmed/28933013.
9. Markota M, Rummans TA, Bostwick JM, Lapid MI. Benzodiazepine use in older adults: dangers, management, and alternative therapies. Mayo Clin Proc [Internet]. 2016 [cited 2017 Dec 9];91(11):1632–9. Available from: http://linkinghub.elsevier.com/retrieve/pii/S0025619616305092.
10. Lanctôt KL, Amatniek J, Ancoli-Israel S, Arnold SE, Ballard C, Cohen-Mansfield J, et al. Neuropsychiatric signs and symptoms of Alzheimer's disease: new treatment paradigms. Alzheimer's Dement Transl Res Clin Interv [Internet]. 2017 [cited 2017 Dec 9];3(3):440–9. Available from: http://www.ncbi.nlm.nih.gov/pubmed/29067350.
11. Theleritis C, Siarkos K, Katirtzoglou E, Politis A. Pharmacological and nonpharmacological treatment for apathy in Alzheimer disease. J Geriatr Psychiatry Neurol [Internet]. 2017 [cited 2017 Dec 9];30(1):26–49. Available from: http://www.ncbi.nlm.nih.gov/pubmed/28248559.
12. Kai K, Hashimoto M, Amano K, Tanaka H, Fukuhara R, Ikeda M. Relationship between eating disturbance and dementia severity in patients with Alzheimer's disease. Ginsberg SD, editor. PLoS One [Internet]. 2015 [cited 2017 Nov 26];10(8):e0133666. Available from: http://www.ncbi.nlm.nih.gov/pubmed/26266531.
13. Abdelhamid A, Bunn D, Copley M, Cowap V, Dickinson A, Gray L, et al. Effectiveness of interventions to directly support food and drink intake in people with dementia: systematic review and meta-analysis. BMC Geriatr [Internet]. 2016 [cited 2017 Nov 26];16(1):26. Available from: http://www.ncbi.nlm.nih.gov/pubmed/26801619.

14. Ikeda M, Brown J, Holland AJ, Fukuhara R, Hodges JR. Changes in appetite, food preference, and eating habits in frontotemporal dementia and Alzheimer's disease. J Neurol Neurosurg Psychiatry [Internet]. 2002 [cited 2017 Nov 26];73(4):371–6. Available from: http://www.ncbi.nlm.nih.gov/pubmed/12235302.
15. Nestor PJ. Reversal of abnormal eating and drinking behaviour in a frontotemporal lobar degeneration patient using low-dose topiramate: Table 1. J Neurol Neurosurg Psychiatry [Internet]. 2012 [cited 2017 Nov 26];83(3):349–50. Available from: http://www.ncbi.nlm.nih.gov/pubmed/21507895.
16. Lanska DJ. The Klüver-Bucy syndrome. Front Neurol Neurosci [Internet]. 2018 [cited 2017 Nov 26];41:77–89. Available from: http://www.ncbi.nlm.nih.gov/pubmed/29145186.
17. Gitlin LN, Kales HC, Lyketsos CG. Nonpharmacologic management of behavioral symptoms in dementia. JAMA [Internet]. 2012 [cited 2018 Jan 13];308(19):2020. Available from: http://www.ncbi.nlm.nih.gov/pubmed/23168825.
18. Porsteinsson AP, Drye LT, Pollock BG, Devanand DP, Frangakis C, Ismail Z, et al. Effect of citalopram on agitation in Alzheimer disease. JAMA [Internet]. 2014 [cited 2017 Nov 26];311(7):682. Available from: http://www.ncbi.nlm.nih.gov/pubmed/24549548.
19. Rabins P, Rover B, Rummans T, Schneider L, Trait P. Guideline watch (October 2014): practice guideline for the treatment of patients with Alzheimer's disease and other dementias. Focus (Madison). 2017;15(1):110–28.
20. Reus VI, Fochtmann LJ, Eyler AE, Hilty DM, Horvitz-Lennon M, Jibson MD, et al. The American Psychiatric Association practice guideline on the use of antipsychotics to treat agitation or psychosis in patients with dementia. Am J Psychiatry [Internet]. 2016 [cited 2017 Nov 26];173(5):543–6. Available from: http://www.ncbi.nlm.nih.gov/pubmed/27133416.
21. Sultzer DL, Davis SM, Tariot PN, Dagerman KS, Lebowitz BD, Lyketsos CG, et al. Clinical symptom responses to atypical antipsychotic medications in Alzheimer's disease: phase 1 outcomes from the CATIE-AD effectiveness trial. Am J Psychiatry [Internet]. 2008 [cited 2017 Nov 26];165(7):844–54. Available from: http://www.ncbi.nlm.nih.gov/pubmed/18519523.
22. Food and Drug Administration. FDA public health advisory: deaths with antipsychotics in elderly patients with behavioral disturbances. [Internet]. [cited 2017 Jan 1]. Available from: https://www.fda.gov/drugs/drugsafety/postmarketdrugsafetyinformationforpatientsandproviders/ucm053171.
23. Wang PS, Schneeweiss S, Avorn J, Fischer MA, Mogun H, Solomon DH, et al. Risk of death in elderly users of conventional vs. atypical antipsychotic medications. N Engl J Med [Internet]. 2005 [cited 2017 Nov 26];353(22):2335–41. Available from: http://www.ncbi.nlm.nih.gov/pubmed/16319382.
24. Nielsen RE, Lolk A, Valentin JB, Andersen K. Cumulative dosages of antipsychotic drugs are associated with increased mortality rate in patients with Alzheimer's dementia. Acta Psychiatr Scand [Internet]. 2016 [cited 2017 Nov 26];134(4):314–20. Available from: http://www.ncbi.nlm.nih.gov/pubmed/27357602.
25. Ballard C, Hanney ML, Theodoulou M, Douglas S, McShane R, Kossakowski K, et al. The dementia antipsychotic withdrawal trial (DART-AD): long-term follow-up of a randomised placebo-controlled trial. Lancet Neurol [Internet]. 2009 [cited 2017 Nov 26];8(2):151–7. Available from: http://www.ncbi.nlm.nih.gov/pubmed/19138567.
26. Kales HC, Kim HM, Zivin K, Valenstein M, Seyfried LS, Chiang C, et al. Risk of mortality among individual antipsychotics in patients with dementia. Am J Psychiatry [Internet]. 2012 [cited 2017 Nov 26];169(1):71–9. Available from: http://www.ncbi.nlm.nih.gov/pubmed/22193526.
27. Wolf A, Leucht S, Pajonk F-G. Do antipsychotics lead to cognitive impairment in dementia? A meta-analysis of randomised placebo-controlled trials. Eur Arch Psychiatry Clin Neurosci [Internet]. 2017 [cited 2017 Dec 9];267(3):187–98. Available from: http://www.ncbi.nlm.nih.gov/pubmed/27530185.
28. Solmi M, Murru A, Pacchiarotti I, Undurraga J, Veronese N, Fornaro M, et al. Safety, tolerability, and risks associated with first- and second-generation antipsychotics: a state-of-the-art clinical review. Ther Clin Risk Manag [Internet]. 2017 [cited 2017 Dec 9];13:757–77. Available from: https://www.dovepress.com/safety-tolerability-and-risks-associated-with-first%2D%2Dand-second-genera-peer-reviewed-article-TCRM.
29. Cummings JL, Mega M, Gray K, Rosenberg-Thompson S, Carusi DA, Gornbein J. The neuropsychiatric inventory: comprehensive assessment of psychopathology in dementia. Neurology [Internet]. 1994 [cited 2017 Dec 9];44(12):2308–14. Available from: http://www.ncbi.nlm.nih.gov/pubmed/7991117.
30. Devanand DP, Mintzer J, Schultz SK, Andrews HF, Sultzer DL, de la Pena D, et al. Relapse risk after discontinuation of risperidone in Alzheimer's disease. N Engl J Med [Internet]. 2012 [cited 2017 Nov 26];367(16):1497–507. Available from: http://www.ncbi.nlm.nih.gov/pubmed/23075176.
31. Declercq T, Petrovic M, Azermai M, Vander Stichele R, De Sutter AI, van Driel ML, et al. Withdrawal versus continuation of chronic antipsychotic drugs for behavioural and psychological symptoms in older people with dementia. In: Declercq T, editor. Cochrane database of systematic reviews [Internet]. Chichester: Wiley; 2013 [cited 2017 Nov 26]. p. CD007726. Available from: http://www.ncbi.nlm.nih.gov/pubmed/23543555
32. Sahli ZT, Tarazi FI. Pimavanserin: novel pharmacotherapy for Parkinson's disease psychosis. Expert Opin Drug Discov [Internet]. 2018[cited 2018 Feb 3];13(1):103–10. Available from: http://www.ncbi.nlm.nih.gov/pubmed/29047301.
33. Maust DT, Bonar EE, Ilgen MA, Blow FC, Kales HC. Agitation in Alzheimer disease as a qualifying condition for medical marijuana in the United States. Am J Geriatr Psychiatry [Internet]. 2016 [cited 2018 Jan 13];24(11):1000–3. Available from: http://www.ncbi.nlm.nih.gov/pubmed/27389672.
34. van den Elsen GAH, Ahmed AIA, Verkes R-J, Kramers C, Feuth T, Rosenberg PB, et al. Tetrahydrocannabinol for neuropsychiatric symptoms in dementia: A randomized controlled trial. Neurology [Internet]. 2015 [cited 2018 Jan 13];84(23):2338–46. Available from: http://www.ncbi.nlm.nih.gov/pubmed/25972490.
35. van den Elsen GAH, Ahmed AIA, Verkes R-J, Feuth T, van der Marck MA, Olde Rikkert MGM. Tetrahydrocannabinol in behavioral disturbances in dementia: a crossover randomized controlled trial. Am J Geriatr Psychiatry [Internet]. 2015 Dec [cited 2018 Jan 13];23(12):1214–24. Available from: http://www.ncbi.nlm.nih.gov/pubmed/26560511.
36. De Asis J, Stern E, Alexopoulos GS, Pan H, et al. Hippocampal and anterior cingulate activation deficits in patients with geriatric depression. Am J Psychiatry. 2001;158:1321–3.
37. Borisovskaya A, Augsburger J, Pascualy M. Electroconvulsive therapy for frontotemporal dementia with comorbid major depressive disorder. J ECT [Internet]. 2014 [cited 2018 Feb 3];30(4):45–6. Available from: http://www.ncbi.nlm.nih.gov/pubmed/24901427.
38. Miller A, Pratt H, Schiffer RB. Pseudobulbar affect: the spectrum of clinical presentations, etiologies and treatments. Expert Rev Neurother [Internet]. 2011 [cited 2017 Nov 26];11(7):1077–88. Available from: http://www.ncbi.nlm.nih.gov/pubmed/21539437.
39. Carota A, Bogousslavsky J. Catastrophe reaction and emotionalism. Front Neurol Neurosci [Internet]. 2018 [cited 2017 Nov 26];41:50–60. Available from: http://www.ncbi.nlm.nih.gov/pubmed/29145183.

40. Sami M, Khan H, Nilforooshan R. Late onset mania as an organic syndrome: A review of case reports in the literature. J Affect Disord [Internet]. 2015 [cited 2017 Nov 26];188:226–31. Available from: http://www.ncbi.nlm.nih.gov/pubmed/26368947.
41. Ducharme S, Bajestan S, Dickerson BC, Voon V. Psychiatric presentations of *C9orf72* mutation: what are the diagnostic implications for clinicians? J Neuropsychiatry Clin Neurosci [Internet]. 2017 [cited 2017 Nov 26];29(3):195–205. Available from: http://www.ncbi.nlm.nih.gov/pubmed/28238272.
42. Samus QM, Johnston D, Black BS, Hess E, Lyman C, Vavilikolanu A, et al. A multidimensional home-based care coordination intervention for elders with memory disorders: the maximizing independence at home (MIND) pilot randomized trial. Am J Geriatr Psychiatry [Internet]. 2014 [cited 2017 Nov 26];22(4):398–414. Available from: http://www.ncbi.nlm.nih.gov/pubmed/24502822.
43. Dickerson BC. Dysfunction of social cognition and behavior. Continuum. American Academy of Neurology. 2015;21:660–77.
44. Goldstein M. Dysphasias, dyspraxias and dysexecutive syndromes: the non-memory cognitive impairments. In: Sealfon SC, Stacy CB, Motiwala R, editors. Mount Sinai expert guidelines: neurology. Malden: Wiley-Blackwell; 2016.
45. Aloysi A, Aron E. A 74-year old woman with anxiety and paranoid delusions. Psychiatr Ann. 2012;42(12):471–5.

Diagnosis and Management of Delirium

Claire K. Ankuda and Olusegun Apoeso

A. Chun (ed.), *Geriatric Practice*, https://doi.org/10.1007/978-3-030-19625-7_19

- **Part 1. Competencies**
  - Be able to define the clinical characteristics of delirium
  - List some of the potentially reversible causes of delirium
  - Describe effective delirium prevention strategies in the hospital
  - Describe effective delirium treatment strategies

Case

Ms. S is a 73-year-old woman with a past medical history of hypertension and alcohol and tobacco abuse and recently diagnosed with small cell carcinoma of the lung that has metastasized to the bones. After meeting with her oncologist, she decided to opt out of any cancer-directed chemotherapies and focus on comfort with the months of life she has left. She is very interested in enrolling in hospice and wants to talk to her primary care physician about it.

Ms. S comes into the emergency department presenting with the history of a fall but unable to explain how she feels now or what happened. She indicates that she just feels "funny." An hour later, her daughter and surrogate joins her in the emergency department. She tells you that she's heard her fall a few times in the house. The first time she thinks that the patient hit her left side and ear. She shares her concern that she has been drinking more in the last 2 weeks—drinking a total of two gallons of Jack Daniels over this time period. She has also not been eating much over the last weeks. Before the prior few weeks, she has been able to walk to the liquor store alone, but she now has to pay someone to do it for her. Her last drink was 2 days ago.

In the emergency department, her blood pressure is 156/70 with a pulse of 96. She appears frail and disheveled. She repeatedly tells you she is confused about what happens and that she feels funny but cannot tell you where she is or what day it is. Other than this, she does not answer your questions. Her clothes smell strongly of urine. What is going on?

19.1 Definitions of Delirium

Delirium is a syndrome of altered cognition and attention that is acute, fluctuating, and associated with inattention, disorganized thinking, and altered level of consciousness. Although usually reversible, it's common, frequently missed, and dangerous.

There are several subtypes of delirium that may look very different:

- *Hyperactive delirium:* Also described as agitated, hyperaroused, and hyperalert delirium. It's characterized by restlessness, agitation, increased speech, hallucinations, and delusions. It is common as medication adverse effects as well as alcohol and drug withdrawal. "Sundowning," a clinical state in which people develop hyperactive delirium at night, is common in hospitalized older adults.
- *Hypoactive delirium:* Can also be described as apathetic, hypoalert, or hypoaroused delirium. Hypoactive delirium is more difficult for clinicians to identify. It is characterized by patients being hypoalert and lethargic, quiet, and apathetic. It is common in metabolic disturbances including hepatic encephalopathies, hypoxia, hypercapnia, and certain medications such as anticholinergics. Hypoactive delirium also often occurs most commonly in older adults and in palliative settings. It's difficult to differentiate from states of medication sedation and lethargy associated with end of life.
- *Mixed delirium:* Mixed delirium occurs when individuals fluctuate between hypoactive and hyperactive delirium. Most individuals display daytime sedation with nocturnal agitation and behavioral problems.
- *Delirium tremens:* Delirium tremens is the acute hallucinations and disorientation as a result of alcohol withdrawal. It is accompanied by tachycardia, diaphoresis, hypertension, and hyperthermia. Given that it begins 48–96 hours after last drink and lasts 1–5 days, it is critical to take a thorough alcohol intake history to diagnose delirium tremens.
- *Terminal delirium:* Terminal delirium occurs in the last days of life and is thought to be caused by multiorgan failure. It is distinct from other delirium subtypes in that due to its cause it may not be reversible, and medication treatment strategies are different than for nonterminal delirium.
- *Subsyndromal delirium* has been defined as the presence of some core diagnostic symptoms that do not meet the criteria for diagnostic threshold. Prevalence rates of 30–50% have been reported in intensive care units. A prodromal phase lasting for hours to days can occur before full syndromal delirium becomes evident. This includes sleep disturbances, vivid dreams, frequent calls for assistance, and anxiety.

19

19.2 Background: Prevalence and Importance of Delirium

Delirium can occur at any age, but it occurs more commonly in patients who are elderly and have compromised mental status. Delirium is incredibly common in hospitalized older adults, occurring in 14–56% of elderly patients who are hospitalized [1]. It significantly increases hospital and intensive care unit length of stays [2, 3]. Delirium is present in at least 20% of hospital stays for adults over the age of 65. It has been found in 40% of patients admitted to intensive care units. Prevalence of postoperative delirium following general surgery is 5–10% and as high as 42%

following orthopedic surgery. As many as 80–85% of patients develop delirium near death [14].

Delirium results in increased hospital length of stay and costs [4]. Moreover, delirium often results in significant morbidity, with downstream effects such as functional decline, aspiration, and death [4]. Delirium tremens increases risk of seizure and cardiac events as a result of alcohol withdrawal. Delirium can be a symptom of a medical emergency; thus, it is important to promptly respond to it and assess for possible causes.

Delirium has significant impacts on caregivers as well as patients and is extremely common among nursing home residents. Both hypoactive and hyperactive delirium can be distressing to families, resulting in higher caregiver burden and nursing home placement. Financially, delirium is associated with higher healthcare cost across every setting of care.

The relationship of delirium with other geriatric syndromes such as frailty is complex because the same risk factors for frailty can cause delirium, and episodes of delirium increase the risk of frailty and further poor outcomes.

As stated above, delirium is particularly common at the end of life, where up to 85% of patients experience delirium in the last 2 weeks. Addressing delirium in this setting is critical for the patient and family's quality of life.

19.3 Pathophysiology of Delirium

The mechanism of delirium still is not fully understood. Delirium results from a wide variety of structural or physiological insults. The neuropathogenesis of delirium has been studied in patients with hepatic encephalopathy and alcohol withdrawal. Research in these areas still is limited. The main hypothesis is reversible impairment of cerebral oxidative metabolism and multiple neurotransmitter abnormalities. The following observations support the hypothesis of multiple neurotransmitter abnormalities.

19.3.1 Acetylcholine

Data from animal and clinical studies support the hypothesis that acetylcholine is one of the critical neurotransmitters in the pathogenesis of delirium [4]. A small prospective study among patients who have undergone elective hip replacement surgery showed reduced preoperative plasma cholinesterase activity in as many as one quarter of patients. In addition, reduced preoperative cholinesterase levels were significantly correlated with postoperative delirium [5].

Clinically, good reasons support this hypothesis. Anticholinergic medications are a well-known cause of acute confusional states, and patients with impaired cholinergic transmission, such as those with Alzheimer disease, are particularly susceptible. In patients with postoperative delirium, serum anticholinergic activity is increased.

19.3.2 Dopamine

In the brain, a reciprocal relationship exists between cholinergic and dopaminergic activities. In delirium, an excess of dopaminergic activity occurs. Symptomatic relief occurs with antipsychotic medications such as haloperidol and other neuroleptic dopamine blockers.

19.3.3 Serotonin

Human and animal studies have found that serotonin is increased in patients with hepatic encephalopathy and septic delirium. Hallucinogens such as LSD act as agonists at the site of serotonin receptors. Serotoninergic agents also can cause delirium.

19.3.4 Gamma-Aminobutyric Acid (GABA)

In patients with hepatic encephalopathy, increased inhibitory GABA levels also are observed. An increase in ammonia levels occurs in patients with hepatic encephalopathy, which causes an increase in the amino acids glutamate and glutamine, which are precursors to GABA. Decreases in CNS GABA levels are observed in patients with delirium resulting from benzodiazepine and alcohol withdrawal.

19.3.5 Cortisol and Beta-Endorphins

Delirium has been associated with the disruption of cortisol and beta-endorphin circadian rhythms. This mechanism has been suggested as a possible explanation for delirium caused by exogenous glucocorticoids.

19.3.6 Melatonin

Disturbed melatonin disturbance has been associated with sleep disturbances in delirium [6].

19.4 Other Mechanisms of Delirium

19.4.1 Inflammatory Mechanism

Recent studies have suggested a role for cytokines, such as interleukin-1 and interleukin-6, in the pathogenesis of delirium. Following a wide range of infectious, inflammatory, and toxic insults, endogenous pyrogens, such as interleukin-1, are released from the cells. Head trauma and ischemia, which frequently are associated with delirium, are characterized by brain responses that are mediated by interleukin-1 and interleukin-6 [7, 8].

19.4.2 Stress Reaction Mechanism

Studies indicate psychosocial stress and sleep deprivation facilitate the onset of delirium.

19.4.3 Structural Mechanism

The specific neuronal pathways that cause delirium are unknown. Imaging studies of metabolic (e.g., hepatic encephalopathy) and structural (e.g., traumatic brain injury, stroke) factors support the hypothesis that certain anatomical pathways may play a more important role than others. The reticular formation and its connections are the main sites of arousal and attention. The dorsal tegmental pathway projecting from the mesencephalic reticular formation to the tectum and the thalamus is involved in delirium.

Disrupted blood-brain barrier can allow neurotoxic agents and inflammatory cytokines to enter the brain and may cause delirium. Contrast-enhanced MRI can be used to assess the blood-brain barrier [9, 10].

Visuoperceptual deficits in delirium such as hallucinations and delusions are not due to the underlying cognitive impairment [11]. Visual hallucinations during alcohol-withdrawal delirium are seen in subjects with polymorphisms of genes coding for dopamine transporter and catechol-O-methyltransferase (COMT) [12].

19.5 Diagnosing Delirium (◘ Table 19.1)

To make an accurate diagnosis, periodic application of diagnostic criteria such as CAM or DSM-IV criteria and knowledge of the patient's baseline mental status is imperative.

While delirium is common, it is underdiagnosed, especially in the hospital setting with an estimated one third to two thirds of delirium episodes not identified [1]. The recognition of delirium can be delayed by infrequent observation or documentation. Daily cognitive assessment without formal assessments of attention span and fluctuation may give false results. The physicians depend on nursing notes to identify a fluctuating course, and such information may be less than adequate for developing a timely diagnosis.

For this reason, extensive work has been done to establish useful diagnostic approaches for delirium across healthcare settings. The clinical hallmarks of delirium are decreased attention span and a waxing and waning type of confusion. This can be very difficult for clinicians to diagnose because it requires an understanding of a patient's baseline to assess if their current mental state represents an aberration. For example, in our clinical case, Ms. S is clearly not responding to questions the way she normally does, but this could only be understood through taking a close history from her daughter.

The Mini-Cog can be a predictor of in-hospital delirium. At the time of admission to the hospital, if the older adult patient does not have a history of cognitive impairment, the Mini-Cog can be used to identify patients at high risk for in-hospital delirium.

While the Diagnostic and Statistical Manual of Mental Disorders (DSM) outlines detailed criteria for the clinical diagnosis of delirium (◘ Figs. 19.1 and 19.2) [5], extensive work has been done to translate these criteria to a valid and clinically useful assessment tool, the Confusion Assessment Method (CAM) [6].

The CAM was developed through expert translation of the four DSM-III diagnostic criteria: (1) acute onset and fluctuating course, (2) inattention, (3) disorganized thinking, and (4) altered level of consciousness [6]. The CAM was designed to be administered in 5 minutes or less and has

◘ Table 19.1 Differentiating features of delirium and dementia

Features	Delirium	Dementia
Onset	Acute	Insidious
Course	Fluctuating	Progressive
Duration	Days to weeks	Months to years
Consciousness	Altered	Clear
Attention	Impaired	Normal, except in severe dementia
Psychomotor changes	Increased or decreased	Often normal
Reversibility	Usually	Rarely

A. A disturbance in attention (i.e., reduced ability to direct, focus, sustain, and shift attention) and awareness (reduced orientation to the environment).
B. The disturbance develops over a short period of time (usually hours to a few days), represents a change from baseline attention and awareness, and tends to fluctuate in severity during the course of a day.
C. An additional disturbance in cognition (e.g., memory deficit, disorientation, language, visuospatial ability, or perception).
D. The disturbances in Criteria A and C are not better explained by another preexisting, established, or evolving neurocognitive disorder and do not occur in the context of a severely reduced level of arousal, such as coma.
E. There is evidence from the history, physical examination, or laboratory findings that the disturbance is a direct physiological consequence of another medical condition, substance intoxication or withdrawal (i.e., due to a drug of abuse or to a medication), or exposure to a toxin, or is due to multiple etiologies.

◘ Fig. 19.1 DSM-V classification of delirium

1. Acute onset or symptom fluctuation
2. Inattention
3. Disorganized thinking
4. Altered level of consciousness

For diagnosis, must have 1 and 2 as well as either 3 or 4.

Fig. 19.2 Features of delirium assessed in the CAM-S

since been adapted for the intensive care unit (ICU) setting, through the CAM-ICU [7].

The CAM is comprised of ten items assessing delirium. In a systematic review of validation studies of the CAM across multiple clinical settings (ICU, emergency, and institutional), CAM had an overall sensitivity of 94% (95% confidence interval, CI, of 91–97%) and specificity of 89% (95% CI of 85–94%) [8]. A short form of the CAM, called the CAM-S, has four items and has been demonstrated to be as accurate as the CAM in predicting inpatient length of stay, mortality, and odds of nursing home admission within two cohorts of hospitalized older adults [9].

While the CAM is the most widely used assessment instrument for delirium, several others exist. They include the Delirium Symptom Inventory (DSI) and the Intensive Care Delirium Screening Checklist (ICDSC). The DSI contains 107 items, 44 of which are interviewer observations, making it more useful for in-depth research work than clinical applications [10]. The ICDSC, like CAM-ICU, is designed to assess for delirium in the ICU, but it considers observations collected over 8–24 hours. The CAM-ICU takes data gathered from the patient at one point in time [11].

While CAM assesses for the presence of delirium, it is not intended to assess for severity. Delirium symptom severity can be assessed by the Delirium Detection Scale (DDS) and the Memorial Delirium Assessment Scale (MDAS). The MDAS in particular should not be used to diagnose delirium, only to assess for fluctuations in symptoms after a diagnosis has been made as it does not contain all corresponding clinical indicators of delirium, such as the acuity of symptom onset [12].

19.6 The Management of Delirium

19.6.1 Risk Factors

Dementia is one of the strongest most consistent risk factors. Underlying dementia is observed in 25–50% of patients. The presence of dementia increases the risk of delirium 2–3 times. Low educational level, which may be an indicator of low cognitive reserve, is associated with increased vulnerability to delirium.

Other important independent risk factors:

- Use of physical restraints
- Malnutrition
- Use of a bladder catheter
- Any iatrogenic event
- Use of three or more medications
- Unfamiliar environment
- Dysphoric mood and hopelessness

The first critical principle of delirium management is to identify and reverse any contributing factors. The Hospital Elder Life Program has demonstrated great success in reducing delirium in the hospital setting through providing daily visits to stimulate and orient older adults, correct hearing and vision deficits, promote relaxation and nighttime sleep, mobilize older adults, promote good nutrition, and limit polypharmacy. These approaches can be applied across settings of care. Despite every effort, no cause for delirium can be found in some patients. Components of delirium management include supportive therapy and pharmacological management. Fluid and nutrition should be given carefully because the patient may be unwilling or physically unable to maintain a balanced intake.

Almost any medical illness, intoxication, or medication can cause delirium. Often, delirium is multifactorial in etiology, and the physician treating the delirium should investigate each cause contributing to it. Nonreversible factors, such as age, dementia, disability, and recent surgery, increase the risk of delirium.

Medications are the most common reversible cause of delirium. Nearly any medication can potentially contribute to delirium, and polypharmacy (or the total number of medications) is a risk factor for delirium. Some specific classes of medications have been strongly associated with risk of delirium, especially in frail older adults and those with dementia. Also in older adults, medications at therapeutic doses and levels can cause delirium.

Medications at high risk of inducing delirium are the following:

- Anticholinergics, which include histamine blockers like diphenhydramine and hydroxyzine, antispasmotics, diuretics like furosemide, antiarrhythmics such as digoxin, and oxybutynin
- Benzodiazepines and discontinuation of benzodiazepines
- Opioids, especially at high doses or with rapid changes (although untreated pain can also cause delirium)
- Antidepressants and antipsychotics
- Steroids and discontinuation of steroids

Several potentially reversible causes of delirium such as infection and metabolic abnormality may be harbingers of impending critical illness. Therefore, it is critical to assess for these causes.

Metabolic causes:

- Fluid and electrolyte abnormalities, acid-base disturbances, and hypoxia
- Hypoglycemia
- Hepatic or renal failure
- Vitamin deficiency states (especially thiamine and cyanocobalamin)
- Endocrinopathies associated with the thyroid and parathyroid

Infectious causes:
- CNS infections such as meningitis
- Encephalitis
- HIV-related brain infections
- Septicemia
- Pneumonia
- Urinary tract infections

Structural changes:
- Closed head injury or cerebral hemorrhage
- Cerebrovascular accidents, such as cerebral infarction, subarachnoid hemorrhage, and hypertensive encephalopathy
- Primary or metastatic brain tumors
- Brain abscess

Hypoperfusion states:
- Shock
- Congestive heart failure
- Cardiac arrhythmias
- Anemias

Toxic causes:
- Substance intoxication – alcohol, heroin, cannabis, PCP, and LSD
- Substance withdrawal from alcohol, opioids, and benzodiazepines

Operation-related delirium:
- Preoperative (dementia, polypharmacy, fluid and electrolyte imbalance)
- Intraoperative (meperidine, long-acting benzodiazepines, anticholinergics such as atropine; however, medications such as glycopyrrolate can be used because, in contrast to atropine, they do not cross the blood brain barrier)
- Postoperative (hypoxia, hypotension, drug withdrawal)
- Mild cognitive impairment and vascular risk factors can be independent risk factors for postoperative delirium.

Other causes:
- Postictal state
- Hypoxia
- Hyperthermia

19.6.2 History Taking for Patients with Delirium

The diagnosis and management of delirium rests on a thorough history to identify potentially reversible factors that could be contributing. The diagnosis of delirium is clinical, and no laboratory test can diagnose delirium. Obtaining a thorough history is essential. Specific considerations for history-taking for patients with delirium include:
- Because delirious patients often are confused and unable to provide accurate information, getting a detailed history from family, caregivers, and nursing staff is particularly important.
- Some patients with delirium also may become suicidal or homicidal. Therefore, they should not be left unattended or alone.
- Delirium is mistaken for dementia or depression, especially when patients are quiet or withdrawn.
- Depression symptoms are commonly seen with delirium. In a recent study, patients having symptoms of dysphoric mood and hopelessness are at risk for incident delirium while in the hospital [18]. On the other hand, hypoactive delirium may be mistaken for depression. Up to 42% of patients referred to psychiatry services for suspected depressive illness in the hospital may have delirium [19]. Screening for depression in the presence of delirium is quite challenging.
- Delirium develops in a short period of time (within hours), and an acute change in consciousness or difficulty focusing on what was being said could occur during the interview. Disturbance of the sleep-wake cycle with insomnia, daytime drowsiness, or disturbing dreams or nightmares can also occur. Patients are often unable to remember why they are in the hospital or the events that occurred during the delirious period (for most patients, it is like a blackout period).
- Patients may have false beliefs or thinking (misinterpreting intravenous lines as ropes or snakes) or see or hear things that are not present (picking up things in the air or seeing bugs in the bedclothes). Patients may also misjudge their level of wellness and try to elope from the hospital. Emotional disturbances leading to depression, anxiety, fear, and irritability may be seen in some patients. Delirium in hospitalized seniors may result in the self-removal of catheters or intravenous tubing or attempts to get out of bed, resulting in a fall or injury. (◘ Table 19.2)

Specific tests are dependent on the clinical context. For new onset of delirium without an obvious cause (such as clear relationship to a medication), a reasonable testing approach might include:
- Pulse oximetry is used to diagnose hypoxia as a cause of delirium.
- Chest radiograph is used to diagnose pneumonia or congestive heart failure.
- Electrocardiogram is used to diagnose ischemic and arrhythmic causes.
- Complete blood cell count with differential – helpful to diagnose infection and anemia.
- Electrolytes and glucose – electrolyte imbalance, hypoglycemia, diabetic ketoacidosis, and hyperosmolar nonketotic states.
- Renal, thyroid, and liver function tests – to diagnose liver and renal failure, hyper- and hypothyroidism.
- Urine and blood drug screen – used to diagnose toxicological causes.
- Thiamine and vitamin B-12 levels – used to detect deficiency states of these vitamins.
- Tests for bacteriological and viral etiologies – to diagnose infection.

- Brain imaging if any suspicion of brain metastasis, intracranial ischemia, or bleeds.
- Lumbar puncture if any meningism or headache.
- Drug screen including alcohol level.
- Tests for other infectious causes if necessary or clinically indicated. (These tests are not performed routinely, even though 30–40% of hospitalized patients with HIV infection develop delirium during hospitalization.)
- Serum marker for delirium: the calcium-binding protein S-100 B could be a serum marker of delirium. Higher levels are seen in patients with delirium when compared to patients without delirium.

Table 19.2 Reversible causes of delirium: what to look for

Drugs	Prescription drugs: many, detailed above	What new drugs were started in the hours to days before onset?
	Withdrawal from prescription drugs	What drugs were stopped in the hours to days before onset?
	Illicit	Has a detailed alcohol and drug history been taken?
Infection	Urinary, other	Are there any clinical or testing signs of infections? Has urine been tested?
Hospital environment	Sensory disruptions	Does the patient need glasses or hearing aids?
	Sleep/wake cycles	Can the patient be stimulated more during the day?
		Can disruptions in sleep (lab draws, RN care, noise) be reduced?
		Can the patient be moved to a room with a window?
	Tethers	Can urinary catheters or restraints be removed?
	Immobility	Can the patient walk more during the day?
	Care changes	Are healthcare staff trained to reorient delirious patients?
Symptoms	Pain	Is the patient in pain? If they cannot report pain, are they grimacing?
	Constipation	Have bowel movements been regular?
Metabolic abnormality	Electrolyte imbalance	Have labs been checked recently?
	Malnutrition	How has the patient been eating at home?
	Dehydration	Are they drinking?

- Brain electroencephalogram if there is any concern for seizures and to differentiate delirium from psychiatric illness
  - In delirium, generally, slowing of the posterior dominant rhythm and increased generalized slow-wave activity are observed on electroencephalogram (EEG) recordings.
  - In delirium resulting from alcohol/sedative withdrawal, increased EEG fast-wave activity occurs.
  - In patients with hepatic encephalopathy, diffuse EEG slowing occurs.
  - The type of patterns observed includes triphasic waves in toxicity or metabolic derangement, continuous discharges in non-convulsive status epilepticus, and localized delta activity in focal lesions.

19.7 Environmental/Behavioral Approaches to Delirium Treatment

The first step in treatment is to identify potentially reversible causes of delirium and address them (Table 19.3). In particular, it is critical to assess for potential life-threatening causes of delirium such as infection or metabolic abnormalities and promptly address them. Next, assess for new or contributing medications and deprescribe them if they can be avoided.

There are additional measures that can be used to optimize the hospital environment in particular to prevent and treat delirium regardless of cause. The Hospital Elder Life Program (HELP) addresses six common contributing factors to delirium and has been demonstrated to reduce the number of older adults experiencing cognitive decline during hospitalization by more than two thirds and reduce the number experiencing functional decline during hospitalization by more than half [13]. The components of HELP are

Table 19.3 Components of the Hospital Elder Life Program (HELP)

Delirium risk factor	Intervention
Cognitive impairment	Orientation protocol to orient to day/schedule/place
	Cognitively stimulating activities
Sleep disturbance	Bedtime routine protocol
	Quiet environment at night
Immobility	Early mobilization protocol
Visual impairment	Visual aids and adaptive equipment
Hearing impairment	Hearing amplification devices, earwax disimpaction, communication techniques
Dehydration	Protocol for early identification and rehydration

demonstrated in ◘ Table 19.3 and can be routinely applied to hospital and nursing home- based patient care.

Reorientation techniques or memory cues such as a calendar, clocks, and family photos may be helpful. The environment should be stable, quiet, and well-lighted. One study showed a reduction of sound during the night by using earplugs in the ICU setting decreased the risk of delirium by 53% and improved the self-reported sleep perception of the patient for 48 hours. Family members and staff should explain proceedings at every opportunity, reinforce orientation, and reassure the patient. Support from a familiar nurse and family should be encouraged.

Sensory deficits should be corrected, if necessary, with eyeglasses and hearing aids.

Physical restraints should be avoided. Delirious patients may pull out intravenous lines, climb out of bed, and may not be compliant. Perceptual problems lead to agitation, fear, combative behavior, and wandering. Severely delirious patients benefit from constant observation (sitters), which may be cost effective for these patients and help avoid the use of physical restraints. These patients should never be left alone or unattended.

19.8 Pharmacologic Approaches to Delirium

After non-pharmacologic approaches to delirium have failed, several medications may be used to treat delirium. However, all of these medications have significant risks and therefore should only be used once potentially reversible causes of delirium and non-pharmacological approaches have been optimized. No medications have FDA approval for the treatment of delirium and give to the paucity of data on pharmacologic management of delirium; none have strong evidence.

Delirium that causes injury to the patient or others should be treated with medications. The most common medications used are neuroleptics. Benzodiazepines often are used for withdrawal states. Even though case reports showed evidence that cholinesterase inhibitors may play a role in the management of delirium, larger trials and systematic review did not support this use. Summary of evidence of each medication class is below.

19.8.1 Neuroleptics

These are the medication of choice in the treatment of psychotic symptoms. Older neuroleptics such as haloperidol, a high-potency antipsychotic, are useful but have many adverse neurological effects. Newer neuroleptics such as risperidone, olanzapine, and quetiapine relieve symptoms while minimizing adverse effects. Initial doses may need to be higher than maintenance doses. Neuroleptics can be associated with adverse neurological effects such as extrapyramidal symptoms, neuroleptic malignant syndrome, and tardive dyskinesia. Observational data has shown a higher mortality rate for older adults taking neuroleptics, leading to an FDA black box warning. In order to balance the burden and potential benefit of these medications, they should only be initiated in refractory delirium after environmental and behavioral modifications have been made. Doses should be kept as low as possible to minimize adverse effects, and neuroleptics should be tapered as soon as symptoms are under control and discontinued as soon as possible (◘ Table 19.4).

◘ **Table 19.4** Pharmacologic treatment of delirium

Drug	Dosing	Comments
Haloperidol	0.5–2 mg every 2–12 hours. Advised starting dose: 0.5 mg Q8H. Available PO, IV, IM, SC	Concern for QT prolongation and resulting torsades des pointes, extrapyramidal side effects (tardive dyskinesia, neuroleptic malignant syndrome, dyskinesias). Contraindicated in patients with Parkinson's disease. First line of treatment for terminal delirium [15] Equally effective in hypoactive and hyperactive subtypes of delirium [15]. May add lorazepam(0.5–1 mg every 2–4 hours) for agitated patients [15]
Risperidone	Advised starting dose 0.5 mg Q12H. Available as tablet, rapidly dissolving tablet, liquid, IM	EPS with doses >1 mg/day. May have clinical effect in hypoactive delirium, but equally effective in aggressive agitation. Also helpful with psychotic features
Quetiapine	Dose of 25–200 mg daily	Lower risk for EPS, hence choice medication in patients with Parkinson's disease or Lewy Body dementia. May increase risk for hyperglycemia. Eye exam recommended every 6 months to rule out cataract formation
Clomethiazole		For delirium secondary to alcohol withdrawal
Clozapine	12.5–200 mg daily.	Monitor CBC weekly to rule out agranulocytosis. Also watch out for hyperglycemia and myocarditis. Reserved for refractory cases and should not be stopped
Olanzapine	Dose range from 2.5 to 10 mg. Also available as rapidly dissolving tablet and IM injection	Effective against agitated delirium. May be less effective in hypoactive delirium and older age group

19

Delirium as a result of alcohol or drug withdrawal is managed differently than other causes. In this condition, the goal is to prevent progression of alcohol withdrawal to severe symptoms such as seizure and cardiac events. Benzodiazepines are used to control agitation and should be proactively escalated to manage symptoms. Several protocols for such symptom-triggered therapy exist. In addition, correction of any hypovolemia and infusion of thiamine and glucose should be administered to prevent Wernicke's encephalopathy. Correction of vitamins and minerals such as potassium, magnesium, phosphate, and folic acid supplementation are recommended.

19.8.2 Benzodiazepines

Co-administration of benzodiazepines with neuroleptics is considered only in patients who tolerate lower doses of either medication or have prominent anxiety or agitation. Benzodiazepines may also be used when unknown substances may have been ingested and may be helpful in delirium from hallucinogen, cocaine, stimulant, or PCP toxicity. Use special precaution when using benzodiazepines because they may cause respiratory depression, especially in patients who are elderly, those with pulmonary problems, or debilitated patients.

Lorazepam is a preferable benzodiazepine for the treatment of delirium because it is short acting and has no active metabolites. In addition, it can be used in both IM and IV forms. When patients need to be sedated for longer than 24 hours, this medication is excellent and is commonly used prophylactically to prevent delirium tremens. However, lorazepam, like other benzodiazepines, can have a paradoxical effect of causing or worsening delirium [16]. Therefore, their use should be limited to situations where significant sedation is required, for alcohol withdrawal, or in conditions such as Parkinson's or neuroleptic malignant syndrome where antipsychotics are contraindicated [17].

19.8.3 Cyanocobalamin (Crystamine, Cyomin, Nascobal)

Vitamin B-12 deficiency can cause confusion or delirium in patients in older adults. Deoxyadenosylcobalamin and hydroxocobalamin are active forms of vitamin B-12 in humans. Vitamin B-12 is synthesized by microbes but not by humans or plants. Vitamin B-12 deficiency may result from intrinsic factor deficiency (pernicious anemia), partial or total gastrectomy, or diseases of the distal ileum.

Terminal delirium is distinct in that it is caused by irreversible processes, and the risks/benefits of treatments are weighed differently given the short prognosis. Haloperidol is first line for treatment of terminal delirium. A randomized controlled trial compared the addition of lorazepam to haloperidol alone in 58 hospitalized advanced cancer patients. They found that the combination of lorazepam and haloperidol reduced Richmond Agitation-Sedation Scale scores more than haloperidol alone. While the study used doses of 3 mg IV lorazepam and 2 mg IV haloperidol on the onset of delirium, at our institution we have success with 0.5 mg IV lorazepam Q6H and 0.5 mg IV haloperidol Q8H, increasing doses and offering breakthrough doses as needed.

In summary, the probable etiology of Ms. S' confusional state will include delirium tremens, but a work-up to exclude intracranial pathology from recurrent falls will not be unreasonable. Screening for infections, folate, and B-12 deficiency will also be appropriate. Delirium prevention and early recognition key to the control of high cost associated with increased hospital length of stay and morbidity. Non-pharmacologic management remains the treatment of choice.

References

1. Inouye SK. The dilemma of delirium: clinical and research controversies regarding diagnosis and evaluation of delirium in hospitalized elderly medical patients. Am J Med. 1994;97(3):278–88.
2. Ely E, Gautam S, Margolin R, Francis J, May L, Speroff T, et al. The impact of delirium in the intensive care unit on hospital length of stay. Intensive Care Med. 2001;27(12):1892–900.
3. Francis J, Martin D, Kapoor WN. Prospective study of delirium hospitalized elderly. JAMA. 1990;263:1097–101.
4. Inouye SK. Delirium in older persons. N Engl J Med. 2006;354:1157–65. Available from: http://jama.jamanetwork.com/article.aspx?doi=10.1001/jama.2017.12067.
5. American Psychiatric Association. Diagnostic and statistical manual of disorders. 5th ed. Arlington: American Psychiatric Publishing; 2013.
6. Inouye SK, van Dyck C, Alessi C, Balkin S, Siegal A, Horwitz R. Clarifying confusion: the confusion assessment method. A new method for detection of delirium. Ann Intern Med. 1990;113(12):941–8.
7. Ely EW, Inouye SK, Bernard GR, Gordon S, Francis J, May L, Truman B, Speroff T, Gautam S, Margolin R, Hart RP, Robert M. Delirium in mechanically ventilated patients: validity and reliability of the confusion assessment method for the intensive care unit (CAM-ICU). J Am Med Assoc. 2001;286(21):2703–10.
8. Inouye SK, van Dyck CH, Alessi CA, Balkin S, Siegal AP, Horwitz RI. The Confusion Assessment Method (CAM): a systematic review of current usage. Ann Intern Med. 1990;113(12):941–8.
9. Inouye SK, Kosar CM, Tommet D, Schmitt EM, Puelle MR, Saczynski JS, et al. The CAM-S: Development and validation of a new scoring system for delirium severity in 2 cohorts. Ann Intern Med. 2014;160(8):526–33.
10. Rapp CG, Wakefield B, Kundrat M, Mentes J, Tripp-Reimer T, Culp K, et al. Acute confusion assessment instruments: clinical versus research usability. Appl Nurs Res. 2000;13(1):37–45.
11. Brummel NE, Vasilevskis EE, Han JH, Boehm L, Pun BT, Ely EW. Implementing delirium screening in the ICU: secrets to success. Crit Care Med. 2013;41(9):2196–208.
12. Adamis D, Sharma N, Whelan PJP, MacDonald AJD. Delirium scales: a review of current evidence. Aging Ment Health. 2010;14(5):543–55.
13. Inouye SK, Bogardus ST, Baker DI, Leo-Summers L, Cooney LM. The Hospital Elder Life Program: a model of care to prevent cognitive and functional decline in older hospitalized patients. Hospital Elder Life Program. J Am Geriatr Soc. 2000;48(12):1697–706.
14. Breitbart W, Alici Y. Agitation and delirium at the end of life: "We couldn't manage him". JAMA. 2008;300(24):2898–910.

15. Inouye SK. The confusion assessment method (CAM): training manual and coding guide 2003. Boston: Yale University School of Medicine; 2003.
16. American Geriatrics Society 2015 Beers Criteria Update Expert Panel. American Geriatrics Society 2015 updated Beers criteria for potentially inappropriate medication use in older adults. J Am Geriatr Soc. 2015;63:2227–46.
17. Jin YH, Li N, Mu W, Lei X, Si JH, Chen, J, Shang HC. Benzodiazepines for treatment of delirium in non-ICU settings. Cochrine Library. 22 May 2017.

Assessment of Memory and Function

Matthew Majeske

A. Chun (ed.), *Geriatric Practice*, https://doi.org/10.1007/978-3-030-19625-7_20

Case Example

The patient was a 78-year-old woman referred by her primary care physician for evaluation of memory disturbance and possible depression. She was brought to her appointment by her husband who was somewhat younger and still employed. He reported a 2-year history of memory decline with word-finding difficulty and forgetting names of close relatives. She had attended trade school and was a retired secretary who had always been attentive to her appearance with makeup and stylish dress. She had begun to show disinterest in activities that she had always enjoyed, including socializing with friends, playing bridge, and attending theater. On a few occasions, he had come home to observe she had burned a pot on the stove while trying to prepare a meal. She had given up on crossword puzzles as she found them mentally taxing and spent most of her time watching television. On two occasions, she had become lost in the neighborhood after she had gone out shopping. Her husband was anxious to leave her alone and had begun to experience headaches. Her medical history was significant for gastroesophageal reflux disease and osteoarthritis. The patient had no prior psychiatric history. There was a family history of dementia in her mother. She was of normal height and weight, and her physician reported an unremarkable physical and neurologic examination.

On mental status examination, she was an alert elderly female casually dressed albeit somewhat disheveled with her hair askew and malodorous. She was alert and made good eye contact with the examiner. She was oriented to place, person, and time. She could remember one of three objects after 5 minutes. Asked to subtract 7's from 100, she responded 93, 85, 77, 70, and 63. She could identify the president but not the vice-president, governor, or mayor. She was unable to interpret the proverb "you can't judge a book by its cover…" She reported a normal mood but had a flattened affect. Her replies tended to be brief and unelaborated. She denied hallucinations and no delusions were elicited. She denied suicidal thoughts. When asked to draw a clock showing 11:10, her drawing skewed numbers to the right and lacked proportion. On the Mini-Mental State Exam (MMSE), she scored 20 points out of a possible 30. Case formulation is below.

Cognitive assessment is essential to the geriatric patient. The incidence of neurocognitive disorder rises steeply with age. For example, the prevalence of dementia among individuals 65 years old is 1–2%, rising to 30% among 85-year-old individuals [1]. Delirium may be the only indication of an occult medical condition, e.g., urinary tract infection. Hence, it behooves any clinician treating the elderly to have an approach to cognitive assessment. In this chapter, I review history-taking, the mental status examination, and some standardized instruments that form the basis of the cognitive assessment of older adults.

The *Diagnostic and Statistical Manual of Mental Disorders, 5th Edition* (DSM-5) identifies six neurocognitive domains that form the basis of assessment [1]. These include complex attention, executive function, learning and memory, language, perceptual/motor, and social cognition. Throughout the clinical interview, mental status exam, and the use of standardized instruments, all of these domains should be explored to form a composite impression of the patient. They help differentiate between delirium, mild, and major neurocognitive disorders. The neurocognitive disorders are a decline from a previous level of functioning, in contrast to learning and developmental disorders, which were established early in life. DSM-5 allows for the use of the term dementia, the equivalent of major neurocognitive disorder. The change in nomenclature was established to reflect more accurately the continuum between mild and major forms of cognitive dysfunction, such as is observed in the progression of mild cognitive impairment to dementia, characteristic of Alzheimer's disease.

The clinical interview forms the cornerstone of cognitive assessment. There are a few principles to keep in mind when initially approaching an elderly patient. Because of cognitive and sensory issues (e.g., hearing loss, visual impairment), you may need to proceed more slowly; speak slowly and allow more time for the patient to absorb the information and respond [2]. Maintain good eye contact. A reliable informant and corroborating information are important as many patients may be cautious as to what they reveal to a physician or not remember important details. For this reason, many patients will come to appointments with spouses, family members, or caregivers.

Take note of the appearance of the patient. Does he appear alert and able to attend to the interview? Or is he distractable and unable to answer questions meaningfully? Does the patient apprehend he is visiting a physician for a medical interview? How is his hygiene and is there evidence of self-neglect? Is he properly dressed? Do you observe mismatched clothing, e.g., wearing a heavy coat in hot weather? Is there evidence of agitation (hand-wringing, inability to sit still)?

Elicit a chief complaint. Inquire as to any difficulties with executive functioning, for example, shopping, preparing a meal, and filing income taxes. Is the patient able to formulate, plan, and see through to completion a task? Is there a complaint of memory impairment? Does the patient recall recent events or repeat himself during the interview? It should be noted that cognitive norms can be challenging for individuals of especially high or low educational attainment, due to the presence or absence of cognitive reserve. Typically, elderly individuals with dementia will retain remote memories (e.g., who was president during World War II, autobiographical details) but struggle to form new ones. Does the patient need frequent reminders? Is he able to keep track of lists?

Are there any difficulties with language? Does the patient have word-finding difficulty? Are there grammatical errors in his speech, does he use general rather than specific terms? *Aphasia* is the inability to understand language (receptive aphasia) or to express oneself (expressive aphasia) and is a hallmark of neurocognitive disorders. Is the patient able to dress himself, operate a motor vehicle, use tools and implements? *Apraxia*, also a feature of neurocognitive impairment, is defined as the loss of ability to execute or carry out learned purposeful movements, despite having the desire and physical ability. Does the patient recognize familiar objects and persons? *Agnosia* is the loss of ability to recognize objects, persons, sounds, and smells.

Evaluate social cognition. Does the patient observe social norms and conventions? Is he aware of the feelings of others? Does he stray into topics likely to cause discomfort for others, for example, religion, politics, or sexuality, despite negative feedback? Are decisions taken without regard to risk or safety? Is there evidence of apathy and social withdrawal?

While this chapter focuses on cognition, it should be appreciated that psychiatric symptoms are inextricable from neurocognitive disorders. Mood disturbance is common and many patients will become depressed or apathetic. Inquire about sadness, irritability, or crying spells. Disturbance of the sleep wake cycle is often reported with patients awake and active in the middle of the night, at times with pacing and agitation. Hallucinations, or sensory stimuli without an external stimulus, may be reported, and visual hallucinations are a hallmark of Lewy body dementia and dementia associated with Parkinson's disease. Patients may become paranoid, attributing malign intentions to loved ones or accusing others of stealing funds. Occasionally, patients with dementia report that his spouse is having an affair or an imposter. Some patients with neurocognitive disorder will have preexisting mental illness; however, when psychiatric symptoms occur de novo in old age, neurocognitive impairment is the likely cause.

It is also crucial to assess suicidal thinking in patients with neurocognitive disorder. Some who retain insight into their condition may have a catastrophic reaction. All patients should be asked whether they would wish to be dead, followed by questions about suicidal thoughts, prior attempts, intention, and plan. Occasionally, patients become disinhibited and pose a risk of violence. Any patient with a history of violence or aggression should be queried about such feelings at present. Evaluate the means to carry out such actions, e.g., possession of firearms, hoarded supplies of medication for overdose.

Intact cognition is the underpinning of all daily activities (ADLs), and cognitive decline will reveal itself as these activities become more difficult to negotiate. The history should include questions regarding basic ADLs and instrumental ADLs. Basic ADLs will include dressing and bathing, whereas instrumental ADLs would include grocery shopping and financial management. Functional status becomes especially important because cognitive impairment puts patients at risk for a variety of negative outcomes, including car accidents, mishaps with cooking and firearms, falls, medication noncompliance, fraud, abuse, poor decisions, undue influence related to finances, health, sexual consent, and legal contracts [3]. An inquiry into the patient's functioning rounds out the history that becomes invaluable for treatment planning and working with families. It is also the basis of delineating mild versus major neurocognitive disorder. In mild illness, functioning is preserved but may require compensatory strategies (greater effort, time); in major illness, functioning is adversely effected and such strategies are ineffective (■ Table 20.1).

■ Table 20.1 ADLs and IADLs

Activities of daily living (ADLs)	Instrumental activities of daily living (IADLs)
Able to ambulate inside and outside the home	Meal preparation
Bathing	Maintain bank account, balance checkbook
Dressing	Shopping
Self -hygiene, e.g., brushes teeth	Driving, using public transport

Other aspects of the history will be relevant in determining the diagnosis. Time course can distinguish delirium from dementia. If the neurocognitive disorders can be thought of as syndromes of brain failure, delirium is generally acute whereas dementia is chronic. While there are chronic forms of delirium, the typical presentation will be an acute mental status change as a result of a medical condition or substance intoxication or withdrawal. Symptoms of delirium fluctuate and resolve as the underlying disturbance clears. Dementia by contrast is generally chronic and slowly evolving with persisting deficits. The diagnoses are not mutually exclusive; patients with pre-existing dementia are at greater risk for developing a superimposed delirium.

Social history can elicit important information. Neurocognitive disorders require a decline from a previous level, and so an understanding of premorbid functioning is required. Educational attainment, literacy, and occupational history provide a frame of reference for the patient's current mental state. Some patients will have cultural and language barriers that may adversely affect their performance on the interview, e.g., a lack of familiarity with English proverbs or local politics. A family history of dementia is common in patients with dementia.

It will be apparent from the discussion so far that the mental status examination begins with history-taking. How the patient appears and interacts with the examiner initiates the formal mental status. Is the patient alert and able to engage? Or does he appear unduly sedated or hyper-aroused, unable to attend to and engage in the interview? A clear sensorium is a distinguishing feature between delirium and dementia. Serial 7's (or serial 3's for lower educational attainment) are a good method of evaluating alertness and attention span. Orientation questions are an essential feature of basic cognitive functioning, without which one can rapidly identify neurocognitive impairment. Can the patient state his name, where he is, the month, year, and date? At the outset of the exam, provide the patient with three disparate objects (e.g., apple, honesty, and eyedropper) and ask him to repeat. After a suitable interval (3–4 minutes) during which he is distracted by other questions, ask him to recall the three objects. If the patient is unable to remember, provide a clue. Highly characteristic of dementia is the ability to register items at first but be unable to retain them after a delay. Questions about current events can evaluate recent memory. Ask the patient to discuss recent items in the news, or to name the presidents in reverse order, or identify local politicians. In addition to recent memory, these questions can provide a gauge of intelligence. Vague, nonspecific answers can indicate impairment. During the interview, the examiner will be observing the patient's ability to understand and express language. A task to probe the presence of aphasia is to ask the patient to write a sentence on a piece of paper. Object naming or asking the patient to close his eyes and identify a set of keys placed in his hand will assess the presence of agnosia.

Apraxia can be assessed by asking the patient to imitate a particular motor task, for example "show me what it would look like to beat eggs or wind a watch." Executive function can be probed by asking the patient to carry out a multi-step complex motor task, as in "pick up this piece of paper with your right hand, fold it in half, and put it on the floor." Asking the patient to interpret a proverb is a test of the ability to abstract, a higher cognitive function, and also receptive and expressive language.

Psychiatric symptoms must also be evaluated, as they are intricate parts of several neurocognitive disorders. Frontotemporal dementia frequently features behavior symptoms such as disinhibition or apathy; Lewy body dementia and Parkinson's dementia frequently manifest visual hallucinations. Mood disturbance, particularly depression, is common in the early phase of Alzheimer's dementia; agitation, wandering, and psychotic symptoms may develop in the later stages. Hence, a thorough mental status exam will inquire into psychiatric symptoms. Mood refers to the prevailing feeling state of the patient (sadness, depression, euphoria) whereas affect describes the transient feeling state that exists from 1 minute to the next. Descriptors of affect include labile, tearful, euphoric, blunted, flat, or full range. Hallucinations are sensory experiences without an external stimulus and may manifest in any of the sensory modalities, including auditory, visual, olfactory, gustatory, and tactile. Delusions are fixed and false beliefs that commonly appear in dementia, such as the belief that one's deceased spouse is alive, or that others are intent on stealing the patient's funds. Other disorders of thought content may be perseveration, the tendency to repeat oneself as prior statements are forgotten. The thought process of patients with neurocognitive disorder may become impoverished due to aphasia, with sentences that are brief, unelaborated, or vague. Psychomotor activity should be commented upon. Is the patient calm or agitated? Is there evidence of marked slowing, as in psychomotor retardation?

How is the patient's attitude toward the examiner? Does he apprehend that he is being examined by a physician? Is there undue familiarity or flirtatiousness? Is the patient hostile and guarded? These observations can illuminate social cognition, the understanding of social context and inhibitory mechanisms that can fray in dementia.

There are several rating instruments that can be employed in the assessment of memory and function. They provide a standardized, quantifiable assessment that reduces subjectivity in the evaluation. As discussed above, norms can be challenged by patients with especially low or high educational attainment, illiteracy, or cultural and language barriers. The elderly can also have sensory barriers with hearing or visual impairment.

The Mini-Mental State Exam (MMSE) is the most commonly used bedside scale. It measures basic orientation, ability to recall three objects after a delay, and copying a figure among other items. The MMSE is most helpful in distinguishing normal individuals from those with dementia. It lacks the sensitivity to distinguish normal individuals from those with mild cognitive impairment. It also lacks sensitivity in detecting cognitive impairment in individuals with higher education. There are a total of 30 possible points. 7–12 errors will indicate mild-to-moderate impairment; 13 or more errors will indicate severe impairment.

The clock drawing test is another commonly used measure. The patient is asked to draw a clock indicating a particular time, for example, 11:10. This test measures memory, visual-spatial cognition, and executive functioning. An abnormal test may reveal a lack of anchoring of the numbers or the hands of the clock. The clock drawing test is helpful in distinguishing cognitively normal individuals from those with mild neurocognitive disorder. An abnormal clock, for example, can be observed in patients who otherwise score in the normal range on the MMSE.

The Mini-Cog is a modification of the clock drawing test in that it adds to the drawing the ability to remember three objects after a several minute delay. It helps distinguish older adults with normal cognition from those with dementia. Dementia would be indicated by remembering 0/3 objects at 3 minutes or remembering 1–2 objects at 3 minutes with an abnormal clock drawing.

The Montreal Cognitive Assessment (MoCA) is a more demanding screen. Difficulty is enhanced by the addition of a trails-making task, clock drawing, and copying a figure. By its nature, the MoCA is designed to elicit mild cognitive impairment. The Confusion Assessment Method (CAM) is an algorithm for identifying delirium, derived from the diagnostic criteria, which probes the presence of (1) acute and fluctuating course, (2) inattention, (3) disorganized thinking, and (4) altered level of consciousness. The diagnosis of delirium is established by the presence of (1) and (2) plus either (3) or (4) (◘ Table 20.2).

Returning to the case example, the most likely diagnosis is major neurocognitive disorder (dementia) of the Alzheimer's type. This is the most common type of dementia, comprising 50–75% of all cases. A number of features in the case example point to this formulation. The patient had experienced a gradual decline in memory functioning over a several year period. She is elderly (78), and age is the greatest risk factor for the disease. In addition to memory decline, she exhibited other cognitive impairments, including language (word finding difficulty), executive functioning (inability to safely prepare a meal), and visual-spatial (getting lost in her

Table 20.2 Cognitive screens summary [4–7]

Cognitive screens	Validation	Pros	Cons
MMSE	<24 indicates impairment	Widely used	Not sensitive to MCI
Clock drawing	Varies by scoring	Brief and easy to use	Low specificity
Mini-cog	Algorithm distinguishes demented vs. normal	More sensitive than MMSE	Not sensitive to MCI
MOCA	<26 indicates impairment	More sensitive to MCI	Lacks empirical support as screening tool for MCI

Adapted from Mitchell and Atri [3], p. 474–482

neighborhood). She exhibited behavior changes commonly seen in dementia, e.g., apathy and withdrawal from formerly engaged activities (playing bridge, attending theater). Her presentation revealed a decline in social cognition; formerly, she had always been well groomed and attentive to her appearance, whereas now she was disheveled and did not bathe regularly.

Her mental status examination revealed impairments consistent with dementia. She was able to remember only one of three objects after a delay, and memory disturbance is the hallmark of Alzheimer's dementia. Her inability to perform serial 7's revealed a disturbance in working memory and concentration; one would anticipate with her educational background an ability to perform the task. Her form of thought had become impoverished with an inability to recall basic information such as the identity of local politicians.

The history of cognitive decline was supported by the use of standardized instruments (MMSE, clock-drawing) which revealed impairment. An MMSE score of 20/30 qualifies for at least moderate impairment, and her clock figure revealed visual-spatial and executive-functioning deficits. The cognitive decline qualified for *major* neurocognitive disorder as opposed to mild, based on clear impairment in functioning. In mild disease, functional impairment can be muted with the use of compensatory strategies (e.g., reminder lists, prompts) that this patient now lacked. The patient was alert and had a clear sensorium, and hence delirium was unlikely. A family history of dementia is noted. The patient had no prior psychiatric history, suggesting that her symptoms were most likely due to neurodegenerative disorder rather than a psychiatric illness such as depression.

The case also illustrates the value of having a family informant, as the patient would have been unlikely to remember many details. The husband also is showing signs of caregiver stress, a common scenario in dementia. The disabled patient requires more and more supervision and oversight over time. While Alzheimer's disease is the most common form of dementia, there are other types such as vascular, frontotemporal, Lewy body, and dementia associated with Parkinson's disease. These are deemed unlikely in this case presentation owing to the lack of cardiovascular risk factors that attend vascular dementia (history of stroke, heart disease, hypertension, or diabetes with neurologic impairment). Lewy body or Parkinson's dementia would be expected to reveal the motor symptoms of Parkinson's (slowed movements, tremor) and possibly visual hallucinations. With frontotemporal dementia, one might anticipate an earlier age of onset with a more psychiatric presentation (behavioral disinhibition) and relative sparing of memory function.

Much of the management of this case would lie with marshaling resources and family education. As such, the management of dementia involves care coordination between various disciplines, including primary care, social work, and psychiatry, among others. Her husband would be encouraged to obtain home care to provide supervision and oversight of the patient as well as respite for him. Caregiver support can be accessed through community organizations. The patient would benefit from neuropsychological testing to flesh out the full extent of her impairments. She would be discouraged from cooking, driving, or going out in public alone. As the case illustrates, safety considerations become paramount as demented patients may lack the judgment to navigate risky situations such as driving, cooking, and use of firearms. Consideration would be given to the initiation of a cholinesterase inhibitor such as donepezil to delay the progression of cognitive decline. Behavioral activation might be considered to preserve function for as long as possible.

Putting it all together, the history, mental status examination, and cognitive testing instruments, based on the clinical interview, are the foundation of the assessment of cognition and function. All three elements will probe the patient's level of attention, memory, use of language, perceptual/ motor and social cognition, and executive functioning. An in-depth history will reveal the extent to which neurocognitive impairment impairs function to distinguish between mild and major forms of neurocognitive disorder. As these three elements are elaborated in the clinical interview, case formulation and diagnosis come into focus and allow for treatment, provision of services, and safety planning.

References

1. American Psychiatric Association. Neurocognitive disorders. In: Diagnostic and statistical manual of mental disorders. 5th ed. Arlington: American Psychiatric Association; 2013. p. 591–643.
2. Blazer DG. The psychiatric interview of older adults. In: Thakur ME, Blazer DG, Steffens DC, editors. Clinical manual of geriatric psychiatry. Washington, DC: American Psychiatric Press; 2014. p. 1–15.
3. Mitchell MB, Atri A. Dementia screening and mental status examination in clinical practice. In: Dickerson B, Atri A, editors. Dementia: comprehensive principles and practice. New York: Oxford University Press; 2014. p. 461–86.
4. Folstein MF, Folstein SE, McHugh PR. Mini-mental state. J Psychiatr Res. 1975;12(3):189–98.
5. Borson S, Scanlan J, Brush M, Vitaliano P, Dokmak A. The mini-cog: a cognitive vital signs measure for dementia screening in multi-lingual elderly. Int J Geriatr Psychiatry. 2000;15(11):1021–7.
6. Nasreddine ZS, Phillips NA, Bedirian V, Charbonneau S, Whitehead V, Collin I, Chertkow H. The Montreal Cognitive Assessment, MoCA: a brief screening tool for mild cognitive impairment. J Am Geriatric Soc. 2005;53(4):695–9.
7. Huang LW, Inouye SK. Delirium. In: Thakur ME, Blazer DG, Steffens DC, editors. Clinical manual of geriatric psychiatry. Washington, DC: American Psychiatric Press; 2014. p. 83–97.

Nonpharmacological Management of BPSD: Agitation and Behavioral Problems in Dementia

Christine Chang

A. Chun (ed.), *Geriatric Practice*, https://doi.org/10.1007/978-3-030-19625-7_21

21.1 Competency

Cognitive and Behavioral Disorders #8: Develop an evaluation and nonpharmacological management plan for agitated demented or delirious patients.

21.1.1 How Would You Approach This Case?

Case

You are seeing Mrs. Ava Smith, a 72-year-old with mild Alzheimer's disease (MMSE 21 of 30), hypertension, osteoarthritis, and urinary incontinence who comes to the office with her daughter for "acting up" for past 2 weeks. Daughter reports that she repeats stories and packs her bags, stating that she is "going home." She is up frequently at night, pacing and wandering. The other day, she punched her home attendant.

Medications: donepezil 5 mg daily, hydrochlorothiazide 25 mg daily, lisinopril 10 mg daily, baby aspirin, tolterodine LA 2 mg, and acetaminophen 500 mg once daily.

21.1.1.1 Background

Over 5.4 million Americans [1] over age 65 years and nearly 50 million persons worldwide [2] are afflicted with Alzheimer's disease in 2012. As of 2013, Alzheimer's disease (AD) is the fifth leading cause of death in Americans aging ≥65 years [1]. Dementia presents as a gradual global decline in both cognitive and physical abilities that often leads to the development of "agitation" and other distressing neuropsychiatric symptoms of dementia (NPSD) or behavioral and psychological symptoms of dementia (BPSD) [43]. Caregivers identify BPSD as one of the most challenging and distressing aspects of care [25, 44]. The presence of BPSD, especially physical aggression, is a leading cause of nursing home placement [68]. These behaviors can have an immense impact on the quality of life of both the patient and the caregiver [25, 44]. This chapter has been created to help care providers have a structured approach to the evaluation and management of BPSD.

What Is BPSD (Behavioral and Psychological Symptoms of Dementia)?

BPSD is the *noncognitive* manifestations of dementia. They encompass both behavioral and psychological symptoms of dementia ([39]; Table 21.1). These behavioral symptoms are often labeled as "agitation" and can be characterized as either aggressive or nonaggressive and verbal or physical. Common agitation episodes include verbal outbursts, hitting, and biting and tend to occur during personal care activities—often related to "resistiveness" to care. The psychological symptoms of BPSD include mood and psychotic symptoms as well as sleep disturbances. Common mood symptoms include depression, apathy, anxiety, as well as irritability, euphoria, and disinhibition. Delusions and hallucination are not infrequent psychotic symptoms suffered by those with dementia. These neuropsychiatric symptoms in Alzheimer's disease and other types of dementia are extremely common and are often much more troubling than amnestic symptoms. It is known that 80–90% of patients with dementia develop at least one distressing symptom during the course of illness, often related to disease progression [12, 63]. Lifetime risk of developing any neuropsychiatric symptom is nearly 100%.

Table 21.1 Behavioral and Psychological Symptoms of Dementia (BPSD) is the noncognitive manifestations of dementia

Behavioral	Psychological
"Agitation" Often related to resistiveness to care	Mood symptoms Depression, anxiety, apathy, euphoria, irritability, disinhibition
Physical vs verbal	Psychotic symptoms Hallucinations, delusions
Aggressive vs nonaggressive Verbal outburst, hitting, biting, vs pacing, wandering, hoarding	Sleep disturbances

They encompass both behavioral and psychological symptoms of dementia as outlined below [39]

21.2 Understanding Pathophysiology of BPSD

Neurodegeneration and neuronal apoptosis, especially in the right hemisphere and right frontal lobe, are associated with social and emotional dysregulation and decline in emotional control or motivation [61]. These changes can contribute to anxiety and can manifest as emotional lability, characterized by involuntary episodes of laughing, crying, anguish, or other emotional displays [4, 31]. Anxiety can cause agitation which can lead to aggressive "agitated behaviors" (such as verbal outbursts, combativeness, and other resistive behaviors) as well as nonaggressive "agitated behaviors" (such as wandering and pacing) [12]. Professionals and families must realize that BPSD is *NOT* intentional and is the results of neurocognitive degeneration.

21.3 Approach to Evaluating New or Worsening BPSD

BPSD can arise from a variety of underlying causes in patients with dementia, so identifying the precipitating etiology of the BPSD is critical to effective management. Formal evaluation requires a comprehensive history, physical exam and investigation for the possible underlying etiologies. Always systematically look for reversible causes of BPSD as they are more readily treatable than progression of the dementia (◘ Fig. 21.1). First, obtain a history with clear description of the disruptive "behavior" from the patient and others. Details about the temporal onset, course, and associated circumstance with relationship to key environmental factors in context of the patient's medical, family, and social history can be helpful. Questions to assess for organic causes of delirium (► Appendix 1) as well as common environmental precipitants are important. Acute organic conditions (including new infections, ischemia, electrolyte or endocrine derangements, pain, and even constipation) and medication toxicity can trigger BPSD. In addition, the environment can precipitate BPSD when basic physical needs are not met or with disruptions in the usual routine of the caregiving environment. Over and under stimulation and a new, stressed, or sick caregiver can provoke BPSD as can pain, fear, confusion, or poor sleep. After medical, environmental, and caregiving causes are excluded, it can be concluded that the primary cause for the BPSD is progression of the dementia.

New or Worsening BPSD

↓

Determine the cause of the BPSD
History

Obtain clear description of the behavior from the patient and collateral sources

1. **Assess and treat for organic causes of delirium such as:**
   a. **Acute medical conditions** such as infections (i.e. pneumonia, diarrhea, cellulitis, and UTI), endocrine and electrolyte derangements, angina/heart failure, pain and constipation.

   b. **Medication toxicity or adverse effects of new or existing medications.**
   High-risk medications include psychotropics, opioid pain medications and anticholinergics. Even chronic medications can cause toxicity when patients become dehydrated and septic.

2. **Assess for Environmental causes that commonly precipitate BPSD such as:**
   a. **Unmet physical needs** (i.e. hunger, thirst, fatigue, cold, hot, pain, incontinence)

   b. **Known environmental precipitants** such as:
   - **Disruption in routine** This can occur with a new, sick or stressed caregiver or time zone changes
   - **Overstimulation** (crowded and noisy environments) may cause a patient to become agitated
   - **Understimulation** may cause boredom and sleep disturbances

   After medical, environmental, and care giving causes are excluded, it can be concluded that the primary cause is progression of the dementia

↓

Physical Exam

- Perform a comprehensive physical examination to help identify any organic cause of BPSD (i.e. look for signs of dehydration, infections, heart failure, pain, constipation)

- Assess Mental Status and rule out **DELIRIUM via CONFUSION ASSESSMENT METHOD** (Inouye 2003) (See Appendix 1)
  Pay attention to:
  - Appearance and Behavior
  - Speech
  - Mood, Thoughts and Perceptions
  - Cognitive Function
  - Attention

↓

Lab Testing for all new cases of BPSD should include:

- CBC, electrolytes, calcium, and drug levels (when applicable)
- Brain imaging, EKG, Chest XR, urinalysis and other studies should be based on history and examination

◘ **Fig. 21.1** Approach to evaluating new or worsening BPSD

Next, perform a comprehensive physical examination to help identify any organic cause of BPSD. Be sure to look for signs of dehydration, infections, stroke, heart failure, pain, and constipation. Assess neurological and mental status to rule out delirium via Confusion Assessment Method [28] (▶ Appendix 1). Pay attention to the patient's appearance and behavior, speech, mood, thoughts and perceptions, cognitive function, and attention. Lab testing for all new cases of BPSD should include CBC with differential, electrolytes, calcium, and drug levels (when applicable). Brain imaging, EKG, chest X-ray, urinalysis, and other studies should be based on history and examination.

21.4 Treatment Options for BPSD

All guidelines for the management of BPSD recommend treating the underlying organic precipitant to BPSD and, concomitantly, using nonpharmacological interventions first unless harmful to self or others [3, 14, 18, 22, 29, 37, 46, 51, 60, 62, 81].

21.4.1 Why?

- 40% of BPSD symptoms *spontaneously* resolve; "they come and go."
- Most behaviors do not respond to pharmacological treatment as medication does not address the underlying trigger or pathophysiology.
- Placebo response can be quite substantial for any psychotropic medication.
- No FDA-approved medications for psychosis in AD, and antipsychotics are associated with the Black Box warning (▶ Appendix 2).

Since BPSD presents differently in each individual with dementia, treatment and symptom management should be individualized [30]. Care for the patient with dementia should be patient centered and initially focus on nonpharmacological strategies before relying on pharmacological therapies. Several studies demonstrate that nonpharmacological interventions can decrease BPSD and improve caregiver well-being with fewer side effects when compared with pharmacological therapies. Available comprehensive caregiver education programs commonly teach caregivers about three key concepts:

1. Dementia—the disease, its prognosis, and having realistic expectations
2. General and symptom-targeted patient-centered techniques to *minimize* the development of BPSD (see ▶ Box 21.1)
3. General and symptom-targeted strategies to deal with *present* BPSD and *prevent* future episodes of BPSD (▶ Box 21.2)

The nonpharmacological and pharmacological strategies discussed can be divided into "general" recommendations that help most BPSD symptoms and "symptom-targeted" recommendations that help mitigate distressing mood, psychotic symptom, and sleep-related BPSD symptoms. Common target symptoms include aggression, agitation, insomnia, as well as depression, psychosis, mania, and hypersexuality. Nonpharmacological strategies tend to work better for the former symptoms (aggression, agitation, insomnia) and for less severe forms of the latter. Pharmacologics can be used for persistent, severe, and harmful aggression, mood, and psychotic symptoms. These nonpharmacological strategies will be reviewed below.

21.4.2 Practical "General" Nonpharmacological Tips for Caregivers to Manage BPSD (see ▶ Boxes 21.1 and 21.2)

In addition to understanding the natural history and progression of dementia, caregivers should be educated on what to do should their loved one develops BPSD. Caregivers should be familiar with patient-centered techniques to minimize development of BPSD (see ▶ Box 21.1) and feel comfortable implementing strategies to deal with present BPSD and prevent future episodes of BPSD (▶ Box 21.2).

21.4.3 "General" Patient-Centered Nonpharmacological Techniques to Minimize Development of BPSD (see ▶ Box 21.1)

There are five goals of care when it comes to managing dementia symptoms in older adults. Patients with dementia should experience a sense of control, safety, comfort, pleasure, and feel minimal stress [27]. Recognizing the patient as an individual and meeting their need for identity, occupation, comfort, and companionship can enhance self-worth and reduce BPSD [27]. This is best accomplished by establishing a daily routine of meaningful activities so the resident feels comfortable in their daily activities in a safe, orienting, comfortable environment. Predictability of daily routines is often reassuring and less anxiety provoking. Encouraging patients to independently perform ADLs under supervision for as long as possible ensures autonomy and pride. This may require correction of sensory impairments and simplifying or setting up activities of daily living (ADL) routines to maximize the chance of success. When patients require assistance with their ADLs and instrumental ADLs, caregivers need to make sure that these tasks are completed in a patient-centered manner. Bathing is a problematic area for many. Often agitation and aggression arises when personal care is performed in an insistent, intrusive, impersonal, and task-focused manner. Using a patient-centered approach to bathing that creates a bathing environment focused on patient's comfort and preferences can minimize the development of BPSD [65, 79, 80].

Box 21.1 "General" Patient-Centered Nonpharmacological Techniques to Minimize Development of BPSD

1. **Maintain a structured daily routine** of meaningful activities. Predictability of daily routines is often reassuring and less anxiety provoking
   - **Encourage independence in ADLs**
     - Correct sensory impairments
     - Simplify routines, set up, limit choices
     - Consider finger foods and use of pullovers, velcro, and snaps when feeding and dressing apraxias develop
   - **Perform all ADL/IADLs in a patient-centered manner—especially personal care**
     - Brushing hair and hand massages can be soothing
     - Person-centered showers and towel baths [65, 79, 80] Suggests the following:
       - Create environment based on patient comfort and preference
       - Cover with towels to maintain warmth and modesty
       - Use no-rinse soap and warm water
       - Use gentle massage to cleanse
       - Modify shower spray
   - **Incorporate purposeful therapeutic activities in your structured daily routine.** Activities can include daily exercise ([49]; [72]; [77]), pet [45], art, music [15], and other structured activity therapies
   - **Ensuring adequate sleep** (see ▶ Box 21.3)
2. **Environmental modifications**
   - Keep environment safe, comfortable, and orienting
   - Home-like, familiar surroundings with photos/personal items, and recorded familiar voices will maximize existing cognitive functions via reminiscence therapy [70, 71]
   - Maintain conspicuous displays of clocks and calendars. Links to the outside world through newspapers, radios, and televisions may benefit some mildly impaired patients
   - Have preferred familiar music playing in the background [15]
   - Employ soothing aroma therapy. Lavender on pillow or lotion to skin. Diffusions of *Lavandula angustifolia* or sunflower [57]
   - Bright light therapy to encourage proper sleep-wake cycles and help with sundowning
3. **Behavioral management techniques**
   - **Communication techniques** [41]:
     - Smile
     - Speak slowly, clearly, in nonconfrontational manner. Use a calm and positive tone
     - Simple sentence structure and one-step directions
     - Repeated reminders about conversation content may enhance communication
     - Allow adequate time for response
   - **Memory stimulation**
     - **Reminiscence therapy** ([70]; [71])
     - Familiar environment with personal items like photos, videos, recording of familiar voices and belonging
   - **Sensory stimulation**
     - **Visual:** Personal photos and belongings
     - **Auditory:** Familiar, preferred music (listening vs group activities) [15]
     - **Olfactory:** Lavender, *Lavandula angustifolia* or sunflower, patchouli, rosemary, peppermint [57]
     - **Gustatory:** Offer simple choices and finger foods
     - **Tactile** [13, 47, 76]: touch, massage, stroking, brushing hair, hand massage, hand-under-hand technique [74] and pet-assisted ([45]; [48])

******Physical restraints should be avoided***

Box 21.2 Strategies to Deal with Present BPSD and to Prevent Future Episodes of BPSD

For agitation or aggression that is *NOT* harmful to self or others, use behavioral interventions

1. **Identify precipitating factors and avoid the triggers**
   - Be a sleuth: Do the "ABC's" and avoid triggers—look at the Antecedent Behaviors that lead to a particular Catastrophic Consequence and avoid **it.** Identify the precipitating factor and avoid the triggers
   - Address unmet needs: Make sure that basic needs are met. Patients may "act out" when they are unable to communicate their needs. For example, hunger, thirst, and incontinence can lead to BPSD as well as pain and boredom
2. **Avoid confronting patient about unwanted behaviors, instead use 3 R's (repeat, reassure, and redirect)**
   - Positive reinforcement (by praising, encouraging, or reassuring) to encourage desirable behaviors (Skinner's Operant and Pavlov's Classical conditioned learned responses [66])
   - Redirection-distraction techniques

Physical restraints should be avoided!

"Symptom-targeted" patient-centered nonpharmacological techniques
Adapted from ([3, 5, 7, 8, 9, 14, 18, 19, 20, 23, 24, 26, 27, 29, 31, 34, 35, 37, 42, 50, 51, 55, 60, 62, 65, 67, 73, 81]). ([3, 5, 7, 8, 12, 14, 18, 19, 20, 23, 24, 26, 27, 29–32, 34, 35, 37, 41, 42, 50, 51, 55, 59, 60, 62, 65, 67, 69, 73, 77, 81])

As caregivers plan out their itinerary of structured daily routines, it is important that they remember to incorporate purposeful therapeutic activities that employ behavioral techniques such as memory and sensory stimulation which can improve patient quality of life as well as reduce BPSD. Activities can include daily exercise, sleep and rest, reminiscence [70, 71], pet [45], art, music [15], and other structured activity therapies (see ▶ Box 21.1).

Exercise is important for maintaining physical health, cognition and sleep in all older adults and in patients with dementia. Exercise programs can consist of multiple components, such as daily sessions of aerobic, balance, resistance, and walking. Exercises can be done in a chair or standing. The attention and activity inherent in exercise programs can be an opportunity to improve patient-caregiver interactions. If positive behavioral strategies are used for encouraging exercise participation, exercise may increase opportunities for pleasant interactions between patient and caregiver and conflicts may be reduced. Randomized controlled trials have demonstrated that individuals with dementia who participated in an exercise program for 30 minutes twice a week for at least 3 months have experienced an enhanced level of physical functioning and independence, as well as improvement in their mood; this resulted in a reduction of anxiety and agitation. Thus, a caregiver-supervised exercise program for patients with Alzheimer's disease may yield significant improvements in physical health, affect, and behavioral distress [49, 72, 77].

Finally, ensuring adequate sleep and rest for the patient and caregiver is important for cognition and stress. Caregivers should incorporate this as a purposeful therapeutic activity in the patient itinerary of structured daily routines just like exercise. When patients with dementia develop sleep disturbances, caregivers can use the *symptom-targeted* nonpharmacological approach. This will be discussed later in the chapter (see ▶ Box 21.3).

Modifying the environment is another important way to minimize the development of BPSD. Caregivers should strive to keep the environment comfortable, orienting, and safe. Having preferred familiar music playing in the background [15] with soothing aromas like lavender and lemon balm [57] and having familiar personal items like photos and other belongings are comforting as familiar surroundings will maximize existing cognitive functions via reminiscence therapy [70, 71]. Conspicuous displays of clocks, calendars, and links to world media via newspapers, radios, and televisions may benefit some mildly impaired patients. Patients with dementia may have decreased safety awareness, making them more prone to falls and other accidents. So caregivers should modify the home to minimize such hazards by ensuring adequate lighting and maintaining clutter-free pathways to common areas like the kitchen and bathroom. Finally, bright light therapy may encourage proper sleep-wake cycles and help with sundowning.

Caregivers should utilize behavioral management techniques to minimize the development of BPSD. These include proper communication techniques as well as memory and sensory stimulation. As a patient's cognition starts to decline, basic verbal communication skills will also deteriorate. Caregivers can use certain techniques to better communicate with older adults with BPSD. First, speak slowly and clearly with a calm, positive tone and smile. Use simple sentence structure and one-step directions. Using statements instead of questions when possible can be helpful. Patients should be encouraged to make simple choices. Offering a choice helps maintain individuals' sense of autonomy without confusing them with too many choices. Respecting personal autonomy, when possible, can help to reduce anxiety. It is all right to repeat reminders about conversation content to enhance communication. Also be sure to allow adequate time for response. Talking to older adults as if they were a child should be avoided [41].

Memory and sensory stimulation behavioral techniques can improve memory, mood, self-esteem, and social interaction with reductions in disorientation and anxiety which contribute to BPSD. Caregivers should try to incorporate these into their structured daily routines as "activities" or modify the environment to make it comforting and orienting (see ▶ Box 21.1).

Reminiscence therapy (RT) uses personal photographs or belongings from the past to trigger memories in individuals with dementia in order to improve their sense of self. Caregivers can help patients to remember and relive the emotions and memories of positive past events like birthdays, weddings, and family vacations by using "memory books" which contain memorabilia of positive past events. Memory books and even recorded audio tape stories from family members discussing happy memories have been shown to enhance communication; reduce anxiety, agitation, and wandering; and improve overall quality of life [70, 71] (see ▶ Box 21.1).

Like audio recordings used in reminiscence therapy, familiar songs can stimulate long-term memory, enhance emotional well-being, and reduce anxiety and aggression in patients with dementia. Individuals with dementia can participate in music therapy (MT) by singing or playing an instrument, or they can be passive participants by just listen-

Box 21.3 "Symptom-Targeted" Patient-Centered Nonpharmacological Approach for Sleep-Wake Cycle Disturbance >1 month

Do ABC's to systematically investigate for the potential underlying causes and triggers for insomnia

1. Investigate medications that may be contributing to sleep disturbances via circadian rhythm disruption. Obtain a complete medication list with timing
   - Diuretic given late in day can cause nocturia which can cause poor sleep at night
   - Stimulants/sympathomimetic (nicotine, caffeine, bronchodilators) given late in the day can be activating causing insomnia
   - Anticholinergics, sedating medications (allergy and overactive bladder medications, sinemet, analgesics) given during the daytime may cause daytime sleepiness and napping which can contribute to insomnia
   - SSRI→ can decrease REM which can change the quality of the sleep
2. Complete a sleep diary to assess for patterns or triggers for insomnia
3. R/O primary sleep disorders such as obstructive sleep apnea and restless leg periodic limb movement disorders
4. R/O depression + other psychiatric conditions which can present with sleep disturbances and thus should be treated if persist or severe
5. Look for flares in chronic diseases like congestive heart failure, COPD, diabetes, pain that can contribute to interrupted sleep

ing to preferred familiar music playing in the background. While the literature conflicts, MT is noninvasive, poses little to no risk to patients, requires minimal training, and can be easily implemented by caregivers in the home as well as other patient-care settings [15].

Aromatherapy is a nonpharmacological treatment that is simple to use, safe, and well tolerated. Controlled clinical trials have shown promising results with daily administration of aromatherapy to improve BPSD. Regular use of various aromas (such as lavender, Melissa, geranium, mandarin, sunflower oil, ylang ylang, patchouli, rosemary, and peppermint via various exposure methods including diffusion, lotion, placed under pillows nightly) showed a reduction in physical aggression, verbal agitation, anxiety, and wandering behaviors as well as improve sleep patterns [16, 36, 53, 57].

Food can be a source of stress for older adults with dementia due to all the choices of food and feeding apraxias. Caregivers can alleviate mealtime stress by offering portable finger foods (such as small sandwiches, fruit and cheese trays, muffins, cereal bars, and finger snacks) when patients struggle to use silverware. Offering a couple of food choices helps maintain individuals' sense of autonomy without confusing them with too many choices. With gentle support, set up, and encouragement, caregivers can create a more pleasant dining experience for their loved ones.

Based on the Namaste Care theory, all human beings respond to and benefit from touch close contact [13, 47, 76]. Touch can convey attention, communication, and close contact. Tactile stimulation contributes to a feeling of trust and also promotes relaxation and a sense of calm. Therapeutic tactile stimulation can include gently brushing hair to massages. Providing a hand massage connects the caregiver with the individual in an intimate relationship. Caregivers can utilize the "hand-under-hand" technique, which involves the caregiver placing their hand under the individual's hand while providing guidance [74]. Studies have shown that tactile massage can reduce anxiety and improve cognition, and caregivers have reported feeling closer to older individuals after providing the technique. Allowing the older adult to stroke and interact with pets is another way that tactile stimulation is accomplished [45, 48]. One study showed that pet therapy could reduce agitation and anxiety among older adults with cognitive disorders [45, 48].

21.4.4 General Strategies to Deal with *Present BPSD and Prevent Future* Episodes of BPSD (▶ Box 21.2) [3, 5, 7–9, 14, 18–20, 23, 24, 26, 27, 29, 31, 34, 35, 37, 42, 50, 51, 55, 60, 62, 65, 73, 81]

For agitation or aggression that is *NOT* harmful to self or others, it is helpful for caregivers to have strategies to deal with present BPSD. Two helpful behavioral interventions include the "ABC's" and 3 R's (Repeat, Reassure, Redirect).

21.5 ABC's

When agitation occurs, caregivers must be a detective and do the "ABC's to identify precipitating factors and avoid the triggers. Caregivers should look at the ANTECEDENT BEHAVIORS that lead to a particular CATASTROPHIC CONSEQUENCE and AVOID it as patients with dementia are unable to understand or learn how to prevent it from recurring. Often the detective work will show that there is an UNMET NEED that is making the patient uncomfortable. Since the individual with dementia may not be able to communicate what the problem is, he/she may manifest as "acting out" or agitation. It is thus prudent for caregivers to search for unmet basic needs such as hunger, thirst, fatigue, pain, and incontinence as triggers for BPSD. Sometimes the trigger is not apparent, so caregivers should observe their loved one with dementia to see how they interact with their environment, try to understand how certain situations contribute to the individual's anxiety or aggression, and then try to prevent those situations. The ABC's is also known as functional-analysis-based interventions. Encouraging caregivers to use this patient-centered ABC's behavioral approach is an effective means of increasing their social interaction with individuals with dementia and reduce BPSD [14, 33, 69].

21.5.1 3 R's (Repeat, Reassure, and Redirect)

The 3 R's is another behavioral technique that uses repetition, reassurance, and redirection to diffuse BPSD, especially wandering, aggression, anxiety, and agitation. During episodes of agitation, an individual with dementia may be confused about the situation so simply repeating/reminding in a calm, clear manner what you are doing can diffuse that situation. Because individuals with dementia are unable to "actively" learn, caregivers can employ reassurance (positive reinforcement) to coax loved ones to "learn" new preferred behaviors similar to Skinner's Operant and Pavlov's Classical learned conditioned responses [66]. Redirecting and providing reassurances to older adults allow the caregiver to guide them to an increased sense of safety. As dementia progresses, confronting or reasoning will likely not change behaviors, as individuals with dementia often lose the cognitive ability follow logic or to reason. Instead, caregivers should calmly acknowledge their emotion and redirect the individual using a distraction to address the agitated behavior. Since individuals with dementia have difficulty with multitasking, caregivers can gently redirect an individual's attention to some other distraction such as a change of subject, food and drink, another activity, or a rest period. One technique that may be used for older adults with wandering behavior is the placement of a mirror in front of the exit door. He or she will see their reflection and be redirected to where they came from, reducing exit-seeking behavior [21, 24].

21.5.2 "Symptom-Targeted" Patient-Centered Nonpharmacological Techniques

The "general" nonpharmacological approach with techniques and interventions discussed above (► Boxes 21.1 and 21.2) is effective for most BPSD, especially mild agitation, aggression, pacing, and wandering. "Symptom-targeted" patient-centered nonpharmacological techniques and pharmacologics are reserved for unique BPSD symptoms like sleep disturbances and distressing mood and psychotic symptoms.

Sleep disturbances commonly occur in this population due to physiological changes associated with age and Alzheimer's disease [10, 56, 58, 75]. These changes include:

- Suprachiasmatic nucleus damage which affects:
  - Sleep initiation/maintenance
- Circadian rhythm degeneration which leads to:
  - Increased sleep fragmentation
  - Increased light sleep (Stages 1 and 2)
  - Less restorative sleep (Stages 3 and 4)
  - Decreased total sleep time
- Decreased melatonin secretion
- Decreased hypocretin (orexin) secretion—hypocretin system acts as a stabilizing factor in the sleep-wake flip-flop, keeping it in the waking state
- Decreased REM (due to loss of cholinergic neurons in nucleus basalis)
- Excess hypersomnolence with some apoE4 subtypes

When patients with dementia develop sleep disturbances, caregivers can use the symptom-targeted nonpharmacological approach first as recommended by guidelines ([6, 11, 40, 53, 55, 75]).

21.5.3 Approach to Evaluating Sleep Disturbances in Dementia

Primary care providers can work with the caregiver to do the ABC's (see ► Box 21.2) to systematically investigate for the potential underlying causes and triggers for insomnia (see ► Box 21.3). Medications given at inappropriate times can disrupt the circadian rhythm causing insomnia. It is important to review the medication list and timing to ensure that they are not contributing to the insomnia. Completing a sleep diary can help providers to look for other common triggers like UNMET NEEDS—hunger, incontinence, pain, boredom, as well as flare in chronic conditions like heart failure, COPD, reflux, and osteoarthritis (see ► Box 21.2) which can contribute to napping and insomnia. Finally, a search for other concurrent medical conditions like primary sleep disorders (obstructive sleep apnea and restless leg syndrome) and depression and psychosis (which have sleep disturbance as part of their constellation of symptoms) can be helpful in determining best treatment for insomnia. Triggers should be addressed and nonpharmacological sleep interventions employed as first. Here are the eight nonpharmacological interventions for insomnia that were used in the RCT by McCurry SM et al. [40]. This protocol employed four of the six traditional techniques used to manage insomnia in cognitively intact elders: sleep hygiene, stimulus control, sleep restriction, and circadian rhythm manipulators. Only cognitive behavioral therapy (CBT) and active "relaxation" were not used [40]. The nonpharmacological protocol for insomnia are as follows:

1. Follow structured sleep and rising times that were not to deviate no more than 30 minutes from the selected times (circadian).
2. Encouraged patients not to nap after 1 PM and limit naps to 30 minutes or less (sleep hygiene, circadian, sleep restriction).
3. Walk for 30 minutes, exercise daily (circadian).
4. Bright light therapy (BLT) at dawn/dusk (circadian).
5. Eliminate triggers for nighttime awakenings, i.e., unmet needs. May need to control night time pain, give nightly snack, and take activating meds in the AM (stimulus control).
6. Reduce light/noise levels in their sleeping areas (stimulus control).
7. Switch to decaffeinated drinks and reduce evening fluid consumption (stimulus control).
8. If nocturia affected sleep, encourage toileting schedules at night, use of incontinence pads, and exclude urinary tract infections (stimulus control).

Caregivers who used this protocol showed significantly greater reductions in number of nighttime awakenings, total time awake at night, and depression, and increases in weekly exercise days than control subjects [40].

21.5.4 Bright Light Therapy and Sleep

Light plays a major role in regulating the phase relationships among core body temperature, melatonin rhythm, and the circadian rest-activity cycle. Typically, light exposure is timed to coincide with the beginning and end of the human photoperiod. Currently, there is no accepted gold standard for when light exposure should occur, how long it should be delivered, which light wavelengths are maximally safe and effective, or which method of light delivery is optimal. Morning light exposure is most beneficial for phase-delayed individuals (i.e., those whose sleep onset and morning rising are pushed to later hours) or those who may be suffering from a seasonal depressive disorder. Evening bright light treatment is beneficial for sleep maintenance problems in older adults and for phase-advanced individuals (i.e., those who fall asleep in the early evening and awaken too early in the morning). Some adverse side effects were reported for light therapy (irritability, dizziness, headache), and treatment effects were relatively modest; the authors concluded that whole-day bright light is safe for use and is helpful as part of the nonpharmacological protocols for insomnia [11, 75].

21.5.5 Exercise and Sleep

Exercise is a nonphototic circadian rhythm manipulator and can help produce more restful sleep in older adults. Although regular physical activity may also enhance the sleep of individuals with dementia, no controlled trials looking at the isolated effects of exercise on sleep in dementia have been published thus far. Studies have shown that caregivers can be trained to function as exercise "coaches" for individuals with dementia, and older adults with a wide range of cognitive impairment enjoy participating in structured exercise programs.

Because of the multifaceted nature of sleep disturbances and fragility of older adult patients with dementia, nonpharmacological interventions should always be considered first.

21.5.6 Resources for Providers and Family About Nonpharmacological Approach to BPSD [9, 14, 19, 20, 23, 31, 42, 73, 78, 79, 80]

Most caregivers will not ask for assistance or report behaviors until they have become a crisis—perhaps from embarrassment or fear of being perceived as unable to cope. In order to avoid crisis, primary care providers should be proactive in routinely screening/asking about BPSD. Although studies demonstrate that nonpharmacological interventions can decrease BPSD and improve caregiver well-being with fewer side effects when compared with pharmacologics, teaching caregivers how to manage BPSD can be challenging. Primary care doctors do not have enough time to do this comprehensively in clinic; so often members of the trans-professional team can help. In addition, there are many books and comprehensive caregiver education programs available to teach caregivers about the concepts needed to successfully implement the nonpharmacological approach which are:

1. Dementia—the disease, its prognosis, and having realistic expectations
2. General patient-centered techniques to minimize development of BPSD
3. Strategies to deal with present BPSD and prevent future episodes of BPSD

Here are some resources for providers and caregivers to learn about proactively managing BPSD:

- ► Alz.org—Caring Kind (formerly the Alzheimer's Association, NYC Chapter) ► http://caringkindnyc.org/
- **WeCareAdvisor™** [31]:
  Web-based. Uses the DICE approach to developed patient-centered response to mitigate BPSD
  - D: Describe
  - I: Investigate
  - C: Create
  - E: Evaluate
- **Dementia Care Manager model**: ► www.agingbraincare.org/ ABC Care Protocols by Dr. Callahan at Indiana University
- **The Savvy Caregiver Program**: Developing and testing a transportable dementia family caregiver training program [23]
- **P.I.E.C.E.S.** (Physical, Intellectual, Emotional, Capability, Environment, and Social) method is a framework created to help screen and assess behaviors in an efficient yet comprehensive way. This framework will allow you to better understand the causes behind the behavior and to draw a more accurate and effective intervention plan [9, 59]

21.5.7 Evidence of Efficacy of Nonpharmacological Behavioral Techniques [3, 5, 7, 8, 14, 18, 19, 20, 23, 24, 26, 27, 29, 31, 34, 35, 37, 42, 50, 52, 53, 59, 60, 62, 65, 67, 69, 73, 76, 77, 81]

There are several studies demonstrating the effectiveness of nonpharmacological techniques for management of BPSD. A 2014 systematic review of nonpharmacological interventions for agitation in dementia included randomized trials with at least 45 participants—effective interventions in one or more trials were the implementation of activities, music therapy, person-centered communication skills training for caregivers, and sensory interventions such as massage [37]. For the most part, positive trials demonstrated evidence of short-term benefit. A 2017 systematic overview summarizes RCT evidence for the effects of 17 different pharmacological and nonpharmacological interventions for the management of BPSD. A statistically significant effect in improving global BPSD was seen for functional analysis-based interventions, music therapy, analgesics, melatonin, donepezil, galantamine, and atypical antipsychotics but with caveats. Importantly, the nonpharmacological approaches have a similar effect size for treating global BPSD to the pharmacological approaches. Nonpharmacological approaches did not have any reported adverse events, whereas atypical antipsychotics and cholinesterase inhibitors were reported to have an increased risk of many adverse events in comparison with placebo. While the quality of the evidence base for nonpharmacological approaches is generally lower than for pharmacological treatments, it is noteworthy that the estimates of effect size of these interventions are similar to that of the pharmacological treatments and that the nonpharmacological treatment is not associated with any adverse events. Overall, this 2017 overview provides support for using the nonpharmacological approach of functional-analysis-based interventions as a first-line therapy for BPSD, due to the significant impact on global BPSD measures, moderate-quality evidence, and the lack of adverse events. Music therapy may also be effective in the management of BPSD; however, further high-quality evidence would be useful to strengthen the support for its use.

Take-Home Points
- Always obtain a thorough history about the "disturbance."
- Rule out delirium and other environmental factors contributing to the disturbance.
- Use nonpharmacological interventions for BPSD first.
- Consider "targeted," time-limited pharmacological trials for severe or persistent BPSD symptoms given modest evidence of efficacy and moderate potential for harm.

21.6 Content

If appropriate to topic, please incorporate:
- Interprofessional care
- Normal/abnormal for older adults
- Special considerations for older adults
- Family/caregiver role
- Community resources
- Educational resources
- Hospital vs outpatient (ambulatory and home) vs LTC management differences

Case Conclusion

As the physician, you obtain further history from the patient and daughter and perform a thorough physical. Daughter reports that patient has been more incontinent these days but has had no fevers, chills, flank pain, or hematuria. Patient has been eating a little less as well but reports no nausea, vomiting, diarrhea, or constipation. ROS is otherwise negative. There are no new medications and no changes in the care giving environment.

Physical exam is unremarkable except for temperature 100.1, mild suprapubic tenderness without guarding or rebound or CVA tenderness. Neurological exam is nonfocal though technically difficult. She is oriented only to person and easily distracted.

Labs are unremarkable except for urine with positive nitrites and leukocyte esterase, and CBC with mild leukocytosis with left shift.

Diagnosis: UTI with delirium with BPSD. You treat the patient with an antibiotic and review the nonpharmacological approach as delineated in ► Boxes 21.1 and 21.2.

Appendix 1: Confusion Assessment Method (CAM) Diagnosis of Delirium Requires a Present or Abnormal Rating for Criteria 1 and 2 Plus Either 3 or 4 [28]

Criteria

1. **Acute onset and fluctuating course**:
   - Is there evidence of an acute change in mental status from the patient's baseline? Corroboration with caretakers and family member is usually required.
   - Did this behavior come and go or wax or wane in severity in the last 24 hours?
2. **Inattention**:
   - Does the patient have difficulty focusing attention?
   - Are they easily distracted?
   - Do they have difficulty keeping track of what is being said?
   - Consider asking the patient to recite the days of the week backwards.
3. **Disorganized thinking**:
   - Is the patient's speech disorganized or incoherent?
   - Does the patient ramble or have irrelevant conversation that is unclear with illogical flow of ideas, and unpredictable switching between subjects?
4. **Altered level of consciousness**:
   - Only patients who are calm and alert are considered normal.
   - Patient meet criteria if they are: vigilant (hyperalert), lethargic (drowsy, easily aroused), stuporous (difficult to arouse), or comatose.

Appendix 2: Blackbox Warning for Antipsychotics [17, 64]

- Increased risk of mortality. Rate of death was 1.6–1.7 times that of placebo (3.5 vs 2.3%).
- Death appeared to be heart related or from infections (e.g., pneumonia).
- Often causing diabetes mellitus, hyperglycemia, ketoacidosis, and hyperosmolar states.
- All antipsychotic drugs will now include the same information about this risk in a BOXED WARNING and WARNING section.
- Antipsychotics are *NOT indicated* for the treatment of dementia-related psychosis and are off-labeled use.

References

1. Alzheimer's disease facts and figures. Alzheimer's Dement. 2016;12(4):459–509.
2. Alzheimer's Disease International. Dementia statistics. https://www.alz.co.uk/research/statistics. Accessed 27 Dec 2017.
3. Ayalon L, Gum AM, Feliciano L, Areán PA. Effectiveness of nonpharmacological interventions for the management of neuropsychiatric symptoms in patients with dementia: a systematic review. Arch Intern Med. 2006;166(20):2182–8.
4. Badrakalimnthu VR, Tarbuck AF. Anxiety: a hidden element in dementia. Adv Psychiatr Treat. 2012;18(2):119–28.
5. Bird M, Jones RH, Korten A, Smithers H. A controlled trial of a predominantly psychosocial approach to BPSD: treating causality. Int Psychogeriatr. 2007;19(5):874–91. Epub 2007 Jan 19.
6. Bliwise DL. Sleep disorders in Alzheimer's disease and other dementias. Clin Cornerstone. 2004;6. Suppl 1A:S16–28.
7. Cohen-Mansfield J. Nonpharmacologic interventions for inappropriate behaviors in dementia: a review, summary, and critique. Am J Geriatr Psychiatry. 2001;9(4):361–81.
8. Cohen-Mansfield J, Thein K, Marx MS, Dakheel-Ali M, Freedman L. Efficacy of nonpharmacologic interventions for agitation in

advanced dementia: a randomized, placebo-controlled trial. J Clin Psychiatry. 2012;73(9):1255–61. https://doi.org/10.4088/JCP.12m07918.
9. Collins J, Harris D, LeClair K. Putting the PIECES Together, The PIECES Collaboration Office. Shop for Learning Publishing, 6th Edition. 2010.
10. Cooke JR, Ancoli-Israel S. Normal and abnormal sleep in the elderly. Handb Clin Neurol. 2011;98:653–65.
11. Deschenes CL, McCurry SM. Current treatments for sleep disturbances in individuals with dementia. Curr Psychiatry Rep. 2009;11:20.
12. Drouillard N, Mithani A, Chan PKY. Therapeutic approaches in the management of behavioral and psychological symptoms of dementia in the elderly. B C Med J. 2013;55(2):90–5.
13. Duffin C. How Namaste principles improve resident' lives. Nurs Older People. 2012;24(6):14–7.
14. Dyer SM, Harrison SL, Laver K, Whitehead C, Crotty M. An overview of systematic reviews of pharmacological and non-pharmacological interventions for the treatment of behavioral and psychological symptoms of dementia. Int Psychogeriatr. 2017;16:1–15. https://doi.org/10.1017/S1041610217002344.
15. Fakhoury N, Wilhelm N, Sobota KF, Kroustos KR. Impact of music therapy on dementia behaviors: a literature review. Consult Pharm. 2017;32(10):623–8.
16. Fujii M, Hatakeyama R, Fukuoka Y, et al. Lavender aroma therapy for behavioral and psychological symptoms in dementia patients. Geriatr Gerontol Int. 2008;8(2):136–8.
17. Gill SS, Bronskill SE, Normand SL, Anderson GM, Sykora K, Lam K, Bell CM, Lee PE, Fischer HD, Herrmann N, Gurwitz JH, Rochon PA. Antipsychotic drug use and mortality in older adults with dementia. Ann Intern Med. 2007;146:775–86.
18. Gitlin LN, Kales HC, Lyketsos CG. Managing behavioral symptoms in dementia using nonpharmacologic approaches: an overview. JAMA. 2012;308(19):2020–9.
19. Gitlin LN, Winter L, Dennis MP, Hodgson N, Hauck WW. Targeting and managing behavioral symptoms in individuals with dementia: a randomized trial of a nonpharmacological intervention. J Am Geriatr Soc. 2010;58(8):1465–74.
20. Gitlin LN, Winter L, Dennis MP, Hodgson N, Hauck WW. A biobehavioral home-based intervention and the well-being of patients with dementia and their caregivers: the COPE randomized trial. JAMA. 2010;304(9):983–91.
21. Gu L. Nursing interventions in managing wandering behavior in patients with dementia: a literature review. Arch Psychiatr Nurs. 2015;29(6):454–7.
22. Guideline Adaptation Committee. Clinical practice guidelines and principles of care for people with dementia. Sydney: NHMRC Cognitive Decline Partnership Centre; 2016. Available at: http://www.clinicalguidelines.gov.au/portal/2503/clinical-practice-guidelines-and-principles-care-people-dementia.
23. Hepburn KW, Lewis M, Sherman CW, et al. The Savvy Caregiver Program: developing and testing a transportable dementia family caregiver training program. Gerontologist. 2003;43:908–15.
24. Hermans DG, Tay H, Hla U, McShane R. Non-pharmacological interventions for wandering of people with dementia in the domestic setting. [Systematic Review] Cochrane Dementia and Cognitive Improvement Group Cochrane Database of Systematic Reviews. 2007;4.
25. Hurt C, et al. Patient and caregiver perspectives of quality of life in dementia. An investigation of the relationship to behavioural and psychological symptoms in dementia. Dement Geriatr Cogn Disord. 2008;26:138–46.
26. Husebo BS, Ballard C, Aarsland D. Pain treatment of agitation in patients with dementia: a systematic review. Int J Geriatr Psychiatry. 2011;26(10):1012–8. https://doi.org/10.1002/gps.2649. Epub 2011 Feb 9.
27. Hwang R. Managing difficult behaviors in patients with dementia. Virtual Mentor. 2008;10(6):379–82.
28. Inouye SK. The confusion assessment method (CAM): training manual and coding guide 2003. Boston: Yale University School of Medicine; 2003.
29. Jeste DV, Blazer D, Casey D, Meeks T, Salzman C, Schneider L, Tariot P, Yaffe K. ACNP White Paper: update on use of antipsychotic drugs in elderly persons with dementia. Neuropsychopharmacology. 2008;33:957–70.
30. Kales HC, Gitlin LN, Lyketsos CG. Assessment and management of behavioral and psychological symptoms of dementia. BMJ. 2015;350:h369.
31. Kales HC, Gitlin LN, Stanislawski B, Marx K, Turnwald M, Watkins DC, Lyketsos CG. WeCareAdvisor™: the development of a caregiver-focused, web-based program to assess and manage behavioral and psychological symptoms of dementia. Alzheimer Dis Assoc Disord. 2017;31(3):263–70.
32. Kar N. Behavioral and psychological symptoms of dementia and their management. Indian J Psychiatry. 2009;51(Suppl 1):s77–86.
33. Kok JS, van Heuvelen MJG, Berg IJ, Scherder EJA. Small scale home-like special care units and traditional special care units: effects on cognition in dementia; a longitudinal controlled intervention study. BMC Geriatr. 2016;16:47.
34. Kong EH, Evans LK, Guevara JP. Nonpharmacological intervention for agitation in dementia: a systematic review and meta-analysis. Aging Ment Health. 2009;13:512–20.
35. Kovach CR, Taneli Y, Dohearty P, et al. Effect of the BACE intervention on agitation in people with dementia. Gerontologist. 2004;44:797–806. [PubMed: 15611216].
36. Lin PW, Chan WC, Ng BF, Lam LC. Efficacy of aromatherapy (Lavandula angustifolia) as an intervention for agitated behaviours in Chinese older persons with dementia: a cross-over randomized trial. Int J Geriatr Psychiatry. 2007;22(5):405–10.
37. Livingston G, Johnston K, Katona C, et al. Systematic review of psychological approaches to the management of neuropsychiatric symptoms of dementia. Am J Psychiatry. 2005;162(11):1996–2021.
38. Livingston G, Kelly L, Lewis-Holmes E, et al. Non-pharmacological interventions for agitation in dementia: systematic review of randomised controlled trials. Br J Psychiatry. 2014;205:436.
39. Lyketsos CG, Steinberg M, Tschanz JT, Norton MC, Steffens DC, Breitner JC. Mental and behavioral disturbances in dementia: findings from the cache county study on memory in aging. Am J Psychiatr. 2000;157:708–14.
40. McCurry SM, Gibbons LE, Logsdon RG, Vitiello MV, Teri L. Nighttime insomnia treatment and education for Alzheimer's disease: a randomized, controlled trial. J Am Geriatr Soc. 2005;53(5):793–802.
41. McEvoy P, Eden J, Plant R. Dementia communication using empathic curiosity. Nurs Times. 2014;110(24):12–5.
42. McGonigal-Kenny ML, Schutte DL. Nonpharmacologic management of agitated behaviors in persons with Alzheimer disease and other chronic dementing conditions. J Gerontol Nurs. 2006;32(2):9–14.
43. Mitchell SL. Advanced dementia. N Engl J Med. 2015;372(26):2533–40.
44. Moore M, Zhu C, Clipp E. Informal costs of dementia care: estimates from the national longitudinal caregiver study. J Gerontol B Psychol Sci Soc Sci. 2001;56:S219–28.
45. Moretti F, DeRonchi D, Bernabei V, et al. Pet therapy in elderly patients with mental illness. Psychogeriatrics. 2011;11(2):125–9.
46. National Institute for Health and Clinical Excellence-Social Care Institute for Excellence. Dementia. A NICE-SCIE guideline on supporting people with dementia and their carers in health and social care. London: National Clinical Practice Guideline London; 2007.

47. Nicholls D, Chang E, Johnson A, Edenborough M. Touch, the essence of caring for people with end-stage dementia: a mental health perspective in Namaste Care. Aging Ment Health. 2013;17(5):571–8.
48. Nordgren L, Engström G. Effects of dog-assisted interventions on behavioural and psychological symptoms of dementia. Nurs Older People. 2014;26(3):31–8.
49. Öhman H, Savikko N, Strandberg TE, et al. Effects of exercise on cognition: the Finnish Alzheimer disease exercise trial. J Am Geriatr Soc. 2016;64(4):731–8.
50. Caregiver- and patient-directed interventions for dementia an evidence-based analysis. Ont Health Technol Assess Ser. 2008;8(4): 1–98.
51. Osser D, Fischer M. Management of the behavioral and psychological symptoms of dementia. NaRCAD (the National Resource Center for Academic Detailing) with support from a grant from the Agency for Healthcare Research and Quality to the Division of Pharmacoepidemiology and Pharmacoeconomics of the Brigham and Women's Hospital Department of Medicine. 28 Dec 2013.
52. Ostwald SK, Hepburn KW, Caron W, et al. Reducing caregiver burden: a randomized psychoeducational intervention for caregivers of persons with dementia. Gerontologist. 1999;39:299–309. [PubMed: 10396888].
53. Paniagua MA, Paniagua EW. The demented elder with insomnia. Clin Geriatr Med. 2008;24(1):69–81, vii. Review.
54. Perry E. Aromatherapy for the treatment of Alzheimer's disease. J Qual Res Dementia. 2016;3. https://unforgettable-media-unforgettabletra.netdna-ssl.com/media/attach.... Accessed 26 June 2017.
55. Peter-Derex L, Yammine P, Bastuji H, Croisile B. Sleep and Alzheimer's disease. Sleep Med Rev. 2015;19:29–38.
56. Petit D, Gagnon JF, Fantini ML, Ferini-Strambi L, Montplaisir J. Sleep and quantitative EEG in neurodegenerative disorders. J Psychosom Res. 2004;56(5):487–96.
57. Press-Sandler O, Freud T, Volkov I, Peleg R, Press Y. Aromatherapy for the treatment of patients with behavioral and psychological symptoms of dementia: a descriptive analysis of RCTs. J Altern Complement Med. 2016;22(6):422–8.
58. Prinz PN, Peskind ER, Vitaliano PP, et al. Changes in the sleep and waking EEGs of nondemented and demented elderly subjects. J Am Geriatr Soc. 1982;30(2):86–93.
59. Puxty J, Rivard MF. Behavioural and psychological symptoms of dementia (BPSD): a handbook for family physicians. Ontario College of Family Physicians and P.I.E.C.E. Canada. 2009.
60. Rabins PV, et al. American Psychiatric Association practice guideline for the treatment of patients with Alzheimer's disease and other dementias. Second edition. Am J Psychiatry. 2007;164(Suppl 12):5–56.
61. Rosen HJ, Allison SC, Schauer GF, et al. Neuroanatomical correlates of behavioural disorders in dementia. Brain. 2005;128:2612.
62. Salzman C, Jeste D, Meyer RE, Cohen-Mansfield J, Cummings J, Grossberg G, Jarvik L, Kraemer H, Lebowitz B, Maslow K, Pollock B, Raskind M, Schultz S, Wang P, Zito JM, Zubenko GS. Elderly patients with dementia-related symptoms of severe agitation and aggression: consensus statement on treatment options, clinical trials methodology, and policy. J Clin Psychiatry. 2008;69(6):889–98.
63. Savva GM, et al. Prevalence, correlates and course of behavioural and psychological symptoms of dementia in the population. Br J Psychiatry. 2009;194:212–9.
64. Schneeweiss S, Setoguchi S, Brookhart A, Dormuth C, Wang PS. Risk of death associated with the use of conventional versus atypical antipsychotic drugs among elderly patients. CMAJ. 2007;176: 627–32.
65. Sloane PD, Hoeffer B, Mitchell CM, McKenzie DA, Barrick AL, Rader J, Stewart BJ, Talerico KA, Rasin JH, Zink RC, Koch GG. Effect of person-centered showering and the towel bath on bathing-associated aggression, agitation, and discomfort in nursing home residents with dementia: a randomized, controlled trial. J Am Geriatr Soc. 2004;52(11):1795–804.
66. Staddon JER, Cerutti DT. Operant conditioning. Annu Rev Psychol. 2003;54:115–44. https://doi.org/10.1146/annurev.psych.54.101601.145124.
67. Staedtler AV, Nunez D. Nonpharmacological therapy for the management of neuropsychiatric symptoms of Alzheimer's disease: linking evidence to practice. Worldviews Evid Based Nurs. 2015;12(2):108–15. https://doi.org/10.1111/wvn.12086. Epub 2015 Mar 21.
68. Steele C, Rovner B, Chase GA, Folstein M. Psychiatric symptoms and nursing home placement of patients with Alzheimer's disease. Am J Psychiatr. 1990;147:1049–51.
69. Stein-Parbury J, Chenoweth L, Jeon YH, Brodaty H, Haas M, Norman R. Implementing person-centered care in residential dementia care. Clin Gerontol. 2012;35(5):404–24.
70. Subramanian P, Woods B. The impact of individual reminiscence therapy for people with dementia: systematic review. Expert Rev Neurother. 2012;12(5):545–55.
71. Subramanian P, Woods B, Whitaker C. Life review and life story books for people with mild to moderate dementia: a randomized controlled trial. Aging Ment Health. 2014;18(3):363–75.
72. Teri L, Gibbons LE, McCurry SM, et al. Exercise plus behavioral management in patients with Alzheimer disease: a randomized controlled trial. JAMA. 2003;290:2015.
73. Teri L, McCurry SM, Logsdon R, et al. Training community consultants to help family members improve dementia care: a randomized controlled trial. Gerontologist. 2005;45:802–11. [PubMed:16326662].
74. Tuohy D, Graham MM, Johnson K, Tuohy T, Burke K. Developing an educational DVD on the use of hand massage in the care of people with dementia: an innovation. Nurs Educ Pract. 2015;15(4): 299–303.
75. Urrestarazu E, Iriarte J. Clinical management of sleep disturbances in Alzheimer's disease: current and emerging strategies. Nat Sci Sleep. 2016;8:21–33.
76. Viggo Hansen N, Jørgensen T, Ørtenblad L. Massage and touch for dementia. Cochrane Database Syst Rev. 2006;(4):CD004989.
77. Wong C, Leland NE. Non-pharmacological approaches to reducing negative behavioral symptoms: a scoping review. OTJR (Thorofare N J). 2016;36(1):34–4139.
78. www.agingbraincare.org/. ABC care protocols. The nonpharmacologic protocols.
79. www.alz.org/care/alzheimers-dementia-bathing.asp.
80. www.bathingwithoutabattle.unc.edu/.
81. Zec RF, Burkett NR. Non-pharmacological and pharmacological treatment of the cognitive and behavioral symptoms of Alzheimer disease. NeuroRehabilitation. 2008;23(5):425–38.

Late-Life Insomnia

Hylton E. Molzof, Megan E. Petrov, and Kenneth L. Lichstein

A. Chun (ed.), *Geriatric Practice*, https://doi.org/10.1007/978-3-030-19625-7_22

Introductory Case Study

Mrs. Doe, a 68-year-old Caucasian female, presented with primary complaints of difficulty falling asleep, difficulty maintaining sleep, and daytime fatigue. This problem started approximately 3 years ago following her retirement. She estimated obtaining 6 hours of total sleep time (TST) with extensive sleep onset latency (SOL), and wake after sleep onset (WASO). She routinely goes to bed at 10 pm but is unable to fall asleep until 12 am. Additionally, she reported awakening 2–3 times each night with an inability to return to sleep for approximately 30 minutes. Her wake time is variable. Mrs. Doe described her quality of sleep as generally restless and unrefreshing. During the day, she experiences fatigue, difficulty concentrating, and mild irritability. She stated that she has increased cognitive activity when unable to sleep, during which time her mind races and she worries about a variety of topics. When unable to sleep, she often reads books on her tablet while in bed. Mrs. Doe reported that she has tried a few sleep aids, but these have not been helpful. Some nights she will have 1–2 glasses of wine prior to bed, which she stated helps her fall asleep more quickly. She described her physical health as generally good, with no recent changes in her health status. She has a psychiatric history of mild anxiety and depression. Mrs. Doe reported maintaining good relationships with her husband and children. She is engaged in community activities but admitted that she is not as active during the day as she was prior to her retirement.

22.1 Chapter Overview

Older adulthood is characterized by many physical and health-related changes, including changes in sleep. Normative age-related changes in sleep architecture include greater fragility of sleep and a tendency toward "lightening" of sleep [23, 78]. Although these changes in sleep patterning are a part of the natural aging process, older adults disproportionately report sleep complaints such as difficulty maintaining sleep and early morning awakenings, as illustrated in the case example presented at the opening of this chapter [29, 30]. Several reviews have been conducted on age-related sleep changes and late-life insomnia [5, 53, 74, 89]. This chapter will provide a summary of the prevalence and clinical presentation of insomnia symptoms among older adults as well as an overview of guidelines for the assessment, diagnosis, and treatment of late-life insomnia. Non-pathological, age-related changes in sleep will be briefly reviewed to assist clinicians in distinguishing normative sleep patterns from chronic late-life insomnia.

22.2 Normative Age-Related Changes in Sleep Patterns

22.2.1 Sleep Structure and Continuity

The physiology and organization of sleep have been described previously [16, 44, 83]. In brief, sleep is divided into four stages as defined via polysomnography. Stages N1, N2, and N3 comprise non-rapid eye movement (NREM) sleep, and these stages cyclically occur along with rapid eye movement (REM) sleep every 90–120 minutes over the course of an average 8-hour sleep period. N1 and N2 are described as "lighter" stages of sleep from which it is relatively easier to be aroused into wakefulness. Alternatively, N3 sleep, also known as slow-wave sleep, is known for being more restorative and more difficult from which to awaken. REM sleep is characterized by rapid eye movements, muscle atonia, and vivid dreams.

During the aging process, the structure of sleep alters, generally resulting in sleep that is lighter and more easily disrupted. Compared to younger adults, older adults tend to spend a greater percentage of their total sleep time in lighter stages of sleep (N1 and N2), with a lesser percent of sleep time allocated to N3 and REM [21, 34]. A meta-analysis of 65 studies representing 3577 healthy individuals with ages spanning across the adult lifespan found that the largest age-related changes in sleep occur between young adulthood and 60 years of age with minimal variation thereafter [78]. In this meta-analysis, slow-wave sleep was found to decline by 2% per decade until age 60, while sleep continuity was found to decrease by 3% per decade [78]. This deterioration of sleep continuity may contribute to the common adage that older adults sleep less and require less sleep than younger adults. Total sleep time has been shown to decrease with age, and older adults exhibit average shorter sleep duration [14, 78]; however, the amount of sleep obtained by older adults is still considered to be comparable to younger adults [31].

22.2.2 Circadian Rhythm Changes

The sleep-wake cycle follows a 24-hour circadian rhythm maintained by the hypothalamic suprachiasmatic nucleus. In the course of normal aging, the suprachiasmatic nucleus and related brain areas experience neuronal degeneration, which causes disruption of the sleep-wake rhythm. Attenuated amplitude and advanced phase shift of circadian rhythmicity are commonly observed in older adults and contribute to a biological preference for sleep in the early evening hours and waking in the early morning hours [66, 92]. Although these changes are not pathological, insomnia symptoms and sleep loss can result if older adults resist these age-related circadian changes by attempting to sleep outside of their natural sleep phase.

22.2.3 Daytime Sleep

The degradation in sleep continuity, duration, depth, and circadian rhythmicity has been hypothesized to explain the high prevalence of daytime sleep commonly observed among older adults [62]. It currently remains unclear whether daytime sleep is beneficial due to its contribution to total 24-hour sleep duration or if it is detrimental due to its potential for precipitating insomnia symptoms by decreasing nighttime sleep drive [10, 15]. A study comparing community dwelling older adult "nappers" to "non-nappers" revealed that self-reported sleep duration and quality were not significantly different between groups [81]. However, a study using objectively assessed sleep indicated greater sleep fragmentation increased the odds of napping [36]. The impact of daytime sleep has been shown to extend beyond its direct effects on nighttime sleep. A meta-analysis of nine prospective cohort studies indicated that daytime napping was associated with a greater risk of all-cause mortality [113]. Conversely, a recent population-based study conducted among 2974 older adults found that moderate afternoon napping between 30 to 90 minutes was associated with overall better cognition compared to non-napping, short napping (less than 30 minutes), or extended napping (greater than 90 minutes) [54], suggesting that nap duration may be a crucial factor in distinguishing whether napping is beneficial or detrimental. Further research is necessary to determine if and what aspects of daytime sleep may be pathological.

22.3 Diagnosis of Insomnia

Multiple classification systems – including the Diagnostic and Statistical Manual of Mental Disorders [4], the International Classification of Diseases [108], and the International Classification of Sleep Disorders [3] – provide diagnostic criteria for insomnia. Despite differences in the subtypes of insomnia, there are essentially three components of an insomnia diagnosis: (1) complaint of a sleep difficulty, (2) adequate opportunity to attain sufficient sleep, and (3) daytime functioning impairment complaint. The presence of distress about sleep is particularly important for older adults as many who exhibit poor sleep are not distressed about their sleep [61]. Nighttime insomnia symptoms include difficulty initiating asleep, difficulty maintaining sleep, and early morning awakening with the inability to return to sleep. Common daytime functioning impairment complaints include fatigue, poor concentration, excessive sleepiness, worries about sleep, depressed mood, and impaired cognitive functioning [85]. To meet criteria for diagnosis, these functioning deficits must have a negative impact on social, occupational, or physical functioning [4].

Notably, none of the current classification systems provide specific quantitative criteria for measuring insomnia symptoms. General recommendations for quantitative sleep disturbance criteria have been established, which include ≥31 minutes of sleep onset latency (SOL) or wake time after sleep onset (WASO) experienced 3 nights a week for 6 months or longer [13]. These criteria appear to best differentiate older adults with insomnia (OAWI) from normal sleepers. Quantification of early morning awakenings has received attention in the literature on OAWI [11, 46] but not to the extent of onset and maintenance sleep disturbance.

22.4 Insomnia Epidemiology Among Older Adults

The prevalence of insomnia symptoms has been investigated in numerous samples of older adults across multiple countries and cultures. The estimated global prevalence of insomnia symptoms among older adults varies greatly, ranging from 23% to 70% across studies [11, 29, 38, 46, 52, 60]. The prevalence of chronic insomnia among older adults also exhibits diversity, falling between 12% and 40% [29, 32, 75, 91]. The point prevalence of insomnia among the general population has been estimated to be approximately 16% [57]. Numerous epidemiological studies have indicated that the prevalence and incidence of insomnia increase with advancing age [11, 38, 76]. Using empirically based, quantitative criteria for insomnia, our research group examined prevalence changes across the adult lifespan and found that prevalence of insomnia remained fairly constant until the age deciles 70–79 and 80–89, during which insomnia prevalence doubled [57]. Similarly, 1–4-year incidence rates of insomnia among older adults range between 2.8% and 7.3% across studies [30, 32, 70]. One study examining the cumulative 4–8-year incidence of insomnia concluded that, on average, there exists a 3.6% increase in insomnia incidence per year among individuals aged 65 years and older [69]. Depressed mood and physical illness have been consistently identified as predictors of incident insomnia in older age [52, 96].

Gender differences in insomnia have been widely characterized across the lifespan. A meta-analysis of gender differences in insomnia reported that women were at an overall greater risk for developing insomnia compared to men across all ages [111]. Compared to men, women have also been shown to experience more prominent exacerbation of insomnia symptoms in later life [29, 39, 60, 69, 75]. A study conducted among community-dwelling older adults found that 70% of older men and women reported at least 1 symptom of insomnia [46]. However, women more frequently reported 2 or 3 insomnia symptoms, whereas men more often reported only 1 insomnia symptom [46]. Data from our research group show that insomnia prevalence peaks at 41% in women between the ages of 80 and 89 while men culminate at 23% [57]. Physiological changes associated with menopause, including vasomotor symptoms and declining levels of reproductive hormones, have been implicated as contributing to women's greater susceptibility to developing insomnia [48]. Menopausal hormone therapy has been associated with a modest improvement in sleep quality among women with vasomotor symptoms [19].

Growing evidence has indicated the presence of racial and ethnic differences in insomnia epidemiology, which may contribute to the notable diversity in global prevalence estimates. Ethnicity has been shown to be a significant predictor of insomnia symptoms of sleep onset, maintenance, and early morning awakenings [47]. Our research group completed meta-analyses comparing sleep in White and Black individuals with insomnia symptoms [88]. Results showed that White adults exhibit a significantly higher prevalence of sleep complaints, difficulty maintaining sleep, and early morning awakenings. Epidemiological data on Black adults also suggest they report fewer sleep complaints and insomnia symptoms than White adults, despite Black adults reporting poorer sleep quality, non-restorative sleep, and restless sleep [27, 80]. Recent studies focusing on multi-ethnic comparisons of sleep disturbance revealed that

Black, Hispanic, and Chinese adults each exhibit higher odds of short sleep duration (less than 6 hours per night) compared to White adults [18]. Age-related increases in insomnia severity have also been found to be greater among Hispanic older adults compared to Non-Hispanic White older adults [50].

There has been continued interest regarding whether certain types of insomnia symptoms occur more commonly at different ages. To date, research examining the association between age and type of insomnia remains inconclusive. It has been a widely held belief that sleep maintenance insomnia is more common among older adults [68]. There exists evidence to support this notion [39, 46]; however, this finding may not hold true among individuals with insomnia comorbid with other clinical conditions, such as depression [110]. Our research group found a trend for type of insomnia to correlate with age, but all types of insomnia were common across all age groups [57]. Similarly, in a large epidemiological survey of over 13,000 people between the ages of 15 and 100, age was not found to be associated with type of insomnia [77]. Further research is necessary to elucidate the relationship between age and insomnia type.

Table 22.1 Risk factors for insomnia in later life

Physiological/ biological	Psychological	Social/Behavioral
Medical disorders	Depression	Retirement
Cardiovascular (e.g., CHF)	Anxiety disorders	Nursing home placement
Pulmonary (e.g., COPD)	Psychosis	Hospitalization
Gastrointestinal (e.g., GERD)	Schizophrenia	Bereavement
Chronic pain (e.g., arthritis)	Dementia	↓ Physical activity
Medications		Napping
Antidepressants		Financial strain
Opiates		Low social support
Antihistamines		Worry
β-Blockers		Poor sleep habits
Corticosteroids		Unrealistic sleep beliefs
Alcohol, nicotine, caffeine		
Sleep disorders		
Sleep-disordered breathing		
Restless legs syndrome		
PLMD		
REM behavior disorder		

Adapted with permission from Petrov et al. [114] and Oxford University Press

Note. *CHF* congestive heart failure, *COPD* chronic obstructive pulmonary disease, *GERD* gastroesophageal reflux disease, *PLMD* periodic limb movement disorder

22.5 Clinical Risk Factors of Insomnia

Multiple life factors can precipitate, perpetuate, and exacerbate insomnia symptoms (Table 22.1). We will briefly overview the most common psychosocial factors that may contribute to increased risk for insomnia in older adults. A more detailed discussion will focus on insomnia comorbid with depression and chronic pain.

22

22.5.1 Medical and Psychiatric Illnesses

Medical and psychiatric conditions can disrupt sleep and lead to comorbid insomnia through various mechanisms. Medical conditions are the strongest predictors of the incidence and persistence of insomnia in older adults [39]. Insomnia among older adults has been associated with overall poorer physical and mental wellbeing, chronic fatigue, stroke, cardiovascular disease, pulmonary diseases, anxiety, depression, suicidal behavior, risk of falls and accidents, cognitive decline, and all-cause dementia [1, 22, 31, 49, 51, 79, 104]. Other medical and psychiatric illnesses that are known for their sleep-disruptive properties include pain conditions, gastrointestinal diseases, neurological disorders, genitourinary disorders, endocrine disorders, anxiety disorders, psychosis, dementia, schizophrenia, and primary sleep disorders (i.e., obstructive sleep apnea, restless legs syndrome, periodic limb movement disorder, and REM behavior disorder) [5, 53, 74]. Medications intended to treat medical and/or psychiatric illnesses can also precipitate or exacerbate insomnia. The effect of medication on sleep and alertness is reviewed in depth by Roux and Kryger (2010) [86].

22.5.2 Late-Life Insomnia and Depression

Insomnia commonly occurs comorbid with psychiatric conditions, including depression, across the lifespan. There is particular interest in ascertaining whether untreated insomnia predicts depression incidence and greater depression severity. A recent meta-analysis of 48 studies supported the presence of a bidirectional relationship between sleep disturbance and depression [7]. This study indicated that self-reported sleep disturbance was associated with increased risk for the development, recurrence, and worsening of depression. Similarly, older adults with depression were found to have a higher risk of developing and worsening symptoms of sleep disturbance [7]. Chronic insomnia, specifically, appears to increase the risk of persistent major depression despite treatment by 1.8–3.5 times that of older adult patients with no insomnia [82]. Though the psychological mechanisms underlying the relationship between insomnia and depression remain unclear, older adults' beliefs about sleep and sense of hopelessness may contribute to the relationship between these disorders [90].

22.5.3 Late-Life Insomnia and Chronic Pain

Sleep complaints and poor sleep commonly present in the context of chronic pain [98]. Evidence suggests the relationship between chronic pain and sleep disturbance is bidirectional [97]. When examining objectively assessed sleep and self-reported pain in OAWI, night-to-night variability in sleep has been shown to correspond to day-to-day variability in pain reports, suggesting that the experience of insomnia and pain are sensitive to changes in one another [28]. Pain intensity, anxiety, and depression have been independently associated with insomnia among older adults with chronic pain [26]. Similarly, older adults reporting clinical insomnia more frequently experience intense pain compared to older adults who report no clinical insomnia [25]. Beyond pain factors, there exists an association between severe insomnia and wellbeing, quality of life, outpatient care, total medication costs, and total health-care costs for older adults with chronic pain [25].

22.5.4 Social and Behavioral Changes

Psychosocial, cultural, behavioral, and environmental factors that occur more frequently in our latter years contribute to the development and maintenance of chronic insomnia. Common risk factors for late-life insomnia are retirement, nursing home placement, hospitalization, low social support, loss and bereavement, decreased activity, and chronic stressors and cultural influences specific to nations and regions [107]. These events produce stress that may alter sleep-related behaviors, thus increasing risk for chronic insomnia. For example, one study found self-reported sleep disturbance of older adults who recently lost a spouse was more severe than good sleepers but less severe than OAWI [67]. Institutional settings such as nursing homes and hospitals can also produce sleep disruption. Patients of these institutions have limited exposure to bright light to entrain their circadian rhythms, experience more noise in their environment, and spend more time on bed rest, all of which negatively affect their sleep quality [65, 94]. Lastly, being sedentary has been found to be predictive of acute and persistent insomnia [69]. Regular physical exercise (specifically strength training and walking) paired with individualized social activities has been shown to increase total nocturnal sleep among older adults [84, 104].

22.6 Negative Consequences of Insomnia

Schutte-Rodin and colleagues (2008) [93] delineate five major categories of negative consequences of insomnia: poor quality of life, exacerbation of illness, mood disturbances, subjective sleepiness and fatigue, and cognitive impairments. Insomnia symptoms and daytime sleepiness increase the likelihood of poor quality of life in older adults [109]. This decline in quality of life may be partially attributable to decreases in late-life functioning among OAWI. Insomnia symptoms have been associated with greater odds of having limitations in household activities as well as greater odds of having restricted participation in valued activities [100].

Excessive daytime sleepiness is a common complaint for OAWI. Difficulty initiating sleep, early morning awakenings, and difficulty maintaining sleep are also associated with excessive daytime sleepiness in older adults, with the latter being most strongly correlated [42]. Additionally, increased sleepiness – as demonstrated by frequent napping – has been shown to be a risk factor for falls and hip fractures [101]. Actigraphy-measured poor sleep continuity and short sleep duration have also been identified as risk factors for falls [85].

Decrements in daytime performance of cognitive tasks are often reported by OAWI. Studies in OAWI have revealed that, while performance on simple cognitive tasks is comparable to patients without insomnia, performance on more cognitively demanding tasks is reduced [2]. Objective impairments have been observed in attention, memory span, time estimation, integration of cognitive dimensions, executive-order functioning, and visual-perceptual processing [40, 41]. Insomnia has also been linked to increased risk of all-cause dementia [22]. Specifically, reduced sleep efficiency, greater nighttime wakefulness, greater number of waking episodes, and poor self-reported sleep quality have been associated with subsequent cognitive decline among community-dwelling older men [9].

22.7 Assessment

Clinical guidelines for the evaluation of chronic insomnia in all adults are outlined by Schutte-Rodin and colleagues (2008) [93]. A standard, clinical assessment includes a comprehensive sleep, physical, substance, and mental health history accompanied by a physical and mental status exami-

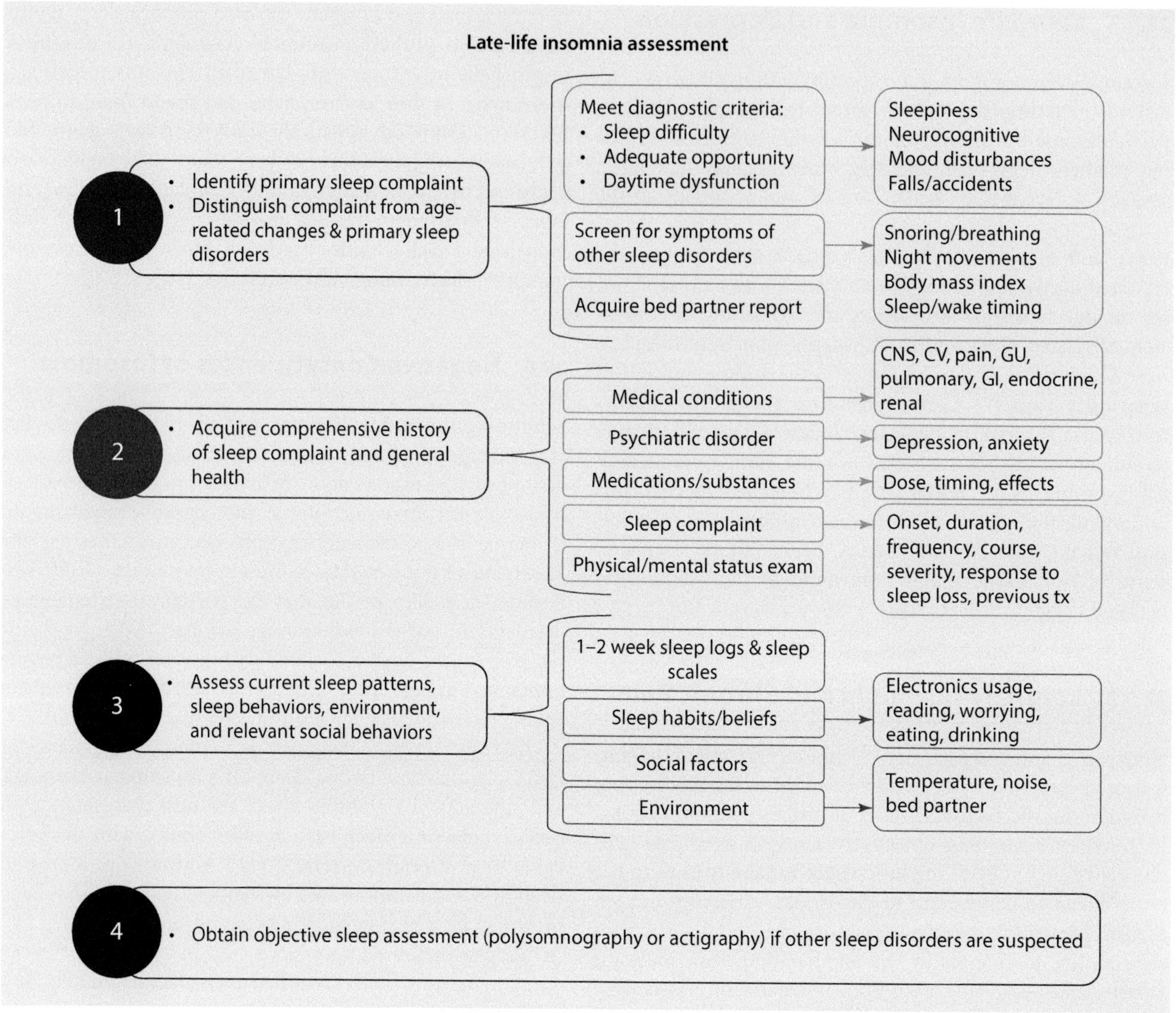

Fig. 22.1 Flowchart of clinical assessment for late-life insomnia. Note. CNS refers to central nervous system; CV refers to cardiovascular; GU refers to genitourinary; GI refers to gastrointestinal [5, 53, 88, 89, 93]. (Adapted with permission from Petrov et al. [114] and Oxford University Press)

nation. Self-reported retrospective and prospective measures of sleep patterns are standard tools of assessment. These measures may include sleep-wake diaries [17], questionnaires, screening tools, and symptom checklists. Objective measures of sleep and daytime sleepiness – such as polysomnography, actigraphy, and the multiple sleep latency test – are generally not recommended, though they may be more indicated for older adults since higher rates of sleep disorders are experienced with advancing age [59]. The following groups may have greater difficulty using traditional sleep logs and questionnaires: nursing home residents, depressed patients, patients with circadian rhythm disturbances, and patients whose activity patterns are suspected to be influencing their sleep [13, 71]. For these groups, wrist actigraphy may be a valuable tool to ascertain sleep disruption. Seven days of actigraphy data is typically considered sufficient to examine meaningful sleep patterns [87].

22

The clinical presentation of insomnia among older adults is often complicated by this age group's higher propensity for medical comorbidities and polypharmacy. During evaluation, it is first important to determine if the insomnia complaint is in excess of normal age-related changes in sleep and not better accounted for by other primary sleep disorders. Useful ways to help rule out alternative primary sleep disorders include assessing movement and restlessness while asleep or relaxed, measuring neck size, assessing snoring and daytime sleepiness through clinical interview, calculating body mass index, and obtaining corroborating reports from bed partners [13, 93]. Precipitating and perpetuating factors of the sleep complaint – including medical, substance-based, psychiatric, environmental, and behavioral – should be thoroughly examined (Fig. 22.1). Schutte-Rodin and colleagues provide six standard categories for assessment, which are outlined as follows [93]:

1. The primary sleep complaint(s) must be identified, such as difficulty initiating sleep, difficulty maintaining sleep, early morning awakenings, and/or non-restorative sleep. The following characteristics of the primary complaint(s) should be determined: duration, frequency, course, distress and daytime impairment severity, agonists and antagonists of the complaint, history of precipitating and perpetuating factors, and previous treatments and treatment responses.
2. Mental and environmental conditions prior to sleep need to be evaluated for the presence of behaviors and attitudes that are counteractive to sleep. Such behaviors and attitudes include using the bed or bedroom as a place for mental stimulation and entertainment (e.g., using electronic devices, exercising, negative interactions with bed partner), and adopting an anxious mindset toward sleep (e.g., hypervigilance, problem-solving/rehearsing in bed, predicting a poor night of sleep).
3. Measurement of the variability in the patient's sleep complaint and sleep-wake schedule allows for the estimation of sleep-wake patterns within the context of the patient's daily life. Sleep-wake diaries are standard tools to quantify parameters of bedtime, wake time, SOL, frequency of awakenings, WASO, time in bed, total sleep time, nap times, and sleep efficiency.
4. Somatic and emotional symptoms occurring during the night provide valuable information regarding differential diagnosis of other sleep disorders, medical conditions, and psychiatric illnesses (e.g., snoring, kicking, reflux, sadness).
5. The five major categories of negative daytime consequences mentioned earlier should also be examined to determine treatable causes of the complaint and outcomes important to the patient.
6. Lastly, the current and personal history of medical and psychiatric conditions and medication/substance usage must be identified. Physical and mental status examinations are also highly recommended.

22.8 Evidence-Based Interventions

There are many evidence-based treatments for insomnia, both pharmacological and cognitive-behavioral, that have demonstrated clinical effectiveness among older adults. These treatments and their empirical support have been laid out extensively in other sources [55, 63]. In the following section, a brief overview of the most common approaches to treating late-life insomnia will be presented. ◘ Table 22.2 highlights specific treatment recommendations for OAWI.

22.8.1 Cognitive-Behavioral Therapy

Cognitive-behavioral therapy (CBT) interventions for insomnia are sometimes implemented in isolation but are more commonly and efficaciously implemented in various packaged multi-component treatments [64]. Their efficacy has been well established in other reviews and meta-analyses [45]. There is evidence that older adults benefit as much from these interventions as their younger counterparts [56, 95]. CBT intervention components are briefly outlined below.

- *Stimulus control* is based on learning principles that suggest the bed and bedroom have become a learned stimulus for arousal and wakeful behaviors through misuse of the bedroom space [12]. The goal is to restore the bed and bedroom as a cue for sleep by confining all sleep behaviors to the bed and removing wakeful behaviors from the bedroom (except sex).
- *Sleep restriction* is an intervention aimed at maximizing sleep efficiency by eliminating time awake in bed through restricting the amount of time allowed for sleep each night [106]. It works by both breaking the associations of the bed with wakefulness and helping the patient build sufficient sleep debt to experience an uninterrupted block of sleep [63].
- *Cognitive therapy* is aimed at reducing cognitive arousal that results from worry about sleep at night, dysfunctional beliefs about sleep, and daytime anxiety about poor sleep [43, 73]. This is typically accomplished through cognitive restructuring, identifying and challenging maladaptive beliefs and thoughts, and helping patients develop realistic alternative thoughts and beliefs [73].
- *Relaxation techniques* help combat mental and physical arousal that may interfere with sleep. Common techniques include progressive muscle relaxation, passive relaxation, breathing strategies, guided imagery, and meditation [55]. For older adults with acute and chronic pain, passive relaxation is recommended as a less intensive strategy [55].
- *Sleep hygiene* aims to provide patients with education about sleep promoting and inhibiting behaviors [64].

22.8.2 Mindfulness-Based Therapy

In recent years, there has been increased interest in utilizing mindfulness-based interventions for the treatment of insomnia. A meta-analysis of six randomized controlled trials suggests that mindfulness meditation may mildly improve total wake time and sleep quality among adults with insomnia [37]. A randomized non-inferiority trial comparing mindfulness-based stress reduction (MBSR) to CBT for insomnia found that MBSR was inferior to CBT for acute improvement of insomnia severity; however, MBSR demonstrated non-inferiority at 3-month post-intervention [33]. Randomized controlled trials conducted specifically among older adults with sleep disturbance found that mindfulness-based interventions produced significant improvements in sleep quality, depressive symptoms, and daytime dysfunction superior to sleep hygiene education or a waitlist control condition [8, 112].

Table 22.2 CBT interventions and special considerations for older adult populations

Intervention	Considerations for elderly populations[a]
Stimulus control: 1. Go to bed only when sleepy 2. Set a fixed morning wake time 3. Eliminate napping 4. Remove all non-sleep behaviors from the bedroom (i.e., reading, watching television, worrying) 5. Leave the bedroom if not asleep within 15–20 minutes and engage in a non-stimulating activity 6. Return to bed only when sleepy again (this applies to the beginning of the night and to awakenings during the middle of the night) 7. Repeat steps 5 and 6 as often as necessary	Sleep may initially get worse before it gets better Telling people to get out of bed to help improve sleep is counter-intuitive for some. Provide adequate rationale to increase buy-in Problem solve ahead of time (i.e., anticipate physical discomfort or difficulty getting out of bed and plan to have measures in place to help alleviate barriers, such as having the patient sit up in bed instead of leaving bed) If stopping naps is a problem, try slowly reducing duration and moving them earlier in the day. Naps should be taken in bed
Relaxation: Progressive muscle relaxation Passive muscle relaxation Deep breathing Meditation Autogenic phrases Guided imagery	Use passive methods instead of progressive muscle relaxation if pain is a concern Allow the patient to choose what best works for them and encourage them to go at their own pace Be aware of the potential for hearing loss when administering relaxation Encourage home practice
Sleep hygiene: Avoid napping Avoid caffeine after noon Avoid nicotine Avoid alcohol within 2 hours of bedtime Avoid heavy meals within 2 hours of bedtime Increase daily exercise, but avoid within 2 hours of bedtime Create an adequate sleep environment (i.e., cool, dark, free of outside noise)	Gradual withdrawal from caffeine, nicotine, or napping and gradual increases in exercise will help the patient find success and build efficacy Developing a baseline for disruptive behaviors can help the patient see how they affect their sleep
Sleep restriction: 1. Gather baseline data on time in bed and total sleep time 2. Prescribe time in bed at the patient's average baseline total sleep time plus 30 minutes 3. Set bedtime and wake time to meet time in bed prescription 4. If average sleep efficiency is >90%, increase time in bed by 15–30 minutes 5. If average sleep efficiency is <85%, decrease time in bed by 15–30 minutes	Help patient identify additional activities to engage in during their newly increased time awake to combat boredom and help improve treatment compliance Emphasize positive changes during treatment to help improve sleep self-efficacy
Cognitive therapy: Cognitive restructuring Correct misconceptions about insomnia and its daytime consequences	Older adults may have more established beliefs about their sleep and may be less flexible when attempting to change them Be concrete when describing principles and provide many practical examples to illustrate concepts

Included with permission from Petrov et al. [114] and Oxford University Press
[a]Many tips for older adults derived from chapters of Lichstein and Morin, 2000

22.8.3 Pharmacological

Numerous pharmacological drugs are used to treat insomnia symptoms in OAWI, including antihistamines, antidepressants, atypical antipsychotics, sedatives, and sedative-hypnotics [102]. Only sedative-hypnotics, which include benzodiazepines (e.g., estazolam, temazepam), non-benzodiazepines (e.g., eszopiclone, zolpidem), melatonin receptor agonists (e.g., ramelteon), orexin receptor antagonists (e.g., suvorexant), and low doses of antidepressants (doxepin), are approved for the treatment of insomnia by the US Food and Drug Administration [6]. There is some evidence that insomnia medications can safely treat OAWI [20], but there remains insufficient evidence regarding the effectiveness of these medications in OAWI [105]. Sedative-hypnotics carry with them the possibility of negative side effects, such as dizziness, increased risk of falls, headaches, fatigue, excessive sleepiness, and interactions with other medications [24, 35].

Recently, some sedative-hypnotics, such as benzodiazepines, have been deemed potentially inappropriate for use in older adults due to the potential for cognitive impairment, delirium, falls, and fractures [58, 103]. In general, CBT has been shown to be more effective than pharmacotherapy for the treatment of late-life insomnia and to have better maintenance of gains in the general population [72, 99].

22.9 Implications for Practice

Insomnia is a highly prevalent problem in older adults that warrants appropriate attention, assessment, and intervention. Despite a more complicated clinical presentation of insomnia, cognitive-behavioral and pharmacological interventions benefit OAWI. However, cognitive-behavioral interventions are more highly recommended as the side-effect profile is minimal, and the persistence of successful treatment outcomes is greater. ◘ Table 22.2 provides a list of special considerations for using CBT for insomnia in older adults. While pharmacological approaches can also be beneficial, caution should be used in prescribing them given the potential for negative side effects. Careful consideration should be given regarding the type of medication that is prescribed to OAWI given that some sedative-hypnotics, such as benzodiazepines, have been deemed potentially inappropriate for use in older adults.

Case Conclusion

Mrs. Doe, a 68-year-old Caucasian female, presents with primary complaints of difficulty falling asleep, difficulty maintaining sleep, and daytime fatigue. During assessment, she indicated several behaviors that may exacerbate sleep difficulties, including increased cognitive activity at bedtime, reading while in bed, alcohol use prior to bed, and electronic use (tablet) at bedtime. Given the onset of Mrs. Doe's sleep difficulties following her retirement, less regularity or activity in her daily schedule may contribute to her present complaint. Mrs. Doe would likely benefit from a multi-component cognitive-behavioral intervention incorporating stimulus control, relaxation, cognitive therapy, and sleep hygiene to foster adaptive sleep-promoting behaviors.

References

1. Abell JG, Shipley MJ, Ferrie JE, Kivimäki M, Kumari M. Association of chronic insomnia symptoms and recurrent extreme sleep duration over 10 years with well-being in older adults: a cohort study. BMJ Open. 2016;6(2):e009501.
2. Altena E, van der Werf Y, Strijers RLM, Van Someren EJW. Sleep loss affects vigilance: effects of chronic insomnia and sleep therapy. J Sleep Res. 2008;17(3):335–43.
3. American Academy of Sleep Medicine. International classification of sleep disorders. 2nd ed. Westchester: American Academy of Sleep Medicine; 2005. p. 1–31.
4. American Psychiatric Association. Diagnostic and statistical manual of mental disorders. 5th ed. Arlington: American Psychiatric Association; 2013.
5. Ancoli-Israel S, Ayalon L, Salzman C. Sleep in the elderly: normal variations and common sleep disorders. Harv Rev Psychiatry. 2008;16(5):279–86.
6. Asnis GM, Thomas M, Henderson MA. Pharmacotherapy treatment options for insomnia: a primer for clinicians. Int J Mol Sci. 2016;17(1):50.
7. Bao YP, Han Y, Ma J, Wang RJ, Shi L, Wang TY, et al. Cooccurrence and bidirectional prediction of sleep disturbances and depression in older adults: meta-analysis and systematic review. Neurosci Biobehav Rev. 2017;75:257–73.
8. Black DS, O'Reilly GA, Olmstead R, Breen EC, Irwin MR. Mindfulness meditation and improvement in sleep quality and daytime impairment among older adults with sleep disturbances. JAMA Intern Med. 2015;175(4):494–501.
9. Blackwell T, Yaffe K, Laffan A, Ancoli-Israel S, Redline S, Ensrud KE, et al. Associations of objectively and subjectively measured sleep quality with subsequent cognitive decline in older community-dwelling men: the MrOS sleep study. Sleep. 2014;37(4):655–63.
10. Boden-Albala B, Bazil C, Moon Y, De Rosa J, Elkind MS, Paik MC et al. Unplanned napping causes seniors vascular events. International Stroke Conference. New Orleans, USA. American Stroke Association; 2008.
11. Bonanni E, Tognoni G, Maestri M, Salvati N, Fabbrini M, Borghetti D, et al. Sleep disturbances in elderly subjects: an epidemiological survey in an Italian district. Acta Neurol Scand. 2010;122(6):389–97.
12. Bootzin RR, Epstein DR. Stimulus control. In: Lichstein KL, Morin CM, editors. Treatment of late-life insomnia. Thousand Oaks: Sage; 2000. p. 185–206.
13. Buysse DJ, Ancoli-Israel S, Edinger JD, Lichstein KL, Morin CM. Recommendations for a standard research assessment of insomnia. Sleep. 2006;29(9):1155–73.
14. Campbell SS, Murphy PJ. The nature of spontaneous sleep across adulthood. J Sleep Res. 2007;16(1):24–32.
15. Campbell SS, Murphy PJ, Stauble TN. Effects of a nap on nighttime sleep and waking function in older subjects. J Am Geriatr Soc. 2005;53(1):48–53.
16. Carley DW, Farabi SS. Physiology of sleep. Diabetes Spectr. 2016;29(1):5–9.
17. Carney CE, Buysse DJ, Ancoli-Israel S, Edinger JD, Krystal AD, Lichstein KL, et al. The consensus sleep diary: standardizing prospective sleep self-monitoring. Sleep. 2012;35:287–302.
18. Chen X, Wang R, Zee P, Lutsey PL, Javaheri S, Alcántara C, et al. Racial/ethnic differences in sleep disturbances: the multi-ethnic study of atherosclerosis (MESA). Sleep. 2015;38(6):877–88.
19. Cintron D, Lipford M, Larrea-Mantilla L, Spencer-Bonilla G, Lloyd R, Gionfriddo MR, et al. Efficacy of menopausal hormone therapy on sleep quality: systematic review and meta-analysis. Endocrine. 2017;55(3):702–11.
20. Cotroneo A, Gareri P, Nicoletti N, Lacava R, Grassone D, Maina E, et al. Effectiveness and safety of hypnotic drugs in the treatment of insomnia in over 70-year old people. Arch Gerontol Geriatr. 2007;44.(suppl:121–4.
21. Crowley K. Sleep and sleep disorders in older adults. Neuropsychol Rev. 2011;21(1):41–13.
22. De Almondes KM, Costa MV, Malloy-Diniz LF, Diniz BS. Insomnia and risk of dementia in older adults: systematic review and meta-analysis. J Psychiatr Res. 2016;77:109–15.
23. Dement W, Richarson G, Prinz P, Carskadon M, Kripke D, Czeisler C. Changes of sleep and wakefulness with age. In: Finch CE, Schneider EL, editors. Handbook of the biology of aging. 2nd ed. New York: Van Nostrand Reinhold; 1985. p. 692–717.
24. Dolder C, Nelson M, McKinsey J. Use of non-benzodiazepine hypnotics in the elderly: are all agents the same? CNS Drugs. 2007;21(5):389–405.
25. Dragioti E, Bernfort L, Larsson B, Gerdle B, Levin LA. Association of insomnia severity with well-being, quality of life and health care costs: a cross-sectional study in older adults with chronic pain (PainS65+). Eur J Pain. 2018;22(2):414–25.

26. Dragioti E, Levin LA, Bernfort L, Larsson B, Gerdle B. Insomnia severity and its relationship with demographics, pain features, anxiety, and depression in older adults with and without pain: cross-sectional population-based results from the PainS65+ cohort. Ann Gen Psychiatry. 2017;16:15.
27. Durrence HH, Lichstein KL. The sleep of African Americans: a comparative review. Behav Sleep Med. 2006;4(1):29–44.
28. Dzierzewski J, Williams JM, Roditi D, Marsiske M, McCoy K, McNamara J, et al. Daily variations in objective nighttime sleep and subjective morning pain in older adults with insomnia: evidence of covariation over time. J Am Geriatr Soc. 2010;58(5):925–30.
29. Foley DJ, Monjan AA, Brown SL, Simonsick EM, Wallace RB, Blazer DG. Sleep complaints among elderly persons: an epidemiologic study of three communities. Sleep. 1995;18(6):425–32.
30. Foley DJ, Monjan A, Simonsick EM, Wallace RB, Blazer DG. Incidence and remission of insomnia among elderly adults: an epidemiologic study of 6,800 persons over three years. Sleep. 1999;22(Suppl 2):S366–72.
31. Foley DJ, Ancoli-Israel S, Britz P, Walsh J. Sleep disturbances and chronic disease in older adults: results of the 2003 National Sleep Foundation Sleep in America survey. J Psychosom Res. 2004;56(5):497–502.
32. Ford DE, Kamerow DB. Epidemiologic study of sleep disturbances and psychiatric disorders. JAMA. 1989;262(11):1479–84.
33. Garland SN, Carlson LE, Stephens AJ, Antle MC, Samuels C, Campbell TS. Mindfulness-based stress reduction compared with cognitive behavioral therapy for the treatment of insomnia comorbid with cancer: a randomized, partially blinded, noninferiority trial. J Clin Oncol. 2014;32(5):449–57.
34. Gillin JC, Ancoli-Israel S. The impact of age on sleep and sleep disorders. In: Salzman C, editor. Clinical geriatric psychopharmacology. 4th ed. Philadelphia: Lippincott Williams & Wilkins; 2005. p. 483–512.
35. Glass J, Lanctot KL, Herrmann N, Sproule BA, Busto UE. Sedative hypnotics in older people with insomnia: meta-analysis of risks and benefits. BMJ. 2005;331(7526):1169.
36. Goldman SE, Hall M, Boudreau R, Matthews KA, Cauley JA, Ancoli-Israel S, et al. Association between nighttime sleep and napping in older adults. Sleep. 2008;31(5):733–40.
37. Gong H, Ni CX, Liu YZ, Zhang Y, Su WJ, Lian YJ. Mindfulness meditation for insomnia: a meta-analysis of randomized controlled trials. J Psychosom Res. 2016;89:1–6.
38. Gureje O, Kola L, Ademola A, Olley BO. Profile, comorbidity and impact of insomnia in the Ibadan study of ageing. Int J Geriatr Psychiatry. 2009;24(7):686–93.
39. Gureje O, Loadeji BD, Abiona T, Makanjuola V, Esan O. The natural history of insomnia in the Ibadan study of ageing. Sleep. 2011;34(7):965–73.
40. Haimov I, Hadad BS, Shurkin D. Visual cognitive function: changes associated with chronic insomnia in older adults. J Gerontol Nurs. 2007;33(10):32–41.
41. Haimov I, Hanuka E, Horowitz Y. Chronic insomnia and cognitive functioning among older adults. Behav Sleep Med. 2008;6(1):32–54.
42. Hara C, Stewart R, Lima-Costa MF, Rocha FL, Fuzikawa C, Uchoa E, et al. Insomnia subtypes and their relationship to excessive daytime sleepiness in Brazilian community-dwelling older adults. Sleep. 2011;34(8):1111–7.
43. Harvey AG. A cognitive model of insomnia. Behav Res Ther. 2002;40(8):869–93.
44. Iber C. The AASM manual for the scoring of sleep and associated events: rules, terminology and technical specification. Westchester: American Academy of Sleep Medicine; 2007.
45. Irwin MR, Cole JC, Nicassio PM. Comparative meta-analysis of behavioral interventions for insomnia and their efficacy in middle-aged adults and in older adults 55+ years of age. Health Psychol. 2006;25(1):3–14.
46. Jaussent I, Dauvilliers Y, Ancelin M, Darigues J, Tavernier B, Touchon J, et al. Insomnia symptoms in older adults: associated factors and gender differences. Am J Geriatr Psychiatry. 2011;19(1):88–97.
47. Jean-Louis G, Magai CM, Cohen CI, Zizi F, von Gizycki H, DiPalma J, et al. Ethnic differences in self-reported sleep problems in older adults. Sleep. 2001;24(8):926–33.
48. Jehan S, Masters-Isarilov A, Salifu I, Zizi F, Jean-Louis G, Pandi-Perumal SR, et al. Sleep disorders in postmenopausal women. J Sleep Disord Ther. 2015;4(5).
49. Kamal NS, Gammack JK. Insomnia in the elderly: cause, approach, and treatment. Am J Med. 2006;119(6):463–9.
50. Kaufmann CN, Mojtabai R, Hock RS, Thorpe RJ, Canham SL, Chen L. Racial/ethnic differences in insomnia trajectories among U.S. older adults. Am J Geriatr Psychiatry. 2016;24(7):575–84.
51. Kay DB, Dombrovski AY, Buysse DJ, Reynolds CF, Begley A, Szanto K. Insomnia is associated with suicide attempt in middle-aged and older adults with depression. Int Psychogeriatr. 2016;28(4):613–9.
52. Kim J, Stewart R, Kim S, Yang S, Shin I, Yoon J. Insomnia, depression, and physical disorders in late life: a 2-year longitudinal community study in Koreans. Sleep. 2009;39(9):1221–8.
53. Krishnan P, Hawranik P. Diagnosis and management of geriatric insomnia: a guide for nurse practitioners. J Am Acad Nurse Pract. 2008;20(12):590–9.
54. Li J, Cacchione PZ, Hodgson N, Riegel B, Keenan BT, Scharf MT, et al. Afternoon napping and cognition in Chinese older adults: findings from the China Health and Retirement Longitudinal Study baseline assessment. J Gerontol A Biol Sci Med Sci. 2017;65(2):373–80.
55. Lichstein KL. Relaxation. In: Lichstein KL, Morin CM, editors. Treatment of late-life insomnia. Thousand Oaks: Sage; 2000. p. 185–206.
56. Lichstein KL, Riedel BW, Wilson NM, Lester KW, Aguillard RN. Relaxation and sleep compression for late-life insomnia: a placebo controlled trial. J Consult Clin Psychol. 2001;69(2):227–39.
57. Lichstein KL, Durrence HH, Riedel BW, Taylor DJ, Bush AJ. Epidemiology of sleep: age, gender, and ethnicity. Mahwah: Lawrence Erlbaum Associates, Inc; 2004.
58. Lie JD, Tu KN, Shen DD, Wong BM. Pharmological treatment of insomnia. PT. 2015;40(11):759–68.
59. Littner M, Hirshkowitz M, Kramer M, Kapen S, Anderson WM, Bailey D, et al. Practice parameters for using polysomnography to evaluate insomnia: an update. Sleep. 2003;26:754–60.
60. Liu X, Liu L. Sleep habits and insomnia in a sample of elderly persons in China. Sleep. 2005;28(12):1579–87.
61. McCrae CS, Rowe MA, Tierney CG, Dautovich ND, DeFinis AL, McNamara JPH. Sleep complaints, subjective and objective sleep patterns, health, psychological adjustment, and daytime functioning in community-dwelling older adults. J Gerontol B Psychol Sci Soc Sci. 2005;60(4):182–9.
62. McCrae CS, Rowe MA, Dautovich ND, Lichstein KL, Durrence HH, Riedel BW, et al. Sleep hygiene practices in two community dwelling samples of older adults. Sleep. 2006;29:1551–60.
63. McCrae CS, Dzierzewski JM, Kay DB. Treatment of late-life insomnia. Sleep Med Clin. 2009;4(4):593–604.
64. McCurry SM, Logsdon RG, Teri L, Vitiello MV. Evidence-based psychological treatments for insomnia in older adults. Psychol Aging. 2007;22(1):18–27.
65. Middelkoop HA, Kerkhof GA, Smilde-van den Doel DA, Ligthart GJ, Kamphuisen HA. Sleep and ageing: the effect of institutionalization on subjective and objective characteristics of sleep. Age Ageing. 1994;23(5):411–7.
66. Monk TH. Aging human circadian rhythms: conventional wisdom may not always be right. J Biol Rhythm. 2005;20(4):366–74.
67. Monk TH, Germain A, Buysse DJ. The sleep of the bereaved. Sleep Hypn. 2009;11(1):219–29.
68. Morgan K. Sleep and aging. In: Lichstein KL, Morin CM, editors. Treatment of late-life insomnia. Thousand Oaks: Sage; 2000. p. 3–36.
69. Morgan K. Daytime activity & risk factors for late-life insomnia. J Sleep Res. 2003;12(3):231–8.

70. Morgan K, Clark D. Longitudinal trends in late-life insomnia: implications for prescribing. Age Aging. 1997;26(3):179–84.
71. Morgenthaler T, Alessi C, Friedman L, Owens J, Kapur V, Boehlecke B, et al. Practice parameters for the use of actigraphy in the assessment of sleep and sleep disorders: an update for 2007. Sleep. 2007;30(4):519–29.
72. Morin CM, Colecchi C, Stone J, Sood R, Brink D. Behavioral and pharmacological therapies for late life insomnia: a randomized controlled trial. JAMA. 1999;281(11):991–9.
73. Morin CM, Savard J, Blais FC. Cognitive therapy. In: Lichstein KL, Morin CM, editors. Treatment of late-life insomnia. Thousand Oaks: Sage; 2000. p. 185–206.
74. Neikrug AB, Ancoli-Israel S. Sleep disorders in the older adult–a mini review. Gerontology. 2010;56(2):181–9.
75. Ohayon M. Epidemiologic study on insomnia in the general population. Sleep. 1996;19(Suppl 1):S7–S15.
76. Ohayon MM. Epidemiology of insomnia: what we know and what we still need to learn. Sleep Med Rev. 2002;6(2):97–111.
77. Ohayon MM, Zulley J, Guilleminault C, Smirne S, Priest RG. How age and daytime activities are related to insomnia in the general population: consequences for older people. J Am Ger Soc. 2001;49(4):360–6.
78. Ohayon MM, Carskadon MA, Guilleminault C, Vitiello MV. Meta-analysis of quantitative sleep parameters from childhood to old age in healthy individuals: developing normative sleep values across the human lifespan. Sleep. 2004;27(7):1255–73.
79. Osorio R, Pirraglia E, Aguera-Ortiz LF, During EH, Sacks H, Ayappa I, et al. Greater risk of Alzheimer's disease in older adults with insomnia. J Am Geriatr Soc. 2011;59(3):559–61.
80. Petrov ME, Lichstein KL. Differences in sleep between black and white adults: an update and future directions. Sleep Med. 2016;18:74–81.
81. Picarsic JL, Glynn NW, Taylor CA, Katula JA, Goldman SE, Studenski SA, et al. Self-reported napping and duration and quality of sleep in the Interventions and Independence for Elders Pilot Study. J Am Geriatr Soc. 2008;56(9):1674–80.
82. Pigeon WR, Hegel M, Unützer J, Fan MY, Sateia MJ, Lyness JM, et al. Is insomnia a perpetuating factor for late-life depression in the IMPACT cohort? Sleep. 2008;31(4):481–8.
83. Rechtschaffen A, Kales AA. A manual of standardized terminology, techniques and scoring system for sleep stages of human subjects. Los Angeles: Brain Information Service; 1968.
84. Richards KC, Lambert C, Beck CK, Bliwise DL, Evans WJ, Kalra GK, et al. Strength training, walking, and social activity improve sleep in nursing home and assisted living residents: randomized controlled trial. J Am Geriatr Soc. 2011;59(2):214–23.
85. Riedel BW, Lichstein KL. Insomnia and daytime functioning. Sleep Med Rev. 2000;4(3):277–98.
86. Roux FJ, Kryger MH. Medication effects on sleep. Clin Chest Med. 2010;31(2):397–405.
87. Rowe M, McCrae C, Campbell J, Horne C, Tiegs T, Lehman B, et al. Actigraphy in older adults: comparison of means and variability of three different aggregates of measurement. Behav Sleep Med. 2008;6(2):127–45.
88. Ruiter ME, DeCoster J, Jacobs L, Lichstein KL. Sleep disorders in African Americans and Caucasian Americans: a meta-analysis. Behav Sleep Med. 2010;8(4):246–59.
89. Ruiter ME, Vander Wal GV, Lichstein KL. Insomnia in the elderly. In: Pandi-Peruman SR, Monti JM, Monjan A, editors. Principles and practice of geriatric sleep medicine. Cambridge: Cambridge University Press; 2010. p. 271–9.
90. Sadler P, McLaren S, Jenkins M. A psychological pathway from insomnia to depression among older adults. Int Psychogeriatr. 2013;25(8):1375–83.
91. Sateia MJ, Doghramji K, Hauri PJ, Morin CM. Evaluation of chronic insomnia: an American Academy of Sleep Medicine review. Sleep. 2000;23(2):237–41.
92. Schmidt C, Peigneux P, Cajochen C. Age-related changes in sleep and circadian rhythms: impact on cognitive performance and underlying neuroanatomical networks. Front Neurol. 2012; 3(118).
93. Schutte-Rodin S, Broch L, Buysse D, Dorsey C, Sateia M. Clinical guideline for the evaluation and management of chronic insomnia in adults. J Clin Sleep Med. 2008;4(5):487–504.
94. Schnelle JF, Cruise PA, Alessi CA, Al-Samarrai N, Ouslander JG. Sleep hygiene in physically dependent nursing home residents. Sleep. 1998;21(5):515–23.
95. Sivertsen B, Omvik S, Pallesen S, Bjorvatn B, Havik OE, Kvale G, et al. Cognitive behavioral therapy vs zopiclone for treatment of chronic primary insomnia in older adults: a randomized controlled trial. JAMA. 2006;295(24):2851–8.
96. Smagula SF, Stone KL, Fabio A, Cauley JA. Risk factors for sleep disturbances in older adults: evidence from prospective studies. Sleep Med Rev. 2016;25:21–30.
97. Smith MT, Haythornthwaite JA. How do sleep disturbance and chronic pain inter-relate? Insights from the longitudinal and cognitive-behavioral clinical trials literature. Sleep Med Rev. 2004;8(2):119–32.
98. Smith MT, Perlis ML, Smith MS, Giles DE, Carmody TP. Sleep quality and presleep arousal in chronic pain. J Behav Med. 2000;23(1): 1–13.
99. Smith MT, Perlis ML, Park A, Smith MA, Pennington J, Giles DE, et al. Comparative meta-analysis of pharmacotherapy and behavior therapy for persistent insomnia. Am J Psychiatry. 2002;159(1): 5–11.
100. Spira AP, Kaufmann CN, Kasper JD, Ohayon MM, Rebok GW, Skidmore E, et al. Association between insomnia symptoms and functional status in U.S. older adults. J Gerontol B Psychol Sci Soc Sci. 2014;69(Suppl 1):S35–41.
101. Stone KL, Ancoli-Israel S, Blackwell T, Ensrud KE, Cauley JA, Redline S, et al. Actigraphy-measured sleep characteristics and risk of falls in older women. Arch Intern Med. 2008;168(16):1768–75.
102. Taylor SR, Weiss JS. Review of insomnia pharmacotherapy options for the elderly: implications for managed care. Popul Health Manag. 2009;12(6):317–23.
103. The American Geriatrics Society 2012 Beers Criteria Update Expert Panel. American Geriatrics Society Updated Beers criteria for potentially inappropriate medication use in older adults. J Am Geriatr Soc. 2012;60:616–31.
104. Varrasse M, Li J, Gooneratne N. Exercise and sleep in community-dwelling older adults. Curr Sleep Med Rep. 2015; 1(4):232–40.
105. Wilt J, MacDonald R, Brasure M, Olson CM, Carlyle M, Fuchs E, et al. Pharmacologic treatment of insomnia disorder: an evidence report for a Clinical Practice Guideline by the American College of Physicians. Ann Intern Med. 2016;165(2):103–12.
106. Wohlgemuth WK, Edinger JD. Sleep restriction therapy. In: Lichstein KL, Morin CM, editors. Treatment of late-life insomnia. Thousand Oaks: Sage; 2000. p. 185–206.
107. Wolkove N, Elkholy O, Baltzan M, Palayew M. Sleep and aging: sleep disorders commonly found in older people. CMAJ. 2007;176(9):1299–04.
108. World Health Organization. The ICD-10 Classification of mental and behavioral disorders. Geneva: World Health Organization; 1993.
109. Yokoyama E, Saito Y, Kaneita Y, Ohida T, Harano S, Tamaki T, et al. Association between subjective well-being and sleep among the elderly in Japan. Sleep Med. 2008;9(2):157–64.
110. Yokoyama E, Kaneita Y, Saito Y, Uchiyama M, Matsuzaki Y, Tamaki T, et al. Association between depression and insomnia subtypes: a longitudinal study on the elderly in Japan. Sleep. 2010;33(12): 1693–702.
111. Zhang B, Wing Y. Sex differences in insomnia: a meta-analysis. Sleep. 2006;29(1):85–93.

112. Zhang JX, Lui HX, Xie XH, Zhao D, Shan MS, Zhang XL, et al. Mindfulness-based stress reduction for chronic insomnia in adults older than 75 years: a randomized, controlled, single-blind clinical trial. Explore. 2015;11(3):180–5.
113. Zhong G, Wang Y, Tao T, Ying J, Zhao Y. Daytime napping and mortality from all causes, cardiovascular disease, and cancer: a meta-analysis of prospective cohort studies. Sleep Med. 2015;16(7):811–9.
114. Petrov MER, Vander Wal GS, Lichstein KL. Late-life insomnia. In: Pachana NA, Laidlaw K, editors. The Oxford handbook of clinical geropsychology. Oxford: Oxford University Press; 2015. p. 527–48.

Functional Assessment/ Self-Care Ability (MOBILITY)

Contents

Assessment of Capability and Capacity

Michele Lee and Katherine Wang

A. Chun (ed.), *Geriatric Practice*, https://doi.org/10.1007/978-3-030-19625-7_23

23.1 Introduction

Over the years, the field of medicine has shifted from paternalism, in which a physician makes decisions based on what he or she believes to be in the patient's best interest, to shared decision-making, in which physicians and patients work together to formulate a treatment plan based on the patient's values. This model of shared decision-making is based on the fundamental principle of patient autonomy: the right of patients to make their own decisions. Informed consent requires that a patient's decisions are voluntary and that the patient possesses decision-making capacity (the ability to understand treatment options and then accept or refuse treatment).

23.1.1 Historical Context

History teaches us the importance of informed consent. During World War II, thousands of prisoners in the Nazi concentration camps were forced to participate in inhumane medical torture such as freezing experiments, ostensibly to learn about hypothermia's effects on the body, or deliberate spread of infectious diseases such as tuberculosis, supposedly to be able to prevent or treat the disease. Prisoners were not told the purpose of the procedures and were powerless to refuse interventions. Many died as a result of these experiments; those that survived were left with severe physical and mental disability and trauma [20]. After the war, these Nazi physicians were put on trial for medical torture. These trials formed the basis for the Nuremberg Code of medical ethics: ten ethical principles about human experimentation that stress that participation must be both voluntary and well-informed [15]. The Nuremberg Code underpins modern-day Institutional Review Board protocols, which review proposed research methods to ensure they are ethical and do not result in coercion.

Similarly, the Public Health Service and the Tuskegee Institute infamously conducted an exploitative study on black men in Alabama from 1932 to 1972 to understand the natural history of syphilis. Participants were told only that they were being treated for "bad blood" and would receive free medical care, but not the true purpose of the study [19]. Though by 1947 penicillin had become readily available as the treatment of choice, researchers still did not offer this curative medication. Shockingly, the study continued for another 25 years, ending only when the Tuskegee Study was publicized in 1972 and received widespread condemnation for unethical study practices [19].

In 1974, the affected families received a settlement of 10 million dollars; remaining participants received the promise of lifetime medical benefits and burial services [19]. Unfortunately, the study caused immeasurable damage and sowed mistrust between black communities and the medical establishment that many argue persists to this day. One study even argues that life expectancy for black men fell by 1.5 years as result of this study [1]. As a result, federally supported studies using human subjects must be reviewed by institutional review boards and obtain proper informed consent from any subjects.

23.2 Informed Consent

In order for a choice to be voluntary, the person must not be manipulated, deceived, or coerced in any way. The patient maintains the right to refuse any medical intervention or treatment that is offered. The physician is obligated to disclose to the patient relevant risks and possible benefits of the proposed medication or intervention, in a way that the patient can understand. The physician's disclosure is considered adequate if the conversation about possible outcomes mirrors that which another reasonable physician would have discussed in the same situation [16]. The framework for the process of informed consent is outlined in ◘ Fig. 23.1.

23.3 Decision-Making Capacity

After being given all the appropriate information, patients must demonstrate decision-making capacity: the ability to understand and appreciate the nature and consequences of a decision regarding accepting or forgoing treatment. For instance, if a

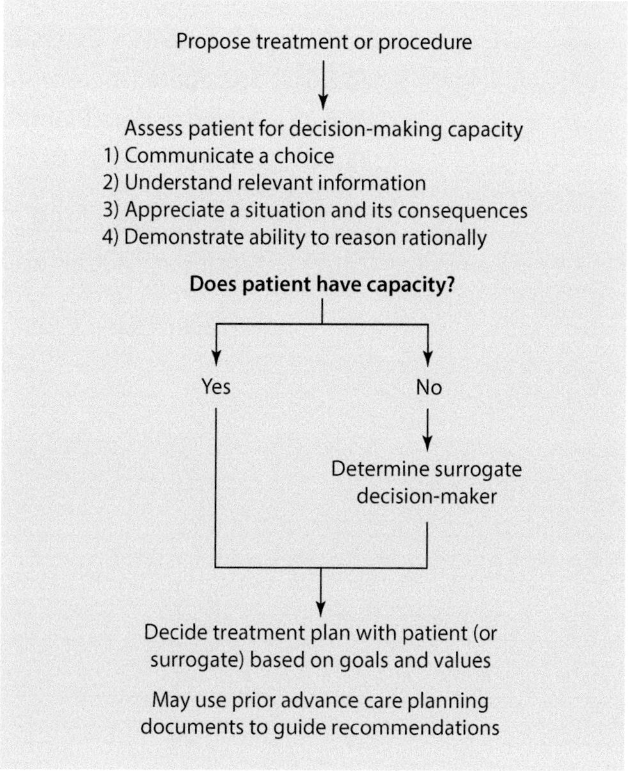

◘ **Fig. 23.1** Process of informed consent: A flow diagram indicating the necessary steps of shared decision-making

patient decides to decline surgery for colorectal cancer, he or she needs to understand that without that treatment the cancer will eventually spread and ultimately cause death.

Physicians determine decision-making capacity through interviews; most of the time, these assessments are being done implicitly with every patient interaction. Patients may prove to have capacity to make some decisions but not others, depending on the complexity of the decision. For example, the decision whether or not to start an antihypertensive is a much simpler choice than whether or not to undergo surgery for colorectal cancer. Therefore, capacity must be assessed for every decision and we must not assume that a patient lacks capacity for all decisions, even if they were deemed to lack capacity for a prior decision.

23.3.1 Capacity and Competency

The terms capacity and competency are similar in that they both can refer to the ability of a patient to make decisions. However, the key difference is that competency is determined by a court [10]. Competency pertains not only to one's ability to make medical decisions but also the ability to participate in other legal matters such as appearing in court or signing a contract. Capacity, on the other hand, is determined by a physician and is decision-specific (◘ Table 23.1).

◘ Table 23.1 Capacity versus competency

Capacity	Competency
Determined by a physician	Determined in court
Refers to one's ability to make decisions regarding one's health including whether to accept or refuse medical interventions	Refers to one's ability to participate in legal matters including signing a contract, creating a living will, or making medical decisions

23.3.2 Risk Factors for Impaired Capacity

Diseases that affect cognitive ability can be associated with a loss of decision-making capacity, but since most diseases have a range of severity, having a particular diagnosis like Alzheimer's disease does not automatically mean one lacks decision-making capacity [2]. Rather, patients should always be assumed to have decision-making capacity unless a thorough evaluation deems otherwise. In addition to neurodegenerative dementias such as Alzheimer's disease, Parkinson's disease, and frontotemporal dementia, psychiatric disorders such as depression and anxiety or reversible conditions such as delirium can impair one's ability to make decisions. It is important for physicians to first treat all reversible conditions such as infection or pain which may be temporarily impairing a patient's cognitive function.

Box 23.1 Reversible Conditions Associated with Delirium/Impaired Capacity

- Pain
- Infection
- Uremia and metabolic derangements
- Hospital-associated delirium
- Medication side effect (particular offenders may be benzodiazepines, opiates, or other sedating medications)
- Substance use

If at any point a physician is concerned about a patient's decision-making capacity, a formal assessment must be performed. Formal assessments are usually done when there is concern about a patient's cognitive ability or when patients go against medical advice and make "unreasonable" decisions where the risk for refusing treatment is an unfavorable outcome. Capacity evaluation may be necessary for a high-stakes decision, such as a surgery for aortic dissection, or a lower-stakes but still important decision such as acceptance of home care.

While clinicians assess capacity informally every day, a more thorough evaluation for decision-making capacity should be prompted by the following scenarios:

1. Patient has an abrupt change in mental status: delirium or acute medical illness may cause a temporary or reversible change in cognition.
2. Patient refuses medical treatment, particularly if reasons are not clear, the refusal is based on misinformation or biases, or the risk of refusing treatment is an unfavorable outcome (e.g., declining amputation for gangrene—risk of death by declining surgery).
3. Patient rapidly consents to high-risk or invasive treatment without careful consideration of risk and benefit.
4. Patient has known risk factor for impaired decision-making such as dementia or mental illness, notable cultural or language barriers, or limited health literacy. Note that having one of these risk factors does not mean that the person automatically lacks capacity, but that a more careful assessment may be required.

Box 23.2 Scenarios That May Prompt Capacity Assessment

- A patient needs assistance with most activities of daily living including toileting and ambulation and is thought to be unsafe at home, but declines any kind of home care.
- A patient has had several minor motor vehicle accidents, but continues to drive.
- A patient declines any medications for uncontrolled high blood pressure.
- A patient continues to smoke despite being on supplemental oxygen at home.
- A patient has been on dialysis for 12 years and decides he would like to discontinue.

23.4 Assessing Capacity

Case: Mr. F

Mr. F is a frail 86-year-old nursing home resident with oxygen-dependent chronic obstructive pulmonary disease (COPD) who presents to the emergency department with new-onset abdominal pain and vomiting. An emergent CT scan reveals a complete small bowel obstruction, and the surgical service recommends urgent surgery. The patient refuses, so the psychiatry service is consulted to evaluate Mr. F's capacity.

During the initial interview, the patient is nauseous, in pain, irritable and appears confused. He is clearly able to communicate the choice of "no surgery," but does he have capacity to make this decision?

To assess capacity, no single approach is universally utilized. The most widely accepted approach involves assessment of four essential elements of decision-making capacity, the abilities to: (1) communicate a choice, (2) understand the relevant information, (3) appreciate a situation and its consequences, and (4) reason rationally (◘ Table 23.2, [2, 3]).

◘ **Table 23.2** Approach to assess decision-making capacity

Essential element	Questions to facilitate assessment	Patients must:
1. Communicate a choice	Which treatment option do you prefer? Do you plan to proceed with the treatment option recommended by your doctor?	Clearly and consistently indicate a preferred treatment option
2. Understand relevant information	Can you explain using your own words what is the problem with your health? Can you tell me what your doctor has told you regarding your health now? Do you know what treatments are available to you? Can you tell me the risks and benefits of having this treatment? Can you tell me the risks and benefits of not having this treatment?	Demonstrate that they understand the current medical situation and the medical interventions available to them
3. Appreciate a situation and its consequences	Do you believe that you need treatment? Can you tell me what the worst possible outcome is for you if you choose that treatment option? What is the best possible outcome? What do you think the most likely outcome is for you if you choose this treatment option? If you decline any therapy, what do you believe will happen to you?	Demonstrate understanding of the most likely outcomes of each treatment option, including no treatment at all
4. Demonstrate ability to reason rationally	Can you explain why you have decided on this treatment option? Can you tell me why the other treatment option that you did not choose is not acceptable to you?	Be able to explain why they prefer one treatment option over another and the values that helped shape their decision

Adapted from Appelbaum, *NEJM* [2]

Box 23.3 Essential Components of Decision-Making Capacity

1. One must be able to communicate a choice.
2. One needs to understand the relevant information presented.
3. One should comprehend the situation and possible consequences.
4. One needs to show ability to reason.

23.4.1 Communicate a Choice

If a patient is unable to indicate a choice, he or she clearly lacks the capacity to make a decision and another individual must be appointed with this responsibility. This is the simplest element, and without this ability, further assessment is not possible. Some patients may be unable to communicate a choice due to impairment of consciousness, psychiatric disease, or memory impairment. Others may be able to make a choice but lack the ability to consistently make the same choice from day to day. Patients always have the right to change their minds, but rapid and inconsistent decisions made without an explanation may indicate lack of decision-making capacity.

Ask: "Could you tell me which treatment option you prefer?"

Case Continued

Mr. F. is given anti-emetics for his nausea and morphine to control his pain. After 20 minutes, he seems much more comfortable and is answering questions appropriately. The surgeons again review the findings of the complete small bowel obstruction found on the abdominal CT scan and stress the importance of urgent surgery. When asked how he would like to proceed, the patient consistently and clearly states that he does not want surgery.

23.4.2 Understand the Relevant Information

Another key component of decision-making depends on the ability to understand the relevant information presented. It is the duty of the physician to ensure that the information they disclose regarding the medical situation, treatment options, and associated risks and benefits are presented in the language and at the appropriate education level that the patient would best understand. For patients whose native language differs from the physician's, an interpreter must be used—in-person if possible, or phone if a live interpreter is unavailable. Family members should not be used to translate; however, it can be helpful to have family and other supportive figures present at this meeting so that they hear the same information.

To properly assess for understanding, it is best to ask the patient to paraphrase in their own words what their medical condition is and what treatments options are available. By asking the patient to summarize the information they were given, physicians can evaluate the patient's comprehension and not just reiteration of the information.

Ask: "Can you explain using your own words what is the problem with your health?"

Case Continued

Mr. F listens to the surgeons discuss the medical situation and possible treatment options including surgery. When asked to explain his current condition he responds, "I have a blockage in my belly and to fix the blockage I need surgery right away." When asked to explain the risks and benefits of the surgery he replies, "the surgery can make the blockage go away, but I could die from the surgery."

Both the surgeons and psychiatrists agree that the patient has a good basic understanding of his illness and treatment choices and continue their assessment of decision-making capacity.

23.4.3 Appreciate a Situation and Its Consequences

Patients should be able to express what they perceive to be the risks and benefits to each treatment option, including no treatment at all, and understand the likely outcomes of each option. No one can be told every possible risk for every option, so it is important to frame the conversation in terms of relative risks and benefits for each patient. Every surgery has the risk of possible death, but in most cases, death is a rare outcome and should not be the sole focus in terms of risk.

To help facilitate discussion and a better understanding of treatment options and potential outcomes, some surgeons now use a communication device known as the Best Case/Worst Case framework [4, 14, 18]. This tool encourages physicians to use visual graphics to help depict the "best case," "worst case," and "most likely" situations the patient may face should they opt for or against surgery. Each scenario is phrased in terms of what the patient is likely to experience with each treatment option; this communication style uses a story to tell the most likely outcome. For instance, for a 92-year-old woman hospitalized with a hip fracture, who has mild cognitive impairment and well-controlled heart failure, a "most likely" outcome of surgery might be spending a few days in the hospital, needing a stay of several weeks in a subacute rehabilitation facility, and then discharge home with the same or perhaps slightly decreased functional status. A "most likely" outcome of nonoperative management might be markedly decreased functional status at home and potential for chronic pain. Use of this framework can help surgeons set tailored expectations for patients about likely outcomes. Both surgeons and patients felt the framework provided clarity about the two proposed options (surgery or not), and helped patients make choices consistent with their values [9]. It is possible that this framework might be adapted to nonsurgical treatment options as well (e.g., dialysis or chemotherapy).

Although a patient may seem to have adequate understanding of the illness, proposed treatment, associated risks and benefits, and alternative approaches, they still may not have the insight to appreciate how this information relates to them specifically. For instance, a patient may be able to recite the mechanism underlying diabetes and the consequences of uncontrolled diabetes, but do not believe that they themselves show signs of advanced diabetes or that they are at risk for future complications. This disconnect may be due to denial or distorted perception of the nature of one's illness. If patients do not believe they have a certain medical condition, they will not understand why they have been recommended for a particular treatment or understand what will happen to them if they refuse therapy. Patients who do not acknowledge their illness cannot appreciate their medical situation or the consequences of receiving care and therefore may lack capacity to make decisions regarding treatment.

Ask:

- "What do you think the most likely outcome is for you if you choose this treatment option?"
- "If you decline any therapy, what do you believe will happen to you?"

Case Continued

*The surgeons explain to Mr. F that death is a possibility of the planned surgery and he is at higher risk due to his age and comorbidities (oxygen-dependent COPD), but stress that if surgery is performed as soon as possible, death during surgery is not the likely outcome. The surgeons explain that if surgery is performed, the most likely outcome is that they will relieve the obstruction, but he will need to stay in the ICU/hospital for days to weeks, and he would leave the hospital for subacute rehabilitation much weaker than he arrived (**Table 23.3**).*

After some discussion, Mr. F appropriately describes his current medical condition by saying "I have a blockage in my belly and can most likely fix it with surgery, but there is a chance I could die because I am older and my lungs have disease. Even if I get the surgery and it is successful, I will probably have to stay in the hospital for a long time and have to go to another place after the hospital to regain my strength. If I don't get surgery, I may have more pain which can be treated with medications or may even die. There is a very slight chance the blockage may resolve on its own, but it's unlikely that this will happen." The physicians agree that Mr. F. understands his current situation as well as the risks of proposed surgery and ask what he has decided to do.

Table 23.3 Abridged best case/worst case

Opts for surgery	
Best case	**Worst case**
Survives surgery Days in ICU, then able to wean from ventilator successfully Needs rehabilitation in facility Will be much weaker; may need long-term placement in facility	Unable to wean from ventilator due to pulmonary disease Other postoperative complications Unable to express wishes or communicate with others Dies in ICU
Opts against surgery	
Best case	**Worst case**
Symptoms controlled Maintains ability to communicate Remains free of invasive therapies Dies in inpatient hospice	Symptoms refractory to medications, requires palliative sedation and cannot communicate Dies in hospital before family can say goodbye

Adapted from Kruser, *J Am Geriatr Soc* [9]

23.4.4 Ability to Reason Rationally

Once a patient makes a decision regarding whether to accept or reject the recommended medical therapy, it is important to ascertain what factors affected the patient's choice. Patients should be able to weigh the risks and benefits of each treatment option, including no treatment, and explain why one treatment option is better than another. The focus should be on the patient's rationale for their choice and not the actual choice itself [3]. Patients may disagree with recommended therapy as long as they can explain why they are willing or unwilling to tolerate some risks. If patients can demonstrate that they understand the consequences of their choices, then they are generally able to make their own decisions, including refusing life-sustaining therapy such as resuscitation, intubation, or dialysis. Some conditions that may hinder rational thought processing are psychotic disorders, extreme anxiety, depression, delirium, or dementia. Careful consideration of any reversible process should be addressed before deeming a patient to lack decision-making capacity.

Ask:

- "Can you explain why you have decided on this treatment option?"
- "Can you tell me why the other treatment option (that you did not choose) is not acceptable to you?"

Case Continued

Mr. F decides to decline surgical intervention for his small bowel obstruction. When asked to explain his reasoning, he replies, "I know that my condition can worsen if I don't do the surgery, but I do not want to undergo an operation where I have a risk of death even if it is a small risk. I cannot imagine being put to sleep and never waking up again. I am comfortable right now and want to continue getting pain medications and medicines to help my nausea. I will hope this blockage goes away on its own, but if it does get worse at least I will be awake and be able to know what is going on."

Since Mr. F clearly demonstrated that he was able to communicate a choice, understand the relevant information, appreciate the situation and its consequences, and was able to reason rationally, he was deemed to have the capacity to refuse surgery. He continued conservative management with aggressive comfort-oriented care in an inpatient palliative care unit.

23.5 Vulnerable Populations

23.5.1 Patients with Dementia

A common challenge exists when assessing capacity in a patient with cognitive impairment. It is of paramount importance to ensure that an individual's rights have not been curtailed because of a prior diagnosis of dementia. It should not be assumed that, because "dementia" or "mild cognitive impairment" is included in a problem list, that the person is incapable of making treatment decisions. Rather, we assume that capacity exists unless it is proven otherwise and, even with obvious impairment, we recognize that individuals may maintain the ability to communicate a clear preference that should help guide treatment.

One study assessed capacity using standards similar to those listed above: evidencing choice, making a reasonable choice, appreciating consequences, giving rational reason for choice, and understanding choice. In the study, patients with mild and moderate dementia (MMSE scores $\geq$19 and 10, respectively) were actually no worse than controls at expressing a treatment choice and making a reasonable treatment choice when the alternative is manifestly unreasonable. Patients with mild and moderate dementia did find it more challenging, however, to appreciate consequences of a choice and demonstrate reasoning. This suggests that, depending on the complexity of the decision at hand, patients with dementia may still maintain ability to contribute to treatment decisions [11].

As stated earlier, capacity is decision-specific; thus, the threshold to demonstrate decision-making capacity may be different depending on the choice. The bar to select a health-care proxy may be relatively low; many patients with cognitive impairment can clearly state that a close relative (or friend, etc.) could make decisions in their stead. On the other hand, demonstrating capacity to consent or refuse a high-risk procedure may be much higher. For instance, an amputation for gangrene may be recommended to prevent sepsis and potentially improve pain; but a patient's desire to salvage a limb is also understandable.

Along these lines, the process of determining consent may be more or less extensive depending on the gravity of the decision at hand. For deciding a health-care proxy, a clinician may make an informal assessment of capacity without devoting much time; a high-stakes decision (for instance, a decision to stop dialysis) demands a more rigorous evaluation, ideally performed by a team.

Some key factors that aid the clinician assessing for decision-making capacity in an individual with dementia:

- Need for collateral information that demonstrates decision-making is consistent with previously stated values and goals. Collateral may be provided by long-time providers like a primary care physician, relatives, or friends.
- Recognize that decisions are not always logic-based but may depend on relationships, culture, and personal values.

Frontotemporal dementia is a unique situation that may merit particular scrutiny when determining capacity. By definition, we see executive functioning impairments, so it stands to reason that the ability to make and communicate a reasoned decision about treatment may be compromised.

Box 23.4 Extra Steps when Assessing Capacity in Person with Dementia

- Give patient as much help as possible to make decision independently
- Communicate information in different way (written, pictures, etc)
- Break information into small chunks
- Think of different ways to describe things (using examples)

Caution must be exercised in assigning too much weight to cognitive testing (such as MMSE or MOCA). While profound impairments on cognitive testing (e.g., MMSE <16) are correlated with impaired capacity, a low MMSE does not guarantee a lack of capacity. By contrast, a normal MMSE does not preclude the possibility of impaired capacity [8, 12].

23.5.2 Patients with Mental Illness

A similar challenge of balancing autonomy and need presents itself in patients with longstanding mental illness. Serious mental illness, such as major depression, bipolar disorder, or schizophrenia, may impair a patient's ability to participate in treatment-related decisions. Many people opt against antipsychotics or other medications due to undesirable side effects; no easy approach exists to determine if involuntary treatment is indicated and how to simultaneously protect against abuse in this vulnerable population [13]. Certain psychiatric diagnoses are associated with increased risk for impaired capacity but do not guarantee it. Schizophrenia in particular places people at higher risk for impaired capacity; one review of 12 studies found that 10–52% of patients with schizophrenia demonstrated impairments on at least one measure of capacity, as compared with 0–18% of controls [7]. Worded differently, however, that means that up to 48–90% of patients with schizophrenia demonstrated no impairments in capacity.

23.6 Alternative Decision-Makers

23.6.1 Surrogate Decision-Making

In the event that a person is deemed not to have capacity and all reversible factors have been treated (e.g., lack of capacity is not a temporary state due to delirium or acute medical illness), decision-making would fall to a surrogate. Typically, a legal guardian would be first, followed by a designated decision-maker such as a health-care proxy or durable power of attorney for health care; if neither of those have been appointed, then a surrogate is identified. Surrogacy hierarchies differ from state to state but usually prioritize a spouse, then other family members.

Box 23.5 Sample Hierarchy of Surrogates (New York State)

1. Legal guardian
2. Health-care proxy
3. The spouse (if not legally separated from the patient) or domestic partner
4. Son or daughter 18 years or older
5. Parent
6. Brother or sister 18 years or older
7. A close friend

23.6.2 Advance Care Planning

Ideally, a patient has engaged in advance care planning and prepared documents that outline preferences for treatment, providing the decision-maker with guidance. Among these documents may be a living will or Physician Orders for Life-Sustaining Treatment (POLST, in some states known as Medical Orders for Life-Sustaining Treatment, or MOLST), which shares preferences about code status, antibiotics, artificial nutrition, and hydration. More innovative work recently has been done to help patients document and share their preferences with loved ones (see box).

Box 23.6 Some Innovative Patient-Centered Advance Care Planning Tools

- PREPARE ► https://prepareforyourcare.org
- The Conversation Project ► https://theconversationproject.org
- Five Wishes ► https://www.agingwithdignity.org
- Go Wish ► http://www.gowish.org
- Advance Directive for Dementia ► https://www.dementia-directive.org/

Unfortunately, there are frequently no available advance directives or the documents that were prepared are not applicable to the present situation. In that case, surrogates are charged with making health-care decisions using the concept of substituted judgment. If uncertain, they should make the decision that is felt to be within the patient's best interests. If surrogates seem to be making decisions at odds with what the patient might have wanted, it is important to try to understand the rationale behind those decisions and offer support for the immense challenge of making decisions on another's behalf.

If no surrogate exists, then the courts may need to appoint a legal guardian to oversee health-care decisions.

23.6.3 Choice to Defer Decision-Making

Even if a person maintains full decision-making capacity, they may voluntarily opt to defer decision-making to another person: a surrogate to make decisions in their stead. In so doing, they often allow some amount of leeway, or flexibility, to the person making decisions. Flexibility gives the decision-maker room to work with providers and potentially change prior medical decisions if something else is better for the patient at the time. Many people opt to grant some flexibility in decision-making because of the level of trust they have in their decision-maker. In other cases, people may limit flexibility because they feel particularly strong about a particular treatment (e.g., resuscitation) or worry that their wishes will not be followed [17].

Box 23.7 Case Study

An example of flexibility in decision-making arose in an inpatient internal medicine unit, where Ms. S, a woman with moderate dementia and osteoarthritis, was admitted with a urinary tract infection. At home, she was ambulatory and required assistance with finances and medication management but lived independently with a part-time caregiver. Ms. S had a prior form filled out in conjunction with her primary care doctor stating her desire to allow a natural death (no resuscitation or intubation). Her daughter was listed as her health-care proxy, and the patient had granted her daughter flexibility in decision-making. In the hospital, Ms. S initially improved with intravenous antibiotics, but on her third day of hospitalization became acutely altered and somnolent. Her blood gas revealed hypercarbia, indicating decreased respiratory rate from the combination of opiates and benzodiazepines she had unfortunately received during the day. Her daughter, in conjunction with providers, recognized that the cause of her respiratory depression was easily fixable and temporarily reversed her code status to allow intubation. The patient was intubated for stabilization; she was successfully extubated the next day. The patient completed a course of antibiotics, returned to her baseline level of function, and was discharged home later that week. Because the cause of her altered mental status was iatrogenic, having flexibility allowed the daughter and providers to feel comfortable reversing the code status temporarily without feeling like they were going against the patient's wishes.

23.7 Conclusion

Respecting patient autonomy—one of the core principles of medical ethics—requires full patient participation in decision-making about medical treatments and therapies. In order to participate in the process of informed consent, patients must demonstrate that they maintain decision-making capacity: the ability to integrate information about their illness and treatment options and decide what treatment would be best for them. Whether the proposed therapy is a blood thinner or a surgery, patients should be permitted to participate in decision-making to the best of their ability. These decisions come up frequently regardless of whether the patient is located at home, in a hospital, or in a nursing home. Physicians should, therefore, feel comfortable doing informal and formal assessments for capacity. Several populations, common in a geriatric practice, demand particular attention: those with dementia or mental illness.

23.7.1 Summary: A Practical Approach to Determining Capacity

The necessary steps for the process of informed consent are described in ◘ Fig. 23.1 and summarized here.

1. **Clinician proposes treatment to patient**, sharing information about the condition, the proposed treatments, and risks and benefits of the treatment. The patient shares his or her preference for treatment.
2. **Clinician and team assess for decision-making capacity** during a structured interview (◘ Table 23.2). The interview focuses on the four key abilities necessary for capacity:
   (a) **Communicating a choice** ("What would you choose?")
   (b) **Understanding relevant information** ("Can you tell me the risks and benefits of having this treatment?")
   (c) **Appreciating the situation and its consequences** ("Regardless of what you choose, do you think it is possible the medicine can benefit you?")
   (d) **Reasoning rationally** ("Can you tell me why you chose this option?")
3. **If decision-making capacity is impaired, a surrogate decision-maker is identified** according to state surrogacy laws.
4. **Patient or surrogate decide treatment plan with clinician**, based on prior stated wishes and advance care planning documents.

Capacity assessments are frequently necessary; to be fully respectful of a patient's rights and autonomy, it is critical to avoid certain common pitfalls. To this end, the National Ethics Committee (NEC) of the Veterans Health Administration (VHA) surveyed over 900 clinicians and ethics committee chairs. The committee identified common myths in capacity assessment and ranked the top 10 most common and important errors. Avoidance of these pitfalls is critical for fair and respectful evaluation of decision-making capacity.

Box 23.8 10 Myths About Decision-Making Capacity [6]

1. Decision-making capacity and competency are the same.
2. Lack of decision-making capacity can be presumed when patients go against medical advice.
3. There is no need to assess decision-making capacity unless patients go against medical advice.
4. Decision-making capacity is an "all or nothing" phenomenon.
5. Cognitive impairment equals lack of decision-making capacity.
6. Lack of decision-making capacity is a permanent condition.
7. Patients who have not been given relevant and consistent information about their treatment lack decision-making capacity.
8. All patients with certain psychiatric disorders lack decision-making capacity.
9. Patients who have been involuntarily committed lack decision-making capacity.
10. Only mental health experts can assess decision-making capacity.

It is common for a patient to demonstrate some impairment but still be able to strongly voice a preference for or against a particular treatment. That patient's preferences should still continue to be incorporated even if he or she is not the sole decision-maker. For complex cases, it is best to work with an interprofessional team who can craft creative solutions that respect the patient's autonomy while also acknowledging the patient's impairment [5]. For instance, in the case of a patient who repeatedly declines subacute rehabilitation despite profound deconditioning during a hospital stay, one solution may be to order home-based physical therapy and train the patient's family and home attendants to do exercises at regularly scheduled intervals throughout the day. While perhaps less activity than might be provided in a rehabilitation facility, the team is respecting the patient's autonomy and desire to return home while still providing necessary services. In sum, a careful and thoughtful assessment of decision-making capacity, regardless of the outcome of that assessment, will lead to a plan of care that respects the patient's values, goals, and preferences.

References

1. Alsan M, Wanamaker M. Tuskegee and the Health of Black Men. Q J Econ. 2018;133(1):407–55.
2. Appelbaum P. Assessment of patients' competence to consent to treatment. N Engl J Med. 2007;357(18):1834–40.
3. Appelbaum P, Grisso T. Assessing patients' capacities to consent to treatment. N Engl J Med. 1988;319(25):1635–8.
4. Best Case/Worst Case. Best case/worst case (BC/WC) communication tool – whiteboard video. [Internet]. Madison: University of Washington; c2016 [cited 2017 Jan 10]. Available from: https://www.youtube.com/watch?v=FnS3K44sbu0.
5. Carrese JA. Refusal of care: patients' well-being and physicians' ethical obligations: "but doctor, I want to go home". JAMA. 2006;296(6):691–5.
6. Ganzini L, Volicer L, Nelson WA, Fox E, Derse AR. Ten myths about decision-making capacity. J Am Med Dir Assoc. 2005;6(3. Suppl):S100–4.
7. Jeste DV, Depp CA, Palmer BW. Magnitude of impairment in decisional capacity in people with schizophrenia compared to normal subjects: an overview. Schizophr Bull. 2006;32(1):121–8.
8. Kim SY, Karlawish JH, Caine ED. Current state of research on decision-making competence of cognitively impaired elderly persons. Am J Geriatr Psychiatry. 2002;10:151–65.
9. Kruser J, Nabozny M, Steffens N, Brasel K, Campbell T, Gaines M, et al. "Best case/worst case": qualitative evaluation of a novel communication tool for difficult in-the-moment surgical decisions. J Am Geriatr Soc. 2015;63(9):1805–11.
10. Leo R. Competency and the capacity to make treatment decisions: a primer for primary care physicians. Prim Care Companion J Clin Psychiatry. 1999;01(05):131–41.
11. Marson DC, Ingram KK, Cody HA, Harrell LE. Assessing the competency of patients with Alzheimer's disease under different legal standards. A prototype instrument. Arch Neurol. 1995;52:949–54.
12. Pruchno RA, Smyer MA, Rose MS, Hartman-Stein PE, Henderson-Laribee DL. Competence of long-term care residents to participate in decisions about their medical care: a brief, objective assessment. Gerontologist. 1995;35:622–9.
13. Rosenbaum L. Liberty versus need – our struggle to care for people with serious mental illness. N Engl J Med. 2016;375(15):1490–5.
14. Schwarze ML, Kehler JM, Campbell TC. Navigating high risk procedures with more than just a street map. J Palliat Med. 2013;(10):1169–71.
15. Shuster E. The Nuremberg Code: Hippocratic ethics and human rights. Lancet. 1998;351(9107):974–7.
16. Soriano R, Fernandez H, Cassel C, Leipzig R. Fundamentals of geriatric medicine a case-based approach. Springer Science+Business Media, LLC, New York, NY; 2007, Chapter 7.
17. Sudore RL, Boscardin J, Feuz MA, McMahan RD, Katen MT, Barnes DE. Effect of the PREPARE website vs an easy-to-read advance directive on advance care planning documentation and engagement among veterans: a randomized clinical trial. JAMA Intern Med. 2017;177(8):1102–9.
18. Taylor LJ, Nabozny MJ, Steffens NM, Tucholka JL, Brasel KJ, Johnson SK, et al. A framework to improve surgeon communication in high-stakes surgical decisions: best case/worst case. JAMA Surg. 2017;152(6):531–8.
19. Tuskegee Study – Timeline – CDC – NCHHSTP [Internet]. Cdc.gov. 2017 [cited 16 December 2017]. Available from: https://www.cdc.gov/tuskegee/timeline.htm.
20. Weindling P, von Villiez A, Loewenau A, Farron N. The victims of unethical human experiments and coerced research under National Socialism. Endeavour. 2016;40(1):1–6.

Developing a Management Plan

Stephanie W. Chow and Lizette Muñoz

A. Chun (ed.), *Geriatric Practice*, https://doi.org/10.1007/978-3-030-19625-7_24

24.1 Introduction to Three Disciplines: Geriatric Medicine, Nursing, and Social Work

Every geriatric patient has her or his own constellation of characteristics, contributing to the design of a uniquely specific management plan [3]. Given the need for interdisciplinary teamwork when providing best quality care for an older patient, it is important to understand a variety of perspectives and management approaches. It is also necessary to understand how each perspective and approach complements the others. A healthcare team may be comprised of any interdisciplinary team combination dependent on the resources available (i.e., doctors, nurses, social workers, care coordinators, physical therapists, pharmacists, etc.). In this chapter, we will discuss developing a comprehensive management plan by using basic strategies in medicine, nursing, and social work.

24.1.1 Medicine

In 2017, the American Geriatrics Society promoted a simplified approach to defining the most important tenets of geriatric medicine. Dubbed the "5Ms," geriatricians in the United States and in Canada began highlighting this teaching tool to more easily describe the specialty of geriatric medicine [7]. This approach also offers simplified guidance to outlining a comprehensive plan of care for a complex older patient.

Per the American Geriatrics Society, the **5Ms of geriatrics** is a way to communicate and describe the key core competencies in geriatrics to nongeriatricians: (1) mind, (2) mobility, (3) medications, (4) multicomplexity, and (5) what matters most (◻ Fig. 24.1).

1. **Mind**: Executive function, attention, and emotions are essential in guiding a patient to follow a management plan. It is important to know and understand your patient's cognitive status and the challenges that arise from your patient's potential cognitive impairment. A patient who is unable to attend to your medical interview will be unable to absorb any information provided and consequently be unable to comply with the management plan. Whether or not the cause of cognitive impairment is reversible becomes an important consideration when designing a management plan. That is, *Do you have concerns for dementia, delirium, or depression? Are such conditions reversible or treatable?* If there is concern for cognitive impairment, it is important to communicate the plan to a caregiver or responsible individual. Should your patient deny or refuse caregiver assistance, you will need to assess your patient's capacity for making decisions regarding your management plan and her or his overall healthcare, allowing for patient autonomy whenever safely able.
2. **Mobility**: Assessment for impaired gait and balance is essential in determining your patient's functionality and safety. Ability to navigate independently in the community often contributes to significantly positive quality of life and optimism about one's health. *Can the patient independently transfer? Has the patient fallen in the past 2 weeks? Are there sufficient and appropriate grab bars and safety measures in place at home? Does the patient require an assistive walking device, and is it appropriate?*
3. **Medications**: Potential age-related increase in comorbid conditions may be accompanied by a lengthier medication list in older adults. It is important to reconcile and reduce medication overprescribing and potential polypharmacy frequently. Patients may be noncompliant to medications for many reasons, including low health

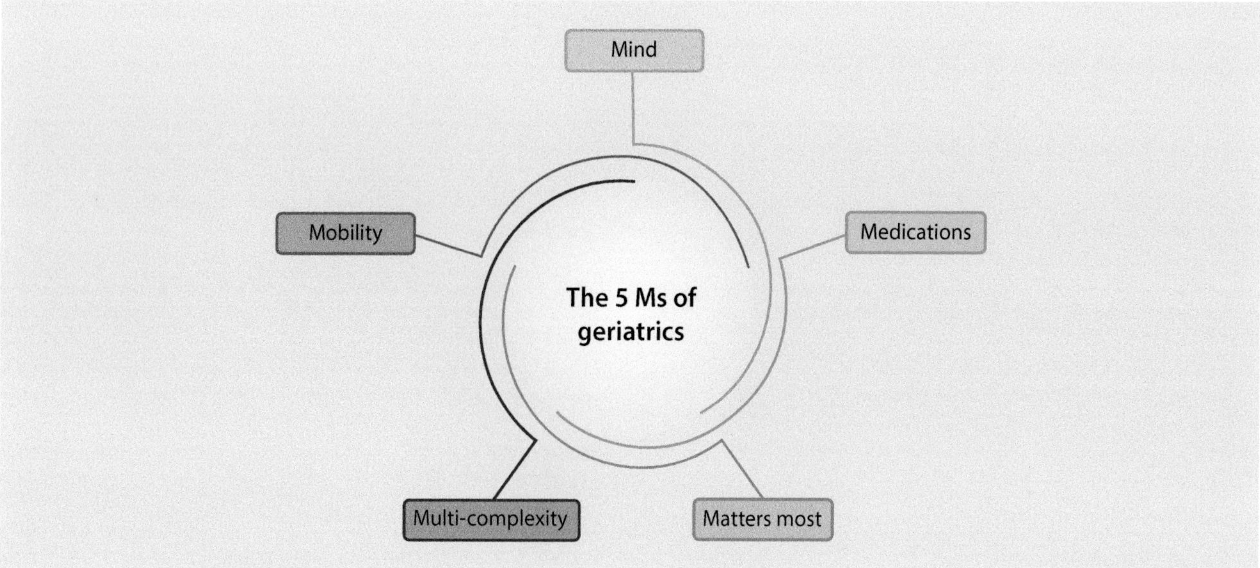

◻ **Fig. 24.1** The 5Ms of geriatrics

literacy, memory or cognitive impairment, cost, or side effects. *Do I have suspicions that the patient may not be taking her or his medications properly? Is there risk for adverse drug interactions?*

4. **Multicomplexity**: Older patients have increased complexity of chronic medical conditions, often invoking greater stress on informal and formal support systems such as family and caregivers, healthcare and living facilities, and other providers. Thorough examination of your patient's ability to accommodate and compensate for these challenges will reveal important key factors to constructing a successful short-term and long-term management plan. *Does the patient have an adequate understanding of her or his chronic diseases, and is she or he prepared and able to self-manage them? If not, who can help?*
5. What **Matters Most**: Patients often cite desire for maintained independence as the most important aspect of remaining healthy. Still, it is important to ask your patient this question as you may encounter unexpected and surprising answers. *What matters most to you in regard to your health and well-being?* Never presume to know the patient's values or goals, especially as these may change over the course of a progressing illness or significant life event. "What Matters Most" should be assessed periodically, with greater frequency dependent on any significant changes in health or life events.

24.1.2 Nursing

Because of the significant differences in nursing level of training, we will focus on the role of the registered nurse for the purpose of contrast between physician, nurse, and social worker.

The American Nurses Association regards the **nursing process** as a critical thinking tool by which nurses deliver holistic and patient-focused care regardless of nursing discipline, allowing for consistent high quality of patient care. The registered nurse uses a comprehensive problem-focused approach that aims to maximize the patient's ability to do the activities that are most important to her or him. "The nursing process complements what other health care professionals do by addressing not only the medical problems, but also human responses – how the person's life is affected by medical problems, treatment plans, and changes in activities of daily life [1, 6]." The nursing process is important in helping nurses interact with patients and is categorized into five phases: **A**ssessment, **D**iagnosis, **P**lanning/Outcomes, **I**mplementation, and **E**valuation, more easily remembered by the acronym **AD-PIE** (Fig. 24.2).

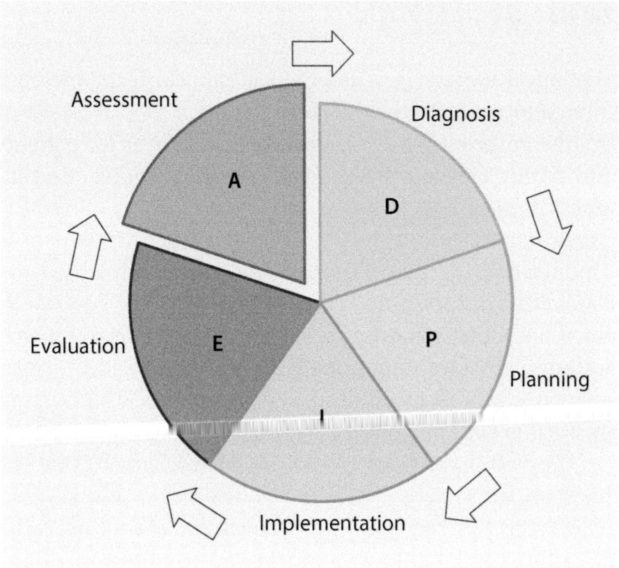

Fig. 24.2 Acronym for five phases of nursing

1. **Assessment**: The assessment encourages the nurse to interact with the patient, family, and caregiver to obtain a comprehensive picture of the patient's needs and goals. During this phase, the nurse will collect and record subjective and objective data which may include the patient's chief complaint, review of systems, past medical history, and surgical history, vital signs, as well as evaluation of psychological, sociocultural, and spiritual domains, physical examination, laboratory testing, and anything else pertaining to patient care (i.e., insurance, transportation, etc.).
2. **Diagnosis**: The nursing diagnosis is the nurse's educated clinical judgment regarding the patient's actual or potential health conditions or needs. A registered nurse may diagnose a medical *condition* but not a *disease*. Each nursing diagnosis is problem focused and based on the patient's signs and symptoms, from which the nurse can formulate a specific short-term or long-term solution for the patient. Nursing diagnoses are most commonly institutionally based, with a predetermined list of nursing diagnoses to select from, and often accompanied by decision-making protocols to guide care [1].
3. **Planning**: During this phase, the nurse identifies and prioritizes the expected or desired outcomes for the patient, focusing on the most severe and highest risk factors first. The nurse may then develop a plan of care via *SMART* goals – that is, goals which are specific, measurable, attainable, realistic/relevant, and time restricted.
4. **Implementation/Intervention**: During the implementation phase, the nurse assesses and reassesses the patient's status to determine if the outcomes are still appropriate and achievable, making any necessary adjustments to realign outcomes and goals.
5. **Evaluation**: The final phase of the nursing process is evaluation. *Have the SMART goals for patient wellness been met?* The nurse evaluates both the patient's status and effectiveness of nursing care, making modifications to the care plan as needed. A patient's condition may be grouped into three possible outcomes: improved, stabilized, or deteriorated/died/discharged.

24.1.3 Social Work

The social worker is a nonmedical clinical team member trained to assist individuals with the psychosocial aspect of healthcare, providing a unique contextual focus for patient- and family-centered care [8]. The social worker aims to identify patient needs and strengths, as well as determine patient goals and priorities. A social worker assessment is conducted in a comprehensive framework known as the *biopsychosocial-spiritual perspective* [6]. This approach recognizes the importance of the "whole person care," accounting for emotional or psychological state; socioeconomic, sociocultural, and sociopolitical status; and spiritual needs and concerns [8].

The National Association of Social Work posits that the standard for social practice in the healthcare setting often reflects a set of guiding principles including self-determination, cultural competency, strengths perspective, person-in-environment framework, social justice, and primacy of the client-social worker relationship. Briefly, this toolbox of principles encourages the patient to self-identify and clarify her or his own goals in a culturally aware and respectful fashion, within the framework or context of her or his physical and social environment. The social worker utilizes the patient's strengths for potential growth and resilience to pursue health goals. Fundamentally, the social worker must first build a therapeutic relationship with the patient, as only after this will a patient and social worker achieve a meaningful working foundation on which to build the aforementioned principles. Finally, social workers aim to promote and advocate for social, economic, political, and cultural values consistent with tenets of social justice [8, 2, 4, 5].

24.2 Biopsychosocial-Spiritual Model (◘ Fig. 24.3)

24.2.1 Biological

The biological or "bio" portion of the biopsychosocial-spiritual assessment addresses the patient's medical issues, age, and developmental and physical characteristics. The patient's health literacy is important in assessing how well the patient understands her or his needs, for example, durable medical equipment, nutrition and diet, substance use/misuse services, and other specialty services.

24.2.2 Psychological

The psychological or "psycho" portion of the biopsychosocial-spiritual assessment explores the patient's mental status, thoughts, behaviors, emotions, and/or history of trauma or abuse. During this time, the social worker

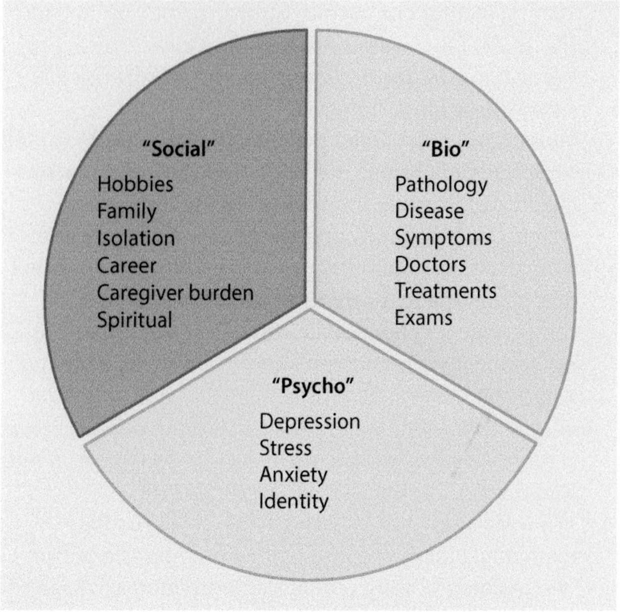

◘ **Fig. 24.3** Biopsychosocial-spiritual model

gains a better understanding of the patient's self-awareness, judgment, and insight, useful in assessing mental health and cognitive status.

24.2.3 Social-Spiritual

The social aspect of the biopsychosocial-spiritual assessment examines the patient's social, cultural, and spiritual aspect that may or may not affect the patient. The social worker explores the patient's current relationship with family and friends, social support, community involvement, religion/spirituality, and finances. This provides insight into the patient's formal and informal supports such as home health aids, caregivers, transportation, insurance, and community services (i.e., Meals on Wheels, Friendly Visitor Program, Senior Centers). Specifically, the spiritual aspect explores the patient's sense of self and purpose, and encourages conversation regarding the patient's values and self-meaning.

The biopsychosocial-spiritual assessment is able to provide the medical provider with a broader perspective of the patient that may have not been captured during a standard medical visit. A social work visit is often able to provide the medical provider with a better understanding of the patient's environment which can impact the way a patient perceives and manages her or his health. This is essential when working with the older population, as this can provide an insight into how the individual has been functioning on a daily basis with or without appropriate support from family, friends, and the community. It allows the social worker to address the patient's needs as well as the medical team's needs and find a unifying plan to meet team goals.

Case Presentation

History of Present Illness

Ms. NG is a 73-year-old Spanish-speaking woman from the Dominican Republic who presents to the geriatrics primary care clinic for knee pain after a fall last night. She has a past medical history of poorly controlled type 2 diabetes, hypertension, osteoarthritis, osteoporosis, gait instability, memory impairment, major depressive disorder, and anxiety. She currently lives alone in a one-bedroom apartment in New York City with daily homecare (4 hours a day, 5 days a week). Ms. NG has a daughter who lives 10 minutes away and will occasionally assist her with health concerns a few times weekly.

Ms. NG complains that she had been feeling lonely, depressed, and anxious last evening, prompting her to leave her apartment to seek help. She reports that she hastily left her apartment to find a neighbor, tripped over the elevated doorframe, and fell forcefully onto her knees. She currently denies any other acute illnesses or concerns.

Review of System

General: Reports feeling a lot of pain over her knees, especially her left knee. Has been unable to sleep due to her pain and feels very tired.

- HEENT: Denies headache, ear aches, or vision changes
- CVS: denies chest pain or palpitations
- Pulm: denies shortness of breath or congestion
- GI: denies nausea, vomiting, diarrhea, or constipation
- GU: denies changes in urination
- Musculoskeletal: reports aching joints throughout her body, especially on top of her knees and lower back, feels general weakness
- Neuro: denies loss of consciousness or lightheadedness; feels generally weaker than her baseline
- Psych: feels depressed and anxious, states her memory is still about the same

Physical Exam

- Vitals: T, 97.6; BP, 96/64; HR, 84; RR, 16; SpO2, 98% RA
- Height, 58 inches; weight, 92 pounds
- General: in moderate distress from knee pain, pleasant, Spanish-speaking, petite elderly woman appearing her stated age
- Eyes: anicteric sclera, extraocular muscles intact, pupils equally reactive to light and accommodation
- Ears/nose/mouth/throat: moist mucous membranes, edentulous without oral lesions
- Cardiovascular: regular rate and rhythm, no appreciable murmurs
- Respiratory: lungs clear to auscultation bilaterally, no work of breathing
- Gastrointestinal/rectal: soft thin abdomen, normoactive bowel sounds present, no masses appreciated
- Musculoskeletal/back: kyphotic spine, right knee moderate patellar tenderness and faint crepitus without appreciable deformity, medial/lateral joint line tenderness, and edema. Knee range of motion reduced bilaterally secondary to knee pain. Unable to complete knee examination secondary to patient's pain.
- Extremity: trace edema bilaterally to both knees, warm
- Neuro: alert and oriented x3, no focal weakness or deficit
- Psych: Mood is pleasant, normal range affect. Speech is soft and clear with normal cadence and rhythm. Thought content reality based with fixation on her loneliness at nighttime. Thought process is linear and logical. No psychomotor agitation observed. No apparent auditory or visual hallucinations. Judgment of her safety at home is poor – she feels she has sufficient safety measures in place despite falling down. Insight into her chronic conditions is also poor – she believes her diabetes is well controlled, but does not check her fingersticks nor can she name her insulin doses.
- Skin: mildly tanned skin, no gross focal lesions
- Function: Stands with one-person assistance and use of chair armrests. Ambulates unsteadily, but independently, slowly, and with difficulty using walking cane, complicated by knee injury.

Radiology

X-ray bilateral knees – bilateral knee osteoarthritis with new nondisplaced right patellar fracture. No other fractures seen.

24.3 Building an Interdisciplinary Geriatric Management Plan

24.3.1 Example Assessment and Plan

Note that the following Table 24.1 *is an example only; each patient may have varying management plans dependent on the treating team.*

Table 24.1 Example assessment and plan

	Medical diagnosis and plan	Nursing diagnosis and plan	Social work plan
Patient assessment	**Mobility** Right patellar fracture Pain control Medication Knee brace/durable medical equipment (i.e., standard walker) Physical therapy referral Consider orthopedic surgery referral	Gait instability and fall risk Pain control counseling Fall risk management	Physical therapy Home safety assessment
	Mobility Osteoarthritis Pain control Medication Assistive walking device Physical therapy and home exercise	Gait instability and fall risk Assistive walking device demonstration	Physical therapy Home safety assessment Assistance with ordering durable medical equipment to reduce fall risk
	Mind Alzheimer's dementia Caregiver and family counseling and education Advance care planning	Memory difficulty, risk for wandering Caregiver and family counseling and education	Informal/formal caregiver supports Medical alert bracelet Application for increased home aid hours Consideration for community programs Advance care planning
	Mind Depression Mental health referral (psychiatry, psychotherapy) Medication consideration	Risk for loneliness, Ineffective individual coping skill Mental health questionnaire/ depression screen	Mental health services Adult day program Psychotherapy/counseling Motivational interviewing
	Medication Polypharmacy Medication review and reconciliation/ simplification, blister packing	Medication noncompliance Medication compliance strategies and education	Formal/informal supports Visiting nurse service
	Multicomplexity Uncontrolled diabetes Medication and diabetes education Hypertension Osteoarthritis Osteoporosis Frailty Dementia Depression Etc.	Medication noncompliance Medication compliance strategies	Visiting nurse service Community diabetes education program Consideration for care coordinator Caregiver support group Home delivery meal program Transportation services
	Matters most Desire for autonomy, independence Cognitive assessment Management plan discussion with possible family meeting Advance care planning/healthcare proxy discussion	Patient and family education and counseling of management plan	Formal/informal supports Community services Advance care planning

Case Conclusion

The above management plan was implemented for Ms. NG with plans to follow-up in 1 week for short-term follow-up. At her return visit, Ms. NG had begun physical therapy at home and was actively working with her daughter and home aid to implement a home exercise program. Ms. NG felt reduced pain and increased **mobility** with her new standard walker. She had no falls during this time. To assist with her **medication adherence**, Ms. NG agreed to blister packing her medications with her local pharmacy. This organized her medications into daily packets, which she would open each day and self administer. Because she had difficulties with her memory at times (**mind**), her home aid would help remind her to take her medications and to exercise daily.

The patient's social worker had initiated a request for increased home aid hours. Visiting nurse services were initiated and patient was receiving twice-weekly visits to ensure management plan compliance with repeated evaluations by nursing to ensure that the current management plan was aligned with team and patient goals using the **AD-PIE** technique.

While not her chief complaint, what **matters most** to Ms. NG is her independence. At the prior visit, the provider and social worker had discussed advance care planning and her memory decline. The team stressed the importance of prioritizing Ms. NG's autonomy, but safeguarding her health and well-being by having advance care documentation in place that was consistent with her wishes. Ms. NG had discussed this paperwork with her caregivers and returned to clinic with the forms completed.

Finally, given Ms. NG's **multicomplexity** of chronic and new conditions, her social worker had initiated applications for supportive community services, considering each of the **biopsychosocial-spiritual** aspects of her health. Program examples included Meals on Wheels, diabetes education program, dementia support group, caregiver burden support group, and mental health counseling.

Ms. NG will return in 1 month for follow-up and is instructed to call the office with any questions or concerns at any time.

Acknowledgment Special acknowledgment to Anne T. Lai, NP.

References

1. Alfaro-LeFevre R. Applying nursing process: a tool for critical thinking. Philadelphia: Lippincott Williams & Wilkins; 2006.
2. Corcoran J, Walsh J. Clinical assessment and diagnosis in social work practice. New York: Oxford University Press; 2006.
3. Heckman GA, Molnar FJ, Lee L. Geriatric medicine leadership of health care transformation: to be or not to be? Can Geriatr J. 2013;6(4):192–5.
4. Jordan C, Franklin C, editors. Clinical assessment for social workers: quantitative and qualitative methods. 4th ed. Chicago: Lyceum Books; 2016.
5. Singer JB, Producer. Bio-psychosocial-Spiritual (BPSS) assessment and Mental Status Exam (MSE) [Episode 2]. Social Work Podcast [Audio podcast]. 2007, January 22. Retrieved from http://socialworkpodcast.com/2007/02/bio-psychosocial-spiritual-bpss.html.
6. Swearingen P. All-in-one care planning resource: medical-surgical, pediatric, maternity and psychiatric, nursing care plans. 2nd ed. St. Louis: Mosby; 2008.
7. Tinetti M, Huang A, Molnar F. The geriatrics 5M's: a new way of communicating what we do. J Am Geriatr Soc. 2017;65(9):2115.
8. Wheeler DP, McClain A, Cox LE, Fritz T, Little V, Otis-Green S, Collins S. NASW standards for social work practice in health care settings; 2016. https://www.socialworkers.org/LinkClick.aspx?fileticket=fFnsRHX-4HE%3D&portalid=0

Safety and Risk Assessment

Karin Ouchida and Parham Khalili

A. Chun (ed.), *Geriatric Practice*, https://doi.org/10.1007/978-3-030-19625-7_25

25.1 Section: Home Safety Assessment

Case: Ms. Smith

Chief Complaint: *"I fell a few times"*

History of Present Illness: *Ms. Smith is an 89-year-old patient with a history of hypertension, atrial fibrillation on long-term anticoagulation, osteoarthritis, spinal stenosis, peripheral neuropathy, hearing loss, and gait instability requiring use of a rolling walker. Over the last year she had 4 emergency department visits for falls at home, in one case possibly related to accidental consumption of extra doses of blood pressure medication. She has difficulty getting to office visits and missed two recent appointments due to problems with her ride-share program. You scheduled a home visit to her apartment to follow-up on her chronic medical issues and identify additional potential risks for further falls and other adverse events. She is very pleased to hear you are coming over, "just like doctors used to when [she] was a little girl," and she promises to whip up a batch of her famous lemon bars.*

Question: What potential risk factors for unintentional injury can you identify based on Ms. Smith's medical diagnoses and history over the last year?

25.1.1 Background and Epidemiology

- In the United States, nearly 40% of women and 20% of men age 65 and older may require assistance for activities of daily living or episodic care needs yet live alone without available help. They are 30% more likely than other groups to experience an unintentional injury in the home [1, 2].
- Older adults are at increased risk for certain *preventable* injuries due to *observable* factors such as physical and cognitive changes, medication side effects, and social and financial barriers to maintaining a safe environment [3–5].
- According to the US Department of Health and Human Services, unintentional injuries accounted for over 85% of all injury deaths among adults age 65 and older in the United States. Of the 90,000 injury deaths occurring between 2012 and 2013, 55% were attributed to falls, 14% to motor vehicle accidents, 8% to suffocation, 4% to poisoning, 2% to fire, and the remainder to less common causes [6].
- **Falls**—Among older adults, falls are associated with direct physical injury such as hip fractures, hospitalization, increased dependence on others, higher likelihood of long-term care placement, and high healthcare costs (approximately $31 billion annually) [7].
- **Fire and burn injuries**—Older adults may underestimate their risk and may be less likely to have working fire and carbon monoxide detectors. In some studies, once a fire or burn is sustained, those 60 and older have a ten-fold higher mortality compared to younger adults [5, 6, 8].
- **Poison exposures**—In part because older adults take more prescription medications, pharmaceuticals are the cause of up to 57% of poisonings, and approximately 91% of all exposures occur at home [9]. Other potentially harmful poison exposures include household products, pesticides, and carbon monoxide.
- **Firearms**—Often overlooked, firearms are an important consideration with respect to home safety risk especially in the setting of depression, other psychiatric illness, or domestic violence [10]. Older adults may be more likely than their younger counterparts to own a firearm. Data from 2004–2009 shows over 17 million adults age 65 own a firearm, most often a handgun [11, 12].
- The CDC's 2001–2003 ICARIS-2 survey found that 21% of gun owners reported having kept the gun *loaded and unlocked* at some point over the prior year, and only 55% of respondents stated that at least one adult member of the household had attended firearm safety training in the past [13].
- In addition, the rate of *suicide by firearm* is highest among individuals age 75 and older, particularly among men, Whites, African Americans, Native Americans, and individuals in rural regions [11, 14].
- **Risk Factors for Unintentional Injury**
- *Physiologic*
  - Physical deconditioning and musculoskeletal conditions
  - Slower reaction times
  - Decreased visual, olfactory, tactile, and hearing sensitivity and acuity
  - Aging-related physiologic changes that increase risk for orthostatic hypotension
  - Cardiac disease (e.g., heart failure, arrhythmia, aortic stenosis)
  - Pulmonary disease (e.g., smoking, COPD, any oxygen requirement)
  - Urologic disease (e.g., urinary incontinence)
  - Neuro-psychiatric disease (e.g., cognitive impairment/dementia, movement disorders, sleep disorders, psychiatric illness)
  - Chronic pain
  - Gait impairment
  - Multi-morbidity
  - Medication effects and side effects
- *Environmental, socioeconomic, and cultural*
  - Neighborhood safety
  - Financial constraints limiting access to home maintenance, safe transportation, and safety equipment
  - Home lighting, flooring, furniture arrangement, and clutter
  - Lack of ambulation assistive devices (when needed)
  - Lack of training on how to use medical devices in the home
  - Gun ownership

25.1.2 Screening

- **General questions**: These are questions that all adults 65 and older should be asked even in the absence of an injury because they have the potential to identify and address salient risk factors.
  - *Have you had a fall in the last 12 months?*
  - *Do you use an assistive device inside or outside your home?*
  - *Do you have any concerns about the safety of your neighborhood?*
  - *Do you have any difficulty getting to and from medical appointments?*
  - *Does your home have working fire and carbon monoxide detectors?*
  - *Do you own a firearm?*
- **Follow-up questions after a fall**: If an injury such as a fall has already occurred, you will likely touch on the topics/questions below as part of your HPI, but go into more depth depending on the type of injury. A "fall history" includes the circumstances of the fall (e.g., where it occurred, the mechanism of the fall, time of day, environment, etc.) [see ► Section VI: Chap. 26].
- **Follow-up questions regarding home environment:**
  - *"Tell me about your home environment…"*
  - *"What type of residence do you live in (apartment, house, etc.)?"*
  - *"Do you have any stairs leading up to your door or stairs in your home?"*
  - *"What is the lighting like? Do you have night lights?"*
  - *"Do you have area rugs?"*
  - *"Do you have clutter? Are their clear pathways for walking in your home?"*

Table 25.1 Selected resources for home safety screening [7, 9, 16, 21]

Consumer Product Safety Commission (CPSC)
General Safety Education
Specific Home Safety Screening Materials
Older Consumer's Safety Checklist
Available from: ► https://www.cpsc.gov/s3fs-public/checklist.pdf
American Association of Retired Persons (AARP)
The largest nonprofit organization providing information and resources for adults age 50 and older
HomeFit Guide, for room-by-room home safety assessments
Information on Medical Alert Systems
Lists of resources for affordable transportation services, adult day care options, hiring a caregiver and other services of interest
Available from: ► https://www.aarp.org/caregiving/home-care/?intcmp=AE-CAR-SUBNAV-CAH
Centers for Disease Control and Prevention (CDC)
Older Adult Falls
Fire Safe Seniors Toolkit
Stopping Elderly Accidents, Deaths and Injuries (STEADI) program materials for patients and providers. Free access to algorithms and Pocket Guides for providers
Available from: ► https://www.cdc.gov/homeandrecreational-safety/index.html
US Health Resources and Safety Administration (HRSA) Poison Prevention Program
Poison prevention and home modification tips
Poison Help emergency line (1-800-222-1222) for assistance from a local poison expert
Open Access: ► https://poisonhelp.hrsa.gov/index.html

25.1.3 Making a House Call

- House call visits may provide valuable first-hand information about the patient's home environment. There are many resources that can provide tools and guidance (see Table 25.1)
- Important but often overlooked details
  - Distance and terrain between the hospital/clinic and the patient's home
  - Neighborhood resources including grocery stores, parks, and other public spaces
  - Sidewalks/curbs, street traffic, and pedestrian signs
  - Distance from the street to the patient's door, number and height of steps, presence of a hand rail
  - Inside the home you can assess the cleanliness, lighting, the presence/absence of clutter and the floor surfaces including presence of area rugs and door sills. Going room by room note:
    - Kitchen—height of cabinets, refrigerator contents, appliances
    - Bedroom—distance to bathroom, height of and type of bed, presence of sleeping pills/sedatives (often kept at bedside)
    - Living room—seating options and height
    - Bathroom—toilet seat height, tub height, presence of grab bars, water temperature
    - Medical devices and medications—oxygen tanks/tubing, assistive devices, medication storage/organization
    - Safety devices—smoke and carbon monoxide detectors, fire extinguishers
    - Fire risks—space heaters, heating blankets, multiple devices plugged into outlets

Question: What aspects of Ms. Smith's neighborhood/home environment should you evaluate?

Case Continued

Ms. Smith's Home Environment Assessment

General Neighborhood and Building

- Apartment not within walking distance of any public transportation, grocery stores, or public parks
- Sidewalk interrupted on many streets, and high volume of traffic on the main street leading to her home
- Street lights are far apart providing limited light at night
- 3 uneven steps leading up to her building with no rails
- Lobby lighting is dim but elevator functioning

Her Apartment

- When you wash your hands, the hot water is scalding hot
- Ceiling light and 1 floor lamp in the corner, appears dim overall
- Several rugs on the ground, wood flooring with raised area in doorways
- Dining table has a small tray with multiple pill bottles; some of them contain what appears to be a mixture of different pills, several bottles have somewhat smudged labels that are difficult to read, and one or two appear to be very old and expired
- Smoke detector/carbon monoxide detector doors open with missing batteries
- Tray of delicious looking lemon bars on the counter; you note the oven is still on
- Large step-in tub without grab bars in the bathroom

Question: Which exam findings might be particularly salient in conjunction with your evaluation of her environment and history?

Focused Exam

- Vital signs: Afebrile. BP 110/68 sitting (HR 64) and 90/60 standing (HR 90), SpO2 99% on room air
- General: Ms. Smith greets you at the door, she is well-groomed and appears happy to see you. She is not using her walker as she guides you into her home to give you "the grand tour"
- HEENT: PERRL, EOMI, symmetrical decrease in hearing bilaterally and no hearing aids in place
- Cardiac: irregularly irregular, normal s1 and s2
- Neurological: alert and oriented to self, place and time, CN II-XII grossly intact, normal tone and strength testing, normal cerebellar testing, normal reflexes, gait is slow and slightly wide based but stable with use of her rolling walker

Laboratory Testing and Imaging (from Ms. Smith's Recent Emergency Department Visits)

- Creatinine 0.72 mg/dL, BUN 22 mg/dL, normal electrolytes
- Wbc 8.0 × 10(9)/L, hemoglobin 12.5 g/dL, MCV 89.4 fL, platelets 224 × 10(9)/L
- AST 23 U/L, ALT 18 U/L, alkaline phosphatase 101 U/L, GGT 12 units/L
- Troponin I < 0.03 ng/mL
- TSH 1.02 mIU/L
- Urinalysis negative
- ECG (12 lead): atrial fibrillation, HR 88, normal axis and intervals, no obvious signs of ischemic changes
- CT scan of the head (non-contrast): no acute infarction or mass; noted mild-to-moderate chronic microvascular changes and mild generalized atrophy without clear signs of ventriculomegaly
- Pelvis and hip x-rays (AP): osteopenia, osteoarthritis bilaterally, no acute fracture or dislocation

Question: What interventions would help improve Ms. Smith's home safety?

Case Conclusion

▪ Assessment and Plan

Ms. Smith is at increased risk of falls and other injuries such as medication side effects and fire/burns. Her physiologic risk factors include the multiple medications she has been prescribed for chronic illness, musculoskeletal conditions and pain, decreased sensory perception, orthostatic hypotension, and atrial fibrillation. The environmental factors that heighten her risk of injury include dim lighting, uneven floors, lack of use of her assistive devices, and the non-working smoke detector. Socioeconomically, she cites difficulty with her ride-share program and she is not close to public transportation.

- **Modify the environment.**
  - Ask building management to install a railing on the entry steps and replace the dim lighting in the lobby.
  - Increase lighting throughout the apartment, remove area rugs and clutter from the floors.
  - Obtain a raised toilet seat and install grab bars in the bathroom.
- **Review her medications and reduce polypharmacy.**
  - Eliminate one of her blood pressure medications because of orthostatic hypotension.
  - Counsel her to dispose of expired medications according to the US Food and
  - Drug Administration guideline [15].
- **Screen for cognitive impairment** (given her ED visit for medication misuse).
- **Burn prevention strategies**
  - Recommend a timer for her oven or appliances with an automatic shut-off feature.
  - Advise her to talk to her building about the water temperature. The US Consumer Product Safety Commission (CPSC) recommends that water heater temperatures be lowered to 120 degrees F to reduce the risk of burns, as burns can even occur within 30 seconds or less at higher temperatures [16].
  - Stress the safety and legal mandate of having working fire and carbon monoxide detectors.
- **Poison prevention strategies**—The US Health Resources and Services Administration (HRSA) poison prevention program recommends keeping household products and medications in their original containers. For Ms. Smith, a pill box might be more helpful but she may need a caregiver to fill it for her or at least check its accuracy each week. She could also ask her pharmacy if her pills could be organized in blister packs.
- **Firearm safety**—If Ms. Smith endorsed having a gun at home or you observed a firearm during your home visit, you could use the "5 Ls" to assess for safety. These include making sure all firearms are "locked," "unloaded," and away from "little" children. You would also want to make sure she is not depressed or

Case Conclusion (continued)

feeling "low" and that she is a "*learned* operator" who has had firearm safety training [13].

- **Fall prevention**
  - **Emphasize the importance of using her assistive device.**
  - **Refer to physical and occupational therapists** to evaluate Ms. Smith's walker and make sure it is the best device for her, i.e., properly fitted and correctly used. Having an assistive device is protective against falls among patients who need one but only when patients also perceive their risk of falls to be significant, have received education, proper fitting/training, and ultimately use the device consistently [17].
  - **Refer to exercise/activity programs at senior or community centers.** Exercise in combination with vision assessment and treatment is strongly associated with reduced falls risks [17–19].
  - **Refer for regular vision and hearing assessments**; also replace hearing aid batteries.
  - **Recommend appropriate footwear** for use inside and outside the home. Some interventions may be intuitive but ineffective, for example, nonslip socks, which appear to be inadequate footwear to prevent falls and may carry risks of spreading infection [20].
  - **Recommend a medical alert device** (usually a bracelet or necklace) so that if she has a fall it will notify a designated individual or 911.
- **Screen for alcohol and other substance use.**
- **Refer to social work** or call her ride-share program to explore her transportation options.
- **Involve other caregivers** or family (as permitted by the patient) to help carry out your recommendations.

25.2 Section: Alcohol and Other Substance Use

Case: Mr. Jones

Chief Complaint: *"I need something for my back."*

History of Present Illness: *Mr. Jones is a 65-year-old man referred by the emergency department to your practice for primary care. His chart notes hypertension, hyperlipidemia, chronic kidney disease, osteoarthritis and lumbar spinal stenosis with several recent emergency department visits for lower back pain. He reports a 5-year history of occasional low back pain dating back to his work as a machinist in a local factory. The factory was shut down 2 years ago, and his pain has steadily worsened since then. He had been planning on retiring at 65, and the sudden loss of his job and reduced pension is a major source of emotional and financial stress. He has sought care at various local urgent cares and emergency departments. Multiple x-rays and an MRI earlier in the year did not show any abnormalities to his knowledge, further frustrating him. He describes the pain as present all the time, achy in character, 7/10 in intensity, located midline in his lower back, non-radiating, and precipitated by bending, twisting and prolonged standing. Six months ago, he could manage the pain with acetaminophen and a heating pad at night. A few weeks ago, his symptoms were exacerbated after he twisted his back and nearly fell walking up slippery stairs. He used up his prescriptions for "really strong" pain medications from his ER visits, and he emphasizes that he subsequently treated his pain over the last 2 months "the old-fashioned way" with "a stiff drink or two." He decided to come today because his pain now makes doing chores difficult without help from his son (who is in the waiting room). He prides himself on being independent.*

Questions: What concerns are raised by Mr. Jones's medical history and recent events? What questions would you want to ask Mr. Jones to clarify his risk for substance use disorder?

Focused Exam

- Vital signs: afebrile, BP 170/90, HR 92, RR 18, BMI 36
- General: +uncombed hair, a few shirt stains, + strong odor of tobacco
- HEENT: PERRL, pupils 3 mm, EOMI, anicteric sclera, no nystagmus, + poor dentition
- Cardiac: RRR, normal s1 and s2, no murmur/gallop/rub
- Lung: distant breath sounds bilaterally, slightly prolonged expiratory phase
- Abdomen: normoactive BS, soft, non-tender, slightly enlarged liver about 1–2 cm below the costal margin
- Skin and extremities: + palmar erythema bilaterally, + gynecomastia
- Musculoskeletal: normal appearing back, decreased range of motion in the lumbar spine, no spinous process tenderness, negative straight leg raise and slump test, normal hip and knee exams bilaterally
- Neurological: alert and oriented to self, place, and time, CN II-XII intact, normal tone and strength, normal cerebellar testing, normal reflexes, normal soft touch sensation and proprioception, no tremor, gait normal
- Psychiatric: mood reported as "not so great I guess," affect flat during interview but brightens a little when discussing his factory job and family (Fig. 25.1 and Fig. 25.2)

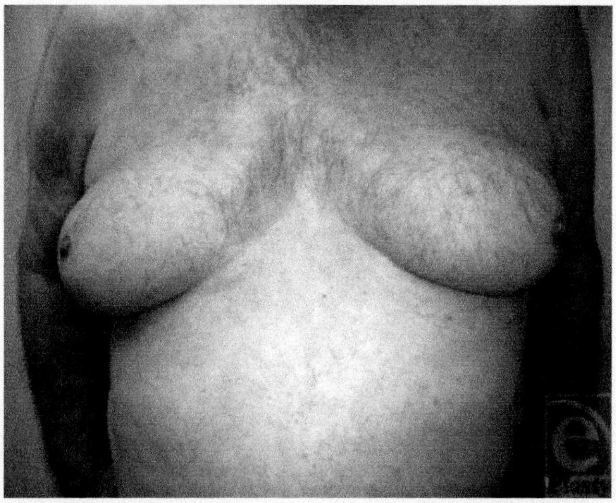

Fig. 25.1 Gynecomastia (Open Access: from Singer-Grannick and Granick, 2009 [22])

Case: Mr. Jones (continued)

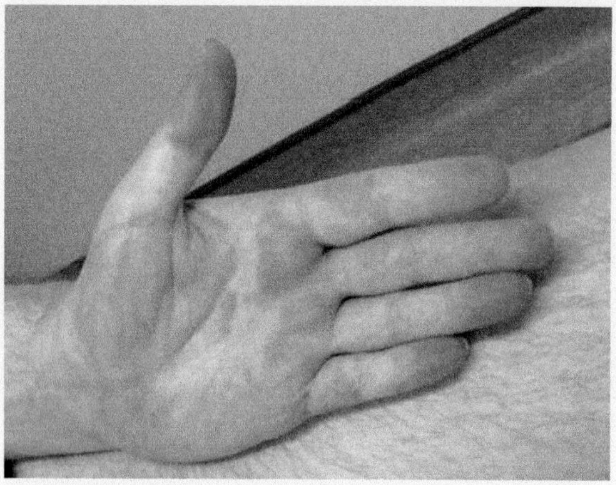

Fig. 25.2 Palmar erythema (Open Access: Open Access: from Norrenberg et al., 2012 [23])

Laboratory Testing and Imaging (from Mr. Jones's Recent Emergency Department Visits)

- Creatinine 1.62 mg/dL, BUN 44 mg/dL with otherwise normal electrolytes
- Wbc 5.6 × 10(9)/L, hemoglobin 10.5 g/dL, MCV 110 fL, platelets 188 × 10(9)/L
- AST 200 U/L, ALT 100 U/L, alkaline phosphatase 128 U/L, GGT 100 U/L
- Chest X-ray (AP view) report: mild COPD
- Lumbar spine X-ray and non-contrast CT scan: diffuse osteoarthritic changes without fracture or dislocation

Question: What physical exam findings and symptoms are associated with substance use and withdrawal?

- **Acute intoxication**
  - Opioids—(i) *mild-moderate*: sedation, slurred speech, miosis (pinpoint pupils); (ii) *severe*: depressed respiratory rate, decreased bowel sounds, significant alteration in mental status
  - Alcohol and sedatives-hypnotics—(i) *mild-moderate*: depressed mental status, disinhibition, poor coordination, slurred speech; (ii) *severe*: gait instability, nystagmus, hypotension and tachycardia depressed respiratory status, even stupor or coma
- **Acute withdrawal**
  - Opioids—(i) *mild-moderate*: mydriasis (dilated pupils), sweating, piloerection, rhinorrhea, lacrimation, restlessness, dysphoria, nausea, emesis, increased bowel sounds; (ii) *severe*: abdominal pain, diarrhea, myalgias, arthralgias, vital sign instability, delirium
  - Alcohol and sedatives-hypnotics—(i) *mild-moderate*: anxiety, restlessness, tremor, nausea and emesis; (ii) *severe*: headache, palpitations, tachycardia, hypertension, delirium-hallucinations and seizures
- **Chronic use**
  - Opioids—(i) *mild-moderate*: somnolence, nausea, pruritus; (ii) *severe*: urinary retention, myoclonus, opioid-induced bowel syndrome (bloating, early satiety, pain and constipation), opioid-induced hyperalgesia
  - Alcohol (including hepatic cirrhosis)—(i) *mild-moderate*: anorexia, weight loss, fatigue, gynecomastia, palmar erythema, cutaneous telangiectasia; (ii) *severe*: jaundice, caput medusa (abdominal wall collaterals), esophageal varices, ascites, splenomegaly, testicular atrophy, Dupuytren's contractures

Question: What laboratory findings are associated with substance use?

- Lab testing may provide insight into recent or heavy substance use but may be of variable utility when used for random screening and lighter use due to factors such as timing of testing, drug half-life, chronicity of use, and lack of ability to distinguish between appropriate and inappropriate use (for prescription drugs).
- Urine toxicology screening
  - The basic drugs of abuse (DOA) test in the United States generally include amphetamine, cocaine, marijuana (THC), natural opioids, benzodiazepines, and phencyclidine (PCP). Synthetic and semi-synthetic opioids (e.g., oxycodone, hydrocodone, and hydromorphone) are not detected by routine screening though specific assays to detect these drugs are also available.
  - Presence of a drug of abuse or one or more of its metabolites does not automatically indicate active intoxication because for each substance there is a period after use during which testing will be positive. This period can vary from 1 to 3 days (e.g., amphetamines, cocaine, opioids) or much longer (e.g., methadone, benzodiazepines, phencyclidine (PCP), ketamine, marijuana).
    - **False positives** due to medication or food may be possible, including: Amphetamines—pseudoephedrine, propranolol, atenolol, levodopa-carbidopa; Opiates—poppy seeds; PCP—dextromethorphan; and Cannabinoids—hemp containing food, Dronabinol.
    - **False negatives** may occur with suboptimal sample procurement, improper handling, and patient subversion techniques (e.g., ingestion of large amounts of water or masking agents), as well as failure of standard immunoassays to detect a drug whose chemical structure is unreactive with the assay (e.g., methamphetamine and MDMA [Ecstasy] may not be detected on routine amphetamine screens).
- Recent alcohol use
  - Blood alcohol content (BAC) is more often tested in acute and emergency care settings, though clinical correlation to serum level may be highly variable and the effect of alcohol may be affected by co-ingestion of other substances.
- Chronic alcohol use including hepatic disease
  - Elevated mean corpuscular volume (MCV) > 100 femtoliters (fL)
  - Elevations in liver enzymes—AST:ALT ratio typically >2.0 but both <300 IU/L
  - Elevated gamma-glutamyl transpeptidase (GGT)

25.2.1 Background and Epidemiology

- Among individuals age 50 and older, the projected prevalence of substance use disorders is expected to increase from 2.8 million in 2002 to 5.7 million in 2020 [24, 25].
- The baby boomers (born between 1946 and 1964) may have higher amounts of substance use and substance use disorders because of different cultural norms regarding psychoactive substances in the 1960s and 1970s and possible varying attitudes toward alcohol and other substance use [26, 27].
- In the 2001–2002 National Epidemiologic Survey on Alcohol and Related Conditions, more than 1 in 5 adults 65 and older reported ever having a substance use

disorder (predominantly tobacco and alcohol use), and 1 in 20 appeared to meet DSM-IV criteria for substance use disorder in the prior year [28].

- American older adults appear to use illicit substances (especially cannabis) more than older adults around the world [29]. Misuse of prescription medications, especially opiates, remains a significant public health concern. While such prescriptions are very commonly obtained from a friend or relative, prescription-opioid users who are at high risk of overdose are also likely to have been prescribed the medication [30].
- Older adults are at elevated risk for harm from lower levels of exposure to alcohol and other substances (such as opiates and benzodiazepines), due to the presence of comorbidities, higher likelihood of requiring multiple medications, generally lower lean body mass and total body water volume, decreased hepatic metabolism, and increased blood-brain barrier permeability [31].
- Though substance abuse disorders (SUDs) can contribute to poor health and social outcomes, few older adults are screened for substance abuse, and only 10–11% of adults with SUDs receive treatment [32, 33].

25.2.2 Definitions

- The **Center for Substance Abuse Treatment** broadly classifies substance use into four categories [34]:
- **Abstinence**—no use of alcohol or illicit substances
- **Low-risk use**—drinking within guidelines (▣ Table 25.2), using medication as instructed, no illicit substances
- **At-risk or unhealthy use**—drinking beyond guidelines, using alcohol and medications that are contraindicated together, unsupervised off-label use of any medicine, use of medications prescribed for someone else, and any use of illicit substances
- **Problem use**—any substance use that leads to medical and psychosocial problems regardless of how much is taken or how often it is consumed
- The **US National Institute on Alcohol Abuse and Alcoholism (NIAAA)** provides estimated levels of alcohol consumption that may correspond to different levels or risk for harm (▣ Table 25.2) [35].
- The ***Diagnostic and Statistical Manual*** **5th Edition (DSM-5)** contains formal criteria for diagnosing Substance use disorder (SUD), including subtypes for alcohol, tobacco, opioids, cannabis, stimulants (including amphetamines and cocaine), anxiolytics, inhalants, and hallucinogens [36].
- Diagnosis requires confirmation of **≥2** symptoms occurring in the last **12** months.
  - Taking the substance in larger amounts or for longer than intended
  - Wanting to cut down or stop using the substance but not managing to do so
  - Spending significant time getting, using, or recovering from use of the substance
  - Cravings and urges to use the substance
  - Recurrent use even when it leads to a failure to fulfill obligations at work, home, or school
  - Continuing to use, even when it causes recurrent social or interpersonal problems
  - Giving up or reducing important social, occupational, or recreational activities due to substance use
  - Using substances again and again, even when it places the individual in physical danger
  - Continuing to use, even when the individual knows that there is a physical or psychological problem that could be made worse by the substance
  - Tolerance, defined as either needing escalating doses of the substance to get the desired effect or markedly diminished effect with continued use of the same amount
  - Development of withdrawal symptoms, which may be reduced by taking the substance
- **Further specifiers include:**
  - Remission status—early (3–12 months) or sustained remission (12 or more months)
  - Use of maintenance therapy
  - Whether the individual is in a controlled environment or not
  - Severity based on number of symptoms—mild, 2–3 symptoms; moderate, 4–5 symptoms; severe, 6 or more symptoms
- **Factors complicating diagnosis of SUD in the older adult:**
  - Physiologic factors, e.g., subtle tolerance, more protracted or atypical signs of withdrawal
  - Decreased ability to assess impact on social behaviors and vocationless self-recognition of problematic substance use due to comorbid cognitive dysfunction
- **Potential risk factors for substance use and SUD** [37]:
  - Sex—male (alcohol), female (prescription drugs)
  - Caucasian ethnicity.
  - Unexpected or forced retirement, transitions in care/living situations, and social isolation (even includes living with non-spousal others)
  - Chronic pain, physical disabilities, or reduced mobility

▣ Table 25.2 NIAAA safe levels of alcohol consumption [35]

Group	Level of consumption at or above which increases risk
Men under age 65	>4 standard drinks on any single day >14 standard drinks per week on average
Women under 65 & **All Adults 65 and older**	>3 standard drinks on any single day More than 7 standard drinks per week on average

1 standard drink [12 grams of ethanol]: 12 oz of beer, or 5 oz of wine, or 1.5 oz of liquor (80-proof)

- Poor overall health status, chronic physical illness, and/or multimorbidity
- Significant drug burden and polypharmacy
- Frequency and pattern of alcohol and other substance use
- Previous and/or concurrent formally diagnosed substance use disorder (SUD)
- Previous and/or concurrent psychiatric illness, bereavement, and avoidance coping style

Question: What screening approaches might be helpful to explore with Mr. Jones and other patients for whom you have increased suspicion for a Substance Use Disorder?

25.2.3 Screening

- **Screening Frequency—The US Preventive Services Task Force (USPSTF)** recommends screening all adults age 18 and older for alcohol misuse and providing brief behavioral counseling interventions to individuals who engage in risky or hazardous alcohol use (Grade B recommendation) [38]. Screening for alcohol and other substances should be considered as part of a routine health assessment as well as whenever there is clinical suspicion of substance use (or misuse).
- **Screening Instruments** (Table 25.3)

Table 25.3 Selected open-access[a] screening instruments for alcohol and substance use among adults [37, 39, 40]

Questionnaire	Substance(s)	Details
AUDIT (10 questions) AUDIT-C (3 questions)	Alcohol	Developed by the World Health Organization (WHO) The most validated instrument Validated among older adults to detect risky use
CAGE-AID (4 questions)	Alcohol and other Drugs	Most common instrument utilized May be less sensitive among binge drinkers and does not distinguish between lifetime and current use [37] CAGE (but not CAGE-AID) validated among older adults
NIDA Quick Screen (1 question) NIDA-modified ASSIST adapted from WHO ASSIST screening test	Alcohol and other Drugs	Developed by National Institute on Drug Abuse (NIDA) Well situated for integration into primary care settings Free access to online tools to calculate a Substance Involvement (SI) score based on the NIDA-modified ASSIST for *each substance endorsed* Risk-level specific recommendations based on SI score Not yet validated for use among older adults, where the sensitivity may differ

[a]Open Access: ► https://www.drugabuse.gov/nidamed-medical-health-professionals/tool-resources-your-practice/screening-assessment-drug-testing-resources/chart-evidence-based-screening-tools-adults

Case Conclusion

Assessment and Plan

- You initiate a **non-judgmental discussion** regarding the intent and consequences of screening for substance use and disorders, emphasizing the desire to both develop a long-term therapeutic relationship and effectively address Mr. Jones' pain and functional status.
  - **The National Institute on Drug Abuse (NIDA)** provides the following sample statement(s): "*Hi, I'm __________, nice to meet you. If it's okay with you, I'd like to ask you a few questions that will help me give you better medical care. The questions relate to your experience with alcohol, cigarettes, and other drugs. Some of the substances we'll talk about are prescribed by a doctor (like pain medications), but I will only record those if you have taken them for reasons or in doses other than prescribed. I'll also ask you about illicit or illegal drug use—but only to better diagnose and treat you.*" [39].
  - Mr. Jones informs you that he drinks 3–4 beers and 2 shots of whiskey per night, 5 nights per week over the last 2 months. He smokes half a pack of cigarettes per day and has done so for almost 40 years. He denies any other substance use.
- **Ask permission to engage other caregivers.**
  - Mr. Jones provides permission to speak with his son, who echoes your concern about Mr. Jones's alcohol use as well as "some type of pain pills."
- **Identify all medications being used.**
  - The prescription drug monitoring program (PDMP) is a state-level intervention aimed at providing prescribers of controlled substances the opportunity to review patients' prescribing histories in real time. Currently 49 states, the District of Columbia, and Guam have legislation authorizing the creation and maintenance of a PDMP.
  - You log onto I-STOP, New York State's PDMP, and note that Mr. Jones had filled a prescription for 10 tabs of oxycodone (5 mg tabs) 4 weeks ago at a nearby pharmacy, as well as 14 tabs of oxycodone-acetaminophen (5 mg/325 mg tabs) 8 weeks ago at another pharmacy.

Case Conclusion (continued)

- **Manage pain and related symptoms.**
  - You prescribe topical lidocaine gel, to be applied to the lower back 2 to 3 times daily. He agrees to try this and avoid opiates, and due to his comorbidities and lab results, he will also avoid nonsteroidal anti-inflammatory drugs (NSAIDs), doses of acetaminophen exceeding 2 grams per day, and accepting prescriptions from other persons. You begin to discuss a Pain Agreement Contract which you will follow-up with him on at the next visit, particularly if controlled substances are potentially prescribed in the future.
  - You refer Mr. Jones to Physiatry and Physical Therapy as well as to the senior/community center for exercise classes and social support. You print him handouts on home exercises and stretching.
  - You engage Mr. Jones in a conversation about tobacco use and cessation, and determine he is precontemplative. He accepts a pamphlet outlining cessation strategies and Nicotine Replacement Therapy.
- **Refer for multidisciplinary mental health, substance abuse counseling, and treatment.**
  - Mr. Jones' screening results suggest a high risk of substance use disorder and harm from his pattern of substance use, so you engage him in a discussion of your concerns and referrals for care.
  - While a thorough discussion of treatment is beyond the scope of this chapter, be aware that a variety of treatment options are available including brief interventions for the primary care setting utilizing motivational interviewing and normative feedback, cognitive behavioral therapy (CBT), supportive therapy models (STM), pharmacotherapy, case management, self-help groups, and other abuse-addiction programs. Despite limited programs and interventions specifically designed for older adults, several studies have demonstrated similar if not better outcomes for older compared to younger adults [41, 42].
  - The Substance Abuse and Mental Health Services Administration (SAMHSA), part of the US Department of Health and Human Services, provides information for many of the above-noted resources, including the Center for Substance Abuse Treatment (CSAT) which hosts a 24-hour National Treatment Referral Line [43].
  - Alcoholics Anonymous and Twelve-Step Facilitation programs may represent an additional resource. Though relatively well known, there are mixed findings in the limited literature regarding the effectiveness of such programs [44, 45].
- **Close follow-up.**
  - Mr. Jones states that while he is not interested in entering any alcohol or substance use programs at this time he is willing to start slowly tapering his alcohol consumption and following up with you in clinic for his pain, substance use, known chronic diagnoses and newly suspected conditions (liver disease and suspected chronic obstructive pulmonary disease). You review with him signs and symptoms warranting a time sensitive call to the clinic and/or assessment in the emergency room, emphasizing that alcohol withdrawal can have serious and life-threatening consequences. On his way out, he tells you that he appreciates your support and feels motivated to improve his health with help from you and his son.

25.3 Section: Sexually Transmitted Infections

Case: Mr. Thomas

Chief Complaint: *"I have a personal problem"*

History of Present Illness: *Mr. Thomas is a 70-year-old patient with a history of controlled hypertension, hyperlipidemia, pre-diabetes, and hypothyroidism. During his scheduled follow-up appointment for his chronic medical issues, Mr. Thomas mentions that he has visualized some irritation and perhaps discharge in the tip of his penis while urinating for the last several days. He denies any urinary frequency, urgency, abdominal pain, rash, or constitutional symptoms. He otherwise says he has been feeling more energetic and socializing more with friends and acquaintances, which is a change for him as he had been more homebound over the last several years after his wife had passed.*

Question: What medical conditions might you be concerned about based on Mr. Thomas's history and symptoms? What would you look for on physical exam?

Focused Exam
- Vital signs: T 37.0C (oral), BP 128/74, HR 76, BMI 25, RR 18, SpO2 100% on room air.
- General: well-groomed and interactive.
- HEENT: PERRL, EOMI, sclera anicteric, mucous membranes moist and without abnormalities.
- Abdomen: normoactive BS, soft, non-tender, non-distended.
- Genitourinary: circumcised penis, subtle erythema of the external urethral opening without purulence, no rash, no testicular edema or tenderness, no local lymphadenopathy.
- Neurological: alert and oriented to self, place, and time.
- Psychiatric: mood is "pretty good except for the problem I told you about."

Review of Laboratory Testing (from Mr. Thomas's Chart and During This Visit)
- Creatinine 0.88 mg/dL, BUN 24 mg/dL, normal electrolytes
- Wbc 7.0 × 10(9)/L, hemoglobin 11.0 g/dL, MCV 82.5 fL, platelets 300 × 10(9)/L
- AST 28 U/L, ALT 26 U/L, alkaline phosphatase 112 U/L, GGT 18 U/L
- A1c 6.0%; TSH 2.1 mIU/L
- Point of care urinalysis: yellow and slightly turbid, notable for >10 WBC per high-power field, negative for RBC, leukocyte esterase, nitrite, or other abnormalities

25.3.1 Background and Epidemiology

- A 2007 longitudinal US study of a probability sample of 3005 of older adults found that nearly a quarter of respondents age 75–85 remained sexually active, despite the proportion of adults reporting sexual activity declining with age [46–48].
- Older adults can still contract sexually transmitted infections (STIs).
  - Centers for Disease Control (CDC) data suggest that in 2011 there were over 12,000 newly diagnosed cases of HIV among adults age 45 and older, including over 1900 individuals age 60 and older [49].
  - 2016 CDC data for newly reported cases of STIs also highlight an increase in chlamydia, gonorrhea, and syphilis rates among older adults for the third year in a row [50].
- Condom use may be significantly lower among adults age 60 and older compared to younger adults [51].
- Older adults may not routinely engage in discussions about STIs with their providers, due to a multitude of factors including potential reticence on the part of both patient and provider to open the dialogue [52–54].

25.3.2 Risk Factors

- Potential physiologic changes can increase the risk of STIs. These may include vaginal dryness and atrophy (increased risk of micro-trauma), decreased progesterone (possible role in increasing risk of vaginal infections), general age- or comorbidity-related changes in immune system response to infection(s), and use of erectile dysfunction medications and progesterone and estrogen creams [55, 56].
- There is considerable regional variation with respect to prevalence of STIs, with lower socioeconomic status often associated with lower likelihood of screening and treatment [57].
- Health literacy and stigma regarding sexual behavior and STIs may also vary by age, region, community, and ethnic and cultural background [57].

25.3.3 Screening

- **Centers for Disease Control and Prevention (CDC)** [49, 50]
  - All adults who are sexually active should engage in a discussion with their healthcare provider about screening risks and benefits.
  - All adults (18–64 years of age) should be screened for HIV at least once in their lifetime.
  - Sexually active older women with risk factors (e.g., new or multiple sex partners, communities with high burden of disease) should have yearly screening for gonorrhea (GC) and chlamydia.
  - HIV+ women should have annual screening for trichomoniasis in addition to GC/chlamydia.
  - Sexually active older men who have sex with men (MSM) should have yearly screening for gonorrhea, chlamydia, HIV, and syphilis (potentially more frequent screening if additional risk factors, such as multiple or anonymous partners, or illicit substance use).
- **Initiating a Dialogue**
  - Healthcare providers can provide a safe, confidential, and judgment-free space for patients.
  - Sample introductory statement: "*Mr. Thomas, I believe that a frank discussion of sexual health and well-being are also important and routine components of a complete medical assessment. I want to reassure you that what we discuss is confidential and will help me provide accurate recommendations for screening to keep you healthy. With your permission I would like to ask about your experiences and provide you an opportunity to discuss concerns or questions you might have.*"
  - Be mindful to use open-ended questions when asking about sexual partners and specific behaviors, avoiding assumptions about the number or biologic sex of partners past or present.
  - Remember to ask about condom use.

Case Conclusion

Follow-Up Discussion

- Mr. Thomas agrees to discuss his sexual health and behaviors. He reports that over the last several months he has been sexually active with several female acquaintances, and most recently, a sex worker about a week prior to his visit today. He did not use condoms during these encounters which did involve penetrative vaginal intercourse. He assumed that he was "safe" because "everything looked okay at first", and he assumed "guys [his] age don't have to worry about that kind of thing."

Plan

- He agrees to testing for gonorrhea, chlamydia, syphilis, and HIV. He also accepts some printed materials from the CDC's website to further educate himself on risk factors and preventive strategies for STIs. He accepts free condoms which your medical office makes available to all patients.

25.4 Section: Elder Mistreatment

Case: Ms. Lee

Chief Complaint: *"I can't breathe."*

History of Present Illness: *Ms. Lee is an 86-year-old woman with a history of dementia, atrial fibrillation on warfarin, congestive heart failure (CHF), hypothyroidism, and diabetes mellitus who presents to the emergency room with shortness of breath, right leg swelling and redness and fever. She has had two recent 48-hour admissions to the hospital for CHF exacerbations where she responded quickly to her home dose of diuretics. After 20 mg of intravenous furosemide in the emergency department, her dyspnea and oxygen level markedly improve. She is started on IV antibiotics for a right leg cellulitis. The ED social worker calls Ms. Lee's son to inform him that she is being admitted and discuss possible short-term rehabilitation since this is her third admission. He becomes angry and insists that she can return home. Review of her outpatient chart shows she has missed multiple follow-up appointments with her primary doctor and cardiologist. She is now admitted to the hospital for acute systolic congestive heart failure, rapid atrial fibrillation and cellulitis.*

- **Social History**

She requires assistance with shopping, meal preparation, medications, and finances. She lives with her adult son and has no home health aide services. She uses a rolling walker.

- **Home Medications**

Furosemide 40 mg daily, levothyroxine 75 mcg daily, digoxin 100 mcg daily, metoprolol 50 mg daily, sitagliptin 25 mg daily, warfarin 2.5 mg nightly

Focused Exam

- Vital signs: afebrile, BP 160/80, heart rate 120 bpm, room air O_2 saturation 92%, BMI 15
- General: dressed in only a thin shirt, sweater, and skirt with bare legs and no coat despite winter weather
- HEENT: ill-fitting dentures
- Cardiac: irregularly irregular, normal s1 and s2, no murmur or rub
- Lung: decreased breath sounds at the lung bases, rales in the mid and upper lung fields bilaterally
- Skin and extremities: 3+ pitting lower extremity edema, 10 cm × 3 cm warm and tender erythematous patch on right lower leg
- Neuro/psych: able to say her name but not oriented to place or date. Restless, picking at the sheets, frequently removing the oxygen tubing

Laboratory Testing and Imaging

- Na^+ 142 mmol/L, K^+ 4.6 mmol/L, Cl^- 100 mmol/L, HCO_3^- 30 mmol/L, BUN 40 mg/dL, Cr 1.5 mg/mL, glucose 300 mg/dL
- WBC 15 × 10(9)/L, Hgb 12.0 g/dL, platelets 320 × 10(9)/L
- BNP: 10,000 and troponin I < 0.03 ng/mL
- INR: 1.2
- Digoxin level 0.0 ng/mL
- TSH 12 mIU/L
- Urinalysis: +glucose
- Hemoglobin A1c: 9% (A1c = 7.2%, 6 months ago)
- ECG: atrial fibrillation with rapid ventricular rate, no acute ischemic changes
- Chest X-ray (PA/Lateral): noted cardiomegaly and signs of pulmonary vascular congestion

? Question: When, how, and what should you assess for elder mistreatment? How common is elder mistreatment?

25.4.1 Screening

- Healthcare providers should adopt "universal precautions" for elder mistreatment and maintain a high index of suspicion. If one type of abuse or neglect is suspected, physicians should screen for all other forms. Physicians must often act as detectives, piecing together the smallest of details to form a larger picture.

25.4.2 Definitions

- The American Medical Association (AMA) classifies elder abuse and neglect as **"acts of commission or omission that result in harm or threatened harm to the health or welfare of an older adult."** The AMA emphasizes mistreatment may be intentional or unintentional. Unintentional mistreatment can be due to a caregiver's ignorance, inexperience, or inability, often stemming from a medical or mental health problems [58].
- Despite the varying definitions of abuse and neglect, agreement exists for the following **six types of mistreatment** (*listed in order of frequency substantiated by Adult Protective Services in the 1998 National Elder Abuse Incidence Study*) [59]. The World Health Organization adds that the "perpetrators" of abuse and neglect are typically persons whom the older adult holds in a position of trust [60].
- **Neglect:** The refusal or failure of a designated caregiver to ensure an older adult's physical and mental well-being. Neglect includes, but is not limited to, the failure to provide basic necessities like food, water, clothing, shelter, and medicine.
- **Self-neglect:** The refusal or failure of an older adult to meet his or her own physical and mental needs resulting in threats to personal health or safety. This includes, but is not limited to, an elder's failure to take medications, adhere to medical treatment or maintain adequate nutrition, personal hygiene, and shelter. In its most extreme form, self-neglect is manifest by domestic squalor, social withdrawal, hoarding behaviors, and refusal to accept help.
- **Psychological abuse:** Verbal or nonverbal acts intended to cause anguish, pain, or distress. This includes, but is not limited to, verbal assaults, insults, threats (including threat of abandonment or institutionalization), intimidation, humiliation, harassment, infantilization, and social isolation.

- **Financial exploitation:** The illegal or improper use of an elder's funds, property, or assets. This includes, but is not limited to, cashing checks without permission, forging an older adult's signature, stealing money or possessions, coercing or deceiving an older adult into signing documents (e.g., contracts, wills, or property deeds), and improper use of conservatorship, guardianship, or power of attorney status.
- **Physical abuse:** Acts intended to cause impairment, physical pain, or bodily injury. Physical abuse includes, but is not limited to, acts of violence such as striking (with or without an object), pushing, shoving, shaking, kicking, pinching, and burning. Additional examples include the inappropriate use of drugs or physical restraints, force feeding, and physical punishment of any kind.
- **Sexual abuse:** Any type of nonconsensual sexual contact including situations in which an older adult is unable to consent.

25.4.3 Background and Epidemiology

- Extrapolating from the best available evidence, the overall prevalence of elder mistreatment in community settings may be as high as 10% [61]. A physician will likely encounter at least one victim of elder abuse for every 20–40 older adults seen [62].
- The original 1998 National Elder Abuse Incidence Study (NEAIS) compared Adult Protective Services records and reports from community agencies who frequently worked with elderly clients. The NEAIS found nearly 80% of incidents were never reported to Adult Protective Services, the major agency tasked with receiving and investigating reports of abuse and neglect [59].
- The New York State Elder Mistreatment Prevalence Study interviewed 4000 older adults by phone and found self-reported rates of mistreatment of 10.8% for neglect, 2.7% for financial abuse, 1.9% for emotional abuse, and 1.8% for physical abuse [63]. Similarly, in a national sample of 5770 cognitively intact individuals, Acierno et al. found comparable annual rates of reported mistreatment (11.4% neglect, 5.2% financial abuse, 4.6% emotional abuse, 1.6% physical abuse, and 0.6% for sexual abuse) [64].
- Financial abuse may be the fastest growing but least often recognized form of elder mistreatment with an estimated $2.9 billion in direct costs [65].
- In long-term care settings, "resident-to-resident" aggression in the form of physical abuse, verbal abuse or sexual aggression is becoming an alarming trend and is actually more common than abuse of residents by nursing home staff [66].
- Physicians should also be aware that elder mistreatment is an independent risk factor for death. A prospective cohort study of 2800 community-dwelling adults age 65 and older found the mortality rate was three times higher in the elder mistreatment group and 1.7 times greater in the self-neglect group. In the group with any elder mistreatment, the survival rate was 9% versus 40% [67].

25.4.4 The Role of Healthcare Professionals

- Despite being ideally suited to detect, manage, and prevent elder mistreatment, physicians and clinicians in general are one of the least likely groups of individuals to report abuse and neglect though they may be the only individuals to come in contact with the abused or neglected adult [68].
- Barriers to physician reporting include insufficient knowledge of assessment protocols and mandatory reporting guidelines, concerns about a negative effect on relationships with patients and caregivers, reluctance to get involved with the legal system, and time constraints.
- Elder mistreatment, especially psychological abuse, financial exploitation, and caregiver neglect are associated with a twofold increase in emergency department use and increased hospitalization [69–71]. Every emergency room visit, admission, and outpatient visit represents a critical opportunity for medical providers to positively impact the lives of both elder mistreatment victims and their caregivers.
- Physicians have the authority and expertise to **(1)** document the presence or absence of mistreatment using the physical exam, labs, and other studies, **(2)** recommend admission or transfer to another setting, and **(3)** order critical services such as home healthcare. For known cases of ongoing abuse in the community, a hospital admission can provide a vital chance to assess and counsel victims away from the influence of abusers and their environments, and to bring new resources to bear on the problem (e.g., psychiatric consultation, social services, physical therapy).

? Question: What risk factors and red flags in Ms. Lee's case raise suspicion for elder mistreatment?

25.4.5 Risk Factors

- Major risk factors for elder abuse and neglect include a shared living situation (except for financial abuse), functional and cognitive impairment, and social isolation from other friends and relatives. The abuser is most likely to be an adult child or spouse, may suffer from mental illness or alcohol misuse, and is generally dependent on the older adult [62, 72]. When older adults present with uncontrolled chronic illness or signs of nonadherence, elder mistreatment should be on the differential diagnosis.
- Red flags for Ms. Lee that may indicate possible elder neglect and/or financial exploitation
  - Multiple admissions for decompensated congestive heart failure

- Rapid positive response to the IV equivalent of her home dose of furosemide
- On physical exam inappropriate attire for the weather, uncontrolled blood pressure, and heart failure
- Laboratory values suggesting nonadherence to warfarin, digoxin, and levothyroxine as well as a major change in her diabetes control compared to 6 months prior

25.4.6 Evaluation: History and Interview

- The presence of any one of the red flags or manifestations in ◘ Table 25.4 should prompt a full assessment for elder mistreatment that begins like any other admission or consultation with a thorough history and physical but with special attention to the patient's functional status and decision-making capacity [58, 72].
- In obtaining the **history**, the physician should **address and document** information from all involved individuals (the older adult, the suspected abuser/neglector, and all collateral sources as described below), and explicitly address functional status as well as social and financial resources [58].

- **Important General Points to Consider**
- It is critical to interview the older adult and the suspected abuser *separately*.
- The older adult's decision-making capacity and willingness to accept help will ultimately determine the intervention strategies employed (◘ Fig. 25.3) [58, 62].
  - The physician can matter-of-factly inform caregivers that hospital/practice policy requires the physician interview each patient privately and provide assurance that time will be allotted to address the caregiver's questions/concerns.
  - For efficiency, another interprofessional team member (e.g., the social worker, nurse, medical

◘ **Table 25.4** Types of elder abuse and assessment strategies for clinicians

Type of abuse	Manifestations	Assessment and notable findings
Physical abuse	Abrasions Lacerations Bruises Fractures Use of restraints Burns Pain Depression Delirium with or without worsening of dementia or dementia-related behavioral problems	Ask directly how injuries were sustained; note findings that are discordant with the mechanism of injury reported Color of bruises does not reliably indicate their age; bruising can occur spontaneously in older adults in the absence of documented or recollected trauma [73].Older adults may bruise spontaneously or without apparent awareness of injury Injuries to the head, neck, and upper arms occur in victims of physical elder abuse, but they must be distinguished from accidental injuries caused by falls and other trauma Jaw and zygomatic fractures are more likely to be sustained in a punch to the face than in a fall (falls typically result in fractures to orbital and nasal bones) Long-bone fractures can occur spontaneously in the absence of physical abuse in patients who are confined to bed Ankles and wrists should be examined for abrasions suggestive of the use of restraints Multiple injuries in various stages of healing should raise the suspicion of abuse (e.g., lacerations healing by secondary intention [i.e., without sutures] and old, unset fractures detected on radiographs) The mouth should be examined for dental fractures and avulsion of teeth A formal assessment for pain should be conducted (this may be difficult in patients with cognitive impairment) Screen formally for depression, ideally with the use of an instrument such as the Geriatric Depression Scale The patient should be assessed for delirium (or worsening of dementia or dementia-related behavioral problems), which can result from pain or other medical problems The interview should be conducted alone with the patient; it may reveal discordant histories or findings inconsistent with the history provided by the caregiver
Verbal or psychological abuse	Direct observation of verbal abuse Subtle signs of intimidation, such as deferring questions to a caregiver or potential abuser Evidence of isolation of victim from both previously trusted friends and family members Depression, anxiety, or both in the patient	Ask specifically about verbal or psychological abuse with questions such as "Does anyone ever yell or curse at you?" "Have you been threatened with being sent to a nursing home?" "Are you ever prevented from seeing friends and family members whom you wish to see?" Assess the size and quality of the patient's social network (beyond the suspected abuser) with questions such as "How many people do you see each day?" "How many do you speak to on the telephone?" "Is there anyone to assist you in the event of accident or emergency?" "Who would that be?" Conduct standardized assessments of depression, anxiety, and cognition, directly or through referral Other types of abuse are often concurrent with verbal abuse Office staff (clinical and front desk) should be encouraged to report verbally abusive behavior to the physician if they observe it

(continued)

Table 25.4 (continued)

Type of abuse	Manifestations	Assessment and notable findings
Sexual abuse	Bruising, abrasions, lacerations in the anogenital area or abdomen Newly acquired sexually transmitted diseases, especially in nursing home residents (and especially in cluster outbreaks) Urinary tract infection	Inquire directly about sexual assault or coercion in any sexual activity Conduct a pelvic examination with a collection of appropriate specimens or refer to the emergency department for comprehensive assessment for sexual assault and collection of specimens. Ideally, forensic evidence should be collected by experienced professionals, such as nurses who have undergone Sexual Assault Nurse Examiners (SANE) training A common form of geriatric sexual assault involves a hypersexual resident with dementia in a long-term care facility assaulting other residents who may or may not also have cognitive impairment [77]. This situation raises fundamental issues about the capacity of older persons with dementia to consent to sexual activity For outpatients with dementia, direct queries to caregivers about hypersexual behavior as part of a larger history regarding dementia-related behaviors Signs of sexual abuse are similar to manifestations of sexual violence in younger adults
Financial abuse	Inability to pay for medicine, medical care, food, rent, or other necessities Failure to renew prescriptions or keep medical appointments Unexplained worsening of chronic medical problems that were previously controlled Nonadherence to medication regimen or other treatment Malnutrition, weight loss, or both, without an obvious medical cause Depression, anxiety Evidence of poor financial decision making provided by the patient, patient history, or others persons Firing of home care or other service providers by abuser Unpaid utility bills leading to loss of service Initiation of eviction proceedings	Ask about financial exploitation with questions such as "Has money or property been taken from you without your consent?" "Have your credit cards or automated-teller-machine card been used without your consent?" "Have people called your home to try and get you to send or wire money to them?" "At the end of the month, do you have enough money left over for food, rent, utilities, or other necessities?" Direct similar questions to caregivers who are not suspected of being the financial abuser Conduct a formal assessment of cognition and mood Be aware that victims may be unwilling to disclose exploitation out of embarrassment Abrupt changes in the financial circumstances of the caregiver in either direction (e.g., sudden unemployment or extravagant purchases) may also herald an increased risk of financial exploitation or exploitation already under way Abuse of the power of attorney is the situation in which an older person is inaccurately designated as lacking financial capacity or being unable to perform necessary financial tasks, or in which a lack of capacity is accurately designated but the person with the power of attorney is abusing the role (e.g., using the money improperly). If misrepresentation of the lack of capacity is suspected, the patient should be interviewed to determine whether he or she should be encouraged to resume personal control of financial matters. If there is concern that the person with power of attorney or healthcare proxy may not be acting in the best interest of the patient, the physician or other members of the interprofessional team should request the necessary documents to ensure that the assumption of fiduciary responsibilities is indeed authorized
Neglect	Decubitus ulcers Malnutrition Dehydration Poor hygiene Nonadherence to medication regimen Delirium with or without worsening of dementia or dementia-related behavioral problems	Examine the skin for pressure injury and skin rashes suggestive of infestations Assess hygiene and cleanliness Assess appropriateness of dress Measure drug levels in serum to assess adherence and accuracy of administration of medicines Measure body mass index and albumin Conduct clinical examination to assess nutrition Measure blood urea nitrogen and creatinine to assess hydration Conduct a directed physical examination to assess the status of chronic illnesses under treatment Interview primary caregiver about his or her understanding of the nature of the patient's care needs and how well care is being rendered Neglect may be intentional or may be unintentional, stemming from an inability to provide care owing to the caregiver's frailty, cognitive impairment, mental illness, or limited health literacy

The table is adapted from Dyer et al. [13]

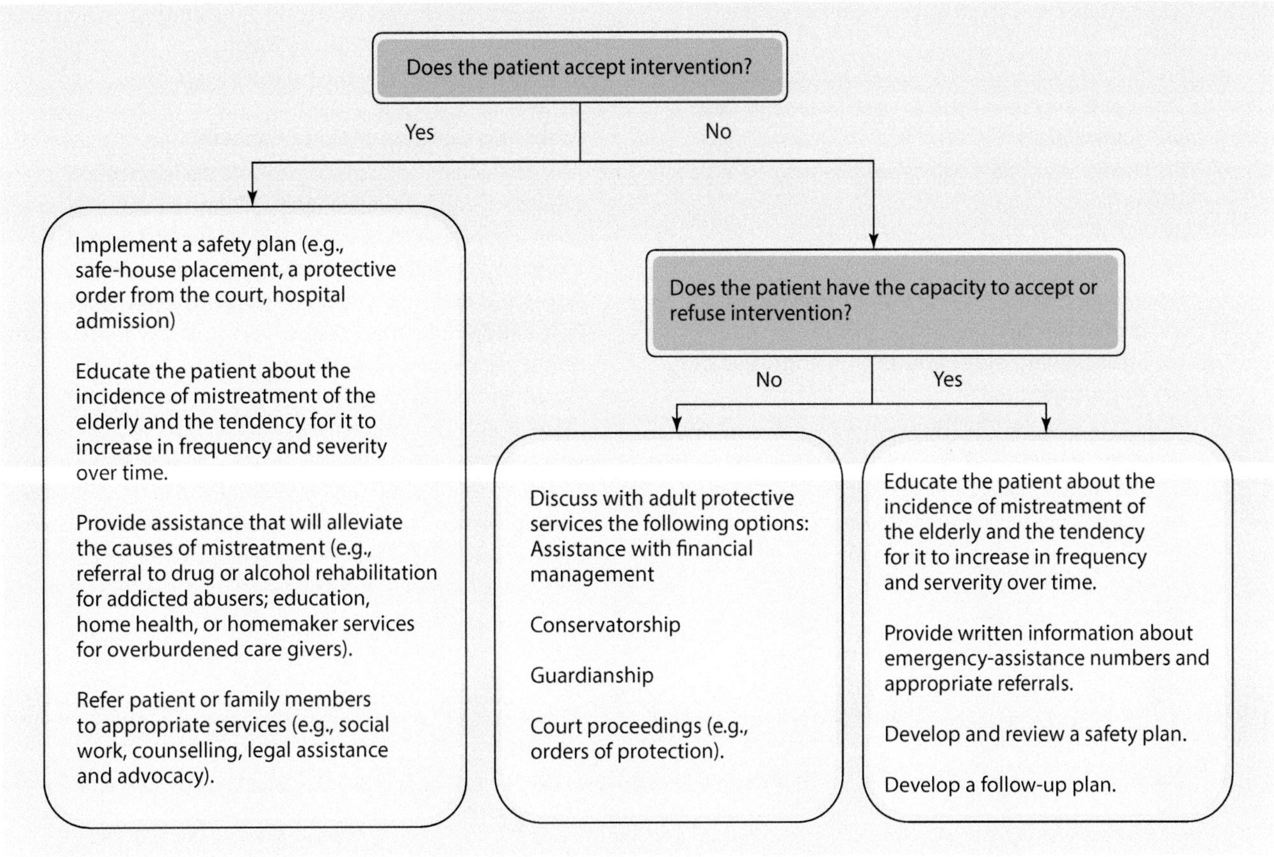

Fig. 25.3 Approach to patient (Adapted from: Lachs MS, Pillemer K. Elder Abuse. *N Engl J Med.* 2015;(373):1947–1956 [72])

trainee) can elicit the caregiver's history while the physician completes the patient interview and physical exam.
- If the suspected abuser refuses to allow the older adult to be interviewed alone, it should raise the examiner's suspicions and should be documented in the medical record.
- Special attention should be paid to how the older adult acts in the caregiver's presence. Note any comments or glances the person gives to the older adult conveying a message to "shut up." Subtle changes in the older adult's demeanor when being interviewed alone can also signal abuse or neglect and should be documented (e.g., withdrawn or depressed affect, quiet speech, poor eye contact).

- Older adults with cognitive impairment or hearing/vision loss can pose additional challenges during but remember these conditions increase vulnerability to mistreatment.
  - Do not assume patients with dementia or sensory impairments cannot adequately report mistreatment. Elder abuse will be missed if the medical team fails to elicit a history directly from the older adult.

Question: What are some ways to open a dialogue with the patient?

- Interview Tips and Considerations: *Speaking with the Patient*
- For all suspected elder mistreatment victims, physicians can build rapport and collect key information by beginning with open-ended questions about the living environment and functional status and then progressing to more specific questions recommended by the American Medical Association [58].
- If elder mistreatment is disclosed (often revealed over multiple conversations), be prepared to validate the patient's experience and listen supportively as you might be the first person the victim has confided in.
- Some victims choose not to disclose or refuse assistance. A victim might refuse help due to a fear of escalating abuse or neglect if the nature of the relationship is altered or exposed.
- **Examples of general questions to begin an interview**
  - *Tell me about your home environment.*
  - *Who lives with you?*
  - *Who, if anyone, helps you with transfers, bathing, toileting, feeding, grooming (ADLs)?*
  - *Who, if anyone helps you with meal preparation, shopping, medications, bills (IADLs)?*
- **Examples of specific questions suggested by the American Medical Association** [3]
  - *Do you feel safe in your home?*

- *Does anyone ever threaten you or verbally assault you?*
- *Has anyone ever touched you without your consent?*
- *Has anyone ever asked you to sign documents you don't understand?*
- *Has anyone ever taken your things without your permission?*
- *Are you afraid of anyone in your home?*
- *Are you alone a lot?*
- *Has anyone ever failed to help you when you were unable to help yourself?*

- **Tips for interviewing older adults with cognitive or sensory impairment** [58]
  - Allot extra time for the interview or break it up over several encounters.
  - Ensure that the patient has his/her assistive devices (e.g., eyeglasses, hearing aid, dentures).
  - Minimize background noise when possible (e.g., draw the curtain, close the door).
  - Position yourself so that you are at eye level (e.g., raise head of the patient's bed, sit in a chair).
  - Speak slowly and clearly; avoid shouting, which may come across as confrontational.
  - Repeat and clarify the patient's responses.

Assessing Decision-Making Capacity

- Any physician can assess a patient's decision-making capacity though for legal purposes and in complex cases, often a psychiatrist is asked to perform and document a capacity evaluation. Remember that physicians can assess and document decision-making capacity whereas only a judge and court of law has the ability to determine *competence versus incompetence.*
- Documenting that a patient is "alert and oriented times three" is not the equivalent of documenting decision-making capacity. To demonstrate capacity, an individual must be able to understand the relevant information or choices being presented, articulate a choice, and provide a reasonable explanation for that choice. Cognitive impairment does not automatically signify a lack of capacity. The assessment of capacity must be decision-specific (e.g., *does this patient have capacity to participate in discharge planning?*).

Case Continued

Ms. Lee is delirious upon admission but after diuresis and treatment with antibiotics, she is able to be interviewed alone in her room. While she cannot list the names of her medications, she knows she takes "heart medications" including "a water pill" as well as "sugar pills and a blood thinner." She states "I know my son doesn't always give me the same number of pills every day. He thinks I'm on too many drugs." She has poor eye contact when discussing her relationship with her son and mumbles that he has never had a steady job and has been living with her for years. He spends much of the day watching TV or on his computer. A call to the home care agency she was referred to after her last hospitalization reveals that her son terminated her nursing, physical therapy and home health aide services after only a week and the agency had referred Ms. Lee to Adult Protective Services because of concerns the son's hoarding created unsanitary conditions. The patient denies any physical, verbal or sexual abuse but does say her son has asked her to sign blank checks and manages their finances.

Question: What are some ways to open a dialogue with a suspected perpetrator?

Interview Tips and Considerations:
Speaking with the Suspected Perpetrator

When interviewing caregivers or suspected perpetrators, the healthcare provider should try to remain nonjudgmental, avoid confrontation, and express empathy for the burden of caregiving. Pay attention to inconsistencies in the explanations provided or frequently changing stories.

- **Helpful questions for caregivers or suspected perpetrators** [58]
  - *How long have you been caring for (the patient)?*
  - *What are your primary caregiving responsibilities?*
  - *Do you feel you have adequate support? Why or why not?*
  - *How are you coping with your responsibilities?*
  - *What is your understanding of the patient's medical conditions and needs?*
  - *Can you tell me in your words what happened? (if physical signs of injury or history of injury)*
- An abuser may not demonstrate aggression in front of the medical providers because he or she does not want any outsider to detect a problem. A caregiver who is neglecting an older adult may attribute signs of neglect like malnutrition, dehydration, uncontrolled chronic diseases, or mood disorders to the patient (e.g., "She refuses to eat or take her medications") or to the aging process (e.g., "Anyone would be depressed in this situation.").

Case Continued

When the ED social worker first meets Ms. Lee's son he appears mildly disheveled, his speech is slightly pressured and his thought process is tangential. He says "My mother belongs at home where I can take care of her. I would never put her in a nursing home. That's where my sister thinks she should live." He perseverates on how hard it is to hire a home health aide "because we only need a few hours a week" and expresses anger toward his sister for "never helping us out." The next day when reviewing Ms. Lee's medications with the medical student, he says "I let her sleep in as much as she wants because of her age" and admits she then misses her morning medications. He doesn't allow her to go to a nearby senior center because he is worried "she will get the flu or something worse." When she appears tired, he withholds her warfarin because he thought it could cause fatigue. The social worker contacts Adult Protective Services and finds out the son was spending large sums of money online shopping and had a significant hoarding problem though the patient's room was kept clean.

Case Continued (continued)

Question: What are other sources of information that should be evaluated?

- Obtain Collateral from Multiple Sources

While the older adult and the reported perpetrator of the abuse or neglect can provide critical history, collateral information from other sources is often necessary to corroborate the validity of the information being presented.

- **Valuable sources of collateral history**
  - The patient's primary care physician or other medical providers
    - Presence and status of chronic illnesses, baseline cognitive and functional status, compliance with visits and medications, previous interaction with caregivers
  - Individuals who live with the older adult (e.g., relatives, friends, personal care workers)
  - Home healthcare providers (e.g., visiting nurse, physical or occupational therapist, social worker, home health aide) who have seen the patient's home environment
    - Presence of clutter or hoarding, adequacy and nutritional content of food, safety of neighborhood, true functional status (e.g., if caregiver says the patient fell out of bed you can ask the physical therapist if that is plausible)
  - Neighbors, friends, additional family members
  - Apartment superintendent or landlord and other building employees (doorman, maintenance worker, etc.)
  - Bank or financial institution officials

25.4.7 Evaluation: Physical Exam and Diagnostic Studies

- Complete Physical Exam

Clinicians should **pay particular attention to and document** the following [58]:

- General appearance (hygiene, cleanliness, and appropriateness of attire).
- Vital signs (orthostatic blood pressure and pulse) and weight.
- Head and neck exam (fit of dentures, oral hygiene/lesions, presence/absence of glasses and hearing aids).
- Full skin exam (ecchymoses, burns, lacerations, abrasions, pressure ulcers).
- Musculoskeletal exam.
- Genitorectal exam (bruising, venereal lesions, inguinal rash, fecal impaction) including rape kit if indicated.
- Mood and affect (in the presence and absence of suspected perpetrator).
- Assessment of cognitive function and decision-making capacity.
- Gait and presence/absence of assistive devices.
- Photographs or body diagrams to document skin findings/injuries and physical evidence (torn/stained clothing, broken glasses, damaged assistive devices).
- Obtain permission from the patient or surrogate.
- Use a ruler or coin to show scale.
- The police will preserve physical evidence that may be used in court.

- Differentiating Signs of Abuse and Neglect from "Normal" Aging

- Some signs of abuse and neglect can be indistinguishable from "normal" changes associated with aging. Other signs of mistreatment may mimic the symptoms or consequences of medical conditions common to the older adult population. For example, bruising or skin tears may be due to thinning skin or use of blood-thinning medications. Multiple fractures may be a consequence of falls, osteoporosis, or underlying malignancy. Pressure ulcers may occur in the absence of neglect in a patient with end-stage dementia, malnutrition, and immobility. Changes in mood and behavior can reflect depression or anxiety independent of elder mistreatment.
- Unlike child abuse, there are no pathognomonic signs of elder mistreatment but certain locations of bruises and injuries may raise concerns. Mosqueda's 2005 study examined the life cycle of bruises in older adults. Ninety percent of accidental bruises occurred on the extremities, and no accidental bruises occurred on the neck, ears, genital area, or soles of the feet [73]. Murphy et al. found that two-thirds of elder abuse injuries are located on the upper extremities and maxillofacial region [74].
- Because the location of bruising and injuries alone is usually insufficient to prove abuse, obtaining a history from the older adult, involved caregivers, and other collateral sources remains paramount.
- When documenting signs of skin breakdown or injury on physical exam, it is critical to describe the location, color, shape, and size of what is visualized as opposed to an overall impression or judgment. For example, bruises can be marked on a standard body diagram with notations for the color, shape, and exact size *instead of being interpreted and documented in the medical record as "old," "fading," or "resolving."* Mosqueda's study looking at the life cycle of bruises in the elderly found that the color of the bruise did *not* predict its age (i.e., some bruises were predominantly yellow during the first 24 hours after onset) [73].

25.4.8 Treatment and Intervention Strategies

- **Document clearly.** When conducting an elder mistreatment assessment, physicians should adopt a "forensic approach" to documentation because there may be legal implications of one's findings. The following should be clearly detailed in the medical record [62].
  - Names of individuals present during the interview and exam and relationship to the patient

- The patient's demeanor and any observed reactions to caregivers
- Verbatim descriptions of events from the patient and caregivers noted in quotation marks
- Timeline of events
- Functional status
- Physical exam including hygiene/dress, cognitive evaluation, and decision-making capacity
- Referrals made (e.g., social work, home care, adult protective services)
- Education provided to the patient and/or caregivers
- Safety plan discussed

- **Involve an interprofessional team early to** benefit from their expertise in safety planning and development of interventions and to share responsibility for various components of the assessment (■ Table 25.5) [75]. Formal interprofessional groups called "Multidisciplinary Teams" or MDTs are increasingly emerging as a critical intervention strategy to address the complex and multidimensional needs of elder mistreatment victims. MDTs bring together representatives from medicine (often a geriatrician, neuropsychologist, and mental health providers), Adult Protective Services, law enforcement, the district attorney's office, and victim advocacy groups [1]. Social workers in inpatient and outpatient/community settings can be instrumental by obtaining collateral information from the patient's caregivers and/or family members, clarifying the patient's current level of social support, and investigating financial resources and community services.
- **Consult experts including geriatricians, psychiatry, and ethics.** Geriatricians can assess functional status

■ **Table 25.5** Groups involved in interprofessional assessment and intervention in cases of suspected elder mistreatment

Group	Role	Comments
Adult Protective Services	Receives mandatory reports of suspected abuse in most states	May serve as guardians in some states
Home healthcare agencies and personnel	Important in both detection and mitigation of abuse	Staff members may be abusers in some situations
Community nongovernmental or nonprofit services and programs for older adults	Provide a variety of programs and services that can mitigate all forms of abuse, including senior centers and home visitation to promote social integration	Some community-service agencies have programs exclusively devoted to preventing elder abuse or dealing with its manifestations (e.g., daily money management and caregiver support)
Police	Often the first responders in cases of elder abuse	Awareness of the importance of training law-enforcement personnel to be sensitive to the needs of older persons is increasing
District attorney's office	Prosecutes cases of elder abuse	Some offices have dedicated units that focus on elder abuse and are separate from domestic-violence units
Housing authority	Handles issues involving eviction, squatting, or misuse of housing for older persons, which are common in cases of elder abuse	Eviction and homelessness can be manifestations of financial exploitation
Legal services agencies	Handle the myriad legal issues that are raised in cases of elder abuse, including decision-making capacity, living wills, and guardianship	Guardians may be financial abusers
Physicians	Play a critical role in identifying mistreatment and making appropriate referrals	Physicians are mandatory reporters of elder abuse in all states that have mandatory-reporting laws
Hospital personnel	Need to be prepared to identify cases of elder abuse	Medical personnel often fail to identify elder abuse, because of clinical and time pressures. The Joint Commission on Accreditation of Healthcare Organizations has guidelines with respect to elder abuse; accreditation may be jeopardized if protocols are absent or inadequate
Nursing homes	Can use excess capacity to house victims safely and provide services, as part of the growing movement in the United States to provide shelter to abused older persons	Elder abuse can occur in long-term care facilities; resident-to-resident abuse is increasingly recognized as the most common form of abuse in such settings
Banks and financial services industry	Critical to the detection of financial exploitation	Institutions in some communities train tellers and other employees to detect exploitation of older persons' finances

and assist with clarifying goals of care. Psychiatrists and geriatric psychiatrists can be especially particularly helpful in assessing a patient's decision-making capacity or determining whether cognitive impairment or a mood disorder is impacting the patient's care. Elder mistreatment cases often involve ethical dilemmas, so if the hospital utilizes an ethicist or ethics committee, a formal consultation can prove invaluable.

- **Consider a home care referral.** Visiting nurses, therapists, and social workers are often utilized as a critical intervention in elder mistreatment to increase the number of "eyes and ears" on the patient and his/her caregivers. While the home health nurse's primary role may be to monitor a wound and instruct a caregiver to perform dressing changes, he can also report back to the outpatient physician on the caregiver's ability and willingness to provide appropriate care and the cleanliness of the home. The physical therapist may perform gait training and muscle strengthening exercises, but she can also alert the physician to red flags for mistreatment such as the patient/caregiver refusing visits, the patient's prescriptions going unfilled, and signs of uncontrolled medical illness.
- **Contact Adult Protective Services.** Adult Protective Services (APS) was established in 1975 and acts as the "first responder" for reports of abuse, neglect, and exploitation of vulnerable adults. Though APS exists in all 50 states, each state may have varying definitions of mistreatment, types of abuse and neglect addressed by state law, eligibility criteria, and settings covered. Despite these differences, all APS agencies generally provide similar services, e.g., investigation of reports of mistreatment, evaluation of client risk and capacity to consent to services, development and implementation of a case plan, client counseling, and assistance with services and benefits. At the time of this writing, New York is the only state without a mandated reporting law [76]. "Good faith reporting" provisions typically protect physicians from liability for having contacted Adult Protective Services or other investigative agencies even if the reports are not substantiated. Even without legal mandates, physicians and mental health professionals have an ethical and moral obligation to report elder mistreatment when there is reasonable suspicion. For patients who reside in a nursing home or long-term care setting, the physician may be required to alert the state Department of Health, APS, and/or the ombudsman.
- **Contact law enforcement if you suspect a crime has been committed and the victim wishes to press charges.** The physician should call 911 and contact the hospital's risk management and legal teams.

25.4.9 Care Transitions Issues

- The essential components of transitional care for all hospitalized patients include physician-to-physician communication across care sites, medication reconciliation, patient education to encourage self-efficacy, and assurance of appropriate social supports.
- Ensuring a safe transition for hospitalized elder mistreatment victims starts with an accurate assessment of baseline and current functional status to determine the appropriate discharge destination and requires communication between the sending (inpatient team) and receiving providers (primary care physician, home health agency, APS). The transfer of information between the inpatient and outpatient providers is especially critical in elder mistreatment cases because often there is suspected (but not confirmed) abuse or neglect. In these situations, patients are often discharged to short-term rehabilitation facilities or to their homes with referrals for home healthcare and an APS evaluation.
- Hospitalists should communicate directly with the patient's primary care provider or the nursing home to alert the receiving physician about abuse and/or neglect concerns. The home care agency must also be informed of the concerns about mistreatment and should know how to contact the outpatient physician if one of its employees witnesses abuse and/or neglect.

Case Conclusion

Ms. Lee is likely the victim of neglect and financial exploitation. Her son is acting as her primary caregiver but does not appear to be able to meet her medical needs. His impairment may stem from mental illness, cognitive impairment and/or low health literacy.

Interventions that can help Ms. Lee (and her son):

- **Clearly document** Ms. Lee's history, the interviews with her and her son, and her exam findings.
- **Obtain collateral information** from Ms. Lee's daughter, the home care agency, and APS.
- **Assess decision-making capacity.** Ask Ms. Lee where she wants to live and assess whether she understands her choices, the pros and cons of each choise, and the consequences of her decision.
- **Involve an interprofessional team** (see ◘ Table 25.4) [72].
- **Communicate with future providers.** If she returns home, contact her primary care physician and refer again for a home health nurse, physical therapy and APS follow-up. If she goes to a rehabilitation facility, contact the social worker there to ensure an APS referral occurs prior to discharge home.
- **Communicate with her son** to provide counseling as to why she medically must have these services and the consequences of discontinuing them (e.g., appointment of the daughter or another individual to serve as her legal guardian responsible for making health and financial decisions for her).

References

1. Jacobson LA, Kent M, Lee M, Mather M. America's aging population. Pop Bulletin. 2011;66(1):1–20.
2. American Burn Association [Internet]. Burn prevention fact sheet/ older adult educator's guide. Chicago; 2012 [cited 2018 Jan 6]. Available from: http://www.ameriburn.org.
3. Runyan CW, Casteel C, Perkis D, et al. Unintentional injuries in the home in the United States. Part I: mortality. Am J Prev Med. 2005;28(1):73–9.
4. Grant EJ. Preventing burns in the elderly: a guide for home healthcare professionals. Home Healthc Nurse. 2013;31(10):561–73.
5. Shields WC, Perry EC, Szanton SL, et al. Knowledge and injury prevention practices in homes of older adults. Geriatr Nursing. 2013;23(1):19–24.
6. Kramarow E, Chen LH, Hedegaard H, Warner M. Deaths from unintentional injury among adults aged 65 and over: UnitedStates, 2000–2013. NCHS data brief, no199. Hyattsville, MD: National Center for Health Statistics. 2015.
7. Centers for Disease Control and Prevention [Internet]. Home and recreational safety. Atlanta. [cited 2018 Jan 6] Available from: https://www.cdc.gov/homeandrecreationalsafety/index.html.
8. Zanni GR. Thermal burns and scalds: clinical complications in the elderly. Consult Pharm. 2012;27(1):16–22.
9. US Health Resources and Services Administration [Internet]. Poison help program: poison exposure data snapshot. Washington, D.C. [cited 2018 Jan 6] Available from: https://poisonhelp.hrsa.gov/index.html.
10. Mertens B, Sorenson S. Current considerations about the elderly and firearms. Am J Public Health. 2012;102(3):396–400.
11. Hepburn L, Miller M, Azrael D, Hemenway D. The US gun stock: results from the 2004 national firearms survey. Inj Prev. 2007;13(1):15–9.
12. US Census Bureau [Internet]. The older population in the United States: 2009. [cited 2018 Jan 6] Available from: http://www.census.gov/population/www/socdemo/age/older_2009.html.
13. Lum HD, Flaten HK, Betz ME. Gun access and safety practices among older adults. Curr Geron Geri Res. 2016; article ID 2980416, 5 pages.
14. Xu JQ, Kochanek KD, Murphy SL, Tejada-Vera B. Deaths: final data for 2007. Natl Vital Stat Rep [Internet]. 2010;58(19). Hyattsville: National Center for Health Statistics; Available from: http://www.cdc.gov/NCHS/data/nvsr/nvsr58/nvsr58_19.pdf.
15. US Food and Drug Association. Disposal of unused medicines: what you should know. Silver Spring. Available from: https://www.fda.gov/Drugs/ResourcesForYou/Consumers/BuyingUsingMedicineSafely/EnsuringSafeUseofMedicine/SafeDisposalofMedicines/ucm186187.htm.
16. Consumer Product Safety Commission [Internet]. Older consumers safety checklist. Bethesda. Available from: https://www.cpsc.gov/s3fs-public/checklist.pdf.
17. Luz C, Bush T, Shen X. Do canes or walkers make any difference? Nonuse and fall injuries. Gerontologist. 2017;57(2):211–8.
18. Tricco AC, Thomas SM, Veroniki AA, et al. Comparisons of interventions for preventing falls in older adults: a systematic review and meta-analysis. JAMA. 2017;318(17):1687–799.
19. Zhang XY, Shuai J, Li LP. Vision and relevant risk factor interventions for preventing falls among older people: a network meta-analysis. Sci Rep. 2015;5:10559.
20. Hartung B, Lalonde M. The use of non-slip socks to prevent falls among hospitalized older adults: a literature review. Geriatr Nurs. 2017;38(5):412–6.
21. American Association of Retired Persons (AARP) [Internet]. Care at home. Washington, D.C. [cited 2018 Jan 6]. Available from: https://www.aarp.org/caregiving/home-care/?intcmp=AE-CAR-SUBNAV-CAH.
22. Singer-Grannick CJ, Granick MS. Gynecomastia: what the surgeon needs to know. Eplasty. 2009;9:e6 (Published online 2009 Jan 15).
23. Norrenberg S, Gangki V, Del Marmol V, Soyfoo MS. Diffuse muscular pain, skin tightening, and nodular regenerative hyperplasia revealing paraneoplastic amyoopathing dermatomyositis due to testicular cancer. Case Rep Rheumatol. 2012:534236. https://doi.org/10.1155/2012/534236. Epub 2012 Dec 17.
24. Colliver JD, Compton WM, Gfroerer JC, et al. Projecting drug use among aging baby boomers in 2020. Ann Epidemiol. 2006;16:257–65.
25. Han B, Gfroerer JC, Colliver JD, et al. Substance use disorder among older adults in the United States in 2020. Addiction. 2009;104:88–96.
26. Johnson RA, Gerstein DR. Initiation of use of alcohol, cigarettes, marijuana, cocaine, and other substances in US birth cohorts since 1919. Am J Public Health. 1998;88:27–33.
27. Substance Abuse and Mental Health Services Administration [Internet]. Results from the 2012 National Survey on Drug Use and Health: summary of national findings. NSDUH series H-46, HHS publication no. (SMA) 13–4795. Rockville; 2013. [cited 2018 Jan 6]. Available from: https://www.samhsa.gov/data/sites/default/files/NSDUHresults2012/NSDUHresults2012.pdf.
28. Lin JC, Karno MP, Grella CE, et al. Alcohol, tobacco, and nonmedical drug use disorders in U.S. adults aged 65 years and older: data from the 2001–2002 National Epidemiologic Survey of Alcohol and Related Conditions. Am J Geriatr Psychiatry. 2011;19:292–9.
29. Degenhardt L, Dierker L, Chiu WT, et al. Evaluating the drug use "gateway" theory using cross-national data: consistency and associations of the order of initiation of drug use among participants in the WHO World Mental Health Surveys. Drug Alcohol Depend. 2010;108(1–2):84–97.
30. Jones CM, Paulozzi LJ, Mack KA. Sources of prescription opioid pain relievers by frequency of past-year nonmedical use in the United States, 2008–2011. JAMA Intern Med. 2014;174:802.
31. Kennedy GJ, Efremova I, Frazier A, et al. The emerging problems of alcohol and substance abuse in late life. J Soc Distress Homel. 1999;8(4):227–39.
32. Park-Lee E, Lipari RN, Hedden SL, Copello EAP, Kroutil LA. Receipt of services for substance use and mental health issues among adults: results from the 2015 National Survey on Drug Use and Health. NSDUH data review. 2016. [cited 2018 Jan 6]. Available from: http://www.samhsa.gov/data/.
33. Duru OK, Xu H, Tseng CH, et al. Correlates of alcohol-related discussions between older adults and their physicians. J Am Geriatr Soc. 2010;58(12):2369–74.
34. Center for Substance Abuse Treatment [Internet]. Substance abuse among older adults: treatment improvement protocol (TIP) series 26. Rockville. [cited 2018 Jan 6]. Available from: https://store.samhsa.gov/shin/content/SMA12-3585/SMA12-3585.pdf.
35. National Institute on Alcohol Abuse and Alcoholism. Helping patients who drink too much: a clinician's guide: updated 2005 edition. Bethesda. [cited 2018 Jan 6]. Available from: https://pubs.niaaa.nih.gov/publications/practitioner/cliniciansguide2005/clinicians_guide.htm.
36. American Psychiatric Association. Diagnostic and statistical manual of mental disorders. 5th ed. Arlington: American Psychiatric Publishing; 2013. p. P491.
37. Kuerbis A, Sacco P, Blazer DG, Moore AA. Substance abuse among older adults. Clin Geriatr Med. 2014;30(3):629–54.
38. Moyer VA. US Preventive Services Task Force. Screening and behavioral counseling interventions in primary care to reduce alcohol misuse: recommendation statement. Ann Intern Med. 2013;159:210.
39. National Institute on Drug Abuse [Internet]. Screening, assessment, and drug testing resources: chart of evidence-based screening tools. Bethesda. [cited 2018 Jan 6]. Available from: https://www.drugabuse.gov/nidamed-medical-health-professionals/tool-resources-your-practice/screening-assessment-drug-testing-resources/chart-evidence-based-screening-tools-adults.
40. Barry KL, Blow FC, Oslin DW. Substance abuse in older adults: review and recommendations for education and practice in medical settings. Subst Abus. 2002;23(Suppl 3):105–31.
41. Brennan PL, Nichol AC, Moos RH. Older and younger patients with substance use disorders: outpatient mental health service use functioning over a 12-month interval. Psychol Addict Behav. 2003;17(1):42–8.

42. Kuerbis AN, Sacco P. A review of existing treatments for substance abuse among the elderly and recommendations for future directions. Subst Abuse. 2013;7:13–37.
43. Substance Abuse and Mental Health Services Administration [Internet]. National helpline. [cited 2018 Jan 6]. Available from: https://www.samhsa.gov/find-help.
44. Ferri M, Amato L, Davoli M. Alcoholics Anonymous and other 12-step programmes for alcohol dependence. Cochrane Database Syst Rev. 2006;(3):CD005032.
45. Kaskutas LA. Alcoholics Anonymous effectiveness: faith meets science. J Addict Dis. 2009;28(2):145–57.
46. Lindau ST, Schumm LP, Laumann EO, et al. A study of sexuality and health among older adults in the United States. N Engl J Med. 2007;357(8):762–74.
47. Nicolosi A, Laumann EO, Glasser DB, et al. Sexual behavior and sexual dysfunctions after age 40: The global study of sexual attitudes and behaviors. Urology. 2004;64(5):991–7.
48. Wang V, Depp CA, Ceglowski J, et al. Sexual health and function in later life: a population based study of 606 older adults with a partner. Am J Geriatr Psych. 2015;23(2):227–33.
49. Centers for Disease Control and Prevention [Internet]. CDC fact sheet: STD trends in the United States (2011 data), (2013b). Atlanta. [cited 2018 Jan 6]. Available from: http://www.cdc.gov/std/stats11/trends-2011.pdf.
50. Centers for Disease Control and Prevention [Internet]. 2016 STD surveillance report, 2016. Atlanta. [cited 2018 Jan 6]. Accessed online at: https://www.cdc.gov/std/stats16/toc.htm.
51. Herbenick D, Reece M, Schick V, et al. Sexual behavior in the United States: results from a national probability sample of men and women ages 14–94. J Sex Med. 2010;7(5):255–65.
52. National Institute on Aging [Internet]. HIV, AIDs, and older people, 2013. Bethesda. [cited 2018 Jan 6]. Available from: http://www.nia.nih.gov/health/publication/hiv-aids-and-older-people.
53. Ports KA, Barnack-Tavlaris JL, Syme G, et al. Sexual health discussions with older adult patients during periodic health exams. J Sex Med. 2014;11(4):901–8.
54. Tilman JL, Mark HD. HIV and STI testing in older adults: an integrative review. J Clin Nurs. 2015;24(15–16):2074–95.
55. Imparato T, Sanders D. STD prevalence demands clinical awareness. Aging Well. 2012;5(1). [cited 2018 Jan 6]. Available from: http://www.todaysgeriatricmedicine.com/archive/012312p14.shtml.
56. Jena AB, Goldman DP, Kamdar A, et al. Sexually transmitted diseases among users of erectile dysfunction drugs: analysis of claims data. Ann Intern Med. 2010;153:1–7.
57. Guo Y, Sims OT. Assessment of recent HIV testing among older adults in the United States. Soc Work Health Care. 2017;56(9):855–64.
58. American Medical Association diagnostic and treatment guidelines on elder abuse and neglect. Chicago: American Medical Association; 1992.
59. National Centre on Elder Abuse (NCEA). National elder abuse incidence study: final report 1998. Administration on Aging and American Public Human Services Association [on-line]. Available at https://www.acl.gov/sites/default/files/programs/2016-09/ABuse Report_Full.pdf. Accessed 14 Feb 2018.
60. WHO. The Toronto declaration on the global prevention of elder abuse. Geneva: WHO; 2002.
61. Laumann EO, Leitsch SA, Waite LJ. Elder mistreatment in the United States: prevalence estimates from a nationally representative study. J Gerontol B Psychol Sci Soc Sci. 2008;63(4):S248–54.
62. Lachs MS, Pillemer K. Elder abuse. Lancet. 2004;364:1263–72.
63. Under the Radar: New York State Elder Abuse Prevalence Study. Lifespan of Greater Rochester, Weill Cornell Medical Center of Cornell University, New York City Department for the Aging [on-line]. Available at http://nyceac.com/wp-content/uploads/2011/05/UndertheRadar051211.pdf. Accessed 24 Feb 2018.
64. Acierno R, Hernandez MS, Amstadter AB, et al. Prevalence and correlates of emotional, physical, sexual, and financial abuse and potential neglect in the United States: The National Elder Mistreatment Study. Am J Public Health. 2010;100:292–7.
65. MetLife Mature Market Institute. The MetLife Study of Elder Financial Abuse: crimes of occasion, desperation, and predation against America's elders. New York: The Institute; 2011. [Online] Available at https://www.metlife.com/assets/cao/mmi/publications/studies/2011/mmi-elder-financial-abuse.pdf. Accessed 24 Feb 2018.
66. Pillemer K, Chen EK, Van Haitsma KS, et al. Resident-to-resident aggression in nursing homes: results from a qualitative event reconstruction study. Gerontologist. 2012;52:24–33.
67. Lachs MS, Williams CS, O'Brien S, et al. The mortality of elder mistreatment. JAMA. 1998;280:428–32.
68. The National Center on Elder Abuse. The 2004 Survey of State Adult Protective Services: abuse of vulnerable adults 18 years of age and older [Online]. Available from https://ncea.acl.gov/resources/docs/archive/2004-Survey-St-Audit-APS-Abuse-18plus-2007.pdf. Accessed on 24 Feb 2018.
69. Dong X, Simon MA. Association between elder abuse and use of ED: findings from the Chicago Health and Aging Project. Am J Emerg Med. 2013:693–8.
70. Franzini L, Dyer CB. Healthcare costs and utilization of vulnerable elderly people reported to adult protective services for self-neglect. J Am Geriatr Soc. 2008;56:667–76.
71. Lachs MS, Williams CS, O'Brien S, et al. ED use by older victims of family violence. Ann Emerg Med. 1997;30:448–54.
72. Lachs MS, Pillemer K. Elder abuse. N Engl J Med. 2015;373:1947–56.
73. Mosqueda L, Burnight K, Liao S. The life cycle of bruises in older adults. J Am Geriatr Soc. 2005;53:1339–43.
74. Murphy K, Waa S, Jaffer H, et al. A literature review of findings in physical elder abuse. Can Assoc Radiol J. 2013;64:10–4.
75. Lachs MS, Pillemer K. Abuse and neglect of elderly persons. N Engl J Med. 1995;332:437–43.
76. The United States Department of Justice. State elder abuse statues [Online]. Available from https://www.justice.gov/elderjustice/elder-justice-statutes-0#SL3. Accessed on 24 Feb 2018.
77. Rosen T, Lachs MS, Pillemer K. Sexual aggression between residents in nursing homes: literature synthesis of an underrecognized problem. J Am Geriatr Soc. 2010;58(10):1970–9. https://doi.org/10.1111/j.1532-5415.2010.03064.x.

Falls Screening, Differential Diagnosis, Evaluation, and Treatment

Kristen DeCarlo and Sara M. Bradley

A. Chun (ed.), *Geriatric Practice*, https://doi.org/10.1007/978-3-030-19625-7_26

Learning Objectives
- Define the epidemiology of falls and associated morbidity and mortality.
- List risk factors for falls in community-dwelling older adults.
- Describe validated fall risk screening and gait assessments for community-dwelling and acute and long-term care patients.
- Discuss evidence-based interventions to prevent falls.

26.1 Epidemiology of Falls in Older Adults

A fall is defined as an unintended event in which a person comes to rest on the ground, floor, or other lower level without known loss of consciousness. Falls in the elderly are a major public health problem worldwide. The incidence of falls in community-dwelling individuals in the United States affects one in three persons aged 65 or older, and the incidence of falls increases to one in two persons aged 80 years or older. Worldwide, persons over 70 years old have an increased risk of fall-related mortality compared to younger people, and the severity of fall-related complications increases with age [1]. Approximately 45–70% of long-term care patients fall annually, and up to 27% of hospitalized patients in acute geriatric wards have incident falls during their hospitalization [2]. Furthermore, almost 60 percent of patients with a fall history in the previous year will sustain a subsequent fall [3].

Falls are the leading cause of fatal and nonfatal injuries among adults aged 65 years or older. Falls may result in injury, ranging from minor insults to major events (◘ Table 26.1). Minor injuries occur in 30% to 50% of falls and include soft tissue injury, bruises, or scrapes. Up to 25% of falls cause major injuries such as traumatic brain injury (TBI) or fractures, and these serious events occur with increased frequency as age advances. TBI is the cause of 46% of all deaths due to falling [4]. The lifetime risk of a hip fracture is 17.5% in women and 6% in men and is associated with high mortality. After hip fracture, the rate of in-hospital, 6-month, and 1-year mortality is 2.7%, 19%, and 26% respectively. Furthermore, only half of those surviving a hip fracture will regain their baseline ability to perform their activities of daily living (ADLs), which include the ability to bathe, dress, groom, toilet, eat, and transfer on their own. Decline after a hip fracture is also seen in instrumental activities of daily living (iADLs), mobility, and cognitive status [5, 6].

◘ Table 26.1 Consequences of falling

Minor injuries Bruises Lacerations	Major injuries Fractures Traumatic brain injury
Long lies Rhabdomyolysis Dehydration Pneumonia Pressure sores	Fear of falling Restriction of activity Social isolation Depression
Pain	Functional disability
Emergency room visits and hospitalizations	Nursing home placement

Approximately half of those who fall are unable to get up on their own afterward. In one prospective cohort study of adults over the age of 90, 80% of those who fell were unable to get up by themselves afterwards, and 30% were on the ground for over an hour. These falls, resulting in long lies, often result in pressure ulcers, rhabdomyolysis, dehydration, and pneumonia [7].

Following a fall, 40% of patients restrict their activity because of the fear of falling again. Fall anxiety is one of many post-fall syndromes, which also includes decreased overall functional status, increased dependence, loss of autonomy, immobilization, and depression [1–4].

The Centers for Disease Control and Prevention (CDC) reported from the Behavioral Risk Factor Surveillance System Survey (BRFSS) that during 2014, there was an estimated 29 million falls in older adults, resulting in approximately 7 million injuries, and 27,000 deaths as a result of falls. Another 2.8 million of patients were treated in the emergency department for fall-related injuries, and of these, an estimated 800,000 required subsequent hospitalization for their injuries [8].

According to the BRFSS in 2014, annual Medicare costs for adult falls were estimated at $31.3 billion, and with an expanding geriatric population, estimates of annual healthcare costs as a result of falls are expected to continue to rise. Furthermore, falls are a leading risk factor for nursing home placement and greater use of medical services [4]. Given the significant incidence of falls in the elderly and high rate of morbidity and mortality associated with falls, appropriate care of older patients requires a thorough evaluation of fall history, fall risk, as well as fall prevention strategies.

26.2 Risk Factors of Falls

Falls in older patients are most often multifactorial due to underlying patient demographics, medical conditions, and neuropsychological and sensorimotor impairments that pose increased fall risk. Falls result from a complex interaction between activities that increase fall risk, environmental hazards, and individual susceptibility. Several classes of medications have also been associated with increased risk of falls. Beyond considering specific fall risk factors, it is also important to remember a fall may actually represent an atypical presentation of disease. See ◘ Table 26.2 for the differential diagnosis of a patient presenting with a fall.

Table 26.2 Differential diagnosis of falls

Category	Diagnosis
Cardiovascular	Arrhythmia Carotid sinus syndrome Myocardial infarction Orthostatic hypotension Postprandial hypotension Syncope Vasovagal syndrome
Cognitive or psychiatric	Delirium Dementia Depression
Endocrine disorders	Adrenal insufficiency Hypothyroidism Thyrotoxicosis
Drugs	Medication effects or polypharmacy Substance abuse
Hematologic disorders	Anemia
Infectious diseases	Infection/sepsis Influenza
Metabolic derangements	Dehydration Hyponatremia Hypoglycemia/hyperglycemia Hypokalemia/hyperkalemia
Musculoskeletal	Deconditioning Gait disorders
Neurologic	Cerebrovascular accident Movement disorders (Parkinson's disease) Peripheral sensory neuropathy Seizure Subdural hematoma Transient ischemic attack Vestibular dysfunction Visual impairment
Renal disorders	Acute kidney injury Chronic kidney disease

26.2.1 Demographic Risk Factors

In community-dwelling older adults, falls are more common with increased age and female gender. The increased incidence of falls in women has been attributed to reduced muscle strength and higher likelihood of psychotropic medication use. Women are also more likely to sustain fall-related fractures, due to higher rates of osteoporosis. Living alone is an additional risk factor for falling among persons living in the community. Since females comprise the majority of the older patient population living in the community, this may be a confounding factor accounting for increased fall rate among women. Of note, men and women have similar fall incidence in hospitals and long-term care facilities [9].

Table 26.3 Risk factors with highest relative risk or odds of falling

Risk factor	RR-OR[a]
Muscle weakness	4.4
History of falls	2.0
Gait deficit	2.9
Use of assistive device	2.6
Visual deficit	2.5
Arthritis	2.4
Impaired ADL	2.3
Depression	2.2
Cognitive impairment	1.8
Age > 80 years	1.7

Adapted from Guideline for the Prevention of Falls in Older Persons. American Geriatrics Society, British Geriatrics Society, and American Academy of Orthopaedic Surgeons Panel on Falls Prevention [11]
ADLs activities of daily living
[a]Relative risk ratios (RR) calculated from prospective studies. Odds ratios (OR) calculated for retrospective studies

26.2.2 Medical Risk Factors

Many underlying medical conditions and impairments have been identified as risk factors of falling in older adults. Individual susceptibility results from the accumulation of small impairments in multiple domains that when challenged make it difficult for an older adult to compensate. While many intrinsic risk factors for falling or experiencing a fall-related injury have been identified, some factors are associated with higher relative risk of falling than others. The risk factors associated with falling are listed in Table 26.3.

One study analyzed the risk factors for falls in community-dwelling older people and found the strongest associations in persons with history of falls, gait problems, assistive device use, vertigo, Parkinson disease, cognitive impairment, stroke history, and antiepileptic drug use [10]. A systematic review found the individual risk factors most highly correlated with falls included history of fall, use of more than four medications or psychotropic medication use, and impairment in strength, gait, or balance. Another analysis found lower extremity muscle weakness increased the odds of falling by four times, gait and balance impairments increased the odds three times, and vision problems, arthritis, cognitive impairment, depression, and age over 80 doubled the odds of falling [11]. Similar to the results found in community-dwelling persons, a study looking at patients in the long-term care setting found the strongest risk factors for falls include history of falls, assistive device use, and moderate disability. In hospitalized patients, the strongest association was found in patients with a history of falls [12].

Adequate balance requires complex integration of sensory and motor systems; therefore vision, muscle strength, and central processing play an integral role in fall risk [9]. Visual impairment, commonly caused by glaucoma, macular degeneration, and cataracts, impairs contrast, depth perception, and visual field range and may result in misjudging obstacles in the environment and increased risk of falls. Normal aging may be associated with some impairments in these sensorimotor systems that contribute to balance, thereby leading to decreased safety and ability to perform daily functional tasks including rising from a chair, turning while walking, using stairs, and transferring.

26.2.3 Environmental Risk Factors

Activities that increase fall risk include climbing a ladder or step stool or walking on an icy sidewalk. Environmental hazards at home include loose carpets, showers or bathtubs without grab bars, stairwells, poor lighting, and cords or clutter in walking paths (◘ Table 26.4). Estimates indicate that environmental hazards are involved in 35–45% of falls; however studies have not been able to conclusively demonstrate this. Environmental hazards in the hospital or nursing home can include wet slippery floors, bedrails, restraints, and tethers such as oxygen tubing, intravenous lines, or catheters that can contribute to falling [9].

There is evidence to suggest that environmental hazards play a more significant role in falls occurring away from the home, where 25% to 50% of all falls occur. Falls away from home often involve stairs, slipping, or tripping hazards, as well as transient hazards that are difficult to anticipate. Elderly persons with robust physical abilities can withstand a wider range of environmental challenges without experiencing a fall, whereas frail persons may experience increased risk of fall even in relatively hazard-free environments.

◘ **Table 26.4** Environmental hazards contributing to falls

Community setting	Hospital and/or long-term care facility
Clutter obstructing paths	Wet or slippery floors
Electric cords	Bedrails
Throw rugs, loose carpet	Restraints
Poor lighting	Intravenous lines
Lack of non-slip bathmats or grab bars	Oxygen tubing
Unsafe footwear	Foley catheters
Stairwells	

26.2.4 Medications

Medication use is an important modifiable risk factor for falls in older adults. Greater number of medications (of any type), certain medication classes, and recent medication dose adjustments have all been associated with increased risk of falling (◘ Table 26.5). Polypharmacy, defined as using more than four medications, is common in older adults and increases fall risk. Medications from drug classes that affect the central nervous system, including neuroleptics, sedatives, hypnotics, benzodiazepines, antipsychotics and antidepressants, are associated with increased risk of fall [10–13]. Antihypertensive medications, in particular vasodilators, are associated with an increased risk of falling. However, beta-blockers do not appear to have a significant effect on fall risk, while diuretics contribute a minimal increased risk of fall [14].

Case: Falls and Gait Instability

History of Present Illness: Mrs. C is a 72-year-old woman with a past medical history of diabetes complicated by peripheral neuropathy, hypertension, atrial fibrillation on anticoagulation, hyperlipidemia, chronic low back pain, and depression, who presents to clinic in the setting of left wrist pain after a recent fall.

Active medication list:

- Warfarin 2.5 mg PO nightly
- Digoxin 0.125 mg PO daily
- Glipizide 10 mg PO daily
- Lisinopril 20 mg PO daily
- Hydrochlorothiazide 25 mg PO daily
- Carvedilol 6.25 mg PO twice daily
- Atorvastatin 20 mg PO nightly
- Citalopram 10 mg PO daily
- Zolpidem 10 mg PO nightly as needed for sleep

Consider the following questions (Part I):

- What questions do you want to ask Mrs. C regarding her fall?
- What historical information do you want to know regarding her fall?

◘ **Table 26.5** Odds of falling by high-risk medication class

Medication class	Odds ratio
Antidepressants	1.68
Neuroleptics and antipsychotics	1.59
Benzodiazepines	1.57
Sedatives and hypnotics	1.47
Antihypertensives	1.24
Non-steroidal anti-inflammatories	1.21
Diuretics	1.07
Beta-blockers	1.01
Narcotics	0.96

Adapted from Woolcott et al. [13]

26.3 Evaluation for Patients with Increased Fall Risk or Fall History

The American Geriatrics Society's (AGS), British Geriatrics Society's (BGS), and American Academy of Orthopedic Surgeons (AAOS) Guidelines for the Prevention of Falls in Older Persons recommend that all older adults be screened annually for falls, as well as any problems with balance or walking. This guideline is based on evidence from a number of studies indicating that fall-related assessments potentially reduce future falls when coupled with patient-centered fall prevention strategies. Fall risk screening is a quality measure included in several programs, including the Centers for Medicare and Medicaid Services (CMS), Physician Quality Reporting System (PRQS), Meaningful Use Incentive Program, Medicare Annual Wellness Visit, and Accountable Care Organization.

26.3.1 Fall History and Screening

The depth of fall risk assessment varies by the target population. A fall risk assessment as part of routine primary care visit for a low-risk patient is brief. A brief evaluation often includes two central questions:

1. Have you fallen in the past year?
2. Do you have trouble with walking or balance?

If the answer to one or more of the above screening questions is positive, according to the AGS and BGS, a more detailed history is warranted including a multifactorial fall risk assessment. High-risk groups include patients with a history of falls and recurrent falls, those reporting balance and walking difficulties, or persons living in long-term care facilities. If initial screening questions are positive or the patient belongs to a high-risk group, a multifactorial fall risk assessment is recommended [11].

Evidence-based measure for the assessment and quality improvement of care provided to older adults called the Assessing Care of Vulnerable Elders (ACOVE) project, created by RAND Health and Pfizer, recommends a multifactorial fall risk assessment for patients reporting a history of two or more falls or one injurious fall in the last year [15]. The United States Preventive Services Task Force (USPSTF) as of 2012 recommends that clinicians consider the benefit of performing an in-depth multifactorial fall risk assessment in community-dwelling adults 65 years and older based on individual patient characteristics (including a positive history of falls or problems with balance and gait, consideration of comorbid medical conditions, and poor performance on the timed "Get Up and Go" test) and does not recommend automatically performing an in-depth multifactorial risk assessment in all patients [16].

A comprehensive historical assessment includes a detailed history regarding the specific circumstances of a prior fall (including witness account when available) and questions focused on identifying potential fall risk factors. This includes a discussion of medical comorbidities, current medications, substance use, environmental risk factors, and general functional status. Identified risk factors may be modifiable (such as muscle weakness, home hazards, or medication side effects) or non-modifiable (such as history of falls, neurologic conditions, and cognitive impairment). Treatment planning for high-risk patients includes a multifactorial intervention based on an individual's specific risk factors [11].

Case: Falls and Gait Instability: Part II

Fall history:

Mrs. C reports she fell 2 days prior to her clinic visit while rushing to answer the phone just as she returned home from the grocery store. She is not sure but thinks she may have tripped on the edge of the rug. She was able to get up on her own, but had left wrist pain immediately. For the past 2 days, she has been icing her wrist and taking acetaminophen 500 mg 1 tablet twice a day for pain.

She had been feeling like her usual self before the fall and denies any recent fever, chills, cough, shortness of breath, urinary frequency, dysuria, constipation, or diarrhea. She did not hit her head or lose consciousness and denies any chest pain, palpitations, or dizziness prior to the fall. She does not use an assistive device and admits she feels unsteady on her feet at times. She lives alone in her apartment except for her two cats and does not have an aide or anyone else who helps her in the home.

She reports one previous fall approximately 1 year ago while walking outside on the sidewalk. No injury occurred at that time. She does not monitor her sugar at home but thinks her last hemoglobin A1c was 6.9. She has not been to her ophthalmologist in the past year. She denies any symptoms from her atrial fibrillation and her blood pressure has been well controlled. She occasionally feels lightheaded when she stands up from the sitting position. Her low back pain bothers her when she stands for a long period but using a heating pad and taking the acetaminophen helps. Her mood has improved since starting citalopram and she continues to use zolpidem for sleep. She denies alcohol use.

Consider the following questions (Part II):

- Based on her history, what risk factors for falling does Mrs. C have?
- What physical exam maneuvers and tests would you like to perform?

26.3.2 Physical Examination

As part of a multifactorial fall risk assessment, the physical examination should include examination of orthostatic vital signs, visual acuity, auditory screen, the cardiac system, musculoskeletal strength and range of motion, neurologic function (including vibration and proprioception), gait, balance, and cognition. Additional aspects of the physical examination in a patient who has a high risk of falls, history of falls, or trouble with balance and gait should focus upon individual risk factors. An example of a multifactorial fall risk assessment is outlined in ► Box 26.1 and a fall screening algorithm in ◻ Fig. 26.1.

Box 26.1 Patient Fall Assessment

- *Fall History*
  - Circumstances of prior fall
  - Associated symptoms
  - Chronic medical conditions
  - Functional status and mobility
  - Medications
  - Substance abuse
- *Physical Examination*
  - Orthostatic vital signs
  - Visual acuity testing
  - Hearing evaluation
  - Cardiovascular exam
  - Musculoskeletal and neurologic exam
  - Gait and balance assessment
- *Recommended Routine Tests*
  - EKG
  - Complete blood count
  - Chemistry panel
  - Drug levels (i.e., digoxin level, INR)
  - TSH
  - Vitamin B12 level
  - Vitamin D 25, OH level
- *As Individual Fall History Indicates*
  - Imaging studies (X-ray, head CT, spine X-ray or MRI, etc.)
  - Cardiac testing for arrhythmia
  - ECHO
  - EEG
  - Vestibular testing

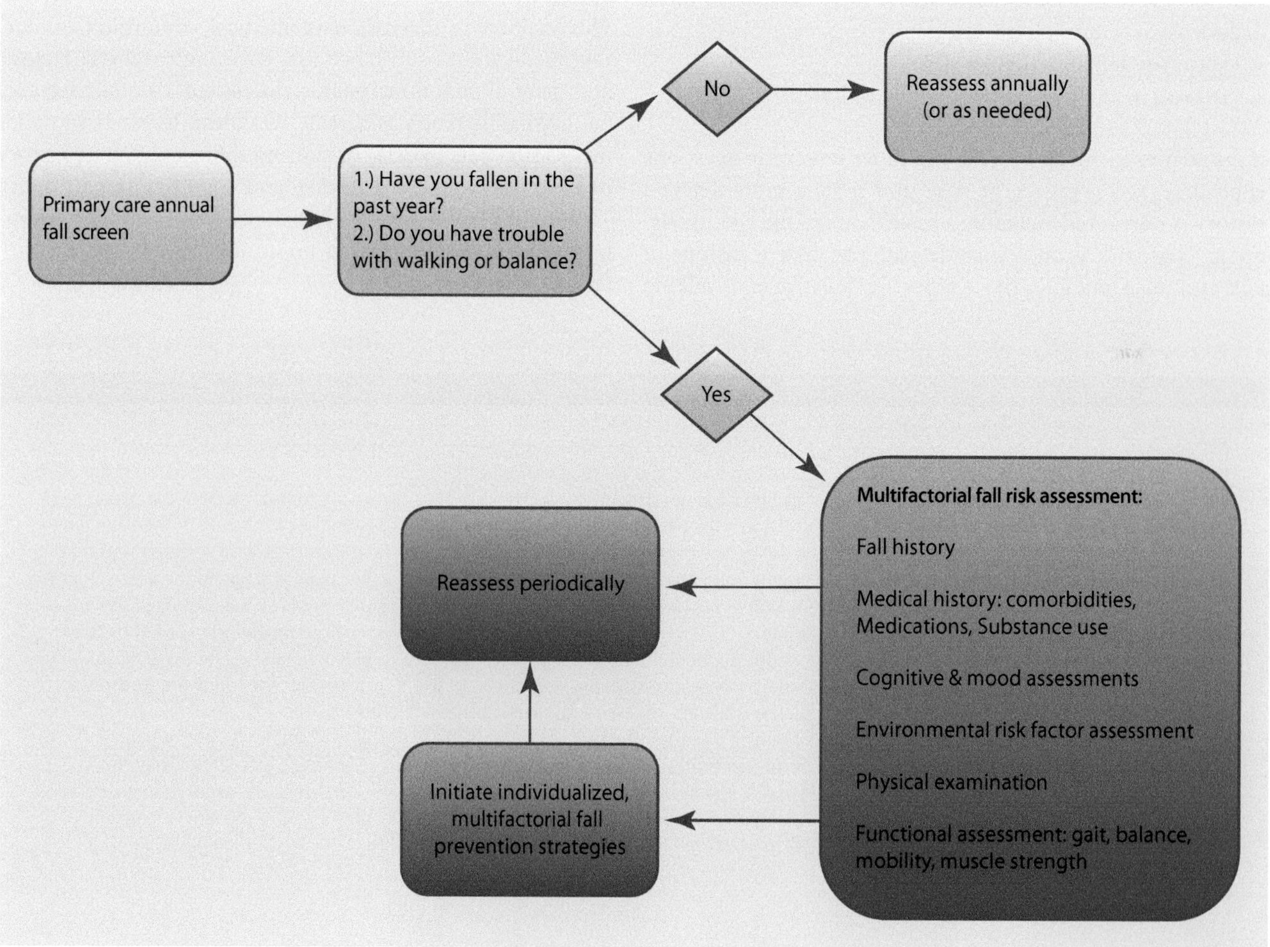

◻ **Fig. 26.1** Screening and evaluation of falls in older adults

Table 26.6 Examples of fall risk screening tools

Setting	Screening tool
Community	"Get Up and Go" test (TUG) Functional Reach Test
Hospital or acute care facility	St. Thomas Risk Assessment Tool (STRATIFY) Hendrich II Fall Risk Model
Long-term care facility or nursing homes	Care Home Falls Screen (CaHFRiS) Morse Fall Scale

26.3.3 Gait and Balance Assessment

While many tools for assessing gait and balance and estimating fall risk in various clinical setting have been developed and validated (Table 26.6), they are not often incorporated into routine clinical care due to time constraints and competing priorities. Two assessment tools that are particularly useful include the "Get Up and Go" test (TUG) and the Functional Reach Test, as each requires only a short time to perform. Older persons who report a fall in the last year or difficulty with balance and gait should be evaluated with one of these assessment tools.

In the "Get Up and Go" test, the patient is asked to rise from a chair, walk 10 feet (3 meters) at a normal pace (with an assistive device if needed), turn around, walk back to the chair, and sit down in their original position. The patient is timed and observed for sitting balance, transfer ability from sitting to standing, postural stability, steppage, stride length, sway, and ability to turn without staggering. Timing from initial getting up to re-seating is measured and compared to the mean time of adults in their age group (for 60–69 years of age, mean test time is 8.1 seconds; for 70–79 years of age, mean test time is 9.2 seconds; and for 80–99 years of age, mean test time is 11.3 seconds) [17]. In prospective and retrospective studies, the TUG has shown some predictive value, where a time of greater than 12 seconds to complete the test indicates impaired functioning in community-dwelling elders. If the patient is unable to complete the test or appears unsteady during examination, it is recommended that the patient be referred to physical therapy for further evaluation. If the examination is normal for age group based on age and overall performance, no further assessment is required. However, if the TUG is abnormal, a complete fall history and physical examination evaluation is warranted if not already performed [11].

The Functional Reach Test is performed using a leveled yardstick horizontally secured to a wall at shoulder height. The patient is asked to stand close to the wall with their arm outstretched horizontally. The patient is directed to reach as far forward as they can without taking a step or losing stability, keeping the arm at shoulder height. The length of fist movement forward from the zero position is measured along the yardstick. The patient should be able to move the fist forward at least 6 inches, and shorter reach distances are associated with increased risk of falling [18]. In one study of community-dwelling persons, the ability to reach less than 8 inches was associated with limited functional balance, with a sensitivity of 73% and specificity of 88% for predicting fallers from non-fallers [19].

Case: Falls and Gait Instability: Part III

Physical Exam:

- Vital signs: T 98.7, BP 136/68, HR 76, RR 14, oxygen saturation 99% on room air
- Orthostatic vital signs: 132/72, HR 74 supine → 124/68, HR 80 standing
- HEENT: pupils equal, round, reactive to light; extraocular movements intact; anicteric, oropharynx clear and mucous membranes are moist, no lymphadenopathy, vision 20/70 (not corrected), bilateral cataracts
- Heart: irregularly irregular rhythm, no rubs, murmurs, or gallops
- Lungs: CTA bilaterally, no wheezes or crackles
- Back: no spinal point tenderness or paravertebral muscle tenderness to palpation
- Abdomen: soft, NT, ND, +BS
- Extremities: trace edema, bruise on left forearm, left wrist mildly tender to palpation, full ROM and no swelling
- Neuro: CN II-XII, slightly decreased proprioception and sensation to light touch in the lower extremities bilaterally, motor strength 4/5 in her lower extremities bilaterally
- Cognitive assessment: Montreal Cognitive Assessment (MOCA), 27/30
- Mood assessment: Patient Health Questionnaire-2 (PHQ-2), 0/2
- Gait assessment: "Get Up and Go" test, ~16 seconds (some difficulty turning), noted to have wide-based gait, decreased stride length
- Balance assessment: 5.5 inches on functional reach testing

Consider the following questions (Part III):

- Based on Mrs. C's history and physical exam, what factors are contributing to her falls?
- What tests (if any) will you order following this clinic visit?
- What are your recommendations for Mrs. C to help prevent future falls?

26.3.4 Diagnostic Evaluation

Expert consensus recommends baseline diagnostic testing for patients at high risk of falling or a history of falls. Complete blood count, serum chemistry, glucose concentration, and thyroid function studies can rule out causes of fall including anemia, dehydration, autonomic neuropathy related to diabetes, and metabolic disease related to thyroid dysfunction respectively. Serum 25-hydroxyvitamin D levels identify the community-dwelling elderly with vitamin D deficiency who would benefit from vitamin D supplementation. Additional testing may be indicated based on individual history and physical examination. Vitamin B12 levels should be obtained to evaluate the etiology of peripheral neuropathy if present. Cardiac monitoring for arrhythmia, electroencephalogram (EEG) looking for seizure activity, or neuroimaging studies to evaluate for ischemic disease or hydrocephalus are only indicated if findings from history or physical examination are highly suggestive of these conditions. Echocardiogram (ECHO) may be considered in patients with heart murmurs thought to contribute to the etiology of a fall. Spine radiographs or magnetic resonance imaging (MRI) may be useful in patients with gait disorders or abnormalities on neurologic examination.

26.4 Fall Prevention: Community-Dwelling Adults

Evidence-based single interventions are strategies that on their own prevent falls in community-dwelling adults, including exercise, medication management, visual interventions, and home safety evaluations and interventions [20]. Multifactorial and multicomponent interventions involve the simultaneous implementation of more than one fall prevention measure, such as physical therapy, home hazard reduction, and medication review.

26.4.1 Single Intervention Strategies in Community-Dwelling Adults

26.4.1.1 Exercise

Multiple randomized controlled trials and meta-analysis show that exercise reduces the incidence of falls in the elderly by 13–40% [21, 22]. Fall prevention exercise programs also reduce fall-related injuries, with a systemic review demonstrating pooled estimates of rate ratios for all injurious falls in ten trials as 0.63 (95% CI 0.51–0.77) for patients enrolled in exercise programs [23]. Thus experts, including the AGS, BGS, USPSTF, and the National Council on Aging, recommend that community-dwelling older adults, in particular those at increased risk of falls or a history of fall, participate in exercise programs as part of a fall prevention strategy.

Various exercise interventions have been studied and are grouped into categories, including gait and balance training, strength training, flexibility, movement, general physical activity, and endurance. In an effort to identify the exercise-based programs that have been adequately studied and proven efficacious, the CDC Injury Center has created the CDC Compendium of Effective Fall Interventions, outlining 14 validated exercise-based interventions for fall prevention, with associated patient resources, and references [24].

Overall, exercise interventions are most effective if they target ≥2 of four exercise components, strength, balance, flexibility, or endurance, where programs that include a focus on balance training are the most effective in preventing falls [20, 22, 25]. Other significant exercise methods include step training, a method of training intentional or reactive steps in response to environmental challenges (i.e., avoiding ice or uneven pavement on a sidewalk). A meta-analysis of seven randomized controlled trials determined the efficacy of step training in reducing the proportion of fallers (rate ratio 0.51, 95% CI 0.38–0.68) and the rate of falls (rate ratio 0.48, 95% CI 0.36–0.65) [26]. Tai chi is a group exercise incorporating elements of strength and balance training and has been widely studied for fall prevention strategies. A systematic review and meta-analysis demonstrated that tai chi practice reduced the rate of falls and injurious falls at 12 months by approximately 43 and 50 percent respectively [27]. Further, analysis of several studies incorporating multicomponent exercise programs demonstrated a reduction not only in the rate of falls but also in the risk of falling (rate ratio 0.71, 95% CI 0.63–0.82, and risk ratio 0.85, 95% CI 0.76–0.96) [22].

26.4.1.2 Medication Management

Polypharmacy and certain medication classes are known risk factors for falls in older patients. One study found an intensive intervention for primary care physicians that included education on medication management, financial incentives, and feedback on prescribing practices resulted in 36% fewer falls and 54% fewer injuries requiring medical attention [28]. Another randomized controlled study of a medication intervention to prevent falls found gradual withdrawal of psychotropic medications in adults aged >65 years reduced the rate of falls by 66% [29].

26.4.1.3 Vitamin D Supplementation

All patients over the age of 65 years with low serum 25-hydroxyvitamin D levels (<10 ng/mL or 25 nmol/L) are at risk of loss of muscle mass and strength and have a higher risk of hip fracture, and vitamin D supplementation may improve bone density and muscle function in such patients[30, 31].

The effect of vitamin D supplementation on fall prevention in the elderly population remains controversial, as previous studies provided evidence that vitamin D supplementation decreased fall risk [32]. A recent Cochrane review in community-dwelling elderly did not find a reduction rate of falls (rate ratio 1.00) or risk of falling (relative risk 0.96, 95% CI 0.89–1.03) in patients taking vitamin D supplementation, but found it may have an effect in patients with low pretreatment vitamin D levels [22].

Although current evidence is not definitive, an AGS Consensus Statement in 2014 concluded that in community-dwelling adults, the goal serum 25-hydroxyvitamin D concentration minimum is 30 ng/mL (75 nmol/L) and vitamin D supplementation of at least 1000 IU per day is recommended to all patients >65 years of age to reduce the risk of fractures or falls [33].

26.4.1.4 Cardiovascular Interventions

In patients with recurrent falls, in the absence of gait and balance problems or other fall risk factors, clinicians should consider a detailed cardiac assessment. Underlying cardiac conditions associated with falls include orthostatic hypotension, carotid sinus syndrome, and vasovagal syndrome [11]. Studies evaluating the efficacy of pacemaker implantation as a fall prevention strategy in patients with carotid sinus hypersensitivity found that persons with a pacemaker insertion had a reduction in fall rate (odds ratio 0.42, 95% CI 0.23–0.75) compared to controls [22, 34].

26.4.1.5 Visual Interventions

Nonsurgical vision correction alone has not been shown to prevent or reduce incidence of falls and may even increase fall risk [11, 21]. A trial of expedited first cataract surgery (4 weeks versus 12 months) showed that the intervention group had a significantly lower fall rate (34% reduction) and a 67% reduced relative risk of fracture from a fall. Further, the number needed to treat with early cataract surgery to prevent one fall was only 19 patients [35]. A follow-up trial of cataract surgery for the second eye reduced falls by a similar amount (32%) in the operated group; however, this reduction did not meet statistical significance [36].

26.4.1.6 Environmental and Home Safety Interventions

A meta-analysis of home safety assessments and interventions found these strategies were effective in reducing the rate of falls (relative risk 0.81, 95% CI 0.68–0.97) and risk of falling (relative risk 0.88, 95% CI 0.8–0.96). These interventions were particularly effective for patients at higher fall risk and when the home safety implementations were conducted by an occupational therapist [22]. The AGS and BGS Guidelines for the Prevention of Falls in Older Persons recommend a home safety assessment and intervention for patients with a previous fall history or at high risk of falls [11].

26.4.2 Multifactorial Interventions in Community-Dwelling Adults

Falls are typically the result of impairments in multiple domains; therefore fall prevention strategies addressing more than one intervention simultaneously have been studied, including multicomponent and multifactorial approaches. Multicomponent interventions include a fixed set of interventions for all patients, where multifactorial interventions are tailored prevention approaches based on individual fall risk assessments [22].

Studies of multifactorial interventions show mixed results regarding fall risk and incidence [37, 38]. Overall, meta-analyses conclude that a multifactorial approach is beneficial for community dwelling older adults if the interventions are provided directly, rather than simply recommendations or referrals [21, 22]. The AGS and BGS guidelines recommend that multifactorial interventions include the following components: gait training (including education for assistive device use), medication review and modification, exercise programs (with balance and gait training as one component), treatment of postural hypotension and cardiovascular disorders, and modification of environmental hazards [11]. ◘ Table 26.7 outlines elements of a multifactorial fall prevention approach with associated interventions and patient education components.

◘ **Table 26.7** A multifactorial intervention for fall prevention in community-dwelling patients

Risk factor	Provider intervention	Patient education
Balance or gait instability	Refer to physical therapy to initiate validated exercise programs (including strength, balance, and gait training) Recommend tai chi Prescribe assistive device and review proper use	Use assistive device as instructed Wear nonskid, well-fitting footwear covering the entire foot, with thin sole and low heel Consider emergency call device
Polypharmacy (≥4 medications)	Prescription review with medication risk assessment Discontinue unnecessary medications (particularly psychotropics if possible) Recommend nonpharmacological treatment when possible	Maintain active medication list (including herbals, supplements, and over the counter prescriptions) Bring medication list to all medical visits Use pillbox to avoid medication errors
Cardiovascular risks (orthostatic hypotension, carotid sinus syndrome)	Orthostatic hypotension Measure orthostatic vital signs Reduce contributing medications Liberalize salt in diet Carotid sinus syndrome Consultation for pacemaker implantation	Orthostatic hypotension Drink sufficient water daily Avoid sudden change in position Wear compression stocking if tolerated
Visual impairment	Inquire about vision Screen for visual acuity Ophthalmology referral Recommend early cataract surgery when indicated	Schedule routine vision testing Do not wear reading glasses when walking Avoid multifocal glasses in outdoor setting (bifocals blur ground-level hazards)
Environmental and home hazards	Perform or refer visiting nurse/occupational therapy to complete home safety assessment Provide check list to patient or caregiver to assess home safety	Ensure well-lit environment (including nightlights) Remove area rugs and slippery throw rugs Remove clutter and ensure clear walking paths are available Install handrails accompanying stairs and grab bars in bathrooms

26.4.3 Population-Based Interventions

Population-based interventions are programs that are designed to incorporate the entire communities into fall prevention strategies. Such interventions range from policy development to education and engagement of local health professionals and organizations to home visits from multidisciplinary medical teams to education and awareness via brochures, television, or web-based initiatives. A Cochrane review of population-based fall prevention strategies found a significant downward trend in fall-related injuries in participating communities, with the relative reduction in fall-related injuries ranging from 6% to 33%. Of significance, in community intervention groups, a 33% decrease in lower extremity fractures was observed [39]. Further studies are needed to establish a standard for public health practices aimed at fall prevention on the community level, as current evidence does not provide a guide for widespread implementation.

26.5 Fall Prevention: Acute and Long-Term Care

Studies of fall prevention strategies in hospitals and long-term care facilities show inconclusive evidence of effectiveness of most fall prevention interventions [40–41]. Evaluating and interpreting these studies poses several challenges, including a wide range of cognitive and physical impairments among patients, as well as variation in types of facilities.

Single intervention exercise strategies for fall prevention in older patients in acute and long-term care facilities demonstrate no reduction in the rate of falls or number of fallers [42]. Subgroup analysis of these studies suggests that exercise may reduce falls in patients with less disability in intermediate-level facilities but may increase falls in patients requiring higher levels of nursing care [42]. While tai chi practice has proven beneficial in fall prevention in the community, studies in nursing home residents did not reproduce these results and no benefit was observed [43].

Available evidence regarding medication management and fall prevention in institutionalized settings suggests a trend toward improved outcomes in intervention groups. Medication review and adjustment as one component of a multifactorial fall prevention program in nursing home patients resulted in a reduction in fall rates, but failed to reach statistical significance [44]. Another study incorporating medication review in conjunction with individualized fall risk interventions showed a 20% reduction in the number of recurrent fallers in the intervention group [45].

In care facilities, studies demonstrate inconsistent results regarding fall rates and vitamin D supplementation. In a systematic review in nursing home facilities, vitamin D supplementation reduced the rate of falls but not the risk of falling [42]. The AGS still recommends vitamin D supplementation of 1000 IU per day for both community-dwelling and long-term care patients >65 years of age to reduce the risk of fractures or falls [33].

Multifactorial interventions have been widely studied in the nursing home setting. Approaches aimed at fall prevention include staff training, environmental modifications, exercise (including balance and strength training), medication management and reconciliation, and occupational therapy evaluations. A meta-analysis of patients in acute and long-term care facilities receiving a multifactorial fall prevention strategy suggested a benefit based on rate of falls (rate ratio 0.78, 95% CI 0.59–1.04) and risk of falls (relative risk 0.89, 95% CI 0.77–1.02), but evidence is not conclusive [42].

In the acute care setting, individual interventions used to prevent falls, including bedrails, restraints, fall-alert bracelets, and bed alarms, have not proven effective in fall prevention strategies and may increase fall risk [41, 42, 46, 47].

26.6 Preventing Fall Complications

While single and multifactorial intervention strategies may help to prevent falls in the community, acute care, and long-term care facilities, these care plans do not prevent falls entirely. Devices have been developed with the aim of preventing falls or injuries from falls in patients at high risk, including assistive devices, hip protectors, and call alarm systems.

26.6.1 Assistive Devices

There are no randomized controlled trials indicating that assistive devices prevent falls. In fact, observational studies find an association between assistive device use and increased risk of falls. This finding likely represents a population of patients inherently at an increased risk of falling, given the need for an assistive device as a result of gait or balance impairment. Additionally, most patients who use an assistive device were never taught proper use by a health-care professional [48].

Health-care providers should routinely assess for proper assistive device use and fit. For a cane, the top of the handle should be at the level of the superior aspect of the greater trochanter or at the break of the wrist when the patient stands upright with arms at their side. Further, when holding a cane, there should be approximately a 15-degree bend at the elbow. Walkers are preferred when balance is poor and a cane does not offer sufficient stability. Front-wheeled walkers allow for a more natural gait and are preferred in patients with cognitive impairment. Rollator walkers or four-wheeled devices allow for a faster gait pace but require increased coordination and processing speed as these devices require use of the brakes [48].

26.6.2 Hip Protectors

Hip protectors are specialized protective garments (pant or undergarment) that contain pads (hard plastic shields or soft foam pads) on the lateral aspect of the hip and leg that are designed to prevent fracture or injury in the setting of a fall. Studies of both community-dwelling and nursing home patients using hip protectors demonstrated no significant reduction of hip fractures after a fall. A significant limitation of these studies is the poor adherence and acceptance of wearing hip protectors among many of the adults in study groups [49]. Use can be considered in very frail high-risk nursing home patients when adherence can be ensured and the patient is willing.

26.6.3 Call Alarm Systems

Approximately half of those who fall are unable to get up on their own afterward, resulting in prolonged time on the ground [7]. Long lies are associated with serious injury, hospital admission, and transition to long-term care facilities. Call alarm systems aim to avoid these long lies in the aftermath of a fall and are generally worn as a necklace or around the wrist. These alert systems can be recommended to those patients at high risk of falling, particularly if they live alone. Their effectiveness is uncertain due to lack of adequate study data.

26.6.4 Osteoporosis

Osteoporosis is a skeletal disorder characterized by compromised bone strength (including bone density and bone quality) that predisposes patients to increased risk of fracture in the setting of a fall. The National Osteoporosis Foundation (NOF) provides universal recommendations that all post-menopausal women and men age 50 years and older receive a diet that includes adequate amounts of calcium intake (1000 mg/day for men 50–70 years old; 1200 mg/day for women 51 and older and men 71 and older), incorporating dietary supplements only if diet is insufficient [50]. Routine screening for low 25-hydroxyvitamin D levels is not necessary, and recommended daily vitamin D intake for all individuals age 50 and older is 800–1000 IU daily (including supplements if necessary) [50].

Bone mineral density (BMD) testing is recommended for all women over the age of 65 years according to the USPSTF. While BMD testing is not currently recommended for men by the USPSTF, the NOF recommends BMD in all men after the age of 70 years and in men with a prior clinical fracture after age 65 [50]. Pharmacologic treatment of osteoporosis is recommended when clinically indicated as per USPSTS and NOF guidelines and should be considered in patients with a history of falls and at high risk of falls if they meet guideline criteria for therapy. Osteoporosis treatment itself does not decrease the risk of falls; however, studies show that bisphosphonate therapy does reduce the risk of hip, vertebral, and non-vertebral fractures [50–52].

26.6.5 Anticoagulation

Approximately 5% of elderly persons have atrial fibrillation and require lifelong anticoagulation therapy to reduce the risk of stroke. The risk of antithrombotic therapy includes serious bleeding events, such as subdural hematoma (SDH) and intracerebral hemorrhage. Head trauma in the setting of fall may lead to SDH or intracerebral hemorrhage, and therefore the risk versus benefit analysis of chronic antithrombotic therapy in elderly patients at risk of fall has been an area of debate. A systematic review showed that patients with atrial fibrillation and average risk of stroke and falling must fall approximately 300 times in a year for the risks of anticoagulation to outweigh its benefits [53]. Overall, in elderly persons with atrial fibrillation and a predisposition to falls with a potential for head trauma, anticoagulation therapy is still rarely contraindicated and should be continued for stroke prevention in spite of fall history or risk of fall [53].

A summary of answers to the clinical case is outlined in ▶ Box 26.2.

Box 26.2 Clinical Case Conclusions

- *Questions to Consider (Part I)*
  - What questions do you want to ask Mrs. C regarding her fall? What historical information do you want to know regarding her fall?
    - Circumstances surrounding fall
    - Associated symptoms leading up to and following fall
    - Review of comorbid conditions
    - Medications
    - Functional status and mobility
    - Substance use
- *Questions to Consider (Part II):*
  - Based on her history, what risk factors for falling does Mrs. C have?
    - Age
    - History of falls
    - Polypharmacy
    - Diabetic neuropathy
    - Depression
    - Orthostasis
    - Poor balance
    - Environmental hazards in the home
  - What physical exam maneuvers and tests would you like to perform?
    - Orthostatic blood pressure
    - Visual acuity assessment
    - Auditory screen
    - Cardiac examination
    - Neurologic testing
    - Cognitive and mood evaluation
    - Gait evaluation including "Get Up and Go" or Functional Reach Test
- *Questions to Consider (Part III):*
  - Based on Mrs. C's history and physical exam, what factors are contributing to her falls?
    - Multifactorial: gait impairment, muscle weakness, poor balance, neuropathy, impaired visual acuity
  - What tests will you order following this clinic visit?
    - CBC, chemistry, glucose, TSH, vitamin D level, EKG
  - What are your recommendations for Mrs. C to help prevent future falls?
    - Exercise: physical therapy, validated exercise program, and/or tai chi
    - Medication reconciliation to decrease polypharmacy
    - Ophthalmology referral for cataract surgery
    - Environment and home safety assessment
    - Podiatry referral

Driving

Kelly Cummings and Helen Fernandez

A. Chun (ed.), *Geriatric Practice*, https://doi.org/10.1007/978-3-030-19625-7_27

Objectives

Upon completion of the chapter, the student should be able to:

1. Recognize the signs/symptoms of an at-risk older driver and understand how to further assess older adults for driving safety.
2. Explain that the goal of assessing for driving safety is to prevent decline in and improve driving function, not to take away a patient's driving privilege unless in case of irreversible loss of driving skills.
3. Discuss the implications of driving cessation and be able to recommend alternative transportation options.

Case (Part 1)

Ed Driver is an 80-year-old man who comes to your clinic accompanied by his daughter, Shelby, due to a minor car accident. It occurred 2 days ago on his way to pick up his grandchildren from school. He appears concerned and states "Doctor, I was backing out of the driveway as I have many times before and accidently hit a parked car on the street. I don't understand how it happened, nothing like this has ever happened before." Mr. Driver states that he didn't see the car at first, and by the time he did he felt as if his legs were stiff and he couldn't reach the brake in time. Shelby, who is also concerned, confirms this was his first car accident and that she has always considered him a good driver.

27.1 Introduction

Driving in older adults is a common concern brought forth by patients and their families in the clinical setting. It is a difficult topic to navigate because it is a balance between a patient's independence and safety. As the population of adults over the age of 65 continues to rise, the number of older drivers will follow. Despite this rise, the National Highway Traffic Safety Administration reported that older adults still have a lower rate of fatal crashes per 100,000 licensed drivers than any other age group, are more likely to be restrained, and have the lowest blood alcohol content levels of all drivers of drinking-involved fatal crashes [1]. However, it is still important to evaluate for driving safety, because older drivers are more likely than younger drivers to suffer injuries or die as a result of motor vehicle crashes because of their increased susceptibility to injury and medical complications. Total traffic fatalities among older adults rose by 13 percent in the years 2007–2016 and were the highest in the 85 and older group [1].

The task of driving is complicated, requiring intact executive and visuospatial function, good visual acuity, and coordinated sensorimotor function. Many common preventable, reversible, and treatable age-related changes and those associated with chronic medical conditions can impair these abilities making driving difficult and potentially unsafe. However, a survey by the CDC found that 1 in 10 older adults reported they would never stop driving and likely overestimate their ability to drive [2]. Driving cessation in older adults on the other hand also has many implications for their independence, sociability, and access to food and healthcare services.

Case (Part 2)

Mr. Driver lives alone ever since his wife passed away 6 months ago. Shelby lives just a few blocks away but works during the day, so Mr. Driver often helps take care of his grandchildren during the week. He is a retired banker and spends his free time playing golf on the weekends. He has been driving for the past 62 years without any traffic tickets, motor vehicle accidents, or near misses and has never gotten lost while driving.

27.2 Clinical Assessment

Assessing older adults for driving safety is challenging and complex. There is no single assessment. There are both normal age-related changes and abnormal changes that can affect the driving ability of an older adult. Often patients may be unaware of these changes and how it affects their ability to drive. Concerns may be brought to the clinician's attention by a caregiver who is concerned about the patient's safety and safety of the public. It is important to focus the evaluation on medical and functional abilities of the patient, not just their age. Although primary care physicians are in the best position to screen for driving fitness, all physicians have a responsibility to discuss driving with their patients. The goal of the clinical assessment is early identification and management of medical conditions, potential driving-impairing medications and functional deficits in order to maintain or improve driving ability and road safety, not to focus only on those patients in which driving cessation should occur.

The American Geriatrics Society in coordination with the National Highway Traffic Safety Administration created a useful algorithm for navigating the assessment of an older driver (◘ Fig. 27.1).

27.2.1 Screening

In the absence of any clinical signs to investigate, annual screening of driving safety should be done after age 65 as part the Annual Wellness Visit [4]. Additionally, driving fitness should be assessed with any new diagnosis or change in chronic medical condition, if a new medication is prescribed or with medication changes, or a change in functional ability. As driving for older adults can be a sensitive topic to discuss, it is important to frame your conversation that your focus is on prevention and optimizing their driving ability, not to stop them from driving.

Begin with simple screening questions:

- Are you still driving?
- If not, have you ever driven? Why did you stop driving?
- Have you ever been in an accident? Even as minor as hitting curbs when parking or backing up.

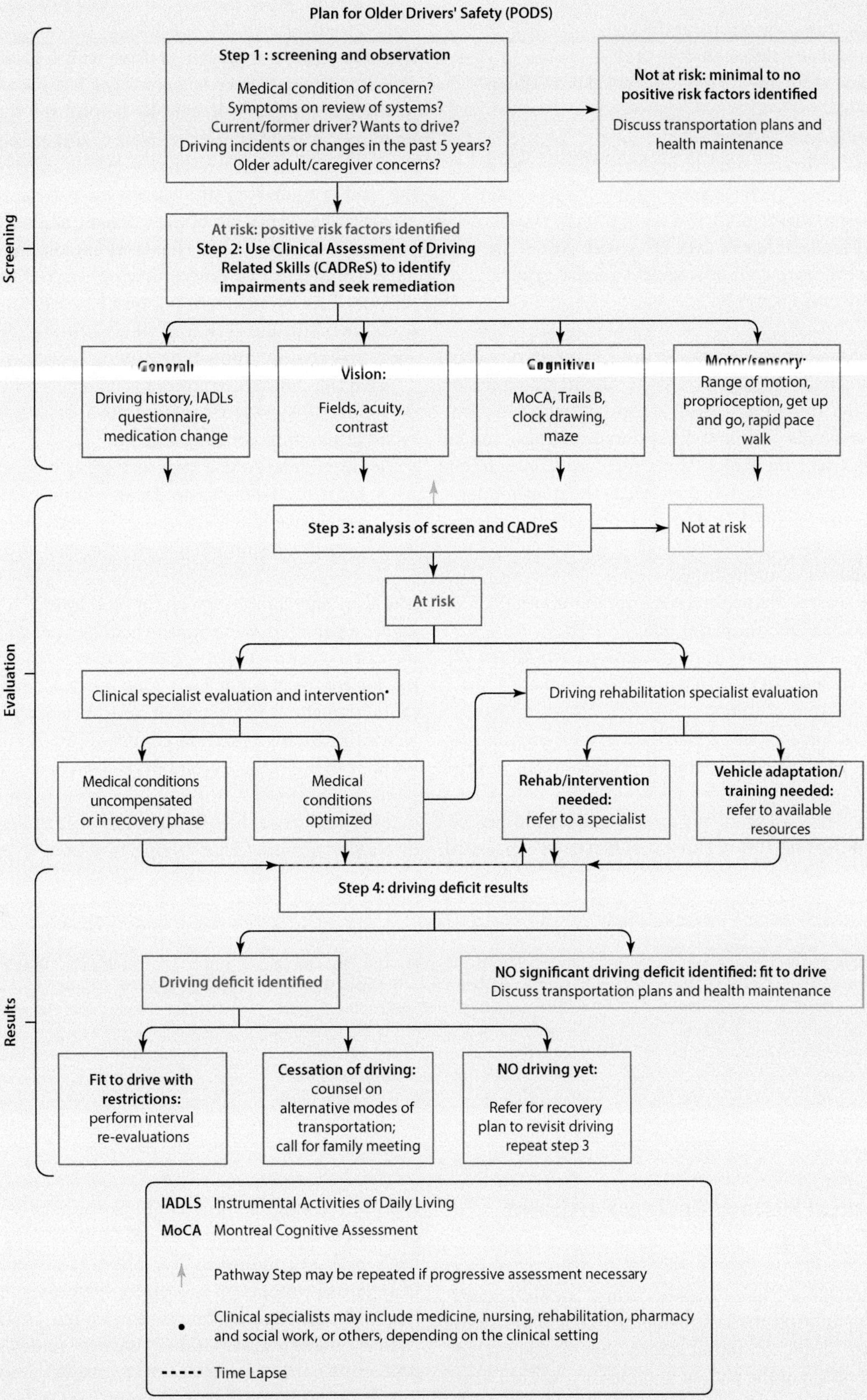
Plan for Older Drivers' Safety (PODS)
Screening
Step 1 : screening and observation
Medical condition of concern?
Symptoms on review of systems?
Current/former driver? Wants to drive?
Driving incidents or changes in the past 5 years?
Older adult/caregiver concerns?
Not at risk: minimal to no positive risk factors identified
Discuss transportation plans and health maintenance
At risk: positive risk factors identified
Step 2: Use Clinical Assessment of Driving Related Skills (CADReS) to identify impairments and seek remediation
General:
Driving history, IADLs questionnaire, medication change
Vision:
Fields, acuity, contrast
Cognitive:
MoCA, Trails B, clock drawing, maze
Motor/sensory:
Range of motion, proprioception, get up and go, rapid pace walk
Evaluation
Step 3: analysis of screen and CADreS
Not at risk
At risk
Clinical specialist evaluation and intervention•
Driving rehabilitation specialist evaluation
Medical conditions uncompensated or in recovery phase
Medical conditions optimized
Rehab/intervention needed:
refer to a specialist
Vehicle adaptation/ training needed:
refer to available resources
Results
Step 4: driving deficit results
Driving deficit identified
NO significant driving deficit identified: fit to drive
Discuss transportation plans and health maintenance
Fit to drive with restrictions:
perform interval re-evaluations
Cessation of driving:
counsel on alternative modes of transportation;
call for family meeting
NO driving yet:
Refer for recovery plan to revisit driving repeat step 3
IADLS Instrumental Activities of Daily Living
MoCA Montreal Cognitive Assessment
Pathway Step may be repeated if progressive assessment necessary
Clinical specialists may include medicine, nursing, rehabilitation, pharmacy and social work, or others, depending on the clinical setting
Time Lapse

Fig. 27.1 Plan for Older Driver's Safety (PODS) (Adapted from Pomidor [3])

- Are there any new dents or scratches you've noticed on your vehicle?
- Any recent traffic violations or tickets?
- Have you had any close calls?
- Do you have difficulty turning the wheel or making turns?
- Do you wear your seatbelt?
- Do you avoid driving at night or during certain weather conditions?
- Where do you drive?
- Do your friends or family ever drive with you?
- Have you ever forgotten how to get to a place you've been many times before?

A full clinical assessment should be done if there's any concern after the screening questions. Other useful resources for assessing for declining traffic skills are use of self-assessment tools both hand-outs or online questionnaires. These can be good options when the patient feels they are a safe driver, but the clinician or family has concern as the questionnaire can give objective feedback that further evaluation is recommended.

Helpful Self-Assessment Tools:
- "Fitness to drive" online screening questionnaire [5]
- Driving Habits Questionnaire [6]
- University of Michigan Driving Decisions Workbook [7] or online version, SAFER Driving [8]

As patients may have impaired insight as to their own driving safety, with a patient's permission the clinician can inquire to a caregiver or family if they have noticed any concerning driving behaviors or ask the same screening questions above. One survey found that 70% of caregivers had been concerned for a year that the older patient was not driving safely most often due to slow reaction time, slow driving, and inattention to road hazards [9]. Specifically, if a caregiver won't drive with the patient or let others drive with him or her, that is a red flag. If a caregiver has concerns but the patient refuses to discuss the topic, it may be helpful for them to review resources available online on how to discuss concerns about driving safety with a loved one, warning signs of unsafe driving, and even driving simulations the patient can do to have an objective evaluation of their driving skills (see list of webpages below). The AARP has a more comprehensive list of 28 warning signs of unsafe driving, ranked from minor to serious. This is important because less serious signs may be overcome with intervention, whereas more serious warning signs may require immediate driving cessation.

Helpful Online Resources for Patients and Caregivers:
- ▶ https://www.aarp.org/auto/driver-safety/driving-tips/
- ▶ https://seniordriving.aaa.com/
- ▶ https://www.nhtsa.gov/road-safety/older-drivers
- ▶ https://www.thehartford.com/resources/mature-market-excellence/family-conversations-with-older-drivers
- ▶ https://www.nia.nih.gov/health/older-drivers

It is also important to screen for "copiloting," a phenomenon where a person drives with the help of a passenger providing directions on how to get somewhere, reading signs, or coaching for common traffic laws. One retrospective cohort study found that about 10 percent of older men with dementia who were still driving relied on copilots [10]. The use of a copilot for driving should prompt the clinician to investigate the patient's cognition further, and if the use is for reading signs or instructions on how to drive, then it should prompt the discussion of immediate driving cessation.

Case (Part 3)

Mr. Driver does not wear eye glasses since having bilateral cataract surgery 2 years ago and wears bilateral hearing aids for sensorineural hearing loss. He has no apparent memory problems or history of falls and ambulates independently. Review of systems reveals that his knee pain has been worse lately and he has been having difficulty falling asleep at night. His medical history is significant for atrial fibrillation, well-controlled chronic obstructive pulmonary disease, osteoarthritis of the knees, and benign prostatic hypertrophy. He used to drink alcohol socially but stopped completely about 5 years ago. He reports prior smoking history of 40 years but quit 20 years ago and denies any illicit drug use. He is independent in all basic and instrumental activities of daily living. His medications include apixaban, albuterol, and ibuprofen as needed, and he has been tolerating the escitalopram that was started at his last visit. He also reports recently trying an over-the-counter sleep aid but states it is not helping.

27.2.2 Medical History Review Pertinent to Driving

Most older adults have one or more chronic medical conditions and take multiple medications putting them at risk for adverse effects. Thus, the initial screen should also include clinical observation of the patient and identifying "red flags" in the patient's history such as medical conditions and medications that may impair safe driving.

There should be a careful review of medical history looking for medical conditions that cause sensory deprivation, impaired physical function, and impaired cognition, specifically, any conditions that could potentially be reversible or optimized with treatment. See ◘ Table 27.1 for a list of "red flag" medical conditions. Similarly, a comprehensive review of systems is important to identify symptoms that may interfere with driving capability, for example, dizziness, vision changes, decreased sensation in the extremities, or movement limited by pain. A survey of over 2000 licensed drivers over the age of 70 found that if a patient had fallen two or more times in the past year, they were 53% more likely to be involved in a motor vehicle crash and two times as likely to have caused the accident [11]. It is important to assess a patient's medication list looking for medications that may

Table 27.1 "Red flag" medical conditions

Ocular and vestibular disease	Cataracts Diabetic retinopathy Macular degeneration Glaucoma Retinitis pigmentosa Ptosis Field deficits Decreased contrast sensitivity Low visual acuity even after correction Sensorineural hearing loss Benign paroxysmal positional vertigo
Cardiovascular disease	Unstable coronary syndrome Arrhythmias Palpitations Congestive heart failure Hypertrophic obstructive cardiomyopathy Valvular disease Peripheral vascular disease
Respiratory disease	Chronic obstructive pulmonary disease Obstructive sleep apnea
Neurologic disease	Dementia Multiple sclerosis Parkinson's disease Peripheral neuropathy Cerebral vascular disease including transient ischemic attack or stroke Spinal cord injury Seizure Syncope Autonomic dysfunction Delirium
Psychiatric disease	Depression Anxiety Insomnia Mood disorders Psychosis Personality disorders Alcohol or other substance abuse
Endocrine disease	Diabetes specifically hypoglycemia attacks Thyroid disorders Adrenal insufficiency Pituitary macroadenoma
Musculoskeletal disease	Arthritis and foot abnormalities Contractures and decreased range of motion Degenerative disc disease or spinal stenosis Inflammation Pain History of falls
Other	Chronic renal failure Cancer and chemotherapy Poor hygiene or lack of grooming

Adapted from Pomidor [3] and Physician's guide to assessing and counseling older drivers [13]

have adverse effects such as drowsiness, confusion, dizziness, or nausea which can impair a person's ability to concentrate and drive safely and could be discontinued. The American Geriatrics Society (AGS) Beers Criteria for Potentially Inappropriate Medication Use in Older Adults is a list of medications to be used in caution in older adults as they have been found to be associated with poor health outcomes, including confusion, falls, and mortality [12]. Examples of at-risk medications include benzodiazepines, narcotics, and sedating antihistamines. Beyond the standard social history questions of tobacco, alcohol, and illicit drug use, the clinician should ask about the patient's physical activity, use of an ambulatory assist device such as cane or walker, and basic and instrumental activities of daily living (ADLs and IADLs). Since activities such as cooking, managing appointments, and financial management share similar cognitive functions as driving, any difficulties or lack of insight related to at least one IADL should warrant further investigation of cognition [3].

Finally, if a patient is diagnosed with a new medical condition or given a medication with potential side effects that can impact driving ability, then they must be counseled on caution with or cessation of driving for a short period while optimizing new medical illness or adjusting medication doses. For example, a patient with an acute congestive heart failure exacerbation on increased doses of their diuretic may be at increased risk for hypotension, dizziness, and even syncope, making it periodically unsafe for them to drive.

Case (Part 4)

On physical exam, Mr. Driver is afebrile, has an irregularly irregular pulse of 82 beats per minute, blood pressure of 132/84, respiratory rate of 16, and pulse oximetry of 96 percent on room air. He is a well-dressed elderly male but appears tired. Cardiopulmonary and abdominal examinations are within normal limits. Visual fields are intact, visual acuity is 20/20, and fundoscopic examination is normal. A Montreal Cognitive Assessment is performed, and he scores 28/30. Examination of his lower extremities shows some crepitus over both his knees. Neurological exam is normal, including 5/5 strength throughout and intact sensation and proprioception. He has normal range of motion in his neck, shoulders, and legs. He is unable to rise from the chair without use of his arms and takes 12 seconds on a Rapid Pace Walk test.

27.2.3 Clinical Exam and Diagnostics

When initial screening reveals an older adult may be at risk for medically impaired driving, the clinician should investigate further. The clinical assessment should be focused on three key areas related to driving fitness and also several of which may decline with age:

- Vision
- Cognition
- Motor and sensory function

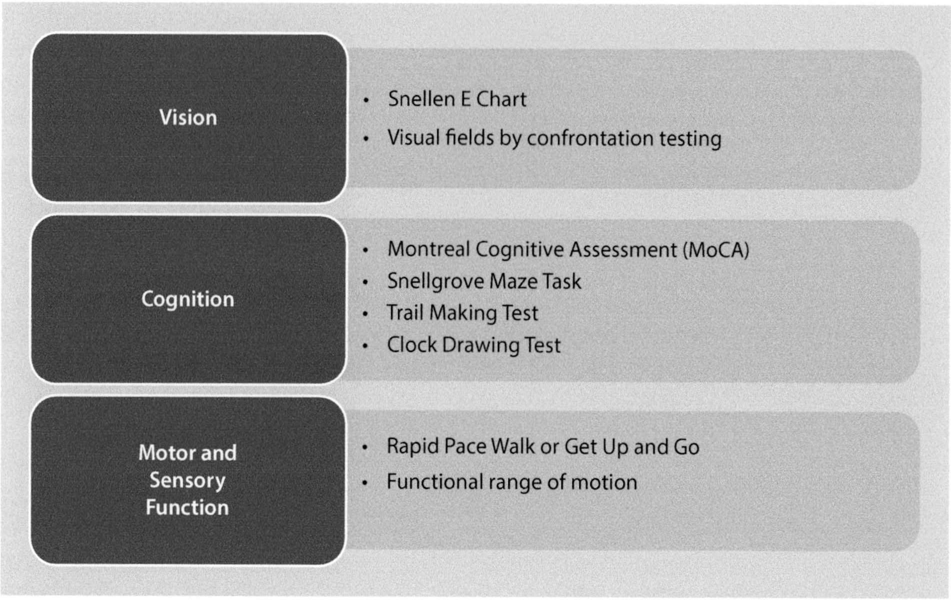

Fig. 27.2 The Clinical Assessment of Driving-Related Skills (CADReS)

The Clinical Assessment of Driving-Related Skills (CADReS), created by the American Medical Association in coordination with the National Highway Traffic Safety Administration, is a toolbox of practical, validated, and office-based assessments of the main areas of function related to driving ability [3, 13]. The components of the CADReS are listed in Fig. 27.2.

27.2.4 Vision

The primary sense needed for driving is vision. In all states, vision testing is required to obtain your driver's license, and many states also require repeat testing for license renewal.

The aspects of vision that should be assessed include:

- Visual acuity
- Visual fields
- Contrast sensitivity

Far visual acuity is measured using the Snellen E chart (refer to ► Chap. 5). Most states require visual testing for license renewal and require a visual acuity of 20/40 for an unrestricted license [3]. Patients with visual acuity worse than 20/40 should restrict driving until vision is corrected. Besides testing far visual acuity with a Snellen chart, it is also important to consider near visual acuity, to ensure patients can read gauges and controls inside of the car. Visual fields are evaluated through confrontation testing (refer to ► Chap. 5). Visual field deficits can be the result of several common age-related eye conditions such as glaucoma or strokes and can affect the ability of drivers to see traffic signs and other cars or nearby pedestrians. There are several recent studies demonstrating that older adults with visual field deficits are at increased risk of motor vehicle crashes [14]. Contrast sensitivity is when a person has difficulty distinguishing objects from the background which can be especially dangerous if driving at night or during certain weather conditions. In older adults, contrast sensitivity has been found to be a valid predictor of crash risk; however, it requires special testing in an ophthalmology office and thus is not included in the CADReS toolbox. It is important to monitor closely for progression of any visual deficits.

27.2.5 Cognition

All the pieces of cognition should be intact in order for an older adult to safely perform the complex task of driving. Cognition is not routinely tested by states for licensure renewal but should be evaluated by physicians taking care of older drivers.

The aspects of cognition that should be assessed include:

- Memory
- Visuospatial skills
- Attention
- Executive function
- Insight

Memory is essential for remembering directions, traffic rules, and how to operate a car and for retaining and processing new information. Visuospatial skills are needed to process distance between other vehicles or objects and predict the time needed to slow or stop. Attention is needed to avoid distraction and be aware of critical stimuli. Executive skills are needed for coordination, problem solving, and planning. Insight is needed for an older adult to be able to recognize and understand any limitations that could affect their driving. In the CADReS toolbox, the Montreal Cognitive Assessment (MoCA) is used as a validated brief cognitive test that measures executive function, memory, language, attention, visuospatial skills, abstract thinking, and orientation (refer to ► Chap. 20). The MoCA includes both the Trails B and Clock-Drawing Test. If a patient scores 18 or less on the MOCA, interventions are recommended [15]. For the Trail-Making Test, a completion time of greater than 3 minutes and any incorrect element on the Clock-Drawing Test are both indications for intervention [16, 17]. The Snellgrove Maze task similarly assesses visual perception, abstract thinking, and executive function and has been validated as a cognitive screen for driving ability in older adults [3].

27.2.6 Motor and Sensory

Driving requires a certain amount of physical strength, movement, and sensory input.

Aspects of motor and sensory function that should be assessed include:
- Mobility
- Range of Motion
- Strength
- Proprioception

Many common musculoskeletal conditions that develop with age such as osteoarthritis may limit an older adult's ability to turn over their shoulder when changing lanes or even be able to put on their seatbelt. The CADReS toolbox tests somatosensory function using the Rapid Pace Walk and/or Get Up and Go (refer to ► Chap. 26) and manual evaluation of range of motion and strength. The Rapid Pace Walk measures lower limb mobility, trunk stability, and balance, and a score of greater than 9 seconds has been associated with increased crash risk [18]. A Get Up and Go Test score of 3 or more is associated with an increased risk of falling which is associated with an increased risk of getting in a motor vehicle accident [3]. Patients should also be assessed for impaired proprioception as it can cause a phenomenon of "pedal confusion" from inability to feel or gauge which pedal they are stepping on.

Case (Part 5)

Mr. Driver agrees to discontinue his use of the over-the-counter sleep aid as well as the ibuprofen and is willing to try melatonin for sleep and acetaminophen for pain instead. He is given a script for physical therapy, and local driving resources are discussed. He has agreed to stop driving until his follow-up visit in a few weeks to assess if his sleep and pain are improved. His daughter arranged for a friend to help with picking her children up for school, and Mr. D's friend is willing to pick him up for golf on the weekends.

27.3 Interventions

Once an older adult is found to be at risk for driving, the first step is to distinguish between a progressive disease and a treatable one. The goal is to treat any reversible medical conditions, optimize functional deficits, and refer to a specialist as needed. It is also important to begin the conversation of driving safety and why you are concerned and plan for a safe transition if driving cessation is necessary. All chronic progressive medical problems should be periodically re-reviewed for relation to driving safety. If evaluation of an older adult did not reveal a driving risk, it still is important to discuss tips for safe driving and any medical conditions that could progress and later impact driving ability, encourage periodic follow-up, and begin planning for alternative transportation options.

27.3.1 Treatment and Optimization

If a condition or functional deficit is identified and potentially correctable, then medical treatment and interventions should be done until the older adult's condition has been optimized; see ◘ Table 27.2. Depending on the severity of the deficit identified in the CADReS, the patient should also be counseled on potentially not driving until further evaluation or treatment is pursued and reassured that you will re-assess their driving fitness once treatment is complete. For example, a person with incorrect corrective lenses, cognitive impairment due to sensorineural hearing loss, and hypoglycemia due to too much insulin may be at similar risk for a motor vehicle crash as someone with Parkinson's disease and dementia. Although in both scenarios it would be recommended for the patient to stop driving immediately, the first scenario could potentially be treated. After medical optimization with new glasses, hearing aids, and lower insulin to avoid hypoglycemia, re-evaluation may find the patient safe to resume driving.

Once an older adult is medically optimized and there is no contraindication to driving, the clinician should still provide education on safe driving tips and become familiar with local alternative options of transportation.

◘ **Table 27.2** Interventions for the three main functional aspects related to driving skills sometimes may require referral to a specialist

Vision	Cognition	Somatosensory
Cataract removal Ensure appropriate corrective lenses Treat underlying cause of vision loss Adaptive devices for low vision Occupational therapy referral for vision training for field deficits Surgical repair of ptosis Educate on driving limitations, such as driving during daytime and good weather only	Evaluate and treat reversible causes of cognitive decline: anemia, vitamin B12/folate deficiency, infection, chronic kidney disease, hypoglycemia, hypoxia, hypothyroidism, liver dysfunction, depression, and side effects of medications Secondary prevention with medical management for h/o vascular dementia and/or stroke Refer to neurology, psychiatry, or neuropsychiatry for further evaluation and treatment as needed	Power steering, power brakes, automatic transmission, back-up mirrors, blind spot sensors Provide effective pain control, but educate on caution of motor vehicle operation with certain pain medications (i.e., opioids, muscle relaxants) Regular physical activity Physical therapy or occupational therapy for mobility, strength, and adaptive tools Podiatry, orthopedics, and vascular referral depending on the issue

27.3.2 Referral to Driving Rehabilitation Specialist

In instances where driving risk is not clear-cut, referral to a driver rehabilitation specialist (DRS) can be helpful. Referral to a DRS may also be useful when a patient has function deficits that are not amenable to medical treatment such as spinal cord injuries. A DRS can directly evaluate how a functional impairment is affecting the actual task of driving. Then, based on their assessment, can make objective recommendations. A DRS is most often an occupational therapist but can also be a physical therapist, kinesiotherapist, psychologist, or driver educator who has undergone specialty training in driving rehabilitation.

A DRS evaluation consists of three aspects:

- Driver observation
- Vehicle assessment
- Interventions if needed

Driver observation consists of many similar clinical assessments already described above in this chapter but also includes a comprehensive on-road assessment. This includes assessment of the older adult's ability to transport themselves into a vehicle if they require an ambulatory assist device and how they adhere to common traffic laws and their awareness and attention to their driving environment. An on-road assessment by a DRS is particularly useful for assessing conditions such as inattention, cognitive impairment, fatigue, or low vision on the actual task of driving. A DRS will also assess the older adult's vehicle to determine if there is a need for modification or special equipment and can even assist with patients interested in purchasing a new vehicle. For example, if the clinical assessment reveals an older adult has limited range of motion in their neck or arms due to chronic osteoarthritis, a DRS may recommend a vehicle with a low-effort power steering, a back-up camera, and blind spot sensors for safe lane changes. Other adaptive devices include installing extra mirrors for poor neck range of motion, a spinner knob on the steering wheel to compensate for poor hand grip, an extended gear shift lever to overcome reduced reach, and enlarged side and rear-view mirrors to compensate for visual field deficits [3]. A DRS can provide close follow-up for re-evaluation of driving safety after an intervention is instituted and can also assist with alternative transportation plans if driving cessation is recommended.

After assessment, a DRS will then give recommendations to the driver. Below are examples of possible recommendations:

- Patient may continue driving with no need for intervention.
- Patient may continue driving but with the following restrictions such as avoiding rush hour or not driving at night.
- Patient should attend a driving instruction course for retraining.
- Patient should be given adaptive devices to overcome a deficit and trained in its use.
- Patient should temporarily stop driving until interventions are performed and patient is reassessed for safety.
- Patient should permanently stop driving, deficit not amenable to intervention.

DRSs referrals can usually be made through local occupational therapy departments and require a prescription detailing the reason for referral. Further resources can be found on the Association for Driver Rehabilitation Specialists and the American Occupation Therapy Association websites [19, 20]. The clinician should discuss with the patient the reasons for referral to a DRS, the goal, and expectations of the referral and assist in determining the expected cost. The cost of a driving rehabilitation program is most often out of pocket and can vary depending on services required. Coverage by Medicare, Medicaid, and private insurances is variable and generally starts around $300–600 for a full initial assessment. However, the cost and benefit of a DRS far outweighs any potential costs of vehicle damage, human injury, or death caused by a motor vehicle crash. If a DRS is not an option in the local area for a patient, other options may include general occupational therapists for evaluation of IADLs, driver's education instructors or programs, or other medical specialists such as a geriatrician.

After an older adult completes assessment and intervention with a DRS, it is important for the referring clinician to follow up with the patient in order to reinforce recommendations and continue planning for alternative transportation options if driving safety changes.

27.3.3 Driving Cessation and Transitions

After initial assessment and optimization, the clinician must consider if it is still safe for the patient to drive. Ideally a discussion about driving safety and a contingency plan would happen prior to a patient losing the ability to drive. Unfortunately, most often the topic of driving ability in an older adult is brought up because a patient or caregiver has already noticed limitations or areas of concern. For example, cognitive impairment due to Alzheimer's disease and vision loss due to dry age-related macular degeneration are progressive, irreversible diseases that severely impair driving ability. In such patients, discussion of immediate driving cessation with a patient and their caregivers is imperative. If driving cessation is recommended, the conclusion should be clearly communicated to the patient and their caregivers and clearly documented in the patient's health record.

One framework that can be helpful when discussing driving cessation with a patient is a six-step protocol for delivering bad news by the acronym "SPIKES" [21].

1. **S**etting up the interview
2. Assessing the patient's **p**erception
3. Obtaining the patient's **i**nvitation
4. Giving **k**nowledge and information to the patient
5. Addressing the patient's **e**motions with empathetic responses
6. **S**trategy and summary

First, ensure you have the right environment and amount of time to discuss driving cessation with the patient. The clinician should have all the information from history and physical function testing to be able to share with the patient the informed decision. As well, with the patient's permission, any necessary caregivers should be present for the discussion.

Next the clinician should try to understand the patient's perception on their driving ability and why driving is important to them. It is particularly important to understand why the patient has refused a driving evaluation or refuses to stop driving. Driving cessation can have several negative consequences such as social isolation, depression, and decreased mobility out of the home [22]. Therefore, it is crucial for the clinician to recognize the impacts of not driving may have on each individual patient and their family. For instance, a patient's only means of obtaining food or getting to doctor's appointments may have been by driving themselves. Or they may be the primary caregiver for someone else who depends on them for transportation. In this step, the clinician also needs to assess the caregiver's understanding of the risks of the patient continuing to drive, why driving cessation is recommended, and the caregiver's ability to assist with alternate transportation options. The clinician should also make sure the patient wants to hear the results of their driving evaluation and who can this information be shared with.

Step four is information sharing with the patient. The clinician should have an agenda for what should be discussed and be prepared to react to emotional responses from the patient. Starting the conversation by giving the patient a warning shot, such as "Unfortunately, I have some bad news to tell you", can lessen the shock that may follow delivering bad news [21]. Next, share information in small pieces, using nontechnical words, and check back frequently to make sure the patient is comprehending the news. Emphasize that your main concern is the health and safety of the patient and that of the public, but also validate and address any concerns the patient has. Make sure to address the patient's emotions with empathetic responses by observing, giving time, exploring, and validating. Showing empathy and sensitivity to a patient's circumstances around driving may help with eventual compliance with your recommendations.

The last step in the discussion of driving cessation is planning and follow-through. After exploring the patient's mobility needs and potential barriers, the clinician should emphasize their goal to help the patient plan for the future and find alternative modes of transportation. Although the feasibility of public transportation may be challenging outside of major cities, in those without a social support system, reliance on local community resources such as buses, trains, taxi cabs, walking, community or volunteer shuttles, Medi-car, or private care services can allow the older adult to remain independent and prevent social isolation. Other members of the healthcare team, social workers, and a geriatric care manager can be useful resources for transportation options as well. As part of follow-through, it is crucial to regularly evaluate compliance and more importantly look for signs of depression and isolation in patients whom driving cessation is recommended. If the plan involves more responsibility on the caregiver for transportation, it is important to regularly assess for caregiver burnout and need of increasing support to maintain safe environment for all involved. Useful resources for caregiver support can be found through the National Family Caregivers Association (▶ http://caregiveraction.org/ or 1-800-896-3650).

Resources for alternative transportation:

- National Center on Senior Transportation
- AARP, AAA, DMV, NHTSA
- University of Michigan Transportation Research Institute
- Rides in Sight
- National Volunteer Transportation Center
- Area Agency on Aging
- Alzheimer's Association
- The Eldercare Locator (800-677-1116 or ▶ www.eldercare.gov/)
- National Association of Social Workers
- Independent Transportation Network (ITN) America
- The Health in Aging Foundation
- Family Caregiver Alliance

A full list of resources can be found in the Clinician's Guide to Assessing and Counseling Older Drivers [3].

27.3.4 Ethical and Legal implications

Driving cessation is a sensitive topic, and many clinicians fear ruining the doctor-patient relationship or discouraging patients from seeking care for new symptoms and are thus reluctant to discuss. However, clinicians have an ethical responsibility to keep the patient and the public safe. Additional ethical considerations are patient confidentiality and autonomy. Nevertheless, in states where physicians are held legally responsible to report unsafe drivers, they are protected to do so as "the duty to protect public health outweighs the duty to maintain a patient's confidence" [23]. In states without strict reporting laws, the physician must first obtain a signed medical release form before disclosing the name of an at-risk driver. Regardless of individual state laws, to respect the doctor-patient relationship, the clinician should inform the patient before reporting them. It may help to explain why you feel their condition does not allow them to drive safely and that you are ethically responsible for both the patient's and publics' safety. If an older adult lacks insight to their driving risk, intervention may require more involvement of caregivers, courts, and state department of motor vehicles. Although it is important to involve caregivers in the discussion of driving safety, a patient must first give the clinician permission to contact caregivers and for it to be clearly documented. Furthermore, patients with capacity have the right to deny permission, and the clinician must respect this decision.

Regulations on driver license renewal and reporting policies for unsafe driver laws vary state by state and can change over time. Some states find physicians legally responsible for reporting unsafe drivers. Thus, it is important for clinicians to be familiar with their state reporting laws. There are six states currently with mandatory reporting requirements: CA, DE, NJ, NV, OR, and PA [3]. Studies found that in these six states, physicians were more likely to report [3]. Health professionals in 18 out of the 43 states with voluntary reporting laws are not protected from liability for civil damages [3]. Each state's licensing requirements for visual acuity may also differ.

The final determination of licensing is legally the responsibility of the state, not the physician. However, the clinician can assist by determining which patients are high risk for driving accident and should be reported.

List of resources for state-by-state policies:

- ► http://lpp.seniordrivers.org/
- ► https://www.iihs.org/iihs/topics/laws/olderdrivers
- ► https://drivinglaws.aaa.com/

27.4 Conclusion

In summary, assessing driving safety in older adults is important for patient and public safety. Obtaining an accurate history of driving abilities, medical symptoms, and diseases and assessing visual, cognitive, and physical function can lead to early identification and intervention of risk factors or conditions that may impair driving skills. Based on the clinical assessment, clinicians should weigh the risks and benefits of driving and determine a recommendation. Whether the recommendation is continued driving but with limitations, temporary driving cessation until further assessment completed or medical condition optimized, or immediate driving cessation, it is important to plan ahead and provide alternative transportation resources. Driving cessation can have serious implications on older adults' social and emotional well-being. When discussing the recommendation for a patient to stop driving, clinicians need to be supportive, sensitive, and empathetic. Overall, assessing driving skills in older adults requires comprehensive evaluation, re-evaluation, and thoughtful management and planning to keep patients safe while also maintaining quality of life. The American Geriatrics Society in coordination with the National Highway Traffic Safety Administration has created a free app called "Safe Older Drivers" that can be downloaded on any smartphone or tablet which contains many resources discussed in this chapter for assessing and counseling older drivers.

References

1. 2016 Older population fact sheet (Traffic Safety Facts. Report No. DOT HS 812 500). Washington, DC: National Highway Traffic Safety Administration's National Center for Statistics and Analysis; May 2018.
2. Naumann RB, West BA, Sauber-Schatz EK. At what age do you think you will stop driving? Views of older U.S. adults. J Am Geriatr Soc. 2014;62(10):1999–2001.
3. Pomidor AE. Clinician's guide to assessing and counseling older drivers. New York: The American Geriatrics Society; 2015.
4. Bhattacharya SB. Assessing well-being in older drivers: Medscape Education Family Medicine; 2018 Available from: https://www.medscape.org/viewarticle/897520_3.
5. Fitness-to-drive screening measure online. University of Florida Institute for Mobility, Activity and Participation.2013 Available from: http://fitnesstodrive.phhp.ufl.edu/us/questionnaire.php.
6. Owsley C, Stalvey B, Wells J, Sloane ME. Older drivers and cataract: driving habits and crash risk. J Gerontol A Biol Sci Med Sci. 1999;54(4):M203–11.
7. Eby D, Molnar LJ, Shope JT. Driving decisions workbook. In: Institute UoMTR, editor; 2000.
8. SAFER driving: the enhanced driving decisions Workbook University of Michigan Transportation Research Institute2006 Available from: http://um-saferdriving.org/firstPage.php.
9. Survey of families and caregivers concerned about the safety of an older driver NYSUT Social Services2013 Available from: https://www.nysut.org/resources/all-listing/2013/april/survey-of-families-and-caregivers-concerned-about-the-safety-of-an-older-driver.
10. Foley DJ, Masaki KH, Ross GW, White LR. Driving cessation in older men with incident dementia. J Am Geriatr Soc. 2000;48(8):928–30.
11. Huisingh C, McGwin G Jr, Orman KA, Owsley C. Frequent falling and motor vehicle collision involvement of older drivers. J Am Geriatr Soc. 2014;62(1):123–9.
12. By the American Geriatrics Society Beers Criteria Update Expert P. American Geriatrics Society 2015 Updated Beers Criteria for Potentially Inappropriate Medication Use in Older Adults. J Am Geriatr Soc. 2015;63(11):2227–46.
13. Wang CC, Kosinski CJ, Schwartzberg JG, Shanklin AV. Physician's guide to assessing and counseling older drivers. Washington, DC: National Highway Traffic Safety Administration; 2003.
14. Dobbs BM. Medical conditions and driving: a review of the scientific literature (1960–2000). Washington, DC: U.S. Department of Transportation National Highway Traffic Safety Administration; 2005.
15. Hollis AM, Duncanson H, Kapust LR, Xi PM, O'Connor MG. Validity of the mini-mental state examination and the montreal cognitive assessment in the prediction of driving test outcome. J Am Geriatr Soc. 2015;63(5):988–92.
16. Staplin L, Gish KW, Sifrit KJ. Using cognitive status to predict crash risk: blazing new trails? J Saf Res. 2014;48:19–25.
17. Freund B, Gravenstein S, Ferris R, Burke BL, Shaheen E. Drawing clocks and driving cars. J Gen Intern Med. 2005;20(3):240–4.
18. Staplin L, Gish KW, Wagner EK. MaryPODS revisited: updated crash analysis and implications for screening program implementation. J Saf Res. 2003;34(4):389–97.
19. Driver rehabilitation provider.: The Association for Driver Rehabilitation Specialists.; Available from: https://www.aded.net/search/custom.asp?id=1984.
20. Find a driving specialist: The American Occupational Therapy Association, Inc.; Available from: https://myaota.aota.org/driver_search/index.aspx.
21. Baile WF, Buckman R, Lenzi R, Glober G, Beale EA, Kudelka AP. SPIKES-A six-step protocol for delivering bad news: application to the patient with cancer. Oncologist. 2000;5(4):302–11.
22. Curl AL, Stowe JD, Cooney TM, Proulx CM. Giving up the keys: how driving cessation affects engagement in later life. Gerontologist. 2014;54(3):423–33.
23. De Bord JBW, Dudzinski D. Confidentiality 2013. Available from: https://depts.washington.edu/bioethx/topics/confiden.html.

Individualized Decision-Making for Preventive Medicine in Older Adults

Lindsey C. Yourman, Jean Y. Guan, and Roopali Gupta

A. Chun (ed.), *Geriatric Practice*, https://doi.org/10.1007/978-3-030-19625-7_28

28

28.1 AAMC Competency

The graduating medical student, in the context of a specific older adult patient scenario, must be able to:

Health Care Planning and Promotion	
15	Accurately identify clinical situations where life expectancy, functional status, patient preference, or goals of care should override standard recommendations for screening tests in older adults.

28.2 Cases

Consider the following two patients who present to establish primary care. While the two patients are of the same chronologic age, they differ substantially in their comorbidities and functional status. We will use these contrasting patient presentations to help illustrate clinical situations where life expectancy, functional status, patient preference, or goals of care should override standard recommendations for screening tests in older adults.

Case 1

Mr. Jones is a 75-year-old male who presents to establish care. Overall, he feels well, "just slower than I used to be."

Past Medical History:

- Coronary artery disease (status-post stent placement 8 years ago and again 2 years ago)
- Ischemic cardiomyopathy (ejection fraction of 30%)
- Atrial fibrillation (diagnosed when patient presented with a stroke 5 years ago)
- Cardioembolic stroke with residual deficits
- Hypertension
- Hyperlipidemia
- Type II diabetes mellitus (complicated by nephropathy, retinopathy, and neuropathy)
- Chronic obstructive pulmonary disease
- Benign prostatic hyperplasia

Medications:

- Aspirin
- Coumadin
- Lisinopril
- Carvedilol
- Nifedipine
- Atorvastatin
- Metformin
- Glargine
- Gabapentin
- Budesonide/formoterol
- Albuterol as needed
- Tamsulosin

Social History:

Mr. Jones lives in an apartment with his wife, who is in charge of all finances, helps with his medications, and all other household chores, "I don't do much around the house." Since his stroke, he has had a caregiver who comes twice a week to help with bathing. He has a shower chair and uses a walker, "I use the walker most when I need something to rest on when I'm out and about."

- Current smoker, 1 pack daily for 50 years. "I've quit in the past, but after my stroke I started up again and haven't been able to drop it again."
- An occasional beer over the holidays.

Physical Exam:

- Vitals: BP 145/81, HR 63, afebrile, weight 210 lbs, height 5′10″ (BMI 30).
- General: Obese, pleasant male, short of breath after walking from the waiting room to the exam room.
- Eyes: Arcus senilis. Pupils equal and reactive to light. Spectacles in place.
- HENT: Well-fitting dentures in place, oropharynx clear. Cerumen impaction bilaterally.
- Cardiovascular: Irregularly irregular. S4 present. 2/6 early-peaking crescendo-decrescendo murmur, loudest at right upper sternal border, without radiation. Jugular venous pressure 9 cm H_2O at 30 degrees. 2+ symmetrical radial and posterior tibial pulses bilaterally.
- Pulmonary: 1 sentence dyspnea. No use of accessory muscles. Distant breath sounds bilaterally, with faint bibasilar crackles. No wheezing.
- Abdominal: soft, nontender
- Neurologic: Cranial nerves II–XII intact. 4+/5 strength left lower extremity (per patient and wife, this is chronic), 5/5 strength remainder of extremities. 2+ patellar reflexes bilaterally, 1+ achilles reflexes bilaterally. Decreased sensation with vibration and monofilament testing bilateral feet to ankles. Coordination intact. No cogwheeling or rigidity.
- Extremities: Chronic venous stasis changes with woody induration. 1 mm pitting edema bilateral lower extremities to mid-shin.
- Skin: Scattered solar lentigo bilateral arms and face. Several old bruises on shins and arms.

Cognitive Evaluation:

- Montreal Cognitive Assessment (MoCA): 17/30 (missed trails B, cube, and clock (0/5); 2/3 on serial 100 s; 1/5 on delayed recall; missed 1 on abstraction and 2 on orientation)
- PHQ-2: 0 points

Gait/Balance Assessment:

- Get Up and Go: Used arms to push out of chair; walked slowly with use of walker with a deliberate, narrow gait. Unsteadiness on turn. Returned slowly to chair and used arms to return to seated position. Some pursed lip breathing at the end of this. The total time it took for him to walk 10 feet and back was approximately 30 seconds.
- Static Balance Tests: No difficulty with feet together. Unable to hold semi-tandem for more than a second. Unable to place feet in proper position for full tandem.

Case 2

Mrs. Smith is a 75-year-old female who presents to establish care. She has no symptoms or concerns.

Past Medical History:
- Hypertension
- Hypothyroidism

Osteoporosis Medications:
- Amlodipine
- Levothyroxine
- Alendronate

Social History:
She has been living alone since her husband of 47 years passed away last year. Before he passed away, she was his primary caregiver. She continues to pay her own bills, does her own grocery shopping, and does not require help with any Instrumental Activities of Daily Living or Activities of Daily Living, "I've always been independent." Enjoys organizing and leading discussions at her book club and going on 2-mile walks with friends several times a week.
- Never smoker.
- One glass of wine at book club, weekly.

Physical Exam:
- Vitals: BP 121/74, HR 72, afebrile, weight 135 lbs, height 5′5,″ BMI 22.5
- General: Well-developed female, appearing younger than stated age
- Eyes: Pupils equal and reactive
- HENT: Thinning hair. Well-fitting dentures in place
- Cardiovascular: Regular rate and rhythm. No extra heart sounds. 2+ symmetrical radial and posterior tibialis pulses
- Pulmonary: Comfortably breathing on room air. Clear to auscultation bilaterally
- Abdomen: Soft, nontender
- Neurologic: Cranial nerves II–XII intact. 5/5 strength bilateral upper and lower extremities. Sensation intact to light touch and vibration throughout
- Skin: Several seborrheic keratoses on arms

Cognitive Evaluation:
- Montreal Cognitive Assessment (MoCA): 27/30 (4/5 delayed recall)
- PHQ-2: 0 points

Gait/Balance Assessment:
- Get Up and Go: Able to rise from chair without use of side arms and it takes her approximately 15 seconds to walk 10 feet, turn, and return to her chair.
- Static Balance Tests: No difficulty with semi-tandem and feet together. Lost balance with full tandem after 5 seconds. Normal for her age.

Considerable uncertainty exists on when and how to screen older adults for diseases such as cancer, cardiovascular disease, and diabetes. In part, this is because the oldest and the sickest patients are often excluded from the studies that provide the evidence-base for screening guidelines. For example, there is a paucity of randomized controlled trial data to guide cancer screening in adults older than 75 years of age [1].

Age-based screening guidelines provide thresholds for screening a geriatrics population with the goal of maximizing benefit over harm. For example, because after age 75, the older adult is generally less likely to benefit from cancer screening, harm from screening may outweigh potential benefit. While age-based guidelines hold value, these guidelines are based on the *average* life expectancy for a given age, that is, they rest on the assumption that two older adults age 76 years old will each live the same number of years before they die. As exemplified by the two patients we will discuss, there is significant heterogeneity in life expectancy for older adults.

A patient's life expectancy matters for decisions about whether to screen for a disease because if the patient is not likely to live long enough to die from the disease, then he or she will not benefit from a screening program. For example, a frail older adult whose life expectancy is shortened by other comorbidities and declining functional status may be more likely to die *with* that colon cancer than *from* that colon cancer. Furthermore, screening tests carry potential harm such as complications from the screening procedure. Clinicians should individualize decisions about screening taking into account the heterogeneity among older adults of the same age and patient preferences.

Using cancer screening as a paradigm, this chapter suggests a five-step person-centered framework for screening decisions for older adults:

1. **Recognize the heterogeneity of aging and factors that influence life expectancy.**
2. **Identify the current societal screening guidelines for older adults and their differences.**
3. **Understand characteristics of screening tests, such as lagtime to benefit, potential immediate harms, and screening biases.**
4. **Elicit patients' preferences and values to guide shared decision-making.**
5. **Consider a patient's predicted life expectancy, likelihood to benefit accounting for test characteristics, and patient preferences when making individualized screening decisions in older adults.**

1. **Recognize the heterogeneity of aging and factors that influence life expectancy.**

"Heterogeneity of aging" refers to the broad range of "phenotypes" among older adults. Multiple studies have examined how the following factors may help account for the large variation in disease and disability that is seen in older adults of the same age group [2]. These factors include:
- Environment
- Childhood diseases
- Health behaviors
- Genetic links

Considering the multitude of factors that influence how we age, it may be less surprising how much life expectancy can vary for patients in the same age group. When median life expectancies are stratified by quartile (see ◘ Fig. 28.1), the heterogeneity of aging and life expectancy is readily apparent [1].

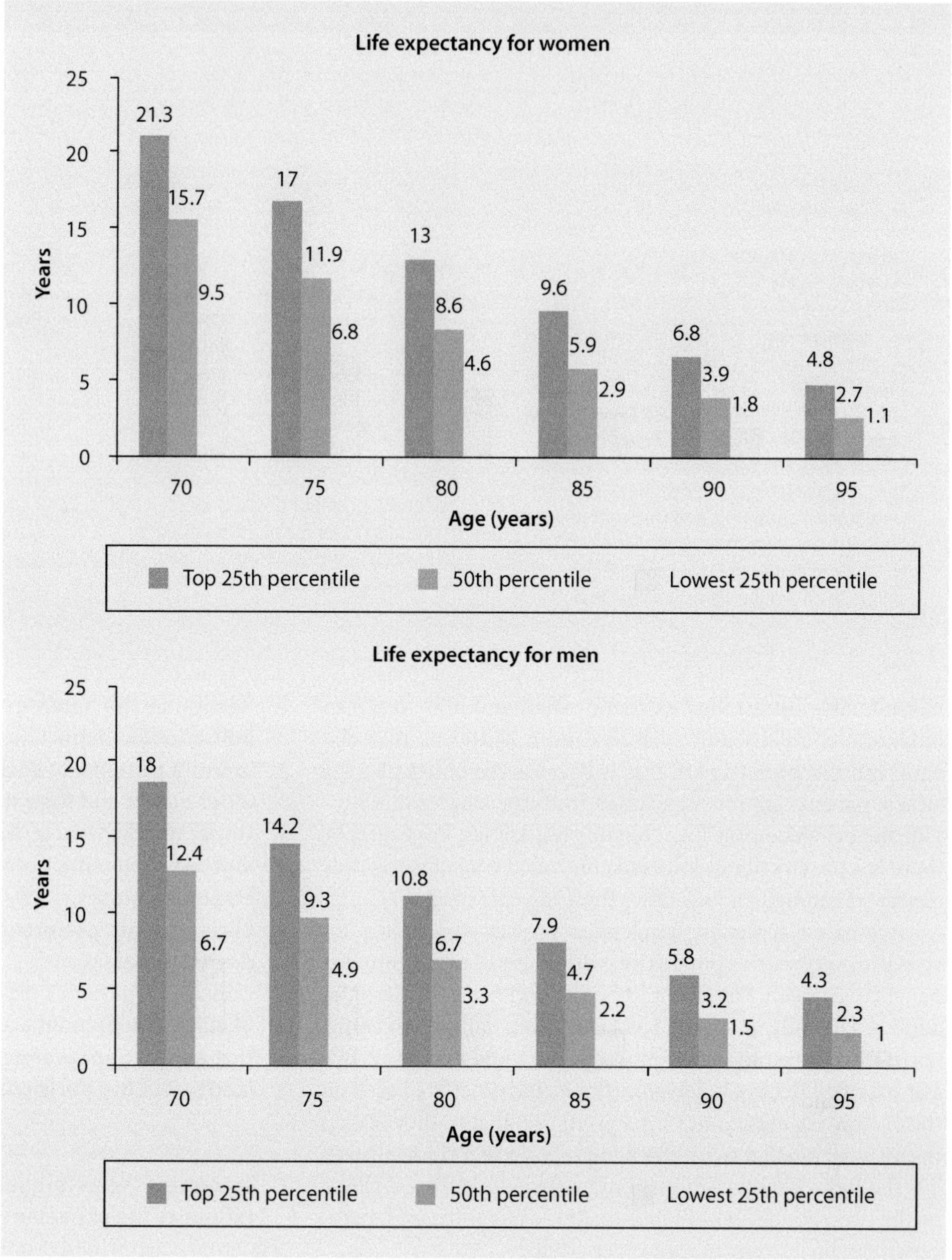

Fig. 28.1 Median life expectancy by quartile of overall health status

28.2.1 Factors That Influence Life Expectancy

Evidence suggests that many factors other than age exert a strong influence on a patient's life expectancy. Such factors include:

- Sex (females live longer)
- Physical function
- Cognitive function
- Comorbid medical conditions (i.e., congestive heart failure, cancer, COPD, diabetes)
- Ethnicity
- Socioeconomic status
- Environmental factors (i.e., diet, exercise, pollution)
- Genetics

28.2.2 No One Has a "Crystal Ball" (and Not All Patients Want One)

A prognosis is a predication about what is most likely to happen to a patient in the future, and the science of prognostication is early in its development. While this chapter provides examples of tools that can help clinicians make predictions about a patient's life expectancy, it is important to remember that these predictions are only probabilities. For example, it would be inappropriate to tell Mrs. Smith, "I have great news, you will live to 92 years old!" A more adept communication would be to tell Mrs. Smith, "It is my assessment than you are in excellent health, and patients who are in excellent health often live well into their 90s." Further, for a variety of personal or cultural reasons, some older adults prefer not to discuss their life expectancy, though studies suggest that many do and the vast majority would like to at least be provided the option to discuss it.

28.2.3 Tools to Improve Prediction of Life Expectancy

Inherent uncertainty of prognostication aside, studies suggest that combining clinical judgment with evidence-based prognostic tools results in more accurate predictions than either alone [3].

Examples of evidence-based prognostic resources include:

- Actuarial tables
- Census reports
- Life expectancy tables
- E-prognosis – ▶ www.eprognosis.org (a compilation of prognostic indices for mortality in older adults with multiple comorbidities)
- Palliative Performance Index (for patients of any age with a terminal cancer)
- Literature that explores mortality rates on the basis of health status

Before using any tool to make a prediction for a patient, it is important to consider whether it was studied in a population that included people similar to your patient, as well as how accurately the tool has performed when tested in other populations [3].

(a) **Life Expectancy Tables Stratified by Overall Health**

Life expectancy graphs provide a general idea of the distribution of median life expectancies for a given sex and age. Clinicians can stratify patients into life expectancy quartiles based on their clinical judgment of whether that patient's health status is above (75th percentile), at (50th percentile), or below average (25th percentile) for their age and sex [1].

Case Application of Lifetable Graphs by Overall Health Status to Predict Life Expectancy for Mr. Jones and Mrs. Smith

For example, a clinician might consider Mr. Jones to be in the lowest quartile due to his functional problems such as needing help with showers, transfers, medications, and other instrumental activities of daily living. He also has multiple medical problems including coronary artery disease, ischemic cardiomyopathy, diabetes, and history of stroke. Using the lifetables graphs, his life expectancy is an estimated 4.9 years (75-year-old male, lowest quartile).

In contrast, Mrs. Smith might be considered in the highest quartile as she is quite functional and has minimal comorbidity. Using the lifetables graphs, her life expectancy is an estimated 17 years (75-year-old female, highest quartile).

In this case example, despite both individuals being the same age, differences in sex and our estimate of quartile ranking based on health status suggest a significantly different life expectancy.

(b) **Life Expectancy Tables Stratified by Functional Status**

After age and sex, function is the strongest predictor of life expectancy [1]. Estimating quartiles can be difficult, so some clinicians stratify patients based on function. One study even used epidemiological data to create life expectancy tables organized into three functional groups associated with different life expectancies:

- Independent
- Mobility Disabled (inability to walk half a mile and/or walk up and down a flight of stairs without help)
- ADL Disabled (needing help with bathing, transferring, dressing, eating, or using the toilet) (See ◘ Fig. 28.2)

Case Application of Lifetable Graphs by Function to Predict Life Expectancy for Mr. Jones and Mrs. Smith

Using life expectancy tables based on that study (see ◘ Fig. 28.1, Functional Status Lifetable Graph), Mr. Jones is considered ADL disabled and would therefore be in the lowest quartile of life expectancy for his age group (4 years). In contrast, Mrs. Smith is considered independent, and would therefore be in the highest quartile of life expectancy for her age group (13 years).

Women	Life expectancy (years)		
Age	Independent	Mobility disabled	ADL disabled
70	16.7	15.7	11.5
75	13.2	12	8.2
80	10.3	9	6
85	8	6.9	4.6

Men	Life expectancy (years)		
Age	Independent	Mobility disabled	ADL disabled
70	12.1	10.7	6.5
75	9.4	7.9	4.4
80	7.2	5.7	3.1
85	5.8	4.4	2.3

◘ **Fig. 28.2** Median life expectancy by quartile of overall functional status. (Data extrapolated from Table 1 of Keeler et al. [20])

(c) **Prognostic Indices**

A prognostic index is a clinical tool that quantifies the contributions that various components of the history, physical exam, and labs make toward a diagnosis, prognosis, or likely response to treatment. In the example of a prognostic index provided in (◘ Fig. 28.3) [1], answering 11 questions (e.g., history of diabetes, difficulty walking several blocks) about Mr. Jones will generate a prediction of his mortality risk within the next 5 years (69%) and 9 years (92%). A compilation of prognostic indices and a guide to interpreting and communicating their results can be found at ► www.eprognosis.org.

2. **Identify the current societal cancer screening guidelines for older adults and their differences.**

Approximately 39.6% of the US population will be diagnosed with cancer at some point during their lifetime [4]. In an effort to promote early detection and decrease mortality, the US Preventive Services Task Force (USPSTF), American Cancer Society (ACS), and other specialty societies have developed cancer screening guidelines. Differences in guidelines exist for various reasons including:

1. *Differences in guideline panel's structure*. Guideline panel members may be comprised of specialists, primary care clinicians, or both. Panels often include other healthcare experts including epidemiologists, public health specialists, or statisticians. The composition of the panel likely influences perspectives through which evidence is interpreted. For example, oncologists, whose clinical practice consists of diagnosed cancer patients and whose

a

I. Age		65–69: 0 points
		70–74: 1 point
		75–79: 3 points
		80–84: 5 points
		85+: 7 points
2. Sex	Female: 0 points	Male: 3 points
3.Weight	BMI: <25 2 points	
Height		
703 X (Weight in pounds/height in inches^2)		
Body mass index (BMI) = ____		
4. Would you say your health in general is		Excellent/very good: 0 points
		Fair/poor: 2 points
5. Have you ever been told by a doctor or health professional that you had		
a. Emphysema/chronic bronchitis?		
	No: 0 points	Yes: 2 points
b. A cancer? (do not include skin cancer unless it was melanoma)		
	No: 0 points	Yes: 2 points
c. Diabetes (include borderline diabetes)		
	No: 0 points	Yes: 2 points
6. Because of a physical, mental, or emotional problem, do you need the help of other persons in handling routine needs such as everyday household chores, doing necessary business, shopping, or getting around for other purposes?		
	No: 0 points	Yes: 2 points
7. By yourself, and without using any special equipment, how difficult is it for you to walk a quarter of a mile—about 3 city blocks?		
	a. Not at all difficult: 0 points	
	b. A little difficult to very difficult: 3 points	
	c. Can't do at all/do not do: 3 points	
8. Which best describes your cigarette use?		
a. Never smoked (less than 100 cigarettes in your entire life): 0 points		
b. Former smoker: 1 point		
c. Current smoker (smoke some days or every day): 3 points		
9. During the past 12 months, how many times were you hospitalized overmight?		
	None: 0 points	
	Once: 1 point	
	Twice or more: 3 points	

b

Result based on score:
Your total score is 20

Five and nine year mortality		
Points	Risk of 5 years mortality (95% CI)	Risk of 9 years mortality (95% CI)
0 – 1	2% (1 – 3)	7% (4 – 13)
2 – 3	4% (3 – 5)	8% (6 – 11)
4 – 5	6% (5 – 7)	16% (13 – 19)
6 – 7	9% (7 – 10)	26% (23 – 29)
8 – 9	13% (12 – 15)	33% (29 – 37)
10 – 11	23% (20 – 25)	52% (48 – 56)
12 – 13	35% (32 – 38)	58% (53 – 62)
14 – 15	43% (39 – 47)	75% (69 – 80)
16 – 17	59% (54 – 63)	83% (76 – 88)
≥18	69% (63 – 73)	92% (86 – 96)

◘ **Fig. 28.3** (**a**, **b**) Sample prognostic index to predict risk of 5- and 9-year all-cause mortality. (Adapted from: Schonberg et al. [18])

exposure is predominantly to witness the benefits of treatment, may be more likely to be biased toward more aggressive screening guidelines. On the other hand, primary care physicians, who more frequently see patients that screen negative for cancer, may be biased toward more conservative screening guidelines.
2. *Differences in weight assigned to evidence.* For cancer screening, scientific evidence and statistics help describe the continuum of benefit versus harm. However, guidelines are essentially value judgments as to where to set thresholds for recommendations.

As previously discussed, age-based guidelines are complicated for older adults given the relative lack of data in this population as well as the variation in screening benefit versus harm based on life expectancy. The following section reviews the current screening guidelines for asymptomatic patients at average risk for malignancy, highlighting those specific to older adults and taking into account life expectancy.

28.2.4 Breast Cancer

For women 75 years or older, the USPSTF recommendation states that the current evidence is insufficient to assess the balance of benefits and harms of screening mammography [5]. The American Cancer Society (ACS) recommends screening should continue as long as the patient is in good health and expected to live 10 years or longer [7]. The American College of Obstetrics and Gynecology (ACOG) recommends offering annual mammography for patients >40 years of age without specification of age-based thresholds or life expectancy [9].

28.2.5 Cervical Cancer

For women age 65 or older, both the USPSTF and the ACS recommend against screening if there has been prior adequate screening and the last three tests have been normal [5, 7]. Also, patients who have had a total hysterectomy (uterus and cervix removed) for reasons not related to cervical cancer and pre-cancer do not need continued testing. All women who have been vaccinated against HPV should still follow screening recommendations.

28.2.6 Colorectal Cancer

The USPSTF, ACS, and American College of Gastroenterology (ACG) recommend screening for patient ages 50–75 years [7]. There are various screening methods available, which the ACG has grouped into cancer prevention tests and cancer detection tests (◘ Table 28.1) [5, 10]. There should be shared decision-making regarding the type of screening test to pursue, as the data does not clearly demonstrate that any one screening strategy is superior to another. The best test is the one that is most likely to promote patient adherence to screening over time [6]. The guideline emphasizes individualized screening for colorectal cancer in adults aged 76–85 years. Adults in this age group who have never been screened for colorectal cancer are more likely to benefit and should be considered for screening. However, screening is most appropriate for patients who are healthy enough to undergo treatment if cancer is detected, and do not have comorbid conditions that would significantly limit life expectancy [6].

◘ **Table 28.1** Cancer prevention and detection tests (if any of the tests other than colonoscopy are positive, need to do colonoscopy) [7]

Cancer prevention tests[a]	Cancer detection tests
Colonoscopy (every 10 years) CT colonography (every 5 years)[b] Flexible sigmoidoscopy (every 5 years) Double-contrast barium enema (every 5 years)	Fecal immunochemical test (FIT) (annual)[c] Guaiac-based fecal occult blood test (FOBT) (annual) Stool DNA test (every 3 years)

[a]Preferred over detection tests per ACG recommendations
[b]Preferred radiographic screening alternative, per ACG recommendations
[c]Preferred cancer detection test, per ACG recommendations

28.2.7 Lung Cancer

The USPSTF recommends annual low-dose computed tomography (LDCT) for all adults 55–80 years of age who have a 30 pack-year smoking history and currently smoke or quit within the last 15 years. Screening should be discontinued once a person has not smoked for 15 years or develops a health problem that substantially limits life expectancy or the ability or willingness to have curative lung surgery [5]. The ACS recommends screening for annual LDCT for patient aged 55–74 years of age who are in good health [7].

28.2.8 Prostate Cancer

The USPSTF recommends against prostate-specific antigen (PSA)-based screening for prostate cancer for men 70 years and older [5]. The ACS recommends shared decision-making for PSA testing starting at 50 years of age [7]. The American Urological Association (AUA) recommends shared decision-making with annual PSA for patients 55–69 years of age. They do not recommend screening in patients ≥70 years old or with less than a 10–15 year life expectancy [11] (◘ Table 28.2).

Table 28.2 Societal recommendations for cancer screening specific to older adults

	US Preventive Services Task Force (USPSTF)	American Cancer Society (ACS) [4]	Specialty Societies
Colorectal cancer	>75 years old: stop screening if life expectancy <10 years		
Lung cancer	55–80 years old with 30 pack-year history and quit in the last 15 years: annual LDCT		
Breast cancer	≥75 years old: likely little benefit to continued screening if life expectancy <10 years	≥55 years: biennial mammograms, but may also opt to continue annually. Continue screening until life expectancy <10 years	
Cervical cancer	≥65 years old with three consecutive negative pap or two consecutive negative pap with contesting within the past 10 years, with most recent test performed 5 years ago: no further screening Hysterectomy with removal of cervix and no history of precancerous lesion: no further screening		
Prostate cancer	PSA testing not recommended	≥50 years old: shared decision-making. Recommend against screening if life expectancy <10 years	55–69 years old: shared decision-making ≥70 years old: stop screening if life expectancy <10–15 years

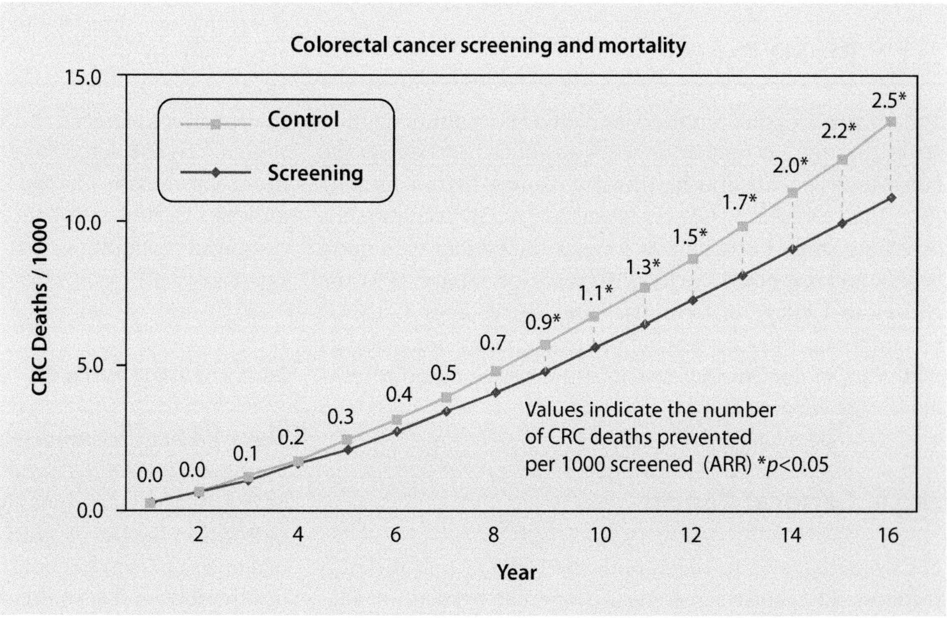

Fig. 28.4 Lagtime to benefit for colorectal cancer screening. (Data extrapolated from Lee et al. [13])

3. **Understand characteristics of screening tests, such as lagtime to benefit, principles of screening, and screening biases.**

"Lagtime to benefit" is defined as the time between the preventive intervention and the time when improved health outcomes are seen [12]. Harm and complications are most likely to occur during the preventive intervention time and benefit is most likely to occur over time. Screening tests differ in lagtime to benefit. For example, studies suggest that on average it takes over 10 years for 1 death from colorectal cancer to be prevented for every 1000 patients screened [13] (see Fig. 28.4). If it generally takes 10 years to benefit from colorectal cancer screening, then harm would likely exceed benefit for an individual with a predicted life expectancy of less than 5 years. Additionally, factors associated with limited life expectancy are also risk factors for complications from interventions, further increasing the risk of harm versus benefit.

Assessing an older patient's life expectancy together with lagtime to benefit may help clinicians identify which patients are more likely to benefit from screening and which patients are more likely to be harmed. The following algorithm has been suggested by experts [12]:

1. Estimate the patient's life expectancy (LE)
2. Estimate the preventive intervention's lagtime to benefit (LtB)
3. (a) If LE >> LtB, the intervention may help and should generally be recommended.
   (b) If LE << LtB, the intervention is more likely to harm and generally should not be recommended.

(c) If LE ~ LtB, the benefits versus harms of the preventive intervention are a "close call" and patient preferences (e.g., the degree of importance placed on the potential benefits and harms) should play the dominant role in decision-making.

While life expectancy and lagtime to benefit are the most important considerations when making screening decisions on an *individual level*, it is also important to understand screening characteristics for *population-based screening strategies*. Fundamental principles of screening include:

(A) *Considerations about the disease for which to be screened*
1. The disease must have an asymptomatic state and progress to a symptomatic state.
2. The disease must be sufficiently prevalent in the population.
3. The disease must cause significant morbidity and mortality.
4. Treatments must be available that will beneficially affect morbidity and mortality.

(B) *Considerations about the tests for the disease*
1. The screening test must be a good test (e.g., sensitivity/specificity, PPV/NPV).
2. The evaluation of the screening program must avoid the common significant biases.
3. The screening test must be cost-effective.

(C) *Considerations about the patient(s) to be screened*
1. The screening test must be acceptable to the patient.
2. The patient must have sufficient life expectancy to derive benefit from the potential life gained by the screening program.

Fundamental principles of screening apply to all populations but certain elements may need special considerations in a geriatrics population. For example, many diseases have a higher prevalence in older adults and can cause significant mortality. However, treatments that beneficially affect morbidity and mortality in the general population may not be beneficial in a population with limited life expectancy. Further, while a screening test may be an accurate test in terms of sensitivity and specificity, it may detect disease that is inconsequential to some populations or give a false sense of increased survival based on potential screening biases.

28.2.9 Screening Biases

28.2.9.1 Overdiagnosis Bias

Overdiagnosis can occur when there is an overestimation of screen-detected cases due to the inclusion of pseudodisease, subclinical disease, or slow growing disease that would not become overt before the patient dies of other causes.

Example: A 76-year-old woman has breast cancer that is unknown to her as she has no symptoms. She may choose to discontinue breast cancer screening, the breast cancer is never diagnosed, and she dies of a heart attack at age 80. She may choose to undergo breast cancer screening, the cancer is diagnosed, she recieves surgery and radiotherapy, and she dies of a heart attack at age 80. This is an example of overdiagnosis bias detected by screening, and treatment ultimately may not have affected her survival.

28.2.9.2 Lead Time Bias

Lead time bias can occur when screening finds an asymptomatic cancer earlier than that cancer would normally have been diagnosed, but the earlier diagnosis does nothing to change the overall disease course or patient mortality. The earlier diagnosis provides the appearance that the screening intervention lead to longer survival, but in actuality, the longer survival was due to the disease being identified earlier.

Example: Two 72-year-old gentlemen with a history of tobacco use have lung cancer. Neither have symptoms. The first patient is diagnosed with lung cancer by a screening test at age 75. He receives treatment and lives up to 80 years old, hence a survival after cancer diagnosis of 5 years. The second patient does not undergo screening, but develops symptoms from lung cancer at age 77 and is diagnosed at that time. He also receives treatment and lives up to 80 years old. However, his survival after cancer diagnosis is only 3 years. Despite both men living to the same age, the screened individual appears to have a longer survival. This is an example of lead time bias (see ◘ Fig. 28.5).

4. **Elicit patients' preferences and values to guide shared decision-making.**

Eliciting patient preferences and values is a key component of shared decision-making. One suggested approach to eliciting these values is a shared discussion about short- and long-term goals. Short-term goals prioritize immediate symptom control and health needs, which may become the only focus for patients with limited life expectancy. Long-term goals include chronic disease management, and preventive care and health promotion, and are more likely to be discussed with healthy older adults.

Some examples of introductory open-ended questions to facilitate these discussions are:

- "What are the values that you hold for your medical care?"
- "What is most important to you in life?"
- "What are your thoughts about cancer screening?"
- "Would you tell me about your past experiences with cancer screening?"
- "What do you hope to gain through screening for ______ cancer?"
- "Discussing cancer screening provides us an opportunity to discuss your overall thoughts and preferences for your medical care. It's important to understand what tests and procedures can do for us, and what we would do with the information these tests would provide. Have you thought about your wishes for how you would like your medical care to help you?"

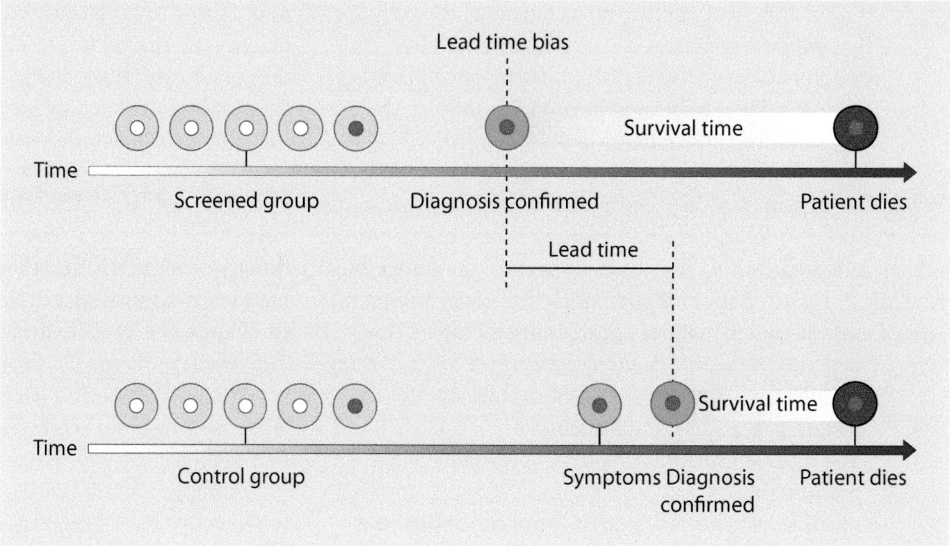

Fig. 28.5 Lead time bias

Shared decision-making usually entails strategies such as ask-tell-ask, in which the clinician (1) asks the patient for his/her understanding about the decision at hand and (2) offers information about the decision such as risks and benefits.

5. **Consider a patient's predicted life expectancy, likelihood to benefit accounting for test characteristics, and patient preferences when making individualized screening decisions in older adults.**

The final step of this framework requires synthesizing all of the information from the previous steps into formulating a final shared decision.

Case Conclusion

Should Mr. Jones and Mrs. Smith be screened for colon cancer?
Final Discussion with Patients:
Clinician: "What do you hope to gain through cancer screening?"
Mr. Jones: "I've got too much on my plate right now to think about another test. I'd love to focus on getting my energy back and getting off some of these medications if possible."
Mrs. Smith: "I want as much time around as possible, I hope to see my grandchildren get married. I don't mind more tests and procedures."

For Mr. Jones, taking into account predicted life expectancy (4–5 years), likelihood to benefit (lagtime to benefit 10 years), and patient preferences, a shared decision with Mr. Jones would likely result in stopping colon cancer screening at this time.

In contrast, a shared decision with Mrs. Smith would likely result in continuing screening given her predicted life expectancy (13–17 years), likelihood to benefit (lagtime to benefit 10 years), and patient preferences.

The decision-making process for these two patients, of the same age but with different health status and goals of care, illustrates how screening decisions in older adults require individualization. This framework can be applied to many other preventive care measures for older adults.

References

1. Walter LC, Covinsky KE. Cancer screening in elderly patients: a framework for individualized decision making. JAMA. 2001;285(21):2750–6.
2. Welch HG, Albertsen PC, Nease RF, Bubolz TA, Wasson JH. Estimating treatment benefits for the elderly: the effect of competing risks. Ann Intern Med. 1996;124:577–84.
3. Justice AC, Covinsky KE, Berlin JA. Assessing the generalizability of prognostic information. Ann Intern Med. 1999:130(6):515–24.
4. https://www.cancer.gov/about-cancer/understanding/statistics.
5. www.uspreventiveservicestaskforce.org.
6. Screening for Colorectal Cancer: US Preventive Services Task Force Recommendation Statement. JAMA. 2016;315(23):2564–75. https://doi.org/10.1001/jama.2016.5989.
7. https://www.cancer.org/healthy/find-cancer-early/cancer-screening-guidelines/american-cancer-society-guidelines-for-the-early-detection-of-cancer.html.
8. https://www.acog.org/Clinical-Guidance-and-Publications/Practice-Advisories/Practice-Advisory-Cervical-Cancer-Screening.
9. https://www.acog.org/About-ACOG/News-Room/Statements/2016/ACOG-Statement-on-Breast-Cancer-Screening-Guidelines.
10. https://gi.org/guideline/colorectal-cancer-screening/.
11. http://www.auanet.org/guidelines/early-detection-of-prostate-cancer-(2013-reviewed-and-validity-confirmed-2015).
12. Lee SJ, Leipzig RM, Walter LC. "When will it help?" incorporating lagtime to benefit into prevention decisions for older adults. JAMA. 2013;310(24):2609–10.
13. Lee SJ, Boscardin WJ, Stijacic-Cenzer I, Conell-Price J, O'Brien S, Walter LC. Time lag to benefit after screening for breast and colorectal

cancer: meta-analysis of survival data from the United States, Sweden, United Kingdom, and Denmark. BMJ. 2013;346
14. Van Zee KJ, Manasseh DM, Bevilacqua JL, et al. A nomogram for predicting the likelihood of additional nodal metastases in breast cancer patients with a positive sentinel node biopsy. Ann Surg Oncol. 2003;10(10):1140–51.
15. Ross PL, Gerigk C, Gonen M, et al. Comparisons of nomograms and urologists' predictions in prostate cancer. Semin Urol Oncol. 2002;20(2):82–8.
16. Justice AC, Covinsky KE, Berlin JA. Assessing the generalizability of prognostic information. Ann Intern Med. 1999;130(6):515–24.
17. Inouye SK, Bogardus ST Jr, Vitagliano G, et al. Burden of illness score for elderly persons: risk adjustment incorporating the cumulative impact of diseases, physiologic abnormalities, and functional impairments. Med Care. 2003;41(1):70–83.
18. Schonberg MA, Davis RB, McCarthy EP, Marcantonio ER. External validation of an index to predict up to 9-year mortality of community-dwelling adults aged 65 and older. J Am Geriatr Soc. 2011;59(8):1444–51.
19. Flaherty JH, Morley JE, Murphy DJ, et al. The development of outpatient clinical glidepaths. J Am Geriatr Soc. 2002;50(11):1886–901.
20. Keeler E, Guralnik JM, Tian H, Wallace RB, Reuben DB. The impact of functional status on life expectancy in older persons. J Gerontol A Biol Sci Med Sci. 2010;65(7):727–33. PMID: 20363833.

Health Promotion and Advance Care Planning (MATTERS)

Contents

Advance Care Planning for Older Adults

Mollie A. Biewald

A. Chun (ed.), *Geriatric Practice*, https://doi.org/10.1007/978-3-030-19625-7_29

29.1 What Is Advance Care Planning?

Advance care planning (ACP) is the process of helping a patient discuss and document wishes for future medical care in the event that they later lose decision-making capacity. Many people lose decision-making capacity when they become seriously ill or are at the end of life, and discussing and documenting preferences ahead of time help a patient's care team, family, and friends respect the patient's wishes for care. This is a process that can be done at any point in care, but ideally starts early, in a setting where a patient has time to think and decision-making is not an emergency. Key elements of advance care planning include identifying a surrogate decision-maker who can make decisions on behalf of a patient who has lost capacity and discussing a patient's preferences for location and focus of medical care in the future.

29.2 What Are the Benefits of Advance Care Planning?

Advance care planning has been shown to have a variety of benefits for the patient, the family or other decision-makers, and the health-care team. Benefits to the patient include increased likelihood that a patient's values and treatment preferences will be respected during serious illness or end of life [4]. Advance care planning has also been shown to increase quality of life during the dying process [17]. Although most people when asked express a wish to die at home, the majority in the United States die in the hospital [15]. Eliciting patient preference on the location they wish to be in when they die can decrease hospitalization at the end of life. Advance care planning has also been shown to increase the likelihood of a patient using hospice services and decrease use of intensive care at the end of life [16].

Benefits to the family of a patient who has expressed wishes for future care include decreased decision-making burden and lower levels of stress and anxiety after a family member's death [5]. For patients who may have multiple family members participating in medical decision-making, having a clear sense of the patient's goals and preferences can decrease the likelihood of conflict between the decision-makers. Finally, health-care professionals have been shown to have less moral distress caring for patients at the end of life when patients have expressed preferences for care [7].

Case Part 1: Edith Jones

Edith Jones is a 70-year-old woman with a history of hypertension who was diagnosed 1 month ago with lung cancer. She comes to the clinic to see her primary care physician, Dr. Hong, for the first time since her new diagnosis. Other than a dry cough, she is feeling well.

Ms. Jones is a retired nurse who lives alone in Queens, NY. She has three grown children. She separated from her husband, Arthur Jones, 5 years ago after he had an extramarital affair, but they remain legally married to one another. Following her cancer diagnosis, she is wondering about prognosis but is not sure how to ask. Her cousin died of cancer on a mechanical ventilator in an ICU a few years ago, and Ms. Jones would never want to be in a similar circumstance, but has never spoken about this with her family as she does not want to worry them.

At the visit, Dr. Hong focuses on making sure Ms. Jones understands her upcoming cancer treatment plan and updating her influenza vaccine. At the end of the visit as Dr. Hong is leaving the exam room, Ms. Jones asks, "do I need to get my affairs in order?" Dr. Hong suggests she make an appointment to come back in 1 week so they can spend dedicated time talking about advance care planning.

29.3 When Should Advance Care Planning Discussions Take Place?

Ideally, the process of advance care planning begins in the outpatient setting with a health-care provider who knows the patient well. A discussion can be triggered by a change in a patient's clinical status, a new diagnosis, or a recent hospitalization. The scope and urgency of the discussion will likely depend on the patient's condition. For example, with a patient who is generally healthy, a conversation may focus on selecting a surrogate decision-maker as a routine part of medical care. In contrast, for a patient who is medically unstable, the discussion might address specific preferences about intubation or other medical treatments being considered by the care team. Advance care planning is a topic that can be readdressed periodically over time.

29.4 Who Should Engage in Advance Care Planning?

Discussing preferences for future medical care is appropriate for all people, as everyone is at risk for serious illness and loss of capacity to make medical decisions. Certain groups of patients are at higher risk of losing capacity. These include older people, particularly those with frailty or multiple medical problems. Patients in the early stages of dementia who are able to express preferences for medical care may benefit from documenting their wishes before their memory loss progresses.

Selecting a health-care proxy can be particularly important for patients whose preferred decision-maker may not correspond to the individual automatically selected as the surrogate by state law. These patients can include those in same sex partnerships, unmarried couples, and single people.

Ideally, ACP discussions should include the patient, any family members or friends the patient wishes to involve, and members of the medical care team. The optimal discussion would include a patient's primary care provider or other practitioner who knows the patient well and is involved over time. This is not always feasible, however, and in a hospital setting, any member of the care team may be involved.

Case Part 2

One week later, Ms. Jones returns to Dr. Hong's office to discuss advance care planning. Dr. Hong explains that advance care planning means thinking ahead about what kind of medical care Ms. Jones would want if her condition worsened.

Dr. Hong explains to Ms. Jones that she can prepare a legal document called a living will that details what types of medical interventions she would or would not want if in the future she were unable to speak for herself.

Dr. Hong also mentions that one of the most important things Ms. Jones can do to help provide guidance to her medical team in the future is to select a health-care proxy. She explains that a health-care proxy is a person that a patient selects who they would trust to make medical decisions on their behalf if in the future they were not able to do so independently. She asks Ms. Jones if there is a person in her life that comes to mind. Ms. Jones mentions that she might want either her youngest daughter who is an ICU nurse or a close friend with whom she worked for many years. She says that she needs time to think about the decision.

Dr. Hong provides Ms. Jones with the health-care proxy form and explains that she can take it home and complete it as long as it is signed by any two witnesses who are adults and who are not the person she chooses as a proxy.

29.5 Documenting ACP Preferences

Advance directives (ADs) are documents that record a patient's wishes for medical care and identify his or her chosen decision-maker. The Patient Self-Determination Act, a federal law passed in 1990 requires hospitals and other health organizations to inform patients of their health-care rights, including the right to prepare an advance directive. ADs become applicable only when a patient loses the capacity to make his or her own health-care decisions.

Many patients have thought about advance directives but have not completed a document or communicated their wishes with their health-care team. A large study of hospitalized elderly patients found that while 76.3% of patients had thought about end-of-life care, only 55.3% had spoken with any member of their care team about their wishes, and only 30.2% had documentation in their chart about their preferences [9]. Another study of community dwelling elders showed that while 88% preferred to die rather than be permanently on a ventilator, only 15% of them had this information listed in their medical record [20]. These studies highlight the importance of asking patients about preferences and encouraging them to document and communicate their wishes.

Substantive vs. Process Directives Advance directives fall into two main categories, substantive and process. In a substantive directive, a patient compiles a list of preferences for care in the event that they are unable to communicate wishes at a future time. Examples of these documents include living wills, a form called Five Wishes (valid only in certain states), and a personal wishes statement. Typically, substantive directives cover topics such as CPR, mechanical ventilation, and other potentially life-sustaining measures. Some include preferences about more specific interventions including whether a patient would want artificial nutrition through a gastric tube or dialysis if he or she developed kidney failure. Topics such as organ donation after death are sometimes addressed as well.

One problem in substantive directives is that it is generally impossible to anticipate the specific clinical scenario a patient might end up in and that the directions contained within may not be relevant to the issues at hand. For instance, many living wills provide specify the type of care to provide if a patient is in an irreversible coma or persistent vegetative state. Many patients who lack capacity are not in a coma or vegetative state, so the guidance provided is not helpful to the medical team. Also, living wills often contain ambiguous language including "extraordinary means" and "unnatural prolongation of life" that require interpretation. For this reason, it is often helpful for patients to complete a process directive, meaning that they designate a person to make medical decisions on their behalf.

A second problem with living wills and other substantive directives is that they are sometimes ignored. A major trial in the 1990s found that living wills had minimal impact on end-of-life care [15]. In addition, many patients are not sure what type of care they would want in a future situation. One study found that 45% of people were not sure what kind of care they would want, even in a hypothetical situation where the outcome of life support would be poor. In this study, Latino and Asian patients and those with limited health literacy were most likely to be unsure what kind of care they would want [13]. Even if a patient initially wants one type of care, this may change over time. For instance, many patients with cancer initially want aggressive treatment, but later in the illness may choose a less aggressive approach. These nuances can be difficult to document clearly in a substantive advance directive.

The second category of advance directives includes process directives. When a patient completes a process directive, they designate a person to make health-care decisions for them if they become incapacitated. In some states, this is known as a health-care proxy (HCP), and in others, it is called a durable power of attorney for health care (DPAHC). A process directive can address some of the disadvantages listed above with substantive directives. The agent is able to make health-care decisions that may not have been anticipated or clear from the substantive directive.

Any patient who has capacity to select a decision-maker can designate or change their HCP. Any person can be selected as HCP, including a family member, friend, or acquaintance, other than the patient's health-care professionals. The HCP form is a legal document signed by the patient and witnessed by any two people other than the person chosen as the decision-maker. Only the patient can select a proxy. A friend or family member cannot designate him or herself as a proxy after the patient has lost capacity. Ideally, the patient will inform the designated person that he or she has been chosen and will inform that person of the patient's wishes for future medical care, but this is not a requirement. Sometimes the medical team will contact an HCP and find that that person was unaware that they had been chosen. In this case, the HCP should do their best to make decisions that are consistent with what they think the patient would have decided for him or herself.

Once a patient has lost capacity, the HCP is the person the medical team will reach out to for decisions regarding invasive procedures and whether to continue or withhold life-sustaining treatments. This can be an overwhelming task for some, so ideally the patient chooses an HCP who is comfortable making such decisions and is familiar with the patient's wishes. A person who is chosen as HCP has the right to decline to participate in decision-making. If a patient loses capacity and has not designated an HCP, a surrogate decision-maker is identified by a hierarchy of family members and acquaintances that is determined by state law. Printable copies of HCP or DPAHC forms for each state can be found online (◘ Fig. 29.1).

◘ **Fig. 29.1** New York State Health Care Proxy

Health Care Proxy

(1) I, ____________________

hereby appoint ____________________
(name, home address and telephone number)

____

____

as my health care agent to make any and all health care decisions for me, except to the extent that I state otherwise. This proxy shall take effect only when and if I become unable to make my own health care decisions.

(2) Optional: Alternate Agent
If the person I appoint is unable, unwilling or unavailable to act as my health care agent, I hereby

appoint ____________________
(name, home address and telephone number)

____

____

as my health care agent to make any and all health care decisions for me, except to the extent that I state otherwise.

(3) Unless I revoke it or state an expiration date or circumstances under which it will expire, this proxy shall remain in effect indefinitely. *(Optional: If you want this proxy to expire, state the date or conditions here.)* This proxy shall expire *(specify date or conditions)*: ____________________

____

____

(4) Optional: I direct my health care agent to make health care decisions according to my wishes and limitations, as he or she knows or as stated below. *(If you want to limit your agent's authority to make health care decisions for you or to give specific instructions, you may state your wishes or limitations here.)* I direct my health care agent to make health care decisions in accordance with the following limitations and/or instructions *(attach additional pages as necessary)*: ____________________

____

____

In order for your agent to make health care decisions for you about artificial nutrition and hydration *(nourishment and water provided by feeding tube and intravenous line)*, your agent must reasonably know your wishes. You can either tell your agent what your wishes are or include them in this section. See instructions for sample language that you could use if you choose to include your wishes on this form, including your wishes about artificial nutrition and hydration.

Fig. 1 (continued)

(5) Your Identification *(please print)*

Your Name ______________________________

Your Signature ______________________________ Date __________

Your Address ______________________________

(6) Optional: Organ and/or Tissue Donation

I hereby make an anatomical gift, to be effective upon my death, of:
(check any that apply)

☐ Any needed organs and/or tissues

☐ The following organs and/or tissues ______________________________

____

☐ Limitations ______________________________

If you do not state your wishes or instructions about organ and/or tissue donation on this form, it will not be taken to mean that you do not wish to make a donation or prevent a person, who is otherwise authorized by law, to consent to a donation on your behalf.

Your Signature ____________________ Date ____________________

(7) Statement by Witnesses *(Witnesses must be 18 years of age or older and cannot be the health care agent or alternate.)*

I declare that the person who signed this document is personally known to me and appears to be of sound mind and acting of his or her own free will. He or she signed (or asked another to sign for him or her) this document in my presence.

Date ____________________	Date ____________________
Name of Witness 1 *(print)* ____________________	Name of Witness 2 *(print)* ____________________
Signature ____________________	Signature ____________________
Address ____________________	Address ____________________
____________________	____________________

NEW YORK STATE | Department of Health

1430 11/15

29.6 How to Discuss Choosing a Health-Care Proxy or Durable Power of Attorney for Health Care?

It is preferable to talk about HCP selection in a one-on-one conversation with the patient, without friends or family members present. This protects the patients from pressure to choose a person who is present. Some clinicians begin the conversation by normalizing the subject: "This is an important topic I bring up with all of my patients." Next, explain what an HCP is, for example, "as your health-care provider, it is important for me to know who I should speak with to make decisions about your care if for any reason you could not speak for yourself. Is there a person you would trust to make health-care decisions for you?" Or "if you were to become so sick that you were not able to make medical decisions, is there a person you would want to speak on your behalf?"

If a patient does choose an HCP, a form should be completed with the patient and HCP's information and signed by two witnesses. One copy should be placed in the medical chart, and a copy should be given to the patient for their records. It is also important to encourage the patient to inform the HCP that they have been chosen and to have a conversation with the selected person about wishes for future medical care. If a patient does not know who to select or does not want to designate an HCP, it can be helpful to explain that if they do not, a surrogate decision-maker will be identified for them based on their state's surrogacy hierarchy.

Case Part 3

Later that evening, Ms. Jones is home alone and starts to feel feverish. Overnight, she feels unable to catch her breath. She calls 911 and EMS comes to evaluate her. She is found to be hypoxic to 85% on room air and tachypneic with a respiratory rate of 30. She is brought to the emergency department where imaging shows a right upper lobe consolidation, and she is started on antibiotics for pneumonia.

Unfortunately, Ms. Jones becomes lethargic and her breathing appears increasingly labored. The emergency physician feels that she may need to be intubated. The resident looks in the medical chart to see whether Ms. Jones ever indicated her wishes regarding CPR and mechanical ventilation and does not find any documents. The medical team determines that Arthur, Ms. Jones's legal husband with whom she has had no contact for 5 years, is the legal surrogate based on New York state law.

The team calls Arthur to ask whether intubation is in line with Ms. Jones's goals of care. He seems surprised to receive the call and says, "I have no idea, just do whatever you think is right."

Ms. Jones is intubated and her endotracheal tube is attached to a mechanical ventilator. She receives medications for sedation and is moved to the medical intensive care unit.

29.7 What Is a Surrogate Decision-Maker?

If a patient loses capacity and has not selected a health-care proxy/durable power of attorney for health care, the medical team can identify a surrogate decision-maker. This is determined by a hierarchy set by state law. In most states, the default hierarchy is in the following order: spouse, adult children, parent, adult siblings, nearest living relative, and close friend [14]. If the patient happens to have a court-appointed guardian, the guardian takes priority. The job of the surrogate is to express to the medical team what he or she thinks the patient would decide if the patient were able to make decisions, using the principle of substituted judgement. If the surrogate is not sure what the patient would want, they should decide based on what they think is in the best interests of the patient. In most states, the following persons are designated to serve as surrogates, in descending order: the spouse (unless divorced or legally separated), an adult child, a parent, and an adult sibling [18].

29.8 What Are Challenges of Surrogate Decision-Making?

A main problem with relying on a surrogate to make decisions is that the surrogate has not been chosen by the patient, and may not be familiar with or agree with the patient's preferences for medical care. An issue that comes up frequently in clinical practice is that there may be multiple surrogate decision-makers who do not agree on care. For instance, if a patient does not have a spouse and has multiple adult children, all of the children have equal right to participate in decisions. It can be logistically complex to incorporate all opinions, particularly if the surrogates do not agree. Another potential issue is that if a patient is still legally married but has not been in a relationship with a former spouse for years, in many cases, the legally married spouse is the legal surrogate, even if the patient has a new partner.

29.9 What Happens When There Is No Surrogate?

Occasionally, a patient loses capacity who has no health-care proxy and no identifiable family or friends. This person may be referred to as "unbefriended." Typically, the medical team does an exhaustive search to identify any acquaintance who might be able to assist with decision-making. If no one can be identified, there are two ways to proceed. One is the legal process of establishing a court-appointed guardian to make decisions. This process can take a long amount of time, and urgent medical decisions may occur before it is possible to establish a guardian. In many states, two physicians together can make decisions regarding medical issues in the absence of HCP or surrogate [14]. If two physicians determine that a treatment will not provide benefit because a patient will die imminently, even with the treatment, life-sustaining therapies can be legally withheld or withdrawn.

Case Part 4

After 3 days of antibiotics in the ICU, Ms. Jones's respiratory status has improved. She is successfully extubated with her daughter Diane at bedside. For the first 24 hours after extubation, she has mild delirium and thinks that she is at home. The next day, her mental status has returned to baseline.

Ms. Jones is moved from the ICU to a general medicine floor. Samira, the third-year medical student on Ms. Jones's team, introduces herself to Ms. Jones and Diane. She asks Diane if she would mind stepping out of the room for a few minutes to speak privately with the patient.

Samira asks Ms. Jones whether she has heard of a health-care proxy before. Ms. Jones recalls that she has and that she had been meaning to select Diane as her proxy. Samira asks her resident to join her in the room to verify and witness the health-care proxy form that they help Ms. Jones complete and then file in the medical chart.

The next day, the medical team and the unit social worker sit down with Ms. Jones and Diane to have a family meeting and discuss goals of care. The resident on the team asks Ms. Jones whether being re-intubated is something she would be willing to go through again if her breathing got worse. Ms. Jones states, "for me, that would be a fate worse than death. I don't want to be hooked up to machines." The social worker asks Ms.

Jones what the most important things to her are, and Ms. Jones lists spending time with her family, being at home, being comfortable, getting stronger, and maintaining independence. Based on these wishes, the resident makes a recommendation that Ms. Jones have a code status of do not resuscitate/do not intubate and that the team pursue discharge to a subacute rehabilitation so that Ms. Jones can try to regain the strength to walk before going home.

The attending physician speaks further with Ms. Jones and Diane, and together they complete a neon pink MOLST form detailing that if her condition worsened, she would want to be re-hospitalized and treated with antibiotics, but that she would never want a feeding tube or to be on a breathing machine again.

29.10 What Is a POLST/MOLST?

One challenge with advance directives is that preferences for care must be communicated and recorded in a way that is easy for health providers to find and interpret when important decisions must be made. The Physician Orders for Life-Sustaining Treatment (POLST) form, in some states called Medical Orders for Life-Sustaining Treatment (MOLST), is a document that contains medical orders, signed by a physician, corresponding to a patient's wishes for care at the end of life. In many cases, the form is printed on neon pink paper to make it quickly identifiable. The form is typically completed after a discussion between the physician and the patient, or if they lack capacity, the health-care proxy or surrogate. The medical orders listed are portable across care sites, meaning that they are valid in settings including the hospital, at home, in a dialysis center, at a nursing home, and in an ambulance. The form lists explicit preferences regarding CPR, limitations on medical interventions, intubation and duration of mechanical ventilation, whether a patient would want to be hospitalized, administration of artificial fluids and nutrition, and use of antibiotics. Preferences for hemodialysis and blood transfusions can also be included. The form is periodically reviewed and renewed by the physicians caring for the patient. A printable copy of the form can be downloaded at ▶ www.POLST.com. Completion of a POLST form is recommended for patients who have an estimated prognosis of 1 year or less. Forms are often completed for nursing home residents (◘ Fig. 29.2).

Case Part 5

Ms. Jones has been home from subacute rehab for a few weeks when she again develops a fever and altered mental status. Her daughter calls 911 and EMS comes to the house. They quickly identify her MOLST form on the refrigerator based on its distinctive color and bring a copy with the patient to a community hospital near her home.

In the ED, she is found to be febrile and obtunded. Chest radiograph is consistent with multilobar pneumonia. The attending physician in the ED feels that the patient may be in the dying process and explains this to Diane. Over the next 2 days, Ms. Jones's condition worsens despite antibiotics. Her family members are at bedside when she dies peacefully later that week.

After the patient's death, Diane expresses to the medical team how relieved she is that Ms. Jones was able to express her preferences regarding code status and care at the end of life so that the family and the team could respect her wishes.

29.11 What Is Code Status?

Patients in the hospital generally have a medical order in their charts stating "full code" or "DNR/DNI." This refers to their wishes for life-sustaining treatment in the event that they lose their pulse or cannot breathe. "Full code" indicates that a patient wishes to receive cardiopulmonary resuscitation (CPR) if they have no pulse in an attempt to restart the heart. It also indicates a wish to be intubated and placed on a mechanical ventilator if they cannot breathe. "DNR/DNI" refers to "do not resuscitate/do not intubate" and means that if a patient loses his or her pulse or ability to breathe, they would not want an attempt at resuscitation. Some consider this to be an order to allow a natural death.

Code status is a topic that some patients are familiar with and may have already decided on, but for others will be unfamiliar. Many patients are familiar with CPR from depictions in television and movies in which the majority of events are depicted as successful [11]. Patients may not realize that in real life, particularly for elderly patients and those with medical comorbidities, the majority do not survive. One major study of patients 65 years and older who received CPR in the hospital found that only 18% survived to discharge [6]. Those patients who do survive often sustain neurologic injury and may not return to prior functional status. Code status is an important topic to discuss with patients and ideally is discussed while the patient is medically stable and not acutely at risk of losing a pulse or the ability to breathe.

A common misconception among patients and families is that choosing to have a DNR/DNI order means that the team will stop providing active care to the patient. In fact, this order is relevant only in the event that a patient does not have a pulse or is not breathing. A DNR/DNI order does not typically change care in any other situation. If a patient with a DNR/DNI order has difficulty breathing, typically the medical team will administer medications and other treatments to ease dyspnea.

29.12 How to Approach Advance Care Planning?

Ideally, advance care planning involves multiple discussions over time with a patient and his or her health-care providers and includes family or friends of the patient's choosing. A patient may be reluctant to discuss future care or lack knowledge about advance care planning, so it is important that the clinician be skilled in communicating about these topics. There are many ways to bring up the topic. The urgency of the discussion, topics covered, and language used will likely depend on the context in which the discussion is taking place. For instance, for an outpatient whose condition is relatively stable, advance care planning may involve a discussion of whether the patient has written a living will and whether they have considered designating a health-care proxy. In contrast, for an unstable patient in the emergency department whose breathing is labored, an urgent discussion of code status and whether to intubate may occur.

29.13 Capacity for Advance Care Planning

Before engaging a patient in a discussion of goals of care, it is important to assess his or her capacity to make medical decisions. In order to have capacity to make a health-care

Fig. 29.2 Pages 1–2 of NYS MOLST form

NEW YORK STATE DEPARTMENT OF HEALTH **Medical Orders for Life-Sustaining Treatment (MOLST)**

THE PATIENT KEEPS THE ORIGINAL MOLST FORM DURING TRAVEL TO DIFFERENT CARE SETTINGS. THE PHYSICIAN KEEPS A COPY.

LAST NAME/FIRST NAME/MIDDLE INITIAL OF PATIENT

ADDRESS

CITY/STATE/ZIP

DATE OF BIRTH (MM/DD/YYYY) ☐ Male ☐ Female eMOLST NUMBER **(THIS IS NOT AN eMOLST FORM)**

Do-Not-Resuscitate (DNR) and Other Life-Sustaining Treatment (LST)

This is a medical order form that tells others the patient's wishes for life-sustaining treatment. A health care professional must complete or change the MOLST form, based on the patient's current medical condition, values, wishes and MOLST Instructions. If the patient is unable to make medical decisions, the orders should reflect patient wishes, as best understood by the health care agent or surrogate. A physician must sign the MOLST form. All health care professionals must follow these medical orders as the patient moves from one location to another, unless a physician examines the patient, reviews the orders and changes them.

MOLST is generally for patients with serious health conditions. The patient or other decision-maker should work with the physician and consider asking the physician to fill out a MOLST form if the patient:

- Wants to avoid or receive any or all life-sustaining treatment.
- Resides in a long-term care facility or requires long-term care services.
- Might die within the next year.

If the patient has a developmental disability and does not have ability to decide, the doctor must follow special procedures and attach the appropriate legal requirements checklist.

SECTION A Resuscitation Instructions When the Patient Has No Pulse and/or Is Not Breathing

Check one:

☐ **CPR Order: Attempt Cardio-Pulmonary Resuscitation**
CPR involves artificial breathing and forceful pressure on the chest to try to restart the heart. It usually involves electric shock (defibrillation) and a plastic tube down the throat into the windpipe to assist breathing (intubation). It means that all medical treatments will be done to prolong life when the heart stops or breathing stops, including being placed on a breathing machine and being transferred to the hospital.

☐ **DNR Order: Do Not Attempt Resuscitation (Allow Natural Death)**
This means do not begin CPR, as defined above, to make the heart or breathing start again if either stops.

SECTION B Consent for Resuscitation Instructions (Section A)

The patient can make a decision about resuscitation if he or she has the ability to decide about resuscitation. If the patient does NOT have the ability to decide about resuscitation and has a health care proxy, the health care agent makes this decision. If there is no health care proxy, another person will decide, chosen from a list based on NYS law.

SIGNATURE ☐ Check if verbal consent (Leave signature line blank) DATE/TIME

PRINT NAME OF DECISION-MAKER

PRINT FIRST WITNESS NAME PRINT SECOND WITNESS NAME

Who made the decision? ☐ Patient ☐ Health Care Agent ☐ Public Health Law Surrogate ☐ Minor's Parent/Guardian ☐ §1750-b Surrogate

SECTION C Physician Signature for Sections A and B

PHYSICIAN SIGNATURE PRINT PHYSICIAN NAME DATE/TIME

PHYSICIAN LICENSE NUMBER PHYSICIAN PHONE/PAGER NUMBER

SECTION D Advance Directives

Check all advance directives known to have been completed:

☐ Health Care Proxy ☐ Living Will ☐ Organ Donation ☐ Documentation of Oral Advance Directive

DOH-5003 (6/10) Page 1 of 4 *HIPAA permits disclosure of MOLST to other health care professionals & electronic registry as necessary for treatment.*

Fig. 2 (continued)

THE PATIENT KEEPS THE ORIGINAL MOLST FORM DURING TRAVEL TO DIFFERENT CARE SETTINGS. THE PHYSICIAN KEEPS A COPY.

LAST NAME/FIRST NAME/MIDDLE INITIAL OF PATIENT ______ DATE OF BIRTH (MM/DD/YYYY) ______

SECTION E **Orders For Other Life-Sustaining Treatment and Future Hospitalization When the Patient has a Pulse and the Patient is Breathing**

Life-sustaining treatment may be ordered for a trial period to determine if there is benefit to the patient. If a life-sustaining treatment is started, but turns out not to be helpful, the treatment can be stopped.

Treatment Guidelines No matter what else is chosen, the patient will be treated with dignity and respect, and health care providers will offer comfort measures. *Check one:*

☐ **Comfort measures only** Comfort measures are medical care and treatment provided with the primary goal of relieving pain and other symptoms and reducing suffering. Reasonable measures will be made to offer food and fluids by mouth. Medication, turning in bed, wound care and other measures will be used to relieve pain and suffering. Oxygen, suctioning and manual treatment of airway obstruction will be used as needed for comfort.

☐ **Limited medical interventions** The patient will receive medication by mouth or through a vein, heart monitoring and all other necessary treatment, based on MOLST orders.

☐ **No limitations on medical interventions** The patient will receive all needed treatments.

Instructions for Intubation and Mechanical Ventilation *Check one:*

☐ **Do not intubate (DNI)** Do not place a tube down the patient's throat or connect to a breathing machine that pumps air into and out of lungs. Treatments are available for symptoms of shortness of breath, such as oxygen and morphine. (This box should ***not*** be checked if full CPR is checked in Section A.)

☐ **A trial period** *Check one or both:*

☐ **Intubation and mechanical ventilation**

☐ **Noninvasive ventilation (e.g. BIPAP), if the health care professional agrees that it is appropriate**

☐ **Intubation and long-term mechanical ventilation, if needed** Place a tube down the patient's throat and connect to a breathing machine as long as it is medically needed.

Future Hospitalization/Transfer *Check one:*

☐ **Do not send to the hospital unless pain or severe symptoms cannot be otherwise controlled.**

☐ **Send to the hospital, if necessary, based on MOLST orders.**

Artificially Administered Fluids and Nutrition When a patient can no longer eat or drink, liquid food or fluids can be given by a tube inserted in the stomach or fluids can be given by a small plastic tube (catheter) inserted directly into the vein. If a patient chooses not to have either a feeding tube or IV fluids, food and fluids are offered as tolerated using careful hand feeding. *Check one each for feeding tube and IV fluids:*

☐ **No feeding tube** ☐ **No IV fluids**

☐ **A trial period of feeding tube** ☐ **A trial period of IV fluids**

☐ **Long-term feeding tube, if needed**

Antibiotics *Check one:*

☐ **Do not use antibiotics.** Use other comfort measures to relieve symptoms.

☐ **Determine use or limitation of antibiotics when infection occurs.**

☐ **Use antibiotics** to treat infections, if medically indicated.

Other Instructions about starting or stopping treatments discussed with the doctor or about other treatments not listed above (dialysis, transfusions, etc.).

Consent for Life-Sustaining Treatment Orders (Section E) (Same as Section B, which is the consent for Section A)

SIGNATURE ______ ☐ Check if verbal consent (Leave signature line blank) DATE/TIME ______

PRINT NAME OF DECISION-MAKER ______

PRINT FIRST WITNESS NAME ______ PRINT SECOND WITNESS NAME ______

Who made the decision? ☐ Patient ☐ Health Care Agent ☐ Based on clear and convincing evidence of patient's wishes ☐ Public Health Law Surrogate ☐ Minor's Parent/Guardian ☐ §1750-b Surrogate

Physician Signature for Section E

PHYSICIAN SIGNATURE ______ PRINT PHYSICIAN NAME ______ DATE/TIME ______

DOH-5003 (6/10) Page 2 of 4 *This MOLST form has been approved by the NYSDOH for use in all settings.*

decision, a patient has to have the ability to understand information about their illness and the proposed options and make and communicate a choice that is consistent with his or her values. A patient may lack the capacity to understand complex medical treatment options, but still have the ability to select a person who they trust to make medical decisions on their behalf. It is common to encounter a situation where a patient with dementia is not able make and communicate a decision about a nuanced treatment like mechanical ventilation, but that same person may be able to easily identify which family member they prefer to serve as HCP.

29.14 What Is the Process for Discussing Goals of Care?

Extensive work has been done by Anthony Back, Robert Arnold, James Tulsky, and others to improve clinicians' communication with patients on prognosis and preferences for care [1]. The following framework for holding an advance care planning discussion is based on their work as well as the SPIKES framework for communicating serious news [2]:

1. Prepare: consider ahead of time who needs to be present for the discussion. Consider details of the patient's medical condition, including treatment options and

prognosis. Decide the setting where the discussion will be held (for instance, at bedside or in a family room if the patient is in a shared room). Decide who will run the meeting if multiple team members will be present. Turn pagers and phones off and have tissues available.

2. Perception: find out what the patient knows about his or her condition and how much he or she wants to know. Potential ways of asking include:
   "What have the doctors told you so far about your condition?"
   "What do you know about your illness?"
   "Some of my patients want to know a lot of medical information, and others do not want to hear medical information directly at all. What do you prefer?"
3. Invitation: ask for permission to share information or continue the discussion.
   "Would it be okay if I provide an update on your condition?"
   "Do you feel comfortable talking about how best to care for you if your condition worsens?"
   "Would it be okay if we talk about the best case and worst-case scenarios, given your illness?"
4. Knowledge: share information in a clear, direct way. Patients may want to know information about treatments and prognosis. Avoid using medical jargon. If a patient wants to know prognosis, it is helpful to ask if there is a particular reason the patient is asking, for instance, hoping to live until a holiday or life event. When discussing prognosis, provide an estimate in a range: "most people in your situation live for a range of time between weeks and months."
5. Respond to emotion: after sharing serious news, check in with the patient to see how the news is received. For instance: "is it surprising to hear this news?" or "I can't imagine what it's like to hear this."
6. Explore the patient's goals: for example, if a patient has just learned that prognosis is limited, it may be helpful to ask: "knowing that time is short, what is most important to you?" or "when you think about the future, what worries you most?" "What does quality of life mean to you?" It is helpful to explore what makes a patient's life meaningful and what activities are most enjoyable. Many patients have preferences about the type of setting they prefer to be in, whether it is home or a facility where they can receive skilled medical care. Common fears include being connected to machines long term, inability to recognize loved ones, and loss of independence, cognitive function, or dignity. Some patients fear having a painful or prolonged dying process.
   - It can be helpful to explore a patient's experience with loss, for instance, whether he or she has known someone who spent time in the ICU on a ventilator. Patients who have had an experience with such care may have a clear opinion of whether they would be willing to undergo the same type of care.
7. Make a recommendation based on the patient's goals. For example, if a patient with cancer expresses a desire to maximize time with family and avoid hospitalization, a recommendation could be "given your wish to be at home and be with your family, I would recommend that we focus our treatments on your comfort and avoid bringing you back to the hospital. I would not recommend putting you on machines if you got sicker as this would mean being in the hospital and being unable to communicate with your family." If a patient expressed that being alive in any condition is the most important thing, a recommendation could be "given your wish to prolong life in any way possible, if your condition worsens, I would recommend that we do everything possible to keep you alive, including trying to sustain your life with machines."
   Specific topics that can be helpful to address include preferences for resuscitation, preferences for life-sustaining treatments at the end of life including artificial nutrition/hydration and mechanical ventilation, and preferences about whether to return to the hospital.

29.15 What Tools Help People Decide on Care Preferences?

While a discussion between a patient and his or her medical providers is an important part of advance care planning and determining goals of care, many tools exist to help patients and families consider their wishes for future care. Many patients do not have much exposure to what different care options look like in reality. One online tool that walks patients through choosing a medical decision-maker and deciding on future care with video and text tools is called PREPARE for Your Care, developed by Dr. Rebecca Sudore, a geriatrician [12]. The site is ▸ prepareforyourcare.org and was rated easy to use by the majority of subjects.

Another tool to help patients think about how they prefer to be cared for is called the Conversation Project. A free downloadable tool in multiple languages is found at ▸ theconversationproject.org. This resource includes questions that help a patient reflect on their preferences for care in the setting of serious illness or at the end of life, how involved they want to be in decision-making, and thoughts on quality versus quantity of life. A study was done at the University of Colorado using this tool to engage third-year medical students in learning about advance care planning [10]. Following use of the tool, more than 90% of the medical students reported having thought about their own preferences for future medical care. Both of these resources are free and may be useful for patients who want additional guidance in advance care planning.

29.16 Who Has Completed an Advance Directive?

Many patients lose the ability to make and/or communicate decisions about medical care during serious illness. In one study looking at adults who died between 2000 and 2006, 70.3% of people lost capacity near the end of life [21]. Fortunately, 67.6% of those who had lost capacity had completed an advance directive. This highlights the large number of patients for whom the medical team may depend on advance care planning and designation of an HCP to guide treatment decisions. A 2017 systematic review of US studies found that 37% of the general adult population had completed an advance directive [19]. Patients who were more likely to have an advance directive included older people, Caucasians, people with a history of chronic disease, and those with a higher education level or socioeconomic status.

29.17 What Barriers Prevent Advance Care Planning?

Barriers to engaging in advance care planning exist on the part of the patient and the clinician and embedded in the medical system [3]. Patients may find the topic anxiety provoking, may be in denial about possible outcomes of an illness, or wish to protect family members from potentially difficult discussions. Clinicians may lack the time to have a conversation about the future, may not have experience or training in such discussions, and may not feel comfortable bringing up the topic. In the medical system, the default if preferences have not been discussed is for life-sustaining treatment, including CPR and mechanical ventilation. Systems to document and communicate patients' wishes are not always standardized across care sites and may be difficult to access or interpret. In order to overcome these barriers, it is important that clinicians receive training and practice in having advance care planning discussions. Standardization of advance directives may help documentation of wishes become more accessible to health-care providers. Increasing public knowledge of advance directives and the importance of selecting a health-care proxy may improve patient engagement in advance care planning.

One inspiring example of a community in which advance care planning has been embraced is that of La Crosse, Wisconsin. The local health system implemented a program called Respecting Choices and used trained facilitators to lead advance care planning discussions that included surrogate decision-makers. The discussions were documented and filed. Local clinicians were educated on the topic. Following this intervention, 90% of people in the community were found to have prepared an advance directive [8]. Ninety-nine percent of advance directives were filed in the medical record at the time of death, and 99% of people received end-of-life care that was consistent with their documented wishes. The goal of advance care planning is to identify how a patient would want to be cared for if his or condition worsens, and the example of La Crosse shows how successful this can be in providing care consistent with a patient's wishes.

References

1. Back A, et al. Mastering communication with seriously ill patients: balancing honesty with empathy and hope. Cambridge: Cambridge University Press; 2009.
2. Baile WF, et al. SPIKES—a six-step protocol for delivering bad news: application to the patient with cancer. Oncologist. 2000;5(4): 302–11.
3. Bernacki RE, Block SD. Communication about serious illness care goals: a review and synthesis of best practices. JAMA Intern Med. 2014;174(12):1994–2003.
4. Bisson JI, et al. Developing a care pathway for advance decisions and powers of attorney: qualitative study. Br J Psychiatry. 2009;194(1):55–61.
5. Detering KM, et al. The impact of advance care planning on end of life care in elderly patients: randomised controlled trial. BMJ. 2010;340:c1345.
6. Ehlenbach WJ, et al. Epidemiologic study of in-hospital cardiopulmonary resuscitation in the elderly. N Engl J Med. 2009;361(1): 22–31.
7. Elpern EH, et al. Moral distress of staff nurses in a medical intensive care unit. Am J Crit Care. 2005;14(6):523–30.
8. Hammes BJ, et al. A comparative, retrospective, observational study of the prevalence, availability, and specificity of advance care plans in a county that implemented an advance care planning microsystem. J Am Geriatr Soc. 2010;58(7):1249–55.
9. Heyland DK, et al. Failure to engage hospitalized elderly patients and their families in advance care planning. JAMA Intern Med. 2013;173(9):778–87.
10. Lum HD, et al. Teaching medical students about "the conversation" an interactive value-based advance care planning session. Am J Hosp Palliat Care. 2017;35(2):324–9.
11. Portanova J, et al. It isn't like this on TV: revisiting CPR survival rates depicted on popular TV shows. Resuscitation. 2015;96:148–50.
12. Sudore RL, et al. A novel website to prepare diverse older adults for decision making and advance care planning: a pilot study. J Pain Symptom Manag. 2014;47(4):674–86.
13. Sudore RL, et al. Uncertainty about advance care planning treatment preferences among diverse older adults. J Health Commun. 2010;15(S2):159–71.
14. Swidler RN. The family health care decisions act: a summary of key provisions, 15 NY St. BA. Health LJ. 2010;32:33.
15. Teno J, et al. Advance directives for seriously ill hospitalized patients: effectiveness with the patient self-determination act and the SUPPORT intervention. J Am Geriatr Soc. 1997;45(4):500–7.
16. Teno JM, et al. Association between advance directives and quality of end-of-life care: a national study. J Am Geriatr Soc. 2007;55(2): 189–94.
17. Tierney WM, et al. The effect of discussions about advance directives on patients' satisfaction with primary care. J Gen Intern Med. 2001;16(1):32–40.
18. Wynn S. Decisions by surrogates: an overview of surrogate consent laws in the United States. Bifocal. 2014;36(1)
19. Yadav KN, et al. Approximately one in three US adults completes any type of advance directive for end-of-life care. Health Aff. 2017;36(7):1244–51.
20. Yung VY, et al. Documentation of advance care planning for community-dwelling elders. J Palliat Med. 2010;13(7):861–7.
21. Silveira MJ, Kim SY, Langa KM. Advance directives and outcomes of surrogate decision making before death. New Eng J Med. 2010; 362(13):1211–8.

Patient Preference, Prognosis, and Decision-Making in Screening and Treatment

Erica Y. Chu

A. Chun (ed.), *Geriatric Practice*, https://doi.org/10.1007/978-3-030-19625-7_30

30

30.1 Geriatric Competencies

At the end of this chapter, the student will be able to:

- 15 - Accurately identify clinical situations where life expectancy, functional status, patient preference, or goals of care should override standard recommendations for screening tests in older adults.
- 16 - Accurately identify clinical situations where life expectancy, functional status, patient preference, or goals of care should override standard recommendations for treatment in older adults.

30.2 Background

Caring for an aging population presents a challenge for medical providers who must apply treatment guidelines to a heterogeneous population of older adults varying widely in prognosis and health preferences. Standard recommendations and guidelines for screening or treatment often revolve around disease-specific information and chronological age, but chronological age for an older adult is often a pale reflection of health status. Variation in functional ability, cognition, comorbidities, and goals of care creates a diverse population in which uniform application of standard treatments does not lead to uniform outcomes. In addition, older adults are often absent or underrepresented in clinical trials, forcing providers to extrapolate from the evidence available to make treatment calls that apply to the older patient. All treatment decisions for an older adult, whether preventive, diagnostic, or therapeutic, must involve an individualized assessment of potential benefits, harms, and values.

Case Part 1

Mr. B is a 65-year-old man with a past medical history of essential hypertension, hyperlipidemia, and paroxysmal atrial fibrillation who presents to establish primary care. During his initial visit, he shares that he is a recently retired newspaper editor who plays tennis, travels frequently with his wife, and easily performs his activities of daily living independently. He manages his own medications and finances without difficulty. He shares with you that his health goals are to pursue any measures that will maintain him in his current state of good health. During his visit, you review with him the age-appropriate cancer screening guidelines for a 65-year-old man. Despite the recommendations of his prior internist, he has never undergone a screening colonoscopy as he felt unable to take time off from his busy career. He asks whether or not you recommend colon cancer screening at this time.

30.3 Screening Interventions: Tailoring to the Older Adult

A high quality screening assessment consists of a test or procedure performed on an asymptomatic individual in order to achieve early detection, early treatment, and thereby better outcomes. In an older adult, the decision to pursue screening tests is often not clear-cut, as the balance between potential long-term gains and short-term harms varies for each individual over time.

30.3.1 Benefits and Harms of Screening

Screening tests are not without potential harms that increase in frequency in older adults. These harms may include complications from the screening test itself or from diagnostic procedures that lead from false-positive results. In the case of colonoscopy screening, patients may not tolerate the bowel prep or sedation, and they face a non-zero risk of procedural complications such as perforation. Patients may have significant anxiety precipitated by the process or results of screening; systematic reviews have found that cancer-specific psychological distress in women after false-positive mammograms may last up to 3 years [1]. Particularly important for older adults, screening interventions may also lead to overdiagnosis and overtreatment of diseases that may have otherwise remained asymptomatic during their lifetimes [2].

Evaluating the long-term gains of screening requires consideration of life expectancy, risk of disease, and time to benefit. For each screening test, there is a lapse of time between the time of screening to the time of benefit, i.e., mortality reduction. For colonoscopy and mammography screening, the estimated lag time to benefit is approximately 10 years [3]. Therefore, not all older adults can be expected to live long enough to see the improvement in survival that screening is intended to provide. For an individual whose life expectancy is limited, the likelihood of harm from screening is greater than potential benefit.

30.3.2 The Role of Prognostication in Screening Decisions

How do providers determine life expectancy and fitness for screening? The health of older adults is often complicated by competing risks to their quality of life and mortality. Navigating these risks is the process of prognostication—to make a prediction regarding life expectancy or other health outcomes in order to guide medical decision-making for providers, patients, and families. For older adults, prognostication requires an understanding of how age, disease, and function interact. Older adults contend with physiologic changes that increase their vulnerability to disease and reduce their ability to heal. They usually face more than one chronic illness and confront changes in mobility or cognition that affect their capacity to live independently. Each of these factors exerts an impact, both independently and synergistically, on quality and duration of life.

To estimate life expectancy, providers have several tools available. Prognostic calculators such as the Lee-Schonberg Index and Suemoto Index (available at ▶ www.ePrognosis.com) can be used to estimate all-cause mortality at 10 years. These indices consider not only demographic data such as age and sex but also functional and cognitive status (expressed as the ability to perform basic and instrumental activities of daily living) and multimorbidity (rated by the presence or absence of specific comorbidities that affect mortality such as diabetes, congestive heart failure, chronic lung disease, and cancer).

Alternatively, providers can estimate individual life expectancy by comparing the general health of their patient to that of the average individual of same age in the United States. Walter and Covinsky calculated the upper, middle, and lower quartiles of life expectancy for US men and women in different age groups [2]. By judging whether or not a patient belongs to the top, middle, or lower quartile of health for the average person in their age-sex cohort, providers can obtain a reasonable estimate of life expectancy.

All published guidelines on age-appropriate cancer screening are not identical, as different expert organizations vary in their judgment of the risks and benefits of screening for older adults and the need to reconcile chronological age with individual health factors. In the example of colon cancer screening, the US Preventive Services Task Force guidelines of 2016 recommend routine screening for adults aged 50 to 75 years old and individualized decision-making for adults 76 to 85 years old [4]. In contrast, the American College of Physicians explicitly recommends against screening in individuals over 75 years old or with a life expectancy of less than 10 years [5]. These subtle differences in the suggested times for screening cessation highlight the complexity of these decisions and the need for shared decision-making.

30.3.3 Patient Preferences in Screening Decisions

Patient preferences should always shape treatment goals for older adults when evidence is incomplete or the application of guidelines is not uniform. Studies have shown that many older adults feel strongly about the continuation of cancer screening regardless of increased risks, although this may be explained less by patient values and more by patient and provider uncertainty when estimating and communicating life expectancy [6]. Further studies are needed to explore patient views on screening cessation, but one framework for conceptualizing patient preferences was delineated by Kotwal and Schonberg, who suggested that by eliciting patient values regarding healthcare, individuals can be classified as "maximizers" or "minimizers" [7]. Patients who have a strong faith in preventive healthcare and focus more on potential benefits may wish to be managed on the most aggressive screening guidelines, whereas those who believe "less is more" espouse health beliefs more in line with a conservative application of guidelines.

In the case of Mr. B, he falls into the age group of 50–75 years old, remains functionally independent and cognitively intact, and expresses a desire to pursue all possible preventive health measures. As his provider, you confidently recommend colon cancer screening based on his life expectancy of over 10 years and his goals of care.

Screening in the Older Adult: Take-Home Points

- Decision to screen should consider risk of disease, harms of screening, prognosis, and patient preferences.
- Benefits of screening decrease and potential harms increase with age.
- Lag time to benefit means that harms are likely to outweigh benefit in patients with decreased life expectancy.

Case Part 2

Mr. B's colonoscopy at age 65 is normal with no polyps or other abnormalities identified. Five years later, Mr. B suffers a stroke leading to left-sided upper and lower extremity weakness. With intensive rehabilitation, he regains the ability to ambulate short distances, but he tires quickly and now requires assistance with many activities of daily living (ADLs). After the stroke, his family also notices increasing short-term memory deficits and assumes responsibility for tasks such as medication management and bill paying. During his annual physical at age 75, Mr. B expresses frustration at the loss of independence he has experienced since his stroke. He finds the frequent visits to different doctors' offices and the rehab center to be burdensome, and he wishes to focus his healthcare on interventions that will help him regain as much function as possible. His daughter accompanies him to the appointment and asks if her father is due for another routine screening colonoscopy.

At age 75, Mr. B's state of health has much evolved since your initial visit with him 10 years ago. Not only has his list of comorbidities increased, but his functional and cognitive abilities have declined to the extent that he is no longer independent in his ADLs. These changes in functional status play a key role in reevaluating prognosis. Whether using the median life expectancies for Mr. B's age-sex cohort or the prognostic calculators available, Mr. B's current life expectancy is less than 10 years. In addition, the changes in health for Mr. B have been accompanied by a shift in his goals of care. His desire to refocus his healthcare around the priority of function indicates that on the spectrum of "maximizers" to "minimizers," he has repositioned his preferences closer to the other end of the continuum. Pursuing colon cancer screening at this time is unlikely to help Mr. B live longer or improve his level of independence. Therefore, you recommend against repeating a screening colonoscopy for Mr. B. Instead, you focus on reducing polypharmacy and referring him to home-based physical therapy.

Case Part 3

Five years later, Mr. B is taken to a local hospital after passing out at home and is admitted with profound anemia and guaiac-positive stools. He undergoes a diagnostic colonoscopy and imaging and is diagnosed with stage III colon cancer. Mr. B undergoes a surgical resection of the mass, is discharged to a subacute rehabilitation center, and is instructed to follow up with his oncologist for adjuvant chemotherapy. Mr. B presents to you for follow-up after his discharge from rehab and asks for your opinion regarding his next treatment steps. Currently Mr. B is able to slowly walk approximately 25 feet with a rolling walker. He requires assistance with dressing and bathing but is able to toilet independently. His family reports that his short-term memory has worsened since his hospitalization, and he sometimes becomes disoriented to the time of day or location. He has lost 15 pounds over the past 6 months and still struggles with poor appetite and low energy. He spends most of his days in his reclining chair, napping or watching television. He shares with you that he is anxious about the prospect of chemotherapy as he continues to feel weak since his surgery. He worries about the potential side effects of chemotherapy and how treatment will affect his time with his grandchildren. He wishes to focus on interventions that will minimize symptoms and maximize the quality of time with his family.

30.4 Treatment in the Elderly: Redefining Appropriate Treatment Options and Outcomes

Just as with screening tests, medical decision-making about therapeutic interventions for older adults is often complex. Medications or procedures that may be standard protocol for a younger population take on a different risk-benefit ratio when applied to the older adult. All patient-centered treatment decisions must account for age-related changes in physiology, potential for treatment toxicities, prognosis, and goals of care.

30.4.1 Prognostication for Therapeutic Interventions

While prognosis in the setting of screening largely focuses on life expectancy from normal aging, clinicians must also predict outcomes of specific diseases and treatment interventions to determine the therapies from which patients are most likely to benefit. As different diseases have different trajectories, a multitude of single disease prognostic tools have been developed. For example, patients diagnosed with cancer may be given median life expectancies determined by the primary type and location of cancer and staging. Clinicians may use the Seattle Heart Failure Model to predict mortality for patients with heart failure, the BODE index to assess survival in COPD, or the MELD score in patients with cirrhosis.

These single disease prognostic tools may be sufficient to assess prognosis for the general population but often offer an incomplete picture for older adults who are rarely seen with only a single disease. Multimorbidity, frailty, and impaired functional status exert powerful effects on illness trajectory and response to treatment for older adults. Therefore, clinicians must use other measures in order to assess an older adult's suitability for different treatments. In the field of oncology, functional ability is rated as "performance status," and two commonly used scales are the Eastern Cooperative Oncology Group performance score (ECOG) and the Karnofsky Performance Status Scale (◘ Tables 30.1 and 30.2).

◘ **Table 30.1** Eastern Cooperative Oncology Group

Grade	ECOG
0	Fully active, able to carry on all pre-disease performance without restriction
1	Restricted in physically strenuous activity but ambulatory and able to carry out work of a light or sedentary nature, e.g., light house work, office work
2	Ambulatory and capable of all self-care but unable to carry out any work activities. Up and about more than 50% of waking hours
3	Capable of only limited self-care, confined to bed or chair more than 50% of waking hours
4	Completely disabled. Cannot carry on any self-care. Totally confined to bed or chair
5	Dead

Modified from Oken et al. [8]

These measures of performance status are used by oncologists to judge whether or not the potential side effects and toxicities of treatment such as chemotherapy are likely to outweigh benefit. In patients who are deemed frail and unlikely to tolerate chemotherapy, clinicians may recommend less intensive, dose-reduced therapies or focus on more palliative strategies.

Treatment of older adults may also be tailored based on the assessment of frailty. While performance status largely focuses on an individual's level of function, frailty also takes into account the physiologic changes seen with aging and disease. Frailty is a geriatric syndrome defined as a state of decreased physiologic reserve producing poor resilience and increased vulnerability to stressors [10]. Frailty represents the concept that "age is just a number," as different individuals of the same chronological age have different physiologic abilities to respond to disease and treatment. There are multiple indices to quantify frailty such as the Fried phenotype, which takes into account strength, mobility, nutrition, self-reported energy levels, and activity (◘ Table 30.3). Although current use of frailty indices has been limited more to research set-

Table 30.2 Karnofsky Performance Status Scale

Score	Karnofsky Performance Status
100	Normal, no complaints; no evidence of disease
90	Able to carry on normal activity; minor signs or symptoms of disease
80	Normal activity with effort; some signs or symptoms of disease
70	Cares for self; unable to carry on normal activity or to do active work
60	Requires occasional assistance, but is able to care for most of own personal needs
50	Requires considerable assistance and frequent medical care
40	Disabled; requires special care and assistance
30	Severely disabled; hospital admission is indicated although death not imminent
20	Very sick; hospital admission necessary; active supportive treatment necessary
10	Moribund; fatal processes progressing rapidly
0	Dead

Modified from Schag et al. [9]

tings rather than clinical practice, there is mounting evidence linking frailty to adverse health outcomes, from all-cause mortality, rates of hospitalization, falls, and disability to treatment complications such as chemotherapy intolerance and postoperative complications [10, 11].

Given the impact of frailty and functional status on health outcomes, clinicians must consider these measures in the development of any treatment plan for older adults. A robust 85-year-old may benefit from treatments that would cause more harm to a frail 65-year-old, and the reverse is true. Any treatment that is considered or offered to an older adult must account for individual needs, vulnerabilities, and prognosis.

Prognostication in the Older Adult: Take-Home Points

- Chronological age is an insufficient basis for treatment decisions.
- Older adults face multiple comorbid conditions, age-related physiologic changes, and shifts in mobility and cognition. To encapsulate the impact of all of these factors, assessments that measure function are the best measures of prognosis for the older adult.

Table 30.3 Phenotypic frailty

Frailty criteria	*Measurement*
Weight loss	≥10-pound weight loss in past year
Weakness	Grip strength in lowest 20% based on sex and BMI
Exhaustion	Self-reported exhaustion
Slowness	Walking speed over 15 feet in lowest 20%
Low activity	Kilocalories per week expended in lowest 20%
Scoring:	
Frailty status	*Number of criteria*
Robust	0
Pre-frail	1–2
Frail	3–5

Modified from Fried et al. [12]

30.4.2 Integrating Patient Preferences, Goals, and Interdisciplinary Care

Eliciting patient preferences, values, and expectations is the final vital piece of developing treatment plans for older adults. Clinicians must recognize that patients may have priorities other than living as long as possible, and quality of life is defined differently by each individual. Understanding patients' motivations and goals allows providers to frame the harms and benefits of any intervention in the context of what is important to the patient and thereby make recommendations that incorporate both evidence-based clinical data and patient values.

In addition, as caring for the frail older adult involves multiple dimensions of health, an interdisciplinary team is best poised to deliver patient-centered care and increase the likelihood of positive treatment outcomes. Primary care providers must rely on the expertise of specialists who possess the most up-to-date clinical experience with disease-specific treatments and prognostic information, whereas internists and geriatricians may perform comprehensive geriatric assessments to shed insight on the patient's functional status and risk of geriatric syndromes. Physical and occupational therapists provide additional evidence and support for cognitive and functional ability, and involvement of social work is critical as older adults may have limited social supports or other challenges to their care in the community. Each of these team members plays a necessary role in ensuring ideal treatment outcomes and quality of life.

30

Case Conclusion

Mr. B's prognosis differs greatly when seen from a disease-specific versus a function-focused lens. Stage III colorectal cancer is a potentially curable disease, and some studies have shown that selected elderly patients in good health obtain the same mortality benefit from adjuvant chemotherapy compared to their younger counterparts without significant increase in toxicities [13]. However, Mr. B's performance status is suboptimal, which is not exclusively the product of his new cancer diagnosis; his functional and cognitive decline began years prior with the onset of stroke. His ECOG score is 3 and his Karnofsky Performance Score is 50, denoting an individual with limited ability to perform self-care who leads a sedentary life. Mr. B also meets frailty criteria with his weight loss, low activity level, slow gait speed, and report of low energy. By all measures of function, Mr. B is at risk for worse health outcomes from his colon cancer and potential chemotherapy compared to younger adults or to non-frail members of his age cohort. Mr. B is also able to express his current health priorities and preferences. His desire to focus on quality of life rather than longevity should reframe all treatment decisions within that paradigm—if chemotherapy extends duration of life but at the expense of side effects and further degradation in function, this is unlikely to be a treatment plan satisfactory to the patient. You agree with Mr. B that given his goals, functional status, and frailty, adjuvant chemotherapy may not be the best course of action. You agree to collaborate with his oncologist to individualize further oncologic care, exploring disease-specific treatments only if they meet Mr. B's goals plus palliative measures to promote symptom management and quality of life.

In older patients with serious illness, clinicians are often faced with balancing the harms and benefits of therapies where potential toxicities are great, the margin of benefit may be slim or uncertain, and the tradeoffs in quality of life may be unacceptable to the patient. Chronological age does not reflect any one older adult's fitness for treatment or goals of care; providers must therefore be willing to deviate from standard treatment protocols to individualize care based on the functional status, prognosis, and preferences of each older adult.

References

1. Walter LC, Schonberg MA. Screening mammography in older women: a review. JAMA. 2014;311(13):1336–47.
2. Walter LC, Covinsky KE. Cancer screening in elderly patients: a framework for individualized decision making. JAMA. 2001;285(21):2750 6.
3. Lee SJ, Boscardin WJ, Stijacic-Cenzer I, Conell-Price J, O'Brien S, Walter LC. Time lag to benefit after screening for breast and colorectal cancer: meta-analysis of survival data from the United States, Sweden, United Kingdom, and Denmark. BMJ. 2013;346:e8441.
4. US Preventive Services Task Force, Bibbins-Domingo K, Grossman DC, Curry SJ, Davidson KW, Epling JW Jr, et al. Screening for colorectal cancer: US Preventive Services Task Force Recommendation Statement. JAMA. 2016;315(23):2564–75.
5. Wilt TJ, Harris RP, Qaseem A; High Value Care Task Force of the American College of Physicians. Screening for cancer: advice for high-value care from the American College of Physicians. Ann Intern Med. 2015;162(10):718–25.
6. Schoenborn NL, Lee K, Pollack CE, Armacost K, Dy SM, Bridges JFP, et al. Older adults' views and communication preferences about cancer screening cessation. JAMA Intern Med. 2017;177(8):1121–8.
7. Kotwal AA, Schonberg MA. Cancer screening in the elderly: a review of breast, colorectal, lung, and prostate cancer screening. Cancer J. 2017;23(4):246–53.
8. Oken MM, Creech RH, Tormey DC, Horton J, Davis TE, McFadden ET, et al. Toxicity and response criteria of the Eastern Cooperative Oncology Group. Am J Clin Oncol. 1982;5(6):649–55.
9. Schag CC, Heinrich RL, Ganz PA. Karnofsky performance status revisited: reliability, validity, and guidelines. J Clin Oncol. 1984;2(3):187–93.
10. Robinson TN, Walston JD, Brummel NE, Deiner S, Brown CH, Kennedy M, et al. Frailty for surgeons: review of a National Institute on Aging Conference on Frailty for Specialists. J Am Coll Surg. 2015;221(6):1083–92.
11. Handforth C, Clegg A, Young C, Simpkins S, Seymour MT, Selby PJ, et al. The prevalence and outcomes of frailty in older cancer patients: a systematic review. Ann Oncol. 2015;26(6):1091–101.
12. Fried LP, Tangen CM, Walston J, Newman AB, Hirsch C, Gottdiener J, Seeman T, Tracy R, Kop WJ, Burke G, McBurnie MA, Cardiovascular Health Study Collaborative Research Group. Frailty in older adults: evidence for a phenotype. J Gerontol A Biol Sci Med Sci. 2001;56(3):M146–56.
13. Kim JH. Chemotherapy for colorectal cancer in the elderly. World J Gastroenterol. 2015;21(17):5158–66.

Special Considerations for Sites/Models of Care

Contents

Sites of Care for the Older Adult: Outpatient, Post-Discharge, Hospice

Dustin E. Suanino and Gary H. Brandeis

A. Chun (ed.), *Geriatric Practice*, https://doi.org/10.1007/978-3-030-19625-7_31

31.1 Geriatric Primary Care Facility

The geriatric primary care clinic is a general medical practice that focuses on the evidence-based management and prevention of illness in the outpatient setting. The practice is geared toward a holistic care approach for the older adult to ultimately improve or maintain function by using a geriatric comprehensive assessment. Ideally the practice has an interdisciplinary team that consists of but is not limited to geriatric-specialized physicians, geriatric nurse practitioners, nurses, geriatric social workers, and administrative assistants. Additionally, some practices will have laboratory technicians, geriatric pharmacists, physical therapists, dieticians, geriatric psychiatrists, neuropsychologists, and more depending on the services the clinic provides.

31.1.1 Eligibility

All community-dwelling people regardless of health status, socioeconomic status, religion, gender, sexuality, or culture who are over 65 years of age have the right to receive outpatient geriatric care. Individual clinics will determine what insurances they will accept, which includes Medicare and Medicaid.

31.1.2 Establishment

The geriatric practice should provide both a comfortable and safe environment for evaluation. In the book *Fundamentals of Geriatric Medicine*, it provides recommendations to optimize the older adult's experience in the clinic specially when the older adult has sensory and functional impairment [1]. Autonomic dysfunction is commonly encountered in older adults and increases vulnerability to excessively cool or warm settings, especially when the patient is dressed appropriately for the outside temperature. Accordingly, the examining rooms should be kept between 70° and 80 °F. Brighter lighting is required for adequate perception of the physician's facial expression and gestures by the older patient whose lenses admit less than half the light they did in youth, due to cross-linking of lens proteins. Presbycusis, which is present in over 50% of older adults, makes background noise more distracting and interferes with the patient's hearing. Even in a quiet setting, the high tone loss of presbycusis makes consonants most difficult to discriminate. Therefore, speaking in a lower than usual pitch helps the patient hear, and facing the patient directly improves communication by allowing lip reading. The patient's eyeglasses, dentures, and hearing aid should always be brought to and used at the visit. Chairs with a higher than standard seat or a mechanical lift to assist in arising are useful for frail older persons with quadriceps weakness, and a broad-based step stool with handrail can make mounting and dismounting the examining table safe. Drapes for the patient should not exceed ankle length so as not to be a risk for tripping and falling.

31.1.3 Scheduled Visit

Initial or follow-up evaluation of the older adult is generally prolonged, especially those with multiple disorders and psychosocial issues affecting their care. Dividing the assessment into more than one visit can spare both patient and physician an exhausting and inefficient prolonged encounter. Other personnel in the practice can help collect information by questionnaires before the visit, from previous records, and from patient and family prior to the physician's contact. Good care should be delivered within a reasonable time allocation consistent with contemporary patterns of primary care. One hour for a new visit and 30 minutes for a follow-up are an absolute minimum in most environments.

During the scheduled visit, the comprehensive geriatric assessment (CGA) is utilized. It is an overall evaluation of the health status of the older adult assessing various components of the patient's life. These domains include cognitive function, affective disorders, sensory impairment, functional status, nutrition, mobility, social support, physical environment, caregiver stress, health-related quality of life, and spirituality. The results from the CGA can help establish a baseline for future comparisons, form diagnoses, monitor treatment, provide prognostic information, and screen for occult conditions. This would subsequently invoke a coordinated team approach to improve quality and efficiency of care from the multidisciplinary team and/or consultants.

Geriatric-trained practitioners are able to delineate between normal aging and atypical signs and symptoms of the older adult to determine diagnoses and management of common and uncommon illnesses. Furthermore, geriatric-trained practitioners are able to manage care of older patients with multiple disorders in order of severity. It is also important for the practitioner to be able to coordinate care to other providers, appointed caregivers, and ancillary staff that participate in the patient's care.

31.1.4 Urgent Visit

Similar to some primary care practices, patients are able to walk-in or schedule an urgent visit to be evaluated, triaged, and if appropriate treated for an acute illness. Escalation of care and transition to an acute care facility can be determined and managed accordingly with the help of the interdisciplinary team.

31.1.5 Home Visit

Some geriatric practices may provide a service to do home visitations if needed. This provides another level of insight into a patient's environment and daily functional status. How mobility may affect function in a particular setting, nutrition, medication use and adherence, and social interactions and support can all be assessed by the practitioner or by a multidisciplinary team from the practice.

31

31.1.6 Availability

Most practices have a call center that is available 24 hours, 7 days a week. Patients can leave messages for the geriatric primary care clinic for non-emergent needs. For emergent needs the call center can also contact the on-call practitioner from the practice to appropriately triage and provide recommendations over the phone.

31.1.7 Continuity

Depending on the practice and the relationship it has with nearby hospitals, geriatric-trained outpatient practitioners may have access to the hospital and follow their patients when they are admitted for higher level of care. This promotes a trusting relationship with the patient and their caregivers. There may even be a decrease or prevention in medical errors given the continuity and insight the provider has on the patient. This can also provide a smoother transition of care back to the geriatric primary care practice after discharge from the hospital.

31.1.8 Consultant

Physicians from any specialty can refer their patients who are 65 years and older to the geriatric primary care practice to be evaluated and managed for geriatric syndromes such as falls, memory impairment, functional impairment, and more. The patients do not necessarily need general medical management because they already have a primary care provider in the community.

31.2 Home-Based Primary Care Programs

The number of patients living with multiple chronic medical conditions continues to rise and place a growing burden on the US healthcare system. By 2030, almost 20% of the US population will be older than 65 years with the greatest increase in those over 85 [2]. A portion of these elderly chronically ill patients suffer from functional and cognitive impairment, making them unable to leave their homes to access routine medical care. The number of these homebound seniors will grow to over three million in the coming decade.

Before the mid-twentieth century, physician home visits were a common practice. In 1930, 40% of all physician visits took place in the home; by 1980 less than 1% did, leaving many homebound patients without regular medical care [3]. Recent increases in Medicare reimbursement for home care visits, coupled with the growing need, have contributed to a slow increase in the number of home care providers and practices over the last decade [4, 5]. They are led either by physicians or by nurse practitioners. Other programs include private individual and group practices, Veterans Affairs Medical Center programs, and initiatives affiliated with health systems or academic medical centers.

In addition to continuity of care, other services that can be provided include urgent medical care, transitional care, and multidisciplinary teams with community partners providing longitudinal, primary care.

31.2.1 Eligibility

All community-dwelling people regardless of socioeconomic status, religion, sexuality, or culture who are over 65 years of age and are considered "homebound" are eligible for home-based primary care. There may be additional eligibility requirements depending on each program such as providing care to a limited radius or safety concerns in the home or neighborhood.

The Medicare definition of "homebound" is a patient who has a condition due to an illness or injury that restricts their ability to leave their place of residence except with the aid of supportive devices such as crutches, canes, wheelchairs, and walkers, the use of special transportation, or the assistance of another person or if leaving home is medically contraindicated. Issues such as poverty, isolation, and poor health literacy complicate the delivery of care.

31.2.2 Scheduled Visits

Unlike primary care practices, given the needs of patients who are confined to the home, this model of care requires more regularly scheduled home visits. Similar to the geriatric primary care practice, the goal is to focus on the evidence-based management and prevention of illness. This model is also geared toward a holistic care approach for the older adult to ultimately improve or maintain function by using a geriatric comprehensive assessment. Interdisciplinary team consists of but is not limited to geriatric-specialized physicians, geriatric nurse practitioners, nurses, geriatric social workers, and administrative assistants. Additionally, some practices will have visiting laboratory technicians, geriatric pharmacists, physical therapists, dieticians, geriatric psychiatrists, visiting practitioners from different disciplines, visiting radiology technicians, and more depending on the services the program provides.

When doing home visitations, it is essential that good care be delivered within a reasonable time frame consistent with contemporary patterns of outpatient primary care.

The comprehensive geriatric assessment should also be utilized similar to that of the geriatric outpatient primary care practice. Doing this in the home provides another level of insight and further activates the interdisciplinary team to optimize a patient's care.

31.2.3 Urgent Visit

Patients or their caregivers can request an urgent visit by calling the call center of the home-based care program. There will be someone available to speak with from the team to triage the concern and if necessary send the on-call provider to evaluate and manage the patient's acute concerns. Escalation of care and transition to an acute care facility if in line with the patient's wishes can be determined and managed accordingly with the help of the interdisciplinary team.

31.2.4 Availability

Home-based primary care will likely have a call center that is available 24 hours, 7 days a week. Patients can leave messages for the home-based care program for non-emergent needs. For emergent needs the call center can also contact the on-call practitioner from the program to appropriately triage and provide recommendations over the phone.

31.2.5 Continuity

Depending on the home-based care program and the relationship it has with nearby hospitals, geriatric-trained practitioners may have access to the hospital and follow their patients when they are admitted for higher level of care. This promotes a trusting relationship with the patient and their caregivers. There may even be a decrease or prevention in medical errors given the continuity and insight the provider has on the patient. This can also provide a smoother transition of care back to the home-based care program after discharge from the hospital.

31.3 Discharge from the Hospital

When a patient is being discharged from the hospital, there are several options of where to go. Everyone's first choice is to go home. This is usually the case, and depending on insurance, services such as visiting nurse and therapy can be arranged for home. Moreover, it is possible now to even receive intravenous therapy at home. In some locals, there are visiting doctor programs that have doctors or non-physician providers (NPPs) go to the patient's house. If a patient cannot go home, there are several alternatives.

31.3.1 Acute Hospital Rehabilitation

Geriatric rehabilitation should start in the acute setting. Many times the patient is too ill to participate, but the planning should still occur. Early mobilization is essential for recovery after or even during the acute illness. This is especially true after a stroke or joint surgery. Unfortunately, this can be difficult if the illness is severe, if dementia is present, or if delirium occurs. Regardless, therapy should be involved early to help with the post-acute setting decisions.

31.3.2 Acute Post-rehabilitation Facilities (Inpatient Rehabilitation Facilities (IRF))

These can be within an acute hospital or freestanding. A patient must have a specific qualifying diagnosis. For example, some of these are stroke, multiple trauma, hip fracture, traumatic brain injury, and burns. While these patients are medically complex, they must be able to participate in therapy services in order to enter an IRF.

These facilities have clinicians in-house along with full-time nursing. Clinician visits are required at least five days/week. The patient must also be able to participate in at least two therapies – speech-language pathology (SLP), physical therapy (PT), and/or occupational therapy (OT) – 3 or more hours/day for at least 5 days/week. For example, Medicare fully covers the first 20 days, and then days 21–100 require a co-pay. If a patient is unable to go home after an IRF stay, they can transfer to a skilled nursing facility (SNF).

31.3.3 Veterans Health Administration Geriatric Evaluation and Management (GEM) Program

Veterans Administration Medical Centers may have an inpatient GEM or an outpatient GEM in a clinic setting. This service provides comprehensive and interdisciplinary geriatric evaluation. Providing the service is a physician, nurse, occupational or physical therapist, dietitian, or pharmacist and in the inpatient setting a nurse practitioner. When available a geriatrician is part of the team. The inpatient GEM units are either part of the VA nursing home program or be similar to a SNF-type unit. The goal is to provide the veteran and his/her family with a plan of care upon discharge.

31.3.4 Long-Term Acute Care Hospitals (LTACHs)

These facilities were started by the Centers for Medicare and Medicaid Services (CMS) in the 1980s to care for medically complex patients that still needed significant care, but not in an acute setting. LTACHs were reimbursed at a rate less than the acute hospital, but more than nursing homes. The mean length of stay is ≥25 days. This was done to decrease the cost of hospital care. The original intent of these hospitals was for the care and weaning of mechanically ventilated patients.

This was broadened to include multiple comorbidities with an acute chronic condition. In 2007, approximately 400 LTACH existed. Most of these facilities were clustered in the eastern and south-central United States. As the cost of these facilities increased, CMS instituted rules to manage the costs, for example, not allowing new LTACHs to open. While these hospitals admitted very sick patients, studies did not demonstrate that they prolonged survival and they were costly [6, 7]. In order to tighten admission criteria for LTACH, CMS instituted new rules. For example, for a person to be admitted directly from hospital to LTACH; the patient needed to spend at least 3 days in an intensive care unit (ICU) and was on a ventilator for a minimum of 96 hours. Also needed is a primary medical diagnosis such as active infection, stroke, amputation, ventilator weaning, spinal cord injury or burns. In addition to the primary condition, an active additional condition needs to be present such as high-flow oxygen, pleural chest tube, frequent transfusions, or mechanical ventilation. With these new regulations, it is anticipated that the number of LTACH will decrease. A clinician and nurse needs to be onsite at all times. Medicare pays in full for the first 20 days, and then a co-payment is needed for days 21–100.

31.4 What Is a Nursing Home?

In the past a nursing home was a place where someone lived who needed help to care for themselves. Today, the definition has expanded to encompass various types of care. In addition, names have changed with a change from nursing home to nursing facility. For example, instead of just nursing home or nursing facility in the title, often there are other descriptors such as rehabilitation center or care center. Officially, the CMS lists two area of care – SNF and nursing facility (NF). These facilities provide 24-hour nursing care in addition to as-needed therapy services. According to 2012 Nursing Home Data Compendium, nationally, women comprise two-thirds of nursing home residents, with 42% being age 85 or older and 85% being greater than age 65 [8]. In this section, different models of nursing homes/facilities will be described.

31.4.1 Skilled Nursing Facility (SNF)

These facilities are usually housed within the nursing home or facility and have beds or units designated for this level of care. They are often called subacute rehabilitation (SAR) or post-acute care (PAC) units. Therefore, the SNF or the SAR part of the facility is much different from the NF or long-term care or custodial care. Today, the SNF can be an extension of the hospital. Most people who enter a SNF come directly from the hospital. They have a skilled need that allows their insurance to pay for the stay. A skilled need is defined as a skilled nursing need and/or skilled therapy need that is needed daily. These skilled needs can include nursing needs such as continuation of intravenous antibiotics after a severe infection or intravenous fluids, monitoring the recovery from a hospitalization for heart failure, new ostomy, stage 3 or 4 pressure ulcers/injury, or other complex wounds requiring nursing level monitoring and care. In addition, SNF entrance criteria can be met if the person requires rehabilitation from a licensed therapist after a stroke or a joint replacement, for example.

The length of stay in a SNF varies depending on the reason the person is admitted to the SNF and their progress with treatment. Insurance coverage often plays a role for length of stay. For example, the maximum length of stay in a SNF is up to 100 days. Often, it is much less if the skilled need is no longer applicable. Although the reason for admittance into a facility is medical, usually the first question asked is about finances. While the practitioner wants to focus on the medical and functional needs of the newly admitted patient, the patient and/or family is concerned with the question of who and how long is insurance going to pay for the stay. While this is a simple question, the answer can be complex and confusing, depending on one's insurance. If one has just straight Medicare, 100% of the cost is covered for the first 20 days. After that, a mandated co-pay is instituted of $164.50 per day for days 21–100 (2018 rate). This rate is set by CMS and must be charged. If the person has no other insurance, they (not the family) are responsible. If the person has a policy, often called Medigap insurance, it will pay the co-pay. If the person has Medicaid as a secondary insurance, Medicaid will cover the co-pay, but depending on the state, may not pay the facility. If the person has a commercial insurance, they usually cover the entire amount for as long as the skilled need is present. The nursing facilities need to provide weekly updates to the insurance company, and they determine when the skilled need is over. There are other plans for dual eligible (Medicare and Medicaid) and Medicare Advantage that have their own rules. Although uncommon, some people have commercial long-term care insurance policies to help defer the cost of SNF and/or NF.

31.4.2 Nursing Facility (NF)

While most patients enter a nursing home via the SNF route, some can enter directly into the nursing home as long-term care (LTC) or custodial residents. Most of the patients entering the SNF go home, but many do not. Studies have varied on the actual number that returns home. For instance, for patients admitted to a SNF after a hip fracture, 33% transitioned to long-term care [9]. In addition, once they are in long-term care, one-quarter are hospitalized within the first year [10]. Others have looked at the percent of hospitalized residents who enter a SNF and them become long-term varies by region and by age of admission to the SNF. For those aged greater than 85, 12% remained in the nursing home 6 months after admission from the hospital [10]. The reasons that they do not go home usually are that the level of care that the person needs cannot be provided in the home. This is due to change in functional ability of the person and inadequate resources to accommodate the needs. While nursing homes are predominately for the elderly, there can be variety of ages and medical conditions living under one roof. This applies both to the SNF environment and more so to LTC. While the patients (residents) living in the home may be elderly – the range can be from 65 to over 100. Some homes have younger patients with functional and/or cognitive deficits. Along with multiple medical problems, there are also a range of cognitive status from intact to severe dementia. Regardless of the medical diagnoses and/or the cognitive abilities, the functional capability of the patient is often paramount. Therefore, maintaining the highest level of function for the patient may be the ultimate goal of care. In the LTC environment, the goals of care may change toward a more palliative approach rather than attending to disease-specific goals. This may culminate in end-of-life discussions with the patient and family. In the NF, activities are tailored for the need of the person. The goal changes from rehabilitation in the SNF to establishing programming that is aimed at the person's cognitive and functional state.

31.4.2.1 The Role of the Physician

Every patient who enters a nursing home must have a physician assigned to them. In some nursing homes, it will be the person's community physician, but more often it will be a physician that is practicing in the home who will be assigned to the patient. While patients have a choice of physicians, the actual physician that will take care of the person in the nursing home is often determined by whom is credentialed in that facility, credentialed with the insurance plan of the patient, and affiliated with the hospital that the patient is affiliated and who is available.

Moreover, many nursing homes have nurse practitioners and less so physician assistants (NPP). While each nursing patient/resident has an attending physician assigned to them, the person may be seen more often by NPP.

By regulation the physician needs to see the patient on admission to perform the admission visit (there is no set time when this has to occur), then monthly for first 3 months, and then every 60 days (NPP and physician may alternate). These are the minimum. Regardless of regulations, most facilities have policies that set when a patient must have a physician or NPP visit. However, a patient can be seen as often as medically necessary.

Regarding patient care, the nursing home physician needs to wear several hats. First, when admitting a patient to the SNF from the hospital, a plan of care needs to be designed to address the reason for the hospitalization. In addition, other comorbidities need to be addressed. For example, a patient is admitted to the hospital for heart failure and then after several days of in-hospital dieresis transfers to the SNF. The SNF has to continue the heart failure treatment but also needs to address the other medical problems the person has such as diabetes, lung disease, osteoarthritis, and/or hypertension. Moreover, a plan for therapy needs to be established including mobility and attention to activities of daily living (ADLs). Therefore, the physician needs to be versed not only in acute medical care (heart failure) but also in chronic care (osteoarthritis affecting mobility) and the interplay of both. For example, when admitting a patient to the nursing home, the admitting orders not only need to include the specific medical treatments for the reason for admission (such as medications for heart failure) including medications and laboratories but also need to address advanced directives, rehabilitative services, treatments, consultations, and discharge planning.

For the NF or long-term care patients, the physician needs to be able to recognize and treat in the nursing home an exacerbation of chronic medical problems. For example, when a long-term patient develops a pneumonia, the physician needs to have not only the knowledge to treat the condition but also the knowledge of what is available to treat the patient. For example, how long will it take to obtain phlebotomy, how long for an x-ray to be completed and results available, and can intravenous therapy be instituted or are antibiotics available. The physician must work with a team in addition to the NPP. Practitioners in the nursing home include physical therapists, occupational therapists, speech-language therapists, social workers, certified nursing assistants, dieticians, recreational therapists, pharmacists, consultants, and of course nurses. The physician must be able to incorporate ideas and recommendations from all these disciplines in order to establish care for the patient.

The physician practicing in nursing homes must be aware of the rules and regulations promulgated by CMS and the individual states. Antibiotic stewardship has become a formal program for nursing homes that is monitored on both the national and state level. Practitioners are being monitored for antibiotic prescription orders with the goal of reducing unneeded or unnecessary antibiotic use. Consultant pharmacists review medications for each patient on a monthly basis and leave suggestions for the physician. Whether the physician agrees with the suggestion or not, it must be answered in a timely fashion.

In summary, the physician practicing in a nursing home needs to able to care for acute medical problems and chronic medical problems and the interaction of both. While this training occurs in a geriatric fellowship, there are insufficient numbers of geriatricians to fulfill the need for all nursing homes. Therefore, other physicians are in nursing homes – internal medicine, family medicine, and hospitalists (in the role of "SNFist"). In addition to the medical problems of the patient, there needs to be a knowledge base for federal and state regulations, diagnostic testing capability of the facility, palliative care, psychosocial needs of the patient and the family, and discharge planning for the patient.

While patients admitted to nursing homes today are similar to those who were cared for in a hospital in the past and/or being transferred to the nursing home from the hospital and even directly from the emergency department, the physician must be confident and capable in his/her skills without having the luxury of instantaneous labs, radiology, or consultation. Each nursing home is required to have a medical director. Currently, the medical director must be a physician. The medical director role is separate from the attending physician role. The time spent in the medical director role must be distinct from time spent in patient care. Most medical directors also have a practice in the nursing home that they are medical directors. The role of the medical director is to work with the director of nursing and the administrator of the home to evaluate and ensure that quality care is being provided. Some of the specific duties include oversight to the home in clinical areas, reviewing policies and procedures of the home, monitoring the practice of clinicians in the home, involvement in the state survey process, root cause analysis of hospitalizations to determine if a hospitalization was avoidable, educating the staff on current clinical issues, and representing the home in the community. AMDA (formerly known as the American Medical Directors Association; now known as PALTC (the Society for Post-Acute and Long-Term Care)) has guidelines for medical directors. Furthermore, a physician can become a certified medical director (CMD) from PALTC. While being a CMD is not required to be a medical director, the training that accompanies the obtaining of a CMS is invaluable to carry out the duties of a medical director. These duties include management skills and knowledge of quality assurance and performance improvement (QAPI) processes.

31.4.3 Models of Nursing Homes

Many nursing homes were built and remain in the model of a hospital: long corridors with semiprivate rooms and appear institutional. However, that is changing with the emphasis on home.

Some examples are Eden, Green House, and Comfort Matters program. These programs combine both the physical space that the person lives with changes in staff training to emphasize the individual.

31.4.3.1 Eden Alternative®/Green House Project®

Dr. Bill Thomas started a project called the Eden Alternative® to make nursing homes more homelike. To become an Eden nursing home, staff needs to be trained and embrace the concepts there needs to be companionship with others, with pets. The home needs to be resident-centered rather than staff-centered. The nursing home has to undergo a culture change.

Building on the Eden philosophy, the Green House Project began to change the physical structure of nursing home to be more homelike. For instance, each unit has a small number of rooms (12 residents per home, mostly private) with its own kitchen and common area and staff that not only cooks but also provides direct care [11].

31.4.3.2 Comfort Matters®

Another model of care is Comfort Matters® that trains staff in the care of dementia patients. For example, while the traditional nursing home strives to keep people out-of-bed during the day and involved in activities, the Comfort Matter approach is that if the person wants to go to bed in the afternoon, he/she is allowed to go to bed. Staff is trained to attempt to ascertain the needs of the person, even if the person is not capable of expressing the need verbally due to dementia.

31.4.3.3 Dementia Care Units

Some homes have specialized dementia care units that are designated after meeting certain requirements. The Joint Commission has specific requirements that must be met for a home/unit to be called a "memory care unit." Some states have regulations for training of staff and for the physical plant, such as accessible and safe outdoor space for the cognitively impaired. For instance, older and inner-city facilities may have difficulty fulfilling the requirements. While the majority of the residents in a nursing home have cognitive impairment, the home cannot be designated as dementia care unit if it has not complied with the regulations [12].

31.4.4 Assisted Living Facilities (ALF)

For some an ALF is an alternative to a nursing home. Rather than being alone in one's own home and/or bring services in for the individual, an ALF provides both personal services and a community setting. Therefore, an ALF may be considered more of a social model of care rather than a medical model, such as a nursing home, that is more attractive to people. Yet, people entering an ALF can be very frail and in need of services that maybe comparable to nursing home residents. An ALF is usually less restrictive than a nursing home. However, these facilities are heterogeneous in nature. While states may have some regulations as to what is called an ALF, they differ so that one facility in one state may be very different that one in another state. In other words, they are less regulated than nursing homes. While some people feel that there should be more regulations or oversight for ALFs, many and the ALF providers do not. ALF should be considered places to live with a variety of services as opposed to a nursing home or facility that provides defined services (such as 24-hour nursing care). Most ALF provide housekeeping, meals, and laundry, assistance with dressing and bathing, and assistance with medications and nursing. The amount and availability of these services vary depending on the individual ALF. These homes are based that the elders living in the facility are there for social programs with varying amounts of medical care.

The large majority of ALF is privately owned and was developed without government funding. ALF can be large apartment-type buildings with common dining and activity areas, or they can be smaller homes that have a few rooms. Most units in these buildings will have kitchens and bathrooms and are furnished by the resident. They are less intuitional in appearance than a nursing home. They can be freestanding or be within or associated with a nursing home. Some even have special care units such as memory impairment units. Often, these special care units need to adhere to state guidelines to be advertised as such. The guidelines will include requirements for physical space and for training for the providers on the special care unit.

The ALF usually offers a basic package of services that is included in the monthly fee/rent. For example, it may include 45 minutes a day for aide in dressing, assistance with showering, three meals per day, and reminders to take medications. If a person needs assist to manage medications, that may be available at an additional charge. ALF usually have a nurse available during the day to assist and check vital signs and weights. The ALF may have programs tailored to the needs of its residents such as activities appropriate for cognitively impaired residents [13]. In 2017, the average cost of assisted living in New York State is $4186/month. However, the range is from $2550 to $6550, depending on the location. Special dementia care units can add about $1150 to the monthly cost [14]. While approximately 80% of ALF residents pay privately, about 20% have some Medicaid coverage [14]. Some states do have Medicaid waiver slots for ALF, but they are very limited. In addition, Medicaid reimbursement is often far less than the costs of providing the services in the ALF.

31.4.5 Home Services

Patients can go home from the hospital with services at home. Visiting nurses can come into the home to assess the needs and help with the transition. They also can arrange for other services such as physical and/or occupational therapy. The advantage to the patient is that the person is home, but the intensity of the service is less than in a facility. Also, the coordination between the service providers may not be as strong as when they are working together at one time. Medicare will pay for rehabilitation at home, but there is a dollar cap for the various services provided.

31.5 What Is Hospice?

Hospice is from the Latin word *hospitium* which means place of entertainment, lodging, inn, or guest house. The term originally dates back to the medieval ages where it was considered a "rest house for travelers" especially the houses of refuge and shelter kept by monks in the passes of the Alps. According to the National Hospice and Palliative Care Organization site, hospice today was first applied in 1948 by a physician named Dame Cicely Saunders who cared for dying patients and eventually established the first modern hospice called the St. Christopher's Hospice in London, England, in 1967. She then introduced the idea of a holistic-specialized care for the dying in the United States during a 1963 visit with Yale University. This led to a chain of events, which resulted in the development of hospice care as we know today [15].

31.5.1 Philosophy of Care

In 2014, hospice cares for more than 1.65 million Americans and their families every year, which continues to grow. Hospice is a philosophy model for quality, compassionate, person-centered, and cost-effective care for people with life-limiting serious illness or injury with a prognosis of 6 months or less. This service is available to patients with any terminal illness regardless of age, religion, gender, sexuality, disability, or culture. In 2015 close to 65% of Medicare hospice patients were 80 years of age or older (Table 31.1).

The focus is on caring, not curing. It is also not "giving up," nor is it a form of euthanasia or physician-assisted death. The care involves an interdisciplinary team that provides the medical, emotional, spiritual, and financial support that is tailored to the person's needs and wishes. The hospice team includes but is not limited to a physician, a nurse, a social worker, volunteers, and a chaplain to name a few. Members of the hospice staff develop a care plan that meets the patient's individual needs and make regular visits to assess the patient and provide additional care or other services. The care is available "on-call" after the administrative office has closed 7 days a week, 24 hours a day, in which someone would respond to a call for help within minutes if necessary. Support is also provided to the person's loved ones as well since they typically serve as the primary caregiver and, when appropriate, help make decision for the terminally ill individual. The National Hospice and Palliative Care Organization research shows that 94% of families who had a loved one cared for by hospice rated the care as very good to excellent.

Table 31.1 Percentage of patients by age

Age category (years)	Percentage
<65	5.4
65–69	7.5
70–74	10.0
75–79	12.7
80–84	17.0
>84	47.4

Modified from the National Hospice and Palliative Care Organization (NHPCO) [16]

Table 31.2 Location of death for hospice enrollees

Location of death	2014 (%)	2013 (%)
Patient's place of residence	58.9	66.6
Private residence	35.7	41.7
Nursing home	14.5	17.9
Residential facility	8.7	7.0
Hospice inpatient facility	31.8	26.4
Acute care hospital	9.3	7.0

Modified from the National Hospice and Palliative Care Organization (NHPCO) [16]

Albeit being defined as a home care delivery model, hospice is designed to take place in multiple settings and may change depending on the nature of a patient's disease progression, medical needs of the patient, and plan of care established between the patient and the hospice. The hospice settings include patient's private residence, standalone facilities, hospice residence, long-term care facilities, or hospice inpatient facilities. Federal regulations stipulate that payment for inpatient care is limited. Hospitalization or inpatient hospice are time limited and only for management of acute symptoms or for patients who are actively dying. Because patients require differing intensities of care during the course of their disease, the Medicare Hospice Benefit affords patients four levels of care to meet their needs: routine home care, continuous home care, inpatient respite care, and general inpatient care. In 2014, 93.8% were provided at the routine home care level (Table 31.2).

Core hospice services include skilled nursing services, physician services, volunteer services, counseling services (including bereavement counseling), spiritual care, dietary counseling, and social services. Noncore services, defined as services that may be outsourced by the hospice provider, include physical therapy, occupational therapy, speech-language pathology, home health care, homemaker services, administration and provision of drugs, biological agents, medical supplies, continuous home care, respite care, and other services (Fig. 31.1).

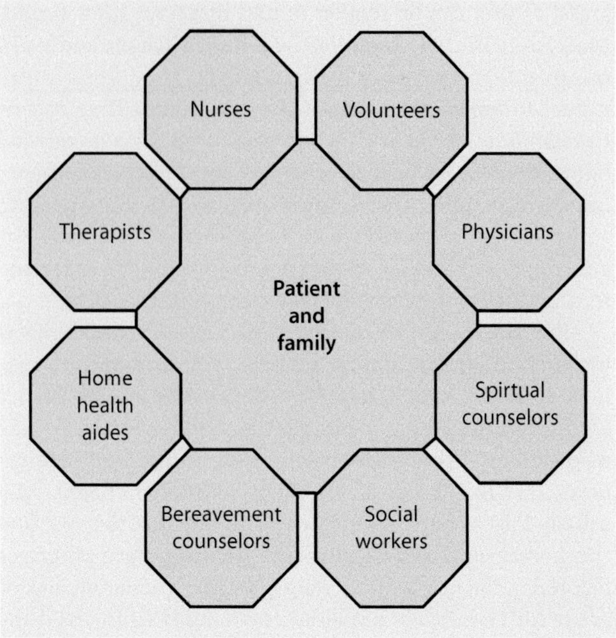

Fig. 31.1 Interdisciplinary hospice team approach in end-of-life care. (Modified from the National Hospice and Palliative Care Organization (NHPCO) [16])

31.5.2 Regulated Insurance Benefit

Hospice is also a regulated insurance benefit. After passing the Tax Equity and Fiscal Responsibility Act (TEFRA) in 1982, the Medicare Hospice Benefit (MHB) was enacted by Congress and is the predominant source of payment. Specifically, 89% of hospice patient care days annually are paid by a flat per diem rate that covers all aspects of the patient's care related to the life-limiting prognosis, including all services delivered by the interdisciplinary team, drugs, medical equipment, and supplies. This is one of Medicare's smallest program and is used by only 47.3% of Medicare decedents in 2013 according to the Medicare Payment Advisory Commission (MedPAC). Those who receive the services are covered by the MHB, with the remaining patients covered by private insurance (9%), Medicaid (5%), and other sources (2%) such as managed care insurance, private pay, or charity care [16]. The extent to which this percentage reflects underuse of hospice is unknown, because of low usage likely reflects a combination of barriers to hospice care and patient preferences not to receive such care before death. Potential barriers include lack of knowledge regarding hospice care, hospice admission criteria, and ineligibility for hospice care under MHB.

31.5.3 Hospice Eligibility Criteria

Patients are eligible to receive hospice care reimbursed under the MHB if they meet the following criteria: (1) the individual is eligible for Medicare part A (hospital insurance); (2) the individual has a life expectancy of 6 months or less if the disease follows its expected course, as certified by two physicians; and (3) the individual forgoes Medicare reimbursement for ongoing therapy or curative medical treatment related to the terminal diagnosis.

The advantage of the MHB and its eligibility criteria is that it offers a comprehensive benefit to a defined population of patients, provided in different care settings by an interdisciplinary health-care team. The disadvantage of the current eligibility criteria is that it is difficult for individuals with uncertain prognosis or those who may be availed of more complex treatment options to access hospice in a timely manner. For example, prognostic difficulty remains a barrier to hospice referral [17–19], particularly for individuals with non-cancer-related diagnoses.

Although dramatic growth has taken place in the number of individuals receiving hospice services, many patients and families enroll in hospice too late in the course of their disease to use the benefit fully. Almost one third of individuals who enroll with hospice die within 1 week of enrollment [16], and the mean length of stay in hospice care in the United States still hovers around 21 days.

It is also important for patients and families to realize that if they do not meet the hospice eligibility criteria, alternative palliative care options are available. There are no federal or commercial insurance benefits specific to palliative care; thus there exist no formal eligibility criteria. Palliative care is available to patients who continue to benefit from life-prolonging treatments, and access to palliative care is not dependent on prognosis. As the disease progresses and when eligible, individuals could transition to hospice care.

31.5.4 Duration of Hospice

Hospice eligibility requirements should not be confused with length of service. A patient in the final phase of life may receive hospice care for as long as necessary when a physician certifies that the patient continues to meet eligibility requirements. Under the MHB, two 90-day periods of care (a total of 6 months) are followed by an unlimited number of 60-day periods. The length of service (LOS) can be influenced by a number of factors including disease course, timing of referral, and access to care. The median LOS in 2014 was 17.4 days, and the average LOS was 72.6 days. Only 10.3% of patients remain under hospice care for longer than 180 days (▣ Fig. 31.2).

31.5.5 Benefits of Hospice

Hospice enrollment saves money for Medicare and improves care quality for Medicare beneficiaries across a number of different lengths of service according to research from Mount Sinai's Icahn School of Medicine in March of 2013 [20]. Furthermore a 2007 Duke University study showed that hospice care reduces Medicare program expenditures during the last year of life by an average of $2309 per hospice patient [21]. Medicare costs for hospice patients were lower than non-hospice Medicare beneficiaries with similar diag-

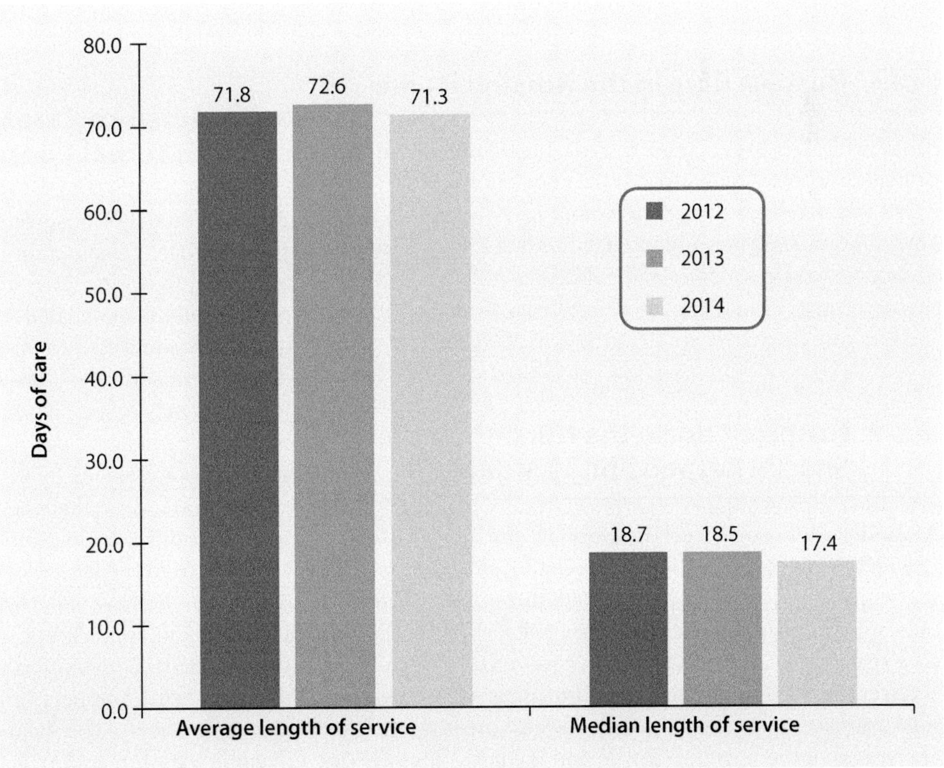

▣ **Fig. 31.2** Length of service by year. (Modified from the National Hospice and Palliative Care Organization (NHPCO) [16])

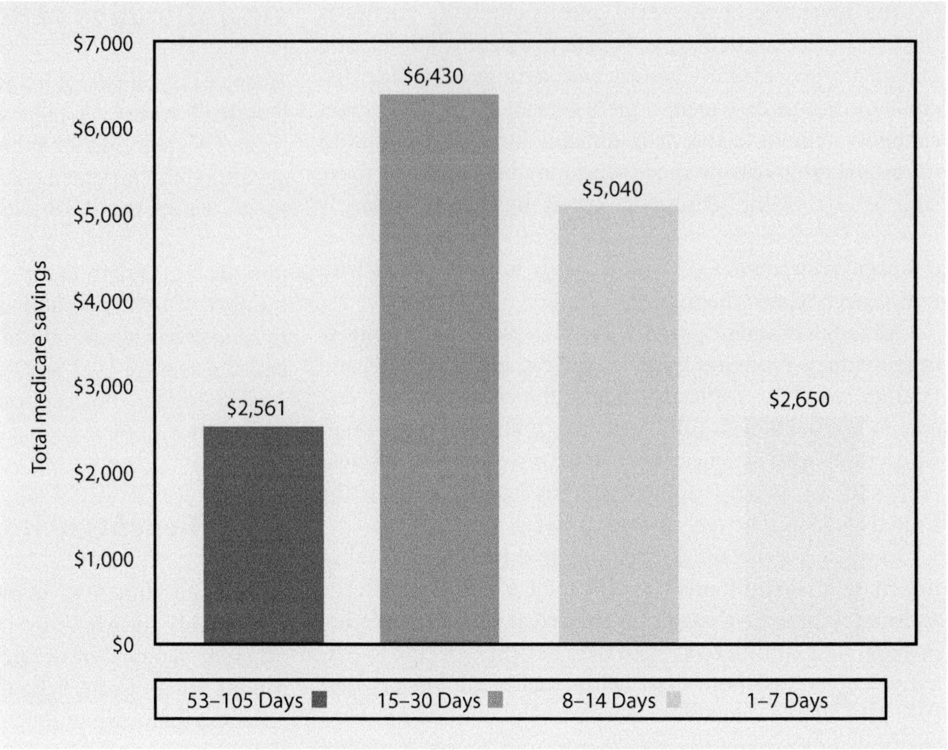

Fig. 31.3 Total Medicare savings between hospice and non-hospice groups. (Modified from the National Hospice and Palliative Care Organization (NHPCO) [16])

noses and patient profiles (Fig. 31.3). Hospice enrollment is associated with fewer 30-day hospital readmissions and in-hospital deaths. It is also associated with significantly fewer hospital and ICU days [8].

31.5.6 Hospice Care in the Nursing Home

Nationwide 25% of people die in a nursing home, and this percentage is expected to increase as the population ages [15]. The MHB was extended to nursing homes in 1989, and by 2004, 78% of US nursing homes contracted with at least one hospice agency for services. Miller and colleagues [22] reported that the percentage of nursing home residents receiving hospice services rose from 14% in 1999 to 33% in 2006.

31.5.7 Hospice Care in the Nursing Home: Shared Responsibility Model

A model of hospice care delivery in the nursing home includes shared responsibility between the nursing home and the hospice agency. When a nursing home resident is enrolled in hospice, the hospice agency is responsible for providing all care that is related to the resident's terminal illness. These services include nursing visits, additional personal care, spiritual counseling and social work services, medications that are related to the terminal illness, and medical supplies. The nursing home continues to provide room and board and long-term care services. Financial disincentives exist however for nursing homes to transfer patients who were admitted under the Medicare skilled nursing facility (SNF) benefit to the MHB because reimbursement to the nursing home for patients on the MHB is much lower than reimbursement for SNF benefit.

31.5.8 Hospice Care in the Nursing Home: External Consultation Team Model

Another model of hospice care includes having an external palliative care consultation team. The team is typically based at a community hospice or palliative care organization or occasionally is associated with hospital palliative care program. An administrator from the nursing home or a resident's primary care provider requests a consultation. Residents may or may not be hospice-eligible. The consultant bills under Medicare part B and thus the costs for these services are not incurred by the nursing home.

There are some challenges with having an external palliative care consultation team model. First the teams are not available in every location. It is difficult to staff teams with clinicians who have expertise in palliative care and an understanding and appreciation of the nursing home setting. To ensure financial viability, consultation services must be able to access large numbers of patients in one facility to maximize efficiency [23]. Given that reimbursement typically is through Medicare part B, it is focused on physician and nurse practitioner visits, which hinders more comprehensive interdisciplinary care.

31.5.9 Hospice Care in the Nursing Home: Internal Teams and Units Model

A study showed that 27% of US nursing homes report that they have implemented specialized programs or staff trained in hospice or palliative care [22]. There are no standard elements across these programs, although they generally encompass staff training, advanced care planning, and symptom management. Some authors have described benefits such as decrease in the use of unnecessary medications following admission of residents to a nursing home-based palliative care unit. Specialized dementia "comfort care" units were found to be associated with higher staff satisfaction, less observed resident discomfort, and lower costs than standard nursing home care.

Other advantages include infusing palliative care principles into daily nursing home care; clinicians' daily interaction with residents may facilitate timely detection of clinical changes; and place expertise and authority for the residents' quality of care. The biggest challenge is the lack of resources and financial disincentives for nursing homes to invest in this type of care for training and additional time necessary to deliver high-quality care.

References

1. Soriano RP, Fernandez HM, Cassel CK, Leipzig RM. Fundamentals of geriatric medicine: a case-based approach. New York: Springer; 2007.
2. U.S. Census Bureau. An aging nation: the older population in the United States (Report No. P25-1140). 2014. Retrieved from https://www.census.gov/prod/2014pubs/p25-1140.pdf.
3. Goldman DP, Shang B, Bhattacharya J, et al. Consequences of health trends and medical innovation for the future elderly. Health Aff (Millwood). 2005;24(suppl 2):W5R5–W5R17.
4. Ornstein K, Smith KL, Boal JB. Understanding and improving the burden of unmet needs of informal caregivers of homebound patients enrolled in a home-based primary care program. J Appl Gerontol. 2009;28(4):482–503.
5. Smith KL, Soriano TA, Boal JB. Brief communication: national quality-of-care standards in home-based primary care. Ann Intern Med. 2007;146(3):188.
6. Kahn JM, Benson NM, et al. Long-term acute care hospital utilization after critical illness. JAMA. 2010;303(322):253–2259.
7. Munoz-Price LS. Long-term acute care hospitals. Clin Infect Dis. 2009;49:438–43.
8. Center for Medicare & Medicaid Services. Nursing home data compendium 2012 edition. https://www.aanac.org/docs/reference-documents/nursinghomedatacompendium_508.pdf?sfvrsn=2.
9. Bonar SK, Tinetti ME, Speechley M, Cooney LM. Factors associated with short-versus long-term skilled nursing facility placement among community-living hip fracture patients. J Am Geritar Soc. 1990;38:1139–44.
10. Goodwin JS, Howrey B, Zhang DD, Kuo YF. Risk of continued institutionalization after hospitalization in older adults. J Gerontol A Biol Sci Med Sci. 2011;66A(12):1321–7.
11. Zimmerman S, Bowerrs BJ, Cohen LW, et al. New evidence on the Green House model of nursing home care: synthesis of findings and implications for policy, practice, and research. Health Serv Res. 2016;51(1):475–96.
12. Rowles GD, Teaser PB, editors. Long-term care in an aging society theory and practice. New York: Springer Publishing; 2016.
13. Han K, Trinkoff AM, et al. Variation across US assisted living facilities: admissions, resident care needs, and staffing. J Nurs Sch. 2017;49(1):24–32.
14. Paying for Senior Care. https://www.payingforseniorcare.com/financial-assistance/new-york.html. Accessed 12/14/2017.
15. Center for Advance Palliative Care. Improving palliative care in nursing homes. 2008. [PDF file]. Retrieved from https://media.capc.org/filer_public/95/b8/95b84a49-7151-427d-be72-200b634eed5b/3123_1606_nursinghomereport-rev.pdf.
16. National Hospice and Palliative Care Organization. Hospice care [Internet]. Alexandria: National Hospice and Palliative Care Organization; 2015 [updated 2017 Apr 3; cited 2018 Jan 4]. Available from: https://www.nhpco.org/about/hospice-care.
17. Brickner L, Scannell K, Marquet S, Ackerson L. Barriers to hospice care and referrals: survey of physicians' knowledge, attitudes, and perceptions in a health maintenance organization. J Palliat Med. 2004;7:411–8.
18. Fox E, Landrum-McNiff K, Zhong Z, Daweson NV, Wu AW, Lynn J. Evaluation of prognostic criteria for determining hospice eligibility in patients with advanced lung, heart, or liver disease. SUPPORT Investigators: Study to Understand Prognoses and Preferences for Outcomes and Risks of Treatments. JAMA. 1999;282:1638–45.
19. Simpson DA. Prognostic criteria for hospice eligibility. JAMA. 2000;283:2527.
20. Kelley AS, Deb P, Du Q, Aldridge Carlson MD, Morrison RS. Hospice enrollment saves money for Medicare and improves care quality across a number of different lengths-of-stay. Health Aff (Project Hope). 2013;32(3):552–61.
21. Taylor DH Jr, Ostermann J, Van Houtven CH, Tulsky JA, Steinhauser K. What length of hospice use maximizes reduction in medical expenditures near death in the US Medicare program? Soc Sci Med. 2007;65(7):1466–78.
22. Miller SC, Han B. End-of-life care in U.S. nursing homes: nursing homes with special programs and trained staff for hospice or palliative/end-of-life care. J Palliat Med. 2008;11:866–77.
23. Miller SC, Lima J, Gozalo PL, Mor V. The growth of hospice care in U.S. nursing homes. J Am Geriatr Soc. 2010;58(8):1481–8.

Acute Care in the Home Setting: Hospital at Home

Barbara Morano, Joanna Jimenez-Mejia, Martine Sanon, Carmen Morano, and Linda V. DeCherrie

A. Chun (ed.), *Geriatric Practice*, https://doi.org/10.1007/978-3-030-19625-7_32

32.1 Background

Could a large urban Health System be serious when it took out a one-page ad in the New York Times on July 22, 2015 with the headline "If our beds are filled, it means we've failed"? In fact, they were very serious and with their focus on population health management, patients are receiving most of their care outside of the traditional hospital setting. One such way they are accomplishing this is through a model of care developed to substitute hospital level care in the home. Hospital at Home (HaH) was developed at Johns Hopkins University in 1995 as a response to the evidence that hospitals may not be the ideal setting for many patients [13]. The hazards of hospitalizations, especially for the older adult, are well documented and can include falls, delirium, functional decline, and other hospital-acquired infections [9]. Additionally, poor transitions both within the hospital setting and at discharge can contribute to lengthier hospital stays, emergency department visits, and readmissions [5]. Home is a site of care that patients prefer and has been shown to be cost saving [12, 14, 15].

32

32.2 Competencies

The Hospital at Home model of care is a multidisciplinary model incorporating medicine, nursing, and social work as the main components. Each discipline has its own competencies that vary greatly in number and content. For purposes of this chapter, the following discipline-specific competencies will be addressed:

32.2.1 Medical Student Geriatric Competencies (AAMC Minimum Geriatrics Competencies 2007)

32.2.1.1 Hospital Care for Elders

Identify potential hazards of hospitalization for all older adult patients (including immobility, delirium, medication side effects, malnutrition, pressure ulcers, procedures, peri- and postoperative periods, transient urinary incontinence, and hospital-acquired infections), and identify potential prevention strategies (22).

Communicate the key components of a safe discharge plan (e.g., accurate medication list, plan for follow-up), including comparing/contrasting potential sites for discharge (25).

Explain the risks, indications, alternatives, and contraindications for indwelling (Foley) catheter use in the older adult patient (23).

Conduct a surveillance examination of areas of the skin at high risk for pressure ulcers and describe existing ulcers (26).

32.2.1.2 Cognitive and Behavioral Disorders

In an older patient with delirium, urgently initiate a diagnostic work-up to determine the root cause (etiology) (6).

Develop an evaluation and non-pharmacologic management plan for agitated, demented, or delirious patients (8).

32.2.1.3 Self-Care Capacity

Identify and assess safety risks in the home environment, and make recommendations to mitigate these (11).

32.2.1.4 Nursing [20] (All Competencies Listed Are for Master-Level Nurse Practitioners)

Assesses the patient's and caregiver's educational needs to provide effective, personalized healthcare

Collaborates with both professional and other caregivers to achieve optimal care outcomes

Coordinates transitional care services in and across care settings

32.2.2 Social Work Competencies

The Education Policy and Accreditation Standards (EPAS) of the Council on Social Work Education (CSWE) adopted 10 Core Competencies for Social Work Practice [7]. CSWE has subsequently developed core competencies in the areas of Geriatric Social Work Practice and Person Centered Care, among others. In a revision to the 2008 core competencies, the 2015 EPAS CSWE adopted the EPAS Standards, reducing the number of core competencies to nine [8], some of which include Engage Diversity and Difference in Practice (CC #2); Engage with Individuals, Families, Groups, Organizations, and Communities (CC#6); and Assess individuals, Families, Groups, Organizations, and Communities (CC#7). The eighth core competency, "Intervene with Individuals, Families, Groups, Organizations and Communities" specifies the following practice behaviors that relate to the role of the HaH social worker:

1. Critically choose and implement interventions to achieve practice goals and enhance capacities of clients and constituencies.
2. Apply knowledge of human behavior and the social environment, person-in-environment, and other multidisciplinary theoretical frameworks in interventions with clients and constituencies.
3. Use inter-professional collaboration as appropriate to achieve beneficial practice outcomes.
4. Negotiate, mediate, and advocate with and on behalf of diverse clients and constituencies.
5. Facilitate effective transitions and endings that advance mutually agreed-on goals.

32.3 Hazards of Hospitalization

The acute hospitalization is often considered a sentinel event for many older adults. As described in greater detail in the following chapter, the acute care hospital setting can be an extremely dangerous environment for vulnerable patients, especially those with advanced age, baseline cognitive impairment, functional limitations, or frailty. An unintended consequence of acute hospitalization places vulnerable older adults at greater risk for decline in healthcare quality of life even once the acute medical issue or complication that led to the admission is resolved [9]. While the hospital has been seen as the traditional model for the delivery of acute medical care, it is not an ideal care environment for many patients [15]. Older adults are at greater risk for iatrogenic events such as nosocomial infections, pressure sores, falls, and delirium [18]. These adverse events often lead to increased hospital length of stay and more complex discharge planning or suboptimal transitions in care at the time of hospital discharge. Older adults often require transitions to skilled nursing facilities (SNF) or long-term care facilities (LTC), rather than home after an acute hospital stay, putting older adults at risk for readmission to the hospital due to their inability to live independently [15]. Identifying acute care models outside of the hospital setting can help mitigate these adverse outcomes.

Older adults tend to have more complex medical comorbidities, greater illness severity, and limited cognitive and functional reserves to overcome the stress of an acute illness. While hospitalization in this population is often necessary, it is difficult to ignore the major risk this entails for the patients. The combination of usual physiological changes of aging and increased susceptibility to stress resulting in hospitalization from an acute illness, often results in an irreversible functional decline that overshadows the actual cure or repair of the illness for which they were admitted [9]. These factors, combined with a prolonged length of hospital stay, result in loss of baseline functional reserves which has a negative impact on long-term patient outcomes, prognosis, and quality of life.

32.4 Hospital at Home Model

Hospital at Home, a relatively new model of care, provides an alternative to hospitalization; essentially providing acute care for patients outside the traditional hospital setting. This model provides a means of treating elderly patients whose care preference is to be at home, where they have lower risk of adverse events and also for patients who are averse to being in the hospital. To substitute entirely for an inpatient admission, HaH must possess three elements:

1. Providing care that substitutes entirely for an inpatient acute admission
2. Providing the same intensity of medical and nursing care similar to that provided in the hospital
3. Providing care that cannot be offered routinely in the community [16]

Every Hospital at Home program also must fit in to the culture and workflow of the institution (see ◘ Fig. 32.1). Some

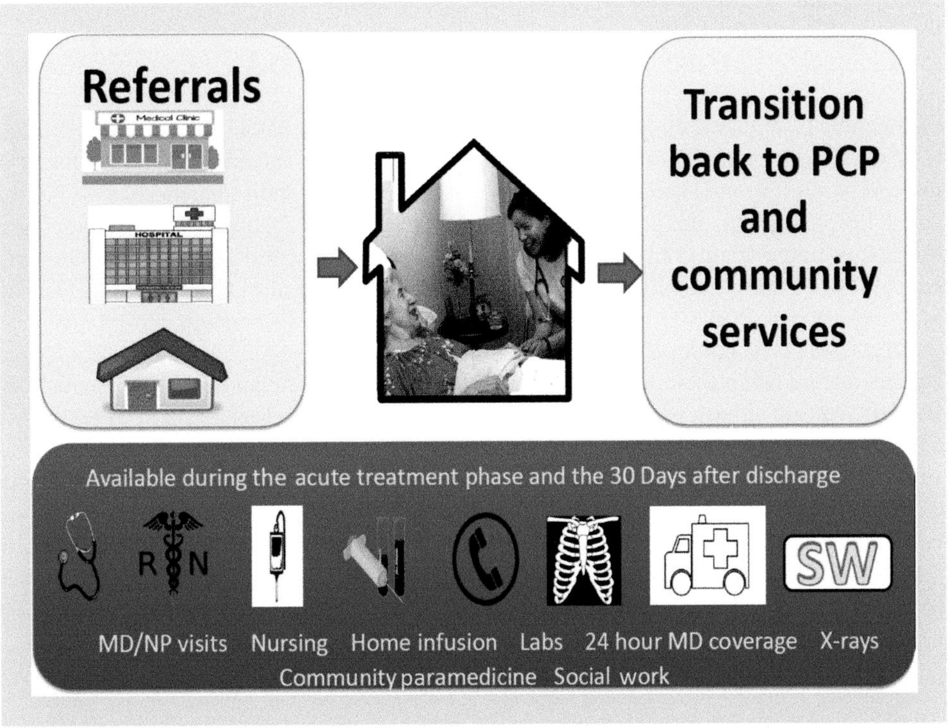

◘ Fig. 32.1 The Hospital at Home model

programs may use emergency department (ED) physicians as the primary source of referrals, others can use hospitalists, and others may do their own case finding as an effective means to recruit patients. Most HaH programs focus on eight admission diagnoses but often expand qualifying diagnoses over time. The basic eight diagnoses include community-acquired pneumonia, urinary tract infection, congestive heart failure, diabetes, chronic obstructive lung disease, asthma, cellulitis, and venous thromboembolism. The Hospital at Home provider is ultimately the decision-maker for program eligibility. Eligibility is based on insurance payer, address, safety issues, and other specific medical exclusion factors. If eligible, informed consent is obtained and patients are then fully evaluated by the hospital-at-home physician in the emergency department at which time medical orders are written. It should be noted that patients can be admitted directly from home or an ambulatory setting, in which case the provider will perform this evaluation in the home setting. If admitted from the ED or observation unit, patients are usually transported home by ambulance. Those patients requiring oxygen therapy are sent home with a portable oxygen tank pending delivery of a concentrator. Once the patient arrives home, the hospital-at-home nurse will conduct a full assessment and provide nursing care as specified in the order set. This can include infusion, wound care, vital signs, etc. The patient will continue to have intermittent nursing visits at least daily. All medications and related supplies associated with the acute diagnosis are delivered to the home. Home radiology, laboratory, and other diagnostic studies are provided by vendor contracts.

The hospital-at-home physician or advanced practice nurse provider makes at least daily home visits or a video-assisted visit and is available 24 hours a day for urgent or emergent calls. At many HaH programs, there is the ability for 24-hour visits, and at the Mount Sinai Health System (MSHS) in New York, that is provided through community paramedics. These are non-911 specifically trained paramedic staffed ambulances that can be dispatched by the HaH team to evaluate patients and coordinate with HaH providers for care while the paramedic is in the home. During the entire hospitalization, the patient is followed by the same hospital-at-home team until his or her condition is stable enough for discharge, at which time care is reverted to the primary care physician.

The MSHS HaH model follows patients for a 30-day transitional period after their home hospitalization, ensuring they are connected back to their primary care. Nursing and Social work triage patients and follow them at different intervals during that time. Providers and community paramedicine are available to the patients as well to avoid unnecessary ED visits or hospitalizations.

The ability to provide acute care outside of the hospital in a safe and comforting home environment essentially eliminates the risks of the hazards of hospitalization. Previous studies have highlighted the quantitative and qualitative benefits of acute care outside of the hospital and its impact on patient outcomes. "Although less procedurally oriented than acute hospital care, hospital-at-home care met quality standards at rates similar to those of acute hospital care, with a shorter length of stay, lower cost for hospital-at-home care than for acute hospital care and fewer complications" ([15], p. 798). Providing acute hospital-level care in a patient's home for carefully selected patients via HaH has been shown to improve patient safety, enhance quality, increase efficiency, reduce variations in practice, and reduce the costs of providing acute care for select medical illnesses [12, 14, 15]. Furthermore, patients and family members' satisfaction was higher in the home setting than among those offered usual hospital care, reflecting the convenience of the model [14].

The benefits of a Hospital at Home model of care are considerable for this population, but several factors must be taken into consideration when identifying the appropriate patient. There are obvious limitations to what can be provided in the home versus a fully staffed and equipped acute care hospital. However, when recognizing the unique challenges an acute hospitalization places on this patient population, the advantages are promising. In order to guarantee success in this program, it is essential to assess each individual patient through a comprehensive interdisciplinary approach, including identifying the appropriate diagnosis, recognizing the capabilities of an interdisciplinary team, partnering with family and caregiver support systems, and having a good understanding of the patients' overall goals of care. The Hospital at Home model is able to ensure a patient-centered approach and can accommodate several care pathways.

32.4.1 Case Examples (See ◘ Fig. 32.2)

Below are examples of three HaH pathways that have proven feasible and successful at MSHS. However, as ◘ Fig. 32.2 indicates, there are a number of other pathways that are in the piloting or developing stage as a result of an identified need in the Health System. The flexibility of the model to address identified needs makes it attractive to Health System leadership.

Acute Hospital at Home This pathway addresses acute medical issues that can be safely treated at home with the proper care team, coordination, family and caregiver support, and access to community resources.

Short-term (3–5 day) acute inpatient-level care at home with a 30-day transition period.

Common diagnoses include pneumonia, urinary tract infection, cellulitis, venous thromboembolism, and dehydration.

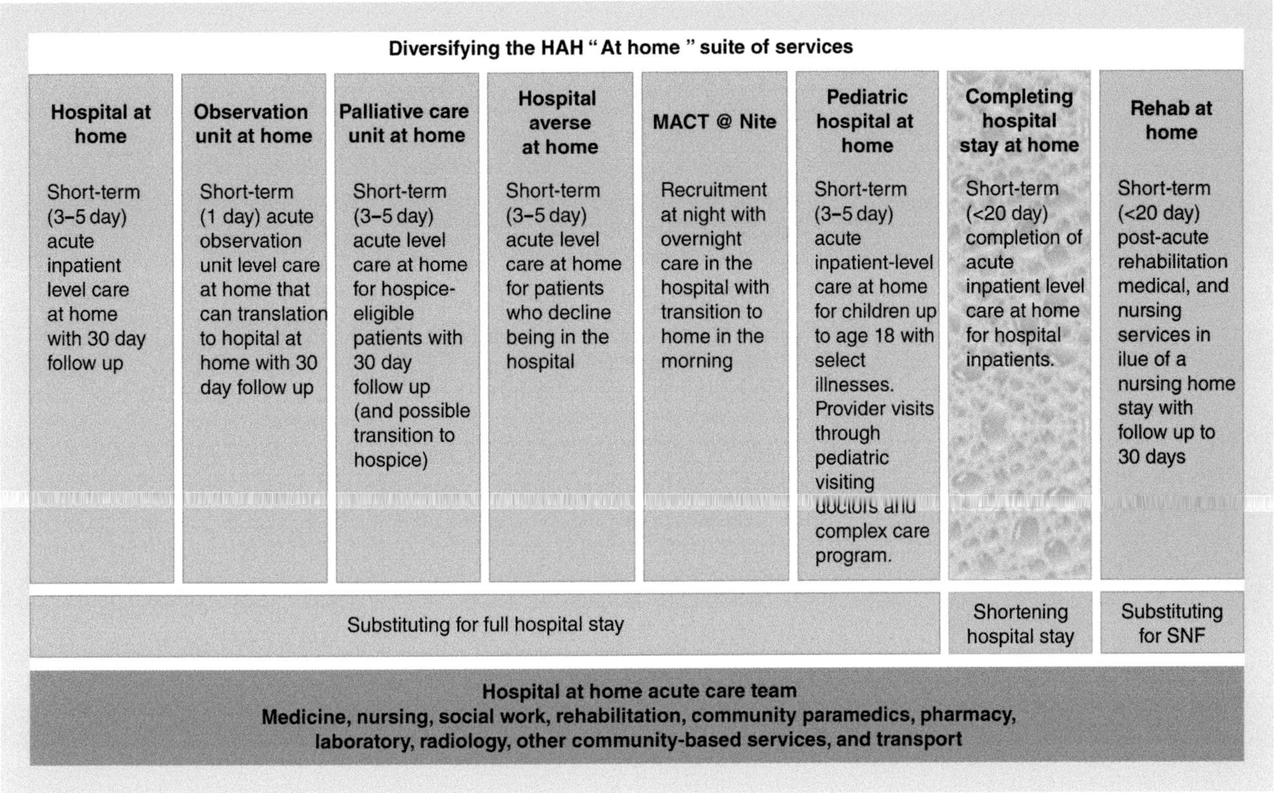
Diversifying the HAH "At home" suite of services
Hospital at home
Short-term (3–5 day) acute inpatient level care at home with 30 day follow up
Observation unit at home
Short-term (1 day) acute observation unit level care at home that can translation to hopital at home with 30 day follow up
Palliative care unit at home
Short-term (3–5 day) acute level care at home for hospice-eligible patients with 30 day follow up (and possible transition to hospice)
Hospital averse at home
Short-term (3–5 day) acute level care at home for patients who decline being in the hospital
MACT @ Nite
Recruitment at night with overnight care in the hospital with transition to home in the morning
Pediatric hospital at home
Short-term (3–5 day) acute inpatient-level care at home for children up to age 18 with select illnesses. Provider visits through pediatric visiting doctors and complex care program.
Completing hospital stay at home
Short-term (<20 day) completion of acute inpatient level care at home for hospital inpatients.
Rehab at home
Short-term (<20 day) post-acute rehabilitation medical, and nursing services in ilue of a nursing home stay with follow up to 30 days
Substituting for full hospital stay
Shortening hospital stay
Substituting for SNF
Hospital at home acute care team
Medicine, nursing, social work, rehabilitation, community paramedics, pharmacy, laboratory, radiology, other community-based services, and transport

Fig. 32.2 Diversifying the HaH "At Home" Suite of Services

Case

JG is an 87-year-old male with a history of hypertension, hyperlipidemia, coronary artery disease, atrial fibrillation, congestive heart failure, pacemaker, and diabetes type 2 who presented with cough productive of green sputum, fever, shortness of breath, and general weakness for the past 3 days. Per his grandson, patient had stopped taking his furosemide for about 1 week prior to presentation, though for unclear reasons. Patient's only contact is his grandson, who currently reports patient having a fever. Brain Naturietic Peptide (BNP) was elevated. Chest x-ray was significant for left lower lobe pneumonia. Patient ambulates with a walker, and has mild dementia. He needs assistance with all activities of daily living, but is well supported by family. JG requires hospital admission for treatment of community-acquired pneumonia and intravenous diuresis for his CHF. During JG's previous hospitalization for surgery 3 years ago, he developed delirium and was eventually discharged for rehabilitation at a skilled nursing facility (SNF). JG is fearful about being hospitalized. JG and his grandson accept the option of Hospital at Home as it provides them with optimal medical treatment while remaining home.

In this pathway, the HaH model of care is able to provide the equivalent hospital level of care in the comfort of the home setting. The patient must meet hospital admission criteria for the specific diagnosis, but be stable enough that all care needs can be met within the home environment. Extended interdisciplinary team members including physicians, nurses, nurse practitioners, social workers, and physical therapists are available to make home visits to oversee the patient's care and progress for the duration of the acute illness. With advancement in technology, further diagnostic lab testing, chest x-ray, and electrocardiogram can also be facilitated in the home, as well as 24-hour availability to reach a provider. The familiar, less disruptive, and comforting environment of home, as opposed to the disorienting emergency department and hospital, provides an atmosphere free of restraints and tethers and restricted hospital diets. Patients are able to navigate in their home environment as they see fit and less likely to develop a significant debility with resultant transition to a SNF.

Hospital Averse This pathway is an appropriate option for the patient who would prefer not to be in a hospital or emergency department but accepts the need for acute medical treatment.

Short-term (3–5 day) acute-level care at home for patients who decline being in the hospital, with a 30-day transitional period.

Common diagnoses include pneumonia, urinary tract infection, cellulitis, and congestive heart failure.

Case

GW is a 68-year-old male with morbid obesity, osteoporosis, chronic pain, severe arthritis, diabetes, hypertension, peripheral vascular disease, and lumbar stenosis who was admitted to the program with right lower extremity cellulitis and edema. He had failed a treatment of oral antibiotics and is referred to the ED by his Primary Care Provider (PCP) for evaluation of his leg and to rule out Deep Vein Thrombosis (DVT) and intravenous (IV) antibiotics. The ultrasound was negative for DVT and the Vascular Medicine team recommended no surgical intervention but hospital admission for IV antibiotics for his cellulitis. Because of poor experiences in the past, the patient is adamant that he did not want to be admitted to the hospital even though he understood that he had an infection that requires treatment. He is confident he can manage at home which is set up with all the appropriate equipment needed to manage his chronic issues and would rather continue oral antibiotics even though they have not been as effective.

In this scenario, the patient is aware of his acute illness and the treatment option that is recommended. The standard of care for this patient would require continued treatment in the hospital for stronger and more effective IV antibiotics. This patient had the capacity to state his choices and understand the treatment options recommended and was able to express the risk and benefits of home-based alternative treatment. He understood the risk of refusing a hospital admission meant the treatment for his infection would be suboptimal as he had failed oral antibiotics in the past. In this *Hospital Averse* option, the program was able to provide the care the patient needed to treat his infection with IV antibiotics and avoid a prolonged acute care hospitalization. With the assistance of a coordinated interdisciplinary team, the patient was able to return home the same evening from the ED, and received his antibiotic therapy twice a day at home with ongoing care at discharge provided through a certified home health agency.

Palliative Care at Home This pathway is appropriate for the high risk, vulnerable patient, still pursuing acute medical care at the end of life. This can serve as a bridge to hospice for patients who have a terminal diagnosis, or at the end of life who need symptom management, but are still hopeful to treat potentially reversible illness (i.e., acute infection).

Short-term (3–5 day) acute-level care at home for hospice-eligible patients with 30-day follow-up (and possible transition to hospice).

Common diagnoses include aspiration pneumonia, UTI, and community-acquired pneumonia.

32

Case

CL is an 86-year-old man with a history of bioprosthetic aortic valve replacement, hyperlipidemia, degenerative joint disease of the spine, and dementia, who was hospitalized 2 months prior with sepsis from methicillin-susceptible *Staphylococcus aureus* (MSSA) bacteremia with a prolonged hospital course complicated by a pressure ulcer to the sacrum, back pain, and delirium. No clear source of the MSSA bacteremia was found, but was highly suspicious for endocarditis. He was discharged to a SNF and treated with 6 weeks of intravenous antibiotics. At a routine follow-up visit with his PCP, a screening culture was noted to be positive again for *Staphylococcus aureus*. He was referred back to the ED for hospital admission which the patient and family were hesitant about since they did not want any invasive high-risk interventions such as heart surgery. The patient was nonambulatory and was made DNR/DNI recently. After a consultation with the specialists, including infectious disease, cardiothoracic surgery, and palliative care, the recommendation was for conservative management of his infection with antibiotics and symptom management. The patient and family understood that the infection would not be cured without the high-risk surgery, but that due to his frail state, was not an option. Patient stated his preference was to return home with a trial of antibiotics and continue conversations about his goals of care. As the patient became more symptomatic, and no longer responded to antibiotics, he was eventually transitioned to home hospice with the assistance of the Hospital at Home program.

This pathway offers a patient-centered approach to care that aligns patient's goals of care with a trial treatment for an acute illness and a treatment plan that incorporates a palliative care approach to a patient at the end of life. It honors the patient's wishes of being home, accepting the diagnosis, and a prognosis that is short. As symptoms become more difficult to manage, the resource of a home-based hospice program was added.

The above cases and various pathways highlight the advantages of this care model: specifically, the range of services available, such as the availability of a 24-hour clinical team with the ability to demonstrate flexibility in clinical care options and at the same time offering a patient-centered approach to care. This model has an impact at the institutional level by clearing out an overcrowded ED and inpatient beds and responds to the broad needs of patients and healthcare providers. This model of providing acute care outside of the hospital is a feasible option especially if it meets the needs of the appropriate patient it is targeted to. It is important to have a clear understanding of the patient's goals of care and clarity about not only the benefits but some of the limitations to how care can be delivered in the hospital versus home. All of these options require the collaboration from family and caregivers, a robust interdisciplinary team, community resources through certified home care nursing services, hospice, and house calls programs and a supportive health system to leverage the resources necessary to make the program effective and sustainable.

32.4.2 Providers of Care and Daily Assignments

The HaH program cares for patients of high complexity levels. An interdisciplinary team is essential in delivering high-quality care to a patient population with multiple needs. By integrating different clinical disciplines in one team, HaH is able to offer a holistic approach to address the clinical and psychosocial needs of patients and their families. The core clinical team involves physicians, nurse practitioners, registered nurses, social workers, community paramedics, physical therapists, occupational therapists and speech therapists, and lab technicians. An ancillary team of administrative staff including a program coordinator, program manager, nurse manager, and administrative assistants help coordinate the program's daily operations. The whole team functions under the guidance of a medical director:

Physicians Physicians who function as HaH hospitalists have a central role in the Hospital at Home program as they are responsible for identifying, screening, and enrolling patients who are appropriate for the program. In order to accomplish that, physicians perform in-depth assessments of potential HaH patients in the emergency department or ambulatory or home setting. Enrolling an appropriate patient requires close collaboration with the ED or ambulatory medical teams, patients' primary care providers, and family or caregivers. After obtaining consent for enrollment, physicians create a plan of care often integrating multiple disciplines required for a successful recovery at home.

Nurse Practitioners Nurse practitioners (NPs) are the main providers in the home setting as they execute the plan of care on a daily basis making adjustments when necessary. NPs collaborate closely with the physicians, registered nurses, and other members of the team to ensure all patients' needs are met during the acute and post-acute phases of enrollment.

Registered Nurses Nursing services are vital in HaH. The program relies heavily on nursing skills to provide home infusions, medication reconciliation and management, patient and caregiver teaching, wound care, and other nursing procedures.

Social Workers Social workers have an essential role in assessing patients' home safety, support system, and the resources that may need to be in place for a successful hospital-at-home admission and discharge. Social workers are even more important during the post-acute period to ensure all psychosocial needs are met and patients can safely remain in the community, connected to community-based enduring resources.

Physical Therapists The integration of physical therapists into patient care both during the acute and the post-acute periods enhances the patient's functional status, improves independence with activities of daily living, and therefore improves the patient's quality of life in the community. Physical therapy can also help to prevent readmissions related to physical deconditioning and falls.

Clinical Nurse Manager A clinical nurse manager is responsible for overseeing the nursing staff, coordinating daily staff scheduling and assignments, as well as determining the program's capacity for admissions. The nurse manager is also involved in monitoring patients in the post-acute phase, triaging of patient-related calls, overseeing the scheduling of tests/consultants, addressing any medical needs that may arise, and ensuring formal hand-offs to community-based services.

32.4.3 Determining Staff Workload and Program Admission Capacity

In the inpatient setting, staff workload is normally based on patient acuity. Hospital admission capacity is highly dependent on the number of staff and number of beds available. On the other hand, the HaH program staff workload and program capacity are intertwined and require a complex equation involving multiple components. While treating patients in their home eliminates the challenges of overcrowding and bed availability hospitals often face, the volume of patients that can be safely admitted to a HaH program is affected by not only patient acuity but also the geography of the admissions, the type of home visits required, and the resources and staffing of the program.

32.4.4 Patient Acuity

A patient's specific diagnoses and illness severity level often influence the level of their needs. A stable patient may require intravenous administration of antibiotics once or twice daily. On the other hand, a patient who is severally ill may require administration of antibiotics, intravenous hydration, wound care, frequent phlebotomy, and other nursing procedures. Increasing a patient's medical needs implies lengthy visits and therefore decreased workload capacity.

32.4.5 Home Visit Type

Initial home visits are generally the most complex and time-consuming. During the initial assessment, providers and nurses can spend a great deal of time in goals of care and plan of care discussions with caregivers. Medication reconciliation, a detailed and in-depth assessment of a patient's medications, also takes place during the first home visit. Follow-up home visits tend to be more problem focused and predictable in terms of length of time. Similarly, discharge visits tend to be straightforward and predictable since the focus is mainly on patient and family education.

32.4.6 Patient Geography

Every HaH program must develop geographic boundaries in order to optimize capacity. In highly urban settings, the boundaries may seem quite small compared to a more suburban or rural area. However, commute times need to be factored in to geographic boundaries. A good rule of thumb is limiting commuting to 1 hour each way since commute time adds on to home visit time and decreases the overall efficiency of the team.

32.4.7 Patient Census

In the hospital setting, a census is an official count of the total number of patients admitted to the facility over a period of time [2]. For staffing and sizing hospital units, the midnight census is the standard indicator of workload [2]. Similarly, HaH utilizes census data to define workload and predict staffing needs. However, a unique feature of the HaH program is its ability to simultaneously admit patients from different settings (e.g., clinics, hospitals, and homes). This, in addition to the variability in length of stay, leads to high fluctuation in the number of HaH-enrolled patients throughout the day. Regular census checks throughout each shift are of vital importance in determining program admission capacity. Determining the workload and capacity for a Hospital at Home program requires a complex formula that must consider the program's current census, patient acuity, geography, type of home visit, number of staff, and resources available. Since admissions can happen from numerous hospitals, ambulatory settings, and a patient's home simultaneously, daily patient volume can be unpredictable. In addition, patients can be discharged from the program, transferred to hospice, or escalated to the hospital at unexpected times. Therefore, frequent census checks and daily huddles are of vital importance for keeping track of the program's capacity and staff workload as well as for enhancing coordination within the clinical team.

32.4.8 Post-acute Care

In recent years, post-acute care has become an essential component of the healthcare delivery system. According to data from the Center for Health Information and Analysis (CHIA), the persistently high 30-day readmission rates among many US hospitals come with an estimated cost of about $26 billion annually, and $17 billion is attributed to preventable admissions [4]. The Medicare Payment Advisory Commission (MedPAC) has estimated that 12% of readmissions are potentially avoidable [17]. Therefore, reducing hospital readmissions is a national priority. The literature shows that some of the biggest causes of readmission within 30 days of hospital discharge include [1]:

- Lack of understanding of the discharge instructions by patients and/or caregivers
- Delayed post-discharge follow-up
- Lack of information sharing and/or miscommunication between inpatient and outpatient providers
- Medication incidents oftentimes due to lack of medication reconciliation or noncompliance with medication regimen
- Lack of support system at home

Although not initially included in the Johns Hopkins Hospital at Home model, more recent models have included a post-acute period of varying lengths, usually between 30 and 60 days beginning upon discharge from the acute episode, to complete recovery from the acute episode, in order to ensure a safe and high-quality transition to the patient's primary care clinician. During this post-acute period, the team works on the implementation of evidence-based transitional care interventions to promote patients' well-being. The interventions include in-depth home assessments, education, medication management oversight, care coordination, and thorough communication with providers and caregivers to help address any identified warning signs before they become emergencies. The HaH post-acute period engages patients and their families to help them understand the clinical, psychosocial, and environmental factors that may impact their recovery.

During the post-acute period, the following are interventions employed to reduce escalations and/or readmissions:

- 48-hour post-discharge call
- Follow-up home visits
- Medication reconciliation
- Patient and caregiver education
- 24/7 support
- Multidisciplinary collaboration
- Care coordination
- Integration and referral to community-based resources
- Insuring patient has followed up with primary care provider and/or specialist

32.4.9 Results

HaH has shown to have some promising results of improved patient's satisfaction, lower complications, and reduced cost [10]. Considering the national 30-day hospital readmission rate is 18.4% [11], a HaH post-acute intervention has the ability to significantly reduce readmission rates. In a meta-analysis it was shown to be 24% less [3] and a 21% reduction in mortality.

32.5 Conclusion

Hospital at Home is a relatively new model of care that is in the middle of a large expansion with more and more payers agreeing to cover the services. It is an excellent location to learn about many of the medical student, social work, and nursing competencies in what has been considered a nontraditional setting for this learning.

References

1. Alper E, O'Malley T, Greenwald J. Hospital discharge and readmission. Up-to-date. 2017. Retrieved from https://www.uptodate.com/contents/hospital-discharge-and-readmission.
2. Beswick S, Hill PD, Anderson MA. Comparison of nurse workload approaches. J Nurs Manag. 2010;18(5):592–8.
3. Caplan GA, et al. A meta-analysis of "hospital in the home". Med J Aust. 2012;197(9):512–9.
4. Center for Health Information and Analysis. Performance of the Massachusetts health care system: a focus on provider quality. 2015. Retrieved from http://www.chiamass.gov/assets/Uploads/A-Focus-on-Provider-Quality-Jan-2015.pdf.
5. Coleman EA, Berenson RA. Lost in transition: challenges and opportunities for improving the quality of transitional care. Ann Intern Med. 2004;141:533–6.
6. http://www.commonwealthfund.org/publications/newsletters/quality-matters/2011/august-september-2011/in-focus.
7. Council on Social Work Education (CSWE). Educational policy and accreditation standards. 2008. Retrieved May 06, 2016, from http://www.cswe.org/NR/rdonlyres/2A81732E-1776-4175-AC42-65974E96BE66/0/2008EducationalPolicyandAccreditationStandards.Pdf.
8. CSWE Commission on Accreditation Standards. EPAS handbook. Pub. Council on social work education. 2016. Retrieved May 10, 2016, from https://www.cswe.org/Accreditation/Standards-and-Policies/EPAS-Handbook.
9. Creditor MC. Hazards of hospitalization of the elderly. Ann Intern Med. 1993;118:219–23.
10. Cryer L, Shannon S, van Amsterdam M, Leff B. Costs for hospital at home patients were 19 percent less, with equal or better outcomes compared to similar inpatients. Health Aff. 2012;31:1237–43.
11. Felix HC, Seaberg B, Bursac Z, Thostenson J, Stewart MK. Why do patients keep coming back? Results of a readmitted patient survey. Soc Work Health Care. 2015;54(1):1–15. https://doi.org/10.1080/00981389.2014.966881.
12. Frick KD, et al. Substitutive Hospital at Home for older persons: effects on costs. Am J Manag Care. 2009;15(1):49–56.
13. Kohn LT, Corrigan JM, Donaldson MS. To err is human: building a safer health system. Washington, DC: National Academy Press; 2000.
14. Leff B, et al. Satisfaction with hospital at home care. J Am Geriatr Soc. 2006;54(9):1355–63.
15. Leff B, Burton L, Mader SL, et al. Hospital at home: feasibility and outcomes of a program to provide hospital-level care at home for acutely ill older patients. Ann Intern Med. 2005;143(11):798–808.
16. Leff B, Montalto M. Home hospital-toward a tighter definition. J Am Geriatr Soc. 2004;52(12):1241.
17. McIlvennan CK, Eapen ZJ, Allen LA. Hospital readmissions reduction program. Circulation. 2015;131(20):1796–803. https://doi.org/10.1161/CIRCULATIONAHA.114.010270.
18. Montalto M. The 500-bed hospital that isn't there: the Victorian Department of Health review of the Hospital in the Home program. Med J Aust. 2010;193(10):598–601.
19. Mueller SK, Sponsler KC, Kripalani S, Schnipper JL. Hospital-based medication reconciliation practices: a systematic review. Arch Intern Med. 2012;172:1057.
20. Nurse Practitioner Core Competencies Content. The National Organizations of Nurse Practitioner Faculties (NONPF). 2017. Retrieved from http://www.nonpf.org/?page=14.
21. The Joint Commission. Medication reconciliation: sentinel event alert. 2006. Retrieved from http://www.jointcommission.org/SentinelEvents/SentinelEventAlert/sea_35.htm.

Hazards of Hospitalization

Martine Sanon

A. Chun (ed.), *Geriatric Practice*, https://doi.org/10.1007/978-3-030-19625-7_33

Case

Mrs. F is an 80-year-old female admitted with dyspnea, worsening lower extremity edema, and a recent fall. She lives with elderly husband and has a home aide 8 hours of the day. She has a past medical history of HTN, CAD, mild vascular dementia, osteoarthritis, and gait instability and walks with cane and rolling walker. Her daughter (who lives out of state) has been doing their finances for the past 2 years. She is able to perform all of her ADLs and only intermittently incontinent. She walks with a walker due to arthritis. Her husband and aide help her with her ADLs due to her osteoarthritis

- **Hospital Course**

Mrs. F is admitted to the medicine service and transferred to a telemetry bed. She is treated with IV diuretics and supplemental oxygen, and a bladder catheter was placed in the ED. She is given one dose of diphenhydramine by the cross-covering intern on her first night in the hospital because she was unable to sleep. She had poor oral intake for the first 2 days and had periods of agitation requiring haloperidol.

After 2 days of ongoing treatment and diuresis of 2.5 L, her breathing improved, but the nurse notes she developed a stage II sacral pressure ulcer. By day 3, Mrs. F develops suprapubic pain and tachypnea in the middle of the night and does not recognize her surroundings. She tries to stand up because she feels like she needs to urinate forgetting she had a urinary catheter. The bed alarm sounds, telemetry leads tangle in her blankets, and her urinary catheter gets caught on her leg. She falls as the aides rush into the room. She is found to have developed a catheter-associated urinary tract infection and sustains a contusion and abrasion to her R knee. She is treated with IV antibiotics for 3 days requiring a 1:1 sitter in the setting of confusion. An additional 2 days of hospitalization is required as attempts are made to find a subacute rehab facility since she is no longer safe to return home due to worsening physical debility, deconditioning, and generalized weakness.

By day 4, her delirium cleared; she needed two persons to get her out of bed to chair. Day 5, the social worker and physical therapist met with Mrs. F and her family. Discharge plan was to a subacute rehabilitation facility for physical therapy and wound care. Day 7, she was discharged to a facility. After 4 weeks of therapy, Mrs. F was unable to recover her ability to walk independently. She was transitioned to a skilled nursing facility for long-term care.

33.1 Functional Decline and Debility

Definition

- Functional impairment is defined as difficulty performing or requiring the assistance of another person to perform one of the activities of daily living (ADLs).
- Hospitalization-associated disability refers to patients who have a new disability in activities of daily living (ADLs) at hospital discharge that they did not have before the onset of the acute illness.

Prevalence

- ~50% of people 85 years of age and older require assistance in one or more ADLs; as many as 25% of older community-dwelling adults have at least one impairment in IADL [2].
- Many hospitalized older people are discharged with ADL function that is worse than their baseline function. It has been reported that nearly 25–35% of older adults admitted to the hospital for treatment of acute medical illness lose independence in one or more ADL [1].

Etiology and Risk Factors

- The combination of usual physiological changes of aging, increased susceptibility to stress, acute illness, hospitalization, and prolonged immobility and bedrest often results in an irreversible functional decline despite the cure or repair of the illness for which they were admitted [5].
- For older adults, hospitalization for an acute medical illness frequently precipitates a disability in ADLs. Risk factors for loss of independence in ADLs during hospitalization include advanced age, cognitive impairment, and IADL impairment at admission (Sager, Gill 6–8).

Special Consideration for Older Adults

- ADL impairment is a stronger predictor of hospital outcomes (functional decline, length of stay, institutionalization, and death) than admitting diagnosis, diagnosis-related group, and other physiologic indices of illness burden. ADL impairment is also a risk factor for nursing home placement, ER visits, and death among community-dwelling adults.
- This loss of baseline functional reserves is often difficult to recover and often impacts long-term patient outcomes, prognosis, and quality of life.
- The oldest patients are at particularly high risk of poor functional outcomes because they are less likely to recover ADL function lost before admission and more likely to develop new functional deficits during hospitalization [3].
- Immobility and functional decline in older hospitalized adults can lead to adverse events such as falls, pressure ulcers, and deep vein thrombosis in the hospital setting.
- Hospitalized seniors lose up to 5% of their muscle strength daily [5].
- New functional impairment impacts care transitions. Older adults often require transitions to skilled nursing facilities (SNF) or long-term care facilities (LTC), rather than home, after an acute hospital stay, or readmission to hospital as they are unable to safely manage in the community.
- Compared with more active and mobile hospitalized counterparts, immobile seniors are six times more likely to be discharged to long-term care facilities and 34.3 times more likely to die in hospital [2].

Table 33.1 Assessing patient's functional status

Activities of daily living (ADLs)	Instrumental activities of daily living (IADLs)
Bathing	Administering own medication
Dressing	Grocery shopping
Toileting	Preparing meals
Transfers	Using the telephone
Grooming	Driving and transportation
Feeding	Handling finances
	Housekeeping
	Laundry

Modified from: Katz [8]

Assessment

- *It is important to* ***identify the patient factors associated with an increased risk of developing disability associated with acute illness and hospitalization*** [12].
- It is important to assess baseline functional status of older hospitalized adults and implement strategies to preserve functional status, as this has significant prognostic implications for older adults after an acute hospitalization [9] (Table 33.1).

33.1.1 Minimum Functional Assessment in Hospitalized Older Adults

33.1.1.1 Functional Domain Assessment on Admission Daily Assessment

ADLs

For each ADL, the following elements should be assessed at admission and before onset of illness:

- **Difficulty with ADL:**
  - On the day of admission, did you have any difficulty bathing or taking a shower?
  - Did you have any difficulty bathing before the onset of the problem that led to your being hospitalized?
- **Ascertainment of equipment use for walking:**
  - Walking (cane or walker) or bathing (shower chair and rails)
- **If patient reports difficulty, assess need for help**:
  - "On the day of admission, did you need the help of another person to bathe?
  - "How about before this illness?"
    - *If the patient needs help, assess adequacy of help:
      - "What help do you need? Who helps you? Do you get enough help?"
- **Ask nurse or nursing assistant at bedside the extent of help** they are providing for bathing, dressing, transferring, using the toilet, eating, and walking.
- **Review nursing and physical/occupational therapy notes.**

33.1.2 Mobility

Observe by asking the patient the following:

- To sit up in bed without assistance
- To get out of bed and stand
- To walk a few steps, using a cane or walker as necessary

Cognitive function

- Administer Mini-Cog
- Three-item recall
- Clock function (Table 33.2)

Hospital Management by Interprofessional Team

- Clinicians can help to prevent hospitalization-associated disability in patients by implementing certain functional status assessment in the hospital focused on evaluation of ADLs, mobility, and cognition [4].
- Inpatient interdisciplinary team members including the RN, MD, PT, and PCA can help recognize risk factors and implement preventative strategies. Minimum functional and cognitive assessments should be incorporated into assessments as described.
- It is important to recognize the risk factors and risk stratification tools that identify older adults at highest risk of hospitalization-associated disability and implement changes to prevent further functional decline.
- Appropriate actions to prevent immobility and falls include increasing exercise and activity levels, improving the hospital environment, and decreasing the use of psychotropic medications.
- These interventions require collaborative efforts from the interprofessional care team, including physicians, nurses, patient care assistants, physical therapists, nutritionists, etc. to ensure patient is able to maintain functional reserve.
- Disability associated with hospitalization has profound effects on the patient and family long after hospital discharge. Rehabilitation interventions may take time, and patients often do not return to their baseline, and this also requires a lot of caregiver support [1].
- Whether patients will be able to live at home depends not only on their capacity but also on their social support, resources, and environment. Planning for a patient's return to home should include assessing whether the patient can successfully accomplish ADLs alone or with available support and recognizing that many patients able to perform these activities before acute illness may be unable to perform them upon returning home [4].

Table 33.2 Minimum functional assessment in hospitalized older adults

Functional domain	Assessment on admission	Daily assessment
ADLs: taking a bath or shower; getting dressed; transferring (getting out of bed and out of a chair); using the toilet; eating; and walking across a room	For each ADL, the following elements should be assessed at admission and before onset of illness: Difficulty with ADL: "On the day of admission, did you have any difficulty bathing or taking a shower? Did you have any difficulty bathing before the onset of the problem that led to your being hospitalized?" Ascertainment of equipment use for walking (cane or walker) or bathing (shower chair and rails) If patient reports difficulty, assess need for help: "On the day of admission, did you need the help of another person to bathe? How about before this illness?" If the patient needs help, assess adequacy of help: "What help do you need? Who helps you? Do you get enough help?"	Ask nurse or nursing assistant at bedside the extent of help they are providing for bathing, dressing, transferring, using the toilet, eating, and walking Review nursing and physical/occupational therapy notes
Mobility	Observe by asking the patient the following: To sit up in bed without assistance To get out of bed and stand To walk a few steps, using a cane or walker as necessary	Repeat on daily rounds
Cognitive function	Administer the Mini-Cog Give the patient 3 items to remember (i.e., bird, paper, watch) Ask the patient to draw a clock, setting hands to show 11:10 (patient should draw circle, place numbers, place hands) Ask patient to recall the 3 words Score 2 points for correct clock and 1 point for each correct word; ≥3 points indicate a passing score	Assess for delirium on daily interview with patient, and consider: Orientation: "What day of the week is it?" Inattentiveness (does the patient have difficulty focusing, is patient easily distractible) Unclear thinking (does the patient seem to ramble; is the flow of speech unclear, tangential, or difficult to follow) Assess these parameters for fluctuation over time Review nursing notes looking for evidence of these features

Modified from: Covinsky et al. [4]
Abbreviation: *ADL* activities of daily living

Role of the Family and Caregivers

- Frail older hospitalized patients represent a vulnerable population who are at increased risk of functional losses resulting from both the acute illness and potentially modifiable processes of hospital care.
- It is important to identify the patient factors associated with an increased risk of developing disability associated with acute illness and hospitalization.
- Family members and caregivers play a tremendous role in helping to prevent this significant decline. They know the patient's baseline; they are able to advocate for patient's basic needs (i.e., toileting in the bathroom, patience with meals, advocating for mobility, and getting patient out of bed).
- Family and caregivers should feel empowered to promote mobility especially for patients who had good functional status before illness.
- Extended team members should prioritize basic ADL tasks such as getting patient out of day during the day, assistance with toileting, and making use of physical therapy and occupational therapy to complement the acute clinical care.
- Preventing the development of further disability in activities of daily living is an important goal as the patient recovers from an acute illness and often requires collaboration with family and the extended clinical care team.

33.2 Delirium

Definition

- Delirium is defined as an acute, fluctuating syndrome associated with altered attention, awareness, and

cognition, often due to an underlying medical condition [13–15, 20, 21, 23, 26].
- Delirium can be classified as hyperactive, hypoactive, or mixed. Hyperactive delirium, often associated with an agitated patient, represents only 25% of the delirium cases. Hypoactive delirium, often referred to as the "quiet" delirium, is associated with poorer prognosis as it is less often recognized [13–15, 20, 21, 23, 26].
- It is extremely common in hospitalized older adults and should be considered a medical emergency as this may be the only presentation of a life-threatening condition [23].

Prevalence
- One third of general medical patients who are 70 years of age or older have delirium, the condition is present in half of these patients on admission and develops during hospitalization in the other half.
- Delirium is the most common surgical complication among older adults, with an incidence of 15–25% after major elective surgery and 50% after high-risk procedures such as hip fracture repair and cardiac surgery [25].
- Among patients undergoing mechanical ventilation in the intensive care unit (ICU), the cumulative incidence of delirium, when combined with stupor and coma, exceeds 75% [16].
- Delirium is present in 10–15% of older adults in the emergency department. The prevalence of delirium at the end of life approaches 85% in palliative care settings [14, 22].

Etiology and Risk Factors
- Delirium is usually multifactorial and results from the complex interrelationship between a vulnerable patient and exposure to precipitating factors or noxious insults [13–15, 20, 21, 23, 26].
- Risk factors for the persistence of delirium include advanced age, pre-existing dementia, multiple coexisting conditions, and the use of physical restraints [14].
- Risks for delirium can be divided into predisposing and precipitating factors. Patients at high risk of delirium because of multiple or severe predisposing factors need minimal precipitators to provoke a delirium episode. Alternatively, a patient with few predisposing factors would require multiple or severe triggers to provoke delirium [20].

Predisposing Risk Factors
- Advanced age (>80)
- Male gender
- Dementia
- ADL impairment
- Sensory impairment (blindness, deafness)
- High medical comorbidity
- Severity of physical illness*
  - Urinary catheterization*
  - Polypharmacy*
  - Low albumin*
- Prolonged ED/hospital stay

Precipitating Factors Associated with an Acute Hospitalization
- Drug use
- Medications
  - Sedatives-hypnotics
  - Narcotics
  - H2 blockers
  - Anticholinergics
- Electrolytes
- Lack of drugs (withdrawal)
  - Infection
    - Fever/hypothermia, urinary, pneumonia
- Reduced sensory input
- Intracranial problems
- Urinary retention and fecal impaction
- Myocardial problems (Table 33.3)

Special Consideration for Older Adults
- While delirium is often considered a transient and reversible condition, in many patients, global cerebral function may never return to baseline [23].
- Delirium in older adults may be the only presentation of an acute illness and can represent the early signs of serious and often fatal condition among older patients [26].
- Delirium has been associated with a number of poor immediate- and long-term outcomes including the increase risk of falls, length of hospital stay, hospital costs, duration of mechanical ventilation, degree of cognitive impairment, functional impairment after a hospital stay, long-term care facility placement, and mortality [14].
- Substantial additional costs accumulate after hospital discharge because of the need for institutionalization, rehabilitation services, formal home healthcare, and informal caregiving [20].

Assessment
- Delirium is unrecognized in as many as 32–66% of cases [17, 19].
- Advances in diagnosis can improve recognition and risk stratification of delirium. Assessment for and prevention of delirium should occur at admission and continue throughout a hospital stay.
- The Confusion Assessment Method (CAM) has been the gold standard in identifying delirium. This besides

Table 33.3 Summary of risk factors for delirium

Predisposing factors	Precipitating factors	Delirium-inducing medications
Comorbidities	Acute insults	High risk
Alcoholism	Dehydration	Anticholinergics (e.g., antihistamines, muscle relaxants, antipsychotics)
Chronic pain	Fracture	
History of baseline lung, liver, kidney, heart, or brain disease	Hypoxia	Benzodiazepines
	Infection	Dopamine agonists
Terminal illness	Ischemia (e.g., cerebral, cardiac)	Meperidine (Demerol)
Demographic factors		Moderate to low risk
Age older than 65 years	Medications	Antibiotics (e.g., quinolones, antimalarials, isoniazid, linezolid [Zyvox], macrolides)
Male sex	Metabolic derangement	
Geriatric syndromes	Poor nutrition	Anticonvulsants
Dementia	Severe illness	Antidizziness agents
Depression	Shock	Antiemetics
Elder abuse	Surgery	Antihypertensives (e.g., beta blockers, clonidine [Catapres])
Falls	Uncontrolled pain	
History of delirium	Urinary or stool retention	Antivirals (e.g., acyclovir [Zovirax], interferon)
Malnutrition	Environmental exposures	Corticosteroids
Polypharmacy	Intensive care unit setting	Low-potency antihistamines (e.g., histamine H_2 blockers, urinary and gastrointestinal antispasmodics)
Pressure ulcers	Sleep deprivation	
Sensory impairment	Tethers	Metoclopramide (Reglan)
Premorbid state		Narcotics other than meperidine
Inactivity		Nonsteroidal anti-inflammatory drugs
Poor functional status		Sedatives-hypnotics
Social isolation		Tricyclic antidepressants

Modified from: Kalish et al. [23]
Information from references ([4]; [13]; [24]; [25])

assessment has been validated in various clinical settings including the ED, ICU, and general medicine wards and can help establish the diagnosis based on the presence or absence of the four features (an acute change in mental status, inattention, and either disorganized thinking or altered level of consciousness [14] (Fig. 33.1).

Hospital Management by Interprofessional Team

- A well-integrated approach to care by physicians, nurses, other providers, and even family members helps to prevent the complications and poor outcomes often seen in delirium. This is the first step in addressing all modifiable contributors to delirium that are identified during the course of the hospitalization [14].
- All members of the patient's clinical team, including the physicians, nursing staff, patient care assistants, and family members/caregivers, should be familiar with how to recognize and treat delirium [23].
- Environmental factors are also important in delirium management. The hospital ward should be well lit during the day and dark and quiet at night. Interventions to improve orientation and reduce sensory deprivation include clocks, calendars, and encouragement of patients to wear eyeglasses and hearing aids.
- Family members should be encouraged to visit and provide orientation and reassurance.
- Getting the patient out of bed to a chair, and preferably walking, can prevent atelectasis, deconditioning, and pressure ulcers. Monitoring of food and fluid intake can identify those at risk for malnutrition and dehydration.

Fig. 33.1 Confusion Assessment Method (CAM). (Modified from: Kalish et al. [23])

1. Acute onset and fluctuating course
   Is there evidence of an acute change in mental status from the patient's baseline? Did this behavior fluctuate during the past day (that is, did it tend to come and go or increase and decrease in severity)?
2. Inattention
   Does the patient have difficulty focusing attention; foe example, being easily distracted or having difficulty keeping track of what was being said?
3. Disorganized thinking
   Is the patient's speech disorganized or incoherent; for example, rambling or irrelevant conversation, unclear or illogical flow of ideas, or unpredictable switching from subject to subject?
4. Altered level of consciousness
   Overall, how Would you rate this patient's level of consciousness: alert (normal); vigilant (hyperalert); lethargic (drowsy, easily aroused); stupor (difficult to arouse); coma (unarousable)?

Note: The diagnosis of delirium requires a present/abnormal rating for criteria 1 and 2, and either 3 or 4.

Some patients with delirium may require aspiration precautions and monitoring.

- Prevention of delirium using non-pharmacologic approaches is documented to be effective, while pharmacologic prevention and treatment often reserved for agitated delirium remain controversial [26].
- Treatment of delirium should focus on identifying and managing the causative medical conditions, providing supportive care, preventing complications, and reinforcing preventive interventions. This requires efforts by the entire interprofessional team.
- Pharmacologic interventions should be reserved for patients who are a threat to their own safety or the safety of others and those patients nearing death [23].

Role of Family and Caregivers

- Caregivers should be educated on risk factors, preventive measures, as well as signs and symptoms of delirium and conditions that would indicate the need for immediate evaluation.
- Certain medications, sensory impairments, cognitive impairment, and various medical conditions are a few of the risk factors associated with delirium.
- Preventive interventions such as frequent reorientation, early and recurrent mobilization, pain management, adequate nutrition and hydration, reducing sensory impairments, and ensuring proper sleep patterns have all been shown to reduce the incidence of delirium, regardless of the care environment.
- Encouraging family members and caregivers to be present during the hospitalization and promoting involvement in daily activities such as meal times or during procedures can help mitigate the risk of delirium in the hospital.

33.3 Malnutrition

Definition

- Malnutrition is a general term used to refer to any condition in which the body does not receive enough nutrients for proper function [36].
- It can be a result of starvation, in which a person has an inadequate intake of calories, or it may be related to a deficiency of one particular nutrient or due to the inability to properly digest or absorb nutrients from the food they consume, as it may occur with certain medical conditions and acute medical illness [36].
- Malnutrition among the hospitalized elderly population is often multifactorial, with physiologic, pathologic, sociologic, and psychologic factors that can impact nutritional deficiency [31]. An acute illness, disease, and disability are associated with higher rates of malnutrition.
- Malnutrition may range from mild to severe and life-threatening.

Prevalence

- The incidence of malnutrition has been estimated to be 11–44% in the general hospital population, and this number increases to 29–61% in the elderly [34].
- Undernutrition (defined as intake of less than 50% of calculated energy requirements) during a hospital stay occurs in 21% of older adults and is associated with increased inhospital mortality and 90-day mortality compared to patients who have higher level of caloric intake [41].
- Malnutrition present on hospital admission is associated with functional decline at 3 months after hospital

discharge, nursing home placement, and increased mortality in the year after hospital discharge [29].

Etiology and Risk Factors

- Many changes associated with the process of aging can contribute to malnutrition [34]. The *anorexia of aging* refers to physiologic decline in food intake as people age, regardless of chronic illness and disease. This normal physiological change is due to alterations in neurotransmitters and hormones that affect the central feeding drive and the peripheral satiation system [30, 33, 38, 39].
- Body composition also changes with age. The loss of lean body mass and the decreased basal metabolic rate observed with advanced age also may influence appetite and food intake [31, 32, 40].
- Even a 10% loss of lean tissue in healthy adults has been shown to impair immunity, increase infection risk, and be associated with increased mortality [34].
- Aging is frequently associated with decreases in taste acuity and smell, deteriorating dental health, which may all affect nutrient intake. Sensory decline in both olfaction and taste decreases the enjoyment of food, leads to decreased dietary variety, and promotes increased dietary use of salt and sugar to compensate for these declines [27, 31, 32, 40].
- Disorders of the gastrointestinal system—ranging from problems with dentition and swallowing to dyspepsia, esophageal reflux, constipation, and diarrhea—are related to poor intake and malabsorption of nutrients. Many diseases (e.g., thyroid, cardiovascular, and pulmonary disease) often lead to unintentional weight loss through increased metabolic demand and decreased appetite and caloric intake [27].
- Older adults are more likely to suffer from chronic illnesses such as diabetes, hypertension, congestive heart failure, and coronary artery disease which are treated with dietary restrictions and with medication that affects food intake [27].
- Furthermore, older adults tend to take more medications to manage their chronic medical issues which can also affect nutritional status through side effects (e.g., anorexia, nausea, and altered taste perception) and through alteration of nutrient absorption, metabolism, and excretion [31] (◘ Tables 33.4 and 33.5).

Special Consideration for Older Adults

- Poor nutritional status and malnutrition in the elderly population have significant implications during an acute hospitalization.
- Malnutrition and unintentional weight loss contribute to progressive decline in health, reduced physical and cognitive functional status, increased utilization of healthcare services, premature institutionalization, and increased mortality.
- Malnutrition has also been associated with an increased length of stay, treatment costs, and readmission to hospital rates [34].

◘ **Table 33.4** Risk factors for malnutrition

Medical factors	Lifestyle and social factors	Psychological factors	Additional risk factors in hospital
Poor appetite Poor dentition, other oral problems, and dysphagia Loss of taste and smell Respiratory disorders, for example, emphysema Gastrointestinal disorders, for example, malabsorption Endocrine disorders, for example, diabetes, thyrotoxicosis Neurological disorders, for example, cerebrovascular accident, Parkinson's disease Infections, for example, urinary tract infection, chest infection Physical disability, for example, arthritis, poor mobility Drug interactions, for example, digoxin, metformin, antibiotics, etc. Other disease states, for example, cancer	Lack of knowledge about food, cooking, and nutrition Isolation/loneliness Poverty Inability to shop or prepare food	Confusion Dementia Depression Bereavement Anxiety	Food service—sole nutritional supply is hospital food, limited choice, presentation may be poor Slow eating and limited time for meals Missing dentures Needs feeding/supervision Inability to reach food, use cutlery, or open packages Unpleasant sights, sounds, and smells Increased nutrient requirement, for example, because of infections, catabolic state, wound healing, etc. Limited provision for religious or cultural dietary needs Nothing by mouth or miss meals while having tests

Modified from Hickson [34]

Table 33.5 Malnutrition in the elderly

Factors influencing nutritional inadequacy in the elderly population			
Physiologic	Pathologic	Sociologic	Psychologic
Decreased taste	Dentition	Ability to shop for food	Depression
Decreased smell	Dysphagia, swallowing problems	Ability to prepare food	Anxiety
Dysregulation of satiation	Diseases (cancer, CHF, COPD, diabetes, ESRD, thyroid)	Financial status low socioeconomic	Loneliness
Delayed gastric emptying	Medications (diuretic, antihypertensive, dopamine agonist, antidepressant, antibiotic, antihistamine)	Impaired activities of daily living skills	Emotionally stressful life events
Decreased gastric acid	Alcoholism	Lack of interactions with others at mealtime	Grief
Decreased lean body mass	Dementia		Dysphoria

Modified from: Evans et al. [104]
CHF congestive heart failure, *COPD* chronic obstructive pulmonary disease, *ESRD* end-stage renal disease

Table 33.6 Validated screening and assessment tools

Malnutrition Screening Tool (MST)	For older adults in hospital setting
Mini Nutritional Assessment (MNA)	For older adults in community or hospital setting
Mini Nutritional Assessment—Short Form	For older adults in all setting

Modified from: ► https://www.agingresearch.org/app/uploads/2017/12/AAR20Malnutrition20Tip20Sheet2072014.pdf, ► https://www.ncoa.org/assesssments-tools/malnutrition-screening-assessment-tools/, ► https://www.agingresearch.org/app/uploads/2017/12/AAR20Malnutrition20Tip20Sheet2072014.pdf

Assessment

- There are a number of validated screening and assessment tools (Alliance for Aging Research) ► https://www.ncoa.org/assesssments-tools/malnutrition-screening-assessment-tools/ [37] (Table 33.6).

Hospital Management by Interprofessional Team

- As previously mentioned, the causes of malnutrition in older hospitalized adults are often multifactorial. It is important to recognize the medical, social, and psychological factors to the patient's overall nutritional state [34].
- Acute illnesses may also contribute by increasing nutritional requirements and altering metabolism. Hospitals have the ability to provide an additional resource of specialists in nutrition, dietary, and speech therapy who can help address the nutritional needs for patient.

Box 33.1 Interventions to address nutritional deficiencies

- Remove or substantially modify dietary restrictions (i.e., liberalize the patient's diet)
- Ensure that patients are equipped with all necessary sensory aids (glasses, dentures, hearing aids)
- Ensure that the patient is seated upright at 90 degrees preferably out of bed and in a chair
- Ensure that food and utensils are removed from wrapped or closed containers and are positioned within the patient's reach
- Remove or minimize unpleasant sights, sounds, and smells
- Allow for a slower pace of eating; do not remove the patient's tray too soon
- If the patient must be fed, allow adequate time for chewing, swallowing, and clearing throat before offering another bite. Rapport between patient and feeder is critical
- Patients with dementia or cognitive impairment may need to be reminded to chew and swallow and may benefit from availability of "finger foods"
- Encourage the family to be present at mealtime and to assist in the feeding

- Conversations that may arise in the hospital setting include palliative care measures, ("comfort feeds"), appetite-stimulating medication, or enteral feeding if appropriate.
- It is important to note that no drug has received US Food and Drug Administration approval for treating anorexia in the geriatric population [31].
- The primary clinical team should be mindful of interventions appropriate for addressing nutritional deficiencies (► Box 33.1).

Role of Family and Caregivers

- Nutrition care plans should result from interdisciplinary teamwork and involve both patient and family/caregivers. Family members and caregivers play an important role in addressing the nutritional needs of hospitalized elders, as they know the patient best, aware of food preferences, snacks, and how and what they eat.
- Cultural preferences and individual choices are important to optimizing nutrition status in frail elders and allow team to address expectations and provide nutritional education.
- Clinical teams should provide patient/caregiver education to ensure adequate nutrition after discharge [28].

33.4 Pressure Ulcers

Definition

- A pressure ulcer (PU) is a localized injury to the skin and/or underlying tissue usually over a bony prominence, as a result of pressure or pressure in combination with shear [71].
- Pressure ulcers may also be referred to as pressure injury, pressure sore, or bedsore [55].

Prevalence

- The incidences of pressure ulcers are reported to be 0.4–38% in acute care, 2.2–23.9% in long-term care, and 0–17% in home setting and are associated with higher mortality, increased hospital length of stay, and increased total cost [44].

Etiology and Risk Factors

- Usual changes in older person's skin place them at greater risk of developing PU. Farage et al. describe these usual changes including thinning epidermis, reduction in the natural water and fat emulsion on the skin and stratum corneum, decreased global lipid content, decreased subcutaneous fat, and changes in amino acid composition, which may all lead to decreased structural instability.
- Additionally there is slower recovery of transepidermal water loss. These usual changes occur via intrinsic aging as well as exogenous insults such as immobility and incontinence, which may predispose the older patient to injury from pressure, moisture, infection, and shear.
- The dermo-epidermal junction flattens by almost a third beginning in the sixth decade which reduces resistance to shearing forces and increased vulnerability to insult [53, 60]. There is an accompanying decrease in vascularity and cellularity which leads to a lower supply of nutrients and oxygen.
- Importantly, these changes lead to an increased recovery time from mechanical depression or injury from minutes in younger skin to over 24 hours in aging skin [53, 63].

Special Consideration for Older Adults

- Pressure ulcer incidence is an indicator of quality in long-term and acute care [46].
- PU in older patients increases mortality by as much as 400%, also associated with an increase in the frequency and length of hospitalization, and decreases quality of life [48].

Assessment

- Assessment and documentation should include risk factors such as impaired mobility, poor nutrition [48, 73], decreased sensation, urinary and fecal incontinence [48], pre-existing stage I ulcer, increased body temperature, and older age [49, 63, 70].
- Assessment should also include a head-to-toe skin and tissue assessment as soon as possible "but within 8 hours of admission," on an ongoing basis, and increase in frequency with any deterioration in clinical condition paying close attention to areas of bony prominence such as the sacrum, back, heels, trochanter, elbows, and occiput [42, 46, 48, 71].
- A validated risk assessment tool is recommended [71, 72] though studies have suggested there is no statistically significant difference in pressure ulcer incidence using different validated assessment tools versus clinical judgment alone [68].
- Pressure ulcers are staged by the most common staging method [48], the NPUAP system, the depth of tissue damage from I to IV with stage (or "category") I as the most superficial and stage IV as the deepest.
- When the wound bed is not visualized or covered with necrotic tissue, it is staged "unstageable." A deep tissue injury is a "purple or maroon localized area of discolored intact skin or blood-filled blister due to damage of underlying soft tissue from pressure and or shear" [71].
- Stage I refers to an area of non-blanchable erythema, stage II refers to superficial skin loss, stage III penetrates into fat, and stage IV penetrates to muscle, bone, and connective tissue [71] (▫ Table 33.7).

Hospital Management by Interprofessional Team

- The basic tenets of PU management include risk assessment, skin assessment, prevention, and treatment [43, 49, 61, 71].
- An interdisciplinary team approach should be considered in preventing and managing PU in the older adult. Nursing and nursing assistants are at the forefront of this management turning and positioning the patient, physicians and nurse practitioners contribute to managing comorbid conditions, pharmacists can help guide better medication choices for the older patient, physical and occupational therapists can help the patient with mobility in and out of the bed, registered dieticians must be consulted to know the correct kilocalorie and protein requirements for the older patient with PU, and speech and language pathologists

Table 33.7 Characteristics of pressure ulcers

Characteristics of pressure ulcers, by stage	
Stage I	Intact skin with non-blanchable redness
Stage II	Partial thickness loss of dermis; no fat visible
Stage III	Full-thickness loss, fat may be visible
Stage IV	Full-thickness loss with exposed bone, tendon, or muscle
Unstageable[a]	Base is covered with slough or eschar. Debridement required to stage

Modified from: Javaheri and Bluestein [58]. Bluestein and Javaheri [45]
[a]Deep tissue injury should be suspected when there is a blood-filled blister or a localized purple- or maroon colored area. A more detailed pressure ulcer staging system is available at ► http://www.npuap.org/pr2.htm

can help evaluate the older patient's ability to swallow safely and help navigate nutritional goals consistent with the patient's goals of care.

- Guidelines for preventing PU include:
  - Repositioning [43, 48, 56, 61, 63, 71]
  - Maintaining clean, dry skin [49, 60, 71] with a pH balanced cleanser and the use of emollients [60, 71]
  - Nutritional supplementation [62, 71]
  - Viscoelastic foam support surfaces, overlays, and Australian medical sheepskin [61, 63, 64, 71, 72]
  - Prophylactic multilayer silicone foam dressings [55, 65–67, 69, 71]
- Evidenced-based PU treatments include similar interventions for prevention, such as positioning and foam support surfaces in addition to other interventions with a similar low-quality evidence base.
- Treatment guidelines from the NPAUP [71] include appropriate pain management, wound cleansing, wound debridement, treatment of infection, wound dressings [43, 46, 48, 55, 76], high-protein nutritional supplementation [62, 63, 73, 74, 76], recombinant platelet-derived growth factor, electrical stimulation [76], electromagnetic agents [43], pulsed radio frequency energy, negative pressure wound therapy [43], and air-fluidized beds (Smith et al. 2016).

(Elder Care Updated May 2005) Javaheri, A and Bluestein, D. Pressure Ulcers in Older Adults. Elder Care: A Resource for Interprofessional Providers. ► www.aging.arizona.edu. June 2009 (updated May 2015) (Tables 33.8 and 33.9)

Table 33.8 Summary of dressing for pressure ulcers [50–52]

Dressing	Suited for	Comments
Transparent film	Stages I–II	Retains moisture; facilitates autolytic debridement; not for infected wounds or fragile skin
Foam	Stages II–IV	Mostly nonadherent; absorbs light and heavy exudates; recommended for fragile skin
Hydrocolloid	Stages I–IV	Not for heavy exudate; molds easily
Hydrogel	Stages II–IV	Relieves pain; good for deep wounds (fills dead space) and infected wounds; not for dry eschar
Alginate	Stages II–IV	Absorbs moderate to heavy exudate; good for deep wounds (fills dead space) and infected wounds; not for dry eschar

Modified from: Bluestein and Javaheri [47], Bergstrom [45]

Table 33.9 Debridement methods

Method	Performed with	Comments
Sharp	Scalpel or scissors	Fastest method. Indicated when infection is present
Mechanical	Whirlpool Wet-to-dry gauze	Saline-moistened wet-to-dry gauze can be used for debridement, but not for routine dressing changes
Enzymatic	Collagen-based	Santyl®
	Papain-urea-chlorophyllin copper	Panafil®
Autolytics	Dressings	Some dressings are autolytic. See Table 33.3

Modified from: Bluestein and Javaheri [47], Javaheri and Bluestein [58], Bergstrom [45]

Role of Family and Caregivers

- Special recommendations for older adults in the NPUAP [71] guidelines include considering the patient's cognitive status, using appropriate pain assessment tool (e.g., FLACC if the patient is nonverbal) [61], differentiating PU from other skin injuries (e.g., skin tear), setting goals consistent with those of the patient, including the family and caregivers in the care plan, educating the patient and family about skin changes in aging, and considering the condition of the patient when repositioning (e.g., critically ill or actively dying) [61].
- Caregivers and family members play a key role in the healing process after a pressure ulcer has developed. They should be educated on preventative strategies that

can be incorporated as basic care to daily routines even after a hospitalization such as:
- Promoting frequent changes in positioning at least every 2 hours. This includes alternating from standing to sitting and moving from one side of the body to the back and then to the other side when lying down.
- **Protecting at-risk areas with extra cushioning.** For example, putting pillows between the legs in bed and using special mattress overlays or chair/wheelchair cushions that are proven to decrease pressure over time can be very useful [75, 77].
- **Regular (at least daily) skin checks of at-risk areas.**
- **Keeping skin lubricated (lotions and creams make the skin more resilient) and free of excess moisture, which increases the risk of skin breakdown.** Barrier creams should be used regularly after every adult brief change to promote skin integrity.
- **Provide nutritious meals that include protein, vitamins, and minerals.** Inadequate nutrition can slow or stop healing and regenerative processes [59, 62].

33.5 Adverse Drug Effects

Definition
- An **adverse drug event** (ADE) is an injury resulting from medical intervention related to a **drug**. This includes medication errors, **adverse drug** reactions, allergic reactions, and overdoses.
- ADEs can happen anywhere: in hospitals, long-term care settings, and outpatient settings.
- Medication-related problems can occur during care transitions from one setting to another and represent a challenge for older adults with complex medication regimens and multiple comorbidities [109].

Prevalence
- Adverse drug reactions (ADR) account for about 10% of all hospital admissions [127].
- 15 percent of hospitalized patients 70 years of age and older experienced at least one ADE, of which more than half were judged preventable [100].
- A meta-analysis of observational studies found that older adult patients were four times more likely to be hospitalized for an adverse drug reaction (ADR) than younger adults.
- Drug-related hospitalizations account for 2.4–6.5 percent of all medical admissions in the general population; the proportion is much higher for older patients [115, 122, 123].
- It is estimated that 88 percent of the ADE hospitalizations among older adults were preventable, compared with 24 percent among young persons [97].

Etiology and Risk Factors
- Older adults are at greater risk for ADR because they are often prescribed and fill more medication than any other group [105].
- With normal aging, there is a decrease in functional reserve with a general loss of total body water, decrease in organ volume, and increase in body fat [103]. Changes in receptor sensitivity, adaptive response, and adherence and under- or overdosing may also lead to ADR [128]. Though aging is a normal process and not pathologic in and of itself, these changes predispose the older adult to ADR.
- Risk factors for developing an ADR include comorbidity, polypharmacy, female gender, specific conditions (e.g., renal failure), decreased function [126], and age-related changes in pharmacokinetics and pharmacodynamics [99, 110, 111].
- ADR increase "exponentially with the number of drugs taken" and may be caused by different types of interactions including drug-drug, drug-disease, drug-herbal, drug-alcohol, drug-food, and drug-nutritional status [126].

Special Consideration for Older Adults
- Older adult patients are vulnerable to medication errors and ADEs due to their multiple comorbidities, diminished physiologic reserve, and more frequent use of multiple drugs [115].
- Adverse drug reactions (ADR) in the older population have been associated with significant morbidity and mortality. ADR effects can include dizziness, lightheadedness, increased risk for falls and fractures, and changes in cardiac conduction, as noted with EKG changes such as prolonged QT interval [99, 126].
- ADR and polypharmacy may predict hospitalization, nursing home placement, death, hypoglycemia, fractures, impaired mobility, pneumonia, and malnutrition [126].
- Older adults are at increased risk of "prescribing cascades." Prescribing cascades occur when a new drug is prescribed to treat symptoms arising from an unrecognized ADE related to an existing therapy [98, 119, 124].
- Drug-induced symptoms in an older person can be easily misinterpreted as indicating a new disease or attributed to the aging process itself rather than the drug therapy.

Assessment
- Medication reconciliation is a process that identifies medication discrepancies, informs prescribing decisions, and prevents medication errors that could harm patients [98, 116, 119, 120, 130].
- A thorough medication reconciliation at various transitions during acute care can reduce discrepancies and decrease actual and potential ADEs [119].

Interventions were most effective that involved pharmacy staff intensively and that targeted high-risk patients.

- A thorough medication reconciliation process should include three steps [107]:
  - Verification: Reviewing the patient's medication use history and developing an accurate list of medications
  - Clarification: Ensuring that the medications and doses are appropriate and using the current list when writing medication orders
  - Reconciliation: Identifying any discrepancies between medications ordered for patients and those on the list, making appropriate changes to the orders, documenting any changes, and communicating the updated list to the next provider within or outside the hospital
- A designated clinician should review the medication list at each patient encounter and every care transition with specific consideration for the use of each medication prescribed, its indication, dose, directions, drug interactions, and side effects when reviewing medications.
- Certain classes of high-risk medications, such as anticoagulants, antihyperglycemic agents, sedatives, narcotics, antibiotics, antipsychotics, and chemotherapeutic agents, are among the leading drug classes associated with ADEs in adults [31, 108].
- These drugs have several common features including narrow therapeutic windows, the potential for idiosyncratic physiologic responses, and variable dosing regimens. Several of the medications require close monitoring and dose adjustment, with the potential for calculation and timing errors.

Hospital Management by Interprofessional Team

- Multidisciplinary approach is important in preventing medical errors.
- Comprehensive medication management involves multiple team members, including the physician, nurse, and pharmacist in the hospital and in the community.
- It is important to be mindful of the high-risk medications which have been consistently associated with ADEs. Specific classes of medications include anticoagulants, antihyperglycemic agents, sedatives, narcotics, antibiotics, and antipsychotics, and chemotherapeutic agents are among the leading drug classes associated with ADEs in adults [31, 108].
- With each care transition, it is important to verify indication of every medication and discontinue any unnecessary drugs. The risk of ADEs increases with the number of medications taken [118].
- Drug-induced side effects are common in older adults and should be considered when a patient presents with a new complaint. Clinicians should discontinue or reduce the dose of medications thought to cause significant adverse effects.
- Clinicians should consider the possibility of a medication inducing new symptoms. It may be necessary to discontinue the inciting drug and replace with an alternative therapy.
- Avoid treating side effects with another drug.
- Be mindful of drug-drug interactions involving commonly used medications (i.e., the risk of bleeding with warfarin therapy is increased with co-administration of NSAIDs).
- It is important to adjust dosing based on age and creatinine clearance in geriatric populations. Due to decreased muscle mass in older adults, serum creatinine levels may not adequately reflect renal function. As a general rule, the initial dose for starting medications in older adults should be significantly reduced and titrated up as tolerated by monitoring side effects or drug levels [117].
- The individual clinician should review the medication list at each patient encounter and adjust medications accordingly to decrease risk of ADEs. This approach includes avoiding high-risk drugs, unnecessary drugs, drugs causing side effects, and drug-drug interaction and adjustments for the patient's creatinine clearance (◘ Table 33.10).

Role of Family and Caregivers

- Patient and caregiver education is extremely important in preventing medication errors. Patients should also be provided written information on the medications when discharged from the hospital.
- For older adults with cognitive impairment and polypharmacy, it is often helpful to explore services available, such as visiting nurses who can assist with medication management and collaborating with outpatient pharmacies to help facilitate proper distribution of medications and safer methods to ensure ADE do not occur.

33.6 Hospital-Acquired Infections

Definition

- Hospital-acquired infection (HAI) is defined as a localized or systemic condition that results from an adverse reaction to the presence of an infectious agent or its toxin; that occurs during a hospital admission; for which there is no evidence the infection was present or incubating at admission; and that meets body site-specific criteria [87].

Prevalence

- The geriatric population is at risk for developing health-care-associated infections especially when hospitalized. This can lead to increased morbidity, mortality, and further complications from hospitalization [79, 80, 86, 93, 129].

Table 33.10 Certain classes of medications have been implicated with more ADE [96, 113, 114, 121, 125, 126]

Drug class	ADE
PPI	Increased risk of osteoporotic fractures of the hip and spine
	Increased risk of developing *Clostridium difficile* infection
	Increased risk of vitamin B12 deficiency
Diabetic medications	Hypoglycemia is associated with increased emergency room visits [102], cardiac ischemia, and in severe episodes development of dementia
	Older adults with an hemoglobin A1c lower than 7% are at an increased risk of falls
	Caution with older adults on beta blockers as this medicine may block the sympathetic response and conceal the symptoms of hypoglycemia
Anticoagu-lants	Bleeding
	Lower risk for ICH with NOAC versus VKA even with falls
	Higher risk of GIB especially with dabigatran
	Risk of GIB increased significantly higher in adults aged
	Drug-drug and drug-food interactions are higher with VKA than NOAC
	NOAC must be adjusted for renal clearance (Karami chael, Kundu, Ng)
Antibiotics	Many require dose adjustments based on renal function
	Nephrotoxicity
	Hearing loss
	Seizure
	Tendon rupture
	Delirium

33

- The >85-year-old age group constitutes a definable group at increased risk for nosocomial and other healthcare-associated infections [89]. In 2010, over 75% of hospital deaths occurred in patients older than 65 years old, and over 27% were older than 85 years old [83, 84, 91, 94].
- One attributed cause is the prevalence of infections such as pneumonia and urinary tract infections. Of these diseases, bloodstream infections (BSIs) are one of the most severe and are associated with high morbidity and mortality rates in older patients [88]. Other types of infection commonly implicated include surgical site infections, soft tissue infections, and other sites.
- The emergence of drug-resistant healthcare infections continues to plague this vulnerable population. These pathogens include MRSA, VRE, and penicillin-resistant pneumococci [90].

Special Consideration for Older Adults

- The geriatric population behaves atypically when presenting with signs and symptoms pertaining to infection [86].
  - Typical features of fever and chills are not reliable markers for infection [80].
    - Older patients have a lower body temperature than that of younger people, and their tolerance to thermal extremes is more limited.
    - Conversely, patients may have fever without infections complicating the decision to administer antibiotics.
- Acute change in mental status or disturbance of consciousness is one of the common atypical presentations in the geriatric patient [84]. Other non-specific manifestations include functional or mobility decline and subtle disturbances in circulation to include hypotension or lactic acidosis without compensatory tachycardia or overt toxemia. Pre-existing cognitive impairment affects the diagnosis even further when patients present with acute delirium.
- They could have positive urine cultures without active signs of infection. It becomes difficult to differentiate asymptomatic bacteriuria versus a true UTI.
- UTIs remain to be the most frequent nosocomial infection in geriatric units [85]. There are two ways by which UTIs arise in catheterized patients: intraluminal ascent and within the space between the catheter surface and the urethral mucosa. In women the latter is favored by virtue of its anatomical proximity to the rectum. The removal of a urinary catheter does not completely protect the individual from infection. About 11% of patients develop bacteriuria within the first 24 hours [92].
- Candida superinfection or a completely stand-alone infection. This develops in 5–10% of catheterized patients and may represent either colonization or an early marker for candidemia [92].
- A 2017 retrospective study by Girard et al. [82] found that nosocomial UTIs (NUTIs) were significantly more frequent among female patients, rehabilitation patients, immunosuppressed patients, and patients with urinary retention with high post-void residual urine volume, history of UTI in the previous 6 months, and functional dependency.
- Furthermore NUTIs were more prevalent in those patients who had a urinary catheter notwithstanding the type (intermittent, indwelling, or suprapubic). Hence the occurrence of NUTI is an important issue in both catheterized and non-catheterized patients that highlights the need for effective prevention programs targeted to both cohorts.
- It is important to underscore that since hospital UTIs are complicated, a single-agent antimicrobial therapy may not be enough. Moreover, treatment may require an

extended course of antibiotics. Relapse is not an uncommon occurrence in geriatric patients treated for UTI.
- Catheter-related bloodstream infections (CR-BSIs) are infections attributed to the use of intravascular catheter.
  - The primary pathogens implicated are *Staphylococcus epidermidis*, *Staphylococcus aureus*, *Pseudomonas aeruginosa*, *Klebsiella* sp., and *Enterobacter*. There are characteristics in the geriatric population that predispose them to developing CR-BSIs. See ◘ Table 33.11 [78]. The retrospective study by Gavazzi [81] showed that community-acquired bloodstream infections are more frequent in the age group older than 85 years.
  - For nosocomial bloodstream infections, *E. coli* and *Staphylococcus aureus* were common pathogens. Mortality was independently associated with the presence of MRSA in both nosocomial and community-acquired bloodstream infections.

◘ Table 33.11 Reasons geriatric patients in ICU are at increased risk for CR-BSIs

Geriatric characteristic	Geriatric response
Increased age	Decreased immunity
Renal compromise	Delays antibiotic filtration or effects amount of antibiotic prescribed
Decreased cardiac output	Lower antibiotic effectiveness
Vascular problems	Inhibit antibiotics from getting to needed areas of the body
Comorbid diseases (COPD, diabetes, hypertension, and pneumonia)	Can affect vasculature and immunity. Multiple lines increase potential CR-BSI
Multiple concurrent medications (steroids, ASA, and NSAIDs)	Can mask signs/symptoms of infections
Increased INR[12]	
	Enhances blood and fluid around CVC insertion site aiding the environment for CR-BSI
Emergently placed CVC (ED, ICU)	
	Increased risk of infection
Thin skin/fragile veins	
	Limit access points and/or lead to vein disruption, infiltration, extravasation
Confusion, dementia, Alzheimer disease	Aids in body movement and positioning at catheter insertion site
Coughing, vomiting, and/or ventilator support	Blood movement in catheter tip and fibrin formation at the tail of the catheter

Modified from: Chermecky et al. [78]
Abbreviations: *ASA* acetylsalicylic acid or aspirin, *COPD* chronic obstructive pulmonary disease, *CR-BSI* catheter-related bloodstream infections, *CVC* central venous catheter, *ED* emergency department, *ICU* intensive care unit, *INR* international normalized ratio, *NSAIDs* nonsteroidal anti-inflammatory drugs

Assessment

- The more common healthcare-associated infections (HAIs) include central line-associated bloodstream infections, catheter-associated urinary tract infections, and ventilator-associated pneumonia. Infections may also occur at surgery sites, known as surgical site infections. The prolonged or inappropriate use of antibiotics can lead to *Clostridium difficile* infections.
- Many of these hospital-acquired infections are preventable, and it is important that clinical teams follow standard protocols to prevent these infections from occurring. This requires daily assessment for the need of central line catheter and urinary catheter or even the use and indication of antibiotic therapy. It is important to be mindful of the date of insertion and the anticipated duration of catheters or antibiotic. Proper precautions with proper hand hygiene and the use of personal protective equipment (PPE) when indicated are fundamental in preventing the spread of infection. It is also extremely important to remove all unnecessary catheters when they are no longer indicated.
- The CDC provides a number of targeted assessment tools to assist institutions in the prevention of HAI. Many institutions have implemented strategies to ensure specific protocols are in place to manage and ensure the prevention of catheter-associated urinary tract infection (CAUTI), central line-associated bloodstream infection (CLABSI), ventilator-associated event (VAE), surgical site infection (SSI), and Clostridium difficile infection (CDI).

Hospital Management by Interprofessional Team

- Institutional settings such as nursing homes and other facilities are equally at risk for developing healthcare-associated infections. Recognition of this hazard of hospitalization has prompted the generation of guidelines aimed toward infection control programs, antimicrobial therapy use, and surveillance activity against drug-resistant pathogens and prevention of nosocomial infections and complications.
- Early goal-directed therapy with antimicrobial agents is a key strategy in treating infections and preventing complications such as sepsis. However, there are significant risks and adverse consequences of inappropriate antibiotic therapy in the elderly including drug interactions, side effects, renal impairment impacting drug dosages and host clearance, and risks associated

with opportunistic superinfection such as *Clostridium difficile*.
- As much as it is vital to proactively treat these infections, it is equally important to practice preventative measures especially from a nursing care standpoint. These high priority activities include handwashing, surface disinfection, flushing, minimal catheter manipulations, dressing management, and minimal use of lines.
- Steps can be taken to control and prevent HAIs, and this requires coordinated efforts by the interdisciplinary care team. Research shows that when healthcare facilities, care teams, and individual doctors and nurses are aware of infection problems and take specific steps to prevent them, rates of some targeted HAIs (e.g., CLABSI) can decrease by more than 70 percent.

Role of Family and Caregivers
- Family members and caregivers should be considered patient advocates in the prevention of HAI. They should be informed of the indication for the use of the catheters and its anticipated duration.
- It is important that they are educated on proper hand hygiene protocols and recommended PPE should be provided.

33.7 Physical and Pharmacologic Restraints

Definition
- **Physical restraint** is defined as the direct application of physical force to a patient with or without the patient's permission to restrict his or her freedom of movement [142]. The types of restraints include protective and restrictive devices such as jackets, cloths, wrist devices, ankle devices, and mittens tied with straps. Its use has the potential for negative patient outcomes to include loss of dignity, violation of patient's rights, psychological impairment, physical harm, and, the worst of them, death [136, 137].
- **Chemical restraint** is the use of pharmacologic agents to control the behavior of an agitated patient. A common recommendation is to use antipsychotics as first line and minimize use of benzodiazepines known to cause paradoxical excitation or agitation in the older adult [136, 137].

Prevalence
- The utilization of physical restraints in the older adult population is a common practice especially in institutional settings such as the hospital, psychiatric facilities, and nursing homes [142]. In the acute care setting, physical restraints are used in the emergency rooms, medical floors, and intensive care units (ICUs).
- The incidence in the ICU setting ranges from 20% to 50% in non-ventilated patients and up to 80% in ventilated patients [132, 138, 143].
- In the emergency rooms, previous studies have cited the use of physical restraints in 0.3–4% of patients [134, 144]. The incidence of both physical and chemical restraints increases with advanced age.

Risk Factors
- Delirium is the most common indication for using both physical and chemical restraints; however, delirium has also been shown to be worsened by use of physical restraints [139].
- Patients who demonstrate behavioral changes such as confusion, agitation, and disorientation in an acute care setting can pose a challenge to nursing staff in managing these behaviors as they can interfere with medical and nursing treatments [141].
- Patient characteristics that are associated with the use of restraints include cognitive impairment, older age, functional dependence in activities of daily living (ADLs), history of falls, polypharmacy, and previous history of restraint use [131].

Special Consideration for Older Adults
- Physical or chemical restraints may be indicated when environmental or behavioral modifications are not practical or deemed ineffective especially for severe behavioral changes that interrupt medical therapy or present a threat to self or staff.
- A study by Michaud et al. [140] supporting the early use of pharmacological treatment in the ICU setting showed shorter duration of use of physical restraints and less time receiving mechanical ventilation compared with those who did not. This is especially helpful in patients who test positive for delirium within 24 hours of being screened for it.
- The downside to using antipsychotics is that in the elderly, adverse reactions may occur to include extrapyramidal symptoms and prolongation of the QTc interval leading to arrhythmia, sedation, ataxia, and worsening confusion in some patients [135].
- The use of physical restraints has the potential for negative patient outcomes to include loss of dignity, violation of patient's rights, psychological impairment, physical harm, and, the worst of them, death.

Hospital Management by Interprofessional Team
- Specialized dementia units have been observed to be more successful than traditional nursing homes to reduce the use of restraints [133].
- It has also been reported that restraints are helpful in keeping patients safe and preventing falls [133].
- In general, the standard management for disruptive behaviors related to delirium is primarily non-pharmacological. This includes but not limited to periodic redirection, reorientation, family visitation, use of one to one sitters, low-level lighting, environmental manipulation, adequate repositioning while lying on the hospital bed, early ambulation, proper

use of sensory aids, continence training, optimal hydration, and nutrition. The success in its application involves collaborative teamwork among the different providers from the doctors to the nurses and the support staff.

- Neuman's systems model is a conceptual framework by which nursing staff's role could be more streamlined regarding interventions for the disruptive older adult patient. This model views the patient as a dynamic system of physiological, psychological, sociocultural, developmental, and spiritual variables [131]. The theory accounts for how patients react with both internal and external environmental stressors and how providers coordinate activities that will help patients respond better to these stressors.
- The intervention of this study focused on education of all staff regarding the use of nonrestraint interventions to manage disruptive behaviors in the acute care setting. See ► Box 33.2 by Nandel Smith (2001) for nonrestraint interventions.

Box 33.2 Restraint options and intervention categories

- *Environmental*
  - Noise
    - Eliminate/decrease noise
    - Play soothing music
  - Lighting
    - Provide day/night lighting
    - Open blinds during the day
    - Leave nightlight/bathroom light on with door closed at night Temperature
    - Control temperature (assess hot versus cold)
  - Bed
    - Leave side rails up × 2, × 3
    - Bed alarm
    - Make call light accessible
  - Treatments (equipment)
    - Evaluate need for intravenous fluids versus intermittent needle therapy
    - Evaluate need for Foley catheter or offer bedpan/urinal frequently
    - Camouflage tubes, dressings, etc.
  - Supportive devices/restraint options
    - Mittens united
    - Intravenous sleeve
    - Freedom splint
    - Activity apron
- *Physical*
  - Nutrition
    - Assess for thirst/hunger
    - Provide ice chips
    - Provide mouth care
  - Comfort
    - Administer medications for pain, itching, nausea, indigestion, etc.
    - Provide repositioning/realignment
    - Offer back rub
  - Sleep patterns
    - Napping throughout the day
    - Caffeine, especially at supper or bedtime
  - Activity
    - Range of motion
    - Out of bed per physician orders
    - Obtain physical therapy consult for ambulation strengthening
- *Physiological*
  - Drug interactions/side effects/toxicity
    - Pain medications
    - Sleeping pills
    - Antihypertensives/diuretics
    - Glycemic agents
  - Infections
    - Urinary tract infections
    - Pneumonia
  - Pulmonary
    - Respiratory distress
    - Hypoxia
    - Obtain respiratory consult
  - Metabolic
    - Electrolyte imbalances
- *Psychological*
  - Cognitive level
    - Provide frequent reorientation
  - Communication barrier
    - Anticipate needs
  - Fatigue
    - Provide rest periods
    - Short naps
  - Anxiety/fear
    - Family support system
    - Stagger visits
    - Provide reassurance
  - Depression/boredom
    - Provide stimulation
    - Obtain occupational therapy consult

Modified from: Smith et al. [141]

Role of Family and Caregivers

- An important member of the team is the caregiver or family member who can help reorient the delirious patient.
- The use of physical and/or chemical restraints is reserved as the last resort especially around patient's safe well-being, staff safety, and treatment administration.
- As previously mentioned, the standard management for disruptive behaviors related to delirium is primarily non-pharmacological. This includes but not limited to periodic redirection, reorientation, and encouraging family visitation.
- Hospitalization, the stress of an acute illness, unfamiliar setting, etc. can contribute to confusion and agitation. Having family and caregivers at the bedside can help mitigate the use and/or need of unnecessary restraints.

References

Functional Decline

1. Boyd CM, Landefeld CS, Counsell SR, Palmer RM, Fortinsky RH, Kresevic D, Burant C, Covinsky KE. Recovery of activities of daily living in older adults after hospitalization for acute medical illness. J Am Geriatr Soc. 2008;56(12):2171–9. https://doi.org/10.1111/j.1532-5415.2008.02023.x.
2. Brown CJ, Friedkin RJ, Inouye SK. Prevalence and outcomes of low mobility in hospitalized older patients. J Am Geriatr Soc. 2004;52(8):1263–70.
3. Covinsky KE, Palmer RM, Fortinsky RH, Counsell SR, Stewart AL, Kresevic D, Burant CJ, Landefeld CS. Loss of independence in activities of daily living in older adults hospitalized with medical illnesses: increased vulnerability with age. J Am Geriatr Soc. 2003;51: 451.
4. Covinsky KE, Pierluissi E, Johnston CB. Hospitalization-associated disability: "She was probably able to ambulate, but I'm not sure". JAMA. 2011;306(16):1782–93. https://doi.org/10.1001/jama.2011.1556.
5. Creditor MC. Hazards of hospitalization of the elderly. Ann Intern Med. 1993;118(3):219–23.
6. Gill TM, Allore HG, Holford TR, Guo Z. Hospitalization, restricted activity, and the development of disability among older persons. See comment in PubMed Commons below JAMA. 2004;292(17): 2115–24.
7. Gill TM, Allore HG, Gahbauer EA, Murphy TE. Change in disability after hospitalization or restricted activity in older persons. JAMA. 2010;304(17):1919–28. https://doi.org/10.1001/jama.2010.1568.
8. Katz S. Assessing self-maintenance: activities of daily living, mobility, and instrumental activities of daily living. J Am Geriatr Soc. 1983;31:721.
9. Mahoney JE. Immobility and falls. Clin Geriatr Med. 1998;14(4): 699–726.
10. Malone ML, Capezuti E, Palmer RM. (2015). Acute care for elders. A model for interdisciplinary care. Flood KL, et al. Geriatrics models of care. Bringing best practice to an aging America (pp 25-45).
11. Russo CA, Elixhauser A. Hospitalizations in the elderly population, 2003. Statistical Brief #6. Healthcare Cost and Utilization Project (HCUP) Statistical Briefs [Internet]. Rockville: Agency for Health Care Policy and Research (US); 2006 May.
12. Sager MA, Franke T, Inouye SK, Landefeld CS, Morgan TM, Rudberg MA, Sebens H, Winograd CH. Functional outcomes of acute medical illness and hospitalization in older persons. Arch Intern Med. 1996;156:645–52.

Delirium

13. Ahmed S, et al. Age Aging. 2014;43(3):326–33.
14. Edward R, Marcantonio MD. Delirium in hospitalized older adults. N Engl J Med. 2017;377:1456–66.
15. Elie M, et al. Delirium risk factors in elderly hospitalized patients. J Gen Intern Med. 1998;13(3):204–12.
16. Ely EW, Shintani A, Truman B, et al. Delirium as a predictor of mortality in mechanically ventilated patients in the intensive care unit. JAMA. 2004a;291:1753.
17. Han JH. Delirium in older emergency department patients: recognition, risk factors, and psychomotor subtypes. Soc Acad Emerg Med. 2009;16:193–200.
18. http://aging.arizona.edu/sites/aging/files/fact-sheet-pdfs/delirium_0.
19. Hustey F, et al. The prevalence and documentation of Impaired mental status in elderly emergency department patients. Ann Emerg Med. 2002;41(5):678–84.
20. Inouye SK. Delirium in older persons. N Engl J Med. 2006;354:1157–65. https://doi.org/10.1056/NEJMra052321.
21. Inouye SK, Bogardus ST, Charpentier PA, Leo-Summers L, Acampora D, Holford TR, Cooney LM. A Multicomponent intervention to prevent delirium in hospitalized older patients. N Engl J Med. 1999;340(9):669–76.
22. Inouye SK, Westendorp RG, Saczynski JS. Delirium in elderly people. Lancet. 2014;383:911–22.
23. Kalish VB, Gillham JE, Unwin BK. Delirium in older persons: evaluation and management. Am Fam Physician. 2014;90(3):150–8.
24. Marcantonio ER. In the clinic: delirium. Ann Intern Med. 2011;154(11):ITC6–1. 8.
25. Marcantonio ER. Postoperative delirium: a 76-year-old woman with delirium following surgery. JAMA. 2012;308:73–81.
26. Oh ES, Fong TG, Hshieh TT, Inouye SK. Delirium in older persons: advances in diagnosis and treatment. See comment in PubMed Commons belowJAMA. 2017;318(12):1161–74. https://doi.org/10.1001/jama.2017.12067.

Malnutrition

27. Ahmed T, Haboubi N. Assessment and management of nutrition in older people and its importance to health. Clin Interv Aging. 2010;5:207–16.
28. Avelino-Silva TJ. Omar Jaluul malnutrition in hospitalized older patients: management strategies to improve patient care and clinical outcomes. Int J Gerontol. 2017;11:56–61.
29. Covinsky KE, Martin GE, Byth RJ, Justice AC, Sehgal AR, Landefeld CS. The relationship between clinical assessments of nutritional status and adverse outcomes in older hospitalized medical patients. J Am Geriatr Soc. 1999;47:532–8.
30. Endoy MP. Anorexia among older adults. American Journal for Nurse Practitioners. 2005;9(5):31–8.
31. Evans C. Malnutrition in the elderly: a multifactorial failure to thrive. Perm J. 2005;9(3):38–41.
32. Fávaro-Moreira NC, Krausch-Hofmann S, Matthys C, et al. Risk factors for malnutrition in older adults: a systematic review of the literature based on longitudinal data. Adv Nutr. 2016;7(3):507–22. https://doi.org/10.3945/an.115.011254.
33. Heersink JT, Brown CJ, Dimaria-Ghalili RA, Locher JL. Undernutrition in hospitalized older adults: patterns and correlates, outcomes, and opportunities for intervention with a focus on processes of care. J Nutr Elder. 2010;29(1):4–41. https://doi.org/10.1080/01639360903574585.
34. Hickson M. Malnutrition and ageing. Postgrad Med J. 2006;82(963):2–8. https://doi.org/10.1136/pgmj.2005.037564.
35. https://www.agingresearch.org/app/uploads/2017/12/AAR20Malnutrition20Tip20Sheet2072014.pdf \.
36. https://www.medicinenet.com/script/main/art.asp?articlekey=88521.
37. https://www.ncoa.org/assesssments-tools/malnutrition-screening-assessment-tools/.
38. Huffman GB. Evaluating and treating unintentional weight loss in the elderly. Am Fam Physician. 2002;65(4):640–50.
39. Morley JE. Pathophysiology of anorexia. Clin Geriatr Med. 2002;18(4):661–73, v.
40. Senior health: how to prevent and detect malnutrition - Mayo Clinic. https://www.mayoclinic.org/healthy-lifestyle/caregivers/in-depth/senior-health/art-20044699.
41. Sullivan DH, Sun S, Walls RC. Protein-energy undernutrition among elderly hospitalized patients: a prospective study. JAMA. 1999;281(21):2013–9.

Pressure Ulcers

42. Ashby RL. A pilot randomized controlled trial of negative pressure wound therapy to treat grade III/IV pressure ulcers [ISRCTN69032034]. Trials. 2012;13(1) https://doi.org/10.1186/1745-6215-13-119.
43. Aziz Z. Electromagnetic therapy for treating pressure ulcers. Cochrane Database Syst Rev. 2015;(9) https://doi.org/10.1002/14651858.CD002930.pub6.

44. Bauer K, Rock K, Nazzal M, Jones O, Qu W. Pressure ulcers in the United States' inpatient population from 2008 to 2012: results of a retrospective nationwide study. Ostomy Wound Manage. 2016;62(11):30–8.
45. Bergstrom N. United States. Treatment of pressure ulcers guideline panel. Treatment of pressure ulcers. Rockville: U.S. Dept. of Health and Human Services, Public Health Service, Agency for Health Care Policy and Research; 1994.
46. Bergstrom N. The National Pressure Ulcer Long-Term Care Study: outcomes of pressure ulcer treatments in long-term care. Journal of the American Geriatrics Society (JAGS). 2005;53(10):1721–9. https://doi.org/10.1111/j.1532-5415.2005.53506.x.
47. Bluestein D, Javaheri A. Pressure ulcers: prevention, evaluation, and management. Am Fam Physician. 2008;78(10):1186–94.
48. CADTH. Canadian Agency for Drugs and Technology in Health. Dressing materials for the treatment of pressure ulcers in patients in long-term care facilities: a review of the comparative clinical effectiveness and quidelines; 2013.
49. Demarre L. Factors predicting the development of pressure ulcers in an at-risk population who receive standardized preventive care: secondary analyses of a multicenter randomized controlled trial. J Adv Nurs. 71(2):391–403. https://doi.org/10.1111/jan.12497.
50. Dumville JC. Alginate dressings for treating pressure ulcers. Cochrane Database Syst Rev. 2015a;(5) https://doi.org/10.1002/14651858.CD011277.pub2.
51. Dumville JC. Hydrogel dressings for treating pressure ulcers. Cochrane Database Syst Rev. 2015b;(2) https://doi.org/10.1002/14651858.CD011226.pub2.
52. Dumville JC. Negative pressure wound therapy for treating pressure ulcers. Cochrane Database Syst Rev. 2015c;(5) https://doi.org/10.1002/14651858.CD011334.pub2.
53. Farage MA. Characteristics of the aging skin. Adv Wound Care (New Rochelle). 2013;2(1):5–10. https://doi.org/10.1089/wound.2011.0356.
54. Francis K. Disposable versus reusable absorbent Underpads for prevention of hospital-acquired incontinence-associated dermatitis and pressure injuries. J Wound Ostomy Continence Nurs. 2017;44(4):374–9. https://doi.org/10.1097/WON.0000000000000337.
55. Gefen A. Clinical and biomechanical perspectives on pressure injury prevention research: the case of prophylactic dressings. Clin Biomech (Bristol). 2016;38:29–34. https://doi.org/10.1016/j.clinbiomech.2016.08.005.
56. Gillespie BM. Repositioning for pressure ulcer prevention in adults. Cochrane Database Syst Rev. 2014;(4) https://doi.org/10.1002/14651858.CD009958.pub2.
57. https://nursingandhealth.asu.edu/sites/default/files/pressure-ulcers.pdf.
58. Javaheri A, Bluestein D. Pressure ulcers in older adults. Elder care: a resource for interprofessional providers. www.aging.arizona.edu. June 2009 (updated May 2015).
59. Koretz RL. Does enteral nutrition affect clinical outcome? A systematic review of the randomized trials. Am J Gastroenterol. 2007;102(2):412–29. https://doi.org/10.1111/j.1572-0241.2006.01024.x.
60. Kottner J. Maintaining skin integrity in the aged: a systematic review. Br J Dermatol. 2013;169(3):528–42. https://doi.org/10.1111/bjd.12469.
61. Langemo D. Evidence-based guidelines for pressure ulcer management at the end of life. Int J Palliat Nurs. 2015;21(5):225–32. https://doi.org/10.12968/ijpn.2015.21.5.225.
62. Langer G, Fink A. Nutritional interventions for preventing and treating pressure ulcers. Cochrane Database Syst Rev. 2014, Issue 6. Art. No.: CD003216. https://doi.org/10.1002/14651858.CD003216.pub2
63. Lozano-Montoya I. Nonpharmacologic interventions to prevent pressure ulcers in older patients: an overview of systematic reviews (the Software ENgine for the assessment and optimization of drug and non-drug therapy in older persons [SENATOR] definition of optimal evidence-based non-drug therapies in older people [ONTOP] series). J Am Med Dir Assoc. 2016;17(4):370.e371–10. https://doi.org/10.1016/j.jamda.2015.12.091.
64. McInnes E. Support surfaces for pressure ulcer prevention. Cochrane Database Syst Rev. 2015;(9) https://doi.org/10.1002/14651858.CD001735.pub5.
65. Moore ZEH. Dressings and topical agents for preventing pressure ulcers. Cochrane Database Syst Rev. 2013;(8) https://doi.org/10.1002/14651858.CD009362.pub2.
66. Moore ZEH. Repositioning for treating pressure ulcers. Cochrane Database Syst Rev. 2015;1 https://doi.org/10.1002/14651858.CD006898.pub4.
67. Moore ZEH. Risk assessment tools for the prevention of pressure ulcers. Cochrane Database Syst Rev. 2019;(2) https://doi.org/10.1002/14651858.CD006471.pub3.
68. Moore ZEH, Cowman S. Wound cleansing for pressure ulcers. Cochrane Database Syst Rev. 2013;(3) https://doi.org/10.1002/14651858.CD004983.pub3.
69. Moore ZEH, Webster J. Dressings and topical agents for preventing pressure ulcers. Cochrane Database Syst Rev. 2013, Issue 8. Art. No.: CD009362. https://doi.org/10.1002/14651858.CD009362.pub2
70. Mudge AM. CHERISH (collaboration for hospitalized elders reducing the impact of stays in hospital): protocol for a multi-site improvement program to reduce geriatric syndromes in older inpatients. BMC Geriatr. 2017;17(1) https://doi.org/10.1186/s12877-016-0399-7.
71. National Pressure Ulcer Advisory Panel. European Pressure Ulcer Advisory Panel and Pan Pacific Pressure Injury Alliance. In: Haesler E, editor. Prevention and treatment of pressure ulcers: quick reference guide. Perth, Australia: Cambridge Media; 2014.
72. Park KH. The efficacy of a viscoelastic foam overlay on prevention of pressure injury in acutely ill patients: a prospective randomized controlled trial. J Wound Ostomy Continence Nurs. 2017;44(5):440–4. https://doi.org/10.1097/WON.0000000000000359.
73. Posthauer ME. The role of nutrition for pressure ulcer management: national pressure ulcer advisory panel, European pressure ulcer advisory panel, and pan pacific pressure injury alliance white paper. Adv Skin Wound Care. 2015;28(4):175–88. https://doi.org/10.1097/01.ASW.0000461911.31139.62.
74. Reddy M, Gill SS, Kalkar SR, Wu W, Anderson PJ. Treatment of pressure ulcers: a systematic review. JAMA. 2008;300(22):2647–62. https://doi.org/10.1001/jama.2008.778.
75. Saha S, Smith MEB, Totten A, Fu R, Wasson N, Rahman B, Motu'apuaka M, Hickam DH. Pressure ulcer treatment strategies: comparative effectiveness. Comparative effectiveness review No. 90. (Prepared by the Oregon Evidence-based Practice Center under contract No. 290-2007-10057-I.) AHRQ Publication No. 13-EHC003-EF. Rockville: Agency for Healthcare Research and Quality; 2013. www.effectivehealthcare.ahrq.gov/reports/final.cfm.
76. Smith MEB. Pressure ulcer treatment strategies: a systematic comparative effectiveness review. Ann Intern Med. 2013;159(1):39–50. https://doi.org/10.7326/0003-4819-159-1-201307020-00007.
77. Teno JM. Feeding tubes and the prevention or healing of pressure ulcers. Arch Intern Med. 2012;172(9):697–701. https://doi.org/10.1001/archinternmed.2012.1200.

Hospital Infections

78. Chermecky C, Macklin D, Blackburn P. Catheter-related bloodstream infections (CR-BSI) in geriatric patients in intensive care units. Crit Care Nurse Q. 2015;38:280–92.
79. Crossley KB, Peterson PK. Infections in the elderly. In: Mandell GL, Bennett JE, Dolin R, editors. Principles and practice of infectious diseases. 5th ed. Philadelphia: Churchill Livingstone; 2000. p. 3164–9.
80. Gavazzi G, Krause KH. Ageing and infection. Lancet Infect Dis. 2002;2:659–66.

81. Gavazzi G, Mallaret MR, Couturier P, Iffenecker A, Franco A. Bloodstream infections: differences between young-old, old, and old-old patients. JAGS. 2002;SO:1667–73.
82. Girard R, Gaujard S, Pergay V, Pornon P, Martin-Gaujard G, Bourguignon L. Risk factors for urinary tract infections in geriatric hospitals. J Hosp Infect. 2017;9:74–8.
83. Hall MJ, Levans S, DeFrances C. Trends in inpatient hospital deaths: National Hospital Discharge Survey, 2000-2010. NCHS Data Brief. 2013;118:1–8.
84. Heppner HJ, Cornel S, Peter W, Philipp B, Katrin S. Infections in the elderly. Crit Care Clin. 2013;29:757–74.
85. Heudorf U, Boehicke K, Schade M. Health-care association in long term care facilities (HALT) in Franfurt am Main, Germany, January to March 2011. Euro Surveill. 2012;17.
86. Juthani-Mehta M, Quagliarello VJ. Infectious diseases in the nursing home setting: challenges and opportunities for clinical investigation. Clin Infect Dis. 2010;51:931–6.
87. Klevens RM, Edwards JR, Richards CL, Horan TC, Gaynes RP, Pollock DA, Cardo DM. Estimating health care-associated infections and deaths in US hospitals, 2002. Public Health Rep. 2007;122: 160–6.
88. McBean M, Rajamani S. Increasing rates of hospitalization due to septicemia in the U.S. elderly population. 1986-97. J Infect Dis. 2001;183:596–603.
89. Strausbaugh LJ, Joseph CJ. Epidemiology and prevention of infections in residents of long term care facilities. In: Mayhall CG, editor. Hospital epidemiology and infection control. 2nd ed. Philadelphia: Lippincott Williams and Wilkins; 1999. p. 1461–82.
90. Strausbaugh LJ, Crossley KB, Nurse BA, Thrupp LD, SHEA Long Term Care Committee. Antimicrobial resistance in long-term care facilities. Infect Control Hosp Epidemiol. 1996;17:129–40.
91. van Duin D. Diagnostic challenges and opportunities in older adults with infectious diseases. Clin Infect Dis. 2012;54:973–8.
92. Wagenlehner FM, Naber KG. Hospital acquired urinary tract infections. J Hosp Infect. 2000;46:171–81.
93. Yoshikawa TT. Epidemiology and unique aspects of aging and infectious diseases. Clin Infect Dis. 2000;30:931–3.
94. Zalacain R, Torres A, Celis R, Blanquer J, Aspa J, Esteban L, et al. Community acquired pneumonia in the elderly: Spanish multicenter study. Eur Resp J. 2003;21:294–302.

Adverse Drug Events

95. American Geriatrics Society. Updated Beers criteria for potentially inappropriate medication use in older adults. J Am Geriatr Soc. 2015;63(11):2227–46. https://doi.org/10.1111/jgs.13702.
96. Beckett CL. Special considerations of antibiotic prescription in the geriatric population. Clin Microbiol Infect. 2015;21(1):3–9. https://doi.org/10.1016/j.cmi.2014.08.018.
97. Beijer HJ, de Blaey CJ. Hospitalisations caused by adverse drug reactions (ADR): a meta-analysis of observational studies. Pharm World Sci. 2002;24:46.
98. Boockvar KS, Carlson LaCorte H, Giambanco V, et al. Medication reconciliation for reducing drug-discrepancy adverse events. Am J Geriatr Pharmacother. 2006;4:236.
99. Bowie MW. Pharmacodynamics in older adults: a review. Am J Geriatr Pharmacother. 2007;5(3):263–303. https://doi.org/10.1016/j.amjopharm.2007.10.001.
100. Boockvar KS, Teresi JA, Inouye SK. Preliminary data: an adapted hospital elder life program to prevent delirium and reduce complications of acute illness in long-term care delivered by certified nursing assistants. J Am Geriatr Soc. 2016;64(5):1108–13. https://doi.org/10.1111/jgs.14091. Epub 2016 May 10.
101. Bucşa C, Farcaş A, Cazacu I, Leucuta D, Achimas-Cadariu A, Mogosan C, Bojita M. How many potential drug–drug interactions cause adverse drug reactions in hospitalized patients? Eur J Intern Med. 2013;24(1):27–33. https://doi.org/10.1016/j.ejim.2012.09.011.
102. Budnitz DS, Lovegrove MC, Shehab N, Richards CL. Emergency hospitalizations for adverse drug events in older Americans November 24, 2011. N Engl J Med. 2011;365:2002–12.
103. Corsonello A. Age-related pharmacokinetic and pharmacodynamic changes and related risk of adverse drug reactions. Curr Med Chem. 2010;17(6):571–84.
104. Evans RS, Lloyd JF, Stoddard GJ, et al. Risk factors for adverse drug events: a 10-year analysis. Ann Pharmacother. 2005;39:1161.
105. Faulkner CM. Unique aspects of antimicrobial use in older adults. Clinical infectious diseases. Clin Infect Dis. 2005;40(7):997–1004.
106. Gray SL, Sager M, Lestico MR, Jalaluddin M. Adverse drug events in hospitalized elderly. J Gerontol A Biol Sci Med Sci. 1998;53:M59.
107. Greenwald JL, Halasyamani L, Greene J, et al. Making inpatient medication reconciliation patient centered, clinically relevant and implementable: a consensus statement on key principles and necessary first steps. J Hosp Med. 2010;5:477.
108. Gurwitz JH, Field TS, Judge J, et al. The incidence of adverse drug events in two large academic long-term care facilities. Am J Med. 2005;118:251.
109. Haver AE, Sakely H, McGivney MS, Thorpe C, Corbo J, Cox-Vance L, Klatt P, Schleiden L, Balestrino V, Coley K. Geriatrics care team perceptions of pharmacists caring for older adults across health care settings. Ann Long Term Care. 2017;25:14–20.
110. Hines LE, Murphy JE. Potentially harmful drug–drug interactions in the elderly: a review. Am J Geriatr Pharmacother. 2011;9(6):364–77. https://doi.org/10.1016/j.amjopharm.2011.10.004.
111. Hutchison LC, Apos, Brien CE. Changes in pharmacokinetics and pharmacodynamics in the elderly patient. J Pharm Pract. 2007;20:4+.
112. Kaiser Family Foundation, 2017. Retail prescription drugs filled at pharmacies (Annual per Capita by Age). https://www.kff.org/other/state-indicator/retail-rx-drugs-by-age/?currentTimeframe=0&sortModel=%7B%22colId%22:%22Location%22,%22sort%22:%22asc%22%7D.
113. Karamichalakis N, Georgopoulos S, Vlachos K, Liatakis I, Efremidis M, Sideris A, Letsas KP. Efficacy and safety of novel anticoagulants in the elderly. Journal of Geriatric Cardiology : JGC. 2016;13(8):718–23. https://doi.org/10.11909/j.issn.1671-5411.2016.08.011.
114. Kundu A. Minimizing the risk of bleeding with NOACs in the elderly. Drugs Aging. 2016;33(7):491–500. https://doi.org/10.1007/s40266-016-0376-z.
115. Lazarou J, Pomeranz BH, Corey PN. Incidence of adverse drug reactions in hospitalized patients: a meta-analysis of prospective studies. JAMA. 1998;279:1200.
116. Lee JY, Leblanc K, Fernandes OA, et al. Medication reconciliation during internal hospital transfer and impact of computerized prescriber order entry. Ann Pharmacother. 2010;44:1887.
117. Mangoni AA. Age-related changes in pharmacokinetics and pharmacodynamics: basic principles and practical applications. Br J Clin Pharmacol. 2004;57(1):6–14.
118. Mihajlovic S, Gauthier J, MacDonald E. Patient characteristics associated with adverse drug events in hospital: an overview of reviews. Can J Hosp Pharm. 2016;69:294.
119. Mueller SK, Sponsler KC, Kripalani S, Schnipper JL. Hospital-based medication reconciliation practices: a systematic review. Arch Intern Med. 2012;172:1057.
120. National Patient Safety Goal on Reconciling Medication Information (NPSF.3.06.01). The Joint Commission, 2017. Available at:

https://www.jointcommission.org/assets/1/6/NPSG_Chapter_HAP_Jan2017.pdf. Accessed on 18 Oct 2017.
121. Ng KH, Hart RG, Eikelboom JW. Anticoagulation in patients aged ≥75 years with atrial fibrillation: role of novel oral anticoagulants. Cardiol Ther. 2013;2(2):135–49. https://doi.org/10.1007/s40119-013-0019-y.
122. Onder G, Pedone C, Landi F, et al. Adverse drug reactions as cause of hospital admissions: results from the Italian Group of Pharmacoepidemiology in the elderly (GIFA). J Am Geriatr Soc. 2002;50:1962.
123. Pirmohamed M, James S, Meakin S, et al. Adverse drug reactions as cause of admission to hospital: prospective analysis of 18 820 patients. BMJ. 2004;329:15.
124. Rochon PA, Gurwitz JH. Optimising drug treatment for elderly people: the prescribing cascade. BMJ. 1997;315:1096.
125. Salazar JA. Clinical consequences of polypharmacy in elderly: expect the unexpected, think the unthinkable. Expert Opin Drug Saf. 2007;6(6):695–704. https://doi.org/10.1517/14740338.6.6.695.
126. Sera LC. Pharmacokinetics and pharmacodynamic changes associated with aging and implications for drug therapy. Clin Geriatr Med. 2012;28(2):273–86. https://doi.org/10.1016/j.cger.2012.01.007.
127. Tamblyn R. A 5-year prospective assessment of the risk associated with individual benzodiazepines and doses in new elderly users. J Am Geriatr Soc. 2005;53(2):233–41.
128. Waring RH. Drug metabolism in the elderly: a multifactorial problem? Maturitas. 2017;100:27–32. https://doi.org/10.1016/j.maturitas.2017.03.004.
129. Wier LM, (Thomson Reuters), Pfuntner A, (Thomson Reuters), Steiner C. (AHRQ). Hospital Utilization among Oldest Adults, 2008. HCUP Statistical Brief #103. Rockville: Agency for Healthcare Research and Quality; 2010, December. http://www.hcup-us.ahrq.gov/reports/statbriefs/sb103.pdf.
130. Wong JD, Bajcar JM, Wong GG, et al. Medication reconciliation at hospital discharge: evaluating discrepancies. Ann Pharmacother. 2008;42:1373.

Restraints

131. Chinn PL, Kramer MK. Theory and nursing: a systematic approach. 3rd ed. St. Louis: Mosby Year Book; 1991.
132. Ely EW, Shintani A, Truman B, et al. Delirium as a predictor of mortality in mechanically ventilated patients in the intensive care unit. JAMA. 2004b;291:1753–62.
133. Karlsson S, Bucht G, Eriksson S, Sandman PO. Factors relating to the use of physical restraints in geriatric care settings. J Am Geriatr Soc. 2001;49:1722–8.
134. Knott JC, Taylor DM, Castle DJ. Randomized clinical trial comparing intravenous midazolam and droperidol for sedation of the acutely agitated patient in the emergency department. Ann Emerg Med. 2006;47:61–7.
135. Kohen I, Preval H, Southard R, Francis A. Naturalistic study of intramuscular ziprasidone versus conventional agents in agitated elderly patients: retrospective findings from a psychiatric emergency service. Am J Geriatr Pharmacother. 2005;3:240–5.
136. Kow JV, Hogan DB. Use of physical and chemical restraints in medical teaching units. J Can Med Assoc. 2000;162:339–40.
137. Kruger C, Mayer H, Haastert B, Meyer G. Use of physical restraints in acute hospitals in Germany: a multi-centre cross-sectional study. Int J Nurs Stud. 2013;50:1599–606.
138. McNicoll L, Pisani MA, Zhang Y, Ely EW, Siegel MD, Inouye SK. Delirium in the intensive care unit: occurrence and clinical course in older patients. J Am Geriatr Soc. 2003;51:591–8.
139. McPherson JA, Wagner CE, Boehm LM, et al. Delirium in the cardiovascular ICU: exploring modifiable risk factors. Crit Care Med. 2013;41:405–13.
140. Michaud CJ, Thomas WL, McAllen KJ. Early pharmacological treatment of delirium may reduce physical restraint use: a retrospective study. Ann Pharmacother. 2014;48:328–34.
141. Smith NH, Timms J, Parker VG, Reimels EM, Hamlin A. The impact of education on the use of physical restraints in the acute care setting. J Contin Educ Nurs. 2003;34:26–33.
142. Swickhamer C, Colvig C, Chan S. Restraint use in the elderly emergency department patent. J Emerg Med. 2013;44:869–74.
143. Thomason JWW, Shintani A, Peterson JF, Pun BT, Jackson JC, Ely EW. Intensive care unit delirium is an independent predictor of longer hospital stay: a prospective analysis of 260 non-ventilated patients. Crit Care. 2005;9:R375–81.
144. Zun LS. A prospective study of the complication rate of use of patient restraint in the emergency department. J Emerg Med. 2003;24:119–24.

Prevention of Hazards of Hospitalization

Claire Davenport and Rebecca J. Stetzer

A. Chun (ed.), *Geriatric Practice*, https://doi.org/10.1007/978-3-030-19625-7_34

34.1 Competency

Medical students will learn how to recognize individuals at risk for hazards of hospitalization and to prevent and decrease them.

Patient Case Continued from the Previous Chapter, "Hazards of Hospitalization"

This case is carried over from the previous chapter and begins when Mrs. F is admitted to the hospital. Changes in the approach to the case that prevented hazards of hospitalization are noted in italics.

Mrs. F is diagnosed with congestive heart failure and admitted to the medicine service. The intern completes a thorough history and physical in the ER and learns about her almost 60-year marriage, the close relationship with her aide, Eileen, and her love for gardening. Mrs. F is planning to start a small flower garden with Eileen's help, right off the front walk so Mrs. F can easily access it while using her walker. The intern shares this with the team and they frame the care plan within these goals, keeping both their and her focus on getting her home in gardening shape.

The admitting team writes admission orders, including IV diuretics and supplemental oxygen. *Review of the EKG showed no new or concerning changes from her prior EKGs, so the team opted for a non-telemetry bed, according to the quality improvement project in their hospital to decrease unnecessary use of telemetry.* On exam, in addition to basilar rales and lower extremity edema, the intern noted some subtle suprapubic tenderness, and 750 cc of retained urine was subsequently found on bladder scan. *According to hospital policy on indwelling foley catheter use, the bladder was decompressed* via *straight catheterization, a specimen was sent for urinalysis, and a plan was in place to monitor for recurrence with ultrasound.*

The nurse calls physical therapy to bring a walker since Mrs. F did not arrive with hers. On further evaluation of her gait, she needed one-person assistance to stand and was able to walk with the walker with contact guard. Fall precautions are initiated.

After 2 days of ongoing treatment and diuresis, her breathing improved. *Because of Mrs. F's risk factors, including cognitive impairment and increased frailty, delirium precautions were put in place. Her walker was available to her at the bedside, she participated in physical and recreational therapy daily, her husband and Eileen kept framed pictures of them and her daughter on the bedside table, a sleep protocol that utilized chamomile tea, calming music and lowering lights was instituted when she had difficulty sleeping, and anticholinergic medications were discontinued. Her ability to stand improved, but her gait remained slow. For this reason, a commode was placed at the bedside to avoid a fall due to rushing to the bathroom.*

When Mrs. F wakes up in the middle of the night to urinate, she reaches for her walker and ambulates to the commode. A bed alarm goes off at the nurses station and the aid rushes in to assist her, while reminding her to use the call bell.

Mrs. F is discharged home after 4 days in the hospital with a follow-up plan that includes a phone call within 24 h from the transitional care team with a scheduled appointment within 1 week, weight tracking and nutrition planning with the local heart failure clinic, medication list and education for her husband regarding Mrs. F's sleep routine and avoidance of over-the-counter sleep aids. Additionally, Mrs. F is referred for Meals on Wheels to help with the afternoon meal on the days her aide is not there. Mr. F is referred to the Alzheimer's support group and the local chapter of the Alzheimer's Association, in an effort to assist with his caregiver's burden.

34.2 Background

Caring for hospitalized older patients is a complex task. Older adults are a vulnerable group, and are likely to have underlying frailty and multiple chronic conditions. Both the acute conditions prompting hospitalization and their treatments impact other existing conditions. Furthermore, as described in the previous chapter, there are risks associated with simply being in the hospital, which increase with the degree of frailty. The interplay of these factors places older adults at increased risks for prolonged and complicated hospital stays, loss of independence, institutionalization, and death.

Understanding the challenges older adults face in the hospital setting provides an opportunity for minimizing and preventing negative outcomes. Successful hazard reduction requires both adoption and standardization of best practices, as well as individualized treatment plans tailored to patients' unique circumstances.

34.3 Hazards of Hospitalization

Over half of hospitalized patients in the USA are over 65 years old. Elders have more frequent hospitalizations with longer stays, higher complexity of medical conditions, and higher mortality rate [1–4]. The reasons for older adults' increased vulnerability to hospital hazards are due to a combination of intrinsic and extrinsic factors. Intrinsic factors include the physiologic changes of aging, as well as the complicated and often intersecting pathophysiologic impairments due to disease state. Extrinsic factors include hospital practices such as mobility restriction, prolonged use of "tethers" such as catheters, intravenous lines and heart monitors, high-risk medications, restricted diets, and altered sensory input. The hospital environment may therefore accelerate disability.

Elders have intrinsic vulnerabilities we can use to identify frailty, and prevent frail patients hazards of hospitalization. First, we need to identify which patients exhibit frailty.

34.4 Homeostenosis

Homeo*stasis* is the stable, balanced state of an organism. Homeo*stenosis* refers to the diminished capacity to maintain homeostasis when stressed. It is a consequence of limited physiologic reserve and blunted compensatory mechanisms. It amounts to decreased "wiggle room," or fewer reserves in response to stress. It leaves patients at higher risk for complications from small insults and increased vulnerability to hospital-associated conditions (◘ Fig. 34.1).

Homeostenosis is the manifestation of many of the normal physiologic changes of aging, as well as the increased incidence of many (and usually multiple) chronic medical conditions noted in ◘ Table 34.1.

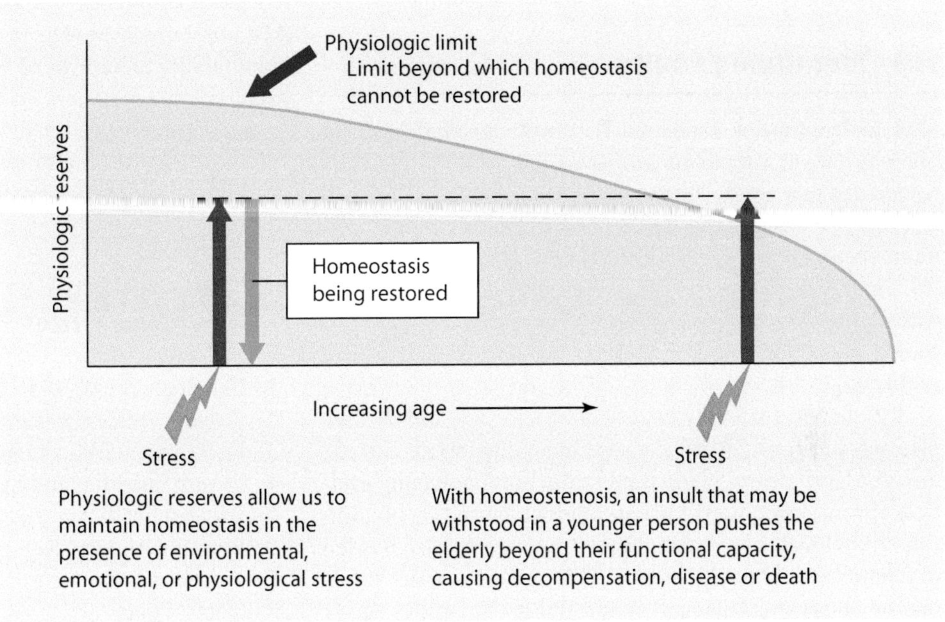

◘ **Fig. 34.1** The combination of frailty and stresses encountered during hospitalization result in hospital-acquired conditions and poor outcomes

◘ **Table 34.1** Physiologic changes of aging contributing to homeostenosis system

	Change	Consequence
Body composition	Muscle tissue replaced by fatty or fibrous tissues	Weakness Impaired mobility Falls
Renal	Loss of cells Decreased blood flow Increased water, decreased salt excretion	Decreased waste removal (including medications) Propensity for dehydration
Cardiovascular	Decrease in beta receptor responsiveness Stiffening of heart and blood vessels Decreased maximum heart rate and cardiac output	Blunted heart rate response to stress, in times of illness, and with standing, increasing fall risk Propensity toward diastolic dysfunction, leaving less tolerance of volume overload as may occur when giving IV fluids for treatment of non-cardiac conditions
Pulmonary	Decreased chest wall compliance and elastic recoil Diminished diaphragm strength Impaired mucocilliary clearance	Intolerance of hypoxemia Increased susceptibility to infection and progression to respiratory failure
Gastrointestinal	Impaired swallow coordination Decreased colonic motility	Dysphagia and aspiration Constipation, risk for bowel obstruction
Immunologic	Decreased barrier integrity due to alterations in skin and mucosa Altered cytokine response Decreased humoral antibody response to infection Blunted febrile response	Increased susceptibility to infection More subtle presentation of infection, making diagnosis more difficult

Organ resilience is based on multiple co-dependent physiologic processes, creating redundancy within an interdependent system. As damage accumulates in each organ, they lose that redundancy and the organs begin to act as though in series. Perturbation in one then affects the entire system. There is a loss of ability to adapt and maintain equilibrium. The individual is at increased risk of adverse outcomes [5]. Loss of the ability to maintain equilibrium, or those with profound homeostenosis, is considered frail.

34.5 Identifying Frailty

Frail patients are at increased risk from hospital hazards. There is not yet a standard definition, but frailty is generally recognized as a constellation of weakness, slowness, reduced activity, low energy, and unintended weight loss. It is common, occurring in up to 10% of community-dwelling elders [6]. The presence of frailty may manifest as the inability to withstand a stress, such as acute illness prompting hospitalization, or multiple small stressors resulting in a fall or failure to thrive.

Risk factors for frailty include advancing age and chronic diseases, but frailty itself is a separate entity. Some chronic diseases have a particularly high frailty burden; having multiple chronic conditions increases vulnerability [7]. In addition, individuals age differently and tolerate disease burden differently [8]. Thus, evaluating frailty gives us more information about an individual's vulnerability than either age or a listing of chronic conditions [9].

Although a well-recognized entity, frailty can be difficult to define or measure. There are dozens of validated, published scales. The Fried phenotype scale is probably the best recognized [10]. It was demonstrated to have reliable prediction of disability, falls, hospitalization, and mortality. It defines frailty as the presence of 3 or more of the following: unintentional weight loss more than 4.5 kg over a year, weakness (lowest twentieth percentile for grip strength), self-reported exhaustion, low physical activity, and slowed walking speed. Other markers of frailty include loss of lean muscle mass, or sarcopenia, [11] being underweight, [12], inability to perform ADLs and iADLs, depression, and impaired cognition [13, 14].

There is also ongoing research to identify frailty biomarkers. These include increased C-reactive protein, anemia, low albumin, glucose intolerance and insulin resistance, increased cortisol, low vitamin levels, and ultrasound-measured muscle quality [15–17]. These, and other biomarkers, are being incorporated into laboratory-based frailty indices [18, 19].

Although there have been attempts to validate frailty markers to inpatients [20], they can be difficult to apply in the hospital, as patients may not be able to participate in performance measures [21] and previous functional levels may not apply. There is also increasing interest and research in the assessment of frailty to predict surgical outcomes [22].

34.6 Using Frailty to Identify Vulnerable Patients in the Hospital

Although there is no standard for measurement of frailty, especially in the hospital setting, being aware that patients may have underlying frailty and looking for some telltale signs can help anticipate vulnerabilities. For example, the Hospital Admission Risk Profile (HARP) score uses age, IADL score and an abbreviated MMSE to help identify high-risk patients, and has been shown to predict hospital-acquired ADL disability as well as in-hospital mortality [23]. Baseline vulnerability to hazards of hospitalization can best be anticipated when admission assessments include assessment for frailty markers such as functional status, physical activity, falls, baseline ADLs and iADLs, cognitive status (including decision-making capacity, if appropriate), and social support.

34.7 Preventing Hazards of Hospitalization for Frail Older Patients

1. Develop a preliminary management plan.
2. Provide sensory and social stimulation.
3. Encourage mobilization.
4. Ensure nutrition and hydration.
5. Support healthy and safe elimination and excretion.
6. Promote healthy sleep hygiene.
7. Ensure appropriate prescriptions.
8. Control pain.
9. Promote good communication in hospital settings.
10. Early discharge planning.

Instituting geriatric care practices in the hospital can prevent hazards of hospitalization and the sequelae [2]. A cascade of hazards can occur following a single adverse event (◘ Fig. 34.2). Rather than being hazard-specific, geriatric care practices reduce a multitude of HOH including delirium, falls, pressure ulcers, unnecessary procedures, hospital-acquired infections, and medication mistakes [1, 3, 4, 24–28{Covinsky, 2011 #5, 29].

Preventing hazards of hospitalization requires person-centered care in addition to the classical disease-based approach. The older patient may be extremely sensitive to changes in their environment, daily routines, and medications. Therefore, the hospital environment and the processes that interrupt the sleep-wake cycle, usual meals, and other routine activities may become triggers for hazards. In addition, due to lack of reserves, medical mistakes affect older people more severely and potentially result in disabling injury [30]. The goal of geriatric care is to both improve the individual's reserves, pushing the physiologic limit farther out as well as to avoid the stressors triggering decompensation. This results in a stabilization of the person's trajectory, despite the onset of acute illness (◘ Fig. 34.3).

1. **Develop a preliminary management plan.** A preliminary management plan incorporates frailty, baseline

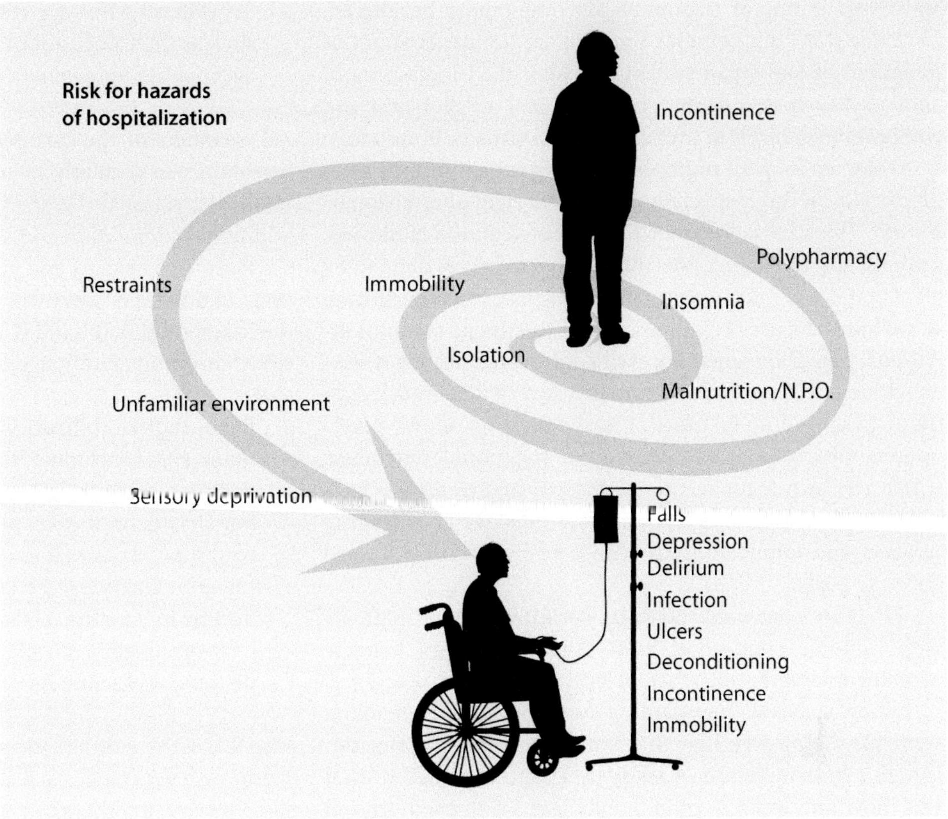

Fig. 34.2 Risks for hazards of hospitalization: multiple small insults culminate into a variety of negative outcomes

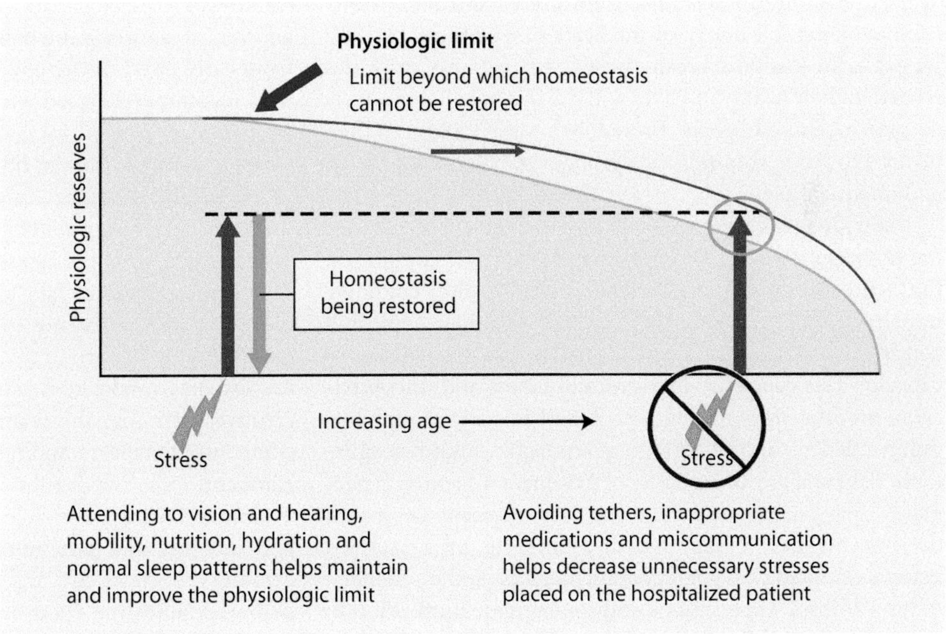

Fig. 34.3 Adopting best practices reduce hazards of hospitalization by improving reserves and reducing stresses

functional status, cognitive assessment, and patient preferences into workup and treatment choices. Prognostic tools such as eprognosis.com or the Charleston Comorbidity Index help the clinician to evaluate and communicate outcomes. Goal-oriented care is developed collaboratively between the provider, the patient, and any caregivers. Established goals, progress, or setbacks are tracked daily.

Hospitalization is frequently a difficult and scary time. This is especially true of older adults who are facing not only treatment of the acute disease crisis but also the effect of both the disease process and the hospitalization on their mobility, independence, and where they live. For fit patients with minimal medical conditions, the goals of care are usually straight forward, and disease-based guidelines direct our care. For frail patients, guidelines may not be appropriate, and expectations of treatment outcomes must be altered. Care decisions are complex and require a balancing act as treatment of one organ system may alter the functioning of another. Reaching a seemingly simple goal of "get better and go home" may result in higher risk of hazards in hospitals.

Older adults with multiple and complex conditions get a lot of medical care, especially during and right after hospitalization. This care is frequently fragmented across clinicians, settings, and diseases. Care without targeted goals defined by what matters to patients both increases the perceived burden as well as decreases compliance with treatment recommendations, especially when not well coordinated among different clinicians. Approaching care in a way that acknowledges the risks and ultimate goals of hospitalization allows development of a care plan focused on functional outcomes, which can help focus recommendations and minimize hazards. Furthermore, we can be more effective in engaging patients and family in their own care by working toward concrete goals.

What are reasonable goals to work toward? For patients with multiple conditions, what outcome defines benefit? Most people agree on a set of universal health outcomes, including survival, maintaining function, and controlling symptoms. However, how that translates to health priorities is highly individualized. A study by Tinetti et al. asked what was most important to older adults faced with the trade-off between the risks of hypertension and falls. About half prioritized avoiding strokes and heart attacks and half prioritized avoiding fall injury or medication symptoms [31]. To set goals, the healthcare team must clarify patients' priorities related to their health and lives and use this to collaboratively develop meaningful goals. These collaborative goals can then be used to guide communication about the illness trajectory and treatment plan.

Individualized treatment plans incorporate understanding of the patient's baseline function and chronic conditions, the acute illness, and healthcare goals. Frailty, cognitive impairment, sensory impairment, and multiple comorbid conditions combine to decrease the body's compensatory capacity. This can result in even mild illness and uncomplicated hospital stays having a profound impact on mobility, independence, and discharge placement. Acknowledging these risks and any uncertainty of treatment outcomes is necessary for patients and families to participate in shared decision-making. Using this discussion to move toward patient-centered care goals enables patients (and physicians) to have realistic expectations and can increase motivation to follow treatment plan recommendations.

2. **Provide sensory and social stimulation.** The hospital can be an isolating and confusing environment for people. Patients with cognitive impairment deprived of sensory engagement and/or socially isolated or dementia are at highest risk for delirium. Obtain and document the baseline cognitive status and iADLs of every older patient – even when they do not have altered sensorium. Document the most recent Montreal Cognitive Assessment (MoCA), Mini Mental Status Exams (MMSE) or Mini-cog results. Delirium assessment tools such as the Confusion Assessment Method (CAM) are appropriate for evaluation of acute changes.

All members of the care team including supportive family members can regularly re-orient patients. If patient is amenable, recreational therapy or volunteer service can provide additional stimulation and support.

Perform a hearing and vision assessment within your history taking and physical exam. Eyeglasses and hearing devices should be placed within reach of the patient. If possible, encourage familiar pictures or other items at the bedside.

3. **Encourage mobilization.** Mobilization can prevent many HOH including hospital-associated disability, delirium, pressure ulcers, contractures, subcutaneous bursitis, incontinence, postoperative complications, readmissions as well as depression, and helplessness [32–40]. Thirty five percent of older adults experience a decline in baseline ADLs after hospitalization, and they have prolonged recovery times [38–41]. Assess and document baseline ADL and activity level at admission

Physical activity orders include out of bed to chair or ambulation with assistance each shift. Orders focus on liberalizing safe movement rather than simply stating bed rest for patients who are unable to ambulate. Ensure easy access to assistive walking devices, clear pathways, gait belts, sturdy equipment, and rest areas along the hallway. Some patients may benefit from early physical therapy consultation. Physical therapists may recommend scaled exercises for frail older adults and adoption of gradual increase in physical activity over the course of hospitalization. Interventions may be active or passive range of motion exercises, isotonic exercise [42].

Support patient mobility and exercise with verbal encouragement and elicit the support of family members in patient rehab efforts. Fear of falls and other factors may come into play when patients do not adhere to early mobilization protocols [43]. It is important to ask about any recent falls, as they are also macroindicators of frailty [44]. It can help to identify creative ways that the team can support the individual to overcome their fears and feel more confident in their environment.

Patients who are unable to transfer will require specific bed mobility and skin nursing care orders. These include keeping skin clean, dry, and moisturized, keeping the patient hydrated, adjusting room temperature, repositioning using pillows and pads at pressure points such as the heels, and monitoring closely for any skin changes. Patients who are incontinent may need more frequent checks. Specific interventions include dynamic splinting or serial casting to prevent contractures. Spasticity can be addressed with medications or surgical release. Disuse osteoporosis can be addressed with standing frame, progressive tilt table conditioning, and other general exercise programs [45–47]. All members of the team will need to be vigilant for any skin changes (◘ Table 34.2).

Table 34.2 Geriatric-specific order set: instituting geriatric care practices in the hospital can prevent hazards of hospitalization and their sequelae

Order	Comment
Admit to: Physician, floor/ward, telemetry	Include special instructions, such as room near nursing station for delirium/fall risks
Acute diagnoses	Include delirium if applicable
Chronic conditions	The presence of multiple chronic conditions affects health status, prognosis, and patient goals. Awareness of these helps with thoughtful evaluation and treatment decisions
Frailty markers: Baseline ADLs/IADLs: independent/assist/dependent Cognitive status: admission screen Baseline activity level Falls in the last year Social support (name, contact information): Malnutrition Depression screen: PHQ-2 or GDS	ADL/IADL dependence, cognitive impairment, malnutrition and depression all increase the risk for iatrogenic events during hospitalization [48]. Cognitive status can be screened with a Mini-cog, or more detailed assessment done with a MoCA
Condition: stable/guarded/critical	
Capacity to make medical decisions: yes/no	Reassess daily if due to delirium
Healthcare proxy (name and contact information): Social work consult if no established healthcare proxy	Previously designated by patient to make healthcare decisions, becomes "activated" when a physician determines a patient is incapable of making medical decisions. Specific legal regulations vary by state. Unbefriended patients without capacity may benefit from ethics consultation
Goals of care:	
Advanced directives: code status, other care limitations	Ask and confirm previous documentation of wishes, initiate discussion of preferences and complete orders as appropriate
Goals of hospitalization	Includes both treatment of the acute condition as well as discharge disposition and functional goals. *For example, recover from myocardial infarction, ambulate to the bathroom, discharge to home*
Discharge planning	Begins at admission. Be clear about functional requirements for planned discharge location. To go home alone, the patient must be able to independently ambulate, eat, toilet, shower, and dress
Vital signs	Orthostatics if relevant
Activity level: Up in chair during day Out of bed for meals To bathroom with assist (vs ad lib) Ambulation orders (i.e., 3 times daily with assist) Place home assistive ambulatory devices (i.e., cane or walker) within reach at the bedside ∗PT consult as needed	Avoid bed rest whenever possible, reassess daily and maximize activity increasing expectation of daily activities over the course of hospitalization
Nursing orders: Assist with glasses and hearing aids Water within patient's reach Feeding assist Skin integrity – daily assessment, out of bed, scheduled position changes if bed-bound Reassess need for catheter, monitor, IV daily	Best practices to avoid delirium are really best practices for hospitalized elders. Using a delirium-prevention approach will help avoid many of the hazards of hospitalization

(continued)

Table 34.2 (continued)

Order	Comment
Elimination and excretion orders Bowels: Daily assessment of bowel movements Standing stool softeners/laxatives with prn orders depending on patient's baseline Bladder: Remove catheters as soon as possible Scheduled toileting Q2h while awake Bedside commode if mobility limiting toileting	Care of bowels and bladder are a critical, and often overlooked, aspect of patient care. Bowel care includes maintaining activity, fluid goals, attention to changes from baseline
Sleep protocol: Lighting bright during day hours, room dark and quiet at night with night light Avoid scheduled medications, vital signs or lab draws between 9 pm and 6 am whenever possible Relaxing music, massage, warm milk, or non-caffeinated tea at bedtime. Melatonin 3 mg an hour before usual sleep with an additional tablet an hour after time of usual sleep as needed	Pay particular attention to timing of medication orders such as diuretics (if twice daily schedule the second dose in the early afternoon to avoid nocturia) and antibiotics (if ordered "four times a day" instead of "every 6 h," nurses can avoid middle-of-the-night doses
Diet orders: Swallow evaluation Consistency, feeding instructions if indicated Dentures Fluid goals per shift Dietician consult for preferences and supplements, especially if baseline malnutrition [49]	Avoid "NPO" whenever possible, reassess at least twice a day. In most cases, dietary restriction does more harm than good. Nursing bedside swallow evaluation vs speech therapy consult if significant dysfunction suspected Fluid goals: maintenance requirement is approx. 30 cc/kg/24 h. Calculate and divide by shift
Allergies	Include reaction whenever possible
Medications: Est CrCl: Home medications	List estimated creatinine clearance by the Cockraft-Gault equation as a reminder for renal dosing of medications Medication reconciliation may require collateral history from caregiver and a call to the outpatient pharmacy for what is actually being taken. Nursing home or rehab patients may have a medication administration record sent with them in a folder. High-risk medications may have been chosen as a last report, discussion with PCP is helpful. Medications that are to be stopped may need to be weaned off to avoid withdrawal symptoms
Labs/ancillary studies	Consider what is going to be done with the information before ordering the test. Is it going to help achieve the patient's goals? Unless emergent schedule between 08:00–21:00 to avoid unnecessary disruptions in sleep
DVT prophylaxis	Combined with anticoagulation, intermittent pneumatic compression devices may reduce the risk of VTE in post-surgical but not medical patients [50]. There is more compelling evidence for use after a stroke. However, they are a form of tether and may contribute to delirium and falls

Refs. [23, 51]

In the hospital, there are a multitude of interventions that prevent freedom of movement. Urinary catheters, intravenous lines, and sequential compression devices may act as tethers preventing mobility. Restraints are acceptable only when there is no safer alternative and there is a significant risk of self-harm or injury. They may be used only for brief period for an emergent intervention or at the patient's request [52–54].

4. **Ensure good nutrition and hydration.** Disordered nutrition and hydration may contribute singly or interact cumulatively with other adverse factors to result in HOH (Fig. 34.4) [25, 55–58]. For example, patients with BUN/Cr ratio greater than or equal to 18 are at higher risk of delirium [58]. In one study, over 40% of hospitalized older patients exhibit clinical findings of dehydration on admission, and it was still present in

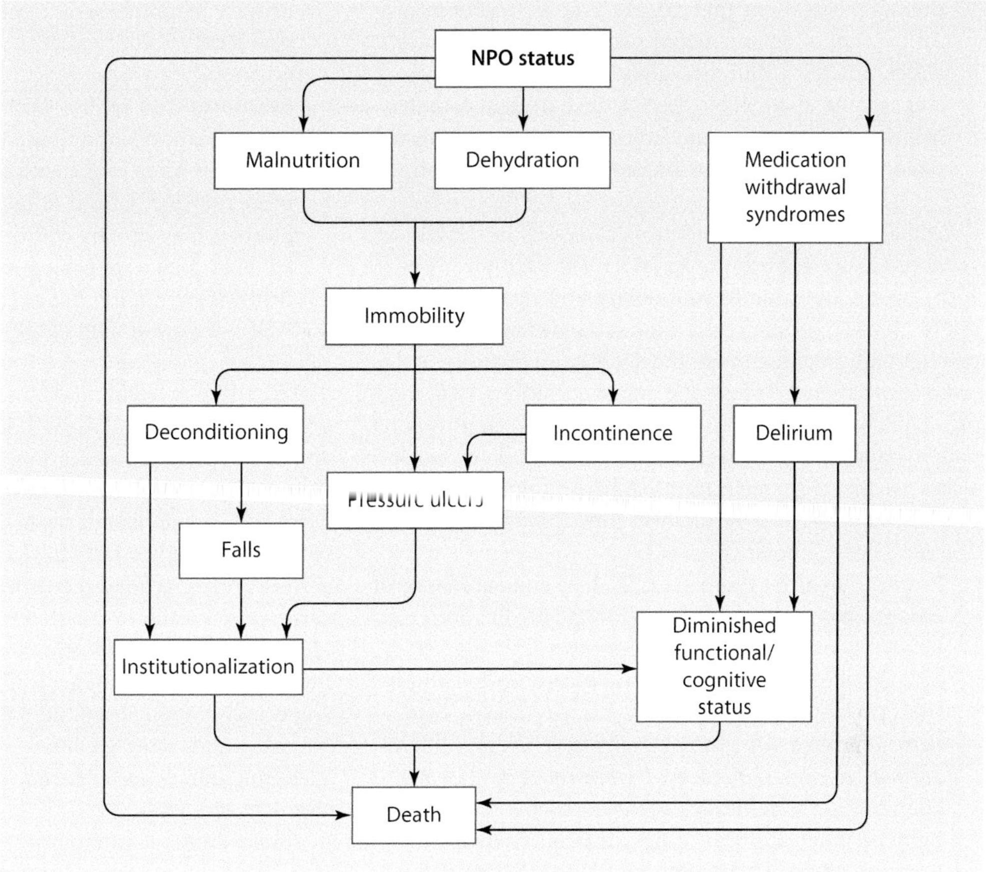

Fig. 34.4 NPO status is Notable for Poor Outcomes: the cascade of comorbidities that can be triggered by NPO status, leading to profound morbidity and mortality

over 60% of those patients 48 h after admission. Patients with dehydration were 6 times more likely to die than hydrated patients, and those who were still deyhdrated at the 48-h mark had the worst outcomes [59]. Even with appropriate measures in place, the older individual may have decreased hypothalamic sensitivity to osmolarity and increased salt wasting and therefore may need encouragement to take in enough fluids to remain intravascularly replete. Initial screens for nutrition and hydration should be performed on all at-risk patients.

Evaluation should include the subjective and objective findings and be supported by meaningful laboratory data. For example, a patient who reports poor appetite may show a 10% weight loss when reviewing prior weights, physical exam may display sarcopenia, abdominal obesity, or skin tenting, and the serum albumin or total lymphocyte count may be low [60]. The plan should then reflect the collected information and describe interventions.

Interventions with respect to malnutrition may begin with an initial bedside dysphagia screen, performed by the physician or other practitioner, to prevent delays in oral intake. Depending on the technique used and clinical setting, bedside screens are 63–96% sensitive for safe oral intake [61–63]. Defer screening patients who are unable to remain alert for testing, have a feeding or tracheostomy tube, require a head elevation of less than 30 degrees, or have known or suspected dysphagia due to a weak cough, history of frequent aspiration pneumonia, or change in voice quality. A simple screen that a physician or nurse can perform is the 3 Ounce Water Swallow Challenge Protocol which has a 96% sensitivity and 46.4% specificity for dysphagia [63]. Sit patient upright at 80–90 degrees and ask them to drink 3 ounces of water from a cup or with a straw, in a sequential swallow, without stopping. If there is no coughing, choking, tearing or change in voice quality, they are safe for an unrestricted diet [64].

Taste sensation decreases with age. Therefore, foods that are low in salt or sugar can be bland and result in poor oral intake. Provide older patients with the least restrictive diet possible. Also minimize the time that a patient must have nothing by mouth (NPO, Latin phrase *nil* per os). Start NPO orders at midnight prior to planned procedures and encourage patients to eat dinner and a snack the night before. Ensure return to a diet as soon as it becomes appropriate. The order might state "contact physician for diet order when patient becomes alert following procedure."

5. **Support healthy and safe elimination and excretion.** Issues with the urinary tract are common in older patients and can be exacerbated by hospital practices. Be vigilant to the appropriate indications for urinary catheter placement, which include output monitoring if the patient is unstable, complete urinary retention, incontinence in patients with serious wounds or skin defects in the perineal and sacral areas, terminally ill or perioperatively [65, 66]. Review and consider discon-

tinuing medications that can exacerbate conditions of urinary retention and incontinence, including opiates, anticholinergics, diuretics, alpha-adrenergic agonists, and calcium channel blockers. Utilize straight catheterization when possible, and timed voiding. Treat constipation as a possible contributor to urinary retention.

Constipation in the hospital setting can easily be missed, and yet, it is a major contributor to HOH. For example, a patient with constipation due to immobility and opioid treatment might develop urinary retention and delirium [67]. Ask patients daily and document the quality and quantity of their bowel movements. When starting medications that might precipitate constipation, such as narcotics, preemptively initiate a standing bowel regimen. Bowel stimulants, such as senna, are first-line single agents. Add osmotic agents such as polyethylene glycol if refractory. Bowel softeners, such as docusate, have poor efficacy [68].

6. **Promote healthy sleep**. Restful sleep and avoidance of sedative hypnotic and anticholinergic medications can help prevent HOH including delirium and falls [29, 67, 69]. Up to 60% of older patients with comorbid conditions such as cognitive impairment, psychiatric disorders, neurologic disease, or frailty have sleep problems at their baseline [70]. Sleep disruption in the hospital is common for a multitude of reasons such as alarms, lights, visitors, ambient noises, unfamiliar environment, tests and vitals [29, 71]. For this reason, between 41% and 96% of older hospitalized patients are prescribed sedative hypnotics and subject to their negative sequelae [69].

Improvements in the sleep environment can be accomplished by decreasing alarms, general noise and light burden at night, avoiding unnecessary vitals checks during usual sleeping hours and rescheduling recurrent IV medications during waking hours. Mobilization, cognitive engagement and access to light during the day can promote normal circadian rhythm [29]. Non-pharmacologic nursing intervention can include massage, essential oils, healing touch therapy, relaxing music, warm non-caffeinated tea, or milk. Milk contains naturally occurring tyramine, an amino acid that promotes sleepiness. Nursing shift documentation can track daytime napping, sleep quality and interruptions of sleep with noted interventions.

Sleep aids are associated with increased risk of delirium and falls during hospitalization [29, 67, 69]. Diphenhydramine is highly anticholinergic and not safe as a sleep aid. Melatonin is currently considered more safe and effective in the inpatient setting. Usual starting dose is 3–5 mg an hour or two prior to usual sleep onset, with additional tablet if sleep is not attained.

7. **Ensure appropriate prescriptions**. Adverse drug events (ADEs) are the most common type of iatrogenic injury and disproportionately impact older patients [72]. Inappropriate prescribing is associated with many HOH including delirium, falls, dizziness, syncope, urinary incontinence, cognitive changes, and sleep problems in older patients. Adverse drug events include errors, adverse drug reactions, allergic reactions and overdoses, and are associated with potentially inappropriate medications and medication omissions alike. ADEs are more likely with the addition of three or more new mediations at once. On the other hand, patients may acutely withdraw from medications that are held such as neuroleptics, antidepressants, or benzodiazepines. It has been estimated that 30–50% of ADEs are preventable [72].

The first step in avoiding ADEs in the hospital is confirming what the patient is taking at home. There are frequently discrepancies among medication lists held by the patient, the primary care physician, specialists, prior discharge summaries, and home health agencies. Contacting pharmacies (including mail-order) to learn what prescriptions are actively being refilled, confirming what is being given by caregivers (family or assisted living or nursing home staff) and asking for all medications to be brought in for review all help confirm that the medication list is accurate. Also ask (repeatedly) about over-the-counter medications, vitamins, herbals, and supplements. The multidisciplinary team, including nurses and pharmacists, are important partners in this detective work.

Prescribing, at minimum, should follow the five rights; right medication, right dose, right patient, right time, and right route. Hospital processes that decrease improper administration of prescription medications include barcode technology and requesting independent double-checks as well as supporting open communication between all care providers regarding potentially unsafe drugs or doses [73]. Document the dose, frequency, indication, and benefit of the medications that are ordered. If the prescriber is concerned about specific side effects, document them and verbalize directly with the bedside care team, including the patient and their family.

Appropriate drug selection can be challenging, particularly in the older, frail patient, where drug-drug and drug-disease interactions can result in serious morbidity and mortality. Classes of medications causing increased ADEs in the elderly include anticholinergics, narcotics, psychotropics, sedative hypnotics, digoxin, and anti-hypertensives. Important prescribing considerations include increased higher likelihood of needing to renally dose medications as well as increased incidence of QT prolongation, restricting use of medications such as fluoroquinolones, and some psychotropics. With multiple chronic conditions, there is also increasing polypharmacy, increasing the risk of drug-drug interaction. Pharmacists are excellent resources in sorting out potential interactions, as well as looking for medications added to treat side effects of other medications.

There are a few tools to help guide medication choices. The Beer's list and Screening Tool of Older People's Potentially Inappropriate Prescriptions (or STOPP) list aim to guide prescribers away from potentially inappropriate medication choices. If medications on these lists cannot be avoided, start them at low doses, with slow upward titration, remaining vigilant for adverse effects. Ensure the entire care team is monitoring for changes in mental status, urinary complications, gastrointestinal effects, imbalance, or falls [2].

Awareness of the increased risks of medications in the elderly is critical, but must not lead to avoiding appropriate treatment. The screening tool to alert doctors to tight treatments (or START) helps to alert physicians to treatments that are indicated, but which might be under prescribed. For example, prescribing anticoagulants in the setting of atrial fibrillation, even in certain patients with fall risks, or starting an angiotensive converting enzyme (ACE) inhibitor following acute myocardial infarction. These tools have resulted in a significant improvement in medication appropriateness, reduced prescribing omissions, correct duration, duplications, and costs [74].

Remember to keep patient goals in mind when developing a new drug regimen for long-term use. Forward thinking about the affordability and lower complexity of a treatment regimen can improve adherence. Clear written directions that convey the name of the medications, the dosage and indication can greatly help the patient or their proxy. Multiple checks on drug reconciliation at the time of discharge, as well as dissemination to the primary care provider and pharmacy, can help prevent confusion and additional errors.

8. **Control pain.** Undertreated pain can precipitate delirium, falls, atelectasis and lead to poorer experience of care. Pain is a subjective experience without specific biologic marker, which presents obstacles in this era of evidence-based medicine and reliance on laboratory and imaging tests for many treatment paradigms. There is understandable concern among many physicians that older adults are more likely to have adverse effects from medications used for pain, including constipation, dizziness and balance issues, and addictive behaviors. Patient factor-based approaches to pain can help balance these important considerations.

When taking a pain history, assessment has been standardized by the Joint Commission on Accreditation of Healthcare Organization to include location, radiation, mode of onset, character, temporal pattern, exacerbating and relieving factors, and intensity. Pain scales such as the Simple Descriptive Pain Distress Scale, 0–10 Numeric Distress Scale, or the Faces Pain Rating Scale may be selected and results documented within the medical chart.

Vital signs such as tachycardia, hypertension, and tachypnea can represent untreated pain. Patients might exhibit neuropsychiatric distress, aggression, and increased confusion. Caregivers may be able to alert the team to other pain-related behaviors. Patients with neurologic disorders may show increased spasticity. The physical exam may reveal tenderness, guarding, wincing, or flinching. Point tenderness, associated findings, or diffuse findings should be carefully documented and reassessed during treatment.

Planning pain control incorporates patient-specific goals with expectation setting, depending on the etiology. For mild pain, non-pharmacologic treatment, such as positional changes, splinting, heat/cold packs, massage, and relaxation, may be helpful. Scheduled or PRN acetaminophen can be considered. Moderate nociceptive pain (4–6 on the Numeric Pain Rating Scale or 3–5 on Nonverbal Pain Scale) can be addressed with scheduled medications. Non-steroidal anti-inflammatory medications can be added to scheduled acetaminophen in patients without active or known coronary vessel disease or renal dysfunction. For moderate-to-severe pain, standing weight and pain severity-based opioids, with additional orders for breakthrough pain, remain standard of care with weight-based dosing, as well as consideration of renal clearance and time to efficacy. In some cases, the dose of opioid medication can be titrated using a patient-controlled analgesia (PCA) pump, which may have a basal rate continuous infusion of weight-based dosed narcotic and additional self-administered boluses, with a threshold shut off. Remember to begin bowel regimens on all patients who are newly begun on opioid medications, starting with bisacodyl or other stimulant or osmotic agent, such as polyethylene glycol. Neuropathic pain may respond to neuroleptic medications such as gabapentin.

9. **Communication in the hospital setting.**

Frail older adults may have very complicated hospital courses. They can be wrought with errors, poor outcomes, and unexpected mortality. All of these things can weigh hard on the patient, their family and the medical team. One of the most important methods to increase resiliency for all of the invested parties is to optimize communication.

Informed consent to care may be challenging for older patients who are frail. Consent is necessary prior to interventions and certain treatments as well as code status and healthcare proxy appointment. The four elements of medical decision-making capacity first described by Appelbaum in 1988 are:

> 1. The ability to communicate a choice
> 2. The ability to understand the relevant information
> 3. The ability to appreciate a situation and its consequences and
> 4. The ability to reason rationally [75]

Capacity to make a medical decision is not all or nothing, and a patient may have capacity to make some decisions (such as refusing a blood draw) but not others (such as surgery). In addition, decisions may evolve and change over time.

When patients are cognitively impaired, collateral information can provide information about the history of present illness, the baseline cognitive and functional status and the patient's prior goals and preferences. Besides family members or friends, additional resources for collateral information include nurse managers at skilled nursing facilities and home healthcare aides.

When acceptable to the patient, offer family meetings to improve understanding and support decision-making. Ask what the patient or their family members understand about the medical conditions and listen to their response for areas of confusion and points that will need to be emphasized during the discussion [76]. Document family meetings within the medical record with clearly stated outcomes.

As team leaders, physicians can improve the overall care by ensuring that all members of the team feel comfortable asking questions and expressing concerns. Careful attention to transitions in care can help to prevent some of the medical mistakes that result in HOH. The Joint Commission Center for Transforming Healthcare mandates all hospitals develop uniform handoff methods. The I-PASS handoff bundle includes communication tools and training to improve handoffs reducing preventable adverse events by 30%. Each transition would include information regarding the illness severity, patient summary, action list, situation awareness, contingency planning, and synthesis by receiver [77].

10. **Incorporate early discharge planning.** Acute medical illness can be a sentinel event in the trajectory of an older person, wherein they may need additional support to return home to the community, acute or subacute rehab, or even institutionalization within a nursing home. Early discharge planning refers to the process by which a social worker or other practitioner evaluates a patient's clinical information and discusses with them (or their representative) the plans for safe discharge from the hospital, when the acute illness is resolved. In meta-analysis, early discharge planning reduced hospital readmissions between 30 days and 12 months after discharge and lowered readmission lengths, but did not change the length of stay, mortality, or patient satisfaction. Qualitative data suggest early dc planning associated with greater overall quality of life in the 2 weeks following discharge [78].

Patients or their proxies should be considered full partners in the discharge planning process. Acute medical illness can be a sentinel event in the trajectory of an older person wherein they may need additional support to return home to the community, acute or subacute rehab, or even institutionalization within a nursing home.

Physical therapists in the hospital can be consulted to evaluate patients who have become debilitated in the community, or over the course of hospitalization. The therapist will recommend certain exercises, and assistive devices while the patient is admitted. The therapist will also recommend the patients' likely disposition at time of discharge.

Concerns for patient safety are addressed by the medical team as it is neither ethical nor legal to discharge a patient into an unsafe environment. Patient safety risks could include physical limitations of their home environment as well as patient or caregiver physical, cognitive, or psychological reasons. Therefore, additional training for the caregiver, home safety evaluation, home physical therapy, and referrals to agencies for nursing or home care or additional support organizations in the region may be recommended. Referrals for institutional care require adequate time for insurance processing and acceptance. Follow-up appointments or tests are arranged for ahead of the discharge date and clearly communicated to the patient upon discharge.

34.8 Additional Resources in the Hospital for the Older Patient

Typically, hospitals excel at rapid patient evaluation with treatment focused solely on the acute medical condition and early discharge home. Yet this approach does not necessarily best serve the frail, older patient. At-risk, older patients can be identified with self-reported tools or indicators within the electronic medical record and steered toward specifically elder-friendly treatment. Acutely ill older patients significantly benefit from geriatric-specific models of care, such as geriatric emergency departments, geriatric evaluation and management units (GEM), acute care for the elderly units (ACE), mobile acute care for the elderly units (MACE), hospital at home programs (HaH) and Nurses Improving Care for Healthsystem Elders (NICHE) training [24, 26, 79, 80]. The Hospital Elder Life Program (HELP) relies on volunteers in the hospital, and has been shown to decrease the incidence of delirium [29].

Consultants can also serve to decrease the incidence or effects of HOH on the older adult. Delirium management can include neurology, psychiatry, and geriatrics. Palliative care consultation can be helpful in the setting of advancing chronic, incurable illness, and end-of-life care.

34.9 Preventing Hazards for Older Surgical Patients

Older adults carry a higher burden of surgical care. Forty percent of all inpatient operations are performed on adults 65 and older [81]. There is a much higher risk for mortality and morbidities with emergency surgery, compared with planned surgeries. Fracture from fall on level ground mortality can be as high as 40% [81]. Additionally, older adults can have higher risk of poor outcomes compared to younger patients, particularly in the setting of emergent unplanned surgery. For example, with acute appendicitis, older adults have two times a higher risk of death. Older patients are frequently under-triaged in the setting of acute trauma, which may contribute to poorer outcomes. Prognostication and information sharing with the patient or their healthcare proxy is essential for informed decision-making in the setting of any proposed surgical intervention.

The American College of Surgeons and American Geriatrics Society have published best practice guidelines for preoperative assessment of the older surgical patient [82]. They recommend an assessment of the cognitive ability, including medical decision-making capacity, screening for depression, risk factors for developing postoperative delirium, alcohol dependence or substance abuse, cardiac evaluation (utilizing the American College of Cardiology and American Heart Association), risk factors for pulmonary complications, functional status, history of falls, baseline frailty score, nutritional status, comprehensive medication history and evaluation of polypharmacy, determining patient's treatment goals and expectations, social support system, and appropriate preoperative diagnostic tests.

Frailty is a vital consideration when deciding on surgical options and prognostication. Increased frailty results in poorer outcomes including prolonged length of stay, higher level of care at discharge, readmission, and both 30-day and 1-year mortality [83]. The patient may express that they feel exhausted, or a social screen may reveal social vulnerability.

During surgery, anesthesia should be tailored to the individual; consider regional options when general anesthesia presents considerable risk. After surgery, best practices should be used, and include the selection of appropriate sleep aids, avoidance and discontinuation of unnecessary anticholinergic medications, avoidance of benzodiazepines, monitoring for any signs of drug or alcohol withdrawal, and cautious use of antipsychotic medications (when absolutely necessary, start low and go slow, checking the QTc or JT index). Titrate down and off of antipsychotics when possible and prior to discharge from the hospital.

Palliative surgeries are considered non-curative, but can be essential in the care of a patient with chronic illness. These treatments should be offered in the setting of severe, advancing, incurable illness and may be an important component of patient-centered care [84].

34.10 Preventing Hazards for Older Patients in the Intensive Unit Care Unit

With the increase in the number of intensive care unit beds across the USA, older patients are accessing this level of care more often. Although 50% of people admitted to the ICU are aged 65 and older, the rates of mortality for older patients in the medical or surgical ICU range between 60–80% [85–87]. Patients in the ICU are at higher risk for nosocomial infection, procedures, poor pain control, mobility restrictions, sleep interruption, delirium, increased in-hospital length of stay, and restrictive visiting with friends and family members resulting in increased morbidity. For patients with advanced dementia, mechanical ventilation showed no improvement in outcomes and had the potential to prolong suffering [88]. Rather than severity of illness, outcomes are better when the decision to admit or transfer an older patient to the ICU is based on the patient's baseline cognition, physical status and personalized goals of care [89–91].

Intensive care unit for older adults is associated with long-lasting cognitive impairment, physical disability, psychological effects including post-traumatic distress syndrome, and depression. Collectively, persisting cognitive, physical, and psychological effects of ICU care are called postintensive care syndrome. In one study, 15–50% of older adults had new cognitive deficits, 40% lost one ADL, 80–100% had persistent skeletal muscle impairments 2 weeks after discharge from the ICU.

Postintensive care syndrome has been the focus of a number of interdisciplinary team-based structured mobility programs, such as the ABCDEF bundle and University of Maryland Medical System's Early Mobility. The ABCDEF bundle stands for Assessing Pain, Both spontaneous awakening and breathing trials, Choice of drugs, Delirium: regularly assess for changes in cognitive status/ institute preventative measures/ identify underlying serious illness/ and manage symptoms monitoring/management, Early exercise/mobility, and Family empowerment [92, 93]. These protocols are associated with increased patient activity level; decreased hospital-associated complications, muscle atrophy, and length of stay; and improved level of discharge. Early rehabilitation was shown to decrease days of mechanical ventilation, length of stay in ICU, delirium, and functional loss, while resulting in improved pulmonary function [94].

An ICU admission is an essential time to host family meetings to convey medical information, and support shared decision-making for an older frail adult. Families may struggle with decisions to discontinue life-sustaining measures. Withdrawing supports at this time is considered ethically equivalent to never having started it. When discontinuing ventilator support, it is important to minimize suffering, using a stepwise approach [95]. The medical team may be faced with the double effect, wherein relieving suffering may decrease the time to death. Interestingly, opioids and other sedatives may actually prolong life rather than hasten death, after ventilator withdrawal [96]. Families benefit from opportunities to share their experiences with the patient, receiving information that is clear with explanation of the process of palliation during end-of-life care. They should be encouraged to utilize spiritual support.

34.11 Case Wrap-Up

Thinking in terms of collaborative goals rather than disease-specific outcomes takes the daily focus away from the disease state, and places treatment of the disease within the context of achieving the patient's goals. Mrs. F of course wants her heart failure exacerbation resolved, but what she really cares about is getting back home to her husband, aide, and gardening plans.

When the medical team took a goal-focused approach, collaborating with Mrs. F and her family to form a realistic and achievable goal, the daily care plan focused on measures that needed to be achieved for Mrs. F to go home, including being able to ambulate in the house, get to the bathroom, and get prepared meals ready. The care plan focused on mobility and strength by avoiding bed rest, calling for a physical therapy consult, providing Mrs. F with a walker and a commode by the bed. This also helped Mrs. F avoid pressure ulcers, falls, urinary incontinence, all of which can lead to increased morbidity and possibly institutionalization. Hopefully, her gardening goals will help provide motivation for her ongoing participation with physical therapy, diet and medication adherence when she gets home. Focusing on these goals can also help the healthcare team make treatment decisions when faced with trade-offs.

The previous chapter outlined common hazards of hospitalization. In this chapter, we have reviewed approaches to care that can avoid or minimize these outcomes. Prevention strategies are of necessity multifactorial, and each intervention impacts multiple outcomes. Working together with your medical team to optimize hospital stays for frail older adult can be challenging, but incredibly rewarding. The collaborative approach can result in achieving your patients' personalized goals and the team feels they have offered the patient their best possible chance for success when they return home.

References

1. Creditor MC. Hazards of hospitalization of the elderly. Ann Intern Med. 1993;118(3):219–23.
2. Guiding principles for the care of older adults with multimorbidity: an approach for c. Guiding principles for the care of older adults with multimorbidity: an approach for clinicians: American Geriatrics Society Expert Panel on the Care of Older Adults with Multimorbidity. J Am Geriatr Soc 2012;60(10):E1-E25.
3. Abraham IL, Bottrell MM, Dash KR, Fulmer TT, Mezey MD, O'Donnell L, et al. Profiling care and benchmarking best practice in care of hospitalized elderly: the Geriatric Institutional Assessment Profile. Nurs Clin North Am. 1999;34(1):237–55.
4. Barnes DE, Palmer RM, Kresevic DM, Fortinsky RH, Kowal J, Chren MM, et al. Acute care for elders units produced shorter hospital stays at lower cost while maintaining patients' functional status. Health Aff (Millwood). 2012;31(6):1227–36.
5. Gavrilov LAGN. Handbook of the Biology of Aging. 6th ed. San Diego: Academic Press; 2006.
6. Collard RM, Boter H, Schoevers RA, Oude Voshaar RC. Prevalence of frailty in community-dwelling older persons: a systematic review. J Am Geriatr Soc. 2012;60(8):1487–92.
7. Wald HL. The geometry of patient safety: horizontal and vertical approaches to the hazards of hospitalization. J Am Geriatr Soc. 2017;65(12):2559–61.
8. Nardi R, Scanelli G, Corrao S, Iori I, Mathieu G, Cataldi Amatrian R. Co-morbidity does not reflect complexity in internal medicine patients. Eur J Intern Med. 2007;18(5):359–68.
9. McMillan GJ, Hubbard RE. Frailty in older inpatients: what physicians need to know. QJM. 2012;105(11):1059–65.
10. Fried LP, Tangen CM, Walston J, Newman AB, Hirsch C, Gottdiener J, et al. Frailty in older adults: evidence for a phenotype. J Gerontol A Biol Sci Med Sci. 2001;56(3):M146–56.
11. Malafarina V, Uriz-Otano F, Iniesta R, Gil-Guerrero L. Sarcopenia in the elderly: diagnosis, physiopathology and treatment. Maturitas. 2012;71(2):109–14.
12. Gill TM, Allore HG, Gahbauer EA, Murphy TE. Change in disability after hospitalization or restricted activity in older persons. JAMA. 2010;304(17):1919–28.
13. Searle SD, Mitnitski A, Gahbauer EA, Gill TM, Rockwood K. A standard procedure for creating a frailty index. BMC Geriatr. 2008;8:24.
14. Rolfson DB, Majumdar SR, Tsuyuki RT, Tahir A, Rockwood K. Validity and reliability of the Edmonton Frail Scale. Age Ageing. 2006;35(5):526–9.
15. Howlett SE, Rockwood MR, Mitnitski A, Rockwood K. Standard laboratory tests to identify older adults at increased risk of death. BMC Med. 2014;12:171.
16. Mitnitski A, Collerton J, Martin-Ruiz C, Jagger C, von Zglinicki T, Rockwood K, et al. Age-related frailty and its association with biological markers of ageing. BMC Med. 2015;13:161.
17. Miron Mombiela R, Facal de Castro F, Moreno P, Borras C. Ultrasonic echo intensity as a new noninvasive in vivo biomarker of frailty. J Am Geriatr Soc. 2017;65(12):2685–90.
18. Erusalimsky JD, Grillari J, Grune T, Jansen-Duerr P, Lippi G, Sinclair AJ, et al. In search of 'omics'-based biomarkers to predict risk of frailty and its consequences in older individuals: The FRAILOMIC Initiative. Gerontology. 2016;62(2):182–90.
19. King KE, Fillenbaum GG, Cohen HJ. A cumulative deficit laboratory test-based frailty index: personal and neighborhood associations. J Am Geriatr Soc. 2017;65(9):1981–7.
20. Evans SJ, Sayers M, Mitnitski A, Rockwood K. The risk of adverse outcomes in hospitalized older patients in relation to a frailty index based on a comprehensive geriatric assessment. Age Ageing. 2014;43(1):127–32.
21. Hubbard RE, O'Mahony MS, Woodhouse KW. Characterising frailty in the clinical setting--a comparison of different approaches. Age Ageing. 2009;38(1):115–9.
22. Subramaniam S, Aalberg JJ, Soriano RP, Divino CM. New 5-factor modified frailty index using American College of Surgeons NSQIP Data. J Am Coll Surg. 2018;226(2),173–81
23. Liu SK, Montgomery J, Yan Y, Mecchella JN, Bartels SJ, Masutani R, et al. Association between hospital admission risk profile score and skilled nursing or acute rehabilitation facility discharges in hospitalized older adults. J Am Geriatr Soc. 2016;64(10):2095–100.
24. Fulmer T, Mezey M, Bottrell M, Abraham I, Sazant J, Grossman S, et al. Nurses improving care for healthsystem elders (NICHE): using outcomes and benchmarks for evidenced-based practice. Geriatr Nurs. 2002;23(3):121–7.
25. Covinsky KE, Pierluissi E, Johnston CB. Hospitalization-associated disability: "She was probably able to ambulate, but I'm not sure"JAMA. 2011;306(16):1782–93.
26. Hung WW, Ross JS, Farber J, Siu AL. Evaluation of the mobile acute care of the elderly (MACE) service. JAMA Intern Med. 2013;173(11):990–6.
27. Wald HL, Glasheen JJ, Guerrasio J, Youngwerth JM, Cumbler EU. Evaluation of a hospitalist-run acute care for the elderly service. J Hosp Med. 2011;6(6):313–21.
28. Lowry E, Woodman RJ, Soiza RL, Mangoni AA. Associations between the anticholinergic risk scale score and physical function: potential implications for adverse outcomes in older hospitalized patients. J Am Med Dir Assoc. 2011;12(8):565–72.
29. Inouye SK, Bogardus ST Jr, Baker DI, Leo-Summers L, Cooney LM Jr. The hospital elder life program: a model of care to prevent cognitive and functional decline in older hospitalized patients. Hospital Elder Life Program. J Am Geriatr Soc. 2000;48(12):1697–706.
30. Brennan TA, Leape LL, Laird NM, Hebert L, Localio AR, Lawthers AG, et al. Incidence of adverse events and negligence in hospitalized patients. Results of the Harvard Medical Practice Study I. N Engl J Med. 1991;324(6):370–6.
31. Tinetti ME, McAvay GJ, Fried TR, Allore HG, Salmon JC, Foody JM, et al. Health outcome priorities among competing cardiovascular, fall injury, and medication-related symptom outcomes. J Am Geriatr Soc. 2008;56(8):1409–16.
32. Latham N, Anderson C, Bennett D, Stretton C. Progressive resistance strength training for physical disability in older people. Cochrane Database Syst Rev. 2003;2:CD002759.
33. Callen BL, Mahoney JE, Wells TJ, Enloe M, Hughes S. Admission and discharge mobility of frail hospitalized older adults. Medsurg Nurs. 2004;13(3):156–63; quiz 64
34. Kim SJ, Lee JH, Han B, Lam J, Bukowy E, Rao A, et al. Effects of hospital-based physical therapy on hospital discharge outcomes among hospitalized older adults with community-acquired pneumonia and declining physical function. Aging Dis. 2015;6(3):174–9.

35. Siebens H, Aronow H, Edwards D, Ghasemi Z. A randomized controlled trial of exercise to improve outcomes of acute hospitalization in older adults. J Am Geriatr Soc. 2000;48(12):1545–52.
36. Inouye SK. Delirium in hospitalized older patients. Clin Geriatr Med. 1998;14(4):745–64.
37. Landefeld CS, Palmer RM, Kresevic DM, Fortinsky RH, Kowal J. A randomized trial of care in a hospital medical unit especially designed to improve the functional outcomes of acutely ill older patients. N Engl J Med. 1995;332(20):1338–44.
38. Inouye SK. Delirium in older persons. N Engl J Med. 2006;354(11):1157–65.
39. Boyd CM, Ricks M, Fried LP, Guralnik JM, Xue QL, Xia J, et al. Functional decline and recovery of activities of daily living in hospitalized, disabled older women: the Women's Health and Aging Study I. J Am Geriatr Soc. 2009;57(10):1757–66.
40. Walter LC, Brand RJ, Counsell SR, Palmer RM, Landefeld CS, Fortinsky RH, et al. Development and validation of a prognostic index for 1-year mortality in older adults after hospitalization. JAMA 2001;285(23):2987–94.
41. Brown CJ, Friedkin RJ, Inouye SK. Prevalence and outcomes of low mobility in hospitalized older patients. J Am Geriatr Soc. 2004;52(8):1263–70.
42. Resnick B, Boltz M, Galik E, Pretzer-Aboff I. Restorative care nursing for older adults: a guide for all care settings. 2nd ed. New York: Springer Publishing Company; 2012.
43. Turhan Damar H, Bilik O, Karayurt O, Ursavas FE. Factors related to older patients' fear of falling during the first mobilization after total knee replacement and total hip replacement. Geriatr Nurs. 2018;39:382.
44. Nowak A, Hubbard RE. Falls and frailty: lessons from complex systems. J R Soc Med. 2009;102(3):98–102.
45. Gillespie BM, Chaboyer WP, McInnes E, Kent B, Whitty JA, Thalib L. Repositioning for pressure ulcer prevention in adults. Cochrane Database Syst Rev. 2014;(4):CD009958.
46. Sheila A, Sorrentino LR. Mosby's textbook for nursing assistants. Elsevier Inc: St. Louis; 2012.
47. Grey JE, Harding KG, Enoch S. Pressure ulcers. BMJ. 2006; 332(7539):472–5.
48. Lefevre F, Feinglass J, Potts S, Soglin L, Yarnold P, Martin GJ, et al. Iatrogenic complications in high-risk, elderly patients. Arch Intern Med. 1992;152(10):2074–80.
49. Gazzotti C, Arnaud-Battandier F, Parello M, Farine S, Seidel L, Albert A, et al. Prevention of malnutrition in older people during and after hospitalisation: results from a randomised controlled clinical trial. Age Ageing. 2003;32(3):321–5.
50. Collaboration CT, Dennis M, Sandercock P, Reid J, Graham C, Forbes J, et al. Effectiveness of intermittent pneumatic compression in reduction of risk of deep vein thrombosis in patients who have had a stroke (CLOTS 3): a multicentre randomised controlled trial. Lancet. 2013;382(9891):516–24.
51. Vandenberg E. Omaha, NE: University of Nebraska Medical Center; [The Pearl cards are a short concise review of a particular geriatric topic]. Available from: https://www.unmc.edu/intmed/divisions/geriatrics/education/resources/geri-pearls.html.
52. Flaherty JH, Little MO. Matching the environment to patients with delirium: lessons learned from the delirium room, a restraint-free environment for older hospitalized adults with delirium. J Am Geriatr Soc. 2011;59(Suppl 2):S295–300.
53. Electronic code of federal regulations. Condition of participation: patient's rights.
54. Society AG. Choosing Wisely; [April 23, 2015].
55. Porter Starr KN, McDonald SR, Bales CW. Nutritional vulnerability in older adults: a continuum of concerns. Curr Nutr Rep. 2015;4(2):176–84.
56. Covinsky KE, Martin GE, Beyth RJ, Justice AC, Sehgal AR, Landefeld CS. The relationship between clinical assessments of nutritional status and adverse outcomes in older hospitalized medical patients. J Am Geriatr Soc. 1999;47(5):532–8.
57. Volpato S, Onder G, Cavalieri M, Guerra G, Sioulis F, Maraldi C, et al. Characteristics of nondisabled older patients developing new disability associated with medical illnesses and hospitalization. J Gen Intern Med. 2007;22(5):668–74.
58. Popeo DM. Delirium in older adults. Mt Sinai J Med. 2011;78(4):571–82.
59. El-Sharkawy AM, Watson P, Neal KR, Ljungqvist O, Maughan RJ, Sahota O, et al. Hydration and outcome in older patients admitted to hospital (The HOOP prospective cohort study). Age Ageing. 2015;44(6):943–7.
60. Sullivan DH, Sun S, Walls RC. Protein-energy undernutrition among elderly hospitalized patients: a prospective study. JAMA. 1999;281(21):2013–9.
61. Schepp SK, Tirschwell DL, Miller RM, Longstreth WT Jr. Swallowing screens after acute stroke: a systematic review. Stroke. 2012;43(3):869–71.
62. Lynch YT, Clark BJ, Macht M, White SD, Taylor H, Wimbish T, et al. The accuracy of the bedside swallowing evaluation for detecting aspiration in survivors of acute respiratory failure. J Crit Care. 2017;39:143–8.
63. Brodsky MB, Suiter DM, Gonzalez-Fernandez M, Michtalik HJ, Frymark TB, Venediktov R, et al. Screening accuracy for aspiration using bedside water swallow tests: a systematic review and meta-analysis. Chest. 2016;150(1):148–63.
64. Suiter DM, Leder SB. Clinical utility of the 3-ounce water swallow test. Dysphagia. 2008;23(3):244–50.
65. Meddings J, Saint S, Fowler KE, Gaies E, Hickner A, Krein SL, et al. The Ann Arbor criteria for appropriate urinary catheter use in hospitalized medical patients: results obtained by using the RAND/UCLA appropriateness method. Ann Intern Med. 2015;162(9 Suppl):S1–34.
66. Carolyn V. Gould M; Craig A. Umscheid; Rajender K. Agarwal; David A. Pegues, the (HICPAC) HICPAC. Guideline For prevention of catheter associated urinary tract infections center for disease control, Committee HICPA; 2009 February 15, 2017.
67. Yue J, Tabloski P, Dowal SL, Puelle MR, Nandan R, Inouye SK. NICE to HELP: operationalizing National Institute for Health and Clinical Excellence guidelines to improve clinical practice. J Am Geriatr Soc. 2014;62(4):754–61.
68. Tarumi Y, Wilson MP, Szafran O, Spooner GR. Randomized, double-blind, placebo-controlled trial of oral docusate in the management of constipation in hospice patients. J Pain Symptom Manag. 2013;45(1):2–13.
69. Sterniczuk R, Rusak B, Rockwood K. Sleep disturbance in older ICU patients. Clin Interv Aging. 2014;9:969–77.
70. Rodriguez JC, Dzierzewski JM, Alessi CA. Sleep problems in the elderly. Med Clin North Am. 2015;99(2):431–9.
71. Manian FA, Manian CJ. Sleep quality in adult hospitalized patients with infection: an observational study. Am J Med Sci. 2015;349(1):56–60.
72. Carbonin P, Pahor M, Bernabei R, Sgadari A. Is age an independent risk factor of adverse drug reactions in hospitalized medical patients? J Am Geriatr Soc. 1991;39(11):1093–9.
73. M. G. The five rights: a destination without a map. Pharmacy and Therapeutics. 2010;35(10):542.
74. Gallagher P, Ryan C, Byrne S, Kennedy J, O'Mahony D. STOPP (Screening Tool of Older Person's Prescriptions) and START (screening tool to alert doctors to right treatment). Consensus validation. Int J Clin Pharmacol Ther. 2008;46(2):72–83.
75. Appelbaum PS, Grisso T. Assessing patients' capacities to consent to treatment. N Engl J Med. 1988;319(25):1635–8.
76. Weissman D, editor. Palliative Care Webinar: facilitating goals of care discussions in complex circumstances. In: Medical College of Wisconsin Palliative Care Center: Healthcare Association of New York State; 2015.
77. Graham KL, Marcantonio ER, Huang GC, Yang J, Davis RB, Smith CC. Effect of a systems intervention on the quality and safety of patient handoffs in an internal medicine residency program. J Gen Intern Med. 2013;28(8):986–93.

78. Fox MT, Persaud M, Maimets I, Brooks D, O'Brien K, Tregunno D. Effectiveness of early discharge planning in acutely ill or injured hospitalized older adults: a systematic review and meta-analysis. BMC Geriatr. 2013;13:70.
79. Rubenstein LZ, Stuck AE, Siu AL, Wieland D. Impacts of geriatric evaluation and management programs on defined outcomes: overview of the evidence. J Am Geriatr Soc. 1991;39(9 Pt 2):8S–16S; discussion 7S-8S
80. Leff B. Defining and disseminating the hospital-at-home model. CMAJ. 2009;180(2):156–7.
81. Preston SD, Southall AR, Nel M, Das SK. Geriatric surgery is about disease, not age. J R Soc Med. 2008;101(8):409–15.
82. Mohanty S, Rosenthal RA, Russell MM, Neuman MD, Ko CY, Esnaola NF. Optimal Perioperative Management of the Geriatric Patient: A Best Practices Guideline from the American College of Surgeons NSQIP and the American Geriatrics Society. J Am Coll Surg. 2016;222(5):930–47.
83. Chow WB, Rosenthal RA, Merkow RP, Ko CY, Esnaola NF. American College of Surgeons National Surgical Quality Improvement P, et al. Optimal preoperative assessment of the geriatric surgical patient: a best practices guideline from the American College of Surgeons National Surgical Quality Improvement Program and the American Geriatrics Society. J Am Coll Surg. 2012;215(4):453–66.
84. John Cameron AC. Current surgical therapy. Philadelphia: Elsevier; 2017.
85. Guerra C, Linde-Zwirble WT, Wunsch H. Risk factors for dementia after critical illness in elderly Medicare beneficiaries. Crit Care. 2012;16(6):R233.
86. Boumendil A, Latouche A, Guidet B, Group I-CS. On the benefit of intensive care for very old patients. Arch Intern Med. 2011; 171(12):1116–7.
87. Martinez-Selles M, Datino T, Bueno H. Coronary care unit admission of very old patients with acute myocardial infarction. Heart. 2006;92(4):549–50.
88. Teno JM, Gozalo P, Khandelwal N, Curtis JR, Meltzer D, Engelberg R, et al. Association of increasing use of mechanical ventilation among nursing home residents with advanced dementia and intensive care unit beds. JAMA Intern Med. 2016;176(12):1809–16.
89. Boumendil A, Somme D, Garrouste-Orgeas M, Guidet B. Should elderly patients be admitted to the intensive care unit? Intensive Care Med. 2007;33(7):1252.
90. Mohan D, Angus DC. Thought outside the box: intensive care unit freakonomics and decision making in the intensive care unit. Crit Care Med. 2010;38(10 Suppl):S637–41.
91. Rodriguez-Molinero A, Lopez-Dieguez M, Tabuenca AI, de la Cruz JJ, Banegas JR. Physicians' impression on the elders' functionality influences decision making for emergency care. Am J Emerg Med. 2010;28(7):757–65.
92. Krystal W, CL, Pittas J, Snedeker K, Von Rueden K, Huffines M, Herr D. Critical care medicine: Lippincott Williams & Wilkins: Wolters Kluwer Health, Inc; 2014.
93. Marra A, Ely EW, Pandharipande PP, Patel MB. The ABCDEF bundle in critical care. Crit Care Clin. 2017;33(2):225–43.
94. Adler J, Malone D. Early mobilization in the intensive care unit: a systematic review. Cardiopulm Phys Ther J. 2012;23(1):5–13.
95. Bentue-Ferrer D, Decombe R, Reymann JM, Schatz C, Allain H. Progress in understanding the pathophysiology of cerebral ischemia: the almitrine-raubasine approach. Clin Neuropharmacol. 1990;13(Suppl 3):S9–25.
96. Bakker J, Jansen TC, Lima A, Kompanje EJ. Why opioids and sedatives may prolong life rather than hasten death after ventilator withdrawal in critically ill patients. Am J Hosp Palliat Care. 2008;25(2):152–4.

Managing Medications and Addressing Polypharmacy

Ruth M. Spinner and Savitri Ramdial

A. Chun (ed.), *Geriatric Practice*, https://doi.org/10.1007/978-3-030-19625-7_35

35.1 Definition of Restraints

A restraint is a device that restricts movement. Restraints can be categorized as being physical or pharmacological.

The Centers for Medicare and Medicaid Services (CMS) defines restraints as the following:

> Physical restraints are any manual method or physical or mechanical device, material, or equipment attached to or adjacent to the resident's body that the individual cannot remove easily which restricts freedom of movement or normal access to one's body. Pharmacological restraints are any drug used for discipline or convenience and not required to treat medical symptoms [1].

Case Study

Mrs. M., an 86-year-old woman who is hospitalized, has fallen twice at night. She was admitted 2 days ago with pneumonia and dehydration and is receiving supplemental oxygen at 2 L/min. She is slowly responding to intravenous antibiotic therapy and fluids. Past medical history includes osteoarthritis of the hips and knees, hypertension, mild cognitive impairment, and the use of bilateral hearing aids. Home medications include losartan 50 mg daily and acetaminophen 650 mg three times daily.

Which one of the following is most likely to prevent further falls while in hospital?

1. Soft restraints
2. Prompted toileting
3. Bedrails
4. Urinary catheterization
5. Bed alarms

35.2 History of Restraints

Use of restraints has been dated back at least 300 years. Restraints were used to take action against unruly citizens and in the healthcare setting to calm aggressive psychiatric patients.

Advocacy for appropriate use of restraints started in England in the 1790s striving for mental health patients to be accorded the same rights as promised in the Revolution's Declaration of the Rights of Man, which was written in 1789. This was later followed by the British Parliament in the 1840s establishing a "Lunacy Commission" whose role was to diminish or abolish the use of restraints on patients in their care [2].

The view in America was more of a positive one, deeming restraints beneficial for patients; it was viewed as a procedure ordered by a physician in his or her role as caretaker of the patient. Debates regarding different views on restraints continued on an international basis until the twentieth century.

In 1998, the *Hartford Courant* reported that during the previous 10 years, 140 patients in the United States had died as a result of physical and mechanical restraints [3].

This was followed by at least a decade of administrative and regulatory efforts to curb the use of physical restraints, educate staff involved, closely monitor use at all times, and collect data regarding the rates and incidents for further efforts geared toward reduction.

35.3 Guidelines

Both the Joint Commission and the Centers for Medicare and Medicaid Services (CMS), which accredit most hospitals and psychiatric residential facilities, have established guidelines for use of restraints [1].

Some of their guidelines are:

- All patients have the right to be free from physical or mental abuse, and corporal punishment.
- All patients have the right to be free from restraint or seclusion, of any form, imposed as a means of coercion, discipline, convenience, or retaliation by staff.
- Restraint or seclusion may only be imposed to ensure the immediate physical safety of the patient, a staff member, or others and must be discontinued at the earliest possible time.

These restraint and seclusion regulations apply to:

- All hospitals (acute care, long-term care, psychiatric, children's, and cancer).
- All locations within the hospital (including medical/surgical units, critical care units, forensic units, emergency department, psychiatric units, etc.).
- All hospital patients, regardless of age, who are restrained or secluded (including both inpatients and outpatients).

Both the Joint Commission and CMS limit the use of patient restraints (physical and pharmacological) to situations in which the patient is an immediate danger to himself/herself or others. A restraint can only be ordered by a licensed medical practitioner, which, depending on the state, could include physicians, nurse practitioners, physician assistants, and sometimes psychologists. The restraint should be terminated as soon as the patient shows evidence of having regained self-control. Restraints cannot be ordered pro re nata (as needed).

35.4 Physical Restraints

35.4.1 Prevalence

The highest prevalence of restraint use in healthcare facilities is found in intensive care units, with a prevalence between 8.5 and 39% [4]. Another recent study identified that 76% of mechanically ventilated patients were restrained for a median of 4 days [5] with an overall hospital prevalence of restraint use ranging between 3% and 25% [4].

A study from 2007 of US hospitals showed that 56% of all restraint days were reported in ICUs and that physical restraint prevalence in hospitals was 50 per 1000 patient days [6].

A study done across five countries showed that the prevalence of physical restraint use in nursing homes from 2002 to 2014 varied more than five-fold across the countries, from an average 6% in Switzerland, 9% in the USA, 20% in Hong Kong, 28% in Finland, and over 31% in Canada. Within each country, substantial variations existed across facilities in both physical restraint and antipsychotic use rates, in part due to differences in definitions [7]. (◘ Fig. 35.1).

35.4.2 Types of Physical Restraints

Physical restraints include any device, equipment, or aids designed to confine bodily movements or free body movement to a preferred position, for example, bilateral bedrails, limb or trunk belts, and fixed tables on a chair or chairs that prevent persons from getting up [1] (▶ Box 35.1; ◻ Table 35.1).

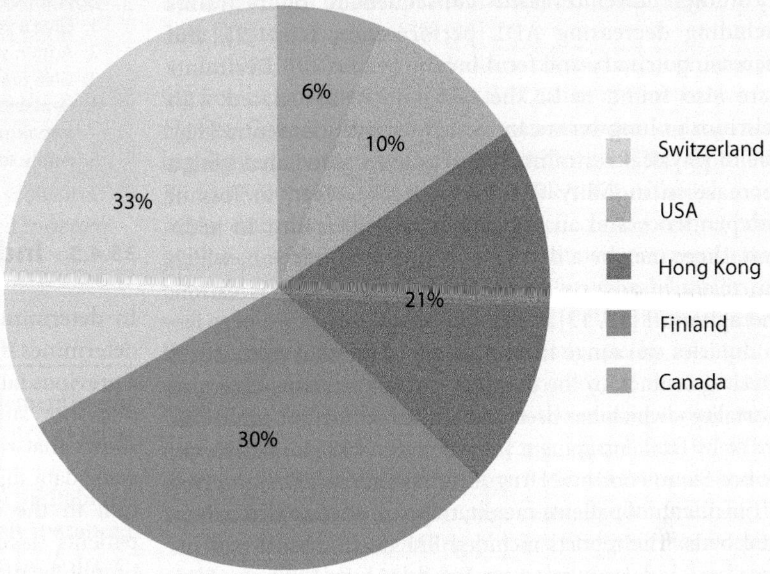

◻ **Fig. 35.1** Prevalence rates of physical restraint use in nursing homes across the globe 2002–2014. (Source: Adapted from Ref. [7])

Box 35.1 Examples of Physical Restraints

Belt in chair, belt in bed (waist, ankle, hands)

Bilateral bedrails

Unilateral bedrail with the other side against a wall

Chair with a table, deep or tipped chair

Special sheets, mittens, sleep suits

Sensor mat, Infrared system

Locked off areas – for example, code-activated elevators, locked floors

Wheelchair brakes locked while seated at the table

◻ **Table 35.1** Different types of physical restraints, examples of use, and risks associated

Type of physical restraint	Example of use	Risks
Belt: chair, wheelchair, bed Body part: waist, ankle, hands	Wheelchair lap belt to attempt to keep someone from standing up or sliding in chair Bed belts to allow needed treatment to be administered (intravenous therapy, tube feedings, artificial ventilation)	Strangulation Limb injury
Bedrails: unilateral, bilateral, full length, or half length (*most common type of restraint)	Attempt to prevent falls from bed during transport or while in bed	Strangulation Fracture Death
Chair with locked table, deep chair, or tipped chair (geri-chair)	Patients at risk of falling or wandering	Falls
Tightened sheets, sleep suits	Tighten sheet over limbs to prevent movement in bed	Confusion Falls
Mittens	Patients that scratch themselves or pull out tubes	Limb injury Confusion
Sensor mat, infrared system	Falls prevention	Falls
Locked floors/wards	To prevent patients with dementia from wandering	Agitation
Wheelchair brakes	Prevention of falls at tables	Falls
Vest, jacket	Restrict limb movement	Limb injury

remained high in nursing homes. The numbers then increased in the mid-1990s with the advent of newer atypical antipsychotics. Cross-sectional studies using national nursing home data found that the rate of antipsychotic use was 27.6% in 2001 [26].

There was a decrease in prescribing of antipsychotic medications following an FDA warning in 2005 of an increase in mortality with use of atypical antipsychotic medications in people with dementia: atypical drug mentions fell 2% overall and 19% among those with dementia [27].

However, an Office of the Inspector General (OIG) report from 2007 still showed widespread off-label use of antipsychotic medications for patients with dementia. The report reviewed antipsychotic medication use and indication listed in Medicare claims data and Minimum Data Set reports from nursing homes from 2007. The report, released in May 2011 [28], showed that 14% of elderly nursing home residents had Medicare claims for atypical antipsychotic drugs. Eighty-three percent of Medicare claims for atypical antipsychotic drugs for elderly nursing home residents were associated with off-label conditions; 88% were associated with the condition specified in the FDA boxed warning.

The prevalence in other countries of antipsychotic use in nursing homes, as shown in studies from 2002 to 2014, ranged from 11% in Hong Kong, between 26 and 27% in Canada and the USA, 34% in Switzerland, and nearly 38% in Finland [7] (◘ Fig. 35.2).

35.5.2 Types of Pharmacological Restraints

Most commonly, pharmaceutical agents used as pharmacological restraints have been antipsychotic medications. Both typical and atypical antipsychotics have been used. More recently, as FDA black box warnings have limited the use of antipsychotic medications, other medications have been used, including, but not limited to, benzodiazepines, mood stabilizers, antihistamines, and other psychotropic medications (◘ Table 35.2).

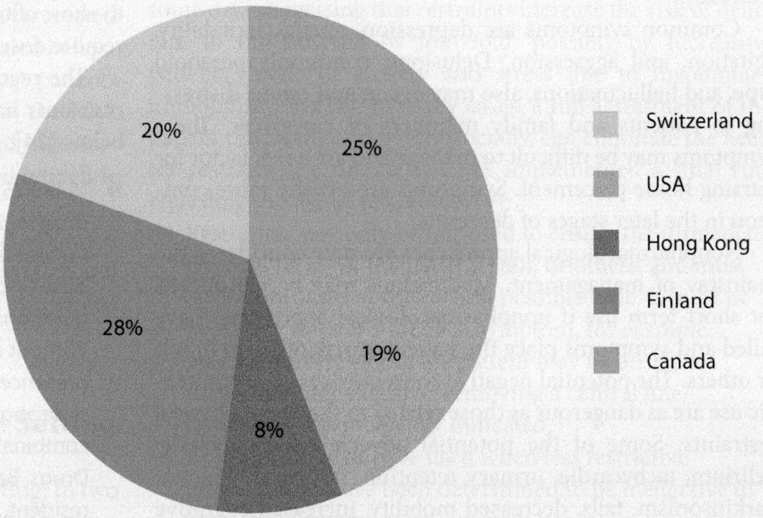

◘ Fig. 35.2 Prevalence rates of pharmacological restraint use in nursing home across the globe 2002–2014. (Adapted from Ref. [7])

◘ Table 35.2 Psychotropic medications used as pharmacological restraints, reasons for use, and the risks associated

Medication	Use	Risk
Benzodiazepines	Agitation	Paradoxical agitation, falls, somnolence
Olanzapine	Hallucinations and delusions	Death, metabolic changes, weight gain, diabetes, cerebrovascular events, hyperlipidemia. Extrapyramidal symptoms
Risperidone	Hallucinations and delusions	Death, cerebrovascular events, extrapyramidal symptoms
Quetiapine	Hallucinations and delusions	Cardiovascular events, death
Haloperidol	Hallucinations and delusions, delirium, aggression in dementia	Death, QT prolongation, extrapyramidal symptoms
Diphenhydramine	Agitation	Anticholinergic side effects
Aripiprazole	Hallucinations and delusions	Cerebrovascular events, death
Dextromethorphan/Quinidine	Pseudobulbar affect	Expensive, limited data on efficacy, falls, diarrhea, urinary tract infection

35.5.3 Risks of Pharmacological Restraints

In 2003, the FDA issued a warning for cerebrovascular adverse events including stroke in dementia patients treated with risperidone vs placebo. In 2005, a meta-analysis showed an increased risk of death with atypical antipsychotic drugs used in the treatment of dementia [29]. In April 2005, the FDA issued an advisory and subsequent black box warning regarding the risks of atypical antipsychotic use among elderly patients with dementia [30]:

> The Food and Drug Administration has determined that the treatment of behavioral disorders in elderly patients with dementia with atypical (second generation) antipsychotic medications is associated with increased mortality. Of a total of seventeen placebo controlled trials performed with olanzapine (Zyprexa), aripiprazole (Abilify), risperidone (Risperdal), or quetiapine (Seroquel) in elderly demented patients with behavioral disorders, fifteen showed numerical increases in mortality in the drug-treated group compared to the placebo-treated patients. These studies enrolled a total of 5106 patients, and several analyses have demonstrated an approximately 1.6–1.7 fold increase in mortality in these studies.

The FDA extended this warning to conventional, or "typical," antipsychotic medications in June 2008, after 2 further studies showed that the risks involved extended to these medications [31, 32]. (◘ Fig. 35.3)

Case Study Continued

Mrs. M. returned to hospital 4 months later, after sustaining a fall while trying to get out of the car. She fractured her hip and subsequently required a right total hip arthroplasty and has now been in a long-term care facility for 6 months.

Since she has been in long-term care, she has declined in Activities of Daily Living (ADL's) – she requires assistance with bathing and toileting, although she is able to feed herself and can groom herself with some assistance. Staff members have noted that over the past few weeks she has been more agitated. Physical examination and laboratory testing have ruled out any acute processes. Several attempts have been made to reorient her, in addition to participating in other activities that she usually enjoys. Despite these measures, she continues to display agitation, which includes hitting staff members when attempts are made to feed, toilet, or bathe her.

What should the next step be?

1. Use of physical restraints during these activities.
2. Haldol IM as needed.
3. Place a PEG tube for feeding.
4. Administer Ativan prior to these activities.
5. Liberalize diet, encourage family and social support during mealtime, trial low-dose antipsychotic medication for short-term use only if risk to herself or others.

35.5.4 Indications for Pharmacologic Management

First-line treatment for the management of agitation and aggression related to cognitive disorders in older adults is non-pharmacologic. There are indications when pharmacological management may be used as a last resort. If other approaches to a belligerent patient have failed, and the patient is at risk of self-harm or harm to others, restraints may be used. Restraints should be used for the shortest duration possible.

35.5.4.1 Delirium

Delirium is an acute confusional state defined as an acute change in mental status with inattention, and either disorganized thinking or altered level of consciousness. There are two presentations to delirium: Hypoactive and Hyperactive. The hyperactive type is less common in older adults. When present, hyperactive delirium can present with agitation and aggression, which if severe, may impede diagnostic and treatment options. In severe cases, when nonpharmacological interventions have failed, pharmacological management may be appropriate to control symptoms. Although antipsychotic or sedating drugs are most commonly used, and they may improve some of the symptoms, they have not been shown to have a benefit on prognosis. Additionally, recent research has demonstrated that antipsychotics and sedatives can prolong the duration of delirium as well as its cognitive changes and may worsen clinical outcomes [33].

35.5.4.2 Dementia

The American Psychiatric Association published practice guidelines on the use of antipsychotics to treat agitation or psychosis in patients with dementia [34]. As discussed above, antipsychotics are not FDA-approved for the treatment of dementia and have many associated risks. When indicated, the drugs may be used when all other options have been exhausted and symptoms are pervasive and place the patient at risk for self-harm or harming others.

Among the guidelines, recommendations include [34]:

- Starting with the lowest dose possible.
- Tapering down the drug when possible.
- Discontinuation after 4 weeks if no significant benefit on an appropriate treatment dose.
- Even with a positive response to treatment, trial a taper of the dosage after 4 months, unless a recurrence occurred with prior attempts.

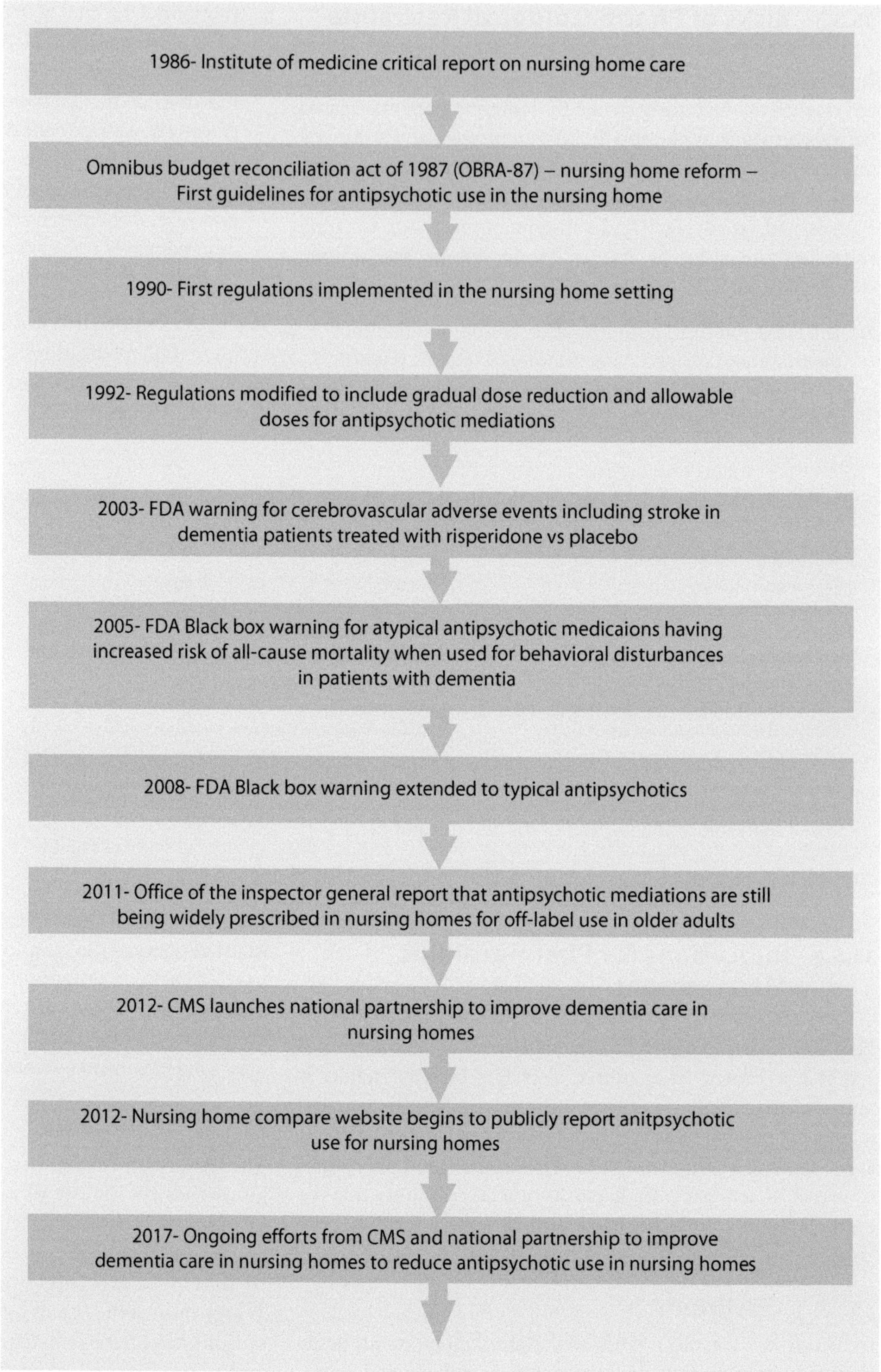
1986- Institute of medicine critical report on nursing home care
Omnibus budget reconciliation act of 1987 (OBRA-87) – nursing home reform – First guidelines for antipsychotic use in the nursing home
1990- First regulations implemented in the nursing home setting
1992- Regulations modified to include gradual dose reduction and allowable doses for antipsychotic mediations
2003- FDA warning for cerebrovascular adverse events including stroke in dementia patients treated with risperidone vs placebo
2005- FDA Black box warning for atypical antipsychotic medicaions having increased risk of all-cause mortality when used for behavioral disturbances in patients with dementia
2008- FDA Black box warning extended to typical antipsychotics
2011- Office of the inspector general report that antipsychotic mediations are still being widely prescribed in nursing homes for off-label use in older adults
2012- CMS launches national partnership to improve dementia care in nursing homes
2012- Nursing home compare website begins to publicly report anitpsychotic use for nursing homes
2017- Ongoing efforts from CMS and national partnership to improve dementia care in nursing homes to reduce antipsychotic use in nursing homes

Fig. 35.3 Timeline showing evolution of guidelines for antipsychotic medications in US nursing home from 1986–2017

Case Study Continued

Mrs. M. became extremely paranoid and combative, and after all nonpharmacological efforts were not effective in relieving her symptoms, she was started on low-dose haloperidol. Her symptoms improved soon after, and she began eating her meals without fear or struggling. She had since been working well with staff and had been receptive to family members. Now, for the past 3 days, she has been refusing oral intake, and she had been biting and spitting on staff. Upon further investigation, her usual caregiver has been re-assigned to a different unit, and several new certified nursing assistants (CNA's) have been assigned to care for her over the past week. What should the next step be:

1. Use physical restraints during meal times.
2. Ask family members to be present during meal time.
3. Reassign her previous CNA.
4. Administer bid dosing of Haldol.
5. PEG tube for feeding.

35.6 Interventions to Reduce Restraint Use

35.6.1 Regulatory

In May 2012, in response to the OIG report CMS launched the National Partnership to Improve Dementia Care in Nursing Homes. The partnership includes federal and state agencies, as well as nursing homes, and advocacy groups, and its mission is to improve the quality of care for nursing home residents with dementia. The partnership promotes person-centered care approaches dementia care and nonpharmacological management using a multidimensional strategy including consistent assignment, exercise, pain management, and activities [35].

With this National Partnership, antipsychotic medication began to be publicly reported on the Nursing Home Compare website [36].

The initial plan of the partnership was to reduce misuse of atypical antipsychotics in nursing homes by 15% by the end of 2012. This goal was not achieved within that time frame, however, it was achieved by 2014.

The partnership regularly reports on antipsychotic use in nursing homes. The reports have shown that in 2011, 23.9% of long-stay nursing home residents were receiving an antipsychotic medication; there has since been a decrease of 35% to a national prevalence in 2017 of 15.5% [35]. CMS recently announced a new goal of a 15% reduction of antipsychotic medication use by the end of 2019 for long-stay residents in those homes with currently limited reduction rates, while continuing to endorse quality improvement initiatives to help achieve this goal.

The Advancing Excellence in America's Nursing Homes campaign, which transferred operation of its project to CMS in 2016, and now the National Nursing Home Quality Improvement (NNHQI) Campaign, is aimed at improvement of the quality of care in nursing homes across the country. Educational objectives have been aimed at organizational improvement and outreach to families and caregivers:

- Fact sheet on Physical Restraint: Knowing the harmful effects of restraints if used inappropriately [37].
- Organizational interventions to decrease medications that can cause unsteady gait, providing night activities for residents with sleep-wake disturbance, encouraging family participation in care-plan meetings to help deliver person-centered care.

35.6.2 Educational Interventions

Educational programs for healthcare professionals include all or any of the following contents:

- Impact of physical restraints, residents' rights and autonomy
- Myths and misconceptions about the use of physical restraints
- Ethical issues
- Legal aspects
- Restraint minimization AP
- Risks and adverse outcomes of physical restraint use
- Management of behavioral
- Alternatives to physical restraints

35.6.3 Organizational Interventions

- Restraint reduction clinical teams or committees to round on patients who are restrained and evaluate for alternative options
- Nursing interventions to provide de-escalation, environmental improvements
- Increased family involvement
- Policies against physical restraints and limiting restraint equipment
- Consistent assignment use to improve person-centered care and knowledge of person-specific triggers for agitation and specific care plans designed to meet these needs

35.6.4 Other Alternative Interventions

- Strengthening and rehabilitation program to help improve falls risk reduction.
- Evaluate for pain and symptom management.
- Focus on reduction of sensory impairment by use of "personal assistance" devices, for example, hearing aids, visual aids, and mobility devices.
- Use of positioning devices such as body and seat cushions and padded furniture, which can reduce use of lap belts.
- Efforts to design a safer physical environment, which can include removal of obstacles that impede movement, placement of objects and furniture in familiar places, ensure that beds are lower and provision of adequate lighting.
- Scheduled toileting and other physical and personal needs, including person-centered care plan for managing thirst, hunger, the need for socialization.
- Design of the physical environment to allow for close observation by staff.
- Reduction of agitation by providing living environments that are relaxing and comfortable, minimize noise, offer soothing music, and appropriate lighting.
- Treating any underlying conditions that may reflect discomfort, pain, or infection, and managing these conditions to avoid escalation of behavioral symptoms.
- Developing a dementia care plan for nursing home residents to determine what specific interventions help calm and minimize restless behavior.
- Determine triggers for agitated behavior.
- Look for patterns of behavior and patterns for falls, which may trigger restraint use.

Case Study Summary

We have seen different instances in which Mrs. M may have received physical or pharmacological restraints in the past. Complications of restraints can be severe, including death from use of both physical and pharmacological restraints. Use of restraints should be used only when other resources have been exhausted. When used, the indication should be appropriately documented and the restraint used only for a limited time. Re-evaluation should take place on a timely basis for effectiveness, indication of use, and for adverse side effects. Proper education, observation, person-centered care, and environmental improvements can reduce use of restraints.

35.7 Educational Resources

1. American Nurses Association. Reduction of patient restraint and seclusion in health- care settings.
   ► http://www.nursingworld.org/restraintposition
2. Hartford Institute for Geriatric Nursing. Try this: avoiding restraints in hospitalized older adults with dementia.
   ► https://consultgeri.org/try-this/dementia/issue-d1
3. Nursing Home Compare
   ► www.medicare.gov/nursinghomecompare
4. National Partnership to Improve Dementia Care in Nursing Homes
   ► https://www.cms.gov/Medicare/Provider-Enrollment-and-Certification/SurveyCertificationGenInfo/National-Partnership-to-Improve-Dementia-Care-in-Nursing-Homes.html

35

References

1. Department of Health & Human Services; Centers for Medicare & Medicaid Services (CMS). CMS Manual System Department of Health & Human Services. https://www.cms.gov/Regulations-and-Guidance/Guidance/Transmittals/downloads/R37SOMA.pdf
2. Masters K. Physical estraint: a historical review and current practice. Psychiatr Ann. 2017;47(1):52–5.
3. Weiss EM. Hundreds of the nation's most vulnerable have been killed by the system intended to care for them; Series: Deadly Restraint. Hartford Courant. 1998. Available from: http://articles.courant.com/1998-10-11/news/9810090779_1_mental-health-deaths-restraint-policy/3
4. Rose L, Burry L, Mallick R, Luk E, Cook D, Fergusson D, et al. Prevalence, risk factors, and outcomes associated with physical restraint use in mechanically ventilated adults. J Crit Care. 2016;31(1):31–5.
5. Agens JE. Chemical and physical restraint use in the older person. Br J Med Pract. 2010;3(1):302.
6. Minnick AF, Mion LC, Johnson ME, Catrambone C, Leipzig R. Prevalence and variation of physical restraint use in acute care settings in the US. J Nurs Scholarsh. 2007;39(1):30–7.
7. Feng Z, Hirdes JP, Smith TF. Use of physical restraints and antipsychotic medications in nursing homes: a cross-national study. Int J Geriatr Psychiatry. 2009;24(10):1110–8.
8. Castle NG, Engberg J. The health consequences of using physical restraints in nursing homes. Med Care. 2009;47(11):1164–73.
9. Mamun K, Lim J. Use of physical restraints in nursing homes: current practice in Singapore. Ann Acad Med Singap. 2005;34(2):158–62.
10. Voyer P, Richard S, Doucet L, Cyr N, Carmichael PH. Precipitating factors associated with delirium among long-term care residents with dementia. Appl Nurs Res. 2011;24(3):171–8.
11. Castle NG, Mor V. Physical restraints in nursing homes: a review of the literature since the nursing home reform act of 1987. Med Care Res Rev. 1998;55(22):139–70.
12. Evans LK, Strumpf NE, Allen-Taylor SL, Capezuti E, Maislin G, Jacobsen B. A clinical trial to reduce restraints in nursing homes. J Am Geriatr Soc. 1997;45(6):675–81.
13. Healey F, Oliver D, Milne A, Connelly J. The effect of bedrails on falls and injury: a systematic review of clinical studies. Age Ageing. 2008;37(4):368–78.
14. Beerens HC, Sutcliffe C, Renom-Guiteras A, Soto ME, Suhonen R, Zabalegui A, Bökberg C, Saks K, Hamers JP. Quality of life and quality of care for people with dementia receiving long term institutional care or professional home care: the European right time place care study. J Med Am Direct Assoc. 2014;15(1):54–61.
15. https://www.fda.gov/downloads/MedicalDevices/ProductsandMedicalProcedures/GeneralHospitalDevicesandSupplies/HospitalBeds/UCM397178.pdf
16. Miles SH, Irvine P. Deaths caused by physical restraints. The Gerontologist. 1992;32(6):762–6.
17. Hamers JP, Bleijlevens MH, Gulpers MJ, Verbeek H. Behind closed doors: involuntary treatment in care of persons with cognitive impairment at home in the Netherlands. J Am Geriatr Soc. 2016;64(2):354–8.
18. Inouye SK, Charpentier PA. Precipitating factors for delirium in hospitalized elderly persons predictive model and interrelationship with baseline vulnerability. JAMA. 1996;275(11):852–7.
19. Federal Register. Part II; Department of Health and Human Services, Centers for Medicare & Medicaid Services; Medicare and Medicaid Programs. 42 CFR Part 482; Medicare and Medicaid Programs; Hospital Conditions of Participation: Patients' Rights; Final Rule. December 8, 2006. www.cms.gov/Regulations-and-Guidance/Legislation/CFCsAndCoPs/downloads/finalpatientrightsrule.pdf
20. Lyketsos CG, Lopez O, Jones B, Fitzpatrick AL, Breitner J, De Kosky S. Prevalence of neuropsychiatric symptoms in dementia and mild cognitive impairment results from the cardiovascular health study. JAMA. 2002;288(12):1475–83.
21. Harris-Kojetin L, Sengupta M, Park-Lee E. Long-term care providers and services users in the United States: data from the national study of long-term care providers. Vital Health Stat. 2016;3(38):10–1.
22. Beers M, Avorn J, Soumerai SB, Daniel EE, Sherman DS, Salem S. Psychoactive medication use in intermediate-care facility residents. JAMA. 1988;260(20):3016–20.
23. Ray WA, Federspiel CF, Schaffner W. A study of antipsychotic drug use in nursing homes: epidemiologic evidence suggesting misuse. Am J Public Health. 1980;70(5):485–91.
24. Department of Health and Human Services. State operations manual (SOM)surveyor guidance revisions related to psychosocial harm in nursing homes. 2016. Available from: https://www.cms.gov/Medicare/Provider-Enrollment-and-Certification/SurveyCertificationGenInfo/Downloads/Survey-and-Cert-Letter-16-15.pdf
25. Borson S, Doane K. The impact of OBRA-87 on psychotropic drug prescribing in skilled nursing facilities. Psychiatr Serv. 1997;48(10):1289–96.
26. Briesacher BA, Limcangco MR, Simoni-Wastila L, Doshi JA, Levens SR, Shea DG, Stuart B. The quality of antipsychotic drug prescribing in nursing homes. Arch Intern Med. 2005;165(11):1280–5.
27. Dorsey ER, Rabbani A, Gallagher SA, Conti RM, Alexander GC. Impact of FDA black box advisory on antipsychotic medication use. Arch Intern Med. 2010;170(1):96–103.
28. Daniel R. Levinson. Medicare atypical antipsychotic drug claims for elderly nursing home resident. https://oig.hhs.gov/oei/reports/oei-07-08-00150.pdf
29. Schneider S, Dagerman KS, Insel P. Risk of death with atypical antipsychotic drug treatment for dementia meta-analysis of randomized placebo-controlled trials. JAMA. 2005;294(15):1934–43.

30. U.S. Food and Drug Administration. www.fda.gov
31. Schneeweiss S, Setoguchi S, Brookhart A, et al. Risk of death associated with the use of conventional versus atypical antipsychotic drugs among elderly patients. Can Med Assoc J. 2007;176(5): 627–32.
32. Gill SS, Bronskill SE, Normand SL, et al. Antipsychotic drug use and mortality in older adults with dementia. Ann Intern Med. 2007;146(11):775–86.
33. Inouye SK, Westendorp RG, Saczynski JS. Delirium in elderly people. Lancet. 2014;383(9920):911–22.
34. Reus VI, Fochtmann LJ, Eyler AE, Hilty DM, Horvitz-Lennon M, Jibson MD, Lopez OL, Mahoney J, Pasic J, Tan ZS, Wills CD, Rhoads R, Yager J. The American psychiatric association practice guideline on the use of antipsychotics to treat agitation or psychosis in patients with dementia. Am J Psychiatry. 2016;173(5):543–6.
35. Advancing excellence in America's nursing home. National partnership to improve dementia care in nursing homes: antipsychotic medication use data report. 2017. https://www.nhqualitycampaign.org/files/AP_package_20171016.pdf
36. Medicare. Nursing home compare. https://www.medicare.gov/nursinghomecompare
37. Advancing excellence in America's nursing home. Fast facts: physical restraints. https://www.nhqualitycampaign.org/files/factsheets/Consumer%20Fact%20Sheet%20-%20Restraints.pdf

Foley Catheter Use and Management of Urinary Symptoms

Cynthia Lien and Neha Naik

A. Chun (ed.), *Geriatric Practice*, https://doi.org/10.1007/978-3-030-19625-7_36

Case

Mr. B is an 88-year-old man with history of benign prostatic hyperplasia (BPH), hypercholesterolemia, cognitive impairment, and Parkinson's disease diagnosed 8 years ago. He complains of urinary frequency, with the urge to void every 2 h and urination three times per night. His medications include tamsulosin 0.4 mg per day, finasteride 5 mg per day, pravastatin 20 mg per day, carbidopa/levodopa 25/100 mg three times per day, and donepezil 5 mg per day. Physical examination reveals a frail-appearing elderly male with stooped posture, gait instability, and cogwheel rigidity of the upper extremities. His mini-mental status exam is 23/30 consistent with mild cognitive impairment. Prostate exam reveals an enlarged prostate gland estimated at 40 g with no asymmetry, nodules, or tenderness. Bladder ultrasound shows pre-void urine volume of 660 mL. His American Urological Association symptom score is 15 consistent with a moderate severity of symptoms.

Due to persistent symptoms on medical therapy, he elected to undergo electro-vaporization of the prostate. Eight days after the procedure, he developed acute urinary retention and presented to the emergency room. He elected to have an indwelling Foley catheter and was instructed to follow up with the urologist for monthly catheter changes. Mr. B lives in a four-story walk up and uses a cane. He had a fall in his home last month, and his friend is concerned that he is unsteady on feet, lives alone, and losing his memory. His friend suggests that he move into an assisted living facility. Over the next 3 months, he fails numerous voiding trials and continues to have monthly catheter changes.

36.1 Background

Aging is associated with an increased prevalence of lower urinary tract symptoms (LUTS) including urinary urgency, difficulty voiding, incomplete bladder emptying and urinary leakage or incontinence in both women and men [2, 4, 31]. Older males are particularly prone to severe symptom burden from LUTS due to prostate enlargement [4]. In fact, urinary symptoms related to prostate enlargement is the fourth most commonly evaluated condition among older men [32]. Women commonly experience symptoms of urgency, weak stream, and nighttime urination or nocturia with advancing age [11]. Urinary incontinence is particularly prevalent among older adults in both the community [2] and nursing homes, and the risk is greater among persons that are older, cognitively impaired, and functionally dependent or physically impaired [52]. As the elderly population continues to expand [63], the overall burden and societal impact of urinary symptoms in older adults are expected to grow both nationally and worldwide [30].

36

36.2 Geriatric Syndromes and Urinary Symptoms

Geriatrics syndromes are common, multifactorial conditions among older adults associated with functional decline and poor quality of life [28]. Cognitive impairment, delirium, falls and functional impairment are among the geriatric syndromes that complicate the assessment and management of genitourinary pathology in older adults. For example, in the setting of a urinary tract infection, cognitively impaired older adults are less likely to report dysuria or urinary frequency and more likely to present with non-specific symptoms such as fatigue, confusion, anorexia, or functional decline [26]. A cognitively impaired adult may not readily communicate signs and symptoms of urinary pathology leading to delays in diagnoses. Acute urinary retention in a cognitively impaired adult may manifest in the form of agitation, behavioral disturbance, elevated blood pressure or abdominal pain. In a functionally impaired older adult, a pressure injury or a fall may be the first presenting sign of urinary incontinence or nocturia. Thus, awareness of these atypical presentations in elderly patients can help to expedite accurate diagnosis and management of urinary symptoms.

Urinary symptoms themselves can also lead to the onset and worsening of geriatric syndromes. For example, urinary incontinence is a known risk factor for falls [14] and fractures [5] among community dwelling older adults and contributes to significant psychological morbidity [3]. Urinary incontinence also contributes to the development of pressure injuries [38] leading to social isolation, pain, worsening functional status and mobility and poor quality of life [23]. The presence of an indwelling catheter, urinary tract infections and urinary retention are all potential precipitating factors of delirium [29]. Given that geriatric syndromes contribute to increased morbidity and mortality, healthcare-related costs and poor quality of life [28] effective management urinary symptoms can improve outcomes in geriatric patients.

36.3 Medications and Urinary Symptoms in Geriatric Patients

Geriatric syndromes not only affect the interpretation of genitourinary pathology in older adults, but also may complicate the treatment course of urinary symptoms. Physiological changes in the elderly can increase the risk of decreased medication clearance and toxicity. Medications commonly used to treat urinary symptoms may contribute to adverse events in the elderly (◘ Table 36.1). For example, α-1-adrenoreceptor blockers (e.g., doxazosin) used to improve urinary flow in BPH may precipitate orthostatic hypotension and dizziness due to its vasodilatory effects and contribute to falls. Anticholinergic medications for overactive bladder such as oxybutynin and tolterodine may also precipitate delirium in the elderly. Thus, optimizing the treatment of urinary

Table 36.1 Common medications for urological conditions with adverse effects in the elderly

Clinical use/therapeutic category	Drug name	Mechanism of action	Risk/adverse events
Benign prostatic hypertrophy (BPH)			
Alpha1-blockers	Doxazosin [Doxazosin®][a] Terazosin [Hytrin®][a] Prazosin [Minipress®][a] Alfuzosin [Uroxandral®] Silodosin [Rapaflo®] Tamsulosin [Flomax®]	Blocks alpha-1 receptor to relax smooth muscle contraction, reduce bladder outlet resistance, and improve urinary flow	Orthostatic hypotension, syncope, bradycardia[a] Increased risk of urinary incontinence, avoid concurrent use of peripheral alpha1-blockers with loop diuretics in older women[a]
Overactive bladder			
Anti-muscarinic agents[a] Beta-3 adrenergic agonist	Oxybutynin [Oxytrol®] Fesoterodine [Toviaz®] Darifenacin [Enablex®] Tolterodine [Detrol®] Solifenacin [Vesicare®] Trospium [Sanctura®] Mirabegron [Myrbetriq®]	Relaxes bladder by inhibiting muscarinic effect of acetylcholine on bladder smooth muscle	Dizziness, somnolence, blurry vision, urinary retention, constipation, diarrhea, nausea, delirium. Avoid in older adults with risk of delirium[a]
Erectile dysfunction			
Phosphodiesterase type 5 inhibitor	Tadalafil [Cialis®] Sildenafil [Viagra®] Avanafil [Stendra®] Vardenafil [Staxyn®, Levitra®]	Blocks cGMP specific phosphodiesterase type-5 (PDE5) in smooth muscle and inhibits cGMP enzymatic degradation Improves penile blood flow due to nitric oxide (NO)-mediated release of cGMP during sexual stimulation, causing relaxation of corpus cavernosum smooth muscle and arteries	Use with caution may exacerbate syncope in individuals with history of syncope or concurrent use of other vasodilators such as nitrates

[a]Fick et al. [18]

symptoms in the elderly requires attention to potential adverse effects and understanding how pharmacotherapy may precipitate or exacerbate geriatric syndromes. Elderly patients are also vulnerable to adverse drug events from other medications, some of which may cause urinary symptoms. Medications with strong anticholinergic properties such as inhaled anti-muscarinic agents for the treatment of chronic obstructive pulmonary disease (COPD) and antihistamines may contribute to acute urinary retention, delirium, and sedation in older adults (Table 36.2). Medication-related adverse events should always be considered in the differential for the evaluation of urinary symptoms in the elderly.

36.4 Genitourinary Anatomy and Aging

36.4.1 Male Genitourinary Anatomy and Clinical Relevance

The bladder wall is comprised of detrusor muscle, a layer of smooth muscle innervated by sympathetic and parasympathetic neurons to regulate bladder contraction. Normally, the bladder can hold a capacity of 400–500 mL. The trigone of the bladder is the triangular area at the base of the bladder formed by two ureteral openings and urethral orifice. In males, detrusor muscle fibers extend to the bladder neck and through the prostatic urethra forming the internal urethral sphincter. The internal urethral sphincter is comprised of smooth muscle responsible for involuntary control of urination and discharge of semen into the urethra. The external sphincter is comprised of paraurethral striated muscle enclosing the entire membranous urethra and facilitates voluntary continence. The dome of the bladder is most vulnerable to rupture when the bladder is full, as it is the weakest and most mobile part of the bladder.

The male urethra is approximately 15–20 cm in length and 8–9 mm in diameter and enables the passage of semen and urine from the bladder to the exterior. The male urethra is subdivided into the anterior and posterior urethra. The posterior urethra extends from the bladder neck distally and includes the prostatic and membranous urethra (Fig. 36.1). The prostatic urethra is the most common site of bladder outlet obstruction as it is prone to compression in prostatic enlargement. The membranous urethra extends from the apex of the prostate to the perineal membrane. At the level of the perineal membrane is the transition point to the anterior

Table 36.2 Common medications with urinary adverse effects in the elderly

Therapeutic category	Drug name	Mechanism of action	Risk/adverse events
Strongly anticholinergic medications[a] **All medications with strong anticholinergic properties may cause risk of urinary retention or incontinence, delirium, falls, confusion, sedation, dry mouth, constipation in elderly**			
Antihistamines Inhaled anticholinergics	Chlorpheniramine [Piriton®] Diphenhydramine [Benadryl®] Hydroxyzine [Atarax®] Meclizine [Antivert®] Promethazine [Phenergan®] Tiotropium [Spiriva®] Ipratropium [Atrovent®]	Antagonizes histamine receptors Causes bronchodilation by inhibition of muscarinic receptors on airway smooth muscle	
Antidepressants	Amitriptyline [Elavil®] Clomipramine [Anafranil®] Desipramine [Norpramin®] Imipramine [Tofranil®] Nortriptyline [Aventyl®]	Variable – inhibits serotonin or norepinephrine reuptake in nerve endings	Sedating, may cause orthostatic hypotension
Antispasmodics	Belladonna alkaloids Dicyclomine Hyoscyamine Scopolamine	Inhibits acetylcholine activity on postganglionic neurons and smooth muscle by blocking muscarinic receptors	Avoid except in short-term palliative care to decrease oral secretions[a]
Antipsychotics	Chlorpromazine Olanzapine [Zyprexa®] Thioridazine	Variable	Increased risk of delirium, mortality risk for use in dementia with behavioral disturbance
Hormone supplement			
Oral and transdermal estrogen, excludes intravaginal estrogen[a] Androgens	Estradiol [Menostar®] Testosterone [Androgel®] Methyltestosterone [Virilon®]		May worsen urinary incontinence, avoid in elderly women[a] Associated potential for cardiac problems, avoid in elderly men[a]

[a]Fick et al. [18]

36

urethra which includes the bulbar urethra, penile urethra, fossa navicularis and urethral meatus. This transition point is prone to injury (rupture, penetration) with catheterization or trauma due to its curved course and because it is a point of fixation. It is estimated that 67% of anterior urethral injuries are related to urinary catheterization [17]. The fossa navicularis is the dilated portion in the glans and lined by squamous epithelium. These cells may become keratinized and contribute to urethral stricture with prolonged instrumentation, trauma, or lichen sclerosus [16].

36.4.2 Female Genitourinary Anatomy and Clinical Relevance

The female urethra is approximately 3–4 cm in length and 6 mm in diameter and connects the bladder neck to the vulvar vestibule at the external urethral meatus. The female urethra has four layers: the mucosa, submucosa, internal urethral sphincter, and external urethral sphincter. The submucosa layer is highly vascular and estrogen-dependent and contributes to maintaining urethral resting tone and closing pressure. In the postmenopausal state, reduced urethral closing pressure may lead to symptoms of stress incontinence. The internal urethral sphincter is comprised of longitudinal smooth muscle extending from the bladder neck to the proximal urethra. The external urethral sphincter is located at the distal end of the urethra and allows voluntary control of micturition (Fig. 36.2). The urethra lies within a layer of fibrous tissue (the periurethral endopelvic fascia) which forms a part of a fibrous network of connective tissue that surrounds all organs of the pelvis and maintains loose connections to surrounding pelvic structures. Elevated intraabdominal pressure during coughing or sneezing causes compression of the urethra against the fascia layer to prevent involuntary urinary flow. Age-associated weakening of the pelvic floor muscles and these support structures can lead to organ prolapse or involuntary urinary leakage.

36.5 Bladder Dysfunction in Aging

Aging is associated with both physiological and pathological changes in bladder structure and function in men and women. Detrusor muscle dysfunction [65] and decreased bladder sensation [8] lead to decreased bladder contractile strength,

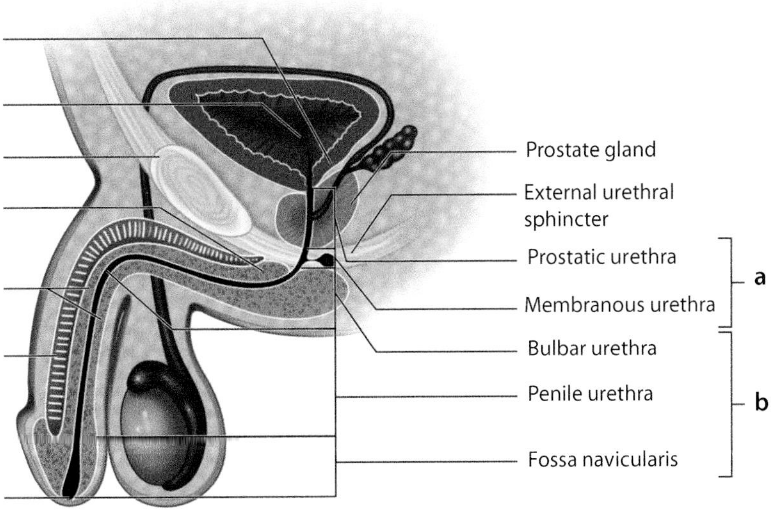

Fig. 36.1 Male genitourinary anatomy – the male bladder lies behind the pubic symphysis and when distended can be readily palpated in the suprapubic region. The trigone of the bladder is the triangular area between the two ureteric openings and urethral orifice. The internal urethral sphincter is formed by converging detrusor muscle fibers extending distally to form the smooth muscle of the urethra. The male urethra is subdivided into anterior and posterior segments. **a** The posterior urethra includes the prostatic urethra and membranous urethra. The prostatic urethra is prone to narrowing with prostate enlargement due to its proximity to the prostate gland. The membranous urethra is surrounded by the external urethral sphincter which is under voluntary control. The membranous urethra is the shortest and least distensible segment of the male urethra. **b** The anterior urethra includes the bulbar urethra, penile urethra, fossa navicularis, and urethral meatus. The anterior urethra serves as a conduit to conduct the passage of urine. The bulbar urethra is prone to straddle trauma and injury due to its proximity to the skin and pelvis. Injury to this region may disrupt the vascular corpus spongiosum resulting in tissue fibrosis and urethral strictures. **c** The membranous urethra and bulbo-membranous junction is prone to trauma during bladder catheterization due to its curved shape, limited distensibility, and narrow diameter

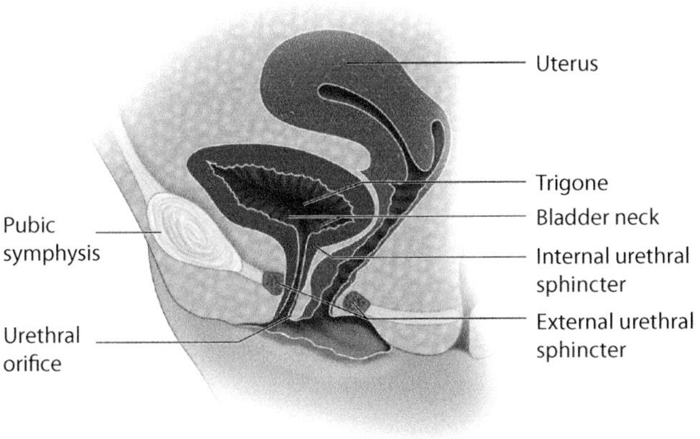

Fig. 36.2 Female genitourinary anatomy – the female bladder lies behind the pubic symphysis and anterior to the uterus and vagina. The bladder is readily palpable in the suprapubic region when distended as in the case of acute or chronic urinary retention. The female urethra lies anterior to the vagina. The submucosa of the female urethra is continuous with the inner longitudinal layer of the bladder wall smooth muscle. The internal urethral sphincter is a dense circular layer of smooth muscle fibers distal to the bladder neck, and distal mid-third of the urethra is surrounded by smooth and striated muscle forming the external urethral sphincter

urinary flow, and bladder capacity [43], resulting in symptoms of disrupted urine storage ("storage symptoms") such retention, frequency, urgency, incontinence, and nocturia. Postmenopausal women are also prone to LUTS due to bladder neck and pelvic floor muscle weakness [39]. An age-related voiding dysfunction, detrusor hyperactivity with impaired contractility (DHIC) is a significant cause of urinary incontinence particularly in institutionalized older women [69]. DHIC is associated with very low detrusor contractions and urethral relaxation, leading to high residual volumes and symptoms of frequency and incontinence in older adults. Among men, this entity can lead to both urinary storage symptoms and voiding symptoms including poor flow, hesitancy, incomplete bladder-emptying and straining [40]. Although many cases can be successfully managed with pharmacotherapy, management strategies may also require intermittent self-catheterization and surgical intervention to relieve bladder outlet obstruction [40].

36.6 Nocturia: A Sign of Underlying Pathology in Older Adults

Nocturia is characterized by the need to wake up at night one or more times to urinate. When an individual is awakened by the urge to urinate, nocturia may be a presenting symptom of underlying bladder dysfunction and systemic illness such as obstructive sleep apnea and congestive heart failure (Table 36.3). Over 50% of men over age 75 and women over 80 in the United States report symptoms of nocturia [41, 45]. The prevalence of nocturia increases with age in both women and men especially after age 65 contributing to interrupted sleep, psychological distress and poor quality of life [12]. The

Table 36.3 Common causes and etiologies of nocturia in older adults

Bladder dysfunction	Etiology
Bladder outlet obstruction Severe detrusor dysfunction with large residual urine volume Detrusor overactivity Bladder irritation Decreased functional bladder capacity Pelvic floor laxity Medications	Benign prostatic hyperplasia, bladder cancer or calculi, hematuria with clots Detrusor hyperactivity with impaired contractility (DHIC), neurogenic bladder Urinary tract infection, urethritis, caffeine Cystocele, uterine prolapse Anticholinergic medications (incomplete bladder emptying), opioid analgesics (incomplete bladder emptying)
Excessive nocturnal urine production	
Edema-forming states Obstructive sleep apnea Neurodegenerative conditions Diabetes mellitus and diabetes Insipidus Hypokalemia and hypercalcemia Medications Chronic kidney disease Excess fluid intake Autonomic neuropathy Idiopathic nocturnal polyuria	Congestive heart failure, venous insufficiency Parkinson's disease, Alzheimer's disease Diuretics, calcium-channel blockers, caffeine, alcohol

Kujubu [37]. Table 19-1, Nocturia in elderly persons and nocturnal polyuria

etiology of nocturia is complex and may include polyuria not limited to sleep hours (global polyuria), urine overproduction during sleep hours (nocturnal polyuria), bladder storage or voiding dysfunction or a combination of etiologies. Global polyuria manifests as increased urinary frequency or increased urine volume in the day or night, and the differential diagnosis may include central diabetes insipidus resulting in abnormal free water storage or polydipsia from psychogenic causes. Nocturnal polyuria may be due to an underlying systemic illness such as congestive heart failure, peripheral edema or venous insufficiency causing increased venous return and cardiac output in the supine position, or iatrogenic causes such as nocturnal fluid, alcohol or caffeine consumption or diuretic use. Obstructive sleep apnea may also result in nocturia as increased airway resistance and intrathoracic pressure during apneic episodes increase atrial natriuretic hormone (ANP) release, resulting in increased water and salt excretion [67]. Bladder dysfunction from a variety of causes (Table 36.3) may also result in nocturia due to reduced urinary storage volume causing leakage or dribbling, urinary frequency, and urgency during sleep hours. Nocturia in an older adult should prompt further investigation of potential underlying anatomical, physiological, and systemic causes (Table 36.3).

36.7 Benign Prostatic Hyperplasia in Men

Anatomical and histological changes in the prostate, bladder, and urethra associated with aging contribute to the development of urinary symptoms in older men. Age-related prostate volume growth due to cellular hyperproliferation of epithelial and stroma cells [9] results in severe LUTS common to older men [4]. Prostate tissue fibrosis from myofibroblast accumulation leads to architectural stiffening and decline in urethral compliance leading to more severe obstructive symptoms [42]. Targeting these processes, 5-α-reductase inhibitors like finasteride and dutasteride and selective α-1 adrenergic receptor blockers like doxazosin and prazosin are effective medications to improve LUTS. 5-α-reductase inhibitors lead to reduced levels of dihydrotestosterone (DHT) in the prostate, the major driver for prostate growth [7] leading to increased epithelial apoptosis and decreased prostate volume. Selective α-1 adrenergic receptor blockers bind to prostatic smooth muscle α-1-A receptors and result in decreased urinary flow rate. Although these medications have been shown to improve urinary flow rate and reduce urinary symptom burden and the risk of acute urinary retention (AUR) [46], AUR still remains a common complication of BPH over time. As the prostate enlarges, bladder outlet obstruction leads to increased voiding pressures and detrusor muscle hypertrophy, causing reduced bladder compliance or bladder hyperactivity and symptoms of dysfunctional urinary storage (urinary frequency, urgency and nocturia). In advanced cases, AUR may develop requiring emergent urinary catheterization.

36.8 Acute Urinary Retention

Acute urinary retention (AUR), a urological emergency characterized by inability to void, typically causes an intense desire to void and suprapubic pain. In severe cases, patients may present with uremia, acute renal failure, and life-threatening electrolyte imbalances. The risk of AUR increases with age [48], and risk factors for acute urinary retention in elderly men include greater LUTS symptom severity, lower peak urinary flow rates, and older age [33, 48]. Prostate volume remains one of the strongest predictors of AUR and the need for BPH-related surgery [55]. Prostate volumes over 40 mL (normal less than 20 mL) are associated with a three-fold increase in the risk of developing AUR over the next 2 years [44].

Assessment of the patient with AUR begins with accurate history-taking and a thorough physical examination to determine the precipitating cause (Fig. 36.3). A prior history of neurological disorder such as spinal cord injury, stroke, parkinson's disease and multiple system atrophy, and history of pelvic or perineal surgery or trauma may contribute to voiding dysfunction. Medications with anticholinergic properties such as antidepressants and antipsychotics (Table 36.2) and also analgesics like morphine may impair

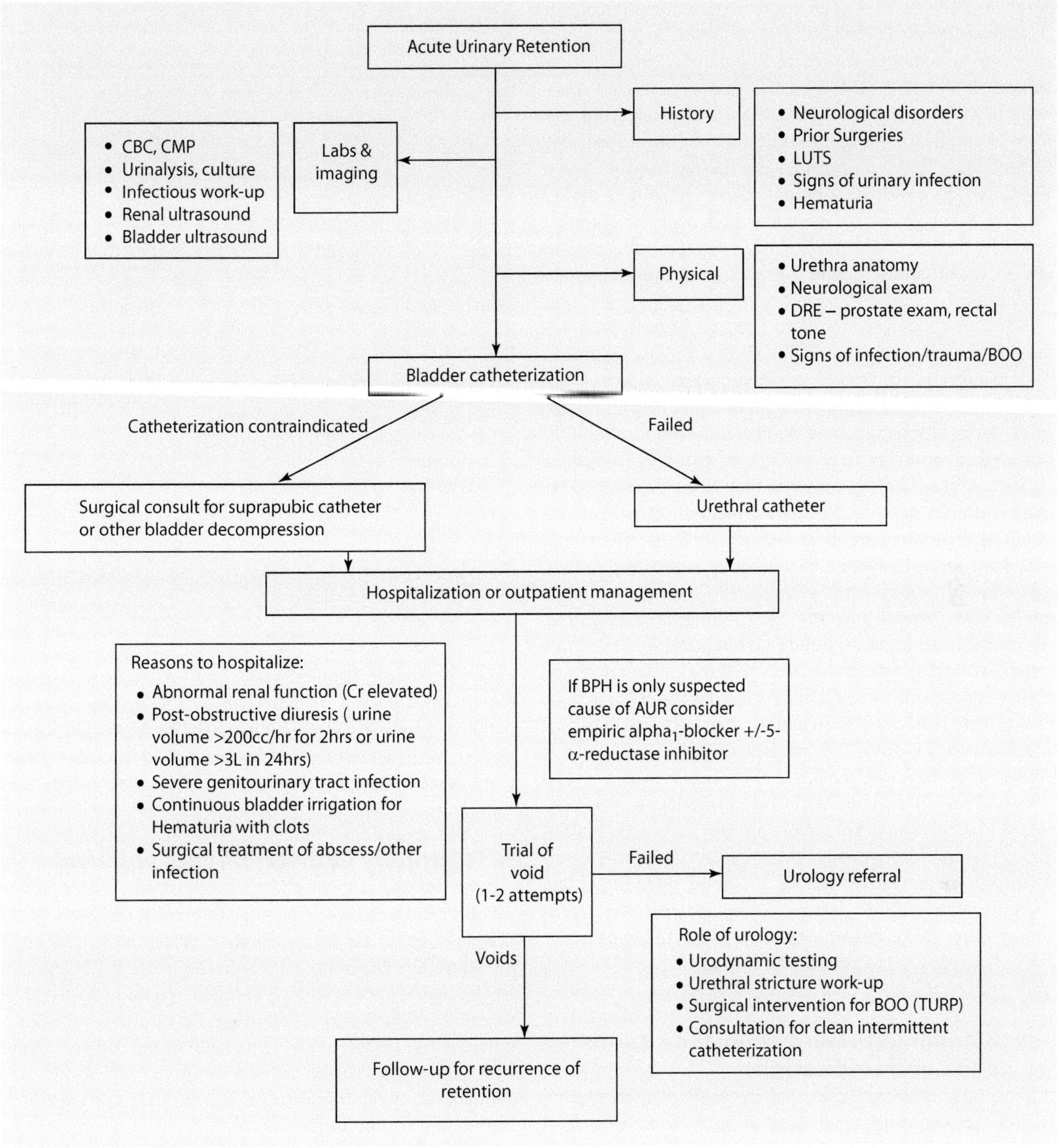

Fig. 36.3 Acute urinary retention work-up algorithm. Suggested algorithm for the management of acute urinary retention. CBC complete blood count, CMP comprehensive metabolic panel, LUTS lower urinary tract symptoms, DRE digital rectal exam, BOO bladder outlet obstruction, Cr creatinine, BPH benign prostatic hyperplasia, TURP transurethral resection of the prostate

detrusor contractiliy and precipitate AUR. Physical examination should be performed to evaluate for any anatomical precipitants such as phimosis or urethral meatus stenosis, strictures, foreign objects and cysocele or prolapse. A digital rectal exam should be performed in males to evaluate for prostate size and pain, as well as an assessment of rectal tone and perineal sensation to consider cauda equina syndrome. Signs of infection such as urethral discharge, epididymitis, and skin lesions to suggest sexually transmitted disease should be explored to rule out pain as an etiology of urinary retention. The urethra should also be examined to ensure safe bladder cahteterization is feasible. The lower abdomen should also be examined for any scar tissue or injury if suprapubic catheterization is considered. A bedside ultrasound is used to assess for bladder urine volume prior to catheterization. Lab work-up may include a complete blood count (CBC) and metabolic panel to evaluate for infection, electrolyte disturbance and renal function. The Prostate-Specific

Antigen (PSA) level is not a reliable marker of malignancy in this scenario as it is elevated with retention, infection, and after instrumentation or prosate palpation. A urinalysis and culture should be performed on a fresh catheterized specimen. If acute prostatitis or prostate abscess is suspected, urinary catheterization is contraindicated for risk of spreading the infection. In this circumstance, a urology consultation is warranted to consider suprapubic catheterization and/or surgical drainage of any infectious collection. A complete sexual history should be performed in patients with prostatis and or epididymitis to rule out gonorrhea and chlamydia infection.

Bladder decompression with urethral catheterization is the first line of treatment for AUR. Once a catheter is successfully placed and the bladder is decompressed without complication, it requires regular observation and cleaning of the insertion site for irritation or skin breakdown and should be removed as soon as it is no longer clinically indicated. Patients with indwelling catheters may either be managed in the community or in the hosptial setting. Indications for hospitalization may include abnormal renal function, hematuria with clots, postobstructive diuresis with high urine output, neurological emergencies such as acute cord compression, and severe urinary infection warranting hospitalization. Abnormal renal function should be further evaluated with a renal ultrasound to evaluate for proximal obstruction and hydronpehrosis. If these features are absent, and there is no concern for anatomical obstruction, a trial of voiding or trial without catheter (TWOC) is attempted. The timing to trial of voiding is variable, and typically may range between several days to weeks. If a second trial of voiding fails, surgical consultation is warranted to explore alternative causes of AUR and to pursue urodynamic testing which is typically performed in the outpatient setting. If chronic retention is suspected, options for urinary drainage include clean intermittent self-cateterization, chronic indwelling catheterization or suprapubic catheter placement.

36.9 Bladder Catheterization: Indications and Contraindications

Bladder catheterization is performed in a variety of clinical settings including in the office, emergency rooms, hospitals, homes and nursing homes. The bladder is accessed with a urinary catheter, a flexible hollow tube that is inserted through the urethra into the bladder. Indwelling catheters are only indicated in specific clinical circumstances (Table 36.4); however, nearly half of the catheterizations are performed without appropriate indications [56]. Indications to keep a Foley catheter should be assessed daily, and catheters should be removed as soon as medically feasible. Examples of common inappropriate usage of urinary catheters include the management of urinary incontinence for nursing home residents or hospitalized patients for convenience [34], for urine sampling in patients that can spontaneously void, and measurement of bladder volume in patients that can spontaneously void. Alternative management strategies are recommended, for instance urinary incontinence is appropriately managed by first exploring the underlying cause, and a bladder ultrasound is a safe alternative to measure urine volume with >90% accuracy [20].

Table 36.4 Common indications and contraindications for indwelling urinary catheterization

Indications	Contraindications
Acute urinary retention[a]	Absolute
Chronic urinary retention	Trauma or injury to the urethra
For example, neurogenic bladder[a], bladder outlet obstruction	Relative
Urinary incontinence refractory to pharmacologic treatment	Recent urinary tract surgery (urethra or bladder neck)
Strict urine output volume measurements	Urethral stricture
Critically ill patients[a]	Presence of artificial sphincter or
Congestive heart failure	Penile prosthesis
Acute renal failure	Combative patient
Intraoperative monitoring[a]	
Hygiene	
Prevent soiling in pressure injuries or open wounds; end-of-life care and comfort[a]	
Hematuria	
Maintain flow for hematuria with clots	
Bladder cancer with outlet obstruction	

[a]Adapted from Cravens and Zweig [13]. Table 1 Indications for Use of Urinary Catheters; p. 1

36.10 Urinary Catheters: Types and Uses

A Foley catheter is frequently used to maintain a closed, sterile drainage system for longer duration (Fig. 36.4). Originally introduced by Dr. Frederic Foley in the 1930s, the Foley catheter has two separate channels or lumens running the length of the catheter, one for urine drainage and the other for balloon inflation and deflation. Once the balloon (or cuff) is inflated with saline, it keeps the catheter secure in the bladder and allows a steady outflow of urine through the drainage lumen. There are different lumen sizes and lengths. French units are used to describe the diameter of the catheter lumen (one French unit is equivalent to 0.33 mm). For example, a 12 French catheter is roughly 4 mm in diameter. Size 16–18 French catheters are commonly used for most adults, whereas larger lumen catheters (20–24 French) may be used for irrigation of blood clots. Three-way Foley catheters are used for continuous bladder irrigation and drainage and contain a small lumen to inflate the cuff, a medium-sized lumen to inject solution for irrigation, and a large lumen for urinary drainage. A straight catheter is typically for one time use to obtain a sterile urine specimen for a urine culture, to determine a post void residual (PVR) volume, or to empty the bladder with clean intermittent self-catheterization. Coudé catheters are curved distally and have a round ball at the tip (Fig. 36.4). Coudé

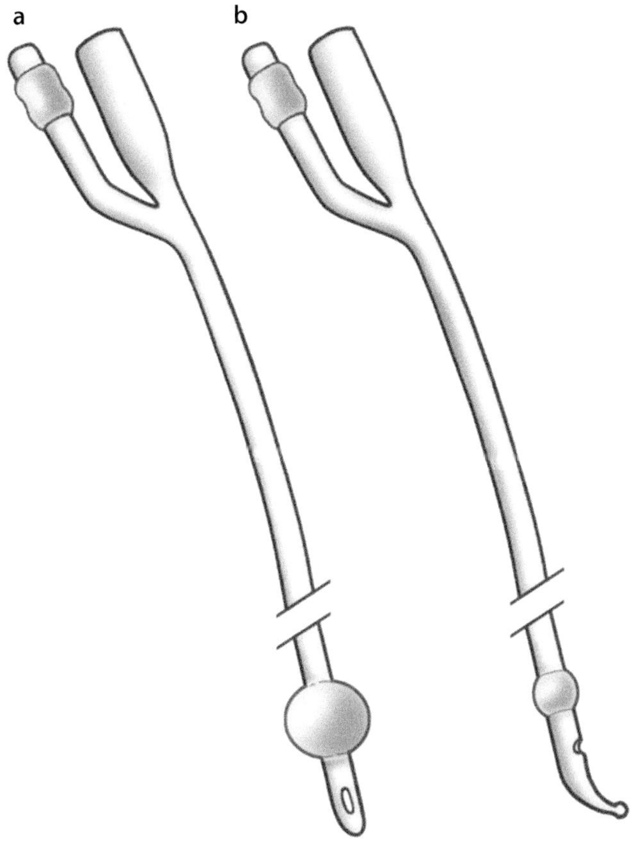

Fig. 36.4 Commonly used urethral catheters. **a** Illustration of the Foley catheter (*left*) **b** Illustration of the Coudé catheter (*right*)

catheters are used when straight tip catheters are difficult to pass, commonly due to urethral strictures, BPH, or urethral narrowing due to radiation or surgery. Condom catheters consist of a flexible, clear sheath fitted over the penis that connects to a drainage tube and bag and does not require urethral insertion. In hospitalized men, condom catheters are associated with reduced risk of bacteriuria, symptomatic UTI, and mortality compared to indwelling urethral catheters [58]. Though it is a useful alternative to urethral catheters in men, condom catheters may cause penile ulceration or dermatitis and are prone to urine leakage and dislodgement.

36.11 Urinary Catheters: Insertion Technique, Management, and Troubleshooting

Indwelling catheters are placed using sterile technique (Figs. 36.5 and 36.6) to maintain a sterile, closed drainage system and avoid ascending infection. Sterile urine specimens may be collected from indwelling catheters through a needle aspiration port, and an anti-reflux valve prevents backflow of contaminated urine in the collection bag into the catheter. Daily urethral examination involves cleaning the genital area to prevent irritation and encrustation and evaluating for catheter-related complications such as blockage and leakage (Table 36.5).

36.12 Complications of Long-Term Indwelling Urinary Catheterization

Complications of long-term indwelling catheters are common and may include recurrent catheter-associated urinary tract infection (CA-UTI), leakage or blockage of urinary flow, urethral irritation and erosion, loss of bladder function, and accidental dislodgement [68]. One in five patients with an indwelling catheter develops bacteriuria, or bacterial colonization of urine, and one quarter of those patients will develop a catheter-associated urinary tract infection (CA-UTI) [56]. In fact, CA-UTIs are the most common nosocomial infection in hospitals and nursing homes [19]. A longer duration of catheterization (>2 days) is associated with significantly higher rates of CA-UTI in the postoperative period [66], and early removal of indwelling catheters is recommended for surgical quality improvement. Although bacteriuria is common and develops at a rate of 3–10% per day of catheterization, only one-quarter of those patients develop symptoms consistent with a CA-UTI [56, 61]. Risk factors for UTI include female sex, older age, diabetes mellitus, bacterial colonization of the drainage bag, and poor catheter care [66]. In patients without symptoms of UTI, antibiotic treatment is only indicated for pregnant women or for patients undergoing urological procedures [51]. Yet, nearly one-third of catheterized patients with asymptomatic bacteriuria are inappropriately treated with antibiotics [64] causing risk of selection for resistant organisms, *Clostridium difficile* colitis infection, and antibiotic-related side effects. Thus, appropriate diagnosis and treatment of CA-UTI [27] and reducing inappropriate urinary catheter use are a national priority [6, 47]. Multidisciplinary, health system-wide, team-based initiatives can effectively reduce the rates of CA-UTIs in acute care settings [22], emergency rooms [50], and nursing homes [49] at regional and national levels.

36.13 Alternatives to Long-Term Indwelling Catheterization

For patients who do not tolerate long-term indwelling catheterization, clean intermittent catheterization (CIC) is a safe alternative to treat voiding dysfunction. CIC is the preferred treatment for voiding dysfunction in neurogenic bladder [15] and well-tolerated among older adults [53]. However, adherence to CIC may be limited by physical barriers such as difficulty with positioning due to imbalance or mobility issues, manual dexterity, visual impairment, cognitive impairment, and psychosocial barriers such as fear of embarrassment, impact on sexual relationships, shame due to stigma and inadequate public facilities [58]. In cases where urethral catheter placement has failed or cannot be safely placed, such as postoperative states, urethral obstruction, or trauma, and self-catheterization cannot be performed, the next step is to consider suprapubic catheter placement. Suprapubic catheterization is associated with fewer cases of asymptomatic bacteriuria and pain compared to long-term

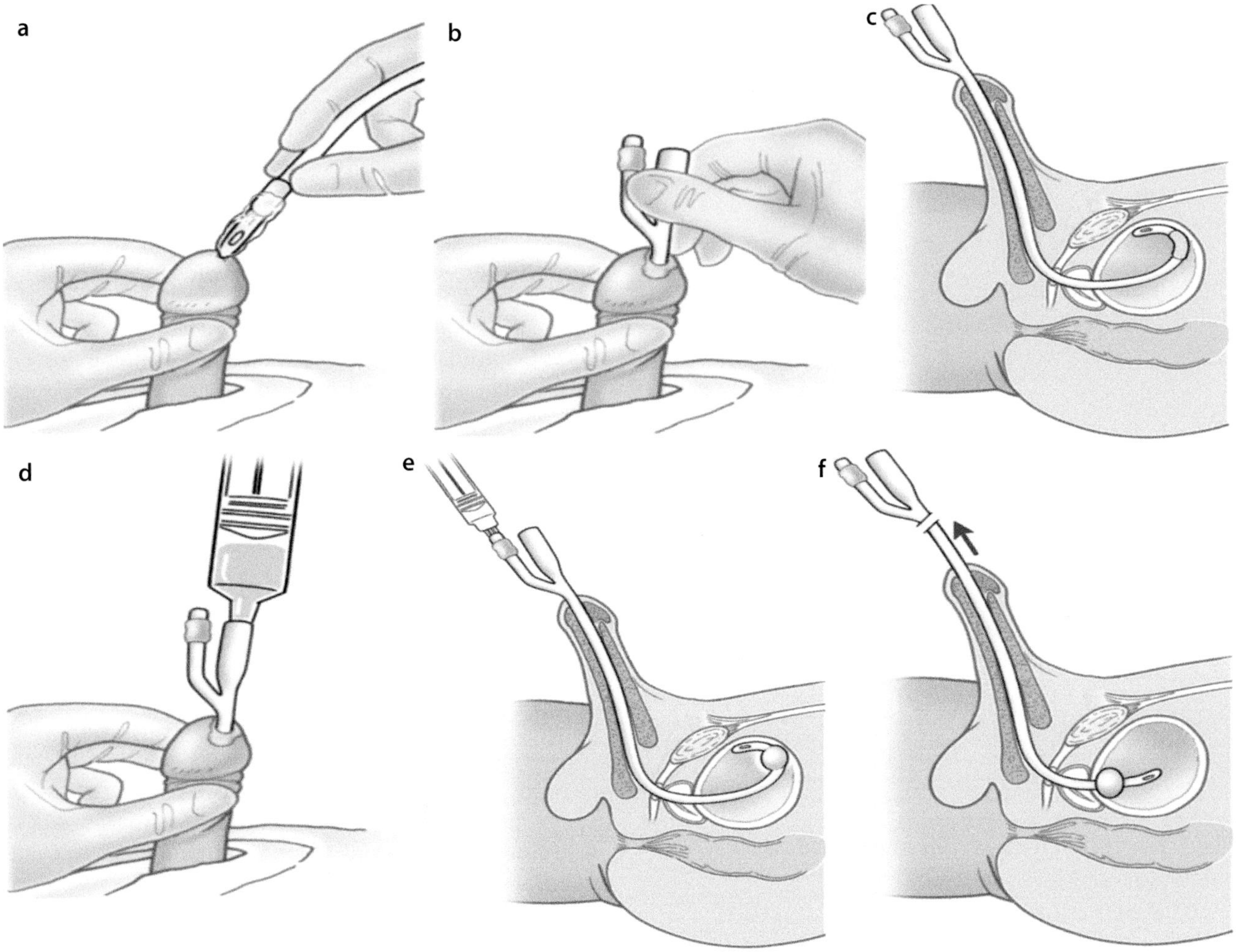

◘ Fig. 36.5 Foley catheter insertion technique. **a** The lubricated catheter is inserted into the urethra. **b** The catheter is advanced until the ports are at the meatus. **c** Cross-section of the male pelvis showing the distal catheter positioned within the bladder. **d** Urine aspiration confirms proper placement of the catheter. **e** The cuff of the tip of the catheter is inflated. **f** The catheter is gently withdrawn to lodge the cuff against the bladder neck. (Source: Reichman [54]. Fig. 142–4, Foley catheter insertion; Copyright ©The McGraw-Hill Companies, Inc. All rights reserved.)

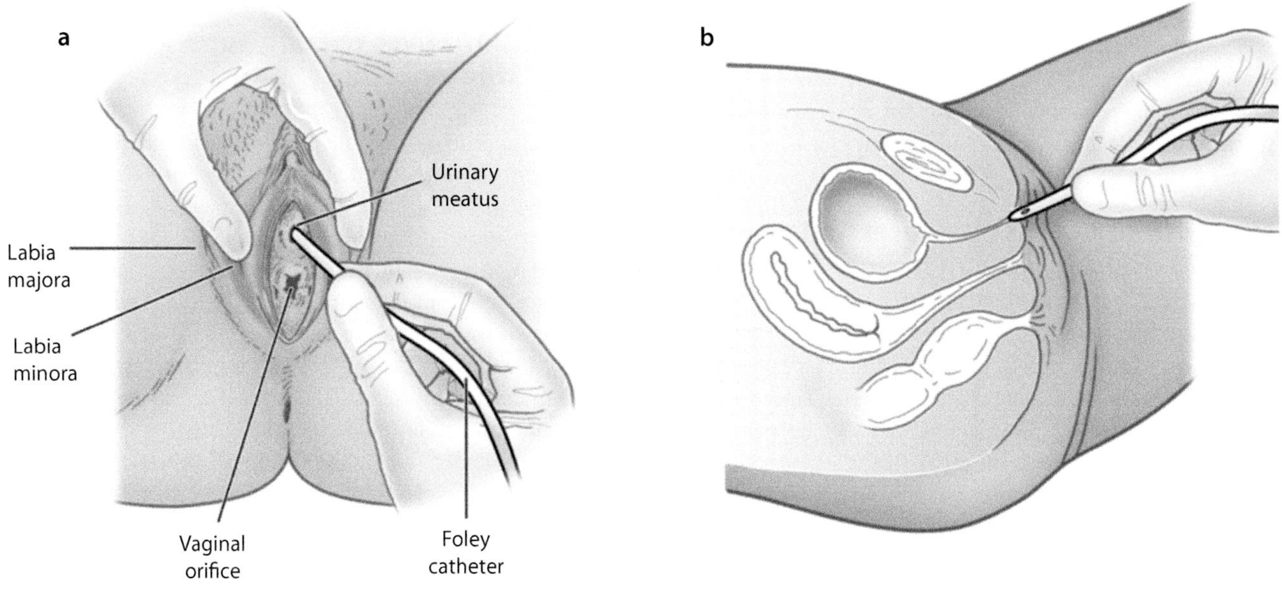

◘ Fig. 36.6 Female urethral catheterization. **a** External view of the genitalia. The catheter is inserted into the urethral meatus and advanced. **b** Midsagittal section of the female pelvis demonstrating catheter insertion. (Source: Reichman [54]. Fig. 142–11, Female urethral catheterization; Copyright ©The McGraw-Hill Companies, Inc. All rights reserved)

Table 36.5 Common problems related to urinary catheters

Problem	Etiology	Troubleshooting
Difficulty with catheter insertion	Incorrect position of catheter tip Difficulty visualizing urethral meatus Urethral meatus stenosis or stricture Penile edema Phimosis Painful catheter insertion	1. Gently apply pressure to suprapubic region 2. Ensure proper position of catheter tip in urethral meatus with adequate lighting 3. 2% lidocaine gel insertion into urethra for pain 4. Consider urology consultation if: No flow after irrigation Resistance with catheter insertion Persistent pain Bleeding
No urine flow/catheter blockage	Kinked tubing Collection bag above level of bladder Constipation/fecal impaction Obstruction due to encrustation, stones, blood clots, biofilm	1. Irrigate with saline 2. Check catheter/drainage bag positioning 3. Replace with new catheter 4. Alternative catheter (e.g., Coudé catheter)
Leakage	Urethral trauma Balloon inflation in urethra Bladder spasms Catheter blockage Urinary flow obstruction due to kinking/twisting of catheter	**Transurethral catheterization is contraindicated if urethral trauma suspected** 1. Irrigate with saline 2. Secure catheter and tubing 3. Consider bladder ultrasound for catheter tip position 4. Exchange catheter
Bleeding	Bladder mass Urinary infection Trauma	**Transurethral catheterization is contraindicated if urethral trauma suspected** 1. Irrigate with saline 2. Evaluate for urinary infection 3. Urology consultation for three-way catheter with irrigation
Skin breakdown/rash	Latex allergy Cellulitis Positioning of catheter tubing	1. Remove catheter, keep site clean and dry 2. If allergy suspected try another catheter material (e.g., silicone, plastic, or Teflon) 3. Consider dermatology or wound care consultation

Adapted from: Ghaffary et al. [21]

indwelling catheterization [36], and for long-term postoperative use (>5 days), the risk of UTI is significantly lower for suprapubic and intermittent catheterization compared to indwelling catheterization [25]. Suprapubic catheter insertion requires surgical intervention, and potential complications include insertion site bleeding, infections, bladder spasms, and technical difficulties such as blockage or leakage resulting in recurrent emergency room visits [1]. Given the risk of long-term complications with both indwelling urethral and suprapubic catheterization and challenges with CIC especially in geriatric patients with cognitive or functional impairment, it is important to consider individual needs, skills, and resources prior to committing to a plan of long-term catheterization.

36.14 Indwelling Catheters in Palliative and End-of-Life Care

The use of indwelling catheters at the end-of-life is indicated for palliation of symptoms associated with urinary retention such as suprapubic or visceral pain from bladder distension [59]. Tumors of the genitourinary tract, urethral stricture associated with radiation, or postsurgical anatomical changes and neurogenic bladder in the late stage of progressive neurodegenerative disease are some conditions which may warrant palliative indwelling catheter insertion. Gross hematuria may result in urinary outflow obstruction from blood clots, and catheterization is used to prevent discomfort associated with urinary retention and bladder distension [24]. Initial management of gross hematuria involves manual irrigation of the indwelling catheter with normal saline to establish clear or light pink urine. If manual irrigation is ineffective, intermittent or continuous bladder irrigation (CBI) is indicated to prevent further clot formation. Indwelling catheters may also be used in patients with urinary incontinence to prevent soiling and worsening of pressure injuries. Although indwelling catheterization may provide symptomatic relief, urethral catheterization is one of the most painful procedures identified in emergency rooms [60], and practitioners must weigh the benefit of symptom relief against the risks of harm associated with catheterization. Topical analgesics like lidocaine 2% gel into the urethra prior to catheter insertion may alleviate catheterization-associated pain [60], and pre-procedure opiates may also help facilitate catheter insertion. Urological intervention may require transfer to an alternate healthcare setting such as to an emergency room, which may not be feasible or consistent with the wishes of patients and families. In these circumstances, medications such as opiates or benzodiazepines are used to alleviate symptoms of distress. Despite the risks associated with catheterization, among patients enrolled in Hospice care the presence of an indwelling catheter has been associated with better pain control [35] and catheterization should be considered an option for effective palliation of urinary symptoms at the end of life.

Case Conclusion

Mr. B has failed numerous trials of voiding at his urologist's office and has been admitted to the emergency room twice in the past month for catheter-related complications including poor flow and leakage. His friend continues to express concern that he lives alone, that his home has started to smell of urine, and that he has fallen multiple times in the home. He has grown more isolated.

Living arrangements and socioeconomic circumstances should be considered in the safe and effective management of indwelling Foley catheters in the older population. In 2016, one in three (29%) community-dwelling adults over age 65 in the United States lived alone, and over half lived with their spouse (56%) [64]. As the proportion of older adults living alone increases with age, a growing number of adults will depend on caregivers for their daily healthcare needs. The decision to place an indwelling Foley catheter in a community-dwelling older adult should also incorporate several key questions:

1. How will the individual maintain hygiene and perform daily catheter evaluation and care?
2. How would an indwelling urinary catheter affect an individual's function and ability to meet his or her daily needs?
3. How will the individual address complications or issues related to the urinary catheter?

The impact of urinary symptoms and catheterization on healthcare utilization and quality of life further underscores the growing need for community-based resources [62] to support the needs of geriatric patients for the safe and effective management of urinary symptoms.

References

36

1. Ahluwalia RS, Johal N, Kouriefs C, Kooiman G, Montgomery BS, Plail RO. The surgical risk of suprapubic catheter insertion and long-term sequelae. Ann R Coll Surg Engl. 2006;88(2):210–3.
2. Anger JT, Saigal CS, Litwin MS. The prevalence of urinary incontinence among community dwelling adult women: results from the National Health and Nutrition Examination Survey. J Urol. 2006;175(2):601–4.
3. Bogner HR, Gallo JJ, Sammel MD, Ford DE, Armenian HK, Eaton WW. Urinary incontinence and psychological distress in community-dwelling older adults. J Am Geriatr Soc. 2002;50(3):489–95.
4. Boyle P, Robertson C, Mazzetta C, et al. The prevalence of lower urinary tract symptoms in men and women in four centres. The UrEpik study. BJU Int. 2003;92(4):409–14.
5. Brown JS, Vittinghoff E, Wyman JF, et al. Urinary incontinence: does it increase risk for falls and fractures? Study of Osteoporotic Fractures Research Group. J Am Geriatr Soc. 2000;48(7):721–5.
6. Bulger J, Nickel W, Messler J, et al. Choosing wisely in adult hospital medicine: five opportunities for improved healthcare value. J Hosp Med. 2013;8(9):486–92.
7. Carson C 3rd, Rittmaster R. The role of dihydrotestosterone in benign prostatic hyperplasia. Urology. 2003;61(4) Suppl 1):2–7.
8. Collas DM, Malone-Lee JG. Age-associated changes in detrusor sensory function in women with lower urinary tract symptoms. Int Urogynecol J Pelvic Floor Dysfunct. 1996;7(7):24–9.
9. Colombel M, Vacherot F, Diez SG, Fontaine E, Buttyan R, Chopin D. Zonal variation of apoptosis and proliferation in the normal prostate and in benign prostatic hyperplasia. Br J Urol. 1998;82(3):380–5.
10. Trautner BW, Cope M, Cevallow ME, Cadle RM, Darouiche RO, Musher DM. Inappropriate treatment of catheter-associated asymptomatic bacteriuria in a tertiary care hospital. Clin Infect Dis. 2009;48(9):1182–8.
11. Coyne KS, Sexton CC, Thompson CL, et al. The prevalence of lower urinary tract symptoms (LUTS) in the USA, the UK and Sweden: results from the epidemiology of LUTS (EpiLUTS) study. BJU Int. 2009;104(3):352–60.
12. Coyne KS, Zhou Z, Bhattacharyya SK, Thompson CL, Dhawan R, Versi E. The prevalence of nocturia and its effect on health-related quality of life and sleep in a community sample in the USA. BJU Int. 2003;92(9):948–54.
13. Cravens DD, Zweig S. Urinary catheter management. Am Fam Physician. 2000;61(2):369–76.
14. Deandrea S, Lucenteforte E, Bravi F, Foschi R, La Vecchia C, Negri E. Risk factors for falls in community-dwelling older people: a systematic review and meta-analysis. Epidemiology. 2010;21(5):658–68.
15. DeFade B, Kennelly M, Deem S. Urological care of the neurologically impaired patient in the outpatient setting. Am Urol Assoc Update Series. 2011;. 30 Lesson 4
16. Dielubanza EJ, Han JS, Gonzalez CM. Distal urethroplasty for fossa navicularis and meatal strictures. Transl Androl Urol. 2014;3(2):163–9.
17. Dobrowolski ZF, Weglarz W, Jakubik P, Lipczynski W, Dobrowolska B. Treatment of posterior and anterior urethral trauma. BJU Int. 2002;89(7):752–4.
18. Fick DM, Semla TP, Beizer J, et al. American Geriatrics Society 2015 updated Beers criteria for potentially inappropriate medication use in older adults. J Am Geriatr Soc. 2015;63(11):2227–46.
19. Foxman B. Epidemiology of urinary tract infections: incidence, morbidity and economic costs. Am J Med. 2002;113(Suppl 1A):5S–13S.
20. Fuse H, Yokoyama T, Muraishi Y, Katayama T. Measurement of residual urine volume using a portable ultrasound instrument. Int Urol Nephrol. 1996;28(5):633–7.
21. Ghaffary C, Yohannes A, Villanueva C, Leslie SW. A practical approach to difficult urinary catheterizations. Curr Urolo Rep. 2013;14(6):565–79.
22. Girard R, Gaujard S, Pergay V, et al. Controlling urinary tract infections associated with intermittent bladder catheterization in geriatric hospitals. J Hosp Infect. 2015;90(3):240–7.
23. Gorecki C, Brown JM, Nelson EA, et al. Impact of pressure ulcers on quality of life in older patients: a systematic review. J Am Geriatr Soc. 2009;57(7):1175–83.
24. Groninger H, Phillips JM. Gross hematuria: assessment and management at the end of life. J Hosp Palliat Nurs. 2012;14(3):184–8.

25. Han CS, Kim S, Radadia KD, et al. Comparison of urinary tract infection rates associated with transurethral catheterization, suprapubic tube and clean intermittent catheterization in the postoperative setting: a network meta-analysis. J Urol. 2017;198(6):1353–8.
26. High KP, Bradley SF, Gravenstein S, et al. Clinical practice guideline for the evaluation of fever and infection in older adult residents of long-term care facilities: 2008 update by the Infectious Diseases Society of America. Clin Infect Dis. 2009;48(2):149–71.
27. Hooton TM, Bradley SF, Cardenas DD, et al. Diagnosis, prevention, and treatment of catheter-associated urinary tract infection in adults: 2009 international clinical practice guidelines from the Infectious Disease Society of America. Clin Infect Dis. 2010;50(5):625–63.
28. Inouye SK, Studenski S, Tinetti ME, Kuchel GA. Geriatric syndromes: clinical, research, and policy implications of a core geriatric concept. J Am Geriatr Soc. 2007;55(5):780–91.
29. Inouye SK, Westendrop RGJ, Saczynski JS. Delirium in elderly people. Lancet. 2014e;383(9920):911–22.
30. Irwin DE, Kopp ZS, Agatep B, Milsom I, Abrams P. Worldwide prevalence estimates of lower urinary tract symptoms, overactive bladder, urinary incontinence and bladder outlet obstruction. BJU Int. 2011;108(7):1132–8.
31. Irwin DE, Milsom I, Kopp Z, Abrams P, Artibani W, Herschorn S. Prevalence, severity and symptom bother of lower urinary tract symptoms among men in the EPIC study: impact of overactive bladder. Euro Urol. 2009;56(1):14–20.
32. Issa MM, Fetner TC, Black L, Grogg AL, Kruep EJ. An assessment of the diagnosed prevalence of diseases in men 50 years of age or older. Am J Manag Care. 2006;12(4). Suppl):S83–9.
33. Jacobsen SJ, Jacobson DJ, Girman CJ, et al. Natural history of prostatism: risk factors for acute urinary retention. J Urol. 1997;158(2):481–7.
34. Jain P, Parada P, David A, Smith LG. Overuse of the indwelling urinary tract catheter in hospitalized medical patients. Arch Intern Med. 1995;155(13):1425–9.
35. Kelly L, Bender L, Harris P, Casarett D. The 'comfortable dying' measure: how patient characteristics affect hospice pain management quality scores. J Palliat Med. 2014;17(6):721–4.
36. Kidd EA, Stewart F, Kassis NC, Horn E, Omar MI. Urethral (indwelling or intermittent) or suprapubic routes for short-term catheterization in hospitalized adults. Cochrane Database Syst Rev [Internet]. 2015 [cited 2018 Feb 05]; (12). Available from: http://onlinelibrary.wiley.com/doi/10.1002/14651858.CD004203.pub3/pdf.
37. Kujubu DA. Nocturia in Elderly Persons and Nocturnal Polyuria. In: American Society of Nephrology Geriatrics Nephrology Curriculum [Internet]. Los Angeles: American Society of Nephrology; 2009. [cited 2017 Dec 15]. Chapter 19. Available from: https://www.asn-online.org/education/distancelearning/curricula/geriatrics/Chapter19.pdf.
38. Lachenbruch C, Ribble D, Emmons K, VanGlider C. Pressure ulcer risk in the incontinent patient: analysis of incontinence and hospital-acquired pressure ulcers from the international pressure ulcer prevalence survey. J Wound Ostomy Continence Nurs. 2016;43(3):235–41.
39. Landi F, Cesari M, Russo A, Onder G, Lattanzio F, Bernabei R. Potentially reversible risk factors and urinary incontinence in frail older people living in community. Age Ageing. 2003;32:194–9.
40. Liu S, Chan L, Tse V. Clinical outcome in male patients with detrusor overactivity with impaired contractility. Int Neurourol J. 2014;18(3):133–7.
41. Lose G, Alling-Moller JP. Nocturia in women. Am J Obstet Gynecol. 2001;185(5):514–21.
42. Ma J, Gharaee-Kermani M, Kunju L, et al. Prostatic fibrosis is associated with lower urinary tract symptoms. J Urol. 2012;188(4):1375–81.
43. Madersbacher S, Pycha A, Schatzl G, Mian C, Klingler C, Marberger M. The aging lower urinary tract: a comparative urodynamic study of men and women. Urology. 1998;51(2):206–12.
44. Marberger MJ, Andersen JT, Nickel JC, et al. Prostate volume and serum prostate-specific antigen as predictors of acute urinary retention: combined experience from three large multinational placebo-controlled trials. Eur Urol. 2000;38:563–8.
45. Markland AD, Vaughan CP, Johnson TM II, Goode PS, Redden DT, Burgio KL. Prevalence of nocturia in United States men: results from the national health and nutrition examination survey. J Urol. 2011;185(3):998–1002.
46. McConnell JD, Roehrborn CG, Bautista O, et al. The long-term effects of doxazosin, finasteride and combination therapy on the clinical progression of benign prostatic hyperplasia. N Engl J Med. 2003;349:2387–98.
47. Meddings J, Rogers MAM, Krein SL, Fakih MG, Olmsted RN, Saint S. Reducing unnecessary urinary catheter use and other strategies to prevent catheter-associated urinary tract infection: an integrative review. BMJ Qual Saf. 2014;23(4):277–89.
48. Meigs JB, Barry MJ, Giovannucci E, Rimm EB, Stampfer MJ, Kawachi I. Incidence rates and risk factors for acute urinary retention: the health professionals follow-up study. J Urol. 1999;162(2):376–82.
49. Mody L, Greene MT, Meddings J, et al. A national implementation project to prevent catheter-associated urinary tract infection in nursing home residents. JAMA Intern Med. 2017;177(8):1154–62.
50. Mulcare MR, Rosen T, Clark S, Viswanathan K, et al. A novel clinical protocol for placement and management of indwelling urinary catheters in older adults in the emergency department, vol. 22. p. 1056.
51. Nicolle L, Bradley S, Colgan R, et al. Infectious Diseases Society of America guidelines for the diagnosis and treatment of asymptomatic bacteriuria in adults. Clin Infect Dis. 2005;40(5):643–54.
52. Offermans MP, Du Moulin MF, Hamers JP, Dassen T, Halfens RJ. Prevalence of urinary incontinence and associated risk factors in nursing home residents: a systematic review. Neurourol Urodyn. 2009;28(4):288–94.
53. Pilloni S, Krhut J, Mair D, Madersbacher H, Kessler TM. Intermittent catheterization in older people: a valuable alternative to indwelling catheter? Age Ageing. 2005;34(1):57–60.
54. Reichman EF. Urethral catheterizationEmergency medicine procedures [internet]. 2nd ed New York: McGraw-Hill Education; 2013 [cited 2018 Feb 05]. Available from: http://accessemergencymedicine.mhmedical.com/content.aspx?bookid=683&sectionid=45343633.
55. Roehrborn CG, McConnell JD, Lieber M, et al. Serum prostate-specific antigen concentration is a powerful predictor of acute urinary retention and need for surgery in men with clinical benign prostatic hyperplasia. PLESS Study Group Urol. 1999;53(3):473–80.
56. Saint S. Clinical and economic consequences of nosocomial catheter-related bacteriuria. Am J Infect Control. 2000;28(1):68–75.
57. Saint S, Kaufman SR, Rogers MA, Baker PD, Ossenkop K, Lipsky BA. Condom versus indwelling urinary catheters: a randomized trial. J Am Geriatr Soc. 2006;54(7):1055–61.
58. Seth JH, Haslam C, Panicker JN. Ensuring patient adherence to clean intermittent self-catheterization. Patient Prefer Adherence. 2014;8:191–8.
59. Sinclair C, Kalender-Rich JL, Griebling TL, Porter-Williamson K. Palliative care of urologic patients at end of life. Clin Geriatr Med. 2015;31(4):667–78.
60. Singer AJ, Richman PB, Kowalska A, Thode HC. Comparison of patient and practitioner assessments of pain from commonly performed emergency department procedures. Ann Emerg Med. 1999;33(6):652–8.
61. Tambyah PA, Maki DG. Catheter-associated urinary tract infection is rarely symptomatic: a prospective study of 1497 catheterized patients. Arch Intern Med. 2000;160:678–82.
62. Tay LJ, Lyons H, Karrouze I, Taylor C, Khan AA, Thompson PM. Impact of the lack of community urinary catheter services on the Emergency Department. BJU Int. 2016;118(2):327–34.

63. West LA, Cole S, Goodkind D, He W. 65+ in the United States: 2010 [internet]. Washington DC: United States Census Bureau; 2014 [cited 2017 Dec 12]. Available from: https://www.census.gov/content/dam/Census/library/publications/2014/demo/p23-212.pdf.
64. United States Department of Health and Human Services. A Profile of Older Americans [Internet]. Washington DC: Administration on Aging; 2016 [cited 2018 Feb 5]. Available from: https://www.acl.gov/aging-and-disability-in-america/data-and-research/profile-older-americans.
65. Van Mastrigt R. Age dependency of urinary bladder contractility. Neuroruol Urodyn. 1992;11:315–7.
66. Wald HL, Ma A, Bratzler DW. Indwelling urinary catheter use in the postoperative period: analysis of the national surgical infection prevention project data. Arch Surg. 2008;143(6):551–7.
67. Weiss JP, Blaivas JG. Nocturnal polyuria versus overactive bladder in nocturia. Urology. 2002;60(5) Suppl 1):28–32.
68. Wilde M, McDonald MV, Brasch J, et al. Long-term urinary catheter users self-care practices and problems. J Clin Nurs. 2013;22(0):356–67.
69. Yalla SV, Sullivan MP, Resnick NM. Update on detrusor hyperactivity with impaired contractility. Curr Bladder Dysfunct Rep. 2007;2(4):191–6.

High-Risk Pressure Ulcers

Lisa A. Perez, Denise Cauble, and Kathryn M. Daniel

A. Chun (ed.), *Geriatric Practice*, https://doi.org/10.1007/978-3-030-19625-7_37

Pressure ulcers (PU) remain a very common, yet preventable comorbidity in the disabled and elderly population. The Agency for Healthcare Research and Quality (AHRQ) estimates 2.5 million persons develop pressure ulcers every year in the United States [1, 2]. In a 12-year period (2000–2012) the National Pressure Ulcer Advisory Panel, European Pressure Ulcer Advisory Panel, and Pan Pacific Advisory Pressure Injury Alliance (2014) reported a prevalence rate of PU (number present at a specific time) of up to 45% in acute care, a significant burden of disease [3]. The elderly represents a high number of these pressure wounds. The incidence (or nosocomial acquisition of PU) in acute care is great, up to 50% in the elderly population. Patients with pressure ulcers acquired in the hospital demonstrate a significant increase in length of stay, cost, and overall mortality rate [4]. AHRQ estimates in 2014 that PU cost between $9.1 and $11.6 billion dollars in the United States [5].

Beginning in 2010, new regulatory guidelines took effect regarding hospital reimbursement for nosocomial (or facility acquired) pressure ulcers. The renewed concern for the prevention and management of this condition emerged across the nation. Hospitals and nursing facilities now are at risk for loss of reimbursement when pressure wounds are linked to care within their facility. This chapter begins with a brief review of the anatomy and physiology of the integumentary system and normal healing. The next section of the chapter describes pressure wound prevention and assessment. The final section of the chapter outlines best practice management of pressure wounds according to wound characteristics.

37.1 Normal Anatomy and Physiology of the Integumentary System

The skin is composed of two layers, the epidermis and the dermis. While its primary purpose is protection, it is also vital to temperature regulation and vitamin D metabolism, and it represents an aesthetic reflection of who we are.

The epidermis is the outer most layer and is formed almost entirely of keratinocytes. These cells are constantly produced at the deepest of five layers called the stratum germinativum. Over the following weeks they rise through the other four layers arriving at the most superficial layer; the stratum corneum at the end of their life cycle. The keratinocytes produce a protein called keratin, which is insoluble in water, provides both a shield from external irritants, and prevents water loss [5]. Melanin-producing melanocytes and Langerhans cells are also located in the epithelium. Both are also important in immune responses.

The dermis is attached to the deepest level of the epidermis via the basement membrane at the dermal–epidermal junction. The dermis is a highly vascular layer, which feeds and supports the epidermis above it. It also houses sensory nerve endings and dermal appendages such as hair follicles, nails, and sweat and sebaceous glands. The dermis is separated into two layers, the deeper reticular dermis and the superficial papillary dermis. The papillary dermis is made of the connective tissue or extracellular matrix that gives skin its strength and elasticity. This superficial region contains the vascular support that feeds the epidermal layer, provides thermoregulation, and allows us to blush. The deeper reticular dermis is located just above the subcutaneous adipose layer or hypodermis. Larger branches of the vascular system are found here as well as fibroelastic connective tissues.

37.1.1 Normal Wound Healing

37.1.1.1 Phases of Wound Healing

From a needle prick on the day of birth, through numerous skinned knees in childhood and various surgical or traumatic wounds across the lifespan, the expectation is that these wounds will heal because the skin is designed to do so. While the days required to accomplish each phase may vary, they generally proceed in the same order. Regardless of etiology, acute wound healing tends to follow a basic four-phase trajectory that begins immediately after wounding occurs.

37.1.2 Types of Acute Wounds

37.1.2.1 Full Thickness

A full-thickness tissue wound refers to the loss of the entire epidermal and dermal structure. These wounds can include subcutaneous fat, muscle, fascia, and bony structures.

37.1.2.2 Partial Thickness

Partial-thickness wounds involve epithelial loss and sometimes partial dermal loss. These superficial wounds heal via epidermal advancement. Since the dermal layer is not completely missing, no granulation tissue growth will be visible in the base; instead, the connective tissue repair of dermis will proceed along with the epithelial resurfacing. Partial-thickness repair does not result in scar formation or pigment loss and proceeds at a much faster rate than full-thickness repair (◘ Fig. 37.1).

37.1.3 Phases of Normal Wound Healing

▪▪ Hemostasis (Day 0)

Hemostasis follows the usual coagulation pathways leading to clot formation. The disruption of vascular structures causes the release of blood into the tissue. The activated platelets release cytokines as well as growth factors that initiate the healing process. These platelets also form the clot, or fibrin matrix that will provide structure for the repair to come.

▪▪ Inflammation (Days 0–7)

The inflammatory phase is initiated by the activated platelets release during hemostasis. These chemoattractants first summon neutrophils to the affected area. Their objective is to

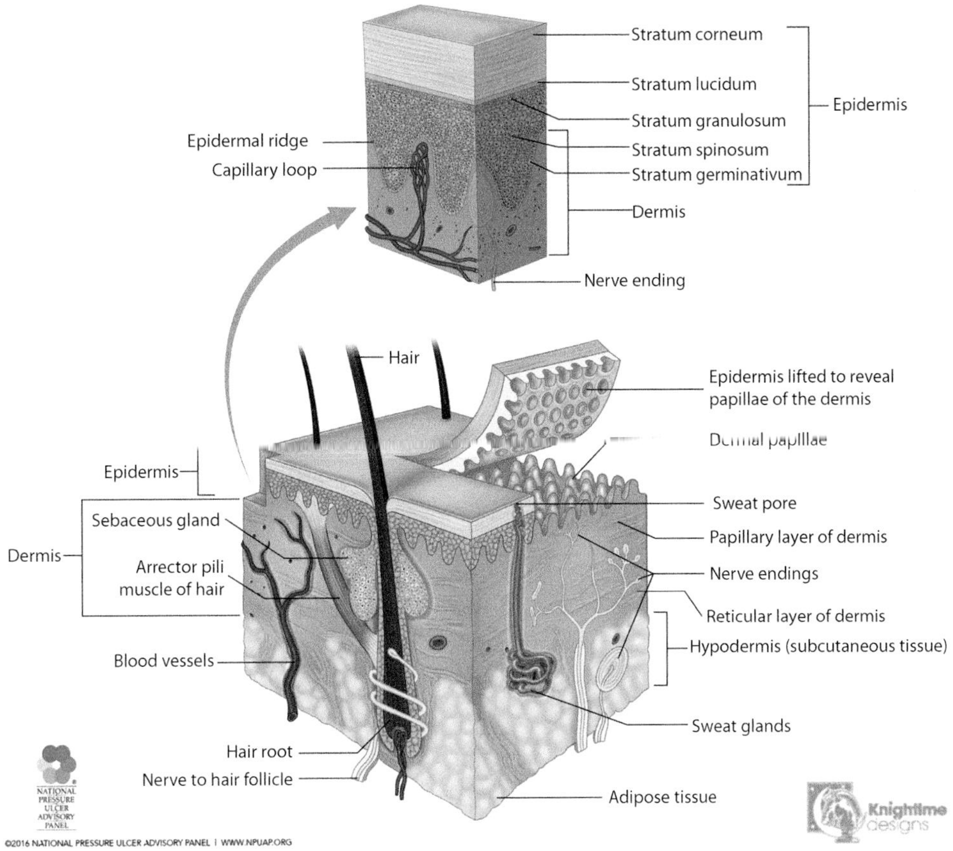

Fig. 37.1 Structures in healthy integumentary system

manage bioburden in the wound bed by attacking and destroying invading bacteria. Once the bacteria are under control, the numbers of neutrophils will decrease, and a surge of macrophages will arrive to eliminate the accumulation of both dead bacteria and spent neutrophils. In turn, the macrophages will release the cytokines that move the wound out of inflammation and into the proliferative phase of healing [5, 6].

▪▪ Proliferation (Days 7–17)

The inflammatory phase centered around ridding the wound bed of necrotic tissue and cellular debris. Once the base is clean, the wound can move into the proliferative or regenerative phase of healing. The main goal here is to fill the defect with scar tissue frequently referred to as granulation tissue and prepare for closure by the epithelium. During the final days of inflammation, fibroblasts begin to migrate to the area from the uninjured dermal layer surrounding the injury. The fibroblasts create new connective tissue such as provisional or type III collagen, while the vascular system creates new blood vessels to supply the newly formed tissue. These new vessels account for the usual beefy red color seen in healthy granulation tissue. Once the defect has been filled with new structures, the wound moves into the remodeling phase of healing [6, 7].

▪▪ Remodeling (Day 20–9 months)

As mentioned above, the fibroblasts synthesize new collagen for the construction of scar tissue. Myofibroblasts are fibroblasts that also contain muscle fibers and can decrease the size of the wound base by contracting and pulling the edges together. These specialized fibroblasts will also help to keep the wound closed during the remodeling or maturation phase of wound healing. The type III collagen laid down during the inflammatory and proliferation phases has little tensile strength and will split apart easily under a moderate amount of tension. The vascular system will also have overproduced new blood vessels during the construction phase. Through a series of apoptosis and vascular trimming, the new tissue will be remodeled over several months. The type III collagen will be removed and replaced with Type I collagen which is stronger and has more stretch. It is important to note, however, that healed full-thickness wounds will never have the strength or elasticity of the original tissue [6, 8].

▪▪ Epithelialization

As we have seen, wound closure is not the end of healing in a full-thickness wound; however, in a partial-thickness wound, epithelialization does mark the end of the healing process. During full-thickness repair, epithelium may be seen to advance any time after inflammation begins. If a wound bed remains moist and at or below the level of surrounding skin, the epithelium will continue to grow over the defect until it reaches the other side. Over growth of granulation, adherence of crust or dried blood will slow down the process in both full-thickness and partial-thickness wound.

Case Study

Mrs. C is an 86-year-old female who has been living alone in a two-story home where she and her family have resided for over 50 years. Six weeks ago, she missed a step while carrying in groceries and fell off the porch. She sustained a fractured right femur head and lay unassisted for several hours prior to transfer to an acute care facility. The patient has a history of atrial fibrillation and was taking Warfarin for anticoagulation therapy. She was also being treated for primary hypertension and osteoporosis. Her BMI has been low for the last 5 years which corresponds with the time of her husband's death. She has few visitors outside of her immediate family whom she corresponds with via phone several times a week but sees only occasionally. She has stopped attending church services due to difficulty with parking and she does not participate in any exercise or social activities outside her home.

Her skin assessment during admission to the emergency department at her local hospital revealed a "large hematoma" over the left hip and thigh, which was attributed to her fall combined with Warfarin use. The right hip fracture was addressed by surgery and her initial recovery went without incident. Within a few days, she was preparing for transfer to an inpatient rehabilitation facility. She began to complain of left hip discomfort, which far outweighed the surgical pain, but no further interventions were ordered regarding the left "hip bruise."

Within 3 days of her transfer to the rehabilitation facility, a wound care specialist was consulted due to the malodorous discharge from the left hip. The patient was transferred to a long-term acute care hospital for ongoing care of an infected and necrotic stage IV pressure injury to her left hip.

An area measuring 27 cm × 18 cm of nonviable tissue was debrided at the bedside. The excised material consisted of necrotic dermis, adipose, and muscle. Negative pressure wound therapy was initiated with an instillation of weak hypochlorous acid to ensure a clean wound base, and an infectious disease consult was initiated for intravenous antibiotic management.

Although Mrs. C had sustained a right hip fracture during her initial fall, she lay on her left hip for several hours while awaiting rescue. The "hematoma" and "large bruise" noted by both medical and nursing staff was likely a deep tissue injury caused by a decrease of arterial flow to the muscle tissue compressed between the ground and her left trochanter. The visible external injury is often referred to as the "tip of the iceberg" since the real trauma occurred deep within the tissue. This case demonstrates that pressure injury may occur over a matter of a few hours in a susceptible person. The patient's rehabilitation was also compromised due to her need for advanced wound care.

37.1.4 Age-Related Factors That Impact Healing

There are multiple reasons why a wound does not follow the usual healing trajectory expected in an acute wound. Wounds with delayed healing are considered chronic wounds. Age itself is not a risk factor for altered healing, but there are skin changes and comorbidities associated with aging that can negatively impact healing. See ◘ Table 37.1 below for a summary of age-related factors that impact healing.

37.1.5 Pressure Injury Definition

Terminology for the description of pressure injury is in transition. The terms pressure wound, pressure ulcer, and pressure injury are all noted and used interchangeably in the literature. The National Pressure Ulcer Advisory Panel (NPUAP) (2016) defines a pressure injury as "localized damage to the skin and/or underlying soft tissue usually over a bony prominence or related to a medical or other device" [16]. Mechanical load as pressure or pressure plus shear being applied to an area of soft tissue and bony prominence is considered to be the primary cause of a pressure injury. When critical capillary closing pressure or the amount of pressure required to produce tissue ischemia is achieved, PU may develop. Time and intensity factors are also an influence; low intensity pressure over a prolonged time or high intensity pressure over a short time can be equally damaging [6]. In the case study presented above, the patient had multiple risk factors that put her at increased risk for a pressure injury.

◘ **Table 37.1** Age-related factors that impact healing and the corresponding results seen in the tissue

Age-related phenomena	Impact on healing
Cellular senescence	Epithelial cells become thicker, keratinocytes replaced at a slower rate
Altered fibroblast function	Reduced ability for fibroblasts to synthesize both type I and type III collagen [5]
Changes in the inflammatory response	Muted allergic and contact reactions Decreased inflammatory reaction Impaired humoral immunity Decreased DNA repair capacity Increased oncogenic activity [5]
Sensation loss	Decreased/delayed sensory perception. Increased risk for repeated trauma or burn injury [5]
Thinning adipose layer, declining collagen content, and loss of elastin	Decreased barrier function Delayer recovery of stratum corneum Dry, flaking corneum Higher pH = increased risk for infection Declined lipid content Decline in sebum production Decreased turgor Increased risk of malignancy [5]
Medications	Corticosteroids, antiplatelet, anti-inflammatory, antibiotics, cytotoxic, nicotine, anticoagulants, immunosuppressive, anti-RA, vasoconstrictors [4]

37.1.6 Pressure Ulcer Frameworks

Causal determinants of pressure ulcers have been proposed since the 1980s. Braden and Bergstrom (1987) described PU development in their landmark work on an individual's intrinsic and extrinsic factors along with pressure and tissue tolerance [12]. They identified decreased mobility and activity and diminished sensory perception as major elements of PU development. They also determined that increased moisture, friction, and shear as extrinsic factors impact the development of PU. Poor nutrition, increased age, decreased arteriole pressure, the amount of interstitial fluid flow, emotional stress, smoking, and skin temperature were noted as individual or intrinsic factors that contribute to the development of PU. This work resulted in one of the first tools developed for use at the bedside to predict the risk of pressure ulcers, the Braden Scale.

The NPUAP/EPUAP mapped an updated causal model in 2009 [16]. The workgroup identified three direct causal factors of PU: immobility, skin/PU status, and poor perfusion. These direct factors are impacted by several key indirect causal factors: poor sensory perception and diabetes (resulting in poor perfusion), as well as moisture and poor nutrition (affecting skin and PU status). Additional indirect risk factors that may influence the development of pressure ulcers include older age, medications, pitting edema, chronic wounds, infections, acute illness, and hyperthermia.

A new conceptual framework for a causal theory of pressure ulcers (PU) was developed by Coleman et al. in 2014 [17]. This framework describes a relationship between the mechanical boundary loads (mechanical load, friction, and shear) and an individuals' physiology, such as the ability to repair, transport and thermal properties, and tissue properties. This framework also incorporates the multiple risk factors that affect the health of skin and tissue. When the mechanical boundary loads are overcome by the individual's susceptibility and tissue tolerance, a pressure injury occurs. By understanding these determinants, healthcare providers can identify an individual's risk factors and weaknesses and implement prevention strategies.

37.1.7 Pressure Ulcer Prevention

37.1.7.1 Risk Factors and Risk Assessment

There are several pressure ulcer risk assessment tools available, but the most popular tool used in the United States is the Braden Scale for Predicting Pressure Sore Risk. It can be used in many levels of patient care. The scale consists of six subscales and the total scores range from 6 to 23. A lower Braden score indicates higher levels of risk for pressure ulcer development. Generally, a score of 18 or less indicates at-risk status. The scale measures sensory perception, moisture, activity, mobility, nutrition, and friction/shear [12]. Most US hospitals require nurses to perform the risk assessment every shift for the most acutely ill patients. At a lower level of care, it may be performed daily or weekly. In nursing homes, it is done on admission, quarterly, and with changes in condition [13].

Once the level of risk has been documented and a thorough skin assessment is completed, interventions for preventing pressure injuries are instituted. Preventing pressure injuries begins with keeping the skin clean and dry. Using a pH balanced or slightly acidic cleanser will maintain the skin's natural acid mantle and decrease potential for infections [2]. The skin should be cleansed promptly after incontinence episodes. The chemical irritants and excess moisture exposure in either urine or feces will result in skin damage that will decrease skin tolerance for pressure or shear [2]. Many institutes are applying a prophylactic dressing to the midsacrum/coccyx to protect the area from moisture and shear forces. Evidence thus far has supported the use of these dressings in critically ill patients but is not yet considered best practice [2].

37.1.7.2 Nutrition

Malnutrition is associated with many adverse outcomes, particularly in the older adult. The Academy of Nutrition and Dietetics defines malnutrition as the presence of two or more of the following characteristics [2]:

- Insufficient energy intake
- Unintended weight loss
- Loss of muscle mass
- Loss of subcutaneous fat
- Localized or general fluid accumulation
- Decreased functional status

Poor nutrition along with poor hydration puts all adults at an increased risk for pressure injury development, but when coupled with hospitalization pressure injuries have been found in as many as 78% of frail elders [14]. The use of nutritional screens upon admission and with any change in condition will alert providers to consult a registered dietitian to perform a comprehensive nutritional assessment and provide recommendations for adequate nitrogen balance and necessary supplements [2]. A positive nitrogen balance and adequate hydration can both protect older adults from developing pressure injuries but will also facilitate the healing process for pre-existing injuries. The addition of Arginine supplements has also been found to reduce the incidence of pressure injuries [2, 15].

37.1.7.3 Repositioning

Repositioning and early mobilization are key factors in pressure injury prevention. Pressure injuries will not occur without a mechanical load on the soft tissue. For those who cannot reposition themselves, assistance must be provided around the clock using a repositioning schedule. For those at greatest risk, the use of pressure redistribution mattresses and chair cushions is also important [2]. Referrals to physical therapy where available will provide expert assessment and increase in activity in a safe yet rapid pace. See ▫ Table 37.2 below for a list of common prevention strategies and rationale.

Table 37.2 Pressure injury prevention strategies

Strategy	Rationale
Prophylactic dressings on heels and sacrum	To reduce friction and shear
Target specific populations prone to PU development	Spinal cord injuries, pediatric, patients using medical devices
Minimize friction and shear	Prompt cleansing after incontinent episodes Use lift equipment in patients with decreased mobility Maintain the head-of-bed position at 30 degrees or lower as tolerated Use a 30-degree side-lying position, turning to right-back-left Utilize a trapeze bar Avoid massage over bony prominences
Minimize pressure	Schedule repositioning for bedbound and chair-bound patients Frequency of turning should be based on the individuals' risk factors, mechanical boundary, and current physiology. Current evidence suggests every 4 h with the use of a pressure-redistributing mattress is as effective as every 2 h on a nonpressure-redistributing mattress
Techniques for repositioning	Frequent small changes using pillows for support Avoid positioning on medical devices Position bariatric patients in a side-lying position, preventing pressure of pannus on skin Avoid positioning on bony prominences
Pressure redistribution for chair-bound individuals	Frequency of reposition is unknown and depends on the anatomy, posture, weight distribution, and mobility. May require assistance There is some evidence that persons who can move to reposition do so every 15 min Maximal time with repositioning should be 2 h Repositioning includes forward leaning, leaning side to side, pressure relief push-ups for 2–3 min, and tilt back in chair 65 degrees Use a chair cushion; gel or pressure redistributing is preferred over foam
Heel pressure injury prevention	Use heel suspension devices Pillows under the calves longitudinally the length of the calf with suspension of the heels Manage plantar flexion
Use of support surfaces	Utilize support surfaces on bed and chairs to redistribute pressure for high-risk patients Manage the microclimate of surfaces to decrease moisture Avoid the use of foam cutouts or rings for pressure redistribution as they can increase pressure to the surrounding tissue Avoid the use of cotton gowns and bed linens Limit extra linen on the support surfaces that may interfere with airflow Use of a standardized algorithm for appropriate choice of a support surface is recommended

Adapted from Wound, Ostomy and Continence Nurses Society [11, 18]

37.1.8 Wound Assessment and Differential Diagnosis

Pressure injury is just one of the major wounds seen in the care of geriatric patients. It is important to recognize the major categories of acute and chronic wounds to create an accurate differential diagnosis. The most common of these wounds are related to pressure, nonhealing surgical, venous insufficiency, peripheral arterial disease, neuropathic or diabetic ulcers, and skin tears. Clues to wound etiology can be collected during a focused patient history and skin assessment. Once etiology is known and treatment has commenced, wound assessment skills remain important for monitoring wound progress, implementing, and managing the appropriate plan of care. See Table 37.3 below for clues to wound etiology and differential diagnosis.

37.1.9 Wound Assessment

There are several factors that place a patient at increased risk for pressure injuries. These risks can be quantified and addressed using a risk assessment tool which was covered in an earlier section of this chapter on risk assessment. A section of skin and soft tissue compressed between a mattress or wheelchair and the skeletal structure can suffer from ischemia due to compression of the blood supply, and buildup of

Table 37.3 Clues to wound etiology and differential diagnosis

	Pathological factors	Location	Manifestation
Pressure injury	Limited mobility Skin and soft tissue compression by medical devices	Bony prominences under medical device	Ischemic damage, color changes Round ulcer (may be irregular) Tunnels or undermining May progress to deep cavern or expose structures Surrounding tissue may be indurated warm or mottled
Venous ulcers	Compromised venous return Edema	Lower extremities	Shallow ulcers Moderate-to-large exudate Good pulses if no arterial disease Surrounding skin may exhibit hemosiderin staining or dermatitis Painful, typically partial relief with elevation
Arterial ulcers	Lower extremity arterial disease with severe tissue ischemia or necrosis	Lower legs, ankles, forefoot and toes	Typically, round with punched out appearance Pale or necrotic base Minimal exudate Pain with activity or elevation
Neuropathic/ diabetic ulcers	Nerve damage leads to sensory loss Repeated trauma results in deformities and ulcers	Plantar foot, metatarsal heads, areas in contact with foot gear	Possible tunnels or undermining May be necrotic Surrounding tissue may be calloused Pins and needles but frequently painless

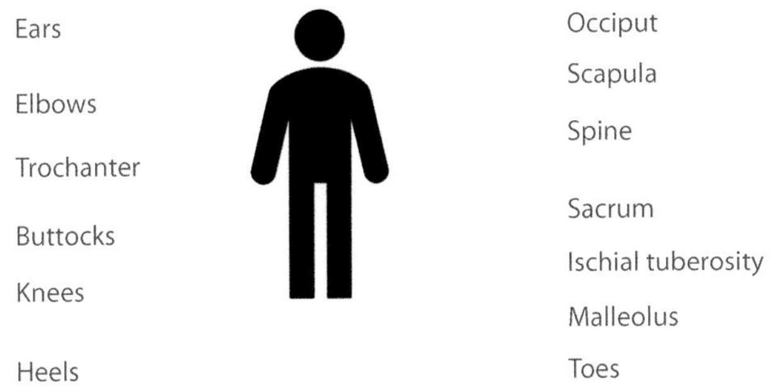
Ears
Elbows
Trochanter
Buttocks
Knees
Heels
Occiput
Scapula
Spine
Sacrum
Ischial tuberosity
Malleolus
Toes

Fig. 37.2 Common sites of pressure injury

waste products, or by deforming the soft tissue and disrupting the capillary beds. In either case, the result is cell death and tissue necrosis [3, 9]. See Fig. 37.2 for a schematic of the most common locations for pressure injuries.

37.1.9.1 Pressure Injury Staging

The National Pressure Ulcer Advisory Panel has developed definitions and illustrations to facilitate appropriate assessment, documentation, and treatment of pressure injuries. There are six pressure injury categories or stages. It is important to note that the staging system is not a continuum. Once the pressure injury stage has been identified, the injury cannot then be identified as a lower stage. For instance, a stage IV pressure injury does not become a stage III or II as it heals. The depth of tissue destruction remains the same even after it has been replaced by scar tissue.

37.1.9.2 Stage 1 Pressure Injury: Nonblanchable Erythema of Intact Skin

Intact skin with a localized area of nonblanchable erythema may appear differently in darkly pigmented skin. The presence of blanchable erythema or changes in sensation, temperature, or firmness may precede visual changes. Color changes do not include purple or maroon discoloration; these may indicate deep tissue pressure injury (Figs. 37.3 and 37.4).

37.1.9.3 Stage 2 Pressure Injury: Partial-Thickness Skin Loss with Exposed Dermis

Partial-thickness loss of skin with exposed dermis. The wound bed is viable, pink or red, and moist and may present as an intact or ruptured serum-filled blister. Adipose (fat) is not visible and deeper tissues are not visible. Granulation tissue, slough, and eschar are not present. These injuries commonly result from adverse microclimate and shear in the skin over the pelvis and shear in the heel. This stage should not be used to describe moisture-associated skin damage (MASD) including incontinence-associated dermatitis (IAD), intertriginous dermatitis (ITD), medical adhesive-related skin injury (MARSI), or traumatic wounds (skin tears, burns, abrasions) (Fig. 37.5).

37.1.9.4 Stage 3 Pressure Injury: Full-Thickness Skin Loss

Full-thickness loss of skin, in which adipose (fat) is visible in the ulcer and granulation tissue and epibole (rolled wound edges) are often present. Slough and/or eschar may be visible. The depth of tissue damage varies by anatomical location; areas of significant adiposity can develop deep wounds. Undermining and tunneling may occur. Fascia, muscle, tendon, ligament, cartilage, and/or bone are not exposed. If slough or eschar obscures the extent of tissue loss, this is an unstageable pressure injury (◘ Fig. 37.6).

37.1.9.5 Stage 4 Pressure Injury: Full-Thickness Skin and Tissue Loss

Full-thickness skin and tissue loss with exposed or directly palpable fascia, muscle, tendon, ligament, cartilage, or bone in the ulcer. Slough and/or eschar may be visible. Epibole (rolled edges), undermining, and/or tunneling often occur. Depth varies by anatomical location. If slough or eschar obscures the extent of tissue loss, this is an unstageable pressure injury (◘ Fig. 37.7).

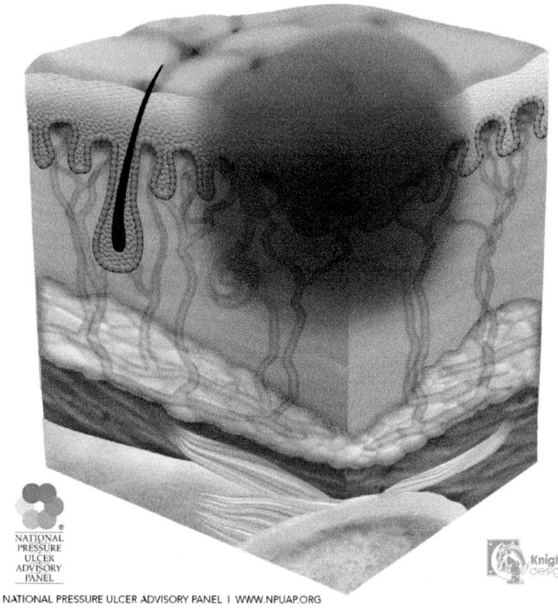

◘ **Fig. 37.3** Stage 1 pressure injury. (Reprinted with permission from National Pressure Ulcer Advisory Panel, European Pressure Ulcer Advisory Panel and Pan Pacific Pressure Injury Alliance [24])

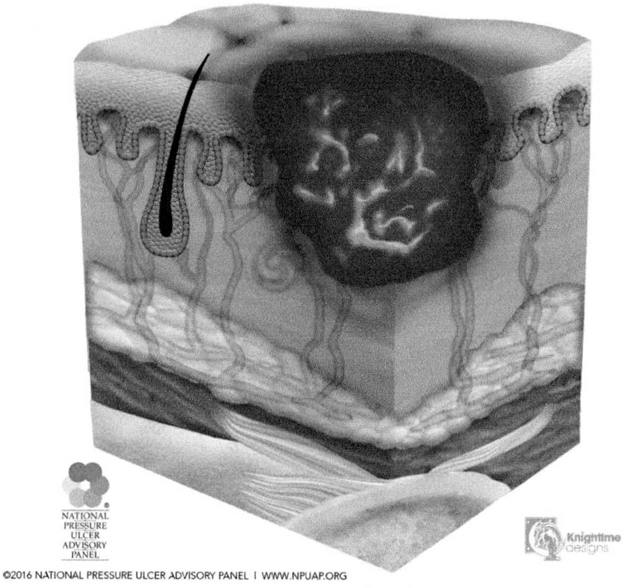

◘ **Fig. 37.5** Stage 2 pressure injury. (Reprinted with permission from National Pressure Ulcer Advisory Panel, European Pressure Ulcer Advisory Panel and Pan Pacific Pressure Injury Alliance [24])

◘ **Fig. 37.4** Blanchable vs. nonblanchable erythema. (Reprinted with permission from National Pressure Ulcer Advisory Panel, European Pressure Ulcer Advisory Panel and Pan Pacific Pressure Injury Alliance [24])

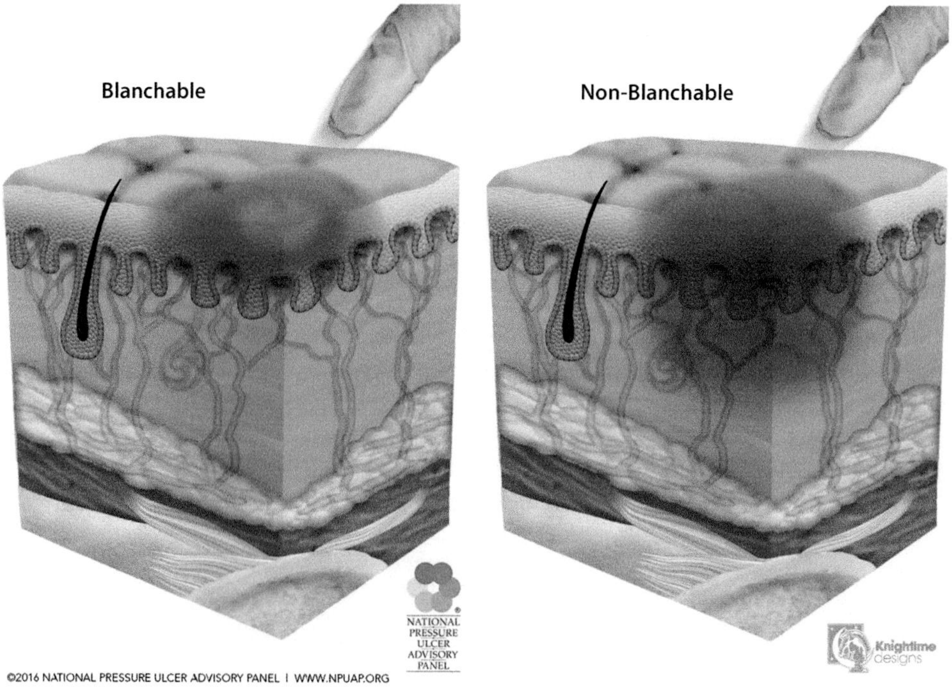

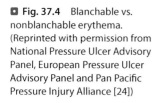

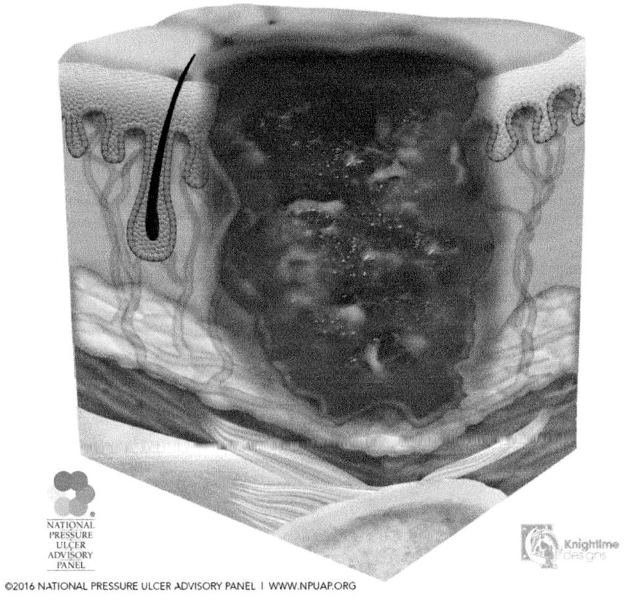

Fig. 37.6 Stage 3 pressure injury. (Reprinted with permission from National Pressure Ulcer Advisory Panel, European Pressure Ulcer Advisory Panel and Pan Pacific Pressure Injury Alliance [24])

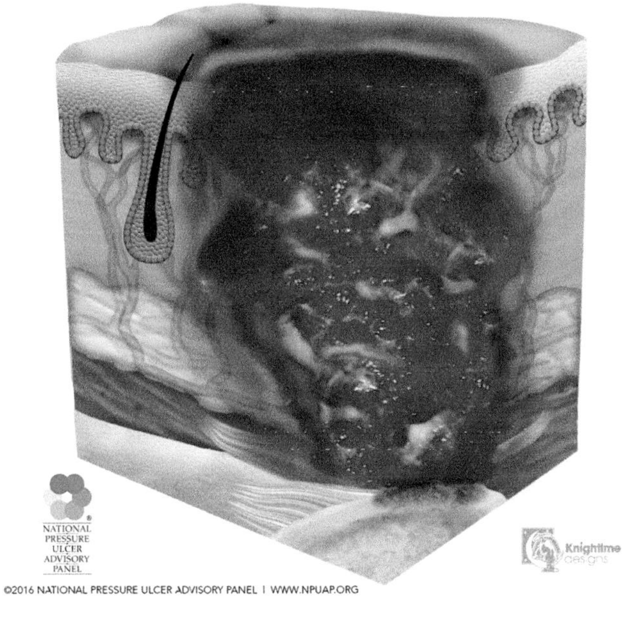

Fig. 37.7 Stage 4 pressure injury. (Reprinted with permission from National Pressure Ulcer Advisory Panel, European Pressure Ulcer Advisory Panel and Pan Pacific Pressure Injury Alliance [24])

37.1.10 Unstageable Pressure Injury: Obscured Full-Thickness Skin and Tissue Loss

Full-thickness skin and tissue loss in which the extent of tissue damage within the ulcer cannot be confirmed because it is obscured by slough or eschar. If slough or eschar is removed, a stage 3 or stage 4 pressure injury will be revealed. Stable eschar (i.e., dry, adherent, intact without erythema or fluctuance) on the heel or ischemic limb should not be softened or removed (Figs. 37.8 and 37.9).

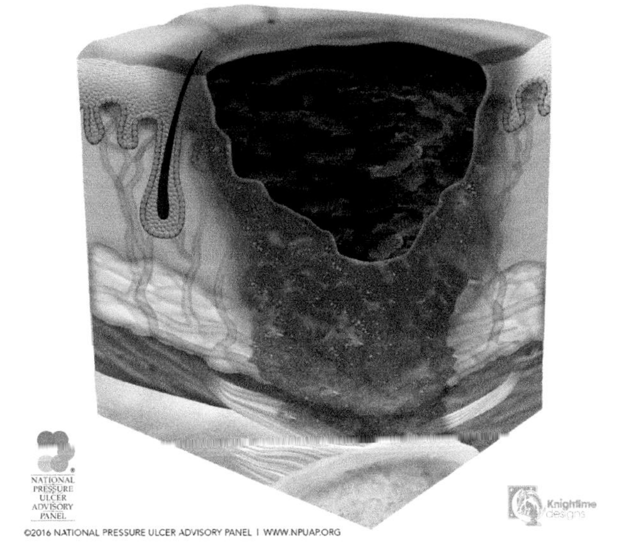

Fig. 37.8 Unstageable – dark-eschar. (Reprinted with permission from National Pressure Ulcer Advisory Panel, European Pressure Ulcer Advisory Panel and Pan Pacific Pressure Injury Alliance [24])

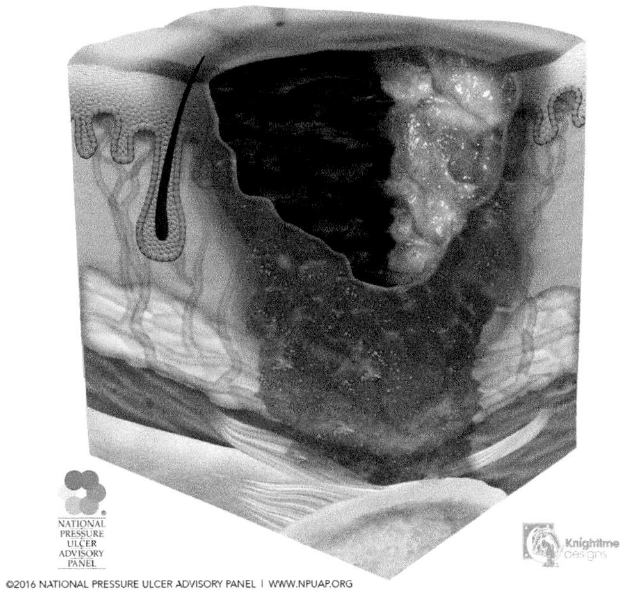

Fig. 37.9 Unstageable slough and eschar. (Reprinted with permission from National Pressure Ulcer Advisory Panel, European Pressure Ulcer Advisory Panel and Pan Pacific Pressure Injury Alliance [24])

37.1.11 Deep Tissue Pressure Injury: Persistent Nonblanchable Deep-Red, Maroon, or Purple Discoloration

Intact or nonintact skin with localized area of persistent nonblanchable deep-red, maroon, or purple discoloration or epidermal separation revealing a dark wound bed or blood-filled blister. Pain and temperature changes often precede skin

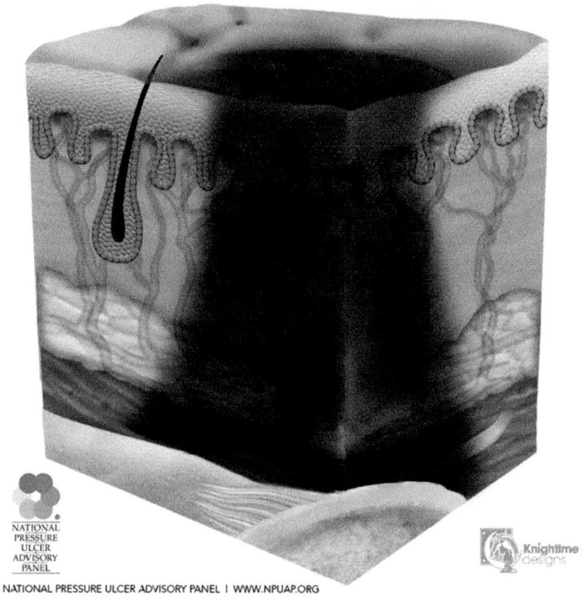

Fig. 37.10 Deep tissue pressure injury. (Reprinted with permission from National Pressure Ulcer Advisory Panel, European Pressure Ulcer Advisory Panel and Pan Pacific Pressure Injury Alliance [24])

color changes. Discoloration may appear differently in darkly pigmented skin. This injury results from intense and/or prolonged pressure and shear forces at the bone–muscle interface. The wound may evolve rapidly to reveal the actual extent of tissue injury or may resolve without tissue loss. If necrotic tissue, subcutaneous tissue, granulation tissue, fascia, muscle, or other underlying structures are visible, this indicates a full-thickness pressure injury (unstageable, stage 3 or stage 4). Do not use DTPI to describe vascular, traumatic, neuropathic, or dermatologic conditions (Fig. 37.10).

37.1.12 Medical Device-Related Pressure Injury

This describes an etiology of a wound: Medical device related pressure injuries result from the use of devices designed and applied for diagnostic or therapeutic purposes. The resultant pressure injury generally conforms to the pattern or shape of the device. The injury should be staged using the staging system. [3]

Once the stage has been established, an accurate description of the wound bed and periwound tissue should be documented. A dedicated pressure injury chart allows for serial assessments and tracking of progress and outcomes. Any assessment should begin with an accurate anatomic location and include exudate, tunneling or undermining, margin attachment, presence of necrotic tissue, pain, and an update of status since last assessment [10]. Most practices use centimeters to measure wounds. A length, width, and depth are included with an assessment but might also include the length of tunnels or undermined regions. See Table 37.4 below for a list of common terms used to describe wound characteristics.

Table 37.4 Pressure injury descriptive characteristics

Characteristic	Definition
Tunnel	A narrow void beginning in one open wound and leading to another opening
Tract	A narrow void originating in the wound bed and leading beneath the intact tissue in the periphery of a wound
Undermined	A cavernous void wider than a tract or tunnel located beneath intact tissue in the periphery of a wound bed. Wound margin will be unattached or rolled in this area
Margins: rolled, attached, or unattached	Rolled or chronic appearing edges have formed an epibole – the epithelium has grown over the edge of the wound and reconnected beneath the wound edge. No further epithelialization will take place Attached margins remain connected to the sides of the wound bed Unattached margins are unsupported and may lie over un-undermined area or tunnel
Exudate	Color: serous, serosanguineous, sanguineous, green, or brown Amount: scant, moderate, large, copious Consistency: clear, purulent, clots Odor: present or not present
Maceration	Overhydrated tissue surrounding a wound bed indicative of high amounts of exudate
Necrotic tissue	Dead, devitalized, avascular tissue may be yellow, gray, brown, or black in color
Slough	Yellow stingy nonviable tissue
Granulation	Moist beefy red viable connective tissue
Status	Improved, unchanged, healing, deteriorating

Adapted from Wound, Ostomy and Continence Nurses Society [11]

37.2 Wound Management

37.2.1 Goals for Wound Management

Topical wound therapy is much more than deciding on a dressing. Individualized care is tantamount to healing. The healthcare provider must consider the overall goal of care before deciding on a course of action for wound management. Usually, the main goal is healing but this is not always the case. Questions that must be raised with the patient and family include whether aggressive wound management is a viable option with an eventual plan of healing or whether a more conservative or palliative approach would be best as in the case of wound chronicity, significant comorbidities, or terminal illness. Is the goal to heal or to provide comfort and symptom control [12]? To establish patient-centered goals, the first action of the healthcare provider is assessment of the patient's goals of care.

37.2.2 Basics of Wound Management

Management of pressure injuries is complex, and many strategies are employed over time. A treatment plan includes (1) management of pressure, friction, and shear, (2) control of comorbidities, (3) pain control, (4) nutrition, and (5) topical wound management. Prevention strategies, as previously discussed, are ongoing to prevent further damage and injury.

A significant area of concern in patients with pressure injuries is incontinence. Uncontrolled urinary and fecal incontinence can cause further breakdown of damaged skin due to maceration. Changes in skin pH and normal skin flora lead to increased alkalinity, triggering the release of cytokines and inducing an inflammatory response [13]. This further causes the skin to be more open to other irritants, such as bacteria. A bladder/bowel program is recommended [11]. Meticulous skin care should be performed after each episode of incontinence with a pH-balanced cleanser with the use of a skin barrier cream. In addition, any incontinence products used should wick the urine and effluent away from the skin.

Another concern in the management of pressure injury is nutrition. Best practices recommend that the clinician assess for adequacy of fluids, calorie, and protein intake: 30–35 Kcals per kg of body weight and 1.25–1.5 g of protein per kg. A significant weight loss, 5% in 30 days, would require additional supplementation though the evidence for this increase is lacking [11]. Kaminski and Drinane (2014) recommend that patients with pressure injuries be monitored for oral and cutaneous signs of micronutrient deficiencies and recommend twice per day doses of vitamin C 500 mg, vitamin D_3 2000 IU, zinc sulfate 220 mg, fish oil 1 g, vitamin B_3 250 mg, glucosmine/chondroitin 600/400 mg, as well as a multivitamin [14].

Pain is a common sequela in individuals with wounds. Untreated pain leads to high stress levels in many wound patients and is believed to increase the inflammatory response by the release of proinflammatory cytokines, thus slowing wound healing. Woo (2012) suggests a multidimensional approach to pain management including a therapeutic alliance with the patient focusing on communication and education [15]. Topics to be addressed should be the commonality of wound pain, the mechanism of pain, and fear of addiction. He also advocates the use of topical medications at the site as well as systemically. Woo recommends using atraumatic type dressings, such as silicone, and using periwound skin protectants. The use of relaxation, imagery, and other psychological methods to control pain is also recommended [15].

37.2.3 Evidence-Based Wound Care

Evidence-based wound care, based on the work of Sackett in 2000, involves using the best available evidence, clinical expertise, and patient preferences [16]. There is a high level of evidence that moist wound healing is best practice; wounds heal better and faster in a moist environment. Moist wound healing is not a new concept. A moist wound environment allows for the cell migration across the wound bed and ultimately the deposit of new tissue for partial and full-thickness wounds. Now there is the opportunity to maintain a moisture balance using innovative wound care dressings needing less time and effort for dressing changes, such as the moisture-retentive dressings that control exudate and prevent desiccation of the wound bed. This is great news, so what is the hold up for wounds healing in a timely manner? We see this lack of healing every day in practice.

In order for a wound to heal, the wound bed must be in optimal condition. Acute wounds generally do not have any problems with healing, for example, a surgical wound progresses through the phases of the wound healing cascade and is epithelialized within the expected time frame of 25 days or less as discussed previously. However, a nonhealing or chronic wound fails to progress due to intrinsic or extrinsic circumstances. The wound bed is not in a condition conducive to wound healing. In this case, best practice recommends returning the wound to an acute state. Now, clinicians should use a systematic approach to wound bed preparation. One such approach is TIME: tissue, inflammation/infection, moisture balance, and epithelial edge advancement [17].

When the tissue in the wound bed is deficient due to defective tissue and adherent debris, debridement or the removal of nonviable necrotic tissue is required. Debridement can be accomplished by various methods including autolytic, mechanical, chemical/enzymatic and surgical (or sharp), larval, hydrosurgery, and ultrasound therapy. Surgical debridement is considered the "gold standard," but research does not show that one form of debridement is better than another. Patient factors, environmental factors, and clinician competence dictate which method is most efficacious to accomplish the goal of a clean wound bed. Debridement is also used to remove biofilm (bacteria embedded in the extracellular matrix of the wound bed). Oftentimes, biofilms cannot be observed and require a wound biopsy to discover and treat.

It is well known that the inflammatory process initiates wound healing. When there is dysregulation of the cellular and molecular components (inflammatory cells, cytokines, growth factors, and elevated levels of proteases), chronic wounds remain in a persistent state of inflammation. This prevents new tissue and blood vessels from forming. Persistent and recurrent infections can occur. In 60–90% of chronic wounds, biofilms develop, preventing the host's natural defenses to act [18]. Several indicators of biofilm require investigation: prolonged infection despite antibiotic treatment, friable granulation tissue in the wound bed (looks funny), and a yellow/white gelatinous material that is easily removed and reforms quickly. Cleansing and debriding are the treatment of choice for biofilm removal.

Wound infections occur across a continuum from contamination to systemic infection. In colonization, microorganisms are present, but are not invasive to the point of an overt infection [19]. Healing is not generally delayed. Likewise, in colonization, the host is not harmed, though there is bacterial growth occurring. Local infection exhibits the signs and symptoms of infection, e.g., friable tissue, wound breakdown and increased size, pain, malodor, erythema, warmth, swelling at the site, or purulent discharge. Note that these signs and symptoms may be subtle or overt.

When wounds infection is spreading, systemic symptoms begin: extending induration and redness, swelling of the lymphatic glands, increasing wound breakdown, malaise, and poor appetite. When left untreated or antibiotics fail, the infection can become systemic. Unfortunately, diagnostic tests for the types and virulence of microbes present can delay proper treatment. Current thoughts on treatment rely on optimizing the host response, reducing the number of microorganisms, and improving the wound environment (TIME). It is recommended that the debridement of biofilm and therapeutic cleansing occur along with topical antibiotics to prevent further biofilm growth [20, 21]. Systemic antibiotics should be carefully chosen to prevent antibiotic resistance.

When acute wounds persist, moisture balance becomes an issue. An inadequate amount of wound fluid leads to cell death and eschar formation. Excess exudate can lead to protein deficiencies, wound edge and periwound skin maceration, and delayed wound healing. There are also increased levels of pro-inflammatory cytokines and proteases that negatively affect the wound bed. It is important to assess the amount and consistency of exudate to identify appropriate treatment modalities, such as antibiotics, topical antiseptics, or specialized wound dressings. Negative pressure wound therapy (NPWT) and absorbent dressings placed directly in the wound bed are frequently used to manage excessive wound exudate [18]. Dressings that do not allow excess fluid on the periwound skin are preferred, and barrier cream should be considered.

Lastly, the wound edge is assessed. In order to heal, the wound edge needs to be in contact with the base of the wound. Wound edge problems that interfere with wound healing include maceration, dehydration, and undermining. When there is significant undermining, migration and epithelialization cannot take place and cause the wound to "stall." Reducing dead space, debriding epibole (rolled edges), and managing exudate improve the condition of wound edges. If current wound treatment is effective, a 20–40% reduction in wound size should occur in the first 2–4 weeks.

37.2.4 Topical Therapy

Providing topical wound treat is a systematic process that begins with assessment. Debridement, cleansing, topical products, and systemic management are the major component included in the process. Research evidence for wound treatment recommendations is available, but the level of evidence is not strong in most cases. There is much work to do! See Table 37.5 below for current wound treatment recommendations.

37

Table 37.5 Current wound care treatment recommendations

Mechanism of action	Guideline recommendations
Debridement – level of evidence = C limited research on debridement mechanisms **Autolytic** – mechanism of action. Collection of phagocytic cells and proteolytic enzymes using a semi-occlusive or occlusive dressing to remove necrotic tissue; enhanced by moist wound healing; slow method; decreased discomfort **Enzymatic** – mechanism of action. Topical collagenase stimulates the breakdown of necrotic tissue; painless. Reduces wound trauma **Mechanical** – removal of nonspecific tissue by physical force; hydrotherapy, irrigation, wet-to-dry dressings; painful; trauma may cause bleeding; time consuming; causes skin maceration **Surgical/sharp** – removal of necrotic tissue using scalpels, scissors, curettes, laser; requires adequate perfusion; fast, tissue selective. May increase the size of wound **Other** – sterile maggots digest devitalized tissue; hydrosurgery, ultrasound	Contraindicated in infected wounds. Frequent dressing changes are needed Apply collagenase directly to wound bed every day; does not harm periwound skin Dry eschar must be cross-hatched Contraindicated in wounds with exposed blood vessels Surgical debridement for extensive necrotic areas to remove tunneling and undermining Performed by physician specialist Conservative sharps debridement removes nonviable tissue only, using sterile instruments; performed by trained wound care specialists; avoid sharps debridement in patients who have bleeding problems or are immunocompromised Maggot treatment may reduce bacterial burden Do not use with hemorrhaging, exposed blood vessels, inadequate perfusion, wounds with sinus tracts or deep cavities, or infections Low-frequency ultrasound assists with removal of purulent drainage and soft tissue debridement; fluid sprays large area outside of wound
Cleansing	**Cleansing solutions** Cleanse the wound at each dressing change using pH balanced skin Cleanser vs. saline. (level of evidence = C) Cleansing with water does not increase infection rate (level of evidence = B) Avoid use of cleansing solutions meant for intact skin as may be cytotoxic to the wound bed Heavy exudative wounds or with debris may benefit from a cleanser with surfactant Cleansing techniques Use of technique dependent on wound condition and may be irrigation, pressurized irrigation (pulsed lavage); gentle swabbing, showering, bathing The recommended pressure for cleansing is between 4 and 15 psi. A 35 ml syringe with a 35-gauge needle or angiocath creates a stream of 8 psi Prevent environmental contamination when using a lavage technique

Table 37.5 (continued)

Mechanism of action	Guideline recommendations
Topical products Dressing selection is based on wound parameters, e.g., exudate. Size, tissue type, location, condition of the periwound, goals for healing, pain reduction and odor control, cost, availability, and ease of use Change dressing type as needed over time and change in condition. Monitor wound at each dressing change. (level of evidence = C) Consider changing dressing type if exudate strike-through is noted between dressing changes	**Protective barrier cream** Protect periwound skin from maceration. Transparent film air exchange through dressing. Use on minimal exudative wound **Foam** Decreased number of dressing changes Decreased cost compared with gauze **Hydrocolloid** Use for stage 2 or 3 injuries with minimal depth, which are not infected **Hydrogel** Used to maintain a moist wound environment. Available in liquid gel or gel pad form **Alginate** Increased absorbency, fewer dressing changes
	Hydrofiber Increased absorbency, fewer dressing changes **Antimicrobial** Limit the use of topical antibiotics due to resistance and hypersensitivity **Silver** Three studies found a greater decrease in wound size, bioburden, and odor Decreased number of dressing changes May stain periwound **Honey** Used in heavily exudating wounds. Three studies revealed a greater heal rate than control **Specialty products** Growth factors (level of evidence = B). Requires daily topical application **Biophysical agents** Electrical stimulation (level of evidence = A) Electromagnetic and phototherapy therapy is available but data is insufficient to make recommendation Low-level laser and ultraviolet light therapy, studies do not support use Ultrasound-limited evidence **Negative pressure wound therapy** Use of subatmospheric pressure via an electronic pump to draw fluid from wound (level of evidence = B) **Hyperbaric oxygen therapy** – no evidence supporting use in PU **Surgical intervention** Myocutaneous flaps are surgery of choice due to blood supply Optimize nutrition Keep area offloaded on a pressure redistribution surface after surgery After incision healed, begin a progressive sitting program High rate of reoccurrence (up to 85%) with increased mortality rates. (eight studies reported) Osteomyelitis is the main cause for flap failure
Systemic management of infection	Ischemic tissues in PU have higher rates of infection Associated with biofilms; PU associated with mortality are likely to have an infected PU, previous stay in an intensive care unit; mechanical ventilation; previous use of antibiotics PU has up to 75% of bacterial colonization with *Staphylococcus aureus* and/ or gram-negative bacillus. Greater than 50% are multidrug-resistant carriers, thus, high risk for bacteremia May not exhibit the classic signs and symptoms of infection Wound cultures – biopsy is the gold standard. The Levine method of swabbing is acceptable if biopsy is contraindicated Bioburden is defined as equal or greater than 10^5 microorganisms cu/cm^2

Adapted from Wound, Ostomy and Continence Nurses Society [11]

It takes a team to effectively care for individuals with pressure injuries [22, 23]. In a unidisciplinary team, the physician, nurse practitioner, or physician assistant provider works with the patient and family to establish a plan of care. In a hospital or a tertiary wound center, many disciplines involved in the care of persons with complex wounds are available. Physicians, nurse practitioners, physician assistants, wound specialists, registered dieticians, physical and occupational therapists, pharmacists, and nurses are all part of the interprofessional team. The team should practice collaboratively and develop the plan of care together with the patient and family, as communication and collaboration are key in the care of complicated wounds to ensure positive outcomes. It is imperative to know the resources available for patients, identify any barriers to comprehensive care, and include this in the plan of care as soon as possible. Utilizing a team approach in wound care may improve outcomes and reduce costs.

Community-dwelling patients depend on their physicians or other primary care providers, for treatment of their skin conditions, including pressure injuries. Small or rural hospitals are often have limited specialty services. Likewise, long-term care nursing facilities are sites where many pressure injuries are treated and managed, but unless this very frail and vulnerable patient is able to leave the nursing facility to attend a nearby wound care clinic, the patients' primary care provider in the nursing facility is the patient's only resource for evaluation and management of this and every problem. Therefore, medical professionals practicing in such settings should be prepared to include wound care evaluation and management skills in their practice.

Primary care providers may be adequate in some settings when there are few comorbidities and the wound is uncomplicated. However, the solo healthcare provider may not have the knowledge of pressure injury prevention or wound management, or the tools at hand to provide comprehensive care for complex pressure injuries and often refers to others, such as a home health agency employing a nurse wound specialist, or to a wound care center. Medical professionals should be familiar with the resources available to patients in their community and work collaboratively with specialists in wound care when needed.

References

1. Wound, Ostomy and Continence Nurses Society-Wound Guidelines Task Force. WOCN 2016 guideline for prevention and management of pressure injuries (ulcers): an executive summary. J Wound Ostomy Cont Nurs. 2017;44(3):241.
2. Berlowitz D, Van Deusen Lukas C, Parker V, Niederhauser A, Silver JLC., Ayello E, et al. Preventing pressure ulcers in hospitals: a toolkit for improving care. 2011.
3. Panel NPUA. Prevention and treatment of pressure ulcers: clinical practice guideline. 2014.
4. Bauer K, Rock K, Nazzal M, Jones O, Qu W. Pressure ulcers in the united states' inpatient population from 2008 to 2012: results of a retrospective nationwide study. Ostomy Wound Manage. 2016; 62(11):30–8.
5. AHRQ. Are we ready for this change. October 2014; Available at: https://www.ahrq.gov/professionals/systems/hospital/pressureulcertoolkit/putool1.html.
6. Pieper B. Pressure ulcers: impact, etiology and classification. In: Bryant R, Nix D, editors. Acute & chronic wounds: current management concepts. 4th ed. Elsevier/Mosby: St. Louis; 2012.
7. Macklebust J, Magnan M. Pressure ulcer prevention. In: Doughty D, McNichol L, editors. Wound, ostomy continence nurses society core curriculum: wound management. Philadelphia: Wolters Kluwer; 2012. p. 333–61.
8. Bates-Jensen B. Assessment of the patient with a wound. In: Doughty D, McNichol L, editors. Core curriculum wound management. 1st ed. Philadelphia: Wound Ostomy and Continence Nurses Society; 2016. p. 38–68.
9. Bly D. A model of pressure, oxygenation, and perfusion risk factors for pressure ulcers in the intensive care unit. Am J Crit Care. 2016;25(2):156–64.
10. Baranoski S, Ayello E, Langemo D. Wound assessment. In: Baranoski S, Ayello E, editors. Wound care essentials. 3rd ed. Philadelphia: Lippincott Williams and Wilkins; 2012. p. 101–25.
11. Wound, Ostomy and Continence Nurses Society. Guideline for prevention and management of pressure ulcers (injuries): WOCN clinical practice guideline series 2. Mt. Laurel: Author; 2016.
12. Hotaling P, Black J. Ten top tips: end of life pressure injuries. Wounds Int. 2018;9(1):18–21.
13. Bryant R, Nix D, editors. Acute and chronic wounds; current management concepts. 4th ed. Saint Louis: Elsevier Mosby; 2012.
14. Kaminski Mitchell V Jr, Drinane JJ. Learning the oral and cutaneous signs of micronutrient deficiencies. J Wound Ostomy Continence Nurs. 2014;41(2):127.
15. Woo KY. Exploring the effects of pain and stress on wound healing. Adv Skin Wound Care. 2012;25(1):38–44.
16. Sackett DL, Straus SE, Richardson WS, Rosenberg W, Haynes RB. Evidence-based medicine: how to practice and teach EBM. 2nd ed. Edinburgh: Churchill Livingstone; 2000.
17. Harries RL, Bosanquet DC, Harding KG. Wound bed preparation: TIME for an update. Int Wound J. 2016;09(13 Suppl 3):8–14.
18. Dowsett C, von Hallern B. The Triangle of Wound Assessment: a holistic framework from wound assessment to management goals and treatments. Wounds Int. 2017;8(4):34–9.
19. Swanson T, Haesler E, Angel D, Sussman G. IWII Wound infection in clinical practice consensus document 2016 update. Wound Pract Res. 2016;24(4):194–8.
20. Wolcott RD, Rhoads DD. A study of biofilm-based wound management in subjects with critical limb ischaemia. J Wound Care. 2008;17(4):145.
21. Wolcott RD, Rhoads DD, Bennett ME, Wolcott BM, Gogokhia L, Costerton JW, et al. Chronic wounds and the medical biofilm paradigm. J Wound Care. 2010;19(2):45.
22. Moore ZEH, Webster J, Samuriwo R. Wound-care teams for preventing and treating pressure ulcers. Cochrane Database Syst Rev. 2015;(9):CD011011.
23. Scarborough P. Understanding your wound care team: defining unidisciplinary, multidisciplinary, and transdisciplinary team models. 2018.
24. National Pressure Ulcer Advisory Panel, European Pressure Ulcer Advisory Panel and Pan Pacific Pressure Injury Alliance. In: Haesler E, editor. Prevention and treatment of pressure ulcers: quick reference guide. Osborne Park: Cambridge Media; 2014.

Transitions of Care, Population Health

Contents

Discharge Planning

Ogechi N. Dike and Grace Farris

A. Chun (ed.), *Geriatric Practice*, https://doi.org/10.1007/978-3-030-19625-7_38

38.1 Introduction: Assessment of Patient's Appropriateness for Discharge

Case

An 81-year-old woman with a past medical history of hypertension is hospitalized for five days with pneumonia complicated by a new diagnosis of atrial fibrillation. While she had resided in an assisted-living facility prior to admission, she reports that she feels much weaker after spending four days on telemetry, mostly in bed. As the team prepares for discharge, what do they need to consider? What is the patient's functional status? What kind of monitoring will she need? Will she be discharged on new medications?

"Discharge planning" describes the process in which a hospitalized patient's care team creates a unique "discharge plan" that details why a patient was hospitalized, what the next steps in the treatment and diagnosis are, and what the patient's discharge destination will be. This chapter will explore the details of the discharge planning process.

The first step in the discharge planning process entails determining whether a patient is suitable for discharge from the acute care setting. This includes identifying whether all inpatient diagnostic work-ups are complete, whether the patient is stable for discharge clinically, and whether an appropriate post-discharge location has been established. If the clinical team determines that all inpatient testing and treatments have been completed and that the remainder of the patient's care plan can be conducted in the outpatient setting, then the team should engage with physical therapy, social work, and case management to identify the most appropriate post-discharge setting for the patient. For example, in the case described above, the patient reports a functional decline. This should be evaluated by physical therapy to determine if she can safely go home or if she will need additional supports either at home or at a skilled nursing facility (SNF).

38.2 Determination of the Appropriate Post-discharge Setting

There are five major types of post-acute care discharge settings: home, home with services, skilled nursing facilities (SNFs), inpatient rehabilitation, and long-term acute care hospitals (LTACH). A discharge to "home" implies that a patient will be going back to where they lived prior to the hospitalization, which might be a house, apartment, assisted living, nursing home, homeless shelter, or "the street" (if a patient is homeless with no regular shelter use). The determination of whether a patient should return "home" is often made in conjunction with an inpatient physical therapy evaluation and consideration of a patient's cognitive function. A physical therapist will individualize the evaluation to a patient's home circumstances, including assessing whether a patient can climb as many stairs as they may have at home and whether the patient has adaptive equipment (e.g., commode, shower seat, etc.) at home to maximize safety and comfort post-discharge. The clinician should determine if a patient's cognitive functioning on discharge would permit them to live independently or if they will require additional support (in terms of medication administration, support for activities of daily living (ADLs)) [10].

If the physical therapist determines that a patient would benefit from additional physical therapy in order to return home safely, the therapist may recommend "home with physical therapy" which is one of the home services included with "discharge home with services." Besides home physical therapy, other patient needs that might require a discharge "home with services" include home infusion needs (e.g., if a patient requires additional days of parenteral antibiotics), nursing needs (a home visiting nurse might be needed to conduct a "home safety evaluation" in which they identify fall risks and safety issues in the home), and visiting social work or palliative care needs.

If the inpatient physical therapy evaluation reveals significant deconditioning and weakness that will prevent a patient from immediately returning home, the physical therapist may recommend discharge to skilled nursing facility (SNF). A skilled nursing facility is what in the United States frequently considered a "nursing home"; except in the post-discharge setting, patients typically are discharged to SNFs for a short course of rehabilitation (usually less than 25 days) [4]. At a SNF, a patient will typically receive 1 hour of physical rehabilitation daily, and other types of care including nursing administration of infusion needs, speech therapy, social work, and palliative services are also available.

Certain patients, particularly those with long critical care stays, may require more extended courses of medical treatment and care. In these cases, long-term acute care hospitals (LTACH) and inpatient rehabilitation may be more appropriate. These settings are equipped to manage complex chronically ill patients, including patients with ventilators, wound vacs, and intravenous medication drip needs (such as furosemide or heparin) as well as patients who will require intensive rehabilitation (e.g., patients who have suffered acute strokes) in the form of physical therapy, speech therapy, and occupational therapy. Clinicians should work with their hospital-based physical therapists and case managers to determine if a patient will require LTACH or inpatient rehabilitation.

38.3 Post-discharge Needs and Medications

As a patient nears discharge, the clinical team should consider whether a patient will require any "durable medical equipment" (e.g., commodes, shower chairs, a wheelchair) on discharge. This decision should be made after discussion with the physical therapist who evaluated the patient. Any recommended "DME" can be ordered via a prescription, but certain larger items (e.g., a hospital bed) may need to be ordered prior to discharge.

Some patients may require ongoing nutrition and IV antibiotics on discharge. When caring for patients who are receiving enteral nutrition ("tube feeds"), parenteral nutrition ("TPN"), or IV antibiotics, it is important to ask who, what, where, and how long the patient will require these products.

When a patient needs tube feeds/TPN/IV antibiotics on discharge, ask:

- **Who?** Who will administer this? A home nurse? A family member? Who will monitor the tests that the patient needs?
- **What?** What product does the patient need? Has the dose stabilized, or will it require monitoring? What type of monitoring will the patient need (i.e., electrolytes or vancomycin levels, kidney function)?
- **Where?** Where should the patient receive these products? At home or in a post-acute care site? The patient's insurance type may affect their ability to receive these products at home.
- **How?** How often will the patient need to have these products administered? How will the patient receive these products? Does the patient have a midline or peripherally inserted central catheter (PICC) in place? Does the patient have a feeding tube? How long will the patient require antibiotics or nutrition support?

Some patients will require home oxygen, although recent studies suggest that home oxygen is less effective than previously thought. If a provider anticipates that a patient will go home with oxygen, it will be important to notify social work and case management so that they can assist with contacting an oxygen delivery company prior to discharge. Typically, a prescription will also be required for home oxygen.

Medication reconciliation is also a vital part of the discharge planning process. Many institutions require medication reconciliation on admission, and on discharge, a process will need to take place to establish which medications are being *started*, which home medications that the patient may have previously taken should be *stopped*, and which home medications should be *continued* or *changed*.

Some medications are high risk and require additional preparation on discharge. For example, anticoagulation medications require planning including whether a patient will need serial INR checks and where this might take place and whether newer oral anticoagulants require a prior authorization in order for a patient to fill them. In the case described at the beginning of this section, the patient has been given a new diagnosis of atrial fibrillation and will likely require anticoagulation on discharge. If she is starting an oral anticoagulant, the team will need to confirm that the patient can fill this on discharge. If she starts warfarin, the team will need to clarify with the patient's primary care doctor where the patient's INR (warfarin monitoring) will be conducted and who will advise her on dosing adjustments.

If a patient has a new diagnosis of diabetes, or is starting insulin for the first time, insulin teaching will be required prior to discharge. Typically, the patient's bedside nurse can conduct insulin teaching with a patient in the days leading up to discharge. With the recent rising costs of insulin, it is extremely important that the clinician confer with social work to determine which insulin regimen a patient's insurance coverage will include.

38.4 Post-discharge Follow-Up After Hospitalization

Close outpatient follow-up with a patient's primary care provider or subspecialist (if the hospitalization was related to the respective comorbidity) is regarded as a crucial aspect of discharge planning. Despite its perceived importance, the ideal interval between hospital discharge and primary care or subspecialty follow-up is unknown. However, there are recommended time intervals for post-discharge follow-up appointments for patients with certain diagnosis. The recommended follow-up for patients admitted to the hospital with an acute congestive heart failure exacerbation is 7–14 days from discharge [12, 17]. For patients admitted to the hospital with an acute COPD exacerbation, the 2017 GOLD guidelines recommend post-discharge follow-up within 1 month of discharge [3]. For medical patients admitted with other diagnoses, the literature suggests that the highest risk patients should receive follow-up within 7 days of discharge [9].

There are clinical and nonclinical patient factors that help providers determine patients at high risk for readmission and who would therefore benefit from early follow-up. Clinical factors that make a patient high risk for readmission are the use of high-risk medications (antibiotics, steroids, anticoagulants, narcotics, antiepileptic medications, antipsychotics, antidepressants, and hypoglycemic agents), polypharmacy, having more than six chronic conditions, and having a diagnosis of either advanced chronic obstructive pulmonary disease, congestive heart failure, stroke, cancer weight loss, depression, or sepsis. Nonclinical factors that increase a patient's risk for readmission to the hospital include prior hospitalization with prolonged length of stay, insurance status (uninsured patients and patients with unsupplemented Medicare and Medicaid), black race, low health literacy, lower socioeconomic status, and discharge against medical advice [2, 5]. Therefore, if a patient has any of these factors, follow-up within 7 days of discharge should be strongly considered (Table 38.1).

38.4.1 Patient Instructions

At discharge, the patient should be provided with verbal and written instructions that help guide them in their transition from the hospital. The average US resident reads at or below an eighth grade reading level, and the average Medicare beneficiary reads at a fifth grade level. Most patient education materials however are written at high school and college reading levels, well above the literacy level of most Americans. To maximize comprehension, a patient's discharge instructions

Table 38.1 Factors that make a patient high risk for readmission to the hospital

Clinical factors	Nonclinical factors

High-risk medications
  Antibiotics
  Steroids
  Anticoagulants
  Narcotics
  Antiepileptic medications
  Antipsychotics
  Antidepressants
  Hypoglycemic agents
Having six or more chronic conditions
Having one of the following diagnoses:
  Advanced chronic obstructive pulmonary disease
  Congestive heart failure
  Stroke
  Cancer weight loss
  Depression
  Sepsis
	Prior hospitalization with prolonged length of stay
	Insurance status
	  Uninsured patients
	  Patients with unsupplemented Medicare and Medicaid
	Black race
	Low health literacy
	Lower socioeconomic status
	Discharge against medical advice

Table adapted from information from Refs. [2, 5]

should be targeted to an eighth grade level at the minimum but should strive for a target reading level of fifth grade which is the recommended level of literacy for patient education materials [1, 15]. There are several tools available which can be used to assess the readability of a document and include the Flesch Reading Ease Scale, Flesch-Kincaid Grade Level, Gunning-Fog Score, Coleman-Liau Index, and Automated Readability Index (ARI). The Flesch Reading Ease Scale and Flesch-Kincaid Grade Level are familiar to most providers as they are the tools used by Microsoft Word to check the readability of documents.

The Flesch Reading Ease Formula uses the sentence length (number of words per sentence) and the number of syllables per word in an equation to calculate the reading ease.[1] The score ranges from 0 to 100. The higher the number, the easier the text is to read. Scores between 90 and 100 are considered easily understandable by an average fifth grader, scores between 60 and 70 are considered easily understood by eighth and ninth graders, and scores between 0 and 30 are considered easily understood by college graduates. The Flesch-Kincaid Reading Grade Level Formula also uses sentence length and syllables per word.[2] The result is a number that corresponds with a US grade level (e.g., a score of 9.3 means that a ninth grader would be able to read the document).

When writing discharge instructions, it is important to keep in mind that the instructions should be written in clear and plain language. The use of jargon, technical, or scientific language should be limited. If the use of jargon or technical terms is necessary, they should be defined first and then explained in language that the patient will understand (e.g., say high blood pressure not hypertension) [13]. Other tips to increase the readability of a patient's discharge instructions include writing in the active vs passive voice, short sentence length (<15 words), and avoidance of multisyllabic words (>2–3 syllables) [8].

The patient's written discharge instructions should be brief and focused on the critical information that the patient and their families need to understand their disease and manage their condition after discharge. The instructions should include the following:

1. Why the patient was admitted.
2. What they were diagnosed with this hospitalization.
3. What was done for them in the hospital.
4. Recommend diet and/or lifestyle modifications after discharge (e.g., low sodium diet, fluid restriction, smoking cessation, daily weight monitoring, etc.).
5. What does the patient need to do after they leave the hospital (i.e., follow-up appointments, get labs, etc.).
6. A list of warning signs or symptoms the patient and their caregivers should look out for at discharge and for which they should call their primary care doctor and/or subspecialist or return to the ER.

Example of patient discharge instruction (Flesch-Kincaid reading level: sixth grade):

> *Dear Mr. Doe*
> *You came to the hospital with a toe infection (gangrene). It was removed by the foot surgeon (podiatrist). You received medicines to treat the infection (metronidazole, ciprofloxacin, and linezolid). Take these medications at home for two weeks. See your foot surgeon in one week. He will change the dressing at that time. Follow-up with the infectious disease doctor in two weeks. Return to the ER if you have fever or worse foot pain.*

The patient instructions should also reference medication changes in an attached medication reconciliation. Information in the medication reconciliation should include:

1. New medications started during the hospitalization
2. Dose changes of medications the patient was on prior to the hospitalization
3. Medications which need to be discontinued after discharge
4. Medications that the patient was taking prior to the hospitalization that may be continued without any changes

In addition to written discharge instructions, patients should also receive verbal discharge instructions. Verbal discharge instructions allow the provider to review the written

---

1 $RE = 206.835 - (1.015 \times ASL) - (84.6 \times ASW)$; RE = readability ease; ASL = average sentence length; ASW = average number of syllables per word.

2 $FKRA = (0.39 \times ASL) + (11.8 \times ASW) - 15.59$; FKRA = Flesch-Kincaid Reading Age; ASL = average sentence length; ASW = average number of syllables per word.

Joint Commission-mandated components	Consensus definition
Reason for hospitalization	Chief complaint (any description of the patient's primary presenting condition); AND/OR History of present illness (a description of a patient's initial presentation to the hospital admission including a description of the initial diagnostic evaluation)
Significant findings	Primary diagnoses (admission/discharge diagnoses noted in the discharge summary)
Procedures and treatment provided	Hospital course (a description of the events occurring to a patient during his/her hospital stay); AND/OR Hospital consults (a description of surgical, medical, other specialty or allied health consults a patient experienced as an inpatient or a specific statement that "no consults" occurred); AND/OR Hospital procedures (a description of surgical, invasive, non-invasive, diagnostic or technical procedures a patient experienced as an inpatient or a specific statement that "no procedures" occurred)
Patient's discharge condition	Any documentation that gives a sense for how the patient is doing at discharge or the patient's health status on discharge

Fig. 38.1 Joint Commission-mandated component definitions. (Modified from Ref. [11])

instructions with the patient and their caregivers and check for understanding of the discharge instructions. Any miscomprehension of the discharge instructions can be clarified in real time by the discharging provider. The intent of this method is to prevent adverse events related to inadequate compression of discharge information. The "teach-back" method can be used by discharging providers to check a patient or caregiver's understanding of their discharge instructions. This method requires the discharging provider to ask the patient to explain in their own words the reason for hospitalization and what they need to do after discharge from the hospital. It is a way to confirm that the provider has explained things in a manner that the patient understands. It is important to remember that this is not a test of the patient's knowledge, but a test of how well the provider explained the concept. If teach-back uncovers a misunderstanding of the discharge instructions and/or reason for hospitalization by the patient or caregiver, the provider will need to explain things again using a different approach. They should perform teach-back again until the patient or their caregiver is able to correctly describe the information in their own words [16].

38.4.2 Discharge Summary

The discharge summary is another critical aspect of the discharge planning process. It is the primary mode of communication between the hospital care team and the aftercare providers. The Joint Commission has several mandated components that must be included in a patient's discharge summary. The elements include reason for hospitalization, significant findings, procedures, treatment provided, and the patient's discharge condition. The elements and their consensus definition are shown in Fig. 38.1.

Other important clinical information to add to the discharge summary includes significant laboratory, radiological and pathology findings, incidental radiographic findings that require non-urgent follow-up, pending test results at discharge, discharge medications, and issues to be addressed at discharge [14].

It is important that the discharge summary is completed in a timely manner in order to reach the primary care provider prior to the patient's scheduled follow-up. Ideally discharge summaries should be completed within 24–48 hours of patient's discharge and no later than 7 days post-discharge [7].

Given the complexity of most hospitalized patients, a discharge checklist is a way to ensure that all of the patient's post-discharge needs as well as communications have been addressed. An example of a discharge checklist endorsed by the Society of Hospital Medicine, which includes both required and optional elements, is shown in Fig. 38.2.

Interprofessional Care: Why Teamwork Matters

Annette M. Hintenach and Judith L. Howe

A. Chun (ed.), *Geriatric Practice*, https://doi.org/10.1007/978-3-030-19625-7_39

39.1 Why Interprofessional Care?

There is mounting and clear evidence that points to the positive outcomes of interprofessional care. Healthcare systems in both the private and public sectors – notably the Veterans Health Administration (VHA) – are mandated to provide team-based care. Interprofessional practice is the preferred method of care delivery in a range of settings, including hospitals, clinics, emergency departments, homes, long-term care facilities, and telehealth. Future clinicians will be in an advantageous position if they understand the principles and approaches of effective teamwork. When delivering geriatric care, interdisciplinary teams are particularly vital [16]. Team-based care refers to "...the provision of health services to individuals, families, and/or their communities by at least two health providers who work collaboratively with patients and their caregivers- to the extent preferred by each patient- to accomplish shared goals within and across settings to achieve coordinated, high-quality care" [20]. Interdisciplinary teamwork is a multilayered process whereby different staff members work collaboratively and share their knowledge, skills, and expertise in order to affect patient care [22]. Interprofessional care encompasses collaboration and coordination to provide wide-ranging levels of care to patients.

Clinicians caring for older persons have been at the forefront of interprofessional care. The first reported interdisciplinary healthcare teams trace back to World War II, where the poor and underserved sought access to healthcare at community health centers [2]. Members of healthcare teams are expected to work collaboratively to better understand the shared objectives of caring for elderly patients and to deliver the highest quality of care [3]. Many older adults have complex healthcare needs which must be addressed by clinicians from several disciplines [14]. For some, this means managing multiple chronic conditions. Common geriatric syndromes such as falls, depression, delirium, dementia, frailty, and urinary incontinence often lead to comorbidities and poor health outcomes among older adults [10]. An interprofessional team approach has been found to improve patient outcomes and patient safety [3]. Geriatrics education and training on interprofessional collaboration can take many forms in geriatrics, from lectures, case discussions, workshops, rotations in geriatric evaluation clinics, and home visits [14, 16, 19].

The importance and benefits of interprofessional teamwork in healthcare have been more clearly demonstrated in the last 15 years [18, 22, 25]. High-profile national initiatives such as the US Department of Health and Human Services (HHS) Agency for Healthcare Research and Quality (AHRQ) funded TeamSTEPPS have been effectively engaging healthcare organizations, leaders, staff, funding agencies, and insurers in advancing the interprofessional practice movement [1]. Other initiatives, such as the Minnesota-based National Center for Interprofessional Practice and Education organization, align interprofessional education and collaborative practice by providing resources, evidence, and leadership through public-private partnerships [23].

In this chapter, we cover the major components and processes of interprofessional team-based care and discuss their impact on patient outcomes. We use the case of Jim Rich, an 84-year-old Korean War Veteran, to illustrate the importance, potential pitfalls, and nuances of effective and compassionate teamwork. In this case, we follow Mr. Rich from his admission to a nursing home to the last days of his life.

Introducing Mr. Rich

Jim Rich is an 84-year-old Veteran who was recently admitted to the nursing home following an above-the-knee amputation of his right leg. After drinking one night, he fell while walking to the bathroom in the dark and fractured his right ankle. He did not seek help for several days, as he did not recognize the severity of the injury. He was admitted to the hospital with a gangrenous right foot, which led to an above-the-knee amputation because of poor circulation. At the time of hospital admission, he was noted to be disheveled and poorly nourished. A psychiatric consult was obtained, and it noted that he appeared to be severely depressed. During the hospital stay, Mr. Rich was started on antidepressants. He was discharged to the nursing home on antidepressant medications and has a scheduled follow-up visit with the psychiatrist. He understands that placement in a nursing home is necessary for rehabilitation and that he will eventually get a prosthesis so that he will be able to walk again. Medicare benefits will probably cover the first 20 days of his stay as well as a portion of the next 80 days as long as he requires skilled services to progress with his rehabilitation.

39.2 The Evidence

Interprofessional collaboration has a number of benefits, including improved quality of care, health outcomes, enhanced systems and processes, and patient safety [17, 28, 29]. Interprofessional care decreases the likelihood of service duplication, reduces the risk for medication errors, and eases patient transitions between sites of care. It also permits healthcare practitioners to practice specific clinical skills at the "top of their licenses," which assists in evenly distributing workload among team members. In healthcare settings, this is particularly important because there may be clinician shortages and overburdened administrative infrastructures, particularly on busy services such as inpatient units, emergency rooms, and outpatient clinics. In the field of geriatrics, collaborative teamwork is especially needed because of the presentation of patients with multiple comorbidities and psychosocial and economic challenges. When team members share ideas, expertise, knowledge, and skills pertinent to their disciplines, the older patient benefits from a collaboration which takes into account the "whole person" with respect to medical, psychosocial, family, and economic needs. It is important to note here that optimal geriatrics teamwork includes family and caregiver input as well.

39.3 History of Interprofessional Practice and Team-based Care

Over the last 20 years, the need for interprofessional care has been demonstrated and reinforced in various forms. VHA has been a leader in developing interprofessional programs and services in the fields of geriatrics, hospice, and palliative care [4]. Additionally, VHA has had a long-standing commitment to workforce development as demonstrated through both interprofessional education and practice [9]. VHA has explored several approaches to integrating interprofessional education into clinical settings, which include offering robust clinical placement settings to associated health trainees, hosting interprofessional palliative care fellowship programs, expanding training and education programs into rural and highly rural areas, and leading an initiative to develop strategies for integrating education into the VHA's model for patient-centered care [9]. The VHA model of interprofessional care, known as the Patient Aligned Care Team (PACT), was initiated in 2010 and is the VHA's form of the patient-centered medical home model being used in the private sector [26]. The PACT model provides Veteran-driven, personalized care in the form of teamlets in an effort to improve care coordination for Veterans.

Although much of the evidence has shown that effective teamwork is fundamental to successful healthcare delivery, there has been less research done that addresses how individual healthcare professionals may contribute to successful teamwork [15]. Education and training needs of team members should be explored, and team-based competencies should be clearly established to help identify what makes effective team members [15]. To best foster interdisciplinary evidence-based practice, there needs to be a paradigm shift among team members across disciplines to move from an individual professional mentality to a synergistic, collaborative approach to care [24].

An Institute of Medicine (IOM) report in 2003 pointed to the pressing need for an overhaul in health professions education because education had not successfully kept up with developing changes in the healthcare system, patient demographics, and practice environments [11]. Subsequent IOM activities addressed five competencies in health professions education, including (1) patient-centered care, (2) interdisciplinary teams, (3) evidence-based practice, (4) quality improvement, and (5) informatics [12]. It was recommended that clinicians "cooperate, collaborate, communicate, and integrate care in teams to ensure that care is continuous and reliable" [12].

In 2008, the Institute of Medicine released *Retooling for an Aging America: Building the Health Care Workforce*, which highlighted a looming healthcare crisis relating to the care of older adults in the United States [13]. The report underscored the lack of geriatrics-trained healthcare specialists needed to care for the expanding aging population and issued a call for action to educate and train healthcare providers and informal caregivers to increase their geriatric competence [13]. The healthcare workforce receives minimal to no geriatrics training, and it is vital that direct practice workers as well as other healthcare professionals, paraprofessionals, and unpaid caregivers have a fundamental knowledge of geriatrics. Recruitment and retention of geriatrics-trained specialists play a pivotal role in this shortage, as does lack of interest and available training and education programs [13]. With regard to medicine, less than 3% of medical students choose to take geriatrics electives in medical school [21]. As students move from medical school through residency programs, there are limited opportunities to complete geriatric fellowships in the United States. The American Geriatrics Society recognizes this shortage as well as the growing need for caring for older patients with multiple chronic conditions and functional limitations in the rapidly aging society.

Several team initiatives have been developed in recent years such as the John A. Hartford Foundation funded Geriatric Interdisciplinary Team Training (GITT) Program, initiated in 1995, geared to improving care for older adults by enriching interdisciplinary training of healthcare trainees in social work, nursing, and medicine [7]. In 2010, the VHA Office of Rural Health Geriatric Scholars Program adapted GITT for rural VHA providers; this program, referred to as Rural Interdisciplinary Team Training (RITT), is now in its eighth year and has trained over 1500 rural clinicians and staff at 106 clinics.

TeamSTEPPS is an evidence-based teamwork model aimed at improving communication and teamwork skills for healthcare professionals, which was launched in 2003. Developed by the U.S. Department of Defense's Patient Safety Program in collaboration with the U.S. Department of Health and Human Services Agency for Healthcare Research and Quality [1], it provides ready-to-use materials and training curriculum for healthcare professionals. Prior to the development of TeamSTEPPS, there was no consensus model of teamwork in healthcare.

Let's revisit the case of Mr. Jim Rich, who was admitted to the hospital after his fall. The geriatrics inpatient team was consulted on the case and found the following upon admission.

Mr. Rich

Past Medical History:

1. Hypertension
2. Forty pack-year history of smoking
3. History of myocardial infarction 8 years ago (after which he quit smoking)
4. Alcoholism for which he has been treated 2–3 times

Allergies: No known allergies

Medications: Sertraline 50 mg qd; amlodipine 5 mg qd; Tylenol #3 1 tab q 6 hr prn pain

Social History: Jim Rich is a retired insurance salesman from a small town who was living alone in an apartment. He has had a long history of alcoholism and has gone through treatment "two or three times" with his wife's support while she was living. Since her death 1 year ago, he has become more and more isolated, drinking heavily alone in his apartment. He has about $5000 in a savings account which he hopes will cover his funeral expenses. He lives on his Social Security check, which is about $1300/month. Mr. Rich has had to borrow money from his daughter at times to make ends meet. His son John and daughter Julie are both married and have responsibilities of their own. At one point in his life, Mr. Rich was active in his community, serving as president of the local Rotary Club, and involved with little league. Now, he mainly watches TV and reads the newspaper.

Review of Symptoms: Stump pain; poor circulation in left leg; constipation; depression; hard of hearing; alcohol abuse

Activities of Daily Living (ADLs): Able to feed, dress, and bathe himself; assistance to toilet × 1; assistance to wheelchair × 1

Instrumental Activities of Daily Living (IADLs): Although able, he exhibits signs of lack of interest in many activities.

Advanced Directives: He has no living will or healthcare proxy.

Environment: Currently lives in nursing home for rehabilitation. Previously lived alone in an apartment.

39

Physical Exam: Weight: 200 lbs. Height: 6′2″ BP: 146/90 P: 80

On exam, Mr. Rich is alert, oriented, and pleasant, although responses are limited to a few words. His only complaint is occasional pain in the amputated leg at night and constipation. His vision is excellent with corrective lenses; he can easily read newsprint. His hearing is moderately impaired on gross exam. Chest is clear. Cardiovascular exam reveals a regular heart rate, no murmur or gallop. Abdominal exam reveals bowel sounds throughout, although he has a large amount of hard stool in his rectum. Examination of his left lower extremity reveals normal proximal pulses, but diminished distal pulses. There is an absence of toe hair on the left foot and a mild rubor when the foot is dangling. The right stump is wrapped with a compression bandage and shows a well-approximated healing incision and some mild edema. The skin over the lower portion of the sacrum is noted to be red and non-blanching.

MMSE: 27/30; Mr. Rich had to be prodded for answers, but usually responded correctly.

39.4 Types of Teams

The gold standard for teamwork has evolved greatly over the years [27]. Depending on the clinical setting, there may be major differences in what healthcare teams look like. The three most common types of healthcare teams are *multidisciplinary teams, interdisciplinary teams, and transdisciplinary teams*. Each type of team serves a specific purpose and function [8, 17]. In this chapter, we will distinguish between multidisciplinary and interdisciplinary healthcare teams and describe their purpose in a healthcare setting.

39.4.1 Multidisciplinary Team

In *multidisciplinary teams*, team members work alongside each other to provide patient care. Team members function within their own discipline, so they are only responsible for completing specific tasks relating to their respective discipline. For example, a physician may be the sole team member to diagnose and treat an illness. That physician may then ask the pharmacist on the team to counsel the patient on medication use and safety. The pharmacist may subsequently refer the patient to the social worker on the team to help coordinate resources in the community. As illustrated, each team member has a designated role in caring for the patient. While each team member is contributing to the overall care of the patient, the roles are clearly distinct among team members. While effective multidisciplinary teamwork is not impossible to achieve, there are some challenges that may arise when utilizing a multidisciplinary approach.

First, team members might layer chart notes, orders, and medications, which may cause confusion and unnecessary work among team members. There may also be an increased risk of uncoordinated care delivered by multiple professions, due to the lack of communication within team members. As a result, patients may suffer due to the lack of proper coordination. Additionally, some of the difficulties that occur in multidisciplinary teams stem from differing attitudes about what constitutes as the best health outcome [6]. Team members from different disciplines may have varying opinions on what an ideal health outcome looks like and often turn to their own profession for guidance, resulting in different allegiances [6].

39.4.2 Interdisciplinary Team

Interdisciplinary teams differ from multidisciplinary teams in several important ways. In an interdisciplinary team, team members have shared responsibility in decision making. Each individual member of the team is contributing to reach a common goal, following the same protocols. Individual disciplines contribute to integrated assessment and care plans for the patient. Communication and collaboration within the team often results in a positive role overlap. With an interdisciplinary team approach, team members must consider the contributions of other team members when making their own contributions. Also, in interdisciplinary teams, clinicians are generally free to work at the "top of their licenses," which refers to working at the maximum extent of training and not spending unnecessary time completing tasks that someone else on the team can perform. This is a critical component of interdisciplinary teams, because it enables healthcare professionals to maximize their time, efforts, and contributions on the team. This is especially important for busy physicians, whose time is often limited due to high patient caseload.

While the interdisciplinary approach to care has increasingly become accepted as the preferred model of care delivery in healthcare settings, interdisciplinary teams may also experience unique challenges. Some examples of possible challenges faced by interdisciplinary team members may include opposing goals and objectives between team members; communication issues both within the team and within the broader senior management of a given organization; mixing of professional roles and responsibilities; issues with morale and motivation; and differing opinions on patient interventions and outcomes [22]. At their highest levels of functioning, interdisciplinary teams may also be referred to as "transdisciplinary." This occurs when team members often cross traditional professional and disciplinary boundaries to work together in providing patient care and share disciplinary roles.

Mr. Rich

One day after Mr. Rich was admitted to the hospital, the geriatrics inpatient team rounded and saw Mr. Rich. At the weekly team meeting the next day, the team sat down to discuss his case and develop a care plan. The team members at the meeting included the physician, registered nurse, social worker, physical therapist, pharmacist, and dietician.

Based on what you know about Mr. Rich at this point in time, think about the following questions:

1. What are the important issues affecting Mr. Rich's health? What are the social issues affecting his lifestyle?
2. What is the team's primary goal for this patient? Which team members should be assigned to dealing with Mr. Rich's various needs?
3. How can the team address Mr. Rich's financial situation?
4. Consider community and family resources. How might they be utilized to improve Mr. Rich's condition?
5. What are the advantages of the team approach for Mr. Rich?

39.5 Team Members

The size of healthcare teams, as well as the team composition varies significantly depending on the healthcare setting and purpose of the team. ◘ Table 39.1 provides a snapshot of disciplines who may work on teams with brief descriptions of required education and training, scope of practice, and typical team roles. There are variances among US states in scopes of practice in some cases; for the purpose of this table, we have used New York State as an illustration.

39.6 Healthcare Settings

Interprofessional care often includes coordination of care services, management of chronic health conditions, or referrals to other providers. There are several types of healthcare settings involved in team practice. Here are the most common settings where interprofessional care is delivered to older adults:

- Hospital/institutional care (inpatient setting)
- Outpatient clinic
- Office
- Managed care organizations
- Hospitals (proving general care, acute care, or specialty care)
- Long-term care facilities (e.g., nursing homes, assisted living facilities)
- Outpatient clinics
- Ambulatory or surgical care centers
- Doctor's offices (generalist or specialty practice)

Now let's revisit Mr. Rich, who was discharged from the hospital to his home 1 month ago. His son, David Rich, is very concerned about his father and has called the hospital geriatrician at least twice a week since he left the hospital. The geriatrician recommends that he try to get an appointment at the nearby VHA medical center where there is a well-known geriatrics clinic. His son calls and is able to get an appointment the next week because of a cancellation. The clinic geriatrician notes that Mr. Rich's weight has dropped from 200 to 188 pounds since he left the hospital 5 weeks ago and that his blood pressure has risen from 146/90 to 180/100. The physician is also worried because Mr. Rich is unkempt, wearing his slippers to the appointment, and smells of alcohol. Also, his stump has not yet healed and he has some yellow discharge from the incision site. In addition, he has a new stage 2 pressure ulcer on his sacrum.

39.7 Geriatrics Healthcare Teams

Geriatrics healthcare teams may vary a great deal in clinical focus. This is usually contingent upon where care is being delivered. Many healthcare settings throughout the United States still do not have existing geriatrics healthcare teams in

Table 39.1 Healthcare team members

Profession	Education	Residency	Scope of practice	Role on team
Physician (MD)	4-year undergraduate degree 4 years of medical school	3–8 years of residency training	Diagnosis, examination, treatment, advisement, or prescription for human disease, ailment, or injury Also performs surgery (if certified to do so)	Provides leadership to other team members in developing and supervising patient's healthcare plan
Physician (DO)	4-year undergraduate degree 4 years of osteopathic medical school	3–4+ years of residency training	Diagnosis, examination, treatment, advisement, or prescription for human disease, ailment, or injury Also performs surgery (if certified to do so)	Provides leadership to other team members in developing and supervising patient's healthcare plan
Physician assistant (PA)	4-year undergraduate degree 2-year physician assistant program	Currently not required	Works under the direction and supervision of a physician to perform various procedures (dependent upon type of practice)	Works with physician to manage patient's healthcare plan and provide guidance to other team members
Nurse practitioner (NP)	4-year bachelor's degree in nursing 1–3-year master's degree (length depends on specialty)	N/A	Works independently to see patients Diagnoses and treats acute illnesses Orders diagnostic testing Prescribes certain medications (varies by state) Performs certain medical exams; supervises and delegates to other nursing professionals (e.g., registered nurses, licensed practical nurses)	Delivers direct care to patients; coordinates interdisciplinary care plan with other team members; helps educate patients about their care plan
Registered nurse (RN)	2-year associate's degree in nursing or 4-year bachelor's degree in nursing* *Now becoming the requirement for most settings	N/A	Performs certain medical exams; supervises and delegates to other nursing professionals (e.g., licensed practical nurses)	Provides direct and indirect care to patients; communicates with physician on the team regarding healthcare plan
Psychiatrist	4-year undergraduate degree 4 years of medical school	4 years of residency training	Medical doctor specializing in mental health Assesses mental and physical aspects of psychological problems	Offers team members unique skills and recommendations for mental health related patient treatment plans
Psychologist	4–5-year bachelor's degree in psychology 2–3-year master's degree in psychology 4–7-year doctoral degree* *Doctor of Psychology (PsyD) or Doctor of Philosophy in Psychology (PhD) depends on career in practice (PsyD) or research (PhD)	2 years of supervised internship (depends on the state)	Assesses behavioral and mental conditions Diagnoses neuropsychological disorders Prevention and treatment of behavioral and mental disorders and dysfunctions	Assists team members with mental health counseling and preventive care as necessary
Pharmacist (PharmD)	3–4 years of undergraduate pre-professional (prerequisite) work 4 years of PharmD program	Residency is not required at this time, although highly encouraged for clinical pharmacists	Conducts health and wellness testing Initiates, monitors, and modifies patient's drug therapy Medication reconciliation	Provides pharmacological recommendations to physicians and other team members Assists team in reducing prescribing errors
Social worker	4-year undergraduate degree in Social Work* 2-year master's degree in social work *Needed for some entry-level social work positions	N/A	Conducts biopsychosocial intake assessments Diagnoses mental, emotional, behavioral, and addictive developmental disorders and disabilities Discharge planning Makes referrals for community resources as necessary Assists with questions regarding entitlement programs	Assists healthcare team in providing biopsychosocial support to patient Provides mental health counseling services as appropriate

Occupational therapist (OT)	2-year associate's degree or 4-year undergraduate degree 2-year master's degree in occupational therapy	N/A	Treats ill, injured, or disabled patients through therapeutic use of everyday activities Helps patients improve, develop, recover, and maintain necessary skills for working and daily living	Assists healthcare team in providing patients with appropriate occupational therapy as needed
Physical therapist (PT)	4-year bachelor's degree in health field 3-year Doctor of Physical Therapy (DPT) degree	Optional 1-year clinical residency for specialty areas of care	Helps patients reduce pain and improve/restore mobility Works with patients to help loss of mobility before it occurs	Assists healthcare team in providing patients with appropriate physical therapy as needed Develops fitness and/or wellness-oriented programs for patients
Dietician	4-year bachelor's degree or higher accredited by the Accreditation Council for Education in Nutrition and Dietetics (ACEND)	Must complete dietetic internship of at least 800 hours of supervised practice	Assesses patient's nutrition needs and food patterns Plans and directs provision of food as appropriate Provides nutrition counseling	Assists healthcare team in assessing and developing nutrition plans for patients
Medical receptionist	High school diploma	–	Answers telephones and patient questions, schedules appointments, registers patients, and updates patient records Provides calm and efficient environment for patients, families, and caregivers	Assists healthcare team with necessary patient information Communicates patient health information to team members as needed Helps coordinate day-to-day schedules of healthcare team members
Family member	–	–	–	Assists healthcare team with developing appropriate, culturally competent, and acceptable treatment plan for patients

Compiled from information from the following sources:
Google. Available from: ▶ https://www.google.com/. Retrieved on December 19, 2017
Physician- Office of the Professions- New York State Education. Available from: ▶ http://www.op.nysed.gov/prof/med/medlic.htm. Retrieved on December 19, 2017.
How To Become A Physician Assistant: Physician Assistant Programs & Careers. Available from: ▶ https://www.learnhowtobecome.org/physician-assistant/. Retrieved on December 19, 2017
Nurse Practitioner- Office of the Professions- New York State Education. Available from: ▶ http://www.op.nysed.gov/prof/nurse/np.htm. Retrieved on December 19, 2017
Nurse Practitioner- New York State Department of Labor. Available from: ▶ https://labor.ny.gov/stats/olcny/nurse-practitioner.shtm. Retrieved on December 19, 2017
How to Become an RN- Education and Career Roadmap. Available from: ▶ https://study.com/how_to_become_a_rn.html. Retrieved on December 19, 2017
NYS Nursing. Available from: ▶ http://www.op.nysed.gov/prof/nurse/. Retrieved on December 19, 2017
How to Become a Psychiatrist in 5 Steps. Available from: ▶ https://learn.org/articles/Psychiatrist_5_Steps_to_Becoming_a_Psychiatrist.html. Retrieved on December 26, 2017
NY State Psychiatrist College Requirements and Program Info. Available from: ▶ https://study.com/ny_state_psychiatrist_college_requirements.html. Retrieved on December 26, 2017
New York Psychology Licensure Requirements. Available from: ▶ https://www.psychologydegree411.com/licensure/new-york/. Retrieved on December 26, 2017
NYS Psychology: License Requirements- Office of the Professions. Available from: ▶ http://www.op.nysed.gov/prof/psych/psychlic.htm. Retrieved on December 26, 2017
Pharmacy School & Pharmacist Careers- How to Become a Pharmacist. Available from: ▶ https://www.learnhowtobecome.org/pharmacist/. Retrieved on December 27, 2017
NYS Pharmacy- Office of the Professions- New York State Education. Available from: ▶ http://www.op.nysed.gov/prof/pharm/. Retrieved on December 27, 2017
NYS Social Work: LCSW License Requirements. Available from: ▶ http://www.op.nysed.gov/prof/sw/lcsw.htm. Retrieved on December 28, 2017
How to Become a Social Worker in New York, NY- Your Initial Steps. Available from: ▶ https://www.socialworklicensure.org/social-worker-steps/become-a-social-worker-in-ny.html#context/api/listings/prefilter. Retrieved on December 28, 2017
NYS Scope of Practice- New York State Society for Clinical Social Work. Available from: ▶ http://www.nysscsw.org/nys-scope-of-practice. Retrieved on December 23, 2017
How To Become an Occupational Therapist. Available from: ▶ http://www.otcareerpath.com/how-to-become-an-occupational-therapist. Retrieved on January 12, 2018
License Requirements: Occupational Therapist & Occupational Therapy Assistant. Available from: ▶ http://www.op.nysed.gov/prof/ot/otlic.htm. Retrieved on January 12, 2018
Occupational Therapists- Bureau of Labor Statistics. Available from: ▶ https://www.bls.gov/ooh/healthcare/occupational-therapists.htm. Retrieved on January 12, 2018
How to Become a Physical Therapist: Physical Therapy Schools and Careers. Available from: ▶ https://www.learnhowtobecome.org/physical-therapist/. Retrieved on January 12, 2018
Who Are Physical Therapists?. Available from: ▶ http://www.apta.org/AboutPTs/. Retrieved on January 12, 2018
Steps to Become a Registered Dietician in New York. Available from: ▶ https://www.nutritioned.org/registered-dietitian-new-york.html#education. Retrieved on January 12, 2018
Dietetics and Nutrition. Available from: ▶ http://www.op.nysed.gov/prof/diet/. Retrieved on January 12, 2018
How to Become a Medical Receptionist. Available from: ▶ http://www.innerbody.com/careers-in-health/how-to-become-a-medical-receptionist.html. Retrieved on January 12, 2018

place. Below are examples of the most common types of healthcare teams present when working with older adults:
- Geriatrics team
- Palliative care team
- Geriatrics palliative care/oncology team
- Pain management team
- Special focus teams (liver, cancer, addiction, etc.)

39.8 Key Elements of Team Effectiveness and Efficiency in Geriatrics Practice

Having clearly defined team goals is one of the most important elements that will drive a team's success. Additionally, having strong communication among team members and understanding professional differences will result in better patient care [5]. Other factors that may impact team effectiveness and efficiency include the following:
- Understanding the agency/organizational mission
- Identifying operational, measurable objectives for all team members
- Ensuring that administrative and clinical systems are in place to ensure successful teamwork
- Having clearly defined tasks and labor division among team members (e.g., assign responsibilities/tasks across the team)
- Team training and education opportunities
- Ongoing team training is necessary
- You can cross-train team members to substitute other roles
- Training for functions

Engaged and effective teams have strong relationships and clearly identified team functions. ◘ Figure 39.1 represents the key components of strong relationships as well as the ideal functions of the healthcare team as identified in the VHA PACT model. As team relationships and functions increase, so will the effectiveness of the team. There are two sides that must work simultaneously together in order to achieve engaged and effective teams. These include *Team Relationships* and *Team Functions*. Components of successful team relationships include civility, respect, psychological safety, and cohesiveness. Components of effective team functions include team purpose and methods, clarity of roles and responsibilities, effective communication, and team responsiveness and awareness.

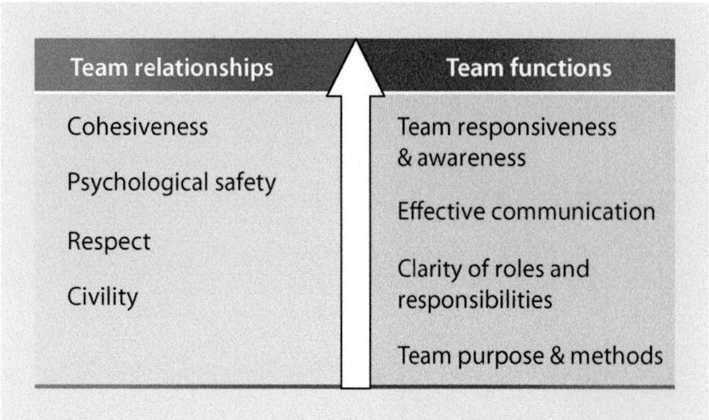

Team relationships
Team functions
Cohesiveness
Psychological safety
Respect
Civility
Team responsiveness & awareness
Effective communication
Clarity of roles and responsibilities
Team purpose & methods

◘ **Fig. 39.1** Engaged and effective teams. (Adapted from the VHA PACT Training Manual train-the-trainer materials, as developed by the VHA National Center for Organization Development, October, 2010)

Mr. Rich

While Mr. Rich was at the VHA geriatrics clinic, he was also seen by the social worker because of Dr. Wallace's concerns about his appearance and his son David's distress about his condition. The next day, at team rounds, Mr. Rich was presented to the team. David is invited to join the discussion about his father and his treatment plan. Dr. Wallace wants Mr. Rich to be placed in a nursing home, but his son, David, is uncertain on what to do, and Mr. Rich's daughter, Julie, has deferred decision making to her brother. Mr. Rich wants to stay in his home.

Think about the following issues and tasks facing the members of the geriatrics team as Mr. Rich continues to decline:
1. What are the important issues facing Mr. Rich and his family at this time?
2. How should the team consider issues of patient autonomy versus beneficence given that Mr. Rich has no living will or healthcare proxy?
3. How can community and personal resources and entitlements be used in developing a plan of care?
4. In developing the care plan, which tasks should be delegated to which team members?
5. What would have happened if Mr. Rich didn't have a team caring for him?

39.9 Team Challenges in Interprofessional Care

Some of the challenges for team members when providing interprofessional care include changing roles of healthcare professionals, varied settings of care, medical hierarchies, and team instability. The most common challenges for team members are related to *cohesion, communication, role clarity, transitions, and phases.*
- **Cohesion**
  - Team cohesion is based on civility, respect, and psychological safety.
  - Team agrees on acceptable behavior(s).
  - Team encourages open and balanced discussion.
- **Communication**
  - Open, honest discussion is important.
  - Team members need to be truthful.

- Team should identify efficient mechanisms for information exchange.
- All team members should have the opportunity to participate in discussions and provide feedback.
- **Role Clarity**
  - Team members should have formally designated roles.
  - Team should understand what roles can be shared among different members.
  - Team members agree how work is to be carried out.
- **Transitions**
  - Team should carve out ample time for effective communication.
  - Lack of understanding along continuum of care results in poor transitions.
  - Team should be able to negotiate between VA and non-VA healthcare systems as necessary.
- **Phases** [5]
  - All teams go through team phases – *forming, norming, confronting, performing, and leaving.*
  - *Forming* – getting to know team members
  - *Norming* – shared expectations among team members
  - *Confronting* – working conflict out with team members
  - *Performing* – team functioning smoothly
  - *Leaving* – team readjustments due to team member turnover

39.10 Physician as a Team Leader

With so many possible members of a healthcare team, team members may occasionally get confused or frustrated by a lack of a clear team leader. Regardless of team size or setting, there should be an established team leader who helps lead the team to make decisions and hold individual members accountable for their contributions (or lack thereof). A leader models team behaviors for other members and encourages junior members of the team to become integrated members of the team, alongside seasoned clinicians. Physicians often assume team leadership roles since they are ultimately responsible for the overall care being provided to the patient. It is important that physician leaders be sensitive to other disciplines and properly manage team conflict, keeping teams current, emerging, and effective. Physicians should model appropriate leadership by working collaboratively with other team members to work efficiently and overcome any challenges that may arise.

So, to conclude the case of Jim Rich, he was admitted to the nursing home, where he died 5 days later. While his death was unexpected, his son and daughter were relieved that he did not die alone in his apartment and that he was no longer suffering. David and Julie were pleased with the team-based care that Mr. Rich had received up until the end of his life and vowed to complete their own advance directives and express their healthcare wishes to their respective families. They made small donations in their father's name to the hospital, outpatient clinic, and nursing home facilities that cared for their father.

Benefits of Interprofessional Care

The benefits of interprofessional care in the case of Mr. Rich include the following:

- Timely, coordinated care
- Ease in transitions of care
- Productive and civil communications among team members
- Input from Mr. Rich's family members

39.11 Looking Ahead to the Future

With the aging of the Baby Boomers, the need for high-quality care is as great as ever. Providing interprofessional care is the cornerstone of successful healthcare delivery. While healthcare teams may vary in their structures and processes, all team members should remain active, participatory, and engaged members of the team. Teams must identify challenges early on and work together to be as effective and efficient as possible. This will help establish and maintain trust within team members. Additionally, team members need to work together to create a culture of open communication and continuous learning from team members. Shared goals and clearly defined values of team members make for strong, cohesive teams. The physician's role as a team leader plays an important part in successful interprofessional care. Managing team dynamics is everyone's responsibility and will help foster a healthy, collaborative environment for all team members to contribute to the care of older adults.

References

1. Agency for Healthcare Research and Quality (AHRQ) [Internet]. Washington, DC: U.S. Department of Health and Human Services; 2017. TeamSTEPPS. Available from https://www.ahrq.gov/teamstepps/index.html.
2. Baldwin DW. Some historical notes on interdisciplinary and interprofessional education and practice in health care in the USA. J Interprof Care. 1996;10(2):173–87.
3. Creditor MC. Hazards of hospitalization of the elderly. Ann Intern Med. 1993;118(3):219–23.
4. Daratsos L, Howe JL. The development of palliative care programs in the Veterans Administration: Zelda Foster's legacy. J Soc Work End Life Palliat Care. 2007;3(1):29–39.
5. Drinka TJ, Clark PG. Health care teamwork: interdisciplinary practice and teaching. Westport: Greenwood Publishing Group; 2000.
6. Firth-Cozens J. Multidisciplinary teamwork: the good, bad, and everything in between. BMJ Qual Saf. 2001;10:65–6.
7. Fulmer T, Flaherty E, Hyer K. The geriatric interdisciplinary team training (GITT) program. Gerontol Geriatr Educ. 2004;24(2):3–12.
8. Hall P, Weaver L. Interdisciplinary education and teamwork: a long and winding road. Med Educ. 2001;35(9):867–75.
9. Howe JL, Daratsos L. Interprofessional practice in the veterans health administration. In: Morano C, editor. Perspectives on interprofessional education and practice. Washington, DC: NASW Press; 2017. p. 209–18.
10. Inouye SK, Studenski S, Tinetti ME, Kuchel GA. Geriatric syndromes: clinical, research, and policy implications of a core geriatric concept. J Am Geriatr Soc. 2007;55(5):780–91.

11. Institute of Medicine. Crossing the quality chasm: a new health system for the 21st century. Washington, DC: National Academies Press; 2001.
12. Institute of Medicine. Health professions education: a bridge to quality. Washington, DC: National Academies Press; 2003.
13. Institute of Medicine. Retooling for an aging America: building the health care workforce. Washington, DC: National Academies Press; 2008.
14. Keijsers CJ, Dreher R, Tanner S, Forde-Johnston C, Thompson S, Education TS. Interprofessional education in geriatric medicine. Eur Geriatr Med. 2016;7(4):306–14.
15. Leggat SG. Effective healthcare teams require effective team members: defining teamwork competencies. BMC Health Serv Res. 2007;7(1):17.
16. Leipzig RM, Hyer K, Ek K, Wallenstein S, Vezina ML, Fairchild S, et al. Attitudes toward working on interdisciplinary healthcare teams: a comparison by discipline. J Am Geriatr Soc. 2002;50(6):1141–8.
17. Lemieux-Charles L, McGuire WL. What do we know about health care team effectiveness? A review of the literature. Med Care Res Rev. 2006;63(3):263–300.
18. Leonard M, Graham S, Bonacum D. The human factor: the critical importance of effective teamwork and communication in providing safe care. Qual Saf Health Care. 2004;13(suppl 1):i85–90.
19. Liston BW, Fischer MA, Way DP, Torre D, Papp KK. Interprofessional education in the internal medicine clerkship: results from a national survey. Acad Med. 2011;86(7):872–6.
20. Mitchell P, Wynia M, Golden R, McNellis B, Okun S, Webb CE, et al. Core principles & values of effective team-based health care. Washington, DC: Institute of Medicine; 2012.
21. Moore MJ, Moir P, Patrick MM. The state of aging and health in America: 2004. Washington, DC: The Merck Institute of Aging and Health; 2004.
22. Nancarrow SA, Booth A, Ariss S, Smith T, Enderby P, Roots A. Ten principles of good interdisciplinary team work. Hum Resour Health. 2013;11(1):19.
23. National Center for Interprofessional Practice and Education (NCIPE) [Internet]; 2017. Available from https://nexusipe.org/.
24. Newhouse RP, Spring B. Interdisciplinary evidence-based practice: moving from silos to synergy. Nurs Outlook. 2010;58(6):309–17.
25. O'leary KJ, Sehgal NL, Terrell G, Williams MV. Interdisciplinary teamwork in hospitals: a review and practical recommendations for improvement. J Hosp Med. 2012;7(1):48–54.
26. Suelzer CJ, Munshi IA, Zipper K, Thayer DS. Using facilitative coaching to support patient aligned care teams. Fed Pract. 2015;32(3):24–8.
27. Tsukuda RA. A perspective on health care teams and team training. In: Siegler EL, Hyer K, Fulmer T, Mezey M, editors. Geriatric interdisciplinary team training. New York, NY: Springer; 1998. p. 21–7.
28. Weaver SJ, Dy SM, Rosen MA. Team-training in healthcare: a narrative synthesis of the literature. BMJ Qual Saf. 2014;23(5):359–72.
29. Zwarenstein M, Goldman J, Reeves S. Interprofessional collaboration: effects of practice-based interventions on professional practice and healthcare outcomes. Cochrane Database Syst Rev. 2009;(3):CD000072.

Chronic Care Management

Siobhan Sundel and David Sundel

A. Chun (ed.), *Geriatric Practice*, https://doi.org/10.1007/978-3-030-19625-7_40

40.1 Introduction

The number and proportion of the US population aged 65 years and older is in a period of rapid growth. An increase in average life expectancy over the past several decades and the aging of the baby boomer generation are two factors driving this trend. The US Census Bureau has projected the percent of the US population aged 65 or older to steadily increase, from 14.5% in 2014 to 23.5% by 2060.[16] At the same time, as advances in medicine over the past century have steadily reduced mortality from infectious diseases, heart attacks and strokes, and even certain cancers, the prevalence of chronic illnesses across the US population has emerged as a looming challenge to the US healthcare system, with 60% of adults in America living with at least one chronic illness [14].

Chronic illnesses – those of slow progression and long duration – are often degenerative and generally incurable. Hypertension, diabetes, and congestive heart failure are but a few of the more pervasive chronic conditions. While the prevalence of chronic illness is widespread within the United States, it is mostly concentrated among the elderly. Over 80% of Americans 65 years and older struggle with multiple chronic illnesses, compared to 42% of all US adults [14].

Those with chronic illnesses often suffer limitations in physical and social functioning. They also utilize the healthcare system most heavily, stressing system resources and driving up healthcare costs significantly. Those with chronic illnesses typically see a higher rate of ER visits, hospitalizations, and rehospitalizations for the same condition [2]. Healthcare costs rise dramatically as the number of chronic conditions increase. While those with five or more co-morbidities make up only 12% of the US adult population, they account for 40% of healthcare spending [14]. The incidence of multiple chronic illnesses increases with age. In 2013, chronic illnesses accounted for 66% of US healthcare costs across the whole population, but 95% of the healthcare costs for those 65 years and older went to chronic diseases [16].

The traditional strength of the US healthcare system has been its ability to respond to episodes of infectious disease or to acute events, such as heart attack and stroke. For many decades, research investment and practice models were structured around reacting to such acute, episodic events of disease-specific illness to produce a cure. In turn, the Medicare fee-for-service reimbursement scheme was designed to work with event-driven periodic care.

However, a healthcare system built around episodic care can be problematic for an older patient with chronic illness requiring coordinated, long-term management. Older patients have different care needs than younger patients [15]. Caring for a geriatric patient is labor and time intensive. Primary and geriatric care is not well reimbursed. This often forces the provider to see patients every 15 minutes, which allows insufficient time to conduct a comprehensive exam for a geriatric patient with multiple chronic conditions. Providers can become overwhelmed with the responsibilities of geriatric care, leading to provider burnout. As well, a patient who must routinely see multiple providers for different conditions can receive inconsistent advice or be prescribed more medications than are therapeutically necessary (polypharmacy). This ultimately results in poor care coordination and fragmented care for an increasingly elderly population [10].

40.2 Adapting to a Model of Chronic Care

By the mid-1990s, it had become apparent that the traditional structure of the healthcare system was ill-designed to effectively manage chronic disease. Deficiencies in the system were identified, such as:

- Time-pressed practitioners unable to perform time-consuming comprehensive exams
- Lack of care coordination within and between provider practices, leading to fragmented care
- Lack of active follow-up on patient progress between visits
- Patients inadequately educated to manage their illnesses
- Provider burn-out due to the demands of a patient population with multiple co-morbidities
- A healthcare financing system designed to reimburse face-to-face caregiving focused on affecting a cure rather than facilitating preventive and long-term management of chronic illness

These concerns led to development of new models of delivering healthcare, with a shift in focus from episodic cure to long-term care. One of the first and most widely accepted of these is the Chronic Care Model (CCM), sometimes called the Wagner model. It was developed by Dr. Ed Wagner and his team at The MacColl Center for Healthcare Innovation in the late 1990s [43]. The MacColl Center website (▶ www.maccollcenter.org) maintains resources for research and practical implementation of the model.

The aim of the CCM is to promote development of collaborative healthcare teams working proactively with patients who are enabled to take more responsibility for their own illness. More effective ongoing management of the patient's chronic conditions can slow the progression of the disease and forestall the development of other co-morbid conditions. This not only assures better quality of life for the patient but reduces the patient's need for increasingly complex and costly healthcare services to deal with increasing disability. Care delivery designed around a collaborative team can relieve primary care providers of much of the stress and frustration of trying to cover complex patients with limited resources.

The CCM seeks to actively encourage patients in self-management of their condition, supported by a healthcare team able to proactively monitor their condition and provide necessary intervention.

Key elements of the CCM are:

- Self-Management Support – enabling patient to assume more responsibility for their own care
- Delivery System Design – using collaborative team-based care

- Decision Support – using evidence-based practice to co-develop care plans with patients
- Clinical Information Systems – using medical electronic records for coordinating care and tracking patient progress
- Community – using community resources and cultural sensitivity in support of the patient's efforts at self-care
- Health System – institutional and government support for collaborative team-based approach and active patient self-management [43]

The fundamental principles outlined in the CCM have been integrated into and adapted for a growing number of practices and incorporated into public policy. It is not a coincidence that the concept of the Patient-Centered Medical Home reflects many of the precepts of the CCM. In 2015, the Center for Medicare and Medicaid Services (CMS) began to reimburse for chronic disease management activities, assuring the financial viability of team-based chronic disease management. And recently the American Medical Association has identified a set of core competencies in chronic care management for undergraduate medical students, based on the elements of the Wagner CCM.

40.2.1 CCM Applied to Geriatrics

Several articles [15, 32] have described the effectiveness of using a team-based approach when providing care to older individuals, as advocated in the CCM. Several geriatric models derived from CCM, such as Programs of All-Inclusive Care for the Elderly (PACE) [17] and Hospital at Home [27], are cited in the literature as providing effective interdisciplinary care coordination. These teams usually consist of attending physicians or geriatric fellows, advanced practice registered nurses (APRNs), social workers, and home health aides. Team members each have unique roles to play in caring for the geriatric patient with chronic conditions. A provider working in a geriatric practice could evaluate the patient for an acute problem, then have the social worker and/or staff nurse meet with the patient to discuss chronic disease self-management issues.

Physical and occupational therapists, behavioral health workers and certified diabetic educators can also be important members of such a team. Team-based care coordination and management of elderly patients with chronic medical problems can lead to improved quality of life for the older individual, decreased stress on caregivers, and reduced cost to the healthcare system by reducing hospital readmissions [40].

Enabling a patient to actively take responsibility for self-management of their chronic illness is a core principle of the CCM. For an elderly patient, possibly with some cognitive decline, there may be limits to how well they can be trained in self-care, and their caregiver will need to be brought into the process. Caregivers are an important resource for the chronically ill geriatric patient and should be seen as integral members of the healthcare team.

It is important to educate the elderly patient or their caregiver about their medication regimen. For example, if the patient has congestive heart failure and is short of breath, the provider may start a diuretic to decrease these symptoms. The patient should understand why they are taking the medication and its common side effects. Providers can also emphasize the importance of taking medications on a daily basis at the same time every day, which a caregiver can oversee.

Medication reconciliation should be done on routine visits, including prescription and over-the-counter medications and herbal supplements. Registered nurses working with providers can perform medication reconciliation with the patient or their primary care giver while the patient is seeing the provider. This helps the provider to determine what prescriptions the patient needs and the pharmacy the patient uses. Many patients use several different pharmacies, including a local pharmacy and a mail order pharmacy. By doing medication reconciliation during routine visits, problems with prescribing to the wrong pharmacy can be avoided.

Team-based care coordination is facilitated by the use of an electronic medical record (EMR) which allows for patient scheduling, referrals, and tracking patient progress. For example, if a patient is seen in cardiology, the APRN can see the progress note and follow-up with recommendations from the cardiologist. Chronic disease management requires frequent office visits or telephone calls; telephone triage can be done by all team members. Patients call frequently with questions about their care and these calls are documented in the EMR. Increasingly, patients and caregivers are able to communicate with their healthcare team using a patient portal system, which most healthcare organizations have adopted. All team members can document in the EMR, promoting better communication across the team and better coverage for the patient. The fact that CMS now provides reimbursement for such non-face-to-face activities incentivizes their adoption.

40.2.2 Third-Party Reimbursement and Chronic Care Management

Historically, government-based initiatives, such as Medicare and Medicaid, have only reimbursed providers for face-to-face encounters. Patients with multiple chronic conditions have generally been left to manage their own symptoms in-between office visits. This has often resulted in poor care coordination and possibly preventable emergency room visits and hospital readmissions, which impacts on the overall cost to the healthcare system. However, this reimbursement scheme has been modified in the last few years to better accommodate the growing need for coordinated long-term care.

In January 2015, CMS created new billing codes that allowed for reimbursement for chronic care management services provided to Medicare beneficiaries with two or more chronic diseases [18]. These guidelines were updated in January 2017 to increase the amount of reimbursement for non-face-to-face time, which includes telephone calls, secure emails, and text messaging [18]. This non-face-to-face time, including the patient consent, can be done by any members of the healthcare team including physicians, nurse practitioners, staff nurses, behavioral health workers, certified diabetes educators, and social workers.

The new codes take into account the patient's chronic conditions and are based on a comprehensive care plan for all team members to use. The time allotted is between 15 and 60 minutes and depends on the complexity of the chronic care management. The comprehensive care plan, which must be done by the provider, should include a current problem list, patient's prognosis and goals, symptoms management, planned interventions including medication management, referral to community or social services, a brief description of how services outside the practice will be coordinated and a schedule of periodic review and revision of the care plan [18]. Reference materials available on the MacColl Center website (▶ www.maccollcenter.org) discuss ways to create effective chronic care teams, as well as discussion of how to structure a practice to maximize the new CMS reimbursement provisions.

40.3 Special Clinical Considerations for Geriatric Chronic Care

There are three aspects of geriatric chronic care management that all practitioners should be familiar with. First, it is important to be aware of the fact that elderly patients do not always present with typical symptoms of common illnesses. Atypical presentation of signs and symptoms can lead to misdiagnosis and wrong treatment, or treatment injurious to a co-morbid condition. A brief review of atypical signs and symptoms appears below, with a case study.

Second, providers should be alert to the influence of certain common conditions associated with aging on the care of a patient with chronic illness. These geriatric syndromes, such as falls, incontinence, and other age-related changes in normal function, can often go undetected and can add further debility to the elderly patient with chronic illness. They can be assessed during routine office visits and treated to improve a patients' quality of life.

The third consideration for clinicians to keep in mind is that standard best practice guidelines for treating various conditions may need to be modified when dealing with geriatric patients with multiple chronic conditions. This is especially true in the area of geriatric prescribing, which becomes more complex, especially where a patient has multiple comorbidities. Medications that may treat one illness may exacerbate symptoms of another. If the patient is followed by several providers for their multiple conditions, the chance of medication errors or polypharmacy (overmedication or redundant prescribing by different providers) is also increased. The American Geriatric Society (AGS) Beers Criteria is introduced below as a useful guide to medications to avoid or to handle with caution when prescribing for geriatric patients. Examples of such considerations as they apply to guidelines for hypertension, diabetes, and heart failure are given below, with case studies highlighting a team approach to care.

40.3.1 Atypical Presentation

Geriatric patients may present with different signs and symptoms than a younger patient with the same illness. Typically, a patient with pneumonia will present with fever, fatigue, and productive cough. An elderly patient with pneumonia might instead present with a dry cough or shortness of breath, fatigue, and no fever – symptoms usually associated with heart failure. Similarly, a younger patient presenting with dysuria might be treated for a urinary tract infection after evaluation with a urine dipstick. An elderly patient might present with increased fatigue and new onset urinary incontinence without dysuria and would require evaluation of vital signs, orientation, and abdominal exam with diagnostic testing including urine analysis, urine culture, serum electrolytes and complete blood count. Atypical presentation in elderly patients is likely due to a combination of factors, including:

- Age-related physiologic changes such as decrease in kidney function [33]
- Age-related loss of physiologic reserve, such as loss of muscle strength otherwise known as sarcopenia [33]
- Interaction of chronic disease and acute illness and patient's underreporting of symptoms [30]

These changes can predispose an elderly patient to be more susceptible to infection or electrolyte imbalances [30]. Elderly individuals frequently require a more intensive work-up when compared to a younger patient. In order to arrive at an accurate diagnosis, providers should complete a detailed history from the patient or the caregiver, perform a thorough physical exam with a focus on the chief complaint, and do an appropriate diagnostic work-up, which may include blood tests and radiological imaging.

Failure to make early, accurate diagnosis and deliver proper treatment of metabolic conditions and infections in the elderly may result in increased hospital admissions and greater morbidity and mortality [10]. Team management of atypical presentation can be very effective, with team members assisting in early identification and treatment of atypical signs and symptoms in an elderly patient. The chart below illustrates some of the frequently encountered signs and symptoms of atypical presentation in an elderly patient (◘ Table 40.1).

Perhaps the best way to explain atypical presentation is by case study.

Case Study #1: Atypical Presentation

MH is an 89-year-old female with HTN, COPD and dementia. Over a three-week period, MH complained of the increased fatigue and weakness, dizziness when standing and tunnel vision. She experienced labored breathing and felt like she could not catch her breath. When talking to her son on the phone, she denied any fever or chills. However, she did sound more confused and was unable to remember when she last ate, drank or had a bowel movement. MH had no appetite or thirst. She was an active member of her church community but during this time she withdrew from normal social contacts and activities. MH did not want to go to urgent care, stating she preferred to stay in bed.

A close friend, a retired nurse, took MH to the emergency room; she was concerned MH might have congestive heart failure based on her symptoms of labored breathing, tunnel vision, lack of fever and cough. Patient had complete blood count with differential and chest x-ray and was diagnosed with pneumonia and dehydration. MH was treated with oral steroids, antibiotics and intravenous hydration. She was hospitalized for 1 week and was discharged with home healthcare and a close follow-up appointment with her primary care provider.

This case study is a classic presentation of atypical signs and symptoms in an elderly patient. MH had increased fatigue, lack of appetite and increased confusion which probably contributed to dehydration and worsening debility.

Table 40.1 Typical vs. atypical signs and symptoms

Typical presentation	Atypical presentation in elderly patients
Fever – temperature >38 °C (100.4 °F) [35]	Afebrile [35]
Cough with sputum production [34] Shortness of breath [34] Purulent sputum [34]	Absence of cough [30] Anorexia [30] Change in mental status [30] Functional decline [30]
Dysuria [31] Urinary frequency [31] Urinary urgency [31]	No complaint of dysuria [30] Altered mental status [30] New onset urinary incontinence [30]

40.3.2 Geriatric Syndromes

Caring for an older adult can be challenging. In addition to multiple chronic medical problems, and atypical presentation, older adults often develop geriatric syndromes. Geriatric syndromes are common conditions that occur in the elderly. They have multiple causes, involving multiple organ systems, with multiple risk factors [23], and are frequently misdiagnosed or undertreated. Commonly seen geriatric syndromes are listed in Table 40.2.

Geriatric syndromes are frequently associated with poor health outcomes and functional decline [24] and may impact or worsen normal age-related changes [23]. Elderly patients with geriatric syndromes may require a more extensive work-up than a younger patient with one chief complaint [15]. These syndromes have many causes and elderly patients maybe predisposed to developing geriatric syndromes based on their risk factors and other co-morbidities. Chronic conditions, in combination with geriatric syndromes, may significantly impact an elderly patient's functional status and their ability to effectively manage their health [29]. Urgent visits to different providers to evaluate these syndromes may result in duplication of diagnostic tests, polypharmacy, and worsening of patient's underlying medical conditions.

Ideally, patients with geriatric syndromes should be seen frequently by the same providers (i.e., doctor or APRN) which

Table 40.2 Commonly seen geriatric syndromes

Geriatric syndrome	Common causes	Risk factors
Falls	Dizziness Medication Polypharmacy Chronic conditions: Osteoarthritis, Parkinson's disease	Age Gender Vision and hearing problems Environmental hazards Dementia Gait and balance impairment Deconditioning Pain Frailty
Dizziness	Inner ear problem Vertigo Low blood pressure Neurological disorders Medication Hypoglycemia Anemia	Age Polypharmacy Kidney disease Diabetes
Urinary Incontinence	Age Menopause Enlarged prostate Medication Neurological disorders	Age Gender Obesity Family history Smoking
Delirium	Electrolyte imbalance Infection Anemia Hypoxemia Use of physical restraints Indwelling catheters	Polypharmacy Alcohol abuse Functional, cognitive or sensory impairment Depression History of delirium

can increase the likelihood of identifying the cause and evaluating the severity of the syndrome. Factors to mitigate geriatric syndromes could result in preventing or diminishing their impact on elderly patients [15]. While geriatric syndromes are not chronic diseases, their prevalence, functional impact on elderly patients and their association with a reduced quality of life indicate these syndromes should be evaluated along with chronic conditions during routine office visits [29].

Geriatric syndromes can have life-altering impacts on an elderly person. For example, a simple fall can have serious consequences, leaving someone who lived independently and was able to perform all activities of daily living (ADL) beforehand to end up with limited mobility and needing homecare. Osteoporosis or osteopenia, conditions that weaken the bone, make it easier for a simple fall to result in broken bones, which may require surgery and months of rehab. A lengthy stay in a hospital bed increases the risk of the patient developing pneumonia, which can prove fatal for a weakened elderly individual [9]. Even if the patient successfully completes rehab and returns home, a previously independent person may now need assistance with ADLs and require expensive renovations to their living space for safety and accessibility. This is illustrated in the following case study.

Case Study #2: Geriatric Syndromes: The Impact of a Fall

SF was an 85-year-old female living independently in a senior community. She required no assistance with activities of daily living (ADL) or instrumental activities of daily living (IADL). As SF was watching television 1 day, she got up suddenly from a chair and tripped on her carpet. She fell into the television cabinet, hitting her head, right wrist and right knee. In great pain, she was able to crawl to the phone, called 911 and was transported to a local hospital. She had sustained a fracture of her right wrist and complex fracture of her right femur.

SF was transported to a regional medical center for emergency surgery with a trauma surgeon. After surgery, she developed hyponatremia and elevated white blood count. She was hospitalized for 1 week, and then transferred to a sub-acute rehabilitation (SAR) center. While in SAR, she developed an upper respiratory infection, which was treated successfully, but which delayed her continuing physical therapy. She remained in SAR for 100 days, maxing out her Medicare-covered time in the SAR.

Upon SF's return home, she had to make renovations in her apartment, installing grab bars, a walk-in shower and new raised toilet. She was dependent on a walker to move around. Upon discharge from the SAR, SF was referred to visiting nurse, who ordered physical and occupational therapy, which allowed her to transition from the walker to a cane. She also paid privately for a home health aide for 34 hours per week, as SF now needed assistance with four of the six ADLs, including bathing, toileting, dressing, and transferring (walking) and needed assistance with all IADLs (cleaning and maintaining the house; managing money; moving within the community and preparing meals). The entire situation left her with persistent heightened anxiety and insomnia. Her primary care provider had to put her on Venlafaxine, which helped. Her life had changed drastically due to one fall.

40.3.3 Clinical Guidelines: Special Considerations for Elderly Patients

Clinical guidelines representing evidence-based best practice standards often exist for treating specific chronic illnesses. These guidelines provide algorithms for diagnosis, treatment options, and follow-up. However, the recommendations in these guidelines may be generalized to the broader patient population and thus fail to take into account special considerations that may apply to elderly patients, especially those presenting with multiple co-morbidities. Ignorance of these special considerations may lead to misdiagnosis, treating the wrong condition, or treating the right condition in a way that exacerbates a co-morbid illness. Awareness of these issues can prevent harm to the patient and avoid possible legal liability for the practitioner.

This section will first consider issues in geriatric prescribing and introduce a useful tool to help in selecting the right medications for geriatric patients. This is followed by discussion of how these special considerations for elderly patients apply within the guidelines for hypertension (HTN), type 2 diabetes mellitus (DM), and congestive heart failure (HF), by way of example. The importance of collaborative teams in managing patients with these conditions is also discussed.

40.3.4 Geriatric Prescribing

Elderly patients are more vulnerable to possible toxic effects of medications and sometimes less responsive to the therapeutic benefits, due to physiological changes of aging [38]. The AGS Beers Criteria for potentially inappropriate medication use in older adults (Beers Criteria) is a clinical tool developed by Mark Beers in 1991 and updated by the American Geriatric Society in 2019 [8]. The Beers Criteria lists medications that are inappropriate or to be used cautiously in older adults, medications that may interact adversely in older adults, and medications that should be adjusted based on older adults' kidney function [8]. It is used in conjunction with guidelines, evidence-based practice, and provider experience. A copy of the full Beers Criteria is available at ► https://www.americangeriatrics.org/.

40.3.5 Hypertension

While there are many hypertension guidelines available, this chapter has relied on those put out by the American College of Cardiology (ACC) and the American Heart Association (AHA) Task Force, published in 2017 [46]. Guideline recommendations for blood pressure are shown in Table 40.3. These blood pressure readings should be taken on at least two separate occasions [46] although, according to Kithas and Supiano [26], blood pressure should be checked on three separate occasions over a period of 4–6 weeks.

Nonpharmacological interventions have been shown to be effective in lowering blood pressure [36] and should be considered before starting medication. Recommendations for nonpharmacological interventions include:

- Low sodium diet, DASH diet (Dietary Approaches to Stop Hypertension) [26]
- Increased intake of potassium [46]
- Limited alcohol use [26]
- Increased physical activity and weight loss [26, 46]
- Smoking cessation [36]

The Trial of Nonpharmacologic Intervention in the Elderly (TONE) found that modest reductions in sodium intake and weight loss (average 4 kg) led to a 30% reduction in the need to restart antihypertensive medication in the intervention group [45].

These recommendations may be challenging to implement in an 80-year-old patient who has always added salt to their food, is unable to exercise due to osteoarthritis or balance problems, and has limited money to purchase fresh fruits and vegetables. In addition, certain ethnicities use seasonings which may have high sodium content, an example of this is adobo seasoning used in the Hispanic community, and present a practical application of the CCM's injunction about cultural sensitivity.

Team members can provide education for this patient on diet recommendations and exercise, as well as teaching the patient or their caregiver how to check their blood pressure at home. The patient might also be referred for home physical therapy by their provider and the social worker could offer information on food stamps and programs that provide healthy food in the patient's community.

Table 40.3 Blood pressure guidelines: normal vs. hypertensive

Status of patient's blood pressure	Blood pressure reading (mm Hg) (systolic/diastolic)
Normal	120/80
Elevated	120–129/<80
Stage 1 hypertension	130–139/or/80–89
Stage 2 hypertension	≥140/or/≥90
Normal for adults ≥60 years	<150/90 (JNC 8)

Whelton et al. [46]

If nonpharmacological interventions fail to lower blood pressure in 2–6 months, then initiating antihypertensive therapy is recommended as primary prevention for individuals who are at risk for developing atherosclerotic heart disease and for secondary prevention for those individuals at risk for recurrent cardiovascular events [46]. There are numerous blood pressure medications including:

- Thiazide or thiazide type diuretics
- Angiotensin converting enzyme (ACE)
- Angiotensin receptor blocker (ARB)
- Calcium channel blocker (CCB)

In addition to the medications listed above, secondary agents include other types of diuretics, beta-blockers, direct renin inhibitors, alpha blockers, centrally acting drugs, and vasodilators [46].

Primary recommendations on antihypertensive agents might not apply to an elderly patient who has urinary incontinence or hyperkalemia, since diuretics cause increased urination and ACE or ARB can cause hyperkalemia. There are other considerations for elderly individuals with co-morbidities such as DM or HF. An individual with HF would benefit from a diuretic, whereas one with DM should be on an ACE or ARB to prevent or decrease albuminuria. According to the guidelines, for a patient with HTN and HF or HTN and DM, optimal blood pressure is <130/80 [46]. However, this reading might be too low for an elderly individual with multiple co-morbidities, causing them to feel dizzy or lightheaded and possibly leading them to suffer a bad fall.

When adjusting blood pressure medication, it is important to assess how the patient feels on a certain medication and whether they are experiencing side effects. The patient should have close follow-up in 1–2 weeks to review blood pressure readings and possible side effects. In the case of diuretics, ACE and ARB, diagnostic blood tests such as creatinine and serum potassium are especially helpful. If a patient complains of dizziness or lightheadedness, orthostatic blood pressure and pulse should be taken during the office visit.

In general, elderly individuals are often at risk for orthostatic hypotension (defined as a drop in systolic blood pressure of 20 mm Hg or decrease in diastolic blood pressure of 10 mm Hg within 3 minutes of standing) due to various factors such as medication, anemia, lack of adequate hydration, and possible metabolic or infectious disease process [28]. Performing orthostatic blood pressures when elderly patients complain of dizziness, lightheadedness, or weakness can help the provider to determine whether the medication needs to be adjusted or discontinued.

ACC/AHA HTN guidelines recommend treatment for a blood pressure goal of 130/80 or less for non-institutionalized community-dwelling individuals 65 years or older, if the blood pressure is over 130/80 [46]. However, for elderly individuals with multiple co-morbidities and limited life expectancy, patient preference and the judgment of the provider should be taken into consideration.

40.3.6 Diabetes Mellitus (DM)

The diagnosis of DM is based on the patient meeting any one of the following criteria:

- Fasting plasma glucose ≥126 mg/dl
- 2-hour plasma glucose ≥200 mg/dl after an oral glucose tolerance test
- Hemoglobin A1c ≥6.5%

American Diabetes Association [7]

The American Diabetes Association (ADA), reflecting principles of CCM, recommends patient-centered communication that takes into account patient preferences and patient's health literacy and addresses any cultural barriers to care [6]. The ADA also supports team-based care aligned with the components of the CCM to enable greater self-care by the patient [6]. Management of DM requires evaluation of the social, medical, and emotional aspects of an elderly patient, which is best achieved using a team approach [7].

There are several points to consider in elderly patients with DM:

- Does the patient have other co-morbidities which may impact on DM [7]?
- Is this a new diagnosis for an elderly patient who has had undiagnosed DM for years and is experiencing complications [39]?
- Is this a new diagnosis with no or minimal complications [39]?

Elderly patients with DM have a higher incidence of dementia, which impacts on their ability to monitor glucose and be compliant with medication and diet [47]. Team members can improve patient's compliance with frequent phone calls and close follow-up. This is emphasized in the case study listed below where team members worked closely together to coordinate care for a patient with DM and dementia.

Case Study #3: DM with Dementia

- Patient's daughter calls the nurse triage line, stating patient's finger stick is 400. Patient has dementia and lives with his daughter.
- Nurse in the practice calls patient's daughter to ask about patient's symptoms, food intake and medication compliance. The daughter realizes that patient has been more tired recently and finger sticks have been elevated for several days. Nurse recommends an urgent visit to the practice and contacts social work to arrange transportation.
- Patient is scheduled for a visit with the urgent provider, who sees the patient, orders diagnostic tests including glucose and urine analysis and urine culture.
- In office, patient complains of fatigue and vital signs are stable. Patient's glucose = 450, urine analysis indicates urinary tract infection, the urgent provider orders Novolog insulin to be administered in the office, e-prescribes antibiotic for possible urinary infection and orders intravenous fluid. Patient's finger stick = 200 after intravenous hydration and Novolog insulin.
- Patient is discharged with a follow-up appointment later in the week.

In 2017, the American Association of Clinical Endocrinologists (AACE) / American College of Endocrinology (ACE) published a consensus statement on the management of DM which featured as key components, lifestyle modification and weight loss. Goals for A1c and blood glucose should be based on age, co-morbidities, life expectancy, years of having DM, risk of hypoglycemia/hyperglycemia, patient motivation and compliance, cost of medication, and diabetes supplies [21]. The APRN, staff nurse, and a certified diabetic educator on the healthcare team can educate the patient or their caregiver in how to check their blood sugar with a glucometer and the importance of maintaining a log of finger sticks vs. meals and exercise.

Lifestyle modification involves all members of the healthcare team and includes medical nutrition therapy (MNT), physical activity and behavioral support, promotion of sleep hygiene, and tobacco cessation [21]. Goals of MNT are to promote healthy eating patterns based on an individual's personal and cultural preferences, health literacy, and access to healthy foods [6]. An evaluation of patient's living situation and social support at home are important considerations when determining goals of MNT and medication.

- Social work and nursing staff can help to determine patient's food preferences and social workers can explore patient's living situation and make appropriate referrals as needed.
- During a patient interview, social work can evaluate the patient's ability to afford healthy foods, which in general cost more than processed foods.
- Community resources available for elderly patients include Meals on Wheels, local senior centers, and the US Department of Agriculture's Older Americans Nutrition Program [25]. When possible, patients would benefit from a referral to a certified diabetes educator or nutritionist in order to receive additional education on food choices.

Physical activity is another component of lifestyle modification and one which patients should be encouraged to do. Physical activity can reduce blood glucose, blood pressure, and hyperlipidemia [21]. A standard recommendation is 150 minutes per week of moderate intensity exercise such as walking and weight training [6]. Nursing staff can provide patients with information on a home exercise program and social work can offer information on exercise programs and gym memberships available to seniors. For example, several insurance companies have developed the Silver Sneakers program, which provides free exercise classes at local facilities to enrolled seniors. Social workers can also provide information on behavioral support and smoking cessation, including community groups dedicated to healthy lifestyle and smoking cessation programs.

Elderly patients with DM should also be evaluated for depression [7]. Depression is common in the elderly and can affect the patient's quality of life and healthcare use [42]. Providers, nursing, and social work staff can screen for depression and make appropriate referrals if positive, although new CMS reimbursement codes will cover a behavioral health worker as well.

If lifestyle modification fails in decreasing A1c for elderly individuals, then drug therapy should be initiated. The ACCE supports an A1c ≤6.5% for most patients. Although a range of ≥6.5–8.0% is recommended if a lower A1c would cause an adverse outcome [21], older individuals who have long-standing DM and are at risk for cardiovascular disease were found to have increased mortality with A1c <6.0% [1].

The American Diabetes Association target A1c treatment goals and recommendations for older individuals are shown in ◘ Table 40.4:

Elderly patients with DM are at risk for episodes of hypoglycemia or hyperglycemia. This is a particular concern with an individual who has dementia with multiple co-morbidities. Team members can work closely with patient caregivers to monitor fluctuations in glucose. Less stringent guidelines, as listed above, are more appropriate for these patients.

Important considerations when prescribing diabetic medication for the elderly include determining the patient's renal function by measuring the glomerular filtration rate or creatinine clearance. Cost of medication and medication frequency should be taken into account when prescribing for an older patient. The Beers Criteria can help guide clinicians in medications to avoid in elderly patients [8].

The American Diabetes Association recommends metformin (Glucophage) as an initial treatment of elderly individuals with diabetes. Metformin is generally well tolerated and can be given once a day. It should be avoided in elderly individuals with advanced kidney disease and heart failure [13]. Insulin therapy is another option, but it requires that the patient or caregiver have visual, cognitive, and manual dexterity [7].

There are a number of medication options for treating DM, some of which should not be prescribed for older adults. Patients with a history of heart failure should not be prescribed thiazolidinedione (Actos or Avandia) since this medication can cause fluid retention [13]. Insulin secretagogues such as sulfonylureas (Amaryl, Glucotrol) can cause hypoglycemia. Elderly patients should therefore be prescribed short-acting sulfonylureas to decrease the incidence of hypoglycemia [13]. Another medication, α-glucosidase inhibitors, such as acarbose, should be avoided in elderly patients with creatinine clearance ≤24 ml/min and can cause gastrointestinal side effects such as diarrhea and gas [13]. Dipeptidyl peptidase 4 inhibitors (Januvia, Tradjenta) are generally well tolerated but are expensive and may not be covered by patient's insurance [7].

◘ **Table 40.4** ADA recommendations for target A1c

Individual	Impairments or co-morbidities	Target A1c
Healthy individual	Limited co-morbidities Cognitively intact and functional	<7.5%
Individual with:	Multiple co-morbidities Impairment in 2+ IADLs Mild-to-moderate cognitive impairment	<8.0%
Individual with poor health	End-stage disease Dependent in 2+ ADLs or Moderate to severe cognitive impairment	<8.5%

ADA [7]

Case Study #4: Elderly Female with HTN, DM, and Mild Cognitive Impairment

BY is an 85-year-old African American female patient who recently moved to New York City to live with her daughter. In addition to the diagnoses listed above, patient has osteoarthritis, glaucoma and history of frequent falls. Her daughter brings her to the initial appointment in the geriatric outpatient practice.

- BY is interviewed by the medical student working with primary care provider (PCP). Patient is on amlodipine for HTN and Glipizide XL for DM. Patient's blood pressure is 170/90. She scores 25/30 on Mini Mental Examination and denies depression. Her blood glucose = 300 in the practice.
- PCP refers the patient to the staff nurse, who discusses diet with BY and her daughter.
- PCP also orders 2 units of Novolog insulin to be given immediately.
- Patient admits to eating ice cream several times per week and does not check her blood glucose at home. Staff nurse refers patient to social work to discuss available resources in the community, such as local senior centers and Meals on Wheels.
- PCP orders visiting nurse to see patient at home to review using glucometer and medication compliance. PCP also discontinues amlodipine and starts an ACE inhibitor, Lisinopril 5 mg daily because ACE inhibitors have been shown to decrease protein levels in the urine.
- BY and daughter leave the practice with a follow-up appointment with the APRN in 2 weeks and referrals to visiting nurse service, nutritionist and ophthalmology.
- PCP reviews patient's test results the following day. Patient's A1c = 9,

GFR >60.00 mL/min/1.73 m2. PCP contacts patient's daughter and discusses stopping Glipizide XL and starting Glucophage 500 mg twice a day; prescription is sent to pharmacy.
- Visiting nurse sees patient the following week and contacts PCP, stating patient has difficulty performing glucose checks and will need supervision by the daughter. Daughter agrees to check patient's glucose daily and record results. Visiting nurse reviews dietary restrictions with patient and daughter and provides a weekly pill box for patient use.
- BY starts metformin and complains of nausea. Daughter calls triage line and speaks with the staff nurse who states this is a common side effect and should resolve within a few weeks.
- BY continues medication and sees the APRN in 2 weeks. Blood pressure is 150/90 and glucose in practice = 150. APRN increases Lisinopril to 10 mg daily and orders basic metabolic blood test, patient's potassium = 4.5 and GFR is within normal limits.
- Patient is seen again in 2 weeks and blood pressure = 130/80, blood glucose = 120; potassium = 4.8, GFR is within normal limits. BY states nausea has resolved, is attending a senior center at lunchtime and is only eating ice cream once a week.

40.4 Heart Failure (HF)

HF patients complain of shortness of breath, fatigue, fluid retention, weight gain, and decreased exercise tolerance [3, 48]. There is no single diagnostic test for HF. Diagnosis is based on patient's symptoms, health history, and physical exam. Two blood tests that may be useful in diagnosing HF are the brain natriuretic peptide (BNP) and N-terminal pro-B-type natriuretic peptide (NT-pro BNP) [48]. These tests are helpful both in excluding the diagnosis of HF and in establishing prognosis and severity of HF [49]. However, elevation of these test results may be due to other underlying conditions such as obesity, renal failure, and atrial fibrillation, to name a few (HF 2017 guidelines). Some of the risk factors for HF include HTN, DM, atherosclerotic heart disease, and metabolic syndrome [48].

The two types of HF are (1) HF with preserved ejection fraction (EF) and (2) HF with reduced EF [48]. The American College of Cardiology and the American Heart Association (ACC/AHA) and the New York Heart Association (NYHA) have provided stages and classifications of the degree of HF, respectively. The ACC/AHA categorizes heart failure in four stages with Stage 1 having modifiable risk factors while Stage 4 is considered refractory heart failure requiring specialized interventions [48]. In comparison, the NYHA classifies heart failure in four categories beginning with asymptomatic heart failure with no limits on physical activity and progressing to symptomatic heart failure seen with any physical activity [48].

Managing heart failure requires a combination of medication compliance and lifestyle modification through diet and exercise. Patients can be taught how to modify their lifestyle by learning to apply principles of self-care. Many outpatient multidisciplinary heart failure programs focus on teaching patients to improve self-care and compliance [4]. Patients need to understand how to monitor their weight and their symptoms, restrict sodium and understand the benefit of taking their medications daily [48].

A team approach to providing care to elderly HF patients encompasses the following elements:

- Assessing patient's social support to promote treatment adherence and a healthy lifestyle [37]
- Patient education with emphasis on self-management and medication adherence. Education should include symptom monitoring, weight gain and changes in functional status [37]
- Increased access to care, especially during times of acute episodes
- Sodium restriction of 1500 mg/dl, according to the American Heart Association. This recommendation is based on the stage of HF (i.e., A and B); usually a greater degree of sodium restriction is required for more advanced stages of HF (i.e., C and D) [48]
- Promoting physical activity, weight loss and when possible, referring patient to cardiac rehabilitation [48]
- Avoidance of certain medications which may exacerbate heart failure such as nonsteroidal anti-inflammatory drugs (NSAIDS) and some cancer drugs [37]
- Encourage smoking cessation and avoidance of alcohol [41, 44]

Managing HF effectively is important for the patient as well as the healthcare organization. The CMS has developed risk-standardized 30-day core measures which establish "best practice" standards for acute myocardial infarction, heart failure, and pneumonia. The agency collects data on these core measures, since patient readmissions within 30 days can be expensive and are considered a negative event for the patient [19]. Measuring readmission rates in hospitals can motivate hospitals to invest in interventions that will improve care. The core measures also help to assess whether the patient is ready for discharge and can facilitate transition from the inpatient to the outpatient setting [19]. These measures are updated annually and have been endorsed by the National Quality Forum. Since October of 2012, hospitals with an excess of readmissions for these conditions began receiving decreased reimbursement from CMS [19].

Pharmacological therapy is often required for HF patients. Medication categories include diuretics, angiotensin-converting enzyme (ACE) inhibitor, angiotensin receptor blocker (ARB), beta-blockers, angiotensin receptor-neprilysin inhibitor, I_f channel inhibitor, aldosterone receptor antagonists, hydralazine and isosorbide dinitrate, and digoxin [49]. When prescribing medication for elderly HF patients, providers should consider at least three key points: (1) cost of medication, (2) frequency of medication, and (3) polypharmacy. Special considerations for three of the more commonly used HF medications (diuretics, ACE inhibitors, and beta-blockers) are discussed below.

Diuretic therapy is usually the initial treatment for an elderly patient experiencing symptoms of HF, including fluid retention, shortness of breath and weight gain [48]. Loop diuretics such as furosemide are more potent than thiazide diuretics for HF patients. Diuretics should be used cautiously and at a low dose when initially prescribed. Patient's renal function should be evaluated before and after initiating diuretics. Diuretic therapy can decrease potassium and magnesium levels which could lead to cardiac arrhythmias [48].

Patients should also be evaluated for hypotension, which may occur with diuretic therapy. In particular, elderly HF patients starting diuretic therapy should be evaluated for dizziness and orthostatic hypotension, which might be related to dehydration. While initiating diuretic therapy, close follow-up within 1–2 weeks is recommended.

ACE inhibitors can decrease mortality and hospitalizations in HF patients [48]. Prior to starting an ACE inhibitor, elderly patients with HF should have serum electrolytes checked, since this medication can cause hyperkalemia and worsen renal function [48]. Patients should start at a low dose with follow-up in 1–2 weeks to check renal function and potassium, as well as patient's response to therapy [48].

A life-threatening adverse side effect of ACE inhibitors is angioedema. If this occurs, the patient should discontinue medication immediately and be evaluated in an emergency room or urgent care practice [48]. Dry cough is a common side effect of ACE inhibitors, which could aggravate a patient's preexisting chronic obstructive pulmonary disease (COPD) symptoms. If this occurs, patient may need to stop the ACE inhibitor and start an ARB [48]. ARBs are prescribed when patients cannot tolerate ACE inhibitors. As with ACE inhibitors, elderly patients with HF should start at a low dose and follow-up in 1–2 weeks to check renal function and potassium, since ARBs can cause hyperkalemia and worsening renal function.

Beta-blockers are also prescribed for HF patients. Three beta-blockers (carvedilol, bisoprolol, and metoprolol XL) have been found to decrease morbidity and mortality in chronic HF with reduced EF [48]. As with other medications, when prescribing for elderly HF patients, a low dose is best. Patients should be monitored for fluid retention, worsening HF, fatigue, bradycardia or heart block and hypotension [48]. Elderly HF patients should be seen 1–2 weeks after starting beta-blockers to check blood pressure, heart rate, and signs of fatigue and fluid retention. Beta-blockers should be used cautiously in patients with reactive airway disease such as asthma or COPD [48].

In caring for elderly HF patients, a team approach works best. Providers and nursing and social work staff play key roles in coordinating care for HF patients. A case study might best emphasize these points.

Case Study # 5: Team Collaborative Care of HF and HTN

- An 80-year-old male with worsening shortness of breath and fatigue is seen by his primary care provider. Patient takes furosemide 40 mg twice a day, has no weight gain but blood pressure is 150/90 and patient's lungs sound clear to auscultation.
- The provider starts patient on an ACE inhibitor, Accupril 5 mg daily.
- Patient meets with the staff nurse to discuss possible side effects of the medication and review low sodium diet.
- Provider receives a call from the pharmacy that medication is not covered by insurance; medication is changed to one that is covered, Lisinopril 5 mg daily. Staff nurse relays this information to the patient.
- Two days later, patient's son calls stating patient is very dizzy. Son contacts the social worker to arrange for transportation and patient is seen by the urgent provider.
- Patient's orthostatic blood pressure is 140/80 supine and 120/70 standing, with heart rate of 60. Urgent provider orders blood test to check renal function and potassium, potassium level is 5.0 mEq/L and creatinine is 1.5 mg/dl. Lisinopril is decreased to 2.5 mg daily.
- Patient returns the following week to see the APRN. At this visit, patient denies dizziness and is not orthostatic by blood pressure; creatinine is at patient's baseline and potassium = 4.5 mEq/L.

40.5 Conclusion

The US healthcare system is undergoing a fundamental shift in how good chronic care is defined, practiced, and financed, driven by demographic and epidemiological forces. Healthcare practitioners across practically all disciplines of medicine will need to develop competency in the special issues involved in the effective care of a growing population of elderly patients who will often have multiple chronic illnesses. The purpose of this chapter has been to provide a brief overview of key issues surrounding this shift.

It should be noted that at this time, the number of new physicians entering the healthcare system has been declining, and even fewer are specializing in geriatrics. It is expected that by 2025, the demand for physicians will exceed supply by a range of between 46,000 to 90,000 [11]. As well, fewer graduates from medical schools are pursuing careers in geriatrics, due to relatively poor reimbursement and the prospect of being overwhelmed with the complexities of managing older patients with multiple co-morbidities [12]. In fact, provider burnout is one of the main reasons for the decline in the number of medical students specializing in primary care and geriatrics [20].

As the number of medical student admissions declines, however, there has been an increase in the number of APRNs entering programs and pursuing careers in primary care and family medicine [5]. APRNs include nurse practitioners, clinical nurse specialists, nurse anesthetists, and midwives. In fact, approximately 89% of APRNs have been educated to practice in primary care, including adult and geriatric health, family medicine, pediatrics, and women's health [5].

APRNs working closely with physicians allow for a more comprehensive approach to patient care. The attending physician can see the patient every 3–4 months for routine follow-up, while the APRN will see the patient in-between those visits. The APRN focuses on chronic disease management and education for such conditions as hypertension, congestive heart failure, and diabetes. APRNs can also order and interpret diagnostic testing and prescribe medication. APRNs see patients for routine follow-up, urgent evaluation, or follow-up after discharge from the hospital.

With the growing number of geriatric patients needing chronic care management, physicians and APRNs working collaboratively in the context of healthcare teams will be able to provide more cost-effective comprehensive care to this population. Improved comprehensive management of geriatric patients with chronic conditions can slow the progression of their illness and its attendant disability and reduce the number of emergency room visits, hospital admissions, and readmissions.

Since the introduction of the Wagner CCM, many of its core principles have been adapted to a variety of medical environments. For instance, outpatient primary care services are sometimes supplemented by Visiting Doctors, a multidisciplinary team that provides primary care to homebound patients. The team may consist of attending physicians, an APRN, a social worker, and an administrative assistant. Team members can see patients monthly and discuss ongoing issues with the patients they follow. The Visiting Doctor model of care is particularly important for the patient unable to leave their home, yet still needing ongoing care for complex medical problems. Providers are able to order x-rays and ultrasounds to be done in the patient's home, thereby allowing for a more comprehensive work-up on a patient's signs and symptoms (January 2, 2018 email from S Sonica to S Sundel).

While the CCM originally was focused on chronic care management in an outpatient primary care setting, inpatient acute care geriatric services have also begun to include care coordination and chronic care management for this population. Many of these services are known as Mobile Acute Care for the Elderly [22]. Historically, acute care for elderly patients occurred on one unit in the hospital; however as census decreased and providers found elderly patients on all floors, the MACE team was created. Team members can include a board certified geriatrician, geriatric fellows, pharmacist, APRN, social worker, and consultants in physical therapy, occupational therapy, speech therapist, and nutrition.

Alternatively, some hospitals employ a consult service, consisting of a board certified geriatric physician and geriatric fellows to follow inpatient geriatric patients. These inpatient teams work closely with providers in outpatient practices, subacute rehabilitation (SAR), and nursing homes to promote the patient's safe transition from the hospital to the home, SAR, or nursing home.

As we go forward, the face of healthcare delivery in the USA is changing in a number of significant ways: from episodic treatment to chronic care, from fragmented to coordinated care, incentivized by a change in the healthcare third-party payment system. The promotion of increased patient self-management of chronic illness and the expansion of a collaborative team-based approach to chronic care will allow primary care providers the opportunity to employ their limited time more productively, while increasing both the quality and cost-effectiveness of care afforded to the growing number of geriatric patients with chronic illness.

References

1. Action to Control Cardiovascular Risk in Diabetes Study Group, Gerstein HC, Miller ME, et al. Effects of intensive glucose lowering in type 2 diabetes. N Engl J Med. 2008;358:2545–59. https://doi.org/10.1056/NEJMoa0802743.
2. Agency for Healthcare Research and Quality [Internet]. Chronic disease management can reduce admissions; 2014 March [cited 2018 January 13]. Available from: https://innovations.ahrq.gov/perspectives/chronicdisease-management-can-reduce-readmissions.
3. Ahmed A. Defeat – Heart failure: a guide to management of geriatric heart failure by generalist physicians. Minerva Med. 2009;100(1):39–50.
4. Albert NM, Collier S, Sumodi V, Wilkinson S, Hammel JP, Vopat L, et al. Nurses' knowledge of heart failure education principles. Heart Lung. 2002;31(2):102–12. https://doi.org/10.4037/ajcc2013212.
5. American Association of Nurse Practitioners [Internet]. Nurse practitioners in primary care. Alexandria, VA: American Association of Nurse Practitioners; [cited 2018 January 14]. 2p. Available from: https://www.aanp.org/.
6. American Diabetes Association. Standards of medical care in diabetes – 2016 abridged for primary care providers. Clin Diabetes. 2016;34(1):3–21. https://doi.org/10.2337/diaclin.34.1.3.
7. American Diabetes Association. Standards of medical care in diabetes – 2017. Clin Diabetes. 2017;40(1):1–142. https://doi.org/10.2337/dc17-S003.
8. American Geriatrics Society 2019 Beers Criteria Update Expert Panel. American geriatrics society 2019 updated beers criteria for potentially inappropriate medication use in older adults. J Am Geriatr Soc. 2019;67(4):674–94. https://doi.org/10.1111/jgs.15767.
9. American Thoracic Society[Internet]. Top 20 pneumonia facts – 2018; 2018 [cited 2018 January 13]. Available from: https://www.thoracic.org/patients/patient-resources/resources/top-pneumonia-facts.pdf.
10. Anderson G. Chronic care: Making the case for ongoing care [Internet]. Princeton, NJ; 2010. [cited 2017 December 5]. 43p. Available from the Robert Wood Johnson Foundation website: https://www.rwjf.org.
11. Association of American Medical Colleges [Internet]. The complexities of physician supply and demand 2017 update: Projections from 2015 to 2030. Washington, DC: Association of American Medical Colleges; 2017 February [cited 2018 January 7]. 68p. Available from: https://aamc-black.global.ssl.fastly.net/production/media/filer_public/a5/c3/a5c3d565-14ec-48fb-974b-99fafaeecb00/aamc_projections_update_2017.pdf.
12. Bagri A, Tiberius R. Medical students perspectives on geriatrics and geriatric education. J Am Geriatr Soc. 2010;58(10):1994–9. https://doi.org/10.1111/j.1532-5415.2010.03074.x.

13. Bansal N, Dhaliwal R, Weinstock RS. Management of diabetes in the elderly. Med Clin North Am. 2015;99(2):351–77. https://doi.org/10.1016/j.mcna.2014.
14. Buttorff C, Ruder T, Bauman M. Multiple chronic conditions in the United States [Internet]. Santa Monica, Calif: Rand Corporation; 2017. [cited 2017 Dec 5]. 33 p. Available from: https://www.rand.org/pubs/tools/TL221.html.
15. Carlson C, Merel SE, Yukawa M. Geriatric syndromes and geriatric assessment for the generalist. Med Clin North Am. 2015;99(2):263–79. https://doi.org/10.1016/j.mcna.2014.11.003.
16. Centers for Disease Control and Prevention [Internet]. The state of aging and health in America 2013. Atlanta, GA: Centers for Disease Control and Prevention, US Dept. of Health and Human Services; 2013 [cited 2017 October 5]. Available from: https://www.cdc.gov/aging/pdf/state-aging-health-in-america-2013.pdf.
17. Center for Medicare and Medicaid Services [Internet]. Quick facts about programs of all-inclusive care for the elderly (PACE); 2011 [cited 2017 November 29]. Available from: https://www.medicare.gov/your-medicare-costs/help-paying-costs/pace/pace.html.
18. Center for Medicare and Medicaid Services [Internet]. Chronic care management changes for 2017; 2016 December [cited 2017 December 5]. Available from: https://www.cms.gov/Outreach-and-Education/Medicare-Learning-Network-MLN/MLNProducts/Downloads/ChronicCareManagementServicesChanges2017.pdf.
19. Center for Medicare and Medicaid Services [Internet]. Outcome measures; 2017 October [cited 2017 Dec 7]. Available from: https://www.cms.gov/Medicare/Quality-Initiatives-Patient-Assessment-Instruments/HospitalQualityInits/OutcomeMeasures.html.
20. Drummond D. Physician burnout. Fam Pract Manag. 2015;22(5):42–7.
21. Garber AJ, Abrahamson MJ, Barzilay JI, Blonde L, Bloomgarden ZT, Bush MA. Consensus statement by the American association of clinical endocrinologists and american college of endocrinology on the comprehensive type 2 diabetes management algorithm – 2017 executive summary. Endocr Pract. 2017;23(2):207–38. https://doi.org/10.4158/EP161682.CS.
22. Hung WW, Ross JS, Farber J, Siu AL. Evaluation of the mobile acute care of the elderly service. JAMA Intern Med. 2013;173(11):990–6. https://doi.org/10.1001/jamainternmed.2013.478.
23. Inouye SK, Studenski S, Tinetti ME, Kuchel GA. Geriatric syndromes: clinical, research, and policy implications of a core geriatric concept. J Am Geriatr Soc. 2007;55(5):780–91. https://doi.org/10.1111/j.1532-5415.2007.01156.x.
24. Karoukian SM, Schiltz N, Warner DF, Sun J, Bakaki PM, Smyth KA, et al. Combinations of chronic conditions, functional limitations, and geriatric syndromes that predict health outcomes. J Gen Intern Med. 2016;31(6):630–7. https://doi.org/10.1007/s11606-016-3590-9.
25. Kirkman MS, Jones Briscoe V, Clark N, Florez H, Haas LB, Halter JB. Diabetes in older adults. Diabetes Care. 2012;35(12):2650–64. https://doi.org/10.2337/dc12-1801.
26. Kithas PA, Supiano MA. Hypertension in the geriatric population. Med Clin North Am. 2015;99(2):379–89. https://doi.org/10.1016/j.mcna.2014.11.009.
27. Klein S., Hostetter M, McCarthy D. The hospital at home model: bringing hospital-level care to the patient [Internet]. The Commonwealth Fund; 2016 August; 25: 1–11. Available from: http://www.commonwealthfund.org
28. Lanier JB, Mote MB, Clay EC. Evaluation and management of orthostatic hypotension. Am Fam Physician. 2011;84(5):527–36.
29. Lee PG, Cigolle C, Blaum C. The co-occurrence of chronic diseases and geriatric syndromes: the health and retirement study. J Am Geriatr Soc. 2009;57(3):511–6. https://doi.org/10.1111/j.1532-5415.2008.02150.x.
30. Liang SY. Sepsis and other infectious disease emergencies in the elderly. Emerg Med Clin North Am. 2016;34(3):501–22. https://doi.org/10.1016/j.emc.2016.04.005.
31. Michels TC, Sands JE. Dysuria: evaluation and differential diagnosis in adults. Am Fam Physician. 2015;92(9):778–88.
32. Munshi MN, Segal AR, Suhl E, Ryan C, Sternthal A, Giusti J, et al. Assessment of barriers to improve diabetes management in older adults. Diabetes Care. 2013;36(3):543–9. https://doi.org/10.2337/dc12-1303.
33. Navaratnarajah A, Jackson SHD. The physiology of aging. Medicine. 2017;45(1):6–10. https://doi.org/10.1016/j.mpmed.2016.10.008.
34. Niederman MS. Community acquired pneumonia. Ann Intern Med. 2015;163(7):ITC1–17. https://doi.org/10.7326/AITC201510060.
35. Norman DC. Fever in the elderly. Clin Infect Dis. 2000;31(1):148–51. https://doi.org/10.1086/313896.
36. Oza R, Garcellano M. Nonpharmacologic management of hypertension: what works? Am Fam Physician. 2015;91(11):772–6.
37. Ponikowski P, Voors AA, Anker SD, Bueno H, Cleland JGF, Coats AJS, et al. 2016 ESC Guidelines for the diagnosis and treatment of acute and chronic heart failure. The task force for the diagnosis and treatment of acute and chronic heart failure of the European society of cardiology (ESC). Eur Heart J. 2016;37(27):2129–200. https://doi.org/10.1093/eurheartj/ehw128.
38. Pretorius RW, Gataric G, Swedlund S, Miller JR. Am Fam Physician. 2013;87(5):331–6.
39. Selvin E, Coresh J, Brancati FL. The burden and treatment of diabetes in elderly individuals in the U.S. Diabetes Care. 2006;29(11):2415–9.
40. Shepperd S, doll H, Angus RM, Clarke MJ, Iliffe S, Kalra L. Avoiding hospital readmission through provision of hospital care at home: a systematic review and meta-analysis of individual patient data. CMAJ. 2009;180(2):175–82. https://doi.org/10.1503/cmaj.081491.
41. Suskin N, Sheth T, Negassa A, Yusuf S. Relationship of current and past smoking to mortality and morbidity in patients with left ventricular dysfunction. J Am Coll Cardiol. 2001;37(6):1677–82.
42. Tran HT, Leonard SD. Geriatric assessment for primary care providers. Prim Care. 2017;44(3):399–411. https://doi.org/10.1016/j.pop.2017.05.001.
43. Wagner EH. Chronic disease management: what will it take to improve care for chronic illness? Eff Clin Pract. 1998;1:2–4.
44. Wannamethee SG, Whincup PH, Lennon L, Papacosta O, Shaper AG. Alcohol consumption and risk of incident heart failure in older men: a prospective cohort study. Open Heart. 2015;2(1):1–9. https://doi.org/10.1136/openhrt-2015-000266.
45. Whelton PK, Appel LJ, Espeland MA, Applegate WB, Ettinger WH Jr, Kostis JB, et al. Sodium reduction and weight loss in the treatment of hypertension in older persons: a Buttorf et al. 2017omized controlled trial of nonpharmacologic interventions in the elderly (TONE). JAMA. 1998;279(11):839–46.
46. Whelton PK, Carey RM, Aronow WS, Casey DE Jr, Collins KJ, Dennison Himmelfarb CD, et al. ACC/AHA/AAPA/ABC/ACPM/AGS/APhA/ASH/ASPC/NMA/PCNA guideline for the prevention, detection, evaluation, and management of high blood pressure in adults: executive summary: a report of the American College of Cardiology/American Heart Association Task Force on Clinical Practice Guidelines. Hypertension. 2017;71:481p. https://doi.org/10.1016/j.jacc.2017.11.006.
47. Xu WL, von Strauss E, Qiu CX, Winblad B, Fratiglioni L. Uncontrolled diabetes increases the risk of Alzheimer's disease: a population based cohort study. Diabetologia. 2009;52(6):1031–9. https://doi.org/10.1007/s00125-009-1323-x.
48. Yancy CW, Jessup M, Bozkurt B, Butler J, Casey DE Jr, Drazner MH, et al. ACCF/AHA guideline for the management of heart failure: a report of the American College of Cardiology Foundation/American Heart Association Task Force on Practice Guidelines. Circulation. 2013;128(16):1810–52. https://doi.org/10.1161/CIR.0b013e31829e8807.
49. Yancy CW, Jessup M, Bozkurt B, Butler J, Casey DE Jr, Colvin MM, et al. ACC/AHA/HFSA focused update of the 2013 ACCF/AHA guideline for the management of heart failure: a report of the American College of Cardiology/American Heart Association Task Force on Clinical Practice Guidelines and the Heart Failure Society of America. Circulation. 2017;136(6):e137–61. https://doi.org/10.1161/CIR.0000000000000509.

Registries/Data in Population Health Management

Ania Wajnberg and Bernard F. Ortega

A. Chun (ed.), *Geriatric Practice*, https://doi.org/10.1007/978-3-030-19625-7_41

41.1 Introduction

Case Example

Dr. S, medical director of an outpatient geriatric practice, wants to make sure that all patients who are seen in the ER are seen promptly for follow-up after discharge back to the community. Dr. S is aware that the literature supports rapid outpatient follow-up after an ED visit or hospitalization and that this is a high-risk time for her geriatric patients. She decides to approach her institution's analytics department to find out how she can ensure that no patients slip through the cracks for a post-discharge phone call and visit.

41.2 What Is Population Health Management?

The landscape of healthcare delivery is changing more today than it ever has before. There have been exponential advances in diagnostic and treatment technologies, and a growing public concern over the accessibility, equity, and cost of healthcare has made healthcare policy and legislation a larger fixture in regular conversation. The need to deliver patient-centered, high-quality care at lower costs – or what has been bundled as the triple aim [1] – is becoming increasingly clear.

One strategy to achieve this triple aim of healthcare improvement is by effectively and efficiently managing population health – or the health outcomes of a group of individuals, including the distribution of such outcomes within the group [2]. Population health management has been defined by a leading outcomes management provider as the "aggregation and analysis of patient data and the actions through which care providers can improve both clinical and financial outcomes for any given group of patients." [3] To achieve effective population health management, several capabilities must be developed and deployed in symbiosis with each other. First, payment structures and contracts with the organizations that finance healthcare (i.e., health insurance companies, trade and labor unions, and government payors) must be aligned with the delivery of value- and quality-based healthcare versus volume. Second, the systems that deliver healthcare must be nuanced enough to provide just the right amount of care in the right setting. The Agency for Healthcare Quality and Research (AHRQ) has defined quality healthcare as "doing the right thing, at the right time, in the right way, for the right person – and having the best possible results" [4]. Or more specifically in this context, healthcare delivery systems must have the ability to provide evidence-based screening, diagnostics, and treatment to the community they serve. Third, in order to help ensure that patients are given just the right amount of care as in a timely manner, the employment of data and registries is critical. Registries are population focused, purpose driven, and designed to derive information on health outcomes defined before the data are collected and analyzed. This is distinct from the electronic medical record in that EHRs are focused on the collection and use of an individual patient's health-related information [5]. Registries should be collectively decided upon and able to produce ongoing, actionable results and outcomes measurements.

41.3 Why Population Health Management?

In addition to the AHRQ definition of quality healthcare, the Institute of Medicine has also created guidelines to improve quality and value within healthcare systems [6]. Population health management can move systems toward safe, effective, patient-centered, equitable, and timely guidelines and clinical interventions. The literature consistently shows a relatively small percentage of the population driving most of the cost in healthcare (Figs. 41.1 and 41.2), though more recent literature reveals that this top percentile cohort of high-need, high-cost patients can turn over with time and can be difficult to predict [7].

Of particular note in a geriatric context, many of these costly patients are frail elderly and older patients with multiple chronic conditions, making geriatric understanding and services critical in any successful population health enterprise.

41.4 What Are Registries?

A registry is an organized system that uses observational study methods to collect uniform data (clinical and other) to evaluate specified outcomes for a population defined by a particular disease, condition, or exposure and that serves one or more predetermined scientific, clinical, or policy purposes. Registries are focused on populations and are designed

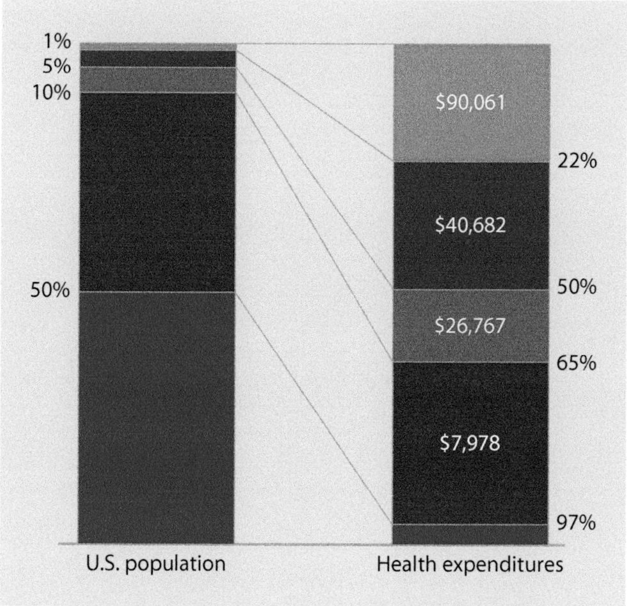

Fig. 41.1 Distribution of healthcare expenditures for the US population, according to magnitude of expenditure, 2009 references. (Adapted from: Blumenthal et al. [11])

41

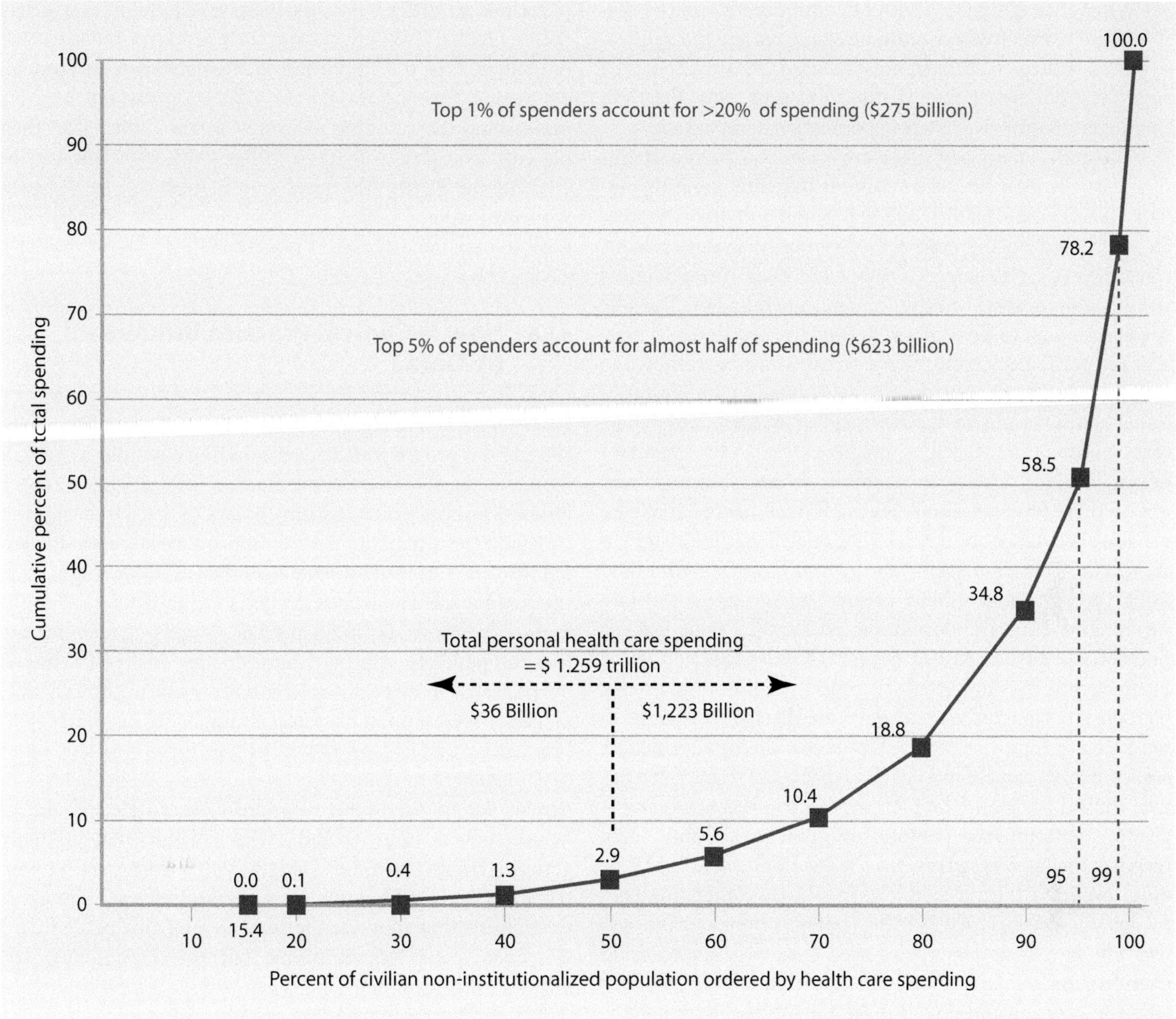

Fig. 41.2 Cumulative distribution of personal healthcare spending, 2009. (Adapted from: Shoenman [12])

to fulfill specific purposes defined before the data are collected and analyzed [5]. Data can be collected from various sources including electronic medical records, payor claims, or other central sources and analyzed to achieve the goals particular to a practice, clinical program, or payor.

41.5 Why Are Registries and Data Important in Population Health Management?

As we begin to conceive our roles differently, expanding from 1:1 patient management to population health, it becomes important to stratify populations to allow for effective targeting and program resource utilization. All geriatric patients do not need end-of-life care or home visits, for example, and we must optimize our data registries to allow for clinical relevance. Although there are many reasons to use registries including research, grants, etc., here we will focus on using registries for population management. It is important to note that usually, these types of risk stratification systems are used to drive clinical targeting for select programs, many of which are designed to avoid hospitalizations and/or SNF for our geriatric patients. Given the high rates of complications from institutionalization in geriatric patients, doing this well becomes even more important than for a healthier or younger population.

Recent changes in the landscape of healthcare, including a shift in financial reimbursement toward delivery systems assuming more financial risk, and the resulting focus on care delivery innovation, have resulted in a wave of new programs that blend traditional face-to-face patient and care team contact with new methods of communication. These programs all intend to focus on proactive monitoring and employing preventive care interventions. Telemonitoring of chronic conditions, teleconsultation of specialty services, home visits, phone calls from centralized nurse care managers, and visits from non-physician care team members are all examples of delivering more "dose" of contact and care to the community.

When managing the health of communities and populations, and to effectively coordinate resources and the delivery of care, a strategic approach must be used. To deliver just the right level of contact dose, at the right time, with the right care teams, requires leveraging population-level data.

Currently, many registries are based on billing claims data. Usually, one can select patients based on certain standard demographic factors (age, sex, number of disease codes, etc.) or based on the presence of certain diagnostic claims categories (e.g., diabetes, COPD, CHF, etc.). These allow a stratification process to begin but are generally not clinically specific enough to drive all programmatic decisions. In geriatrics in particular, certain characteristics have been shown to predict risk that are not usually well coded including functional status, cognitive status, caregiver burden, and symptom burden. In usual outpatient visits or inpatient hospitalizations, claims are focused on disease groups and not on these types of scores (which, if documented at all, are usually in the EMR but not in billing codes). It is important to survey the data your particular system has at baseline and think through the feasibility of supplementing it with more meaningful clinical information relevant to your patient population via the EMR or other standard collection tools. Furthermore, it is important to collect the lists of high-risk patients in a standard way to alert interdisciplinary teams to the patient's high-risk status. Optimally, multiple providers and caregivers can see this "flag" so that it can trigger alternative clinical programs or pathways in the hospitals, emergency departments, outpatient practices, and care management systems. This can also be done via an EMR or other program-specific notification systems. Once these are in place, it becomes easier to select patients from a health system who have a certain type of need (e.g., targeting for mild cognitive impairment) and institute workflows that allow for efficient targeting and care of these patients based on need.

Another category of registry use that has become more common as the United States moves toward value-based care is quality metrics. Quality metrics are usually defined and selected by CMS or by payor plans. Of note, they can be particularly challenging for the geriatric population, as many of them are designed around screening measures that may or may not be relevant for our geriatric or medically complex patients. There are also various disease-specific measures that may not be relevant for our complex geriatric patients – aspirin use, diabetes control, echo for heart failure, etc. Given these complexities, it is important for geriatricians to represent these needs in their institutional IT discussions about the relevance of metrics for these populations and how this can/will be reflected in an EMR or other systematic processes. Registries can be used to identify patients who are missing certain metrics that are relevant to their care and institute workflows to optimize these measures [8].

Finally, and most relevant to geriatric populations under a managed Medicare plan, there are opportunities to optimize revenue for our most complicated geriatric patients by coding their diseases appropriately. Medicare has designed a complex system that rates patients' disease groups and complications in order to assign them a risk value that drives their expected cost per year and their needs for inpatient and outpatient care. It is important that geriatricians and providers caring for our most vulnerable populations learn to understand these coding measures, so they can reflect their patients' complexity in their codes. Although this can be challenging, EMRs and other system tools can be designed with institutional billing or population health management tools to make this as easy as possible [9].

41.6 How Is Clinical Practice Influenced by Data?

Once registries are set up, systems can use these data to make clinical and programmatic decisions. For example, a geriatric inpatient registry may reveal that too few patients receive a follow-up appointment within 14 days of discharge, and this can drive the leadership team to improve access and scheduling for this cohort of patients. Another example might be to realize that a hospital system's geriatric patients have a long average length of stay in local subacute nursing facilities and this can generate improved partnerships between SNF and hospital staff to drive down length of stay or improve quality of care. Yet another example could be to leverage non-physician care team members such as social workers, nurse case managers, and non-clinical coordinators, navigators, or similar patient advocates to address other determinants of health such as housing and social isolation that influence geriatric health outcomes [10]. As you work to set up your registries and dashboards, try to make them as relevant as possible so that they can be used to improve patient care. Consider your organization's current capabilities and limitations in care delivery. When first implementing registries, identify sets of data that can be most readily acted on.

41.7 Measuring Outcomes

Ultimately, the goal of using data and registries in healthcare is to improve patient care. Any dashboard or registry should be able to drive clinical improvements and then measure whether improvements in care were carried out. These outcomes might be clinical or disease-specific (Hgba1c over time, percentage of eligible patients on ACE-I, etc.). They might also be related to system improvement or experience (patient satisfaction, time to next appointment or new appointment availability, etc.). Accurate, relevant, and timely patient data through registries will help determine the most appropriate setting and level of care and is thus a critical ability for any healthcare organization that wishes to be an effective population health manger. To drive improvement, geriatric practices, inpatient services, or systems should work together to design the registry for both clinical utility and ease of tracking performance over time. This will allow for the greatest relevance and for focus on the outcomes most important to the organization and stakeholders.

Case Example, cont.

Dr. S works with her practice manager to ensure that a daily list is sent to her practice of all patients discharged from eight local emergency departments in the preceding 24 hours. Her nurse calls these patients, does a brief clinical assessment, and ensures that the front desk staff schedules these patients for a rapid follow-up appointment. Using EMR data, Dr. S is further able to sort these lists into avoidable and unavoidable ED visits and can particularly highlight patients who had falls or delirium, two areas her practice is working on for quality improvement. This allows Dr. S and her team to optimize care for these patients and ensure that rapid access is used by patients who truly need it.

References

1. http://www.ihi.org/Engage/Initiatives/TripleAim.
2. Kindig D, Stoddart GA. What is population health? J American Journal of Public Health 2003;93(3):380–3
3. Wellcentive. What is population health management? http://www.wellcentive.com/what-is-population-healthmanagement/. Accessed on 17 July 2018.
4. https://archive.ahrq.gov/consumer/qnt/qntqlook.htm.
5. Gliklich RE, Dreyer NA, Leavy MB, editors. Registries for evaluating patient outcomes: a user's guide [Internet]. 3rd ed. Rockville: Agency for Healthcare Research and Quality (US); 2014, Interfacing Registries With Electronic Health Records. Available from: https://www.ncbi.nlm.nih.gov/books/NBK208625/.
6. Institute of Medicine (IOM). Crossing the quality chasm: a new health system for the 21st century. Washington, DC: National Academy Press; 2001.
7. Johnson TL. For many patients who use large amounts of health care services, the need is intense yet temporary. Health Affairs. 2015;34(8):Variety issue.
8. http://www.ncqa.org/Portals/0/HEDISQM/HEDIS2018/Summary%20of%20Changes%20for%20Physician%20Measurement%202018.pdf?ver=2017-12-15-070645-503.
9. https://www.cms.gov/Medicare/Health-Plans/MedicareAdvtg-SpecRateStats/Risk-Adjustors.html.
10. Gale CR, Westbury L, Cooper C. Social isolation and loneliness as risk factors for the progression of frailty: the English Longitudinal Study of Ageing. Age Ageing. https://doi.org/10.1093/ageing/afx188.
11. Blumenthal D. Performance improvement in health care — seizing the moment. N Engl J Med. 2012;366(21):1953.
12. Shoenman JA. The concentration of health care spending. Washington, DC: NIHCM Foundation Data Brief, National Institute of Health Care Management; 2012.

Palliative Care and End of Life

Contents

Management of Pain Symptoms

Megan E. Rau and Emily J. Chai

A. Chun (ed.), *Geriatric Practice*, https://doi.org/10.1007/978-3-030-19625-7_42

Case: Part 1

Opal is a 76-year-old woman with a past medical history of hypertension, hyperlipidemia, obesity, and diabetes mellitus type 2 on insulin. She was also diagnosed 3 years ago with breast cancer and underwent a mastectomy followed by chemotherapy. Opal presents to the outpatient clinic with the chief complaint to left knee pain.

42.1 Prevalence of Pain

The prevalence of pain in the community population age 65 and older is estimated at 25–50%. Persistent pain prevalence among residents in the nursing home is even higher, estimated between 45% and 80% [1, 2].

42.2 Definition of Pain

Pain is an unpleasant sensory and emotional experience associated with actual or potential tissue damage [1, 3]. Pain is subjective and idiosyncratic; its intensity and character are what the patient says they are. Since pain is more than just a physical symptom, it impacts and influences the mood and personality of a person. It can affect a patient's behavior, social life, and interactions [1, 4].

Pain can be subdivided as acute or chronic. Acute pain is sudden in onset and expected to last a short time and is clearly linked to a specific bodily insult or injury. Chronic pain is without apparent biologic purpose that has persisted beyond the normal tissue healing time and typically defined as present for at least 3–6 months [1, 5]. Acute pain may be associated with vital sign changes, whereas chronic pain is often not.

42.3 Types of Pain

42

There are generally three types of pain: nociceptive, neuropathic, and mixed/undetermined pain. It is necessary to distinguish between nociceptive and neuropathic pain because treatment modalities are different between the two types.

Nociceptive pain is due to activation of nociceptive sensory receptors by noxious stimuli resulting from inflammation, swelling, and injury to tissues. Nociceptive pain can be of somatic or visceral origin. Somatic nociceptive pain is well localized in the skin, soft tissues, and/or bone. Patients may describe this type of pain as throbbing, aching, or stabbing [5, 6]. A surgical skin incision can produce somatic nociceptive pain. Visceral nociceptive pain occurs when there is injury to organs (viscera) such as the heart, lungs, gastrointestinal tract, and pelvis. Patients may have difficulty localizing and describing this pain, while others may describe the visceral pain as cramping, tearing, dull, or aching [5, 6]. This can be seen in myocardial infarction, pulmonary embolism, and ischemic bowel among other conditions.

Neuropathic pain is due to irritation of components of the central or peripheral nervous system. Patients describe this type of pain as burning, numbness, pins-and-needles sensation, shooting pain, or lightning-like pain. Common examples of neuropathic pain include diabetes-induced peripheral neuropathy or post-herpetic neuralgia [5–7].

Mixed/undetermined pain is characterized by both components of nociceptive pain and neuropathic pain. This type of pain is common in older pain and may need treatment trials of different medications or combinations of medications before pain improves. Inter-professional team collaboration is often beneficial in treating this form of pain [5].

Characteristics of the three types of pain are further detailed in ◘ Table 42.1.

Case: Part 2

Opal reports her left knee pain started 6 months ago and is worse after she goes shopping or walks to the bus. Due to the pain, she isn't going out as much and is spending more time in her apartment. When she rests and ices her knee, the pain improves. She describes the pain as a dull or aching sensation on the inside of her left knee. She rates her pain as a 3/10 on a bad day and 1/10 if she doesn't do much walking. The pain occurs most days of the week.

42.4 Assessment of Pain

One of the greatest barriers to effective treatment of pain is the inadequate assessment of pain symptoms. Specifically for older adults, assessing how pain is interfering with their function, particularly their ADLs and IADLs, is critical [8]. The pneumonic O, P, Q, R, S, and T can be helpful when asking the patient to characterize their pain (◘ Table 42.2) [8]. A thorough assessment of the nature of their pain and the modalities and medications tried is important in formulating a plan for management. Do not rely solely on electronic medication lists, as they may not be accurate or complete. Ask about over-the-counter medications, and utilize your state's controlled substance prescribing database to determine if opioids have been prescribed in the past [9].

Case: Part 3

Fill in the blanks based on Opal's description of her left knee pain (answers provided at the end of the chapter).

Onset:
Provocative:
Palliative:
Quality:
Region:
Radiation:
Severity:
Timing:

Table 42.1 Characteristics of pain based on type

	Source of pain	Typical description
Nociceptive: somatic pain		
Arthritis, acute postoperative pain, fracture, bony metastases	Tissue injury (bones, soft tissue, joints, muscles)	Well localized, constant, aching, stabbing, gnawing, throbbing
Nociceptive: visceral pain		
Renal colic, constipation, hepatomegaly	Viscera (pericardium, peritoneum, pleura)	Diffuse, poorly localized, referred to other sites, intermittent, dull, colicky, squeezing, deep, cramping
Neuropathic pain		
Cervical or lumbar radiculopathy, post-herpetic neuralgia, trigeminal neuralgia, diabetic neuropathy, herniated vertebral disc, chemotherapy toxicities	Peripheral or central nervous system	Usually constant, sharp, burning, pricking, tingling, electric shock like Associated with other sensory disturbances (paresthesias, allodynia, hyperalgesia)
Mixed/undetermined pain		
Myofascial pain syndrome, somatic symptom pain disorders, fibromyalgia	Poorly understood	No identifiable pathologic etiology or symptoms out of proportion etiology; diffuse musculoskeletal pain, stiffness, and weakness

Modified from Reuben et al. [26]

Table 42.2 Assessment of pain

Assessment of pain (O, P, Q, R, S, T)	
	Example questions
Onset	When did it start? Was there an event that triggered the pain?
Provocative (Aggravating factors)	What makes the pain worse?
Palliative (Relieving factors)	What makes the pain better? What mediations are you taking for the pain? (Ask about both prescription and over-the-counter medications)
Quality	Is the pain burning? Stabbing? Dull? Throbbing? Aching? etc.
Region	Where is the pain? Point with one finger where the pain is the worst Use a pain map
Radiation	Does the pain radiate?
Severity	Use one of these two ways to assess severity: 1. On a scale of 1–10, how do you rate your pain? "0" being no pain and "10" being the worst pain ever 2. How severe is your pain? No pain, mild, moderate, or severe? How do you rate your pain after you take your pain medications?
Timing	When does the pain occur? How long does the pain last? How often do you have the pain? How does the pain affect your daily activities?

42.5 Assessment of Pain in Older Adults with Cognitive Impairment

While some cognitively impaired patients may be able to speak, they may not be able to verbalize the location of their pain and answer all the questions you have regarding their pain [4]. However, these patients can often tell you whether they have pain at the present time. Other patients may not be able to speak at all. Tools have been developed for such circumstances. Pain Assessment in Advanced Dementia (PAINAD) scale is a tool based on five observable behaviors to assess pain symptoms: breathing independent of vocalization, negative vocalization, facial expression, body language, and consolability. Each behavior is scored from 0 to 2 after observing the patient [10]. For example, a patient exhibiting normal breathing is scored a 0, whereas a patient with labored breathing using their accessory muscles is scored a 2. The scores from each category are then added together to obtain a total score. The higher the total score, the more severe the patient's pain, i.e., a total score of 0 is interpreted as no pain and a total score of 10 indicates severe pain.

42.6 Physical Exam

The physical exam is another modality used to assess and characterize pain. Asking the patient to point to the painful area is one method of identifying the location of the pain. The area should be examined for skin changes (redness, bruising, darkening of the skin), swelling (effusions, limb asymmetry), temperature (warm to touch, cold to touch), decreased blood flood (delayed capillary refill), and structural change (tophi, crepitus, joint deviation). It is also important to assess if pain results from non-painful stimuli, active motion, and passive motion and whether palpation causes radiation of pain. Muscle strength and reflexes provide additional clues to the etiology of the pain allowing targeted treatment. Finally, an understanding of how pain is affecting the ability of an older adult to walk, stand from a seated position, or have grip strength can provide you with a more objective target for the pain management.

42.7 Laboratory Tests

Laboratory tests may be beneficial if infections are suspected or if medications considered for management are cleared by the patient's kidney and liver. Routine testing for inflammatory disorders is discouraged unless there is a high index of suspicion for a rheumatologic process provoking the pain.

42.8 Imaging

Imaging should be ordered on a case-by-case basis and is not necessary in every instance of reported pain in the older adult. Unnecessary imaging can lead to overdiagnosis and excessive use of medical resources, as the prevalence of degenerative disease is high in the geriatric population [6]. If a patient presents with red flag signs such as pain after a fall or trauma, a rigid abdomen on exam, history of cancer, and/or new neurological deficit, imaging may be necessary.

Case: Part 4

Upon physical exam of Opal, her vitals are within normal limits, there is no skin redness or increased warm over either knee, and both knees are negative for effusion. Crepitus is present only in the left knee with active and passive range of motion. Opal expresses mild pain upon standing and with walking on the left knee. Laboratory tests reveal no signs of infection, normal kidney function, and normal liver function, and X-ray of the left knee shows joint space narrowing consistent with osteoarthritis. Opal is referred to physical therapy for treatment of her left knee pain.

42

42.9 Principles of Pain Treatment in Older Adults

There is a tendency for undertreatment of pain in older adults. Older adults may minimize or not report their pain; they may have limited health literacy, limited English proficiency, and cognitive impairment or perceive pain as an aspect of getting old. Clinicians may undertreat pain symptoms due to inadequately assessing pain, being hesitant to manage pain due to lack of adequate knowledge of pain management strategies, or misperceptions about opioid medications [1, 4].

When treating pain in the older adult, realistic expectations must be established. The general goal for treatment of pain in the older adult is to improve function, allowing patients to maintain their independence. In many cases it is unrealistic to expect the patient's pain to completely resolve. Treatment is provided to reduce the pain to a manageable level determined by the patient. This is why it is important to know the patient's goals of care, as that will further direct treatment recommendations [9].

42.10 Non-pharmacologic Treatments

Several non-pharmacologic treatments have been shown to decrease chronic musculoskeletal pain in older adults. Physical activities such as regular exercise, physical therapy, and tai chi not only decrease pain but also have the potential benefit of increasing function. Psychosocial treatments may provide pain relief in some patient including massage, heat therapy, cold therapy, and music therapy. Mindfulness-based stressed reduction and cognitive behavioral therapy (CBT) engage older adults to develop coping strategies to help manage their chronic pain [11].

Case: Part 5

Opal returns to your office for follow-up 6 months later. She completed her sessions of physical therapy and increased her total minutes of exercise per week resulting in a 5-pound weight loss. However, over the past 2 months, her left knee pain is worse, and she now relies on her daughter to do the grocery shopping for her. Opal no longer attends church services because walking is too painful. You recommend Opal start taking Tylenol 650 mg by mouth every 6 hours as needed for her pain.

You call Opal to follow up on her pain symptoms a week later. Opal reports she has been taking the Tylenol 650 mg by mouth every 6 hours. The Tylenol is improving her left knee pain and she has resumed going to church services and grocery shopping. Additionally, treatment of her pain has allowed her to resume exercising and she is going to start tai chi classes.

42.11 Pharmacologic Treatment Principles

The consensus when using medications to treat pain in the older adult is to "start low, go slow but do go." This means initiating medications at a low dose and slowly increasing the dose of the medication. This also means that if the medication is not effective upon initial evaluation, you increase the dose. If the patient is still not reaching the pre-established goal of treatment after several increases without side effects, you taper off the medication or decrease the medication to the lowest effective dose. The route of medication delivery is greatly influenced by the setting in which the patient is being treated (i.e., inpatient, outpatient, skilled nursing facility) [6]. It would be much more difficult to give patients intravenous medications in non-monitored settings such as the home. Clinicians must be cognizant of medication costs as well, because many older adults are on a fixed income such as social security or rely on Medicare/Medicaid for their medication coverage [2]. Finally, route of medication delivery is important to consider in geriatric patients as they may have difficulties swallowing (i.e., a patient cannot swallow pills but can swallow liquid medication formulations).

Case: Part 6

Four months later Opal returns to your clinic for an emergency room follow-up appointment. She went to the emergency room because she tripped on the curb and fell. Evaluation showed a broken right radius. Her arm was casted and she was discharged on Tylenol 650 mg every 6 hours as needed by mouth for pain. However, she states the Tylenol is not helping. Her pain is localized in her right forearm and is described as continuous, throbbing, and non radiating. Opal rates her pain as an 8/10 on the pain scale. Upon exam Opal's blood pressure and heart rate are elevated in response to her pain and her right arm is in a cast. She has good capillary refill in her right fingers and they are warm to touch. Review of laboratory tests from the emergency room show normal kidney and liver function.

42.12 Oral and Intravenous Treatments

If non-pharmacologic treatments are not adequate to treat a patient's pain, medications may be required. Analgesic drugs are medications formulated to decrease pain and may be concurrently used with adjuvant drugs [3]. Adjuvant drugs are medications whose primary indication is not for treatment of pain but the drug has pharmacologic properties, which provide an analgesic effect or additive analgesic effect when used with opioids [12, 13]. Determining the intensity of the patient's pain can help guide therapy. If a patient has mild nociceptive pain, initiating treatment with a non-opioid medication (e.g., acetaminophen or a nonsteroidal anti-inflammatory drug) with or without an adjuvant may be sufficient. For continued moderate to severe nociceptive pain, clinicians may consider starting opioid therapy (e.g., morphine, oxycodone, dilaudid, or fentanyl) in conjunction with non-opioid and adjuvant medications [1, 2, 6]. For detailed descriptions of medications, see ◘ Table 42.3.

Of note opioids are a class of medications with opium-like pharmacologic action, whereas opiates refer to the alkaloids found naturally in opium. This should not be confused with the expression narcotics, which is a law enforcement term referring to a variety of substances that dull or distort the senses [14].

42.13 Side Effects of Opioids

When starting an opioid for treatment, it is imperative a bowel regimen is prescribed concurrent to prevent constipation. Treatment to prevent opioid-induced constipation should be continued as long as the patient is prescribed opioid therapy, even if they are taking the opioid only as needed. Tolerance, defined as a decrease in a drug's effect over time due to exposure to the drug, does not develop to constipation [1, 5, 15]. Nausea and vomiting is another side effect of opioid therapy as opioids have a direct effect on the chemoreceptor trigger zone [1, 16]. Short-acting opioids are more likely to cause nausea; however tolerance usually develops within 7 days. Sedation and fatigue are side effects commonly seen upon the initiation or dose escalation of opioid therapy. Tolerance to these side effects usually develops in 1–3 days, and patients should be warned against driving or operating heavy equipment until they know the effect these medications have on them [1]. Delirium is a side effect of great concern in older adults but is most often multifactorial. It is more likely caused by untreated pain or undertreated pain than by use of opioid medications. Other side effects to be aware of include urinary retention, pruritus, dry mouth, and myoclonus. Patient should be assessed routinely for all these side effects while on opioid therapy [2, 9, 14, 16].

Case: Part 7

Given the severe pain from her fracture, you decide to prescribe her morphine. You prescribe a 2-week course of morphine 5 mg orally every 4 hours as needed for pain along with a bowel regimen (senna two tablets at night by mouth). Opal is scheduled for a 2-week follow-up in your clinic for reassessment of her pain.

You call Opal the next day to monitor how her pain is responding to the morphine and assess for any side effects. Opal states after she takes the morphine her pain decreases to a 2/10 and she was able to sleep through the night. She took the morphine three times since filling the prescription and took the senna tablets last night. She had a bowel movement this morning. Opal denies any nausea, vomiting, itching, twitching, or confusion.

42.14 Topical Treatments

Lidocaine is available over the counter in various gel and cream forms. Higher concentrations of lidocaine gels and creams, along with lidocaine patches, are available with a prescription. Lidocaine treats pain through denervation hypersensitivity and decreased systemic absorption through sodium channel blockade. Due to this mechanism of action, patients using lidocaine patches must wear the patch for 12 hours followed by 12 hours without the patch. Topical lidocaine is beneficial in treatment of localized pain in the cases of post-herpetic neuralgia and diabetic neuropathy pain. Patients may find it helpful in treating somatic joint pain as well [17].

Capsaicin is another topical medication available through a prescription. Its mechanism of action was previously thought to be through depletion of substance P at nerve endings. However, more recent evidence shows topical capsaicin works in the skin to reduce pain by defunctionalization of nociceptor fibers and by attenuation of cutaneous hypersensitivity [18].

Topical diclofenac (Voltaren) is classified as a nonsteroidal anti-inflammatory drug (NSAID) that relieves pain by inhibiting both COX-1 and COX-2 locally. Since there is minimal systemic absorption of diclofenac, this topical form can be used in patients with renal impairment [1, 17].

■ **Table 42.3** Pharmacologic treatment of pain

Medication	Mechanism of action	Type of pain	Severity of pain	Starting geriatric dose (opioid-naïve patients)	Route	Considerations and caution	Comments
Anti-inflammatories:							
Acetaminophen (Tylenol)[a]	Inhibits prostaglandin synthesis in the central nervous system Less effect on COX in the peripheral tissues	Nociceptive	Mild pain	650 mg q 6 hrs	PO (tablet, liquid), IV, suppository	Liver dysfunction or heavy alcohol use decrease by 25–50% Renal dysfunction with CrCL <10 dose q 8 hrs	Maximum 3000 mg/24 hrs First-line therapy for persistent pain Included in many OTC medications Does NOT inhibit platelet function
Ibuprofen (Advil, Motrin)[a]	Nonselective NSAID Inhibits prostaglandin synthesis primarily by inhibiting COX that catalyze the first step in prostanoid biosynthesis	Nociceptive	Mild pain	200 mg q 6 hrs	PO	Gastric irritation, *not* recommended in patients with abnormal renal function; abnormal platelet function – all dose dependent Can exacerbate HTN and heart failure Increased risk of cardiovascular events	Avoid using for prolonged periods of time (i.e., 2 weeks) Maximum dose 2400 mg/24 hrs Constipation, confusion, and headache more common in older adults
Naproxen (Aleve)[a] Naprosyn	See ibuprofen	Nociceptive	Mild pain	May require loading dose q 8–12 hrs	PO	Same as ibuprofen	Same as ibuprofen Maximum dose 1000 mg/24 hrs
Partial opioid:							
Tramadol (Ultram)	Binds to the mu-opioid receptor and weakly inhibits the reuptake of NE and serotonin	Nociceptive	Moderate pain	25 mg q 6 hrs PRN	PO	Avoid if CrCL <30 Lowers the seizure threshold	Avoid concurrent use with carbamazepine, SSRI, TCAs, and MAOIs because they can precipitate serotonin syndrome
Short-acting opioids:							
Morphine IR (Roxanol, MSIR)	Inhibits mu, kappa, and delta receptors in the CNS, nerve terminals in the periphery, and on cells in the GI tract Analgesic properties primarily mediated by the mu receptors	Nociceptive	Moderate/severe pain	5 mg PO q 4 hrs PRN 1–2 mg IV PO q 4 hrs PRN	PO (tablet, liquid), SL, IV	Older patients are more sensitive to side effects Do NOT use in severe liver disease Avoid in renal dysfunction CrCL <30 or dialysis patients as toxic metabolites (morphine-6-glucuronide) can accumulate and are not dialyzed off	Found in crude opium Must start bowel regimen to prevent constipation

Oxycodone IR (Roxicodone) Oxycodone-acetaminophen (Percocet)	See morphine	Nociceptive	Moderate/severe pain	2.5 mg q 4 hrs PRN	PO (tablet, liquid)	Caution with renal and liver dysfunction, may need to increase frequency and/or reduce dose	Percocet dosing limited due to acetaminophen
Hydromorphone (Dilaudid)	See morphine IR	Nociceptive	Moderate/severe pain	1 mg PO q 4 hrs PRN 0.2 mg IV q 4 hrs PRN	PO, IV	Preferred opioid in patients with renal dysfunction or on dialysis therapy	No dialyzed but minimal toxicity
Fentanyl	See morphine IR	Nociceptive	Moderate/severe pain	12 mcg q 1–2 hrs PRN	IV	Can be used in liver or renal dysfunction	Short half-life
Long-acting opioids:							
Morphine SR (MS Contin)	See morphine IR	Nociceptive	Moderate/severe pain	15 mg q 12 hrs	PO	See morphine IR	Do NOT crush
Oxycodone SR (OxyContin)	See morphine IR	Nociceptive	Moderate/severe pain	10 mg q 12 hrs	PO	See oxycodone IR	Do NOT crush
Fentanyl patch	See morphine IR Peak effect of the first dose may not occur until 12–24 hrs	Nociceptive	Moderate/severe pain	12.5 mcg patch q 72 hrs	Transdermal	Fever can increase absorption Must be placed over subcutaneous tissue, not the bone	NOT recommended for opioid-naïve patients Drug reservoir is in the skin, not the patch
Anticonvulsants:							
Gabapentin (Neurontin)	Selective inhibitory effect on voltage-gated calcium channels	Neuropathic	Adjuvant	100 mg q 24 hrs titrate q 3–7 days	PO	Dose adjustments required for renal function	Can initially cause drowsiness Maximum dose 3600 mg/24 hrs Side effects include ankle swelling
Pregabalin (Lyrica)	See gabapentin	Neuropathic	Adjuvant	50 mg q 12 hrs	PO	Can titrate to analgesic effect more rapidly	Fewer adverse events than gabapentin Titrate up to 300 mg/24 hrs over several weeks Effect in 3–4 weeks

(continued)

Table 42.3 (continued)

Medication	Mechanism of action	Type of pain	Severity of pain	Starting geriatric dose (opioid-naïve patients)	Route	Considerations and caution	Comments
Anti-depressants:							
Duloxetine (Cymbalta)	Serotonin and NE reuptake inhibitor (SNRI)	Somatic Neuropathic (Chronic MSK pain)	Adjuvant	20 mg q 24 hrs	PO	Reduce dose if CrCL 30–60 Avoid if CrCL <30	Maximum 120 mg/24 hrs Most common side effect is nausea, dry mouth, constipation, diarrhea, urinary hesitancy
Venlafaxine (Effexor)	SNRI	Neuropathic (Chronic MSK pain)	Adjuvant	25 mg q 12 hrs	PO	May increase blood pressure and QTc Withdrawal symptoms may occur if stopped abruptly	Maximum dose 225 mg/24 hrs Monitor for hyponatremia
Nortriptyline	TCA – inhibits the reuptake of NE and serotonin	Neuropathic (Chronic MSK pain)	Adjuvant	10 mg q 24 hrs	PO	Anti-cholinergic and orthostatic hypotension side effects	Best side effect profile of TCAs
Others:							
Steroids (prednisone, dexamethasone, methylprednisolone)	Inhibit prostaglandin synthesis (inflammation) Reduce vascular permeability (tissue edema)	Bone	Adjuvant	Depends on drug	PO, IV	Use with caution in diabetic patient as it increases blood sugar Long-term use can result in adrenal insufficiency if abruptly stopped	Side effects include increased appetite, nausea, sedation, delirium
Calcitonin	Antagonizes effects of parathyroid hormone which results in inhibition of osteoclasts	Spinal compression fractures	Adjuvant	100 mg q 12 hrs	Intranasal	Hypersensitivity with fish allergies	Beneficial for short-term effect on pain
Bisphosphonates (pamidronate, zoledronic acid)	Directly inhibit osteoclast activity	Bone from metastasis	Adjuvant	Depends on drug	IV	Caution with renal dysfunction	Complications include osteonecrosis of the jaw

References [1, 2, 4, 8, 17, 24, 27–29]

[a]Available over the counter (OTC), i.e., without a prescription

COX cyclooxygenase, *mg* milligram, *q quaqua* or every, *hr* hour, *PO* per oral route or by mouth, *IV* intravenous, *CrCL* creatinine clearance, *NSAID* nonsteroidal anti-inflammatory drugs, *HTN* hypertension, *NE* norepinephrine, *PRN* pro re nata or as needed, *SSRI* selective serotonin reuptake inhibitors, *TCA* tricyclic anti-depressants, *MAOI* monoamine oxidase inhibitor, *IR* immediate release, *CNS* central nervous system, *GI* gastrointestinal, *SL* sublingual, *SNRI* serotonin-norepinephrine reuptake inhibitor, *MSK* musculoskeletal pain

42.15 Interventional Pain Treatments

A pain specialist typically performs interventional treatments targeted at the relief of pain. Three common procedures are trigger point injections, pulsed radiofrequency treatment, and nerve blocks.

Trigger point injections are beneficial in myofascial pain syndrome or when patients have active trigger points resulting in pain. The clinician injects 1% lidocaine or 1% procaine into an active trigger point effectively inactivating the trigger point providing prompt symptomatic relief [2, 19, 20].

Pulsed radiofrequency treatment is a procedure where short pulses of radiofrequency waves are delivered through a needle-like catheter targeting specific pain locations. It has been shown to improve cervical radicular pain, trigeminal neuralgia, sacroiliac joint pain, facet arthropathy, shoulder pain, postsurgical pain, radicular pain, and myofascial pain conditions [21, 22].

Nerve blocks are interventional procedures used to treat neuropathic pain in which neurolytic agents are injected directly at the nerve causing the pain. The nerve block can target peripheral nerves such as the median nerve to treat carpel tunnel syndrome or regions of nerves such as the celiac plexus to treat abdominal pain resulting from pancreatic cancer [23–25].

Take-Home Points

- Evaluation and management of pain in the older adults requires a thorough assessment of the characteristics of the pain.
- Cognitively impaired patients who cannot communicate verbally should still be assessed for pain using tools such as PAINAD and receive analgesic treatment.
- A stepped approach to pain treatment is advised starting with non-pharmacologic treatments and escalating to pharmacologic therapies such as opioids.
- When starting pharmacologic treatments in the older adults, "start low, go slow but do go."
- If opioids are initiated, monitor for side effects including constipation, sedation/fatigue, nausea/vomiting, and delirium.
- Always start a bowel regimen concurrently when treating patients with opioids.
- Adjuvant therapies including anticonvulsants, anti-depressants, topical medications, and interventional procedures can be used in addition to opioids to treat pain symptoms.
- Reassessment of pain symptoms, medications, and side effects are required on a regular basis.

Case Conclusion

Opal returns to your office for her 2-week follow-up. Her arm pain is improving and she no longer is taking the morphine tablets; instead she is taking Tylenol 650 mg by mouth every 6 hours as needed if she has pain. She hasn't used any Tylenol in 2 days.

Case: Part 3 Answers

Onset: Past 6 months.
Provocative: Worse after shopping or when she walks to the bus.
Palliative: Improves with resting and ice.
Quality: Dull, aching pain.
Region: Inside of the knee.
Radiation: None.
Severity: Pain is 3/10 on a bad day and 1/10 if she doesn't walk much.
Timing: The pain is most days so she is avoiding going out as much to prevent the knee from hurting.

References

1. Periyakoil VS. Pain management. In: Medina-Walpole A, Pacala JT, Potter JF, editors. Geriatrics review syllabus: a core curriculum in geriatric medicine. 9th ed. New York: American Geriatrics Society; 2016. p. 147–59.
2. Chun A, Morrison RS. Palliative care. In: Halter JB, Ouslander JG, Tinetti ME, Studenski S, High KP, Asthana S, editors. Hazzard's geriatric medicine and gerontology. 6th ed. New York, NY: McGraw-Hill; 2009. p. 373–83.
3. Merskey H, Bogduk N. Pain terms, a current list with definitions and notes on usage. In: IASP Task Force on Taxonomy. Classification of chronic pain. 2nd ed. Seattle: IASP Press; 1994. p. 209–14.
4. Pasero C, McCaffery M. Pain assessment and pharmacologic management. St. Louis: Mosby; 2011.
5. Bain RM. Principles of pain management. In: Soriano RP, Fernandez HM, Cassel CK, editors. Fundamentals of geriatric medicine. New York: Springer; 2007. p. 573–99.
6. Horton JR. Management of pain in older adults. In: Chai E, Meier D, Morris J, Goldhirsch S, editors. Geriatrics palliative care: a practical guide for clinicians. New York: Oxford University Press; 2014. p. 159–69.
7. Baron R, Binder A, Wasner G. Neuropathic pain: diagnosis, pathophysiological mechanisms, and treatment. Lancet Neurol. 2010;9(8):807–19.
8. Reuben DB, Herr KA, Pacala JT, Pollock BG, Potter JF, Semla TP. Geriatrics at your fingertips. New York: American Geriatrics Society; 2017.
9. Dowell D, Haegerich TM, Chou R. CDC Guideline for prescribing opioids for chronic pain—United States, 2016. JAMA. 2016;315(15):1624–45.
10. Warden V, Hurley A, Volicer L. Development and psychometric evaluation of the pain assessment in advanced dementia (PAINAD) scale. J Am Med Dir Assoc. 2003;4(1):9–15.
11. Chou R, Deyo R, Friedly J, Skelly A, Hashimoto R, Weimer M, et al. Nonpharmacologic therapies for acute and chronic low back pain: a review of the evidence for an American Pain Society/American College of Physicians clinical practice guideline. Ann Intern Med. 2007;147(7):493–506.

12. Khan MIA, Walsh D, Brito-Dellan N. Opioid and adjuvant analgesics: compared and contrasted. Am J Hosp Palliat Care. 2011;28(5):378–83.
13. Knotkova H, Pappagallo M. Adjuvant analgesics. Anesthesiol Clin. 2007;25(4):775–86.
14. Ballantyne JC. Opioid therapy for chronic pain. N Engl J Med. 2003;349(20):1943–53.
15. Dupen A, Shen D, Ersek M. Mechanisms of opioid-induced tolerance and hyperalgesia. Pain Manag Nurs. 2007;8(3):113–21.
16. Harris JD. Management of expected and unexpected opioid-related side effects. Clin J Pain. 2008;24(Suppl 10):S8.
17. Harvey RA, Champe PC. Lippinott's illustrated reviews: pharmacology. 4th ed. Philadelphia, PA: Lippincott Williams & Wilkins; 2009. p. 127–70.
18. Anand P, Bley K. Topical capsaicin for pain management: therapeutic potential and mechanisms of action of the new high-concentration capsaicin 8% patch. Br J Anaesth. 2011;107(4):490–502.
19. Alvarez DJ, PG R. Trigger points: diagnosis and management. Am Fam Physician. 2002;15(65):653–61.
20. Nickl S, Terranova LM. Trigger point injections. In: Spinner D, Kirschner J, Herrera J, editors. Atlas of ultrasound guided musculoskeletal injections. Musculoskeletal medicine. New York: Springer; 2014. p. 89–100.
21. Byrd D, Mackey S. Pulsed radiofrequency for chronic pain. Curr Pain Headache Rep. 2008;12(1):37–41.
22. Facchini G, Spinnato P, Guglielmi G, Albisinni U, Bazzocchi A. A comprehensive review of pulsed radiofrequency in the treatment of pain associated with different spinal conditions. Br J Radiol. 2017;90(1073):20150406.
23. Chambers WA. Nerve blocks in palliative care. Br J Anaesth. 2008;101(1):95–100.
24. Goldstein NE, Morrison RS. Evidence-based practice of palliative medicine. Philadelphia: Elsevier Saunders; 2013.
25. Strakowski JA. Ultrasound-guided peripheral nerve procedures. Phys Med Rehabil Clin N Am. 2016;27(3):687–715.
26. Reuben DB, Herr KA, Pacala JT, et al. Table 99. Types of pain, examples, and treatment. In: Geriatrics at your fingertips. 17th ed. New York: American Geriatrics Society; 2015. p. 232.
27. Martin WR. Pharmacology of opioids. Pharmacol Rev. 1983;35(4):283–323.
28. Paice JA, Noskin GA, Vanagunas A, Shott S. Efficacy and safety of scheduled dosing of opioid analgesics: a quality improvement study. J Pain. 2005;6(10):639–43.
29. Sills G. The mechanisms of action of gabapentin and pregabalin. Curr Opin Pharmacol. 2006;6(1):108–13.

Non-pain Symptoms

Belinda Setters and Serena Hsiou-Ling Chao

A. Chun (ed.), *Geriatric Practice*, https://doi.org/10.1007/978-3-030-19625-7_43

Competency 19

Assess and provide initial management of pain and key non-pain symptoms based on patient's goals of care.

43.1 Background Introduction

The appropriate diagnosis and treatment of non-pain symptoms in older patients can be one of the most challenging and important tasks for young physicians to master. Discussing goals of care, prognosis, and quality of life is essential for developing a treatment plan and is especially important when working with older adult and frail patients. This should include obtaining thorough social and functional (daily and instrumental activities) histories. Living arrangements, available caregivers and their limitations, and family and community support should be outlined. Other social and financial resources and stressors should be noted as well as the availability of interdisciplinary care providers such as nurses, social workers, therapists, and chaplains. For many older adult patients with chronic diseases especially toward the end of life, enrollment in a house calls, palliative care, or hospice program (palliative care in the last 6 months of life) is one of the best ways to get interdisciplinary team-based care. These care models not only improve symptom control and patient satisfaction but can extend life for patients with certain diagnoses such as lung cancer [4, 12, 16, 25, 39, 52].

Age-related physiological changes cause older patients to present atypically, often with vague symptomatology. Keeping these changes in mind can help providers avoid pitfalls of caring for older often more frail patients. Evaluating all medications and supplements that patients are taking is critical. Providers should also know patients' hepatic and renal functions in order to make necessary medication dose adjustments. Medical and pharmacy resources such as Micromedex (▶ http://www.micromedexsolutions.com/micromedex2/librarian) and Lexicomp (▶ http://www.wolterskluwercdi.com/lexicomp-online/) are typically available through most medical school or hospital websites and can help determine appropriate dosages (sites accessed July 22, 2019). Discussing possible side effects and what is acceptable or not for the patient and caregiver can help prevent problems with nonadherence and poor symptom control.

Aftercare goals are outlined; documenting and communicating them are critical as patients transition through different sites of care such as home (outpatient office) to hospital. It is not uncommon for a patient's goals and terminal diagnosis to be overlooked in the focus on more acute issues in each care area. Programs focused on ensuring that the patient's goals are acknowledged and emphasized through care transitions have helped reduce these problems and are available in most states now. POLST (Physicians Orders for Life-Sustaining Treatment) is one such program available in 46 states (▶ http://polst.org, accessed July 22, 2019) which uses a shared decision-making model [17] and documents goals clearly to reduce miscommunication and errors as the patient transitions across various sites of care.

Case

Reginald Dwight, a 78-year-old retired musician, presents to your office accompanied by his son for a routine visit. Mr. Dwight complains he feels tired all the time but denies other concerns. A quick chart review reminds you he has a history of hypertensive heart disease with diastolic heart failure, hypothyroidism, and Alzheimer's dementia. Mr. Dwight moved in with his son a year ago and has been increasingly less active, dozing off while watching TV and is restless, frequently getting up out of bed at night. While his memory has declined, he still enjoys playing the piano but is too exhausted to play more than one song. He is in good spirits and wants to go out with family and visit with friends, but this, too, has become difficult for him. Medications include metoprolol, lisinopril, aspirin, furosemide, atorvastatin, levothyroxine, and donepezil.

43.2 Fatigue

Fatigue is extremely common among palliative and multimorbid patients, occurring in ½ to ¾ of them [26, 38]. While its vague nature can make it difficult to define, fatigue is generally described as a symptom characterized by tiredness, low energy, and exhaustion. It results in decreased activity and is not relieved by resting [13].

Much like many symptoms or syndromes in older patients, fatigue can be caused by a wide variety of underlying etiologies as noted in ◻ Table 43.1 [26, 27, 31]. Cancer which occurs in increasing incidence with aging and cardiopulmonary diseases such as heart failure and chronic obstructive pulmonary disease (COPD) are among the common causes of fatigue in older patients. Focusing on methods to improve sleep and conserving energy can be key to addressing symptom management. Cardiopulmonary rehabilitation is often underutilized but can have a significant impact on fatigue management for many such patients [29, 33].

In addition to ensuring quality sleep and energy conservation, addressing medication- related side effects is also important. De-prescribing offending medications can have a tremendous effect on a patient fatigue level and therefore quality of life [5, 21, 28]. Many medications can cause fatigue, several of which are listed in ◻ Table 43.2.

Fatigue is not only a common symptom of cancer, it is one of the most common side effects of chemotherapy regimens [41]. The use of guides such as ePrognosis (▶ www.eprognosis.ucsf.edu, accessed February 8, 2018) can be very helpful in determining which patients should have routine

Table 43.1 Common causes of fatigue

System	Examples
Cardiovascular	Coronary artery disease Heart failure Peripheral vascular disease
Pulmonary	COPD Pulmonary fibrosis
Immunologic	Infections Immune compromise states
Gastrointestinal	Malabsorption Malnutrition GI bleeding
Neurological	Multiple sclerosis Poststroke syndrome Amotrophic Lateral Sclerosis (ALS)
Hematologic	Anemia of chronic disease Iron deficiency anemia
Oncologic	Lung cancer Chemotherapy side effects

Table 43.2 Medications that commonly cause fatigue

System	Drug class	Examples
Cardiac	Beta-blockers	Metoprolol
	ACE inhibitors	Lisinopril
	Diuretics	Furosemide
Immunologic	Antihistamines	Fexofenadine Diphenhydramine
	Antibiotics	Clarithromycin Levofloxacin
Endocrine	Statins	Simvastatin Atorvastatin
	Fibrates	Fenofibrate
Neurologic	Monoamine oxidase	Selegiline
	Muscle relaxants	Metaxalone
	Sleep medications	Zolpidem Zaleplon
Psychiatric	Antidepressants	Sertraline Venlafaxine
	Antipsychotics	Haloperidol Quetiapine
	Anxiolytics	Diazepam Clonazepam
Miscellaneous	Pain medications	Morphine Oxycodone

screens such as colonoscopies or mammograms as well as provide guidance on how to have difficult discussions around invasive testing in light of care goals.

In oncology patients, discussing the patient's goals considering the severity of fatigue is key to aiding the patient in deciding to continue therapy or focus on a more palliative-based approach. Palliative transfusions may be an option to keep fatigue at bay while allowing for more quality time with loved ones or reaching a special life event such as a wedding or birth of a grandchild. They should not be used routinely without a clear indication as transfusion-related risks can be significant and blood resources are limited [53]. Less invasive treatments such as replacing low Vitamin B-12 or iron can also be helpful in patients with such deficiencies. Addressing underlying causes of fatigue can also be helpful as can treating associated psychological and physical symptoms [26, 58]. Not overlooking infectious causes of fatigue in terminal patients is important as patients may experience new or worsening of existing fatigue. [9].

It is important to differentiate the fatigue that occurs at the very end of life as part of the dying process from that of chronic diseases or treatment effects earlier in the disease course. Treatment of symptoms including fatigue in the dying patient should be appropriately focused on the comfort of the patient in the context of care goals.

In the case of Mr. Dwight, there are several possible explanations for his fatigue. He has a history of hypothyroidism, so ensuring his thyroid hormone levels are normal is important as is checking for vitamin deficiency such as B-12, electrolyte abnormalities, renal and liver dysfunction. Reviewing his medication list for possible side effects is also crucial. Mr. Dwight is on several medications that can cause fatigue including a beta-blocker, diuretic, and statin. Adjusting the dose or changing to a different in class or other class medication when possible will often alleviate fatigue symptoms. He appears to have insomnia which is also a common cause of fatigue and given the presenting history, very likely to the main underlying etiology for his fatigue.

43.3 Insomnia

Much like fatigue insomnia, is a very common symptom among palliative patients, occurring in over 70% and is caused by a variety of conditions, often several causes at once [10, 22, 24, 35, 40]. Some common ones are shown in Fig. 43.1. This multifactorial nature lends itself to an interdisciplinary care approach including physical therapy for pain relief, cognitive therapy for anxiety, and depression as well as chaplaincy for spiritual distress. Addressing the different causes of insomnia will improve adherence and symptom control. Tables 43.3 and 43.4 list common nonpharmacological and medication treatments of insomnia, respectively [10, 18, 23, 24].

Hypersomnia may occur separately or in conjunction with insomnia. Dementia can disturb the normal sleep-wake cycle and cause daytime sleepiness [18]. This disturbance in the sleep-wake cycle is a separate phenomenon from the

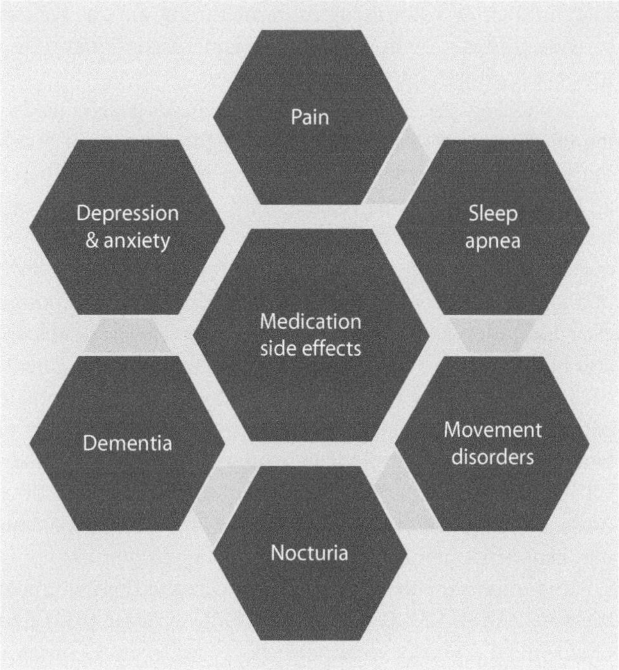

Fig. 43.1 Common causes of insomnia

Table 43.3 Nonpharmacological interventions for insomnia

Therapy	Description
Sleep hygiene	Focuses on activities that create a good sleep experience including: *Maintain a regular bedtime and morning wake time* *Create a comfortable sleep environment* *Avoid excessive amounts of caffeine especially late in the day* *Avoid eating, watching tv, and reading in bed* *Avoid exercise or heavy meals late at night* *Relax before bed, wind down, and only go to bed when sleepy*
Sleep restriction	Limits total time in bed to improve sleep efficiency and quality
Cognitive therapy	Addresses attitudes and beliefs about poor sleep habits
Light therapy	Bright light therapy increases melatonin, improving sleep, and mood
Massage therapy	Like other relaxation techniques, massage can be especially helpful for cancer and chronic pain patients *A family member or sleep partner taught to do simple 30 min massage* *An electronic massager used as directed can also be very effective*

normal changes that may occur to the sleep cycle with aging including earlier onset of nighttime sleepiness, longer latency time to fall asleep and more shallow, fragmented sleep cycles. This can result in more daytime sleepiness and napping.

Prostate hyperplasia and nocturia are also common causes of sleep disturbance and can result in significant sleep deficits. Diuretic medications, especially when taken later in the day can exacerbate these conditions. Other medications such as beta-blockers and serotoninergic antidepressants can cause insomnia in a more direct manner. Decreasing the dose of these medications or stopping them if possible will usually help with insomnia [21]. Educating patients and families about the complexity of insomnia can help establish reasonable treatment goals and cooperation in using a multi-faceted approach to its treatment.

Changes in nonpharmacological habits such as sleep hygiene should be tried before starting medications for the treatment of insomnia [10, 18, 23, 35]. Sleep hygiene encourages good sleep habits such as setting a good environment for sleep (turning off lights, having a comfortable temperature) and avoiding activities that can disturb sleep (caffeine or TV late at night). Warm milk, massage, relaxing music, and setting a scheduled bedtime can also be very helpful in combating sleep disturbances. More information on this and other interventions can be found at the National Sleep Foundation website ► www.sleepfoundation.org (accessed July 22, 2019).

If a patient fails nonpharmacological treatments, the use of supplements such as melatonin and other hypnotics can be useful [18, 24, 35]. Melatonin is available in short- and long-acting formulations. For older and frail patients, starting with a 5 mg or lower dose is recommended. Increasing the dose to achieve desired sleep effect may be needed. If a patient does not respond to melatonin, a trial of other medication such as trazodone or mirtazapine may be useful. While these meds are felt to be safe, serious side effects such as hyponatremia, prolonged QTc on EKG, and serotonin syndrome can occur. Of note, mirtazapine stimulates sleep as a histaminic side effect at lower doses (7.5–15 mg). It also stimulates appetite, so it can be an especially good choice in treating patients with both insomnia and anorexia. Other medication such as benzodiazepine and zolpidem can induce sleep but have severe side effects and are habit-forming. These medications are not recommended for use in older or frail patients for the routine symptom management of insomnia [2].

In Mr. Dwight's case, he was on several medications that were likely contributing to insomnia. He also had several chronic conditions that may be causes. Reductions in doses, or discontinuation if possible, of metoprolol and atorvastatin may be helpful to reduce insomnia symptoms. A work-up to ensure thyroid hormone levels are normal and electrolytes, renal, and hepatic function are normal is also needed. A thorough review of systems and examination should be done to assess for possible malignancy or other related causes such as worsening heart failure.

Table 43.4 Medications used to treat insomnia

Medication		Dosage	Pearls
Melatonin	***Melatonin****	3–6 mg or 5–10 mg	Technically a "supplement," melatonin is purchased in immediate and long-acting formulation over the counter. Long-acting formulation is better at maintaining sleep longer through night Available in gummies for patients with dementia and others who may frequently refuse to take medications and supplements
Melatonin agonist	Ramelteon	8 mg	Should not be used as first line in substitute for melatonin Can cause dizziness and myalgias
Sedating antidepressants	***Trazodone****	25–50 mg	Antidepressant which can be used in doses up to 100 mg for sleep Side effects include orthostasis, priapism, and prolonged QT
	Mirtazapine*	7.5–15 mg	Only effective at lower doses as sedation is a result of histaminic side effect Causes appetite stimulation at low dose which can be especially helpful for patients with both anorexia and insomnia Can also cause serotonin syndrome and hyponatremia especially at higher doses and if used in combination with other serotonin agents
	Doxepin	3–6 mg	Tricyclic antidepressant (TCA) which causes somnolence Should not be taken within 3 hours of eating/mealtime Has antihistaminic and anticholinergic effects which can cause confusion in some patients but generally has lower risk than other TCAs
Nonbenzodiazepine hypnotics	Zolpidem	2.5–5 mg	Can precipitate falls, cause sleep-related behaviors such as sleep walking Available in oral spray and disintegrated tablet and long-acting formulations
Benzodiazepines	Lorazepam	0.5–2 mg	If a benzodiazepine is indicated, a shorter acting one with no active metabolites is strongly preferred, such as lorazepam Very high risk for falls and can cause respiratory suppression especially in patients on opioid pain medications or who have advanced lung disease

Case Continued

Mr. Dwight and his son return to your office 6 months later. He has been sleeping better with the addition of melatonin at night and his fatigue has improved with a decrease in his metoprolol dose. He has started having more difficulty having bowel movements and sometimes goes several days without a movement. He often forgets to eat or drink if his family doesn't prompt him. They frequently come home to his lunch being left on the counter. The patient denies concerns and says he eats just fine, but his son is concerned this is affecting his bowel pattern as well as causing weight loss.

43.4 Constipation

The prevalence of constipation in terminal illness ranges between 7% and 90% [11, 14, 19, 50], with higher rates seen in patients who take opioids to treat pain. Factors associated with constipation include medication side effects, immobility, and worsening oral intake of both fluids and high-fiber foods. Constipation diminishes patients' quality of life through inducing symptoms such as painful abdominal distension, anorexia, nausea, overflowing loose stool, and delirium.

The first step in evaluation is to determine if the cause can be addressed. Stop any medications that are contributing to constipation, if possible. For example, consider using a nonopioid pain agent in place of opioids if constipation is related to the latter. Patients can also try lifestyle changes to treat constipation. If the patient is capable, he/she should attempt to increase daily dietary fiber and fluid intake [42]. He/she should also try toileting immediately after eating meals, to take advantage of the body's natural reflex to defecate following food intake.

If the patient's constipation is due to reasons that cannot be changed (e.g., immobility due to end-stage organ disease), then we can offer medications to facilitate increased bowel movement frequency. Patient preferences and goals should determine what agents we initiate. When choosing between therapies, we must consider several factors including, but not limited to:

- Risk for adverse side effects in the context of the patient's other medical conditions and medications (e.g., magnesium-containing laxatives should be avoided in patients with advanced chronic kidney disease)
- Tolerability (e.g., a rectally administered therapy is preferable in patients with severe nausea and vomiting)
- The patient's current level of oral intake (e.g., bulk-forming laxatives like psyllium require patients to drink a large amount of fluid)
- Availability of others to administer the medication or treatment if necessary

Table 43.5 Medications to treat nausea, by etiology

Cause of nausea	Medication class	Suggested starting dosages	Potential side effects
Cerebral metastases, increased intracranial pressure	Corticosteroids	Dexamethasone 2 mg oral every 8 hours; liquid dose available	Delirium, dyspepsia
Side effects of opioids	Antiemetic agents that are also antipsychotic agents	(a) Prochlorperazine 5 mg oral three times daily 25 mg suppository daily 2.5 mg IV every 4 hours (b) Chlorpromazine 10 mg oral every 6 hour	Extrapyramidal symptoms (dystonias, tremors, akathisia, tardive dyskinesias), constipation
	Prokinetic agents	Metoclopramide 5 mg oral four times a day	Extrapyramidal symptoms (because it is a dopamine receptor antagonist)
Gastric irritation	H_2 blockers	(a) Famotidine 20 mg oral once daily (b) Nizatidine 150 mg oral once daily	Delirium
	Proton pump inhibitors	(a) Lansoprazole 15 mg oral daily (b) Omeprazole 20 mg oral daily (c) Pantoprazole 20 mg oral daily	Increased risk for C. diff infection in the case of prolonged use
Constipation	Osmotic laxatives	(a) Lactulose 15 ml oral daily-twice daily (b) Polyethylene glycol 8.5 g powder mixed in 8 oz water, daily (c) Glycerine one suppository per rectum daily	Abdominal cramps
	Stimulant laxatives	(a) Senna one tablet oral at bedtime (b) Bisacodyl 10 mg suppository per rectum daily	Abdominal cramps
	Enemas	(a) Tap water Twice a week (b) Saline Twice a week	

No single orally administered laxative is superior to others in alleviating constipation in patients receiving palliative care [11]. Whichever agent you choose, start with the lowest possible dose and slowly titrate doses upwards while monitoring for adverse drug reactions (see Table 43.5, "Management of Nausea, By Etiology"). Lactulose is no better than senna [3] although the combination may be effective in constipated patients taking opioids [49]. The combination of docusate plus senna is also no better than using senna alone [51]. Although polyethylene glycol is more effective than lactulose in treating chronic constipation [30], this agent has not been studied in palliative care populations. Many of these laxatives can produce intolerable side effects, including nausea, vomiting, and abdominal pain, necessitating discontinuation if benefits do not outweigh burdens.

If patients are unable to drink large amounts of fluids or swallow pills, then choose agents that can be rectally administered (see Table 43.5). Use tap water or saline enemas if all other measures are either unsuccessful or would cause more harm than comfort [42].

In Mr. Dwight's case, his constipation is likely secondary to his decreased oral intake decreased physical activity and slowed gastrointestinal movement that occurs with aging. He is forgetting to eat lunch and drink fluids when his family is not there to remind him. This is a common problem for dementia patients and can lead to dehydration and renal failure as well as worsening constipation. Reminders to drink fluids throughout the day can be helpful in preventing this. Nursing orders to offer fluids to patients with dementia with medication passes and throughout the day can help patients who are hospitalized or residing in a nursing facility. Adding an osmolotic or stimulant laxative as needed may help this patient.

It should be noted that while Mr. Dwight lives with his family and does not have concerns for food access or financial stressors, many older adults including those at the end of life do. Poverty and socioeconomic factors can impact access to food and other essential needs such as housing and medical access. These should be considered when caring for vulnerable older adults as they can contribute to symptoms and create difficulty for patients to comply with therapy or maintain follow-up appointments. Utilizing local interdisciplinary resources including social work can help address these issues and problem solve around them to create more successful treatment plans.

43.5 Anorexia and Weight Loss

Anorexia and resulting weight loss are common as people with terminal illness approach the end of their lives. For many terminal conditions, weight loss cannot be reversed with improving nutritional intake. Reduced oral intake does not cause suffering for the patient when it occurs as a consequence of terminal illness [42]. However, it can worsen emotional distress experienced by the patient's loved ones. It is important for medical providers to provide patients and their loved ones frequent education that anorexia is an expected consequence of the dying process [36, 43]. Furthermore, we should encourage them to view oral food intake as an activity that provides pleasure, rather than as an activity to provide nutrition. All patients with terminal illness should eat foods that they enjoy, without regard to disease-based dietary guidelines. They should also eat as large or small an amount as provides comfort.

Patients, their loved ones, or specialists may recommend initiating megestrol acetate to improve appetite and stimulate weight gain. Megestrol acetate is only FDA-approved for patients with HIV-associated anorexia [44]. Prescribing it to treat anorexia related to other terminal illnesses would be considered off-label use. Furthermore, megestrol acetate use is associated with increased risk for thromboembolic events, peripheral edema and death [32, 44]. In 2015, megestrol acetate was deemed a medication to avoid in older adults by the American Geriatrics Society Beers Criteria Expert Update Panel. Therefore, we should not prescribe megestrol for older adults with terminal illness, as risks outweigh potential benefits.

In patients with concurrent depression, use of mirtazapine may improve both mood and weight [2, 54]. However, evidence is lacking that mirtazapine results in weight gain in patients without depressed mood [2]. Mirtazapine can also cause the syndrome of inappropriate antidiuretic hormone (SIADH), resulting in hyponatremia. Therefore, this agent should be used with caution, particularly if the patient has declining kidney function and oral intake [2].

While high-calorie nutritional supplements will result in patient weight gain, there is no evidence that their use improves patient's quality of life, functional status, or life expectancy [2]. Furthermore, the top-listed ingredients in many of these supplements are water, corn syrup or corn maltodextrin, and sugar. Therefore, the American Geriatrics Society has recommended that we avoid their use in older adults. Practically speaking, we may consider prescribing high-calorie nutritional supplements if the patient enjoys drinking them and prefers them to other foods or fluids, or if using these supplements reduces caregiver burden because of convenience.

In the case of patients with advanced progressive dementia, placement of a gastric feeding tube should be avoided. This intervention is not associated with improved survival or quality of life [1, 20, 45, 46]. Feeding tubes do not eliminate the risk for aspiration, and placement is associated with adverse events such as bleeding and infection. Instead, we should counsel family members and loved ones to hand feed these patients, with the goal of providing pleasure and comfort.

In our patient's case, progression of his dementia along with heart failure and/or medication side effects are likely contributing to anorexia and weight loss. Nonpharmacological measures noted above along with reminders to eat and drink as noted in the previous section on Constipation may help curb his anorexia and weight loss.

Case Continued

Mr. Dwight continues to slowly decline and requires additional nonskilled in-home care to assist his family in caring for his needs. Despite this, he becomes increasing weak, falling several times and eventually develops worsening anorexia with nausea and vomiting. His family brings him to the emergency department of the local hospital for an evaluation.

43.6 Nausea and Vomiting

Many conditions can lead to nausea and vomiting, including metastases to the brain, increased intracranial pressure, side effects of medications, gastric irritation, or mechanical obstruction of the GI tract [4, 42, 43]. The initial management step is to eliminate medications that may be playing a role, if benefits of these medications do not outweigh burdens. Initiate treatment for the underlying condition, if clinically appropriate. Try nonpharmacological measures, such as ginger products [34] and eating smaller more frequent meals to alleviate nausea.

If the patient continues to have nausea and vomiting, use medications that are targeted to the underlying cause of these symptoms (see ◘ Table 43.5 "Medications to Treat Nausea, by Etiology"; [4, 15, 42, 43]). Always start with the lowest possible dose, and slowly titrate dose upwards in order to minimize intolerable side effects.

Prochlorperazine is commonly included in emergency kits provided by hospice agencies to patients treated in the home [47]. If the patient has intractable vomiting and cannot take oral medications, this agent can be rectally administered via a suppository. Alternatively, the patient could be transferred to an inpatient hospice unit to receive antiemetic therapy intravenously. If a patient has both nausea and terminal delirium, haloperidol has antiemetic properties and can also reduce agitation and psychosis related to delirium ([47]; refer to the chapter focused on delirium).

Case Continued

Mr. Dwight was admitted to the hospital service for dehydration with acute renal insufficiency as well as likely urinary tract infection and delirium. Evaluation found he was severely impacted, having loose stools around this impaction. He was rehydrated, treated with antibiotics and manually dis-impacted. His delirium resolved, but he remained more confused than previously and was very weak. Physical therapy recommended a short course of rehab prior to returning home.

Mr. Dwight went to a local nursing facility for a short-term rehabilitation stay. However, he continued to be more confused and was not able to participate well with therapy. During this time, he also experienced more difficulty "catching his breath" when up walking for exercises. Examination found him to be fluid overloaded with bilateral rales and edematous lower extremities. He did not respond to an increase in his furosemide dosing and began requiring oxygen therapy. He was sent back to the hospital for an IV diuretics and further assessment to rule out other causes of his symptoms.

43.7 Dyspnea

Dyspnea is a common symptom experienced by patients at the end of life, even if they do not have an underlying terminal respiratory disease [7, 37]. The sensation of breathlessness or "air hunger" can arise through multiple mechanisms, including lung irritation by infections or fluid, pain, progressive neuromuscular disease that results in respiratory muscle and diaphragmatic weakness, and worsening anemia.

The initial management step is to treat the underlying etiology of dyspnea, if benefits outweigh risks and the treatment aligns with the patient's goals of care. For example, nebulized albuterol combined with ipratropium and supplemental oxygen may alleviate dyspnea in patients with end-stage chronic bronchitis and hypoxia. Nonpharmacological measures, such as use of hand-held fans, breathing training, and chest wall vibration, may be effective in reducing dyspnea [8, 42].

Opioids are commonly included in hospice emergency kits to treat both dyspnea and pain [47]. Morphine use may result in a short-term improvement in exercise capacity, but the evidence is low quality [7]. Furthermore, its use is associated with increased incidence of nausea and vomiting, constipation, and drowsiness compared to placebo [7]. The advantage of morphine is that it is available in a highly concentrated solution (20 mg per 1 ml) that is readily absorbed by the oral mucosa and therefore can be given to patients who are actively dying. For patients who are alert and suffering from dyspnea, start morphine tablets at 5 mg every 2–4 hours as needed [4, 42]. The initial starting dose of concentrated morphine solution is 5 mg, repeated every 15–30 minutes as needed [42]. Fentanyl does not seem to reduce "air hunger" [7], although it may be preferred over morphine for pain management in patients with advanced kidney disease because its breakdown products are inactive (see ▶ Chap. 42 focused on pain management at the end of life).

Benzodiazepines such as lorazepam are often included in hospice emergency kits [47] to treat both dyspnea and anxiety. There is no strong evidence that benzodiazepines are more effective than placebo in relieving air hunger [48], and its use is associated with increased risk of somnolence. Consider using benzodiazepines as second or third-line therapy for dyspnea if other measures are ineffective [48], and prescribe low doses at the start (e.g., lorazepam 0.5 mg tab or lorazepam 2 mg/1 ml solution 0.25 ml sublingual every 4 hours; [42]).

It was determined that Mr. Dwight was dyspneic from a combination of worsening heart failure and aspiration pneumonitis. Antibiotics were started as he began showing signs of sepsis, and he was put on bi-pap noninvasive pulmonary support; IV diuresis was also pursued.

Case Continued

Mr. Dwight failed to respond to antibiotic therapy for aspiration pneumonitis and aggressive diuresis. A family goals of care meeting was held at the bedside with the palliative care team. His family decided he would not want to be intubated or sustained with aggressive measures as previously expressed. They opted for comfort-based care with hospice services. Mr. White was transferred to the hospice inpatient unit for ongoing symptoms management and aggressive terminal care support including treatment of oral secretions which had worsened during his hospitalization.

43.8 Oral Secretions

As people near the end of life, they experience increased pharyngeal and airway secretions that produce an audible "death rattle," which can be distressing for loved ones to hear. Prevalence of the "death rattle" ranges between 23% and 92% [55]. Reducing cholinergic chemical signaling should in theory reduce secretion production. Common anticholinergic agents prescribed for palliative care and hospice patients include hyoscine hydrobromide, hyoscine butylbromide, scopolamine, atropine, and glycopyrronium bromide. Of note, all of the preceding agents except for glycopyrronium bromide are included in the 2015 AGS Beers Criteria list for agents that should be avoided in older adults, because they are highly anticholinergic [6]. There is mixed evidence regarding the efficacy of anticholinergic agents compared to placebo [55, 57]. This may be explained by the fact that agents can prevent the formation of new secretions but not eliminate secretions already present in the oropharynx. No agent is superior to the others [57].

The initial approach to management should involve repositioning the patient, preferably on the left side, and gentle suctioning of secretions located in the oral cavity. The use of anticholinergic agents can be tried if nonpharmacological measures are ineffective and the presence of secretions is causing suffering for the patient and/or her loved ones. If anticholinergic agents are prescribed, start at the lowest possible doses. Glycopyrronium bromide does not cross the blood-brain barrier; in theory, it should be less likely to cause delirium compared to the other anticholinergic agents. However, it is administered subcutaneously or intravenously, in doses of 0.1–0.4 mg every 4 hours as needed [42]. Therefore, its use may be limited to the inpatient hospital or inpatient hospice settings. For patients in the home setting with trouble swallowing, a scopolamine patch administered every 3 days could be considered, despite its presence on the 2015 AGS Beers Criteria list. Monitor patients closely for the development of side effects, such as delirium, dry mouth, constipation, or urinary retention. Stop medications if side effects are intolerable.

43.9 The Last Hours

It is helpful for medical providers to be familiar with what occurs to people in the last hours of life. Patients and families often rely on their medical providers to teach them about the last moments, in order to psychologically prepare themselves for what is to come. People who face imminent death exhibit features in common, regardless of the underlying terminal disease process or processes. In the last hours to weeks of life, oral intake dramatically declines. With that, urine production lessens and eventually stops. People in the active dying phase become increasingly somnolent, with fewer moments of consciousness. They become immobile and therefore have an increased chance for developing pressure ulcers and constipation. Their breathing becomes irregular, and they sometimes exhibit Cheyne-Stokes breathing, a recurring pattern characterized by quiet, shallow breathing that crescendos to rapid, deep breathing before a dramatic apneic pause. In the last stage, they develop increased oropharyngeal secretions commonly referred to as the "death rattle," fever, mottled extremities, and coma [4, 12, 56].

References

1. AGS Choosing Wisely Workgroup. American Geriatrics Society identifies five things that healthcare providers and patients should question. J Am Geriatr Soc. 2013;61(4):622–31.
2. AGS Choosing Wisely Workgroup. American Geriatrics Society identifies another five things that healthcare providers and patients should question. J Am Geriatr Soc. 2014;62(5):950–60.
3. Agra Y, Sacristan A, Gonzalez M, Ferrari M, Portugues A, Calvo MJ. Efficacy of senna versus lactulose in terminal cancer patients treated with opioids. J Pain Symptom Manag. 1998;15:1–7.
4. Albert R. End-of-life care: managing common symptoms. Am Fam Physician [serial on the Internet]. 2017 [cited February 7, 2018];95(6):356–361. Available from MEDLINE Complete.
5. American Geriatrics Society Expert Panel on the Care of Older Adults in Multimorbidity. Guiding principles for the care of older adults with multimorbidity: an approach for clinicians. J Am Geriatr Soc. 2012;60:E1–E25.
6. American Geriatrics Society 2015 Beers Criteria Update Expert Panel. American Geriatrics Society 2015 updated beers criteria for potentially inappropriate medication use in older adults. J Am Geriatr Soc. 2015;63:2227–46.
7. Barnes H. Opioids for the palliation of refractory breathlessness in adults with advanced disease and terminal illness. Cochrane Database of Systematic Reviews [serial on the Internet]. 2017 [cited February 7, 2018];(10). Available from: Cochrane Database of Systematic Reviews.
8. Bausewein C. Non-pharmacological interventions for breathlessness in advanced stages of malignant and non-malignant disease. Cochrane Database of Systematic Reviews [serial on the Internet]. 2014 [cited February 7, 2018];(4). Available from: Cochrane Database of Systematic Reviews.
9. Buchwald D, Sullivan JL, Komaroff AL. Frequency of 'chronic active Epstein-Barr virus infection' in a general medical practice. JAMA. 1987;257:2303–7.
10. Budhiraja R, Parthasarathy S, Budhiraja P, Habib MP, Wendel C, et al. Insomnia in patients with COPD. Sleep. 2012;35(3):369.
11. Candy B. Laxatives for the management of constipation in people receiving palliative care. Cochrane Database of Systematic Reviews [serial on Internet]. 2015 [cited February 1, 2018];(5). Available from: Cochrane Database of Systemic Reviews.
12. Center to Advance Palliative Care (CAPC). www.capc.org. Accessed 8 Feb 2018.
13. Chai E, Meier D, Morris J, Goldhirsh S. Fatigue. In: Geriatric palliative care. Oxford: Oxford University Press; 2014.
14. Clark K, Currow DC. Assessing constipation in palliative care in a gastroenterology framework. Palliat Med. 2012;26:834–84.
15. Clark K. Metoclopramide for chronic nausea in adult palliative care patients with advanced cancer. Cochrane Database of Systematic Reviews [serial on Internet]. 2013 [cited January 26, 2018];(11). Available from: Cochrane Database of Systemic Reviews.
16. Connor SR, Pyenson B, Fitch K, Spense C, Iwaskai K. Comparing hospice and nonhospice survival among patients who die within a three-year window. J Pain Symptom Manag. 2007;33:238–46.
17. Covinsky KE, Fuller JD, Yaffe K, et al. Communication and decision-making in seriously ill patients: findings of the SUPPORT project: the study to understand prognoses and preferences for outcomes and risks of treatments. J Am Geriatr Soc. 2000;48.:Suppl:S187–93.
18. Deschenes CL, McCurry SM. Current treatments for sleep disturbances in individuals with dementia. Curr Psychiatry Rep. 2009;11:20–6.
19. Erichsén E, Milberg A, Jaarsma T, Friedrichsen MJ. Constipation in specialized palliative care: prevalence, definition, and patient-perceived symptom distress. J Palliat Med. 2015;18(7):585–92.
20. Finucane TE, Christmas C, Travis K. Tube feeding in patients with advanced dementia: a review of the evidence. JAMA. 1999;282:1365–70.
21. Garfinkle D, Mangin D. Feasibility study of a systematic approach for discontinuation of multiple medications in older adults: addressing polypharmacy. Arch Intern Med. 2010;170:1648–54.
22. Glynn J, Gale S, Tank S. Causes of sleep disturbance in a specialist palliative care unit. BMJ Support Palliat Care. 2014;4(Suppl 1):A56.
23. Hayes D Jr, Anstead MI, Ho J, Phillips BA. Insomnia and chronic heart failure. Heart Fail Rev. 2009;14(3):171–82.
24. Hugel H, Ellershaw JE, Cook L, Skinner J, Irvine C. The prevalence, key causes and management of insomnia in palliative care patients. J Pain Symptom Manag. 2004;27(4):316.
25. Kleinpell R, Vasilevskis EE, Fogg L, Ely W. Exploring the association of hospice care on patient experience and outcomes of care. BMJ Support Palliat Care. Published Online First: 16 Aug 2016. https://doi.org/10.1136/bmjspcare-2015-001001.
26. Kroenke K, Arrington ME, Mangelsdorff AD. The prevalence of symptoms in medical outpatients and the adequacy of therapy. Arch Intern Med. 1990;150:1685–9.
27. Kroenke K, Wood DR, Mangelsdorff AD, Meier NJ, Powell JB. Chronic fatigue in primary care. Prevalence, patient characteristics, and outcomes. JAMA. 1988;260:926–34.
28. Kutner JS, Blatchford PJ, Taylor DH Jr, et al. Safety and benefit of discontinuing statin therapy in the setting of advanced, life-limiting illness: a randomized clinical trial. JAMA Intern Med. 2015;175:691–700.

29. Lacasse Y, Golstein R, Lasseron TJ, Martin S. Pulmonary rehabilitation for chronic obstructive pulmonary disease. Cochrane Database of Systematic Reviews. 2006;(4):Art No: CD003793.
30. Lee-Robichaud H. Lactulose versus polyethylene glycol for chronic constipation. Cochrane Database of Systematic Reviews [serial on Internet]. 2010 [cited February 1, 2018];(1). Available from: Cochrane Database of Systemic Reviews.
31. Markowitz AJ, Rabow MW. Palliative management of fatigue at the close of life: "it feels like my body is just worn out". JAMA. 2007;298:217.
32. Marshall LL. Megestrol acetate therapy in geriatric patients: case reviews and associated deep vein thrombosis. Consult Pharm. 2003;18(9):764–73.
33. Martin B, Hauer T, Arena R, Leslie D, Galbraith D, et al. Cardiac rehabilitation attendance and outcomes in coronary artery disease patients. Circulation. 2012;126:677–87.
34. Matthews A. Interventions for nausea and vomiting in early pregnancy. Cochrane Database of Systematic Reviews [serial on Internet]. 2015 [cited February 12, 2018];(9). Available from: Cochrane Database of Systemic Reviews.
35. Mercadante S, Aielli F, Adile C, Ferrera P, Valle A, et al. Sleep disturbances in patients with advanced cancer in different palliative care settings. J Pain Symptom Manag. 2015;50(6):786–92.
36. Milne A. Protein and energy supplementation in elderly people at risk from malnutrition. Cochrane Database of Systematic Reviews [serial on Internet]. 2009 [cited February 5, 2018];(2). Available from: Cochrane Database of Systemic Reviews.
37. Nagar V, Birthi P. Chronic opioid pain management for chronic kidney disease. J Pain Palliat Care Pharmacother [serial on the Internet]. 2015 [cited February 7, 2018];29(1):48–50. Available from: MEDLINE Complete.
38. Narayanan V, Koshy C. Fatigue in cancer: a review of the literature. Indian J Palliat Care. 2009;15:19–25.
39. Polanski J, Jankowska-Polanska B, Chabowski M, Szumanska-Chabowska A. Quality of life of patients with lung cancer. Onco Targets Ther. 2016;9:1023–8.
40. Politis M, Wu K, Molloy S, Bain P G, Chaudhuri KR, Piccini P. Parkinson's disease symptoms: the patient's perspective. Mov Disord. 2010;25(11):1646.
41. Radbruch L, Strasser F, Elsner F, Goncalves JF, Loge J, et al. Fatigue in palliative care patients – an EAPC approach. Palliat Med. 2008;22:13–22.
42. Reuben DB, Herr KA, Pacala JT, Pollock BG, Potter JF, Semla TP. Geriatrics at your fingertips. 19th ed. New York: The American Geriatrics Society; 2017.
43. Ross DD, Alexander CS. Management of common symptoms in terminally ill patients: Part 1. Fatigue, anorexia, cachexia, nausea and vomiting. Am Fam Physician. 2001;64(5):807–14.
44. Ruiz Garcia V. Megestrol acetate for treatment of anorexia-cachexia syndrome. Cochrane Database of Systematic Reviews [serial on Internet]. 2017 [cited February 1, 2018];(7). Available from: Cochrane Database of Systemic Reviews.
45. Sampson E. Enteral tube feeding for older people with advanced dementia. Cochrane Database of Systematic Reviews [serial on Internet]. 2009 [cited February 5, 2018];(2). Available from: Cochrane Database of Systemic Reviews.
46. Sanders DS, Carter MJ, D'Silva J, James G, Bolton RP, Bardhan KD. Survival analysis in percutaneous endoscopic gastrostomy feeding: a worse outcome in patients with dementia. Am J Gastroenterol. 2000;95:1472–5.
47. Sera L, McPherson M, Holmes H. Commonly prescribed medications in a population of hospice patients. Am J Hosp Palliat Care [serial on the Internet]. 2014 [cited February 5, 2018];31(2):126–131. Available from MEDLINE Complete.
48. Simon S. Benzodiazepines for the relief of breathlessness in advanced malignant and non-malignant diseases in adults. Cochrane Database of Systematic Reviews [serial on the Internet]. 2016 [cited February 7, 2018];(10). Available from: Cochrane Database of Systemic Reviews.
49. Sykes N. A clinical comparison of laxatives in a hospice. Palliat Med. 1991;5:307–14.
50. Sykes N. The relationship between opioid use and laxative use in terminally ill cancer patients. Palliat Med. 1998;12:375–82.
51. Tarumi Y, Wilson MP, Szafran O, Spooner GR. Randomized, double-blind, placebo controlled trial of oral docusate in the management of constipation in hospice patients. J Pain Symptom Manag. 2013;45:2–13.
52. Temel JS, Greer JA, Muzikansky A, Gallagher ER, Admane S, et al. Early palliative care for patients with metastatic non-small cell lung cancer. N Engl J Med. 2010;363:733–42.
53. Timothy HM, To LB, Currow DC. Can we detect transfusion benefits in palliative care patients? J Palliat Med. 2016;19:110–1113.
54. Watanabe N. Mirtazapine versus other antidepressant agents for depression. Cochrane Database of Systematic Reviews [serial on Internet]. 2011 [cited February 2, 2018];(12). Available from: Cochrane Database of Systemic Reviews.
55. Wee B. Interventions for noisy breathing in patients near to death. Cochrane Database of Systematic Reviews [serial on Internet]. 2017 [cited February 12, 2018];(4). Available from: Cochrane Databases of Systematic Reviews.
56. Weissman D. Fast Facts and Concepts #3. Syndrome of imminent death. 2005; 3rd ed. May 2015. Available from: https://www.mypcnow.org.
57. Wildiers H, Dhaenekint C, Demeulenaere P, Clement P, Desmet M, Menten J, et al. Atropine, hyoscine butylbromide, or scopolamine are equally effective for the treatment of death rattle in terminal care. J Pain Symptom Manage [serial on the Internet]. 2009 [cited February 5, 2018];38(1):124–133. Available from: MEDLINE Complete.
58. Yennurajalingam S, Bruera E. Palliative management of fatigue at the close of life: "it feels like my body is just worn out". JAMA. 2007;297:295–304.
59. Kroenke K, Spitzer RL, Williams JBW. The PHQ 9: validity of a brief depression severity measure. J Gen Intern Med. 2001;16(9):606–13.
60. Veauthier C, Gaede G, Radbruch H, Wernecke K-D, Paul F. Sleep disorders reduce health-related quality of life in multiple sclerosis (Nottingham Health Profile Data in Patients with Multiple Sclerosis). Int J Mol Sci. 2015;16(7):16514–28.

Psychosocial, Social, and Spiritual Needs of Geriatric Patients

Sheila Barton

A. Chun (ed.), *Geriatric Practice*, https://doi.org/10.1007/978-3-030-19625-7_44

"The good physician treats the disease; the great physician treats the patient."

William Osler

44.1 Introduction

Geriatricians are a heroic lot. They work in a field where their elderly patients have suffered the medical, functional, and cognitive tolls of a long life. The potential for change is limited. Most of the time, there is no way to "fix" the problems that are presented to them because those issues are longstanding and progressive. Information sharing is often difficult due to sensory, cognitive, and/or emotional issues. Finally, older patients may have difficulty adhering to a plan of care due to financial limitations, functional problems, and lack of formal and informal supports. Geriatricians must be part physician, part detective, and part family counselor. In order to be effective, they need to consider multiple plans and view patients in the context of their psychosocial, social, and spiritual needs and motivations. If these needs are not met, chances are that the medical outcome will suffer.

The term "psychosocial" is referenced frequently in the literature as an integral part of geriatric assessment. However, its meaning is often used to reference any interaction between an individual's emotional world and the environment. The basic psychosocial issues of geriatric patients can be classified according to concrete and emotional categories that change over time with the trajectory of the aging process. The term "psychosocial" can refer to any aspect of a patient's emotional/social/living situation that affects safe management in the community: finances, insurance, housing, memory loss, emotional issues, family dynamics, or functional problems.

Abraham Maslow, a psychologist, was one of the first mental health professionals to see human needs and growth on a trajectory that moves from meeting basic physiological and safety needs to meeting higher-level needs for social and psychological fulfillment [1]. Below is a chart using Maslow's hierarchy to illustrate how these needs relate to the world of the older adult. For some, physical and cognitive challenges present barriers to meeting basic needs for health and safety. Mental health issues arise as a consequence of these unmet needs. The chart below illustrates a useful paradigm for analysis of psychosocial needs (Table 44.1).

It is easy for a clinician to become overwhelmed by the scope of an older adult's medical problems combined with the psychosocial and social aspects of her patient's living situation. Medical schools train their students to think about systems (such as GI, cardiology, neurology) and to break those systems down into medical problems and actionable categories. In geriatrics, to a greater extent, the clinician must use a similar method in consideration of the psychosocial context of a patient's medical situation. A fall may be because a patient tripped on a crack in the sidewalk. Or perhaps the patient is a hoarder and fell because of the clutter. Or perhaps the patient is cognitively impaired and became distracted. Or perhaps the patient has low vision and cannot afford glasses because Medicare does not cover glasses. Like the medical systems, the geriatrician does not need to become an expert in each area of psychosocial functioning. Providers need to know enough to look at the psychosocial possibilities, ask the right questions, and identify help from the right sources. Table 44.2 offers examples of geriatric issues and syndromes that may have multiple etiologies.

44.2 Overview

This chapter has three sections and will address the imperative of a team approach to geriatrics, present clinical vignettes illustrating common geriatric problems and their possible resolution, and provide an outline of the special considerations around communication with older patients and their family caregivers.

Table 44.1 Maslow's hierarchy of needs applied to the psychosocial needs of older adults

Maslow's hierarchy of needs	Psychosocial needs of geriatric patients	Barriers to meeting psychosocial needs of geriatric patients	Results of unmet psychosocial needs
Self-actualization	Fulfillment; you have accomplished your life's goals	Cognitive issues, inability to meet current physical, functional, and social needs	Despair, giving up, emotional problems
Esteem	Sense of self; realizing your place in the world, freedom	Dependence, isolation, physical and medical problems, financial problems	Depression, anxiety
Belonging	Social opportunities, friendship, family	Functional issues, sensory issues, multiple losses of friends, family, limited social opportunities, transportation issues	Depression, anxiety, grief
Safety	Accessible, affordable housing; home support services; medical equipment	Inaccessible housing, financial issues, lack of family supports, insurance issues	Falls, safety issues, weight loss, adherence issues
Physiological	Food, shelter, clothing, sleep	Financial issues, lack of family/community supports	Homelessness, falls, weight loss

Table 44.2 Presenting medical problems and psychosocial considerations

Presenting medical problem	Medical reasons	Psychosocial considerations
Fall	Gait instability Vision issues Hearing problems Dementia	Elder abuse Cognitive problem Hoarding/clutter Substance abuse Medication adherence issue
Medication adherence issue	Vision problem Hearing problem Fine motor problems Dementia	Cognitive problem Literacy issue Financial problem Substance abuse Elder abuse Caregiver burden
Depression	Medication issue Gait instability Dementia	Cognitive problem Elder abuse PTSD Financial Grief Isolation Role transition
Weight loss	Cancer GI problems Thyroid medication issue Dementia	Depression Cognitive problem Elder abuse Financial problem
Memory loss	Dementia Stroke Medication non-adherence	Posttraumatic stress Depression
Hygiene problems	Gait instability Sensory problems Incontinence Dementia	Cognitive problem Depression Lack of supports Caregiver burden
Appointment non-adherence	Gait instability Sensory problems Memory loss	Transportation issues Financial issues Depression Caregiver burden

It is important to remember that even in the best situations where "the stars are in alignment" and psychosocial needs are met, a patient's cognitive and/or functional issues may overwhelm all efforts to find a perfect solution.

44.3 The Geriatric Team

Geriatrics is a team sport. Older people face a multitude of physical, cognitive, functional, and psychosocial challenges that interfere with their ability to manage their healthcare and remain independent in the community. A frail senior with functional and cognitive problems cannot follow a treatment plan independently. Likewise, an independent 89-year-old may not be able to afford his medications or deal with the related insurance complications. Psychosocial issues are a significant consideration in producing a successful medical outcome. An interdisciplinary team is critical in providing appropriate care. The geriatric team draws on the expertise of professionals outside of the classic physician/nurse dyad to help with the broad range of psychosocial issues. Ideally, social workers, elder law attorneys, chaplains, psychologists, home health aides, family members, and physical/occupational therapists become partners in the treatment of the geriatric patient (Table 44.3).

44.4 Clinical Vignettes

Listed below are the top ten reasons that a team is required to effectively treat geriatric patients. The vignettes that follow illustrate the complex approach required to resolve them.

Top 10 Psychosocial/Social Issues in Outpatient Geriatrics

1. Functional problems – Problems in ADLs (activities of daily living such as walking, dressing, bathing, feeding, and toileting) and IADLs (instrumental activities of daily living such as bill paying, shopping, laundry, and housework)
2. Cognitive loss
3. Isolation
4. Need for help at home
5. Financial/insurance issues
6. Caregiver/family stress
7. Issues with access to care (transportation, inaccessible housing)
8. Depression/anxiety/psychiatric problems/substance abuse in patient or family
9. End of life issues
10. Elder abuse

44.4.1 Functional Problems

Older adults present with a myriad of slowly progressing problems which impair their ability to function safely and independently. Common presentations are weight loss and falls. The Centers for Disease Control (CDC) cites falls as being the leading cause of injury and death in older Americans, and, per CDC Director Tom Frieden, M.D., M.P.H., "Sadly, falls often herald the end of independence" [2]. Falls lead to more falls unless the reason for the fall is determined and addressed. Recommendations to prevent falls can range from purchasing an emergency call device for someone with balance problems to obtaining help at home for someone who has experienced multiple falls and a serious fall or is at risk for falls.

However, recommendations to obtain help at home often go unheeded due to financial concerns and fear of losing independence.

Table 44.3 The potential geriatric team

Team member	Role
Patient	The center of "team" efforts. Unless a patient lacks the capacity for decision-making, the patient is in charge of all efforts to assist her and can accept or refuse those efforts
Private care manager	Hired by patient or family to manage care for patient at home, facilitate home support services, and refer to community resources
Chaplain	Provides spiritual and emotional support to patient
Elder law attorney	Facilitates financial planning and access to Medicaid system when legal intervention is necessary to access Medicaid funding. Medicaid benefits vary from state to state. Elder law attorneys also assist with advance directives
Family members	Pivotal liaison between patient and medical teams. Can be primary caregiver and perform care management services. Can manage patient's finances and facilitate access to care in community
Geriatrician	Primary care physician and team leader. Provides medical care and outlines care needs.
Geriatric nurse practitioner (GNP)	An expert in nursing care related to chronic medical illnesses. Under the supervision of a geriatrician, provides primary care. Sees patients for focused urgent visits when geriatrician is unavailable
Home health aide (HHA)	Provides day-to-day custodial care to patient at home. Provides information to care team regarding patient's care needs and strengths
Physical therapist/occupational therapist (PT/OT)	Physical and occupational therapists can provide assistance in getting a patient back to baseline level of function after a hospitalization or a period of illness when the patient is deconditioned
Psychologist	Addresses mental health issues of patient. Neuropsychologist provides neuropsychological testing for dementia work-up
Registered nurse (RN)	Provides skilled nursing care in conjunction with medical visit
Licensed social worker (LCSW, LMSW)	Performs psychosocial assessment. Links patient with community resources and entitlements. Provides counseling to patient and family regarding how to maintain patient optimally in the community and avoid hospitalization and emergency department visits
Visiting nurse (VN)	Provides skilled nursing assessment and treatment in the home under the auspices of a certified home health agency

The "patient" is listed first with other members of the team listed alphabetically

Case #1: Falls

Sometimes a Fall Is Not JUST a Fall: Part 1

Ms. J attended an urgent care appointment due to a recent fall. She is an 82-year-old woman with insulin-dependent diabetes mellitus (IDDM), reflux (GERD), and atrial fibrillation (A-Fib). She lives alone in a one bedroom apartment and is independent in all ADLs/IADLs. Her two children live out of state. Her grandson, who is in college, lives nearby. There are bruises on her left wrist and left hip. She states that she tripped on a throw rug in her bathroom and hit her wrist on the sink. X-rays are negative. The urgent provider prescribes ibuprofen.

Two months later, Ms. J comes into the emergency department due to a fall. Her geriatrician happens to be on call and sees her. Patient reports gait instability since her last fall, although this is not evident upon exam. She has bruises on her left arm and wrist. Chart review reveals that she has been seen in multiple urgent care practices within the healthcare system. Inquiry about the details of the fall reveals that her grandson, who abuses drugs, has been taking money from her. He is verbally threatening and on several occasions has been rough with her, grabbing her wrist and arm when she refuses to give him money. She is on a fixed income and can no longer afford the co-pays for her diabetic medications. Ms. J has been trying to compensate by closely monitoring her sugars and eating the right things – but she gets dizzy and ends up on the floor. She doesn't want to get her grandson in trouble, so she has been "doctor hopping." Ms. J agrees to see a social worker.

The social worker convinces Ms. J to involve Adult Protective Services for financial management and an order of protection. The social worker also does a financial screen and finds that patient is above the Medicaid limits. She helps Ms. J apply for the Medicare Savings Program. As part of the Medicare Savings Program, Ms. J automatically obtains full subsidy on her Medicare Part D program and significant savings in paying for her medications. Eventually the social worker obtains Ms. J's permission to involve other family members who purchase an emergency call device for Ms. J and send her grandson to a drug treatment program.

Commentary For a patient with a stable gait who has multiple falls, one possible explanation could be elder abuse. Elder abuse affects approximately one in ten seniors over the age of 60 (National Council on Aging, 2016). The most common form of elder abuse is financial abuse, usually

44

Case #1: Falls (continued)

perpetrated by someone close to the senior without a source of income. It is common for the victim to hide the abuse, out of embarrassment, fear of reprisal, or fear that a loved one will be arrested. Hence, victims will often "doctor hop" so no one provider becomes suspicious. Another clue to signs of physical abuse are "twisting" bruises on the wrist/arm or a handprint where someone has been slapped. Where financial abuse is an issue, a patient may not be able to afford necessities, such as food and/or medications. For patients who have difficulty paying for medications, there are state subsidy programs for pharmaceuticals. Medicare (MC) also provides subsidies for medications through the MC Savings Program and MC D "Extra Help" subsidies.

44.4.2 Substance Abuse

Until recently there has been a serious underestimation of the issue of substance abuse in the elderly [3]. Most of the literature that does exist focuses on alcohol abuse. For our elderly patients who have a recent history of drinking alcoholic beverages to excess, alcohol use may be seen in part as a way to relieve anxiety and depression. Other older adults may have a long history of alcohol consumption and may equate the use of alcohol with socialization. Years ago the three "martini lunch" or the "cocktail hour" was part of the culture. Having a cocktail before dinner was an accepted way to de-stress. In older age, multiple losses and loneliness can create an environment where an individual might use alcohol to self-medicate. Patients suffering from functional and/or cognitive problems may use alcohol to relieve anxiety. However, older patients may have markedly lower capacity to metabolize alcohol.

Case #2: Falls

Sometimes a Fall Is Not JUST a Fall: Part 2

Mr. M is a 76-year-old, widowed retired advertising executive. He has a history of hypertension (HTN), diabetes (DM), and congestive heart failure (CHF). Patient comes to see his PCP after his second fall in 2 months. X-rays are negative. He denies unsteadiness and swears that he is taking his medications regularly. His PCP makes a referral to the Visiting Nurse Service. A visiting nurse and a physical therapist visit the patient's home. Several days later the visiting nurse calls the PCP. Mr. M's apartment is extremely cluttered with artwork, posters, and paperwork from his former advertising days. There are no unobstructed places to walk. There are also empty pizza boxes and food containers strewn around the apt. Five empty bottles of vodka are in the kitchen trash.

Mr. M comes in for an appointment to discuss the visiting nurse's findings. Patient noted that he was in the habit of enjoying a two-martini lunch when he was employed in advertising and when he returned from work he would have a cocktail with his wife before dinner. Since his wife died 3 years ago, Mr. M has been drinking excessively. He admits that "the apartment has gotten the better of him" and the clutter is out of control. He is advised to speak with the social worker about referrals to alcohol treatment and about decluttering programs.

The social worker refers Mr. M to Alcoholics Anonymous and to a local mental health agency for grief counseling. She learns that an eviction notice has been issued to patient due to his hoarding. She also refers Mr. M to Adult Protective Services (APS) for heavy-duty cleaning and to the Legal Aid Society regarding the eviction.

Commentary New-onset hoarding and clutter are common in people who are depressed and alcohol dependent. Alcoholics Anonymous (AA) has been successful in dealing with alcohol abuse. For a lonely senior, AA also provides a social outlet and sense of belonging that remedies social isolation. For those with minimal financial resources, APS provides decluttering services. APS can also intervene in eviction proceedings. Many hospice services provide grief counseling support at no cost. Additionally, for providers who accept Medicare, Medicare Part B will pay at 80% for psychotherapy to address diagnosed depression.

44.4.3 Access to Care

Individuals with functional or sensory problems often have special transportation needs. Due to lack of knowledge about resources or fear of being stigmatized as an "old person," many older individuals do not take advantage of transportation services for the elderly and disabled. Many larger cities have specialized transportation services through their public transportation system, senior citizen centers, and/or religious organizations. Some senior centers also have volunteers to escort patients to medical appointments. Many organizations for the blind or hearing impaired also have volunteers to provide escort services to their clientele.

Case #3: No Shows

Sometimes a Cigar Is Just a Cigar

Ms. B is an 80-year-old retired home attendant. She is a "no show" for her visit today. The PCP notices that this is her third "no show" in 5 months. When contacted, Ms. B states that she has been busy and it slipped her mind. Another appointment is booked and referral is made to the team social worker so that Ms. B can be seen by her during the next medical visit. The PCP suspects that patient may be suffering from memory loss. Ms. B receives a reminder call for her visit.

Ms. B arrives for her appt. The PCP inquires about the no shows. She apologizes and tells you that she cannot use public transportation in the inclement weather because she is afraid of slipping. The winter has been fierce. She can't afford to use taxi service.

The social worker registers Ms. B for a low-cost transportation service for the disabled, which is offered by the city. Patient no longer has issues with attending her appointments.

Commentary It is easy to suspect memory loss in a patient who misses multiple appointments. However, sometimes the explanation is simpler. In geriatric practices, bad weather begets an increase in no shows. Many larger cities have transportation services for senior citizens and the disabled at the cost of public transportation. Additionally, some senior centers and places of worship have vehicles that provide transportation to designated areas for shopping and medical appointments. Finally, many areas of the country with public transportation systems can offer half fare for their senior citizens.

44.4.4 Depression

Depression and anxiety are common in elderly patients given the multiple losses associated with aging: career, financial status, social supports, and functional changes. "More than two million of the 34 million Americans age 65 and older suffer from some form of depression. Symptoms of clinical depression can be triggered by other chronic illnesses common in later life such as Alzheimer's disease, Parkinson's disease, heart disease, cancer and arthritis. More than 55% of older persons treated for mental health services received care from primary care physicians. Less than 3% aged 65 and older received treatment from mental health professionals" [4].

However, according to Butler [5], depression is the most treatable mental health problem in later life. For the patient who is aware of her depressed mood, depression is often missed by the medical provider because of hesitation/embarrassment on the part of the patient. Due to cultural, religious, or other issues, an older patient may consider depression to be a weakness. Untreated depression, however, can have a deleterious impact on quality of life, underlying medical problems, and independence. When a geriatric patient admits to depression, symptoms are often severe and have advanced to the point of affecting a patient's day-to-day life and ability to engage socially.

Depression can be picked up with one question, "Do you often feel sad?" There are many questionnaires to pinpoint level of depression such as the PHQ9 and the Geriatric Depression Scale (see ▶ Appendix A).

Due to the pervasive negative effects of depression on a patient's health and lifestyle, many primary care practices are integrating treatment of depression into their practice. Medicare pays partially for psychiatry. Geropsychiatrists specialize in treatment of mental health issues in older adults. However, the number of geropsychiatrists is small compared to the growing population of older adults.

Case #4: No Shows

Sometimes It Seems Like Sadness

Ms. S is a 78-year-old retired banker who has been a patient in the geriatric practice for 9 years. Medical problems include hypertension, spinal stenosis, osteoporosis, and history of cervical cancer. She has been quite independent. Over the past year and a half, she has been seen monthly due to labile hypertension. She has been missing appointments and receives a reminder call.

Ms. S arrives for her appointment. Patient's blood pressure is quite elevated. It is clear that she hasn't been taking her meds. She appears disheveled and her hygiene is poor. She looks like she lost weight. She scores 18 on the PHQ9 indicating moderate to severe depression. It appears that she may need help at home. Patient refuses, stating that she can't afford it. The PCP prescribes an antidepressant. Referral is made to the social worker.

Conversation with the social worker reveals that patient has been depressed since she lost her younger sister 6 years ago. Initially it wasn't so bad. But in the past year, she finds herself crying at every reminder of her sister's loss. Ms. S states that she sleeps a lot and has stopped going to her book club. She's distracted and is forgetting to give her beloved cat her thyroid medication. She also forgets to take her own medication. Ms. S's only relative, a brother, lives in Canada.

The social worker refers Ms. S for a support group in a local senior center and enrolls patient in transportation through the local department for the aging. The social worker recommends a "blister pack" to help the patient keep track of her medications. A blister pack is a specialized package of medications that is prepared by the pharmacy and labeled with the day and time the patient must take the medications. She also refers patient to Meals on Wheels. The social worker plans to follow up the patient over time in the hope that she will eventually accept help at home.

Commentary Ms. S is showing symptoms of depression, i.e., weight loss, distraction, memory loss, and social isolation. However, depression can also be a symptom of dementia. Patient will be observed over time to determine if memory issues progress. Optimally, Ms. S could use some help at home, but concerns about expense, fearing a stranger in the house, and the symbolic loss of independence can make a senior reluctant to accept help.

44.4.5 Cognitive Decline

"An estimated 5.7 million Americans ages 65 or older may currently have Alzheimer's disease …the number may rise to 14 million by 2050" [6]. It is an expensive disease. "In 2018 the direct costs to American society of caring for those with Alzheimer's will cost $186 billion in Medicare and Medicaid payments" [7]. Signs of dementia include depression, anxiety, weight loss, inability to perform executive tasks such as bill paying, and eventually problems in personal hygiene.

A diagnosis of dementia brings with it a need for extensive planning in terms of support services, financial sustainability, and advanced directives. Initially, for those patients with cognitive and/or functional deficits, a few hours of assistance with bathing or dressing can make the difference between remaining safely at home and suffering a serious safety issue that leads to institutionalization. As functional or cognitive needs increase, so does the need for increasing increments of home supports which can overextend a patient financially.

Where does help come from? Initially, help comes from those who are closest to the patient. As needs progress, assistance must come from outside sources as follows:

- **Informal Supports**: Family/Friends

Statistics show that informal caregivers (family and friends), in staggering numbers, have assumed the responsibility of caregiving. "Of the total lifetime cost of caring for someone with dementia, 70 percent is borne by families – either through out of pocket health and long-term care expenses or from the value of unpaid care. About one in three caregivers is 65 or older" [7].

- **Formal Supports**: Paid caregivers and Medicaid-Funded Home Support Services

Under Medicare, certified home health agencies can provide a few hours of custodial help at home in conjunction with skilled services such as nursing or physical therapy. That provision is designed for patients who have short-term, intermittent needs – usually after a hospitalization. The custodial services stop when the skilled services end.

Medicare also funds hospice services for those patients who have a prognosis of 6 months or less. Hospice is both a program and a philosophy of care that is dedicated to optimizing quality of life for terminally ill patients and their families at home until death. Hospice has an interdisciplinary team which includes a physician, registered nurse, home health aide, social worker, and other disciplines. As a prerequisite for admission to hospice, a patient and family must agree that no curative efforts will be taken to address the admission diagnosis.

For those who financially qualify, Medicaid offers home support services for patients requiring assistance with personal care and/or housekeeping services. Medicaid is an insurance that is subsidized by federal and state governments. It offers financing for medical expenses including help at home. An individual qualifies for Medicaid if they meet the Medicaid income and asset requirements of their state. Elder law is a legal specialty that has become essential in helping functionally and cognitively impaired individuals access the Medicaid benefit. If a patient is not independently wealthy and does not have long-term care insurance, she cannot afford to remain at home without outside funding. Those who are above the Medicaid financial limits can use elder law attorneys to access Medicaid-funded services. The elder law attorney is knowledgeable about Medicaid laws and can assist in qualifying a patient financially for Medicaid. Additionally, the elder law attorney can facilitate advanced directives such as durable power of attorney, which would come into play when a dementia patient is no longer able to manage her finances. There are strict guidelines on how these services are offered and who qualifies for them. In some states, there are opportunities to financially qualify for Medicaid-funded home care through Medicaid surplus programs and pooled income trusts. To obtain information about applying for Medicaid and other resources, patients can talk with social workers available in community and senior centers.

- **Additional Supports**: Community Services, Religious Groups, Caring Kind, and Alzheimer's Association

Community agencies can assist in providing help to people with functional impairments. Home-delivered meals through church groups or social service agencies are of invaluable help to those seniors who are homebound and unable to shop and cook for themselves. Caring Kind and the Alzheimer's Association offer educational seminars and support groups to memory-impaired patients and their families. They also provide counseling regarding services for the memory impaired. The local department for the aging or aging ombudsman also provides advice about where to go for help in obtaining home support and community services.

44.4.6 The Challenges

Patients often refuse to accept help, even the help of a family member. There are many reasons for this, such as:

1. Denial. "I'm not an invalid. I've always coped and I will now."
2. Diminished standing in the family. "I'm the mother. I'm the one who takes care of YOU!"
3. Feelings of loss. Accepting assistance symbolizes a loss of independence and may create the perception that they are on a downward spiral.
4. Fear of theft or abuse. "I don't want strangers in the house."
5. Fear of impoverishment. For those who do not have long-term care insurance or Medicaid, help at home is expensive and, for many, can be unaffordable.
6. Pride. For some accepting Medicaid symbolizes failure. "I've never accepted welfare and I won't now!"

Case #5: Memory Loss

Sometimes Sadness Is Something More

When the PCP sees Ms. S for her next visit, the patient looks better and appears to be taking her medications. A neighbor accompanies Ms. S to her appointment. She tells the PCP privately that the patient has not been paying her rent and has been brought home by other neighbors who find her wandering. The PCP discusses the neighbor's concerns with Ms. S and obtains permission to call her brother. Ms. S and her PCP make the call together and arrange for a family meeting. Ms. S gives her brother durable power of attorney. Under the guidance of the social worker, Ms. S's brother arranges for a private care manager to oversee Ms. S's care, pay bills, and organize daily HHA services. She obtains a medic alert/safe return bracelet for Ms. S through the Alzheimer's Association and refers patient's brother for support groups at the Canadian branch of the Alzheimer's Association. A referral is also made to an elder law attorney for financial planning and a Medicaid application. The elder law attorney organizes patient's finances so that eventually Ms. S is able to obtain daily Medicaid-funded home support services. The care manager remains involved to supervise home support services, to manage medication adherence, to attend MD appointments, and to report back to patient's brother regarding medical updates.

Commentary The Alzheimer's Association provides educational seminars and support services for patients with memory loss and their families. There are chapters worldwide.

44.4.7 Social Needs

It is difficult for older adults to address their need for shelter and socialization because of the increasing levels of support and accessibility required.

Walk-up apartments that were rented in youth become prisons for the functionally impaired older adult. Additionally, the cost of moving can be unaffordable for a senior on a fixed income. According to a report from the Harvard Joint Center for Housing Studies, "by 2035, one out of three U.S. households will be headed by someone over 65. This growth will increase the demand for affordable, accessible housing far beyond what the current supply can meet" [8]. Those functionally impaired adults who reside in inaccessible apartments and houses can become quite isolated with few opportunities for socialization.

Case #6: Weight Loss

When a House Can No Longer Be a Home

Mr. F is an 82-year-old retired doorman with spinal stenosis, sciatica, mild CHF, and hypertension. He has lost 15 lbs in the past 6 months. The medical work-up is negative. Patient is cognitively intact. He has started to use a walker due to sciatic pain. He states that he feels well but doesn't enjoy his food. He denies depression and his PHQ9 = 12 and MMSE = 29/30, which indicates mild depression and a normal mini-mental exam. Patient notes that the only change in his life is that his brother moved away and he misses his company. Patient refuses counseling for depression. The PCP refers Mr. F to the social worker for further exploration of psychosocial issues.

The social worker interviews patient and learns that Mr. F is "down" due to financial issues. Patient's brother had cooked for Mr. F and had contributed to household expenses. Mr. F stated that he can no longer afford the kind of food that he used to eat. He also can't stand up in the kitchen to prepare meals due to sciatic pain. He has become quite isolated and stays home most of the time. Although he could qualify for Medicaid with a spend down to obtain help at home, he refuses to apply, citing "pride." He wants to remain independent as long as possible. The social worker refers Mr. F to Meals on Wheels. She also refers him for food stamps. Finally, they complete an application for a new senior housing development which is subsidized and more affordable, has socialization opportunities, and offers two meals a day. You see patient 6 months later. He has regained the weight and is looking forward to moving.

Commentary Mr. F falls into the category of needing assisted living. Assisted living offers an apartment with home health aides who come in at various times of the day to help with personal care and housekeeping services. Meals are taken in a communal dining room. The prerequisite for admission is the need for help in some area of personal care. Most assisted living programs are financed privately. Home health aides offer care on an as-needed basis and go from apartment to apartment offering care according to the needs of the resident. Meals on Wheels is a benefit offered to homebound seniors throughout the country through local departments of aging, aging ombudsman, religious organizations, and senior centers.

44.4.8 Senior Housing

Senior housing options can vary depending on functional needs and financial abilities:

Independent Living: This is an option for a senior who is independent and wants meals and housekeeping services provided. These are regular apartments in a building with social services, home care, and other supports. There is an option of prepared meals served in a dining room. Residents can participate in senior activities and trips. If a resident needs help with personal care, they can hire an aide from an on-site agency. Some independent living buildings allow their residents to use other homecare providers. Many seniors move into independent living buildings to be closer to their children.

Assisted Living: Again, this is independent living where all of the amenities listed above are provided. In addition, varying increments of help tailored to the individual needs of the residents are available. Care is provided by a staff of home health aides who move in and out of the apartments and help with dressing, bathing, and toileting. The resident must need some help with personal care, and they must be able to walk to the dining room. Most assisted living programs are financed privately.

Nursing Home Care: These are facilities that offer care for the totally dependent patient who has skilled nursing needs and who can no longer have their care needs met in the home environment.

Continuing Care Facilities: These are facilities that provide all levels of care – ranging from independent living to assisted living to nursing home care. There are usually separate buildings or areas on the same campus for each level of service. Continuing care facilities are financed privately and allow an individual to stay in the same facility as their care needs progress.

Case #7: All Options

When Best Efforts Are Not Enough

Ms. C is an 82-year-old retired nurse living alone in a Manhattan apartment. Her daughter brings Ms. C to see the PCP due to concerns about her mother's memory. Ms. C reportedly has a history of hypertension, insulin-dependent diabetes, and breast cancer with mastectomy in 1993. The PCP notes that patient's blood pressure is elevated and her A1C is quite high. Medication adherence is an issue. Ms. C is ambulatory and reports that she is independent. She adamantly denies that she has a memory problem and shares that she is angry at her daughter for bringing her to this appointment. Patient does admit to depression and isolation "because all (her) friends have died." Daughter reports that her mother has gotten lost three times in the past 2 weeks and was brought home by people who recognized her in the street. Since hearing about her mother's wandering, the daughter has been stopping by on a daily basis to help Ms. C She admits to a high level of caregiver stress because she also works and has a family. MMSE = 19 indicating moderate dementia. Aricept and neuropsychological testing are recommended. Patient refuses. Help at home is suggested, as well as a referral to the Visiting Nurse Service for medication adherence issues. Patient agrees to the visiting nurse referral because this is covered by Medicare, but she adamantly refuses "to pay for a stranger to babysit her."

The PCP refers the patient's daughter to the social worker for supportive counseling and resources related to dementia. The social worker refers her to the Alzheimer's Association for educational seminars and caregiver support groups to alleviate caregiver stress. The social worker also financially screens Ms. C for Medicaid. Patient is eligible for Medicaid but refuses to sign off on the application if she has to have a stranger in her home. The social worker introduces the idea of a medical model adult day program which would be funded by Medicaid. The medical model day program would provide socialization and skilled services such as medication administration. The patient agrees to this plan and applies for Medicaid.

Commentary It is important to discuss the full range of options for providing support to patients and families. By providing choices, you are acknowledging the patient's need for autonomy and independence.

44.4.9 Caregiver Stress and Options for Help

"About 34.2 million Americans have provided unpaid care to an adult age 50 or older in the last 12 months" (National Alliance for Caregiving and AARP, 2015). Caregiver burden is often overlooked and underreported. Most caregivers have a job and are responsible for both parents and their own children. The pressures of meeting these obligations can lead to stress-induced health issues; emotional problems, such as depression and anxiety; and financial burden due to absences from work. Caregiver stress can also lead to abuse or neglect of the person receiving care. Practical options to relieve caregiver stress include counseling, support groups, paid help at home, adult day programs, supportive housing, and family medical leave (FMLA). A simple question from the healthcare provider, inquiring about the well-being of the caregiver, can identify the risk of caregiver burnout. Social models of care can be the best recourse because they provide respite for the caregiver and offer a needed outlet for the patient. Depression and anxiety are often alleviated by social engagement.

Social options for care include:

Medical Model Adult Day Programs These day programs are usually attached to a nursing home and provide skilled services such as nursing, OT and PT, and recreational therapy. They are highly structured and each participant is sent to activities tailored to meet her needs. ADPs are funded by Medicaid or private funding – although the fees can be significant. Transportation is included in the fees. Medical model ADPs are set up to meet the needs of the disabled elderly and are not specifically tailored for patients with memory impairment – although most medical model ADPs have memory enhancement programs and service a large number of patients with memory impairments. Meals are provided according to dietary needs. Sessions are usually arranged by half days, i.e., morning program ending in early afternoon and afternoon program ending in evening. These programs offer respite for the caregiver. Additionally, the medical model program enhances medication adherence. The ADP nurses can take sugar levels and administer insulin and other medications. Staff members can also assist patients on a limited basis with toileting, although they do not routinely change diapers.

Social Adult Day Programs There are multiple recreational and social programs. They are privately funded at a much lower cost than a medical model ADP and are usually attached to a senior center. The purpose of the social ADP is enhanced socialization for the memory-impaired patient. These programs are usually run by a social worker or recreational therapist. There are no skilled services, such as nursing. Social model adult day care programs are usually run in half-day increments.

Senior Centers These are usually funded by the local department for the aging and provide activities, low-cost light meals, and celebrations for seniors within their neighborhood. Senior centers do not provide assistance to the functionally or cognitively impaired individual, and the presumption is that the individual will bring her own caregiver.

44.4.10 Spiritual Needs

Understanding a patient's spiritual and religious beliefs is a difficult but an important part of geriatric assessment. Many healthcare professionals hesitate to start such a sensitive conversation. However, spirituality represents the interaction between a patient's belief system and her health. If the topic is handled appropriately, the discussion can lead to a better understanding of a patient's world. If religion and spirituality are important to a patient, it is important that we address this aspect of their life. It is a common perception that older people are more religious and attend formal religious services more often than their younger counterparts. This may be because religious venues offer a form of socialization as well as a means of finding meaning at the end of life.

To understand the role of religion and spirituality in a patient's life, the exploration of four topics is recommended: "History of connection with formal religion; perception of God or lack of God; social network involvement with the faith or spiritual community; potential support services that can come from involvement with religious groups or congregations" [9]. The inquiry can take place in the context of a conversation about the patient's social history.

The following case illustrates opportunities for cultural affiliation and socialization in a faith community.

Case #8: Connection

When Faith Is Not Enough

Ms. C is an 82-year-old woman who comes to see the PCP after her third admission in 3 months for CHF. Six months ago, Ms. C came to NYC from San Francisco to live with her daughter. She notes that she is depressed and feeling quite isolated in her new home. PHQ9 = 16 or moderately depressed. The PCP offers to put her on antidepressants and she refuses, stating that medications won't help. The PCP also recommends that she visit the local senior center. Ms. C states that she tried the senior center and finds that she doesn't "mesh" with the participants. Patient explains that when she lived in San Francisco, she lived in an Italian neighborhood and went to a Catholic church where everyone was Italian. She was quite active in their senior ministry and "life seemed worthwhile." One year she won a prize for her cannoli. Now she lives in a neighborhood where everyone speaks Polish. Even the mass in her local church is said in Polish. She feels alone, like life has no joy. She feels like she is in a foreign land. The PCP refers her to the hospital chaplain. The chaplain happens to be Jewish, but he is familiar with the churches in the area. He calls his friend who is the pastor of a Catholic church in a nearby, mostly Italian, neighborhood. They arrange for Ms. C to take Access-A-Ride so that she can attend their senior ministry and their Italian Mass.

Commentary Chaplains are an asset to any healthcare team. They are educated in the practices of multiple religions and are familiar with the cultural roots of a variety of religious communities. Additionally, they come from a faith-based profession and are not seen as part of the medical establishment, allowing the patient freedom of expression on a spiritual/faith-based level.

The second case illustrates the importance of understanding a patient's religious history and beliefs due to the mind/body connection, no matter how alien to your own beliefs the patient's perspective might be.

Case # 9: Mind/Body

Suspension of Disbelief

Mr. F is a 65-year-old man, originally from the Caribbean, who is a patient on the neurosurgical floor. Patient had spinal surgery s/p MVA. Mr. F is separated with two teenaged children. He runs a restaurant in his neighborhood. Patient's estranged wife appears to be involved and visits regularly along with patient's 85-year-old mother. Mr. F did well immediately after surgery, but on day 3 post-op, he seemed to take a sharp turn for the worse. He stopped eating and communicated minimally. The medical team wonders aloud about mental status changes. Patient's estranged wife sits at the bedside and acknowledges no reason for her ex-husband's decline. The floor housekeeper overhears the team's conversation. He advises that they look under the patient's bed. They find what appear to be amulets and small dolls. The housekeeper, who is from the same country as patient, states that these amulets are "bad" and could be the cause of patient's decline. Privately, the medical team expresses disbelief. However, because this is out of their area of expertise, they call the floor chaplain. She speaks with the patient's wife and parents. The chaplain obtains permission to bring in a religious leader from Mr. F's neighborhood. The minister immediately recognizes the amulets as being "black magic" and performs a ceremony to bless the patient. The minister comes regularly to see patient and Mr. F improves. You later learn from patient's parents of their belief that the estranged wife placed the amulets under the bed in the hopes that their son would die before their divorce was final.

Commentary The interaction between faith and medicine is complicated. A patient's resolve to regain her health can be strengthened or thwarted by their belief system. Spiritual history taking must be comprehensive and non-judgmental in order to elicit the full range of beliefs that may be affecting the patient's health.

44.4.11 Tips for Starting the Conversation with a Geriatric Patient

In order to elicit information about her psychosocial and social experience, the patient needs to be engaged. The quality of that dialog may be influenced by the psychosocial issues themselves. Difficult family dynamics, anger on the part of the patient for being brought to the appointment, fear of losing independence, and other factors such as the patients' hearing deficits may obstruct efforts to obtain insight about her situation. To engage the patient, the following should be considered:

- **Know your patient**

The patient is *your* patient. Get to know that individual. Ask if she can hear you well. If not, consider a voice amplification device. If the patient is cognitively intact, first dismiss the family and ask the patient if it is okay for family members or friends to stay in the room to contribute to the conversation. If she says no, you may be able to obtain permission later. Your goal is to gain the patient's trust.

- **Respect defenses**

Denial is a defense that exists for a reason. It should be respected. A patient in the initial stages of dementia may deny the issue. If there are no safety issues, don't press until you have established a relationship.

- **Avoid medical jargon**

Use the patient's language to describe her condition. For instance, a patient may admit to having a "memory problem" but deny dementia.

- **Speak from a "strengths perspective"**

Focusing exclusively on an older person's weaknesses rather than her strengths can diminish whatever autonomy and abilities the older person has. Resilience and the ability to cope vary from person to person.

- **Simplify communication**

In a situation where the patient lacks capacity due to cognitive or mental health issues and there are multiple family members with differing opinions, ask for one person to represent the group. A family meeting can be scheduled later.

- **Do not rush or interrupt**

"One study found that doctors interrupt a patient within 18 seconds of the initial interview. Once interrupted a patient is less likely to reveal her concerns" [10].

- **Write down take-away points**

It is difficult for any patient to recall everything discussed during an appointment.

- **Enjoy your patients**

We live in an ageist society that moves quickly. Older adults need doctors who will listen. They will sense if you are truly interested in them and be more candid.

44.5 Conclusion

Geriatricians are indeed heroic figures. They routinely enter a complex world where the presenting medical complaints may not be what they seem. An understanding of the psychosocial, social, and spiritual issues of their older patients is essential. All of this takes time, patience, and empathy. However, the other side of the coin is that the world of the older patient is replete with rich history, resilience, and important life lessons. Best of all, geriatric patients have fascinating stories to tell and lend perspective and warmth to those who care for them.

Appendix A

Integrated Beharioral Health Project. California Primary Care Association. Screening Tools for Primary Care. General Resources - Mood and Anxiety Disorders Pages 2–3. Accessed 2/19. ► http://www.ibhpartners.org/wp-content/uploads/2015/12/screeningtool-mandy.pdf

References

1. Maslow A. Toward a psychology of being, a psychology classic. New York: Simon & Schuster; 2012.
2. Centers for Disease Control and Prevention. Press Release. Sept 22, 2016. Falls are leading cause of injury and death in older adults.
3. Center for Substance Abuse Treatment. Substance abuse among older adults, an invisible epidemic. In: Substance abuse among older adults: treatment improvement protocol (TIP). Series No 2. Report No (SMA) 98-3179. Rockville: Substance Abuse & Mental Health Services Administration (US); 1998. p. 1.
4. Common psychological disorders. In: Butler R, Lewis M, Sunderland T. Aging and mental health: positive psychosocial and biomedical approaches. 5th ed. Austin: Pro-Ed, Inc.; 2005. p. 94.
5. Mental Health America. Depression in older adults: more facts. Accessed Feb 2019. Google: https://www.mentalhealthamerica.net/conditions/depression-older-adults-more-facts.
6. Alzheimers Association. 2019-Alzheimer's disease facts & figures. p. 17. Accessed July 2019. Google: http://www.alz.org/media/documents/alzheimers-facts-and-figures-2019-r.pdf.
7. Alzheimer's Assoication. 2019 – Alzheimer's disease facts & figures. p. 31. Accessed July 2019. http://www.alz.org/media/documents/alzheimers-facts-and-figures-2019-r.pdf.
8. Harvard Joint Center for Housing Studies.Projections and implications for housing a growing population: older households 2015–2035. p. 4. Accessed Feb 2019. Google: https://www.jchs/harvard.edu/sites/default/files/harvard_jchs_housing_growing_population_2016_1_0.pdf.
9. Ellor JW. "Spirituality" from handbook of geriatric care management. 4th ed. Burlington, MA: Jones & Barlett Learning Publications. p. 178.
10. National Institute on Aging. Talking with your older patient. Effective communication in talking with the older adult; 2017. Accessed Feb 2019. Google: https://www.nia.nih.gov/health/doctor-patient-communication/talking-with-your-older-patient.

Further Reading

Aldwin CM, Igarashi H, Gilmer DF, Levenson M, editors. Health, illness and optimal aging. Biological and psychosocial perspectives. 3rd ed. New York: Springer Publishing Company; 2018.

Butler RM, Lewis M, Sunderland T, editors. Aging and mental health. Positive psychosocial and biomedical approaches. 5th ed. Boston: Allyn & Bacon; 1998.

Cobb M, Puchalski CM, Rumbold B, editors. Oxford textbook of spirituality in healthcare. Oxford: Oxford University Press; 2012.

Cress CJ, editor. Handbook of geriatric care management. 4th ed. Burlington: Jones and Bartlett Learning; 2017.

Cummings SM, Kropf ND, editors. Handbook of psychosocial interventions with older adults. Evidenced based approaches. New York: Routledge, Taylor and Francis Group; 2009.

Duffy F, Healy JP. Social work with older people in a hospital setting. Soc Work Health Care. 2011;50:109–23.

Langer N. Resilience and spirituality: foundations of strengths perspective counseling with the elderly. Educ Gerontol. 2004;30(7):611.

Meisenhelder JB, Chandler E. Spirituality and health outcomes in the elderly. J Relig Health. 2002;41(3):243.

Stewart M. Spiritual assessment: a patient-centered approach to oncology social work practice. Soc Work Health Care. 2014;53:59–73.

Introduction to Palliative Care

Amanda N. Overstreet

A. Chun (ed.), *Geriatric Practice*, https://doi.org/10.1007/978-3-030-19625-7_45

Case: Mr. S

Mr. S is an 85-year-old man with chronic obstructive pulmonary disease (COPD), osteoarthritis, and mild dementia. He arrives in your outpatient practice for his regular 3-month follow-up visit. He is widowed and lives with his daughter. His daughter mentions that he needs more help at home. He ambulates with a cane but has fallen twice in the last 6 months. Mr. S attributes his functional decline to bilateral knee pain. He needs help with instrumental activities of daily living like cooking and using the telephone. In the last few months, he has also needed assistance for bathing and dressing. He is independent with toileting and eating. He mentions a decrease in his appetite and subsequent weight loss of about 10 pounds. He was hospitalized last month for a few days with a COPD exacerbation and returned home to his daughter's care thereafter.

45.1 Introduction

Changing demographics have influenced healthcare in the United States, and providers need to feel comfortable caring for older adults with life-limiting illness. Palliative care is a relatively modern field of medicine, which focuses on symptom management and psychosocial support for patients living with serious illness. Many people are living into older adulthood and therefore living with at least two chronic medical conditions. A changing life expectancy has also led to changes in the way people die.

The current life expectancy in the United States is approximately 78 years. The most common causes of death are heart disease, cancer, chronic lung diseases, accidents, stroke, and Alzheimer's disease. In contrast to the early 1900s, people are more likely to live to older adulthood and die of a chronic disease (versus death after an acute illness or infection). Today, people are also are more likely to have prolonged periods of functional impairment and symptom burden before death [1]. Many patients require nonpaid family caregivers to help with functional impairment. Two thirds of caregivers for older adults are female and on average 48 years old. Over one third of caregivers are taking care of a parent. When asked why their loved one requires care, the top two problems reported were "old age" and "dementia" [2].

The location of death has also changed over the years, and today older adults are more likely to die in hospitals and nursing homes. The dying process can become prolonged in institutions by technological advances like ventilators, feeding tubes, chemotherapy, and intravenous fluids [1].

45.2 What Is Palliative Care?

Palliative medicine is specialized medical care for people and their families with serious illnesses. It focuses on providing relief from the pain, symptoms, and distress of serious illness. It is a team approach to care involving specialty-trained doctors, nurses, social workers, chaplains, and other specialists focused on improving quality of life. By determining patients' goals of care through skilled communication, treating distressing symptoms, and coordinating care, palliative care teams meet patients' needs and help them avoid unwanted care. Unlike hospice care, palliative care can be provided at the same time as curative treatments; it is appropriate at any age and at any stage of a serious illness [3]. Often even today, physicians continue disease-directed treatment until it is no longer beneficial for patients and then pursue comfort-focused care in the final days. In 2014, approximately 47% of Medicare beneficiaries enrolled in hospice services. Average length of stay in hospice was 88 days in 2014 and medial length of stay was 17 days [4]. As hospice services are appropriate for any patient with a life expectancy of 6 months or less, this implies late referrals to hospice. Today, palliative medicine providers advocate for concurrent palliative care and disease-directed treatment (◘ Fig. 45.1).

Approximately 90% of large hospitals with greater than 300 hospital beds offer palliative care services [5]. Palliative care teams focus on providing patients with relief from symptoms and also on improving quality of life for patients and their families.

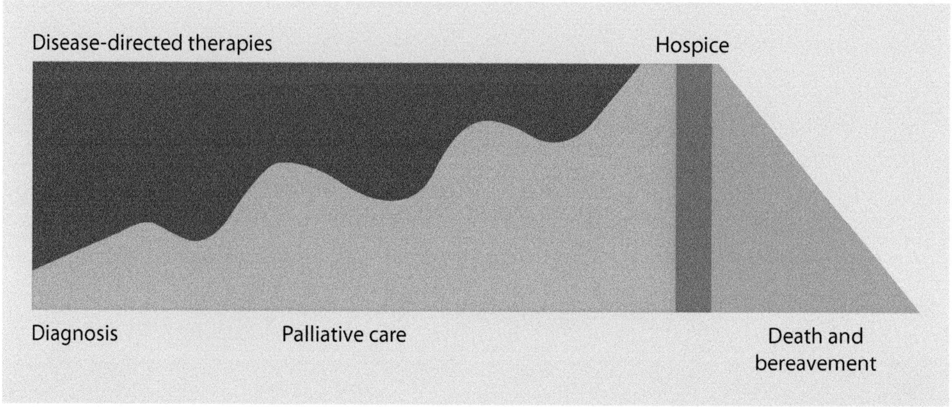

◘ **Fig. 45.1** Model of palliative care delivered concurrently with disease-directed therapies. (Modified from Chai et al. [1])

Palliative care has been shown to improve quality of life for patients with serious illness and their families. The benefits of palliative care consultation are not simply for patients but also for hospital systems. Palliative care consultation has also been shown to reduce hospital readmissions and hospital mortality, as well as reduce hospital length of stay and utilization of critical care services while improving patient/family satisfaction [5].

45.3 Evidence for Palliative Care

Dr. Temel et al. published a sentinel study in 2010 that helped change the way we think about palliative care. The investigators randomly assigned patients with newly diagnosed metastatic non-small-cell lung cancer to receive either early palliative care integrated with standard oncologic care or standard oncologic care alone. Patients randomized to the intervention group saw palliative care providers in the outpatient setting in addition to receiving standard cancer care. These visits focused on illness understanding and education, pain and symptom management, coping with life-threatening illness, and assisting with decision-making. For the first time, patients receiving palliative care not only had improvement in quality of life and mood but also had an increased survival of 2 months compared to standard oncologic care alone [6]. This was an important study in the field because it illustrated that palliative care didn't mean "giving up" on patients and in fact they lived longer.

Hospital-based palliative care consultation has been shown to improve quality of care for patients and has also been associated with significant hospital cost savings. A 2008 study from Dr. Morrison et al. examined data from eight hospitals with established palliative care programs for the years 2002 through 2004. Patients receiving palliative care were matched by propensity score to patients receiving usual care. Patients with a palliative care consultation who were discharged alive had a net savings of $1696 per admission compared to similar patients without a palliative care consultation. Of patients who died, those who died with a palliative care consultation had a net savings of $4908 [7] (◘ Table 45.1).

Case Continued

Is Mr. S appropriate for palliative care?

As Mr. S is living with serious illness and functional impairment, he would certainly benefit from palliative care consultation. He has symptom burden (pain from osteoarthritis, shortness of breath, lack of appetite), and his daughter would benefit from caregiver support. Eliciting his goals of care would help his provider develop the most appropriate treatment plan.

45.4 Palliative Care in Practice

Palliative care requires an interdisciplinary team composed of physicians, advanced practice providers, social workers, chaplains, and volunteers.

◘ **Table 45.1** Outcomes and benefits of palliative care

Patient/family outcomes	Improved symptom control including less pain Equal or longer survival Equal or higher satisfaction with hospital care Care aligned with values and wishes Increased psychosocial and spiritual support Less invasive treatments
Better survival	No data showing worse survival with concurrent palliative care In 2010 study by Dr. Temel, patients lived longer with concurrent palliative care
Hospital outcomes	Lower costs of hospitalization Fewer admissions and readmissions Less ICU utilization Improved patient and family satisfaction with overall hospital care

Adapted from Chapter 43: the Future of Palliative Care [8]

◘ **Table 45.2** Palliative medicine skills

Assessment of decision-making capacity	Symptom management
Prognostication	Care of actively dying patients
Evidence-based palliative care	Advanced communication with patients/families
Advanced pain management	Spiritual assessment
Medical ethics	Withdrawal of life-sustaining treatment

45.5 Palliative Medicine Physicians

Palliative medicine physicians complete medical school and then a residency program (commonly internal medicine or family medicine). Fellowship training in the subspecialty of hospice and palliative medicine is an additional year of training that follows residency training. Fellowship programs are available to graduates of almost any residency program (◘ Table 45.2).

After completing fellowship training, palliative medicine physicians can practice in a variety of settings, including inpatient consults, outpatient work, and hospice medical directorship. Despite the rapid growth in the field, a shortage of palliative medicine providers remains.

45.6 Palliative Medicine Advanced Practice Nurses and Registered Nurses

Advanced practice registered nurse (APRN) is a term that encompasses both clinical nurse specialists and nurse practitioners. Palliative care APRNs serve in many roles, from administration and inpatient consult work to hospice care. Palliative care APRNs often work alongside physicians providing comprehensive pain and symptom management, as well as leading family meetings to discuss goals of care. There are a few avenues to pursue certification in palliative care as an advance practice nurse: graduate education, fellowship training, or immersion courses [9]. Registered nurses are also involved with patient/family education, triage for services, reviewing goals of care, as well as caring for geriatric patients. Registered nurses can also achieve certification in palliative care [9].

45.7 Palliative Care Social Workers

Medical social workers are professionals who assess and care for a patient's social, psychological, financial, and emotional needs. Within palliative care, this is especially important, as patients are often grappling with a serious diagnosis and sometimes a loss of identity. Social workers provide counseling for patients and families coping with serious illness as well as help collaborate with other teams, including a hospice team. Social workers also help patients and families gain access to community and government resources available to them [10].

45.8 Palliative Care Chaplains

Chaplains typically obtain either a bachelor's degree or master's degree and are also ordained by a religious authority. They must also complete clinical pastoral education (CPE) for chaplaincy. Chaplains assist patients with questions about meaning and purpose, feelings of hopelessness, and existential suffering. Chaplains typically see patients as part of an interdisciplinary team both in the hospital as part of a consult team and also as part of a hospice team [11].

45.9 Palliative Care Volunteers

Volunteers can extend the time and services that a palliative care interdisciplinary team provides. Volunteers bring their own skills and life experiences to their work and can support patients and families in many ways. Legacy work is a common way volunteers provide support to patients and families. Legacy work is a form of coping that allows families to complete projects that they can cherish after the patient dies. Volunteers are an integral part of most large palliative care programs [12].

Case Continued

We know that Mr. S would qualify for palliative care consultation, but does he qualify for hospice?

Hospice is a philosophy of care for dying patients that states that the patient must have a terminal illness with an expected prognosis of 6 months or less if the illness runs its normal course. Hospice has been a Medicare benefit since the 1980s. Unlike with palliative care, patients forego curative treatments to enroll in hospice care. Hospice is a piece of palliative care.

As part of the hospice benefit, patients receive care from an interdisciplinary team, including a physician, nurse, chaplain, social worker, and volunteers. Hospice can be delivered in multiple settings, most commonly in a patient's own home. Approximately 95% of hospice care is provided in patients' homes [13]. In addition to receiving hospice services in their own homes, patients can also use their hospice benefit in a long-term care facility or in a general inpatient (GIP) unit. GIP units are hospice facilities for patients with acute symptom needs, often requiring intravenous medications and continuous nursing care. Nurses visit patients at home routinely with the option for continuous care if symptoms are uncontrolled. Hospice also provides durable medical equipment (hospital bed, bedside commode, home oxygen, etc.). Bereavement support is available to the patient's family after death of the patient [14].

45.10 Evidence for Hospice

There is a bias among some healthcare providers that hospice implies "giving up" and that patients will die sooner than if they had continued aggressive medical treatment. In actuality, some hospice patients may live longer than their non-hospice counterparts. A 2007 study examined the survival period for terminally ill patients enrolled in hospice and those not enrolled in hospice. For hospice patients with congestive heart failure, lung cancer, and pancreatic cancer, the mean survival period was significantly longer than similar patients not enrolled in hospice [15].

Similar to the evidence for palliative care, hospice has also been shown to decrease healthcare costs. A 2013 study examined Medicare expenditures for hospice and non-hospice patients. For the patients enrolled in hospice, they had a significantly lower total Medicare expenditure than matched controls. Hospice patients also had fewer hospital admissions, intensive care unit admissions, hospital days, 30-day hospital readmissions, and in-hospital deaths (all $p < 0{:}01$) compared to patients not enrolled in hospice [16].

Case Continued

In order to know whether Mr. S qualifies for hospice, we need to know more about his prognosis.

45.11 Prognostication

Prognostication, or understanding what's to come, is invaluable when helping patients plan for their futures. A life expectancy of 3 months versus 3 years might drastically change a patient's goals. Dying is not an exact science, and physicians

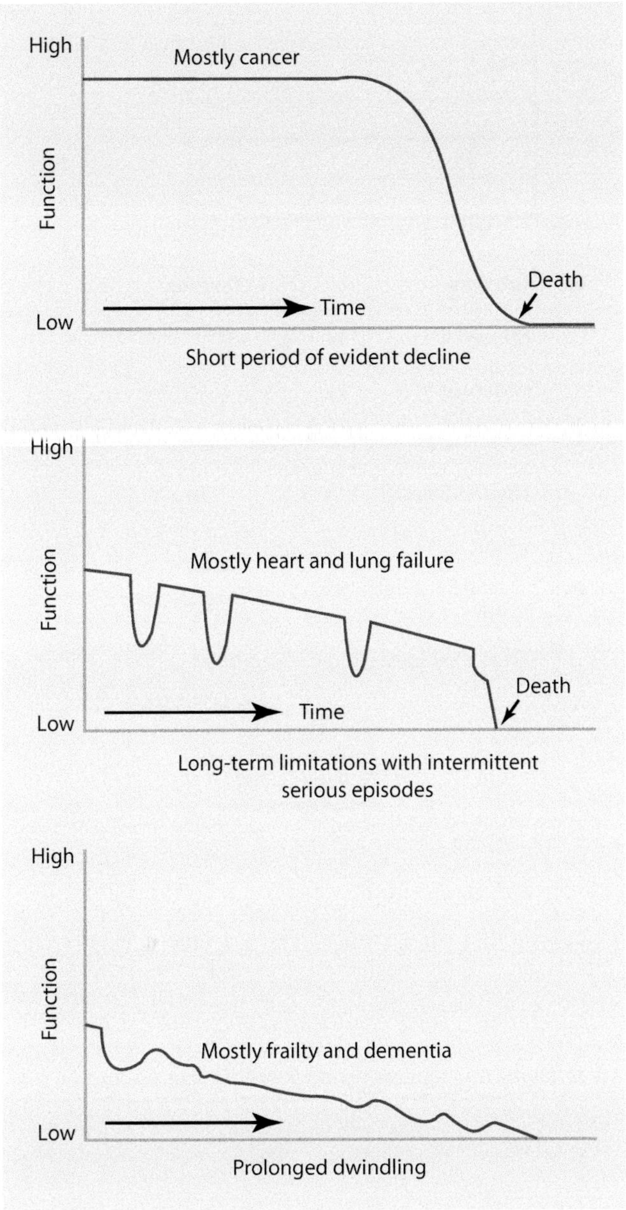

Fig. 45.2 Common trajectories in palliative care. (Modified from Lynn and Adamson [17])

commonly overestimate life expectancy. Several tools exist to aide providers in prognostication. For patients with cancer, their functional decline is usually more rapid and obvious to providers. For patients with chronic conditions like congestive heart failure or chronic obstructive pulmonary disease, their functional decline is usually more insidious with intermittent acute episodes. For patients with dementia, their functional decline can be variable but is often a slow decline over the course of several years. See Fig. 45.2.

Disease-specific tools exist to aide providers in prognostication.

45.12 Prognostication in Congestive Heart Failure

The Seattle Heart Failure Model was derived by retrospectively investigating predictors of survival among 1125 patients with congestive heart failure. Data was used to develop a multivariate risk model, which identifies age, gender, ischemic etiology, New York Heart Association class, ejection fracture, systolic blood pressure, potassium-sparing diuretic use, statin use, allopurinol use, hemoglobin, percent lymphocyte count, uric acid, sodium, cholesterol, and diuretic dose as predictors of survival. This model was validated in total of almost 10,000 patients. The Seattle Heart Failure Model provides an estimate of 1, 2, and 3 years of survival [18] (Fig. 45.3).

45.13 Prognostication in Liver Disease

The MELD (model for end-stage liver disease) score was initially developed in 2001 to estimate survival among patients undergoing elective transjugular intrahepatic portosystemic shunt placement for treatment of portal hypertension. Later, the United Network for Organ Sharing (UNOS) began using the MELD to prioritize patients on their liver transplantation list.

The MELD incorporates creatinine and whether the patient is undergoing dialysis, total bilirubin, INR, and sodium. A score is generated based on these values with corresponding estimated 3-month risk of mortality [19] (Table 45.3).

45.14 Prognostication in Chronic Obstructive Lung Disease

The body mass index, airflow obstruction, dyspnea, and exercise capacity index (BODE index) is a tool to estimate mortality in patients with chronic obstructive lung disease or COPD. Patients are assigned a score based on four variables: percent predicted FEV1, meters walked in 6-minute walk test, MMRC dyspnea scale (0–4), and body mass index (BMI) (Table 45.4).

Points are added for each of the variables and patients are given an index score of 0–10. The table below shows the correlation between BODE index score and mortality for three time intervals [20] (Table 45.5).

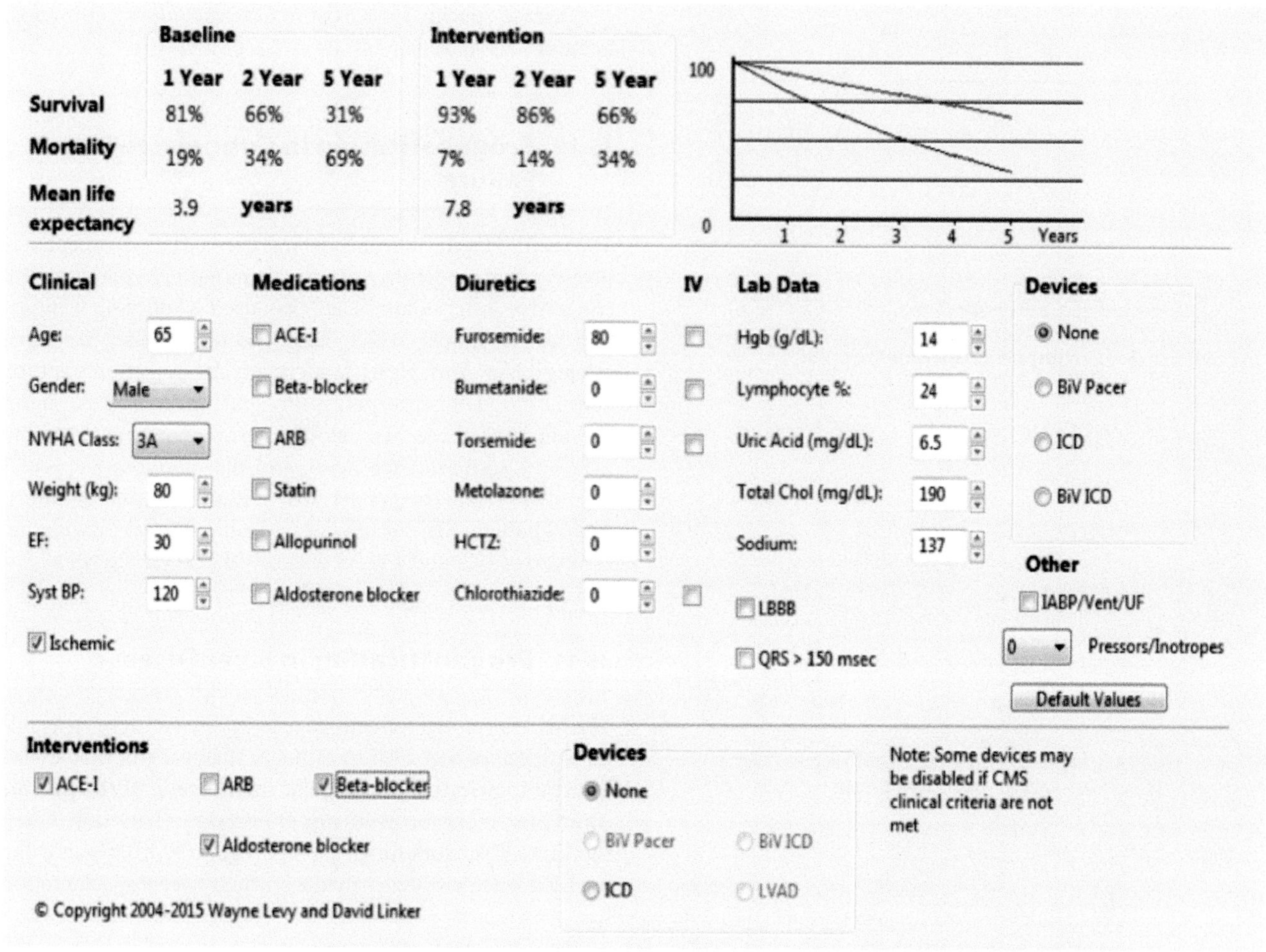

■ **Fig. 45.3** Seattle Heart Failure Model calculator

■ **Table 45.3** MELD (model for end-stage liver disease) score

MELD score	Mortality (%)
≤9	1.9
10–19	6.0
20–29	19.6
30–39	52.6
≥40	71.3

■ **Table 45.4** BODE index

Variable	Points on BODE index			
	0	1	2	3
FEV1 (% predicted)	>65	50–64	36–49	<35
Meters walked in 6 minutes	>350	250–349	150–249	<149
MMRC dyspnea scale	0–1	2	3	4
BMI	>21	<21		

■ **Table 45.5** Mortality in COPD by BODE index score

BODE index score	1-year mortality (%)	2-year mortality (%)	52-month mortality (%)
0–2	2	6	19
3–4	2	8	32
5–6	2	14	40
7–10	5	31	80

45.15 Prognostication in Cancer

There are two scales that oncologists commonly use to determine performance status, called the Eastern Cooperative Oncology Group (ECOG) scale and the Karnofsky Performance Scale (KPS). These scales are used to help determine if patients will benefit from cancer treatment as well as estimate prognosis. A KPS of 30–40 correlates with median survival of 8–50 days, and a KPS of 10–20 correlates with median survival of 7–16 days [21]. Patients who enroll in hospice care typically have a KPS of 50 or less and evidence of clinically widespread disease (■ Table 45.6).

▪ Table 45.6 Comparison of Eastern Cooperative Oncology Group (ECOG) scale and Karnofsky Performance Scale (KPS)

ECOG	ECOG = KPS	KPS
0. Asymptomatic (fully active, able to perform all pre-disease activities without restriction)	ECOG 0 = KPS 100; 90–100	100%: Normal, no complaints, no signs of disease
		90%: Capable of normal activity, few symptoms or signs of disease
1. Symptomatic but completely ambulatory (restricted in physically strenuous activity but ambulatory and able to perform work of a light or sedentary nature, e.g., light housework, office work)	ECOG 1 = KPS 80–90; 70–80	80%: Normal activity with some difficulty, some symptoms or signs
		70%: Caring for self, not capable of normal activity or work
2. Symptomatic, <50% in bed during the day (ambulatory and capable of all self-care but unable to perform any work activities. Up and about more than 50% of waking hours)	ECOG 2 = KPS 60–70; 50–60	60%: Requiring some help, can take care of most personal requirements
		50%: Requires help often, requires frequent medical care
3. Symptomatic, >50% in bed, but not bedbound (capable of only limited self-care, confined to bed or chair 50% or more of waking hours)	ECOG 3 = KPS 40–60; 30–40	40%: Disabled, requires special care and help
		30%: Severely disabled, hospital admission indicated but no risk for death
4. Bedbound (completely disabled. Cannot perform any self-care, totally confined to bed or chair)	ECOG 4 = KPS 20–30; 10–20	20%: Very ill, urgently requiring admission, requires supportive measures or treatment
		10%: Moribund, rapidly progressive fatal disease processes
5. Dead	ECOG 5 = KPS 0	0%: Dead

45.16 Prognostication in Dementia

There are several types of dementia, with Alzheimer's disease being the most common. Dementia can vary in terms of trajectory, but most patients live 7–10 years after diagnosis. The Functional Assessment Staging (FAST) outlines the trajectory of dementia (▪ Table 45.7).

For patients with dementia to enroll in hospice care, they must fall into FAST stage 7 and also have comorbid condition within the last year (aspiration pneumonia, pyelonephritis, septicemia, or multiple stage 3–4 pressure ulcers) [22].

▪ Table 45.7 Functional Assessment Staging (FAST)

Stage	Corresponding function
1	No difficulties
2	Subjective forgetfulness
3	Decreased job functioning and organization
4	Difficulty with instrumental activities of daily living (ADLs)
5	Requires supervision with ADLs
6	Impaired ADLs with incontinence
7A	(a) Ability to speak limited to six words
B	(b) Ability to speak limited to single word
C	(c) Loss of ambulation
D	(d) Inability to sit
E	(e) Inability to smile
F	(f) Inability to hold head up

45.17 Palliative Performance Scale

The palliative performance scale (PPS) helps providers estimate prognosis in patients with cancer but can be extrapolated to estimate prognosis in patients with multiple comorbidities. The PPS uses factors of ambulation, activity level or evidence of disease, self-care, oral intake, and level of consciousness. The PPS is a validated method to estimate median survival in days to either inpatient palliative care unit or inpatient hospice unit (see columns on far right of chart) [23–26]. The PPS is typically used by inpatient palliative medicine providers to help determine prognosis and therefore most appropriate location of care going forward. For example, a patient with an estimated medial survival of 2–6 days (corresponding to PPS of 20%) would likely be best cared for in an inpatient hospice unit or inpatient palliative care unit. Alternatively, a patient with an estimated medical survival of 4–108 days (corresponding to PPS of 60%) would likely qualify for home hospice services and would not require inpatient care (▪ Table 45.8).

Case Continued

For Mr. S, it may be difficult to estimate his prognosis because he has multiple chronic conditions. For patients with more than one life-limiting disease, using tools that compile various prognostication indices may be helpful.

Table 45.8 Palliative performance scale (PPS)

%	Ambulation	Activity-level evidence of disease	Self-care	Intake	Level of consciousness	Estimated median survival in days		
						(a)	(b)	(c)
100	Full	Normal No disease	Full	Normal	Full	N/A	N/A	108
90	Full	Normal Some disease	Full	Normal	Full			
80	Full	Normal with effort Some disease	Full	Normal or reduced	Full			
70	Reduced	Can't do normal job or work Some disease	Full	As above	Full	145		
60	Reduced	Can't do hobbies or housework Significant disease	Occasional assistance needed	As above	Full or confusion	29	4	
50	Mainly sit/lie	Can't do any work Extensive disease	Considerable assistance needed	As above	Full or confusion	30	11	41
40	Mainly in bed	As above	Mainly assistance	As above	Full or drowsy or confusion	18	8	
30	Bedbound	As above	Total care	Reduced	As above	8	5	
20	Bedbound	As above	As above	Minimal	As above	4	2	6
10	Bedbound	As above	As above	Mouth care only	Drowsy or coma	1	1	
0	Death	–	–	–	–			

(a) Survival post-admission to an inpatient palliative unit, all diagnoses [25]
(b) Days until inpatient death following admission to an acute hospice unit, diagnoses not specified [23]
(c) Survival post-admission to an inpatient palliative unit, cancer patients only [24]

The authors of ► ePrognosis.org developed calculators to estimate prognosis in patients in three different settings: living at home in the community, living in a nursing home, and currently hospitalized. The authors use various indices to approximate life expectancy based on the time frame chosen. Physicians can then use these calculators by answering questions about patient's comorbidities and functional status and receive a point score that corresponds to a patient's risk of mortality [27].

Case Continued

To estimate prognosis in our patient, one can use the ePrognosis calculator for patients living at home. The calculator has questions about the patient's other comorbidities and lastly the clinician's best estimate of 1-year mortality. When completing the calculator for Mr. S, the Gagne Index gives us an estimate of 1-year mortality for similar patients. Mr. S has a score of 4 points, which corresponds to a 14.6% risk of 1-year mortality for similar patients.

How should this information be discussed with Mr. S and his daughter?

45.18 Communication

Palliative medicine providers are trained to be experts in communication skills. Providers must be able to give serious news to patients and also to navigate goals of care discussions with patients and their families.

There are various tools to help frame these discussions.

First, providers should be respectful of serious news and how hearing this news will affect their patients and loved ones. Providers should deliver serious news in a straightforward manner while allowing space for and acknowledging emotion [28].

One such tool to help disclose serious news is the SPIKES acronym, a six-step protocol for delivering serious news [29] (Table 45.9).

Responding to emotion can be a difficult skill to master but is incredibly important when delivering serious news. NURSE is an acronym for expressing empathy and responding to emotion [30] (Table 45.10).

Table 45.9 SPIKES protocol

SPIKES	Examples
S: Setting	Determine the "who, what, where" of the meeting. Who should be present? What is the main purpose of the discussion? Where can you find a private, quiet space without interruptions?
P: Assessing the patient's perception	"Tell me what the doctors have told you" This is an open-ended request that doesn't imply that the patient doesn't understand what's going on
I: Invitation	Find out how much the patient wants to know "Are you someone who wants to know details about what's going on or would you rather I simply discuss the big picture?"
K: Knowledge	Giving patient information. Give a warning short before delivering serious news. Speak in short sentences and avoid using medical jargon
E: Responding to emotion	Respond to patient's emotions. Acknowledge the sadness or shock that comes with hearing serious news, (see NURSE acronym below)
S: Strategy and summary	Clarify any of the patient's questions. Discuss next steps and assure the patient that you'll continue to be there for them

Table 45.10 NURSE acronym

N: Name the emotion	"You seem sad" or "you seem angry"
U: Understand the emotion	"I can't imagine how you must be feeling right now"
R: Respect the patient or family	
S: Support	"I will continue to be here for you"
E: Explore the emotion	"Tell me more..."

45.19 Eliciting Goals of Care

After you've delivered serious news, you may need to help elicit the patient's goals of care before determining the best path forward. The first step is to determine what the patient understands about the current situation, and why there is a need to discuss plans moving forward. It's helpful to ask about the patient's hopes and values, as these values can frame future medical treatments. Vital Talk is a non-profit, evidenced-based organization aimed at teaching clinicians communication skills. Their acronym, REMAP, can help guide goals of care discussions [31]. These guides are not meant to be used in total in every discussion but rather as a guide if needed when conversations stall and it's difficult to move forward (Table 45.11).

Table 45.11 REMAP acronym

Reframe why the status quo isn't working	"Unfortunately, your cancer has progressed despite chemotherapy"
Expect emotion and empathize	"I can see you're really sad to hear this news"
Map the future	"When you think about the future, what's most important to you?"
Align with the patient's values	"It sounds like spending time out of the hospital is most important to you"
Plan medical treatments that match patient values	"It seems like the burden of chemotherapy is now too much. Can we talk about other treatments that would help your symptoms?" Discuss hospice if appropriate

Case Continued

You discuss prognosis with Mr. S and his daughter. His life expectancy is likely longer than 6 months, so he would not be eligible for hospice at this point. He says that he would want his daughter to help him with medical decision-making if he were unable. When asked about his goals of care, he wants to spend time at home and avoid hospitalization. His daughter tells you that her goal is to keep Mr. S at home and avoid nursing home placement if possible. You offer support with active listening and reassure Mr. S that you will help align his medical treatments with his goals. How do we translate this discussion into medical documentation?

45.20 Advance Care Planning

Advance directives are medical-legal documents that articulate patient wishes regarding certain medical treatments. The term "advance directive" encompasses several documents, including a living will, healthcare proxy or healthcare power of attorney, and physician orders for life-sustaining treatment (POLST). A POLST document may be called by another name depending on the state (also known as POST or MOLST). An advance directive typically names a healthcare agent who would make medical decisions for a patient if he or she were unable to do so. These are legal documents that state a person's healthcare agent and also their wishes regarding life-sustaining treatment. These documents are very important in a crisis situation, but the discussions leading to completion of an advance directive are often more important. These documents cannot list all scenarios that may arise, and understanding the patient's overall goals of care is often most important. Older adults with life-limiting illness should complete both an advance directive and a POLST form, if possible. POLST forms are signed by a

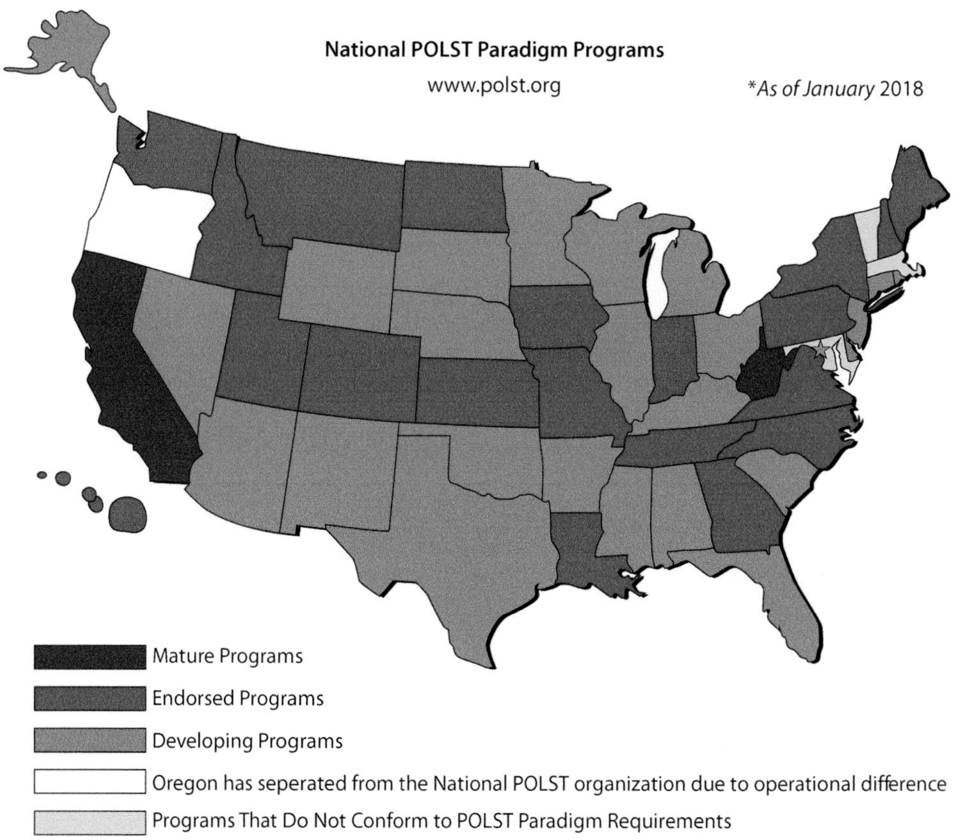

■ **Fig. 45.4** National POLST paradigm programs

physician, and they are medical orders that must be honored by emergency personnel [32].

The POLST form has been adopted by most states, as described in the map below (■ Fig. 45.4).

45.21 Special Topics: Palliative Care for Nursing Home Patients

Nursing homes are facilities that care for patients for a short-term rehabilitation stay or for long-term skilled nursing care. The rehabilitation benefit typically falls under a patient's Medicare Part A coverage, which is the same insurance that pays for acute hospital stays. In contrast, long-term skilled nursing care must be paid out of pocket ("room and board") or with nursing home Medicaid coverage.

In the United States, over 1.4 million people reside in nursing homes [33]. The majority of patients living in nursing homes are female and over the age of 85, and over half have a diagnosis of dementia [34]. These patients are typically medically complex and have limitations in their functional abilities, which is why they require care in a nursing home. As such, almost all patients living in nursing homes would be appropriate for palliative care consultation.

Advance care planning is especially important for patients who live in nursing homes. Many of these patients have dementia and may not be able to make decisions as they arise in the coming months to years after nursing home admission. Providers are encouraged to help patients complete advance directives upon admission, and these documents should be reviewed yearly or whenever the patient has a change in clinical status.

45.22 Summary

Palliative care consultation is appropriate for any patient with serious illness and at any stage of disease. Palliative care has been shown to decrease healthcare costs and improve quality of life for patients and their families. Patients often want to know their prognosis, and this information can guide further medical treatments. Effective communication is an important skill for any provider caring for seriously ill patient.

References

1. Chai E, Meier D, Morris J, Goldhirsch S, editors. Geriatric palliative care. New York: Oxford University Press; 2014.
2. National Alliance for Caregiving and AARP. Caregiving in the U.S. 2009. Available from http://www.caregiving.org/pdf/research/Caregiving_in_the_US_2009_full_report.pdf.
3. Meier D. What is palliative care? Center to Advance Palliative Care. Available from https://www.capc.org/payers-policymakers/what-is-palliative-care/.
4. Medicare Payment Advisory Commission. Report to congress: medicare payment policy. Mar 2016. Available from http://www.medpac.gov/docs/default-source/reports/march-2016-report-to-the-congress-medicare-payment-policy.pdf.
5. Morrison RS, Meier DE. America's care of serious illness: 2015 state-by-state report card on access to Palliative Care in Our Nation's

Hospitals. Available from https://reportcard.capc.org/wp-content/uploads/2015/08/CAPC-Report-Card-2015.pdf.
6. Temel JS, Greer JA, Muzikansky A, Gallagher ER, Admane S, Jackson VA, Dahlin CM, Blinderman CD, Jacobsen J, Pirl WF, Billings JA, Lynch TJ. Early palliative care for patients with metastatic non-small-cell lung cancer. N Engl J Med. 2010;363:733–42.
7. Morrison RS, Penrod JD, Cassel JB, et al. Cost savings associated with US hospital palliative care consultation programs. Arch Intern Med. 2008;168(16):1783–90.
8. Smith TJ, Albrecht TA, Cassel JB. The future of palliative care. In: Coyne PJ, Bobb B, Plakovic K, editors. Conversations in palliative care: questions and answers with the experts. Pittsburgh: Hospice and Palliative Nurses Association; 2017. p. 449–53.
9. Dahlin C. The palliative APRN. In: Coyne PJ, Bobb B, Plakovic K, editors. Conversations in palliative care: questions and answers with the experts. Pittsburgh: Hospice and Palliative Nurses Association; 2017. p. 245–51.
10. Cauthorne VK. Resource utilization. In: Coyne PJ, Bobb B, Plakovic K, editors. Conversations in palliative care: questions and answers with the experts. Pittsburgh: Hospice and Palliative Nurses Association; 2017. p. 235–43.
11. Jacobs MR, Maxwell JP, Walsh J. Palliative care chaplaincy. In: Coyne PJ, Bobb B, Plakovic K, editors. Conversations in palliative care: questions and answers with the experts. Pittsburgh: Hospice and Palliative Nurses Association; 2017. p. 99–107.
12. Bullington J, Yoder C. The role of volunteers in palliative care. In: Coyne PJ, Bobb B, Plakovic K, editors. Conversations in palliative care: questions and answers with the experts. Pittsburgh: Hospice and Palliative Nurses Association; 2017. p. 295–305.
13. Rosielle DA, Turner R. Medicare hospice benefit – part II: places of care and funding. Fast facts #87. Palliative Care Network of Wisconsin. 2007.
14. Rosielle DA, Turner R. Medicare hospice benefit – part I: eligibility and treatment plan. Fast facts #82. Palliative Care Network of Wisconsin. 2007.
15. Connor SR, Pyenson B, Fitch K, Spence C, Iwasaki K. Comparing hospice and nonhospice patient survival among patients who die within a three year window. J Pain Symptom Manag. 2007;33(3):238–46.
16. Kelley AS, Deb P, Du Q, Aldridge Carlson MD, Morrison RS. Hospice enrollment saves money for Medicare and improves care quality across a number of different lengths of stay. Health Aff. 2013;32(3):552–61.
17. Lynn J, Adamson DM. Living Well at the End of Life: Adapting Health Care to Serious Chronic Illness in Old Age. Washington, DC: Rand Health; 2003.
18. Levy WC, Mozzaffarian D, Linker DT, Sutradhar SC, Anker SD, Cropp AB, Anand I, Maggioni A, Burton P, Sullivan MD, Pitt B, Poole-Wilson PA, Mann DL, Packer M. The Seattle Heart Failure Model: prediction of survival in heart failure. Circulation. 2006;113:1424–33.
19. Kamath PS, Wiesner RH, Malinchoc M, Kremers W, Therneau TM, Kosberg CL, D'Amico G, Dickson ER, Kim WR. A model to predict survival in patients with end-stage liver disease. Hepatology. 2001;33(2):464–70.
20. Celli BR, Cote CG, Marin JM, Casanova C, Montes de Oca M, Mendez RA, Pinto Plata V, Cabral HJ. The body-mass index, airflow obstruction, dyspnea and exercise capacity index in chronic obstructive pulmonary disease. N Engl J Med. 2004;350(10):1005–12.
21. Ramchandran KJ, Von Roenn JH. What is the relationship between patient performance status and ability to offer chemotherapeutic treatments? In: Goldstein NE, Morrison RS, editors. Evidence-based practice of palliative medicine. Philadelphia: Elsevier; 2013. p. 287–9.
22. Sing T, Arnold R. Prognostication in dementia. Fast fact #150. Palliative Care Network of Wisconsin. 2006.
23. Anderson F, Downing GM, Hill J. Palliative performance scale (PPS): a new tool. J Palliat Care. 1996;12(1):5–11.
24. Morita T, Tsunoda J, Inoue S, et al. Validity of the palliative performance scale from a survival perspective. J Pain Symptom Manage. 1999;18(1):2–3.
25. Virik K, Glare P. Validation of the palliative performance scale for inpatients admitted to a palliative care unit in Sydney, Australia. J Pain Symptom Manage. 2002;23(6):455–7.
26. Myers J, Kim A, Flanagan J. Palliative performance scale and survival among outpatients with advanced cancer. Support Care Cancer. 2015;23(4):913–8.
27. Yourman LC, Sei JL, Schonberg MA, Widera EW, Smith AK. Prognostic indices for older adults: a systematic review. JAMA. 2012;307(2):182–92.
28. Vital Talk. 2018. Available from https://www.vitaltalk.org/guides/serious-news/.
29. Baile WF, Buckman R, Lenzi R, Glober G, Beale EA, Kudelka AP. SPIKES – a six step protocol for delivering bad news: application to the patient with cancer. Oncologist. 2000;5:302–11.
30. Smith RC, Hoppe RB. The patient's story: integrating the patient and physician-centered approaches to interviewing. Ann Intern Med. 1991;115(6):470–7.
31. Vital Talk. 2017. Available from http://vitaltalk.org/guides/transitionsgoals-of-care/.
32. National POLST Paradigm. Available from http://polst.org/about/
33. National Center for Health Statistics. Nursing home care. 2014. Available from www.cdc.gov/nchs.fastats/nursing-home-care.htm.
34. Harris-Kojetin L, et al. Long-term care services in the United States: 2013 overview. National Center for Health Statistics. Vital Health Stat. 2013;3(37). Available from www.cdc.gov/nchs/data/nsltcp.long_term_care_services_2013.pdf.

Supplementary Information

A. Chun (ed.), *Geriatric Practice*, https://doi.org/10.1007/978-3-030-19625-7

Index

A

B

C

D

E

F

G

H

I

J

K

L

M

N

O

P

Q

R

S

Printed by Printforce, the Netherlands